# Textbook and Color Atlas of Traumatic Injuries to the Teeth

# Textbook and Color Atlas of Traumatic Injuries to the Teeth

## Fourth Edition

Edited by

**J. O. Andreasen**
**F. M. Andreasen**
**L. Andersson**

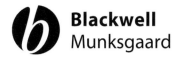

© 1981, 1994 by Munksgaard, Copenhagen, Denmark
© 2007 Blackwell Munksgaard
A Blackwell Publishing Company

Blackwell Publishing editorial offices:
Blackwell Publishing Ltd, 9600 Garsington Road, Oxford OX4 2DQ, UK
  Tel: +44 (0)1865 776868
Blackwell Publishing Professional, 2121 State Avenue, Ames, Iowa 50014-8300, USA
  Tel: +1 515 292 0140
Blackwell Publishing Asia Pty Ltd, 550 Swanston Street, Carlton, Victoria 3053, Australia
  Tel: +61 (0)3 8359 1011

Second edition published 1981 by Munksgaard
Third edition published 1994 by Munksgaard
Fourth edition published 2007 by Blackwell Publishing Ltd

ISBN: 978-1-4051-2954-1

A catalogue record for this title is available from the British Library and the Library of Congress

Set in 9.5pt on 12pt Minion
by SNP Best-set Typesetter Ltd., Hong Kong
Printed and bound by Narayana Press, Odder, Denmark

The publisher's policy is to use permanent paper from mills that operate a sustainable forestry policy, and which has been manufactured from pulp processed using acid-free and elementary chlorine-free practices. Furthermore, the publisher ensures that the text paper and cover board used have met acceptable environmental accreditation standards.

For further information on Blackwell Publishing, visit our website:
www.blackwellmunksgaard.com

# Contents

# Contributors

PER KRAGH ANDERSEN, Cand.Stat., PhD, Med.Dr.
Professor
Department of Biostatistics
University of Copenhagen
Denmark

LARS ANDERSSON, DDS, PhD, Odont.Dr.
Professor of Oral and Maxillofacial Surgery
Department of Surgical Sciences
Faculty of Dentistry
Health Sciences Center
Kuwait University
Kuwait

FRANCES M. ANDREASEN, DDS, Odont.Dr.
Research Associate
Department of Oral and Maxillofacial Surgery and
Center for Rare Oral Diseases
University Hospital, Copenhagen
Denmark

JENS O. ANDREASEN, DDS, Odont.Dr, HC, FRCS
Department of Oral and Maxillofacial Surgery and
Center for Rare Oral Diseases
University Hospital, Copenhagen
Denmark

THOMAS VON ARX, PD.Dr.Med.Dent.
Associate Professor
Department of Oral Surgery and Stomatology
School of Dental Medicine
University of Berne
Switzerland

LEIF K. BAKLAND, DDS
Professor and Chair
Department of Endodontics
School of Dentistry
Loma Linda University
USA

METTE BORUM, DDS, PhD
Director
Municipal Pediatric Dental Service
Hoeje-Taastrup Community
Taastrup
Denmark

DANIEL BUSER, DDS, Dr.Med.Dent.
Professor and Chairman
Department of Oral Surgery and Stomatology
School of Dental Medicine
University of Berne
Switzerland

NICO H.J. CREUGERS, DDS, PhD
Professor and Chairman
Department of Oral Function and Prosthetic Dentistry
Nijmegen Medical Centre, Dental School
Radboud University
The Netherlands

MIOMIR CVEK, DMS, Odont.Dr.
Professor
Faculty of Stomatology
University of Zagreb
Croatia, *and*
Department of Pedodontics
Eastman Dental Institute, Stockholm
Sweden

JON E. DAHL, DDS, Dr.Odont., DSc
Senior Scientist and Professor
Nordic Institute of Dental Materials
Haslum
Norway

JAN W.V. VAN DIJKEN, DDS, Odont.Dr.
Professor
Dental Hygienist Education
Dental School Umeå
Umeå University
Sweden

CRAIG W. DREYER, PhD, MDS, BDS
Senior Lecturer
School of Dentistry
University of Adelaide
Australia

MARIA T. FLORES, DDS
Professor of Pediatric Dentistry
Faculty of Dentistry
University of Valparaiso
Chile

WILLIAM V. GIANNOBILE, DDS, D.Med.Sci.
Najjar Professor of Dentistry and Director
Michigan Center for Oral Health Research
University of Michigan Clinical Center
USA

ULF GLENDOR, DDS, PhD, Med.Dr.
Research Associate
Division of Social Medicine and Public Health Science
Department of Health and Society
University of Linköping
Sweden

FINN GOTTRUP, MD, DMSci
Professor of Surgery
Head of the University Center of Wound Healing
Department of Plastic Surgery
Odense University Hospital
Denmark

CHRISTOPH HÄMMERLE, DMD, Dr.Med.Dent.
Professor
Clinic for Fixed and Removable Prosthodontics
Center for Dental and Oral Medicine and Cranio-
Maxillofacial Surgery
University of Zurich
Switzerland

GIDEON HOLAN, DMD
Director of Postgraduate Program
Department of Pediatric Dentistry
The Hebrew University
Hadassah School of Dental Medicine
Israel

JOHN JENSEN, DDS, PhD
Associate Professor and Chairman
Department of Oral and Maxillofacial Surgery
Aarhus University Hospital
Denmark

QIMING JIN, DDS, PhD
Research Investigator
Department of Periodontics and Oral Medicine
University of Michigan
USA

CEES M. KREULEN, DDS, PhD
Associate Professor
Department of Oral Function and Prosthetic Dentistry
Nijmegen Medical Centre, Dental School
Radboud University
The Netherlands

SVEN F. LINDSKOG, DDS, Odont.Dr.
Professor and Senior Consultant
Department of Oral Pathology
Dental School
Karolinska Institute
Sweden

HENRIK LØVSCHALL, DDS, PhD
Associate Professor
Department of Dental Pathology, Operative Dentistry and
Endodontics
School of Dentistry
University of Aarhus
Denmark

BARBRO MALMGREN, DDS, Med.Dr.
Senior Consultant
Pediatric Department
Karolinska University Hospital
Sweden

OLLE MALMGREN, DDS, Odont.Dr.
Associate Professor
Orthodontic Clinic
Uppsala
Sweden

WAGNER MARCENES, DDS, Odont.Dr.
Professor of Oral Epidemiology
Institute of Dentistry
Queen Mary's School of Medicine and Dentistry
Barts and the London
London
UK

SVEN ERIK NØRHOLT, DDS, Ph.Dr.
Consultant in Oral and Maxillofacial Surgery
Department of Oral and Maxillofacial Surgery
Aarhus University Hospital
Denmark

JAN ÖDMAN, DDS, Odont.Dr.
Consultant Orthodontist
Copenhagen Municipal Pedodontic Service
Trollhättan
Sweden

Kyösti S. Oikarinen, DDS, Odont.Dr.
Professor and Chairman
Department of Oral and Maxillofacial Surgery
University of Oulu
Finland

Ulla Pallesen, DDS
Director of Clinical Teaching
Department of Cariology and Endodontics
School of Dentistry
Copenhagen University
Denmark

Angela M. Pierce, MDS, Odont.Dr., FRACDS, FFOP(RCPA)
Honorary Consultant in Oral Pathology
Division of Tissue Pathology
Institute of Medical and Veterinary Science
Adelaide
Australia

Ulla Rydå, Med. Dr.
Consultant Child Psychiatrist
Jönköping County Council
Jönköping
Sweden

Ole Schwartz, DDS, PhD
Chairman
Department of Oral and Maxillofacial Surgery
University Hospital, Copenhagen
Denmark

Shahrokh Shabahang, DDS, MS, PhD
Associate Professor
Department of Endodontics
School of Dentistry
Loma Linda University
USA

Asgeir Sigurdsson, Cand.Odont, MS
Adjunct Associate Professor
Department of Endodontics
University of North Carolina School of Dentistry, USA, and
Private Endodontic Practice
Reykjavik
Iceland

Martha J. Somerman, DDS, PhD
Dean
School of Dentistry
University of Washington
Seattle
USA

Simon Storgård Jensen, DDS, PhD
Consultant Oral and Maxillofacial Surgeon
Department of Oral and Maxillofacial Surgery
Copenhagen University Hospital
Glostrup
Denmark

Mahmoud Torabinejad, DMD, MSD, PhD
Professor and Advanced Education Program Director
Department of Endodontics
School of Dentistry
Loma Linda University
USA

Sverker Toreskog, DDS
Private Practice
Göteborg
Sweden

Martin Trope, DDS
J. B. Freedland Professor
Department of Endodontics
School of Dentistry
University of North Carolina
USA

Mitsuhiro Tsukiboshi, DDS, PhD
Private Practice, General Dentistry
Aichi
Japan

Richard R. Welbury, MB, BS, PhD, FDSRCS, FRCPCH
Professor of Paediatric Dentistry
Glasgow Dental School and Hospital
UK

Björn U. Zachrisson, DDS, MSD, PhD
Professor and Private Practice in Orthodontics
Department of Orthodontics
University of Oslo
Norway

# Preface

More than thirty years has elapsed since the publication of the first edition of this textbook in 1972. At that time, table clinics were being held, where the theme of treatment was to extract traumatized teeth at the time of injury, and then the problem was solved. Since then, the biology of acute dental trauma has been elucidated through clinical and experimental research and in subsequent editions of this book used as the guiding light in defining treatment strategy.

A disturbing finding from several recent studies is that acute treatment of dental injuries can sometimes lead to inferior healing. This naturally leads to a rethinking of strategy for treatment of the injured patient. Until now, accepted treatment has been to reposition traumatically displaced teeth or bone fragments into an anatomically correct position. However, this procedure itself may further damage already traumatized tissues. This might explain the negative effect of many forceful reductions, as after luxation injuries, particularly upon periodontal healing. Likewise, the idea that an exposed pulp is a diseased and infected pulp which requires immediate or delayed extirpation has not been substantiated in real life. On the contrary, given the right healing conditions, exposed pulp is a survivor. Similarly, root fractured incisors are often removed due to a lack of understanding of the healing capacity of the pulp and periodontium and their respective roles in the healing process.

Previously, acute dental trauma was considered an event encompassing certain treatment problems that could be adequately resolved by proper endodontic, surgical or orthodontic intervention. However, recent new research has altered this view. Now we know that most healing complications following trauma are related to pre-injury or injury factors, and that treatment should be very specific and restricted in order to optimize healing. This edition is devoted to a biologic approach in understanding the nature of trauma and subsequent healing events and how these events can be assisted by treatment interventions.

The study and understanding of healing in hard and soft tissues after trauma is probably one of the most serious chal-lenges facing the dental profession. That this task presently rests with only a handful of researchers is out of proportion with the fact that perhaps half of the world's population today has suffered oral or dental trauma – a paradox that dental trauma is dentistry's stepchild.

In the decade that has elapsed since the third edition of this textbook, the impact of dental implants has been felt. In the wake of esthetically and functionally successful implant therapy, there is a growing tendency towards the approach of: 'If in doubt, take it out' and replace with a dental implant. This mind-set has seriously colored many professionals' perception of conservative therapy, be it active observation or interceptive endodontic therapy. Moreover, it has led to an explosion in the cost of treatment following dental trauma. For the sake of completeness, the chapter on dental implants has therefore been expanded with respect to primary biologic principles, with particular emphasis on problems related to the use of implants following dental trauma. In this regard, it should be borne in mind that trauma patients are most often young patients in whom the placement of an implant is contraindicated because it interferes with growth and development of the jaw. Furthermore, the fact that many families in the world today may live on a few dollars a day brings the cost–benefit aspect of treatment into focus. In such a world, sophisticated treatment modalities that are now available may only be realistic for very few. And then what? This reality is also described.

The enormous impact of a traumatic event on the mental health of the patient has long been ignored. In some situations, the loss of a tooth or parts of teeth may result in a difficult psychological situation, which so far has been completely underplayed and neglected in dental traumatology. This void is addressed in this new edition by a chapter on the psychological impact of dental trauma on the patient. Moreover, a traumatic event, whether crown fracture or tooth loss, usually results in severe esthetic problems. A further chapter is now devoted specifically to esthetic rehabilitation of the traumatized patient.

In this edition, an evidence-based approach to treatment has been chosen. This implies that any treatment procedure must be carefully screened for its effect upon healing processes. Due to the fact that treatment approaches, by their very nature, are usually traumatogenic, treatment principles for traumatized teeth become critical. Randomized clinical studies would be desirable, but inevitably there are practical and ethical problems with this: it would be difficult to ask for signed patient approval to place the patient in group A or B to test the difference between acute treatment procedures.

Acute dental trauma implies severe pain and psychological impact for many of us. There may also be severe economic consequences for trauma victims, especially in less privileged social groups. The dental profession must cope with these problems. One approach could be prevention of dental injuries, but previous efforts in this direction have not always been cost-effective. In this fourth edition, accident-prone sports activities have been identified where mouthguards could be of value.

Statistics from most countries show that one third of all preschool children have suffered a dental trauma involving the primary dentition and 20–25% have suffered a trauma to the permanent dentition. With such statistics it is likely that more than 3 billion of the world's population are trauma victims and, considering the general lack of continuing and serious research into dental trauma, the importance of this area of dentistry cannot be overstated.

It is the authors' hope that a better knowledge of the biology of dental trauma and wound healing will lead to a more intelligent treatment strategy, where the slogan 'Hands off where you can!' to save teeth could mean that the traumatic episode might be a short-lived one and not a protracted story of treatment and re-treatment – not only for the victim of dental trauma, but also for the dental practitioner.

The aim of this textbook is to ignite interest in this stepchild of dentistry, a discipline where all the skills of dentistry are needed to help victims of dental trauma. Please be involved!

Jens O. Andreasen, *DDS, Odont. dr. h.c, Copenhagen*
Frances M. Andreasen, *DDS, dr. odont., Copenhagen*
Lars Andersson, *DDS, dr. odont., Kuwait*

# 1
# Wound Healing Subsequent to Injury

F. Gottrup, S. Storgård Jensen & J. O. Andreasen

*F. Gottrup*

## Definition

The generally accepted definition of wound healing is: 'a reaction of any multicellular organism on tissue damage in order to restore the continuity and function of the tissue or organ'. This is a functional definition saying little about the process itself and which factors are influential.

Traumatic dental injuries usually imply wound healing processes in the periodontium, the pulp and sometimes associated soft tissue. The outcome of these determines the final healing result (Fig. 1.1). The general response of soft and mineralized tissues to surgical and traumatic injuries is a sensitive process, where even minor changes in the treatment procedure may have an impact upon the rate and quality of healing.

In order to design suitable treatment procedures for a traumatized dentition, it is necessary to consider the cellular and humoral elements in wound healing. In this respect considerable progress has been made in understanding of the role of different cells involved.

In this chapter the general response of soft tissues to injury is described, as well as the various factors influencing the wound healing processes. For progress to be made in the treatment of traumatic dental injuries it is necessary to begin with general wound healing principles. The aim of the present chapter is to give a general survey of wound healing as it appears from recent research. For more detailed information about the various topics the reader should consult textbooks and review articles devoted to wound healing (1–23, 607–612).

## Nature of a traumatic injury

Whenever injury disrupts tissue, a sequence of events is initiated whose ultimate goal is to heal the damaged tissue. The sequence of events after wounding is: control of bleeding; establishing a line of defense against infection; cleansing the wound site of necrotic tissue elements, bacteria or foreign bodies; closing the wound gap with newly formed connective tissue and epithelium; and finally modifying the primary wound tissue to a more functionally suitable tissue.

This healing process is basically the same in all tissues, but may vary clinically according to the tissues involved. Thus wound healing after dental trauma is complicated by the multiplicity of cellular systems involved (Fig. 1.2).

During the last two decades, significant advances have been made in the understanding of the biology behind wound healing in general and new details concerning the regulating mechanisms have been discovered.

While a vast body of knowledge exists concerning the healing of cutaneous wounds, relatively sparse information exists concerning healing of oral mucosa and odontogenic tissues. This chapter describes the general features of wound healing, and the present knowledge of the cellular systems involved. Wound healing as it applies to the specific odontogenic tissues will be described in Chapter 2.

## Wound healing biology

Wound healing is a dynamic, interactive process involving cells and extracellular matrix and is dependent on internal as well as external factors. Different schemes have been used in order to summarize the wound healing process. With increasing knowledge of the involved processes, cell types etc., a complete survey of all aspects will be hugely difficult to overview. The authors have for many years used a modification of the original Hunt flow diagram for wound healing (19) (Fig 1.2). This diagram illustrates the main events in superficial epithelialization and production of granulation tissue.

The wound healing process will be described in detail in the following section.

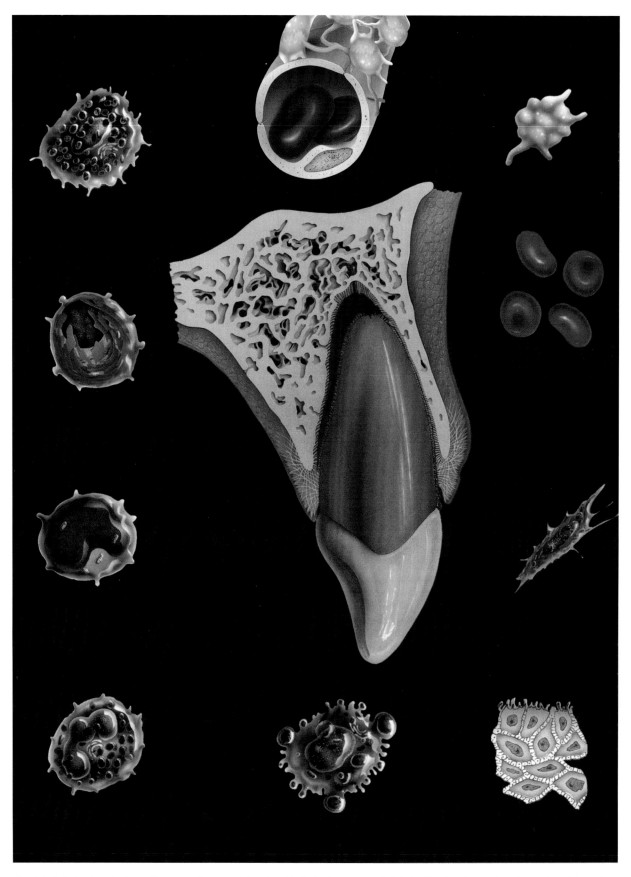

**Fig. 1.1** Cells involved in the healing event after a tooth luxation. Clockwise from top: endothelial cell and pericytes; thrombocyte (platelet); erythrocyte; fibroblast; epithelial cell; macrophage; neutrophil; lymphocytes; mast cell.

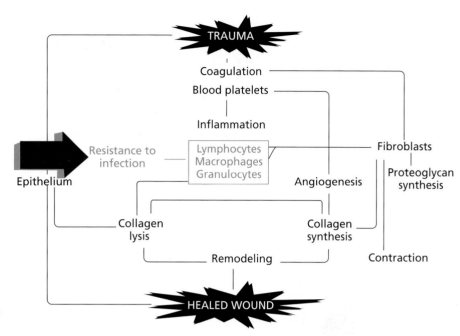

**Fig. 1.2** Modified Hunt flow diagram for wound healing.

## Repair versus regeneration

The goal of the wound healing process after injury is to restore the continuity between wound edges and to re-establish tissue function. In relation to wound healing, it is appropriate to define various terms, such as *repair* and *regeneration*. In this context, it has been suggested that the term *regeneration* should be used for a biologic process by which the structure and function of the disrupted or lost tissue is completely restored, whereas *repair* or scar formation is a biologic process whereby the continuity of the disrupted or lost tissue is regained by new tissue which does not restore structure and function (14). Throughout the text, these terms will be used according to the above definitions. The implication of repair and regeneration as they relate to oral tissues is discussed in Chapter 2.

## Cell differentiation

Cell differentiation is a process whereby an embryonic nonfunctional cell matures and changes into a tissue-specific cell, performing one or more functions characteristic of that cell population. Examples of this are the *mesenchymal paravascular cells* in the periodontal ligament and the pulp, and the basal cells of the epithelium. A problem arises as to whether already functioning odontogenic cells can revert to a more primitive cell type. Although this is known to take place in cutaneous wounds, it is unsettled with respect to dental tissues (see Chapter 2). With regard to cell differentiation, it appears that extracellular matrix compounds, such as proteoglycans, have a significant influence on cell differentiation in wound healing (25).

## Progenitor cells (stem cells)

Among the various cell populations in oral and other tissues, a small fraction are *progenitor cells*. These cells are self-perpetuating, nonspecialized cells, which are the source of new differentiating cells during normal tissue turnover and healing after injury (17–19). The role of these in wound healing is further discussed in Chapter 3.

## Cell cycle

Prior to mitosis, DNA must duplicate and RNA be synthesized. Since materials needed for cell division occupy more than half the cell, a cell that is performing functional synthesis (e.g. a fibroblast producing collagen, an odontoblast producing dentin or an epithelial cell producing keratin) does not have the resources to undergo mitosis. Conversely, a cell preparing for or undergoing mitosis has insufficient resources to undertake its functions. This may explain why it is usually the least differentiated cells that undergo proliferation in a damaged tissue, and why differentiated cells do not often divide (15).

The interval between consecutive mitoses has been termed the *cell cycle* which represents an ordered sequence of events that are necessary before the next mitosis (Fig. 1.3): The cell cycle has been subdivided into phases such as $G_1$, the time before the onset of DNA synthesis. In the S phase the DNA content is replicated, $G_2$ is the time between the S phase and mitosis, and M the time of mitosis (Fig. 1.3). The cumulative length of S, $G_2$ and M is relatively constant at 10–12 hours, whereas differences occur among cell types in the duration of $G_1$ (26).

Cells that have become growth arrested enter a resting phase, $G_0$, which lies outside the cell cycle. The $G_0$ state is reversible and cells can remain viable in $G_0$ for extended periods.

*In vivo*, cells can be classified as continuously dividing (e.g. epithelial cells, fibroblasts), non-dividing post-mitotic (e.g. ameloblasts) and cells reversibly growth arrested in $G_0$ that can be induced to re-enter the proliferative cycle.

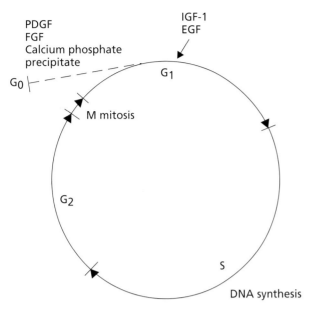

**Fig. 1.3** Cell cycle. $G_0$ = resting phase; $G_1$ = time before onset of DNA synthesis; S = replication of DNA; $G_2$ = time between DNA replication and mitosis; M = mitosis.

Factors leading to fibroblast proliferation have been studied in the fibroblast system. Resting cells are made *competent* to proliferate (i.e. entry of $G_0$ cells into early $G_1$ stage) by so-called *competence factors* (i.e. platelet derived growth factor (PDGF), fibroblast growth factor (FGF) and calcium phosphate precipitates). However, there is no progression beyond $G_1$ until the appearance of progression factors such as insulin-like growth factor-1 (IGF-1), epidermal growth factor (EGF) and other plasma factors (26) (Fig. 1.3).

## Cell migration

Optimal wound repair is dependent upon an orderly influx of cells into the wound area. Directed cell motion requires polarization of cells and formation of both a leading edge that attaches to the matrix and a trailing edge that is pulled along. The stimulus for directional cell migration can be a soluble attractant (*chemotaxis*), a substratum-bound gradient of a particular matrix constituent (*haptotaxis*) or the three-dimensional array of extracellular matrix within the tissue (*contact guidance*). Finally there is a *free edge effect* which occurs in epithelial wound healing (see p. 36) (27, 28).

Typical examples of cells responding to *chemotaxis* are circulating neutrophils and monocytes and macrophages (see p. 23). The chemoattractant is regulated by diffusion of the attractant from its source into an attraction-poor medium.

Cells migrating by *haptotaxis* extend lamellipodia more or less randomly and each of these protruding lamellipodia competes for a matrix component to adhere to, whereby a leading edge will be created on one side of the cell and a new membrane inserted into the leading edge. In that context, fibronectin and laminin seem to be important for adhesion (27).

*Contact guidance* occurs as the cell is forced along paths of least resistance through the extracellular matrix. Thus, migrating cells align themselves according to the matrix configuration, a phenomenon that can be seen in the extended fibrin strands in retracting blood clots (see p. 9), as well as in the orientation of fibroblasts in granulation tissue (29). In this context it should be mentioned that mechanisms also exist whereby spaces are opened within the extracellular area when cells migrate. Thus both fibroblasts and macrophages use enzymes such as plasmin, plasminogen and collagenases for this purpose (30).

During wound repair, a given parenchymal cell may migrate into the wound space by multiple mechanisms occurring concurrently or in succession. Factors related to cell migration in wound healing are described later for each particular cell type.

## Dynamics of wound repair

Classically the events taking place after wounding can be divided into three phases, namely the *inflammation*, the *proliferation* and the *remodeling phases* (5, 13, 20–23, 31). The inflammation phase may, however, be subdivided into a *hemostasis* phase and an *inflammatory* phase. But, it should be remembered that wound healing is a continuous process where the beginning and end of each phase cannot be clearly determined and phases do overlap.

Tissue injury causes disruption of blood vessels and extravasation of blood constituents. Vasoconstriction provides a rapid, but transient, decrease in bleeding. The extrinsic and intrinsic coagulation pathways are also immediately activated. The blood clots together with vasoconstriction re-establish hemostasis and provide a provisional extracellular matrix for cell migration. Adherent platelets undergo morphological changes to facilitate formation of the hemostatic plug and secrete several mediators of wound healing such as platelet derived growth factor, which attract and activate macrophages and fibroblasts. Other growth factors and a great number of other mediators such as chemoattractants and vasoactive substances are also released. The released products soon initiate the inflammatory response.

## Inflammation phase

Following the initial vasoconstriction a vasodilatation takes place in the wound area. This supports the migration of inflammatory cells into the wound area (Fig. 1.4).

These processes take place in the coagulated blood clot placed in the wound cavity. When prothrombin changes to thrombin, cleaving the fibrinogen molecule to fibrin, the clot turns into a fibrin clot, which later becomes the wound crust in open wounds. Fibronolytic activity is, however, also present in this early stage of healing. From plasminogen is produced plasmin which digests fibrin leading to the removal of thrombi. Fibrin has its main effect when angiogenesis starts and the restoration of vascular structure begins.

Neutrophils, lymphocytes and macrophages are the first cells to arrive at the site of injury. Their major role is to guard

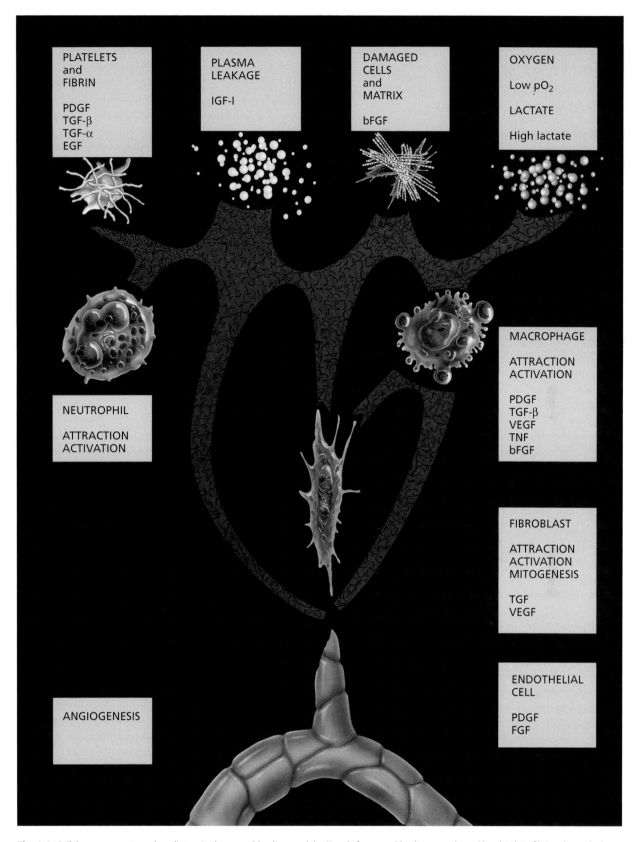

**Fig. 1.4** Cellular components and mediators in the wound healing module. Signals for wound healing are released by platelets, fibrin, plasma leakage, damaged cells and matrix. Furthermore low oxygen tension and a high lactate concentration in the injury site contribute an important stimulus for healing.

against the threat of infection, as well as to cleanse the wound site of cellular matrix debris and foreign bodies. The macrophages appear to direct the concerted action of the wound cell team (Fig. 1.4).

## Proliferative phase (fibroplasia)

This is called the *fibroplasia phase* or *regeneration phase* and is a continuation of the inflammatory phase, characterized by fibroblast proliferation and migration and the production of connective tissue. It starts about day 2 after the tissue trauma and continues for two to three weeks after the trauma in the case of a closed wound. This phase can be extended significantly in the case of an open wound with severe tissue damage, where complete closure will require production of a large amount of connective tissue.

In response to chemoattractants created in the inflammation phase, fibroblasts invade the wound area and this starts the proliferation phase. The invasion of fibroblasts starts at day 2 after injury and by day 4 they are the major cell type in normal healing. Fibroblasts are responsible for replacing the fibrin matrix (clot) with collagen-rich new stroma often called *granulation tissue*. In addition, fibroblasts also produce and release proteoglycans and glycosaminoglycan (GAG), which are important components of the extracellular matrix of the granulation tissue. Vascular restoration uses the new matrix as a scaffold and numerous new capillaries endow the new stroma with a granular appearance (angiogenesis). Macrophages provide a continuing source of growth factors necessary to stimulate fibroplasia and angiogenesis. The structural molecules of newly formed extracellular matrix, termed *provisional matrix*, produce a scaffold or conduit for cell migration. These molecules include fibrin, fibronectin and hyaluronic acid. Fibronectin and the appropriate integrin receptors bind fibronectin, fibrin or both on fibroblasts appearing to limit the rate of formation of granulation tissue.

Stimulated by growth factors and other signals, fibroblasts and endothelial cells divide, and cause a capillary network to move into the wound site which is characterized by ischemic damaged tissue or a coagulum.

The increasing numbers of cells in the wound area induce hypoxia, hypercapnia and lactacidosis, due to the increased need for oxygen in an area with decreased oxygen delivery because of the tissue injury (32, 33).

At cellular level oxygen is an essential nutrient for cell metabolism, especially energy production. This energy is supplied by the coenzyme adenosine triphosphate (ATP), which is the most important store for chemical energy on the molecular/enzymatic level and is synthesized in mitochondria by oxidative phosphorylation. This reaction is oxygen dependent.

*NADPH-linked oxygenase* is the responsible enzyme for the respiratory burst that occurs in leukocytes. During the inflammatory phase of the healing process NADPH-linked oxygenase produces high amounts of oxidants by consuming high amounts of oxygen (34). Successful wound healing can only take place in the presence of the enzyme, because oxidants are required for prevention of wound infection.

Not only phagocytes, but almost every cell in the wound environment is fitted with a specialized enzyme to convert $O_2$ to *reactive oxygen species* (ROS), including oxidizing species such as free radicals and hydrogen peroxide ($H_2O_2$) (35, 36). These ROS act as cellular messengers to promote several important processes that support wound healing. Thus $O_2$ has a role in healing beyond its function as nutrient and antibiotic. Given the growth factors, such as platelet-derived growth factor (PDGF), require ROS for their action on cells (35, 37), it is clear that $O_2$ therapy may act as an effective adjunct. Clinically this has been found in chronic granulomatous disease (CGD) where there are defects in genes that encode NADPH oxidase. The manifestations of this defect are increased susceptibility to infection and impaired wound healing (625).

Simultaneously, the basal cells in the epithelium divide and move into the injury site, thereby closing the defect. Along with revascularization, new collagen is formed which, after 3–5 days, adds strength to the wound. The high rate of collagen production continues for 10–12 days, resulting in strengthening of the wound. At this time healing tissue is dominated by capillaries and immature collagen.

The fibroblasts are responsible for the synthesis, deposition and remodeling of the extracellular matrix, which conversely can have an influence on the fibroblast activities. Cell movements at this stage into the fibrin clot or tightly woven extracellular matrix seem to require an active proteolytic system that can cleave a path for cell migration. Fibroblast derived enzymes (collagenase, gelatinase A, etc.) and serum plasmin are potential candidates for this task (23).

After fibroblast migration into the wound cavity the provisional extracellular matrix is gradually replaced with collagenous matrix. Once an abundant collagen matrix has been deposited in the wound, the fibroblasts stop producing collagen, and the fibroblast rich granulation tissue is replaced by a relatively acellular scar. Cells in the wound undergo apoptosis (cell death) triggered by unknown signals, but doing so the fibroblast dies without raising an inflammatory response. Deregulation of these processes occurs in fibrotic disorders such as keloid formation, morphea and scleroderma. Collagen synthesis and secretion requires hydroxylation of proline and lysine residues. Sufficient blood flow delivering adequate molecular oxygen is pivotal for this process.

Collagen production/deposition and development of strength of the wound is directly correlated to the partial pressure $PO_2$ of the tissue ($P_tO_2$) (38–40). Synthesis of collagen, cross-linking and the resulting wound strength relies on the normal function of specific enzymes (41, 42). The function of these enzymes is directly related to the amount of oxygen present, e.g. hydrolyzation of proline and lysine by hydroxylase enzymes (43).

Recently it has been shown that oxygen also may trigger the differentiation of fibroblasts to myofibroblasts, cells responsible for wound contraction (44).

### Neovascularization/angiogenesis

Early in the healing process there is no vascular supply to the injured area, but the stimulus for angiogenesis is present: growth factors released by especially macrophages, low oxygen and elevated lactate. The angiogenesis starts the day after the lesion. Angiogenesis is complicated, involving endothelial cells and activated epidermal cells. Proteolytic enzymes degrade the endothelial basement membrane allowing endothelial cells from the surroundings of the wound area to proliferate, migrate and form new vessels. The establishment of new blood vessels occurs by the budding or sprouting of intact venoles and the sprouts meet in loops (259, 377; see p. 30). The presence of capillary loops within the provisional matrix provides the tissue with a red granular appearance. Once the wound is filled with new granulation tissue angiogenesis ceases and many of the blood vessels disintegrate as a result of apoptosis. Angiogenesis is dependent upon the extracellular matrix (ECM) (623, 624).

While hypoxia can initiate neovascularization, it cannot sustain it. Supplementary oxygen administration accelerates vessels' growth (35, 45). Vascular endothelial growth factor (VEGF) has been established as a major long-term angiogenetic stimulus at the wound site. Recently the cell response to hypoxia has been further elucidated. Hypoxia inducible factor 1 (HIF-1) has been identified as a transcription factor that is induced by hypoxia (46, 48).

In the presence of normal oxygen tensions HIF-1 transcriptional activity is ubiquinated and degraded (47). HIF-1 seems to upregulate genes involved in glucose metabolism and angiogenesis under hypoxia and in a model of myocardial and cerebral ischemia the factor seems to protect cells from damage. The exact molecular mechanisms of how hypoxia is sensed by the cells are still unknown.

The arrangement of cells in the proliferative phase has been examined in rabbits using ear chambers where wounds heal between closely approximated, optically clear membranes (33, 49). It appears from these experiments that macrophages infiltrate the tissue in the dead space, followed by immature fibroblasts. New vessels are formed next to these fibroblasts which synthesize collagen. This arrangement of cells, which has been termed the *wound healing module*, continues to migrate until the tissue defect is obliterated. The factors controlling the growth of the wound healing module are described on p. 38.

### Epithelialization

Re-epithelialization of wounds begins within hours after injury. If parts of dermis layers are intact, epidermal cells from skin appendages such as hair follicles quickly remove clotted blood and damaged stroma and cover the wound space. This results in fast epithelialization. If dermis is totally destroyed the epithelialization only takes place from the wound edges and epithelialization can continues for a considerable time dependent on wound area.

During epithelialization the cells undergo considerable phenotypic alteration including retraction of intracellular tonofilaments, dissolution of most intercellular desmosomes and formation of peripheral cytoplasmatic actin filaments, which allow cell movement. Furthermore the cells no longer adhere to one another and the basement membrane. This allows migration of the cells dissecting the wound and separating scar from viable tissue. Integrin expression of the migrating epidermal cells appears to determine the path of dissection (23). Epidermal cell migration between collagenous dermis and the fibrin scar requires degradation of extracellular matrix. This is achieved by production of proteinases (collagenases, e.g. MMP-1) and activation of plasmin by activators produced by epidermal cells. In well adapted, non-complicated surgical incisional wounds the first layers of epidermal cells move over the incisional line 1–2 days after suturing. At the same time epidermal cells at the wound margin in open wounds begin to proliferate behind the actively migrating cells. The stimulus for migration and proliferation of epidermal cells is unknown, but the absence of neighbor cells at the margin of the wound (free edge effect), local release of growth factors and increased expression of growth factor receptors may be a suggestion.

During dermal migration from the wound margin a basement membrane reappears in a ziplike fashion and hemidesmosomes and type VII collagen anchoring fibrils form. Epidermal cells firmly attached to the basement membrane and underlying dermis revert to normal phenotype.

The production of epithelial tissue is primarily dependent on the degree of hydration and oxygen. While a moist wound environment increases the rate of epithelialization by a factor of 2–3 (50, 51), the optimal growth of epidermal cells is found at an oxygen concentration of 10–50% (52–54).

### Wound contraction

Wound contraction is a complex process, beneficial because a portion of the lesion is covered by skin despite scar tissue and thus it decreases complications by decreasing the open skin wound area. During the second week of healing, fibroblasts assume a myofibroblast phenotype characterized by large bundles of actin containing microfilaments (55). The stimulus for contraction probably is a combination of growth factors, integrin attachment of the myofibroblasts to collagen matrix and cross-links between collagen bundles (23). Wound contraction seems to be related to the early wound healing period and the effect decreases in time; in chronic unclosed wounds no wound contraction exists.

### Scar contracture

As opposed to the process of wound contraction of skin edges, this is a late pathological process in wound healing. It consists of a contraction of large amounts of scar tissue followed by immobilization of the affected area (e.g. a joint). In scar contracture, the wound area as well as adjacent tissue shrink as opposed to contraction where only the wound area is involved. The morbidity of scar contracture is a major problem in the rehabilitation of severely injured patients.

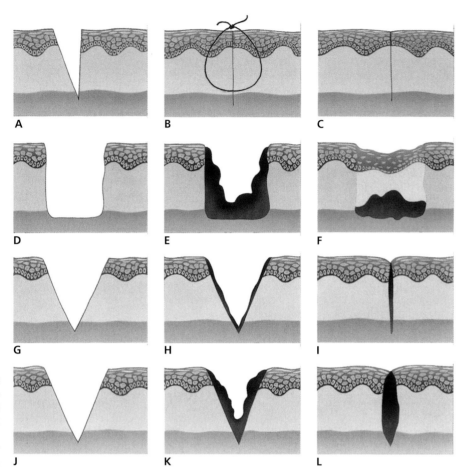

**Fig. 1.5** Wound healing events related to the type of wound and subsequent treatment. A–C: incisional wound with primary closure; D–F: open and non-sutured wound; G–I: delayed primary closure; J–L: secondary closure. From GOTTRUP (56) 1991.

## Remodeling phase

The *remodeling phase* is also called the *moderation phase* or the *scar phase.*

In closed wounds this phase starts 2–3 weeks after closure, while it does not start in open wounds before the wound has healed. Granulation tissue covered by epidermis is known to undergo remodeling earlier than uncovered granulation tissue. The length of this is unknown; some have argued one year but others have claimed the rest of the patient's life.

During this phase the granulation tissue is remodeled and matured to a scar formation. When granulation tissue is covered by epithelium it undergoes remodeling. Similarly a wound covered by a graft will continue the remodeling phase. This results in a decrease in cell density, numbers of capillaries and metabolic activity (55). The collagen fibrils will be united into thicker fiber bundles. There is a major difference between dermis and scar tissue in the arrangement of collagen fiber bundles. In scar tissue, as in granulation tissue, they are organized in arrays parallel to the surface, while in dermis more in basket weave pattern (21). This difference results in a more rigid scar tissue. The collagen composition change from granulation tissue to scar tissue where there is collagen type III decreases from 30% to 10%. In the remodeling phase the biomechanical strength of a scar increases slightly, despite no extra collagen being pro-duced. This increase relates primarily to a better architectural organization of the collagen fiber bundles.

The epidermis of a scar differs from normal skin by lacking the rete pegs, which are anchored within the underlying connective tissue matrix (21). Furthermore there is no regeneration of lost subepidermal appendages such as hair follicles or sweat glands in a scar.

## Types of wound after injury

Wounds can be divided into different types, according to healing and associated wound closure methods (56–58) (Fig. 1.5). This distinction is based on practical treatment regimens while the basic biological wound healing sequences are similar for all wound types.

*Primary healing,* or healing by *first intention,* occurs when wound edges are anatomically accurately opposed and healing proceeds without complication. This type of wound heals with a good cosmetic and functional result and with a minimal amount of scar tissue. These wounds, however, are sensitive to complications, such as infection.

*Secondary healing,* or healing by *second intention,* occurs in wounds associated with tissue loss or when wound edges are not accurately opposed. This type of healing is usually the natural biological process that occurs in the absence of surgical intervention. The defect is gradually filled by granulation tissue and a considerable amount of scar tissue will be formed despite an active contraction process. The resulting scar is less functional and often sensitive to thermal and mechanical injury. Furthermore, this form of healing requires considerable time for epithelial coverage and scar formation, but is rather resistant to infection, at least when granulation tissue has developed.

Surgical closure procedures have combined the advantages of the two types of healing. This has led to a technique of *delayed primary closure*, where the wound is left open for a few days but closure is completed before granulation tissue becomes visible (usually a week after wounding) and the wound is then healed by a process similar to primary healing (59, 60, 435, 614). The resulting wound is more resistant to healing complications (primarily infection) and is functionally and cosmetically improved. If visible granulation tissue has developed before either wound closure or wound contraction has spontaneously approximated the defect, it is called *secondary closure*. This wound is healed by a process similar to secondary healing and scar formation is more pronounced than after delayed primary closure. The different closure techniques are shown in Fig. 1.5. The following section describes the sequential changes in tissue components and their interactions seen during the wound healing process.

## Tissues and compounds in wound healing

### Hemostasis phase and coagulation cascade

An injury that severs the vasculature leads to extravasion of plasma, platelets, erythrocytes and leukocytes. This initiates the coagulation cascade that produces a blood clot usually after a few minutes and which, together with the already induced vascular contraction, limits further blood loss (Fig. 1.6). The tissue injury disrupts the endothelial integrity of the vessels, and exposes the subendothelial structures and various connective tissue components. Exposure of type IV and V collagen in the subendothelium promotes binding and aggregation of platelets and their structural proteins (61, 62). Exposure of collagen and other activating agents provokes endothelial cells and platelets to secrete several substances, such as fibronectin, serotonin, platelet derived growth factor (PDGF), adenosine diphosphate (ADP) thromboxane A and others. Following this activation, platelets aggregate and platelet clot formation begins within a few minutes. The clot formed is impermeable to plasma and serves as a seal for ruptured vasculature as well as to prevent bacterial invasion (62). In addition to platelet aggregation and activation, the coagulation cascade is initiated (Fig. 1.6).

The crucial step in coagulation is the conversion of fibrinogen to fibrin which will create a threadlike network to entrap plasma fractions and formed elements. This fibrin blood clot is formed both intravascularly and extravascularly and supports the initial platelet clot (Fig. 1.6). Extrinsic and intrinsic clotting mechanisms are activated, each giving rise to cascades that will convert prothrombin to thrombin, and in turn cleave fibrinogen to fibrin which then polymerizes to form a clot (63).

The *extrinsic* coagulation pathway is initiated by tissue thromboplastin and coagulation Factor VII, whereas the initiator of the *intrinsic* coagulation cascade consists of Hageman factor (Factor XII), prekallikrein and HMW-kinogen. The extrinsic coagulation pathway is the primary source of clotting, while the intrinsic coagulation pathway is probably most important in producing bradykinin, a vasoactive mediator that increases vascular permeability (64).

Products of the coagulation cascade regulate the cells in the wound area. Thus *intact thrombin* serves as a potent growth stimulator for fibroblasts and endothelial cells (65, 66) whereas *degraded thrombin* fragments stimulate monocytes and platelets (67–69). Likewise *plasmin* acts as a growth factor for parenchymal cells (69). *Fibrin* acts as a chemoattractant for monocytes (70) and induces angiogenesis (64). Other mediators created by blood coagulation for wound healing include *kallikrein, bradykinin,* and *C3a* and *C5a* through a spillover activation of the complement cascade and most of these factors act as chemoattractants for circulating leukocytes. Thus apart from ensuring hemostasis, the clot also initiates healing (Fig. 1.4).

If the blood clot is exposed to air it will dry and form a scab which serves as a temporary wound dressing. A vast network of fibrin strands extends throughout the clot in all directions (Fig. 1.6). These strands subsequently undergo contraction and become reoriented in a plane parallel to the wound edges (71, 72). As the fibrin strands contract, they exert tensional forces on the wound edges whereby serum is extruded from the clot and the distance between wound edges is decreased. Contraction and reorientation of the fibrin strands later serve as pathways for migrating cells (see p. 29).

If proper adaptation of the wound edges has occurred the extravascular clot forms a thin gel filling the narrow space between the wound edges and gluing the wound edges together with fibrin.

If hemostasis is not achieved, blood will continue to leak into the tissue, leading to a hematoma and a coagulum which consists of serum plasma fraction, formed elements and fibrin fragments. The presence of such a hematoma will delay the wound healing and increase the risk of infection (77).

### Coagulation

More extensive blood clot formation is undesirable in most wounds as the clots present barriers between tissue surfaces and force wounds that might have healed without a clot to heal by secondary intention. In oral wounds such as extraction sockets, blood clots are exposed to heavy bacterial colonization from the saliva (74). In this location neutrophil

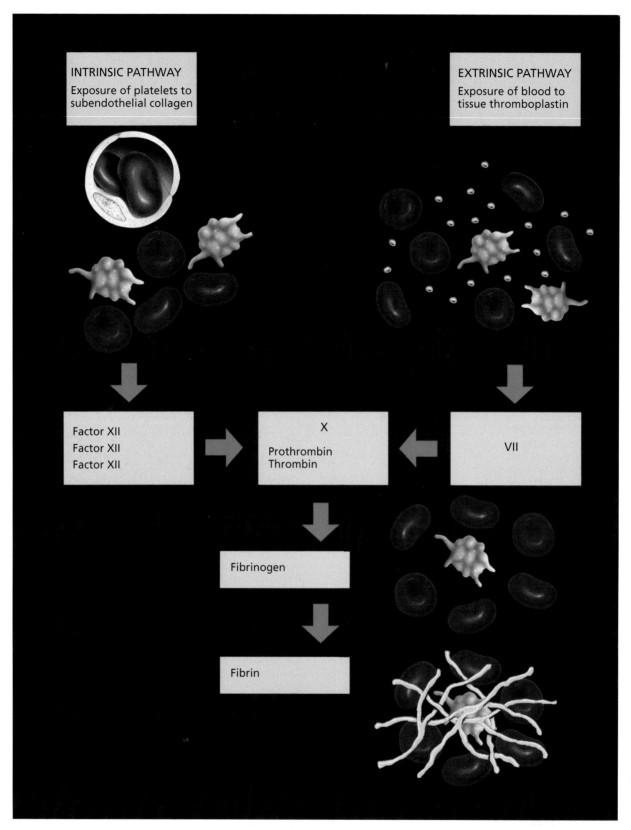

**Fig. 1.6** Extrinsic and intrinsic coagulation cascade.

leukocytes form a dense layer on the exposed blood clot and the most superficial neutrophils contain many phagocytosed bacteria (75).

The breakdown of coagulated blood in the wound releases ferric ions into the tissue which have been shown to decrease the nonspecific host response to infection (76). Furthermore, the presence of a hematoma in the tissue may increase the chance of infection (77).

Clot adhesion to the root surface appears to be important for periodontal ligament healing. Thus an experiment has

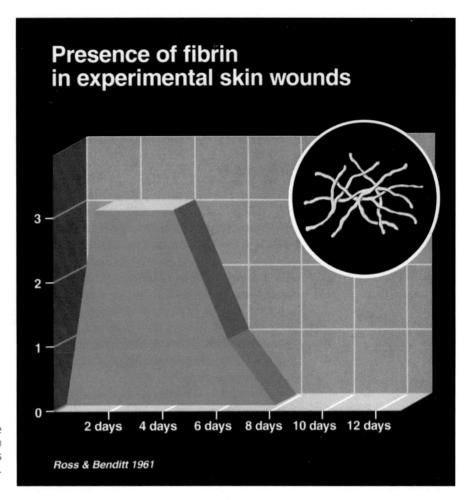

**Presence of fibrin in experimental skin wounds**

*Ross & Benditt 1961*

**Fig. 1.7** Schematic illustration of the presence of fibrin in experimental skin wounds in guinea pigs. The scale is semiquantitative, graded from 0 to 3. From ROSS & BENDITT (73) 1961.

shown that heparin impregnated root surfaces, which prevented clot formation, resulted in significantly less connective tissue repair and an increase in downgrowth of pocket epithelium after gingival flap surgery (78).

## Fibrin

During the coagulation process, fibrinogen is converted to fibrin which, via a fishnet arrangement with entrapped erythrocytes, stabilizes the blood clot (Figs 1.6 and 1.7).

In the early acute inflammatory period extravasation of a serous fluid from the leaking vasculature accumulates as an edema in the tissue spaces. This transudate contains fibrinogen which forms fibrin when acted upon by thrombin (Fig. 1.7). Fibrin plugs then seal damaged lymphatics and thereby confine the inflammatory reaction to an area immediately surrounding the wound.

Fibrin has been found to play a significant role in wound healing by its capacity to bind to fibronectin (63). Thus fibronectin present in the clot will link to both fibrin and to itself (79, 80).

Fibrin clots and fibrinopeptides are weak stimulators of fibroblasts (81), an effect which is prevented by depletion of fibronectin (82). It has also been proposed that an interaction may take place between hyaluronic acid and fibrin which creates an initial scaffold on which cells may migrate into the wound (83).

The extravascular fibrin forms a hygroscopic gel that facilitates migration of neutrophils and macrophages, an effect which possibly reflects a positive interaction between the macrophage surface and the fibrin matrix. Fibrin has also been shown to elicit fibroblast migration and angiogenesis, both of which initiate an early cellular invasion of the clot (63, 64, 84–86).

Fibrin clots are continuously degraded over a 1–3 week period (73, 87, 88). This occurs during the fibrinolysis cascade which is activated by the plasminogen present in damaged endothelial cells and activated granulocytes and macrophages (87–89; Fig. 1.7).

In experimental replantation of teeth in monkeys it has been found that collagen fiber attachment to the root surface was preceded by fibrin leakage, and that this leakage was an initial event in the wound healing response (90).

In summary, the blood clot, apart from being responsible for hemostasis, also serves the purpose of initiating wound healing including functioning as a matrix for migrating connective cells.

## Fibronectin

Fibronectin is a complex glycoprotein, which can be present as soluble plasma fibronectin, produced by hepatocytes, or stromal fibronectin, found in basal laminae and loose connective tissue matrices where it is produced by fibroblasts, macrophages and epithelial cells (91, 92). During wound healing, fibronectin is also produced locally by fibroblasts (93), macrophages in regions where epidermal cell migration occurs (92), endothelial cells (94, 95), and by epidermal cells (96).

Fibronectin plays many roles in wound healing, including platelet aggregation, promotion of re-epithelialization, cell migration, matrix deposition and wound contraction (92, 97).

In wound healing, fibronectin is the first protein to be deposited in the wound (98) and therefore, together with fibrin, serves as a preliminary scaffold and matrix for migrating cells (99) (see p. 29). Thus plasma fibronectin is linked to fibrin which has been spilled from damaged vessels or from highly permeable undamaged vessels (see p. 29) (97, 100). The fibrin–fibronectin complex forms an extensive meshwork throughout the wound bed which facilitates fibroblast attachment and migration into the clot (80, 101–103). Furthermore, soluble fibronectin fragments are chemotactic for fibroblasts and monocytes (104).

Fibronectin appears also to guide the orderly deposition of collagen within the granulation tissue. Thus fibronectin serves as the scaffold for deposition of types III and I collagen (105–109) as well as collagen type VI (109). As dermal wounds age, bundles of type I collagen become more prominent at the expense of type III collagen fibronectin (106). Finally, fibronectin seems to represent a necessary link between collagen and fibroblasts which makes it possible to generate the forces in wound contraction (92, 110).

In endothelium during wound healing, fibronectin is found in the basement membrane and reaches a maximum at approximately the same time as the peak in endothelial cell mitosis occurs, indicating a possible role of fibronectin in endothelial cell migration (111).

In epithelialization, it has been found that fibronectin is implicated in epidermal cell adhesion, migration and differentiation (96, 111–114). Thus migrating epithelial cells are supported by an irregular band of fibrin–fibronectin matrix which provides attachment and a matrix for prompt migration (87, 108).

Clinically, fibronectin has been used to promote attachment of connective tissue to the exposed root and surfaces, and thereby limiting epithelial downgrowth (117–123). Furthermore fibronectin has been shown to accelerate healing of periodontal ligament fibers after tooth replantation (120). This effect has also been shown to occur in experimental marginal periodontal defects in animals (121, 122) as well as in humans (123).

## Complement system

The complement system consists of a group of proteins that play a central role in the inflammatory response. One of the activated factors, C5a, has the ability to cleave its C-terminal arginine residue by a serum carboxypeptidase to form C5a-des-arg which is a potent chemotactic factor for attracting neutrophils to the site of injury (124, 125).

## Necrotic cells

Dead and dying cells release a variety of substances that may be important for wound healing such as tissue factor, lactic acid, lactate dehydrogenase, calcium lysosomal enzymes and fibroblast growth factor (FGF) (126).

## Matrix

### Proteoglycans and hyaluronic acid

All connective tissues contain proteoglycans. In some tissues, such as cartilage, proteoglycans are the major constituent and add typical physical characteristics to the matrix (127).

#### Chondroitin sulfate proteoglycans
Chondrocytes, fibroblasts and smooth muscle cells are all able to produce these proteoglycans. Chondroitin sulfate impairs the adhesion of cells to fibronectin and collagen and thereby promotes cell mobility. Skin contains proteoglycans, termed dermatan sulfates, which are involved in collagen formation.

#### Heparin and heparan sulfate proteoglycans
Heparins are a subtype with an anticoagulant activity. Heparan sulfates are produced by mast cells and adhere to cell surfaces and basement membranes.

*Keratan sulfates* are limited to the cornea, sclera and cartilage. Their role in wound healing is unknown.

*Hyaluronic acid* is a ubiquitous connective tissue component and plays a major role in the structure and organization of the extracellular matrix. Hyaluronic acid has been implicated in the detachment process of cells that allows cells to move. Furthermore hyaluronic acid inhibits cell differentiation. Because of its highly charged nature, hyaluronic acid can absorb a large volume of water (128).

The role of proteoglycans during wound healing is not fully understood (129). Heparin may play a role in the control of clotting at the site of tissue damage. Proteoglycans are also suspected of playing an important role in the early stages of healing when cell migration occurs. Thus *hyaluronic acid* may be involved in detachment of cells so that they can move (130). Furthermore, proteoglycans may provide an open hydrated environment that promotes cell migration (129, 131, 133).

The proliferative phase of healing involves cell duplication, differentiation and synthesis of extracellular matrix components. Thus hyaluronidate has been found to keep cells in an undifferentiated state which is compatible with proliferation and migration (127). At this stage chondroitin and heparan sulfates are apparently important in collagen fibrillogenesis (127) and mast cell heparin promotes capillary endothelial proliferation and migration (132). Furthermore, when endothelium is damaged, a depletion of growth-suppressing heparan sulfate may allow PDGF or other stimuli to stimulate angiogenesis (133).

The combined action of substances released from platelets, blood coagulation and tissue degradation results in hemostasis, initiation of the vasculatory response and release of signals for cell activation, proliferation and migration.

The role of the anticoagulant heparin is to temporarily prevent coagulation of the excess tissue fluid and blood components during the early phase of the inflammatory response.

## Inflammatory phase mediators

The sequence of the inflammatory process is directed by different types of chemical mediators which are responsible for vascular changes and migration of cells into the wound area (Fig 1.6).

### Mediators responsible for vascular changes

Inflammatory mediators such as histamine, kinins and serotonin cause vasodilatation unless autonomic stimulation overrules them.

The effect of these mediators is constriction of smooth muscles. This influences endothelial and periendothelial cells, providing reversible opening of junctions between cells and permitting a passage of plasma solutes across the vascular barrier. These mediators are released primarily during

**Table 1.1** Mediators of vascular response in inflammation. Modified from VENGE (136) 1985.

|  | Mediator | Originating cells |
|---|---|---|
| Humoral | Complement<br>Kallikrein–Kinin system<br>Fibrin |  |
| Cellular | Histamine | Thrombocytes<br>Mast cells<br>Basophils |
|  | Serotonin | Thrombocytes<br>Mast cells |
|  | Prostaglandins | Inflammatory cells |
|  | Thromboxane $A_2$ | Thrombocytes<br>Neutrophils |
|  | Leukotrienes | Mast cells<br>Basophils<br>Eosinophils<br>Macrophages |
|  | Cationic peptides | Neutrophils |
|  | Oxygen radicals | Neutrophils<br>Eosinophils<br>Macrophages |

the process of platelet aggregation and clotting. The best known mediators related to the vascular response are shown in Table 1.1.

### Histamine

The main sources of histamine in the wound appear to be platelets, mast cells, and basophil leukocytes. The histamine release causes a short-lived dilation of the microvasculature (137) and increased permeability of the small venules. The endothelial cells swell and separations occur between the individual cells. This is followed by plasma leaking through the venules and the emigration of polymorphonuclear leukocytes (137–141).

### Serotonin

Serotonin (5-hydroxytryptamine) is generated in the wound by platelets and mast cells. Serotonin appears to increase the permeability of blood vessels, similarly to histamine, but appears to be more potent (139, 140). Apart from causing contraction of arterial and venous smooth muscles and dilation of arterioles, the net hemodynamic effect of serotonin is determined by the balance between dilation and contraction (137, 142).

### Prostaglandins

Other mediators involved in the vascular response are prostaglandins (PG). These substances are metabolites of arachidonic acid and are part of a major group called eicosanoids, which are also considered primary mediators in wound healing (143). Prostaglandins are the best known substances in this group and are released by cells via arachidonic acid following injury to the cell membrane. These include $PGD_2$, $PGE_2$, $PGF_2$, thromboxane A2 and prostacycline ($PGI_2$). These components have an important influence on vascular changes and platelet aggregation in the inflammatory response and some of the effects are antagonistic. Under normal circumstances, a balance of effects is necessary. In tissue injury, the balance will shift towards excess thromboxane $A_2$, leading to a shutdown of the microvasculature (143).

New research suggests that prostaglandins, and especially $PGF_2$, could be endogenous agents that are able to initiate repair or reconstitute the damaged tissue (144). Thus biosynthesis of $PGF_2$ has been shown to have an important effect on fibroblast reparative processes (145), for which reason this prostaglandin may also have an important influence on later phases of the wound healing process. The effect of prostaglandins on the associated inflammatory response elicited subsequent to infection is further discussed in Chapter 2.

### Bradykinin

Bradykinin released via the coagulation cascade relaxes vascular smooth muscles and increases capillary permeability leading to plasma leakage and swelling of the injured area.

### Neurotransmitters (norepinephrine, epinephrine and acetylcholine)

The walls of arteries and arterioles contain adrenergic and cholinergic nerve fibers. In some tissue the sympathetic adrenergic nerve fibers may extend down to the capillary level. Tissue injury will stimulate the release of neurotransmitters which results in vasoconstriction.

## Mediators with chemotactic effects

These mediators promote migration of cells to the area of injury and are thus responsible for the recruitment of the various cells which are involved in the different phases of wound healing (Fig. 1.4).

The first cells to arrive in the area are the leukocytes. The chemotactic effects are mediated through specific receptors on the surface of these cells. Complement activated products like C5a, C5a-des-arg, and others cause the leukocytes to migrate between the endothelial cells into the inflammatory area. This migration is facilitated by the increased capillary permeability that follows the release of the earlier mentioned mediators. Further leukocyte chemoattractants include kallikrein and plasminogen activator, PDGF and platelet factor 4.

Other types of chemotactic receptors are involved when leukocytes recognize immunoglobulin (Ig) and complement proteins such as C3b and C3bi. The mechanism appears to be that B lymphocytes, when activated, secrete immunoglobulin which again triggers the activation of the complement system resulting in production of chemoattractants such as C5a-des-arg (146).

Other mediators involved in chemoattraction will be mentioned in relation to the cell types involved in the wound healing process.

### S. Storgård Jensen

## Growth factors

Growth factors are a group of polypeptides involved in cellular chemotaxis, differentiation, proliferation, and synthesis of extracellular matrix during embryogenesis, postnatal growth and adulthood.

All wound healing events in both hard and soft tissues are influenced by polypeptide growth factors, which can be released from the traumatized tissue itself, can be harbored in the quickly formed blood clot or brought to the area by neutrophils or macrophages.

Growth factors are local signaling molecules. They can act in a paracrine manner where they bind to receptors on the cell surface of neighboring target cells, leading to initiation of specific intracellular transduction pathways; or they can act in an autocrine manner, whereby the function is elicited on the secreting cell itself. Additionally, elevated serum levels have been demonstrated for a few growth factors which may indicate an endocrine effect. Complex feedback loops regulate the production of the individual growth. The effect of each growth factor is highly dependent on the concentration and on the presence of other growth factors. A growth factor can have a stimulatory effect on a specific cell type, whereas an increased concentration may inhibit the exact same cell type. Two different growth factors with a known stimulatory effect on a cell type can in combination result in both an *agonistic*, *synergistic*, and even an *antagonistic* effect.

Growth factors may have the potential to improve healing of traumatized tissues in several ways. First, some growth factors have the ability to recruit specific predetermined cell types and pluripotent stem cells to the wounded area by chemotaxis. Second, they may induce differentiation of mesenchymal precursor cells to mature secreting cells. Third, they often stimulate mitosis of relevant cells, and thereby increase proliferation. Fourth, several growth factors have the ability to increase angiogenesis, the ingrowth of new blood vessels. Finally, they can have a profound effect on both secretion and breakdown of extracellular matrix (ECM) components.

The most important growth factors are listed in Table 1.2 and a brief summary of their characteristics, including their presumed role in wound repair and regeneration is given below.

Dentoalveolar traumas may involve a multitude of tissues like oral mucosa, periodontal ligament, root cementum, dentin, dental pulp, bone, skin, blood vessels and nerves. Only a few clinical studies have evaluated the use of growth factors specifically for oral and maxillofacial traumas (p. 16).

*Platelet derived growth factor (PDGF)* consists of two amino acid chains and comes in homo- and heterodimeric isoforms (AA, AB, BB, CC, and DD, where AA, AB, and BB are the best documented) (147). PDGF binds to two specific receptors: $\alpha$ and $\beta$. Differential binding of the different isoforms to the receptors contributes to the varying effects of PDGF. As the name implies, PDGF is released from platelets, where it is present in large amounts in $\alpha$-granules. Platelets are activated by thrombin or fibrillar collagen. Other sources of PDGF are macrophages, endothelial cells and fibroblasts. PDGF was the first growth factor shown to be chemotactic for cells migrating into the wound area, such as neutrophils, monocytes, and fibroblasts. Additionally, PDGF stimulates proliferation and ECM production of fibroblasts (148) and activates macrophages to debride the wound area (149).

*Transforming growth factors (TGFs)* comprise a large family of cytokines with a widespread impact on the formation and development of many tissues (among those, the BMPs, which are described separately). This factor has earlier been divided into $\alpha$ and $\beta$ subtypes, where the latter is the most important for the wound healing process (150). TGF-$\beta$ is mainly released from platelets and macrophages as a latent homodimer that must be cleaved to be activated. This latent form is present in both wound matrix and saliva.

**Table 1.2** Characteristics of Growth factors involved in healing after dental trauma.

| Growth factor | Originating cells | Target cells | Main effect | Tissue response |
|---|---|---|---|---|
| PDGF | Platelets<br>Macrophages<br>Endothelial cells<br>Osteoblasts | Neutrophils<br>Monocytes<br>Fibroblasts<br>Osteoblasts | Chemotaxis<br>Proliferation | Angiogenesis<br>Macrophage activation |
| TGF | Platelets<br>Macrophages<br>Fibroblasts<br>Lymphocytes<br>Osteoblasts | Fibroblasts<br>Monocytes<br>Neutrophils<br>Macrophages<br>Osteoblastic precursor cells | Chemotaxis<br>ECM production<br>Proliferation | Collagen production (scarring)<br>Down-regulation of other cell types<br>   but fibroblasts<br>Immunoregulation |
| IGF | Hepatocytes<br>Osteoblasts | Fibroblasts<br>Osteoblasts<br>Epithelial cells | Proliferation<br>ECM production<br>Chemotaxis<br>Cell survival | Stimulated DNA synthesis<br>Growth promotion of committed cells |
| EGF | Platelets<br>Salivary glands | Epithelial cells<br>Enamel organ<br>Periodontal ligament fibroblasts<br>Preosteoblasts | Proliferation<br>Chemotaxis<br>ECM production | Epithelialization<br>Tooth eruption |
| FGF | Endothelial cells<br>Macrophages<br>Keratinocytes<br>Osteoblasts | Endothelial cells<br>Fibroblasts<br>Keratinocytes | Proliferation<br>Migration<br>ECM formation | Angiogenesis<br>Epithelialization |
| VEGF | Keratinocytes<br>Macrophages<br>Fibroblasts | Endothelial cells | Proliferation | Angiogenesis |
| BMP | Osteoblasts | Undifferentiated mesenchymal cells<br>Osteoblastic precursor cells<br>Osteoblasts | Differentiation<br>Proliferation<br>ECM production | Bone formation<br>Root cementum formation<br>Dentin formation<br>PDL formation |

ECM, extracellular matrix; PDL, periodontal ligament.

TGF-β is known to be a strong promoter of extracellular matrix production of many cell types (e.g. collagen and mucopolysaccharide) including periodontal ligament fibroblasts. Proliferation of fibroblasts is also induced by TGF-β, whereas mitogenesis of most other cell types is inhibited like keratinocytes, lymphocytes and most epithelial cells. Additionally, TGF-β plays a role in immune and inflammatory regulation. TGF-β is also deposited in bone matrix where it is released during bone remodeling or in relation to traumas and acts chemotactic on osteoblasts. The effects of TGF-β are extremely complex and strongly dependent on the concentration of the growth factor itself, the concentration of other growth factors, and the differentiation state of the target cells.

*Epidermal growth factor (EGF)* was one of the first growth factors to be isolated (151). It is produced by platelets, salivary glands and duodenal glands. TGF-α is today considered to be a member of the EGF family. The receptors for EGF have been found in oral epithelium, enamel organ, periodontal ligament fibroblasts and pre-osteoblasts (152, 153). Stimulation of the EGF receptor causes the cells to become less differentiated and to divide and grow rapidly. In wounds, EGF has been found to encourage cells to continue through the cell cycle. Such a cell proliferative effect has been demonstrated in epithelial cells (154) endothelial cells and periosteal fibroblasts (155). EGF has also been shown to be chemotactic for epithelial cells (156) and to stimulate fibroblast collagenase production (157). In oral tissues it has been shown that EGF controls the proliferation of odontogenic cells (158) and accelerates tooth eruption (159).

*Insulin-like growth factor (IGF)* is a single chain polypeptide which structurally is very similar to proinsulin. Two isoforms, IGF-I and -II are mainly produced in the liver and exert their effects in autocrine, paracrine, and endocrine manners. The endocrine effect is mainly controlled by growth hormone. Osteoblasts also produce IGF that is stored in the bone matrix and acts as paracrine and autocrine (160, 161). IGF alone has hardly any major effect on wound healing (162). Combinations with other growth factors, such as PDGF and FGF, have, however, been shown to have a pronounced stimulatory effect on fibroblast proliferation, collagen synthesis, bone formation, and epithelialization (162).

*Fibroblast growth factors (FGFs)* comprise a growing family of polypeptides, currently consisting of more than 20 members. They are mainly produced by endothelial cells and macrophages. FGFs are mitogenic for several cell types involved in wound healing and support cell survival under stress conditions. FGFs are involved in angiogenesis and epithelialization. FGF-I and FGF-II (earlier known as acidic FGF and basic FGF) are potent stimulators of angiogenesis in the early formation of granulation tissue (days 1–3) by recruiting endothelial cells and inducing proliferation. Neither has a transmembrane sequence and can therefore not be secreted. Instead they are probably released from disrupted cells by tissue damage (163). After release, FGFs interact with heparin and heparan sulfate, with which they can be stored in the extracellular matrix. Here FGF can be activated when injury causes platelets to degranulate and among many other substances release heparin degrading enzymes.

*Vascular endothelial growth factor (VEGF)* is, as far as we know today, the only endothelial-specific growth factor enhancing cell proliferation, and its activity is therefore probably essential for angiogenesis in all tissues during both development and repair. VEGF is produced in large quantities by keratinocytes, macrophages and, to a lesser extent, fibroblasts in the epidermis during wound healing, where it seems to be critical for angiogenesis in the granulation tissue formation from days 4 to 7. Hypoxia, a hallmark of tissue injury, induces VEGF production. Reduced expression and accelerated degradation of VEGF has been shown to cause skin wound defects (163) and addition of VEGF has promoted angiogenesis in skin wounds in diabetic mice (164).

*In vivo*, VEGF has resulted in increased capillary density and bone formation in standardized bone defects in rabbits (165).

No clinical studies have evaluated the effect of VEGF in relation to oral and maxillofacial trauma.

*Bone morphogenetic proteins (BMPs)* are members of the TGF-β superfamily. More than 20 different BMPs have been identified. BMPs are found in bone matrix and in periosteal cells and mesenchymal cells of the bone marrow (166). BMP-2, -4, and -7 (also called osteogenic protein-1 (OP-1)) are the most involved in bone healing, whereas increased BMP-6 has been described in skin wounds. The main task of BMP is to commit undifferentiated pluripotential cells to become bone or cartilage forming cells. BMPs are the only known factors that are capable of forming bone in extraskeletal sites, a phenomenon referred to as osteoinduction (167).

### Experimental data indicating clinical implications of growth factors

#### Angiogenesis

During healing after trauma, *de novo* formation of the disrupted vascular supply is a prerequisite for most of the healing events. This is supported by the finding that hyperbaric oxygen (HBO) is a potent stimulator of healing of both hard and soft tissue healing (168) in sites with a compromised healing potential such as diabetic ulcers and irradi-

ated bone (169, 170). The primary long-term effect of HBO is increased angiogenesis. VEGF, FGF, TGF-β, and PDGF are known to be involved in angiogenesis during wound healing (259). Exactly how these growth factors interact with the extracellular matrix (ECM) environment in the blood clot and in granulation tissue, are, however not known in detail. Revascularization of the dental pulp is necessary, after both tooth fractures and luxation injuries. VEGF, PDGF and FGF have been identified in the soluble and insoluble part of human dentin matrix (171). These may be released during injury and contribute to pulpal wound healing.

### Wounds in the skin and oral mucosa

In most instances, healing proceeds rapidly in healthy individuals. Research has therefore mainly been focused on situations where the healing potential is seriously compromised such as diabetes, malnutrition, and infection. In skin wounds, PDGF is known to be chemotactic to neutrophils, monocytes and fibroblasts. In addition, PDGF is a mitogen for fibroblasts which has led to an FDA approval for the treatment of non-healing ulcers (172, 173). In addition, PDGF stimulates new vascularization of an injured area (174). Exogenously applied TGF-β has been demonstrated to induce fibroblast infiltration in the wound and increased collagen deposition (175), as well as angiogenesis and mucopolysaccharide synthesis (175, 176). This results in an accelerated healing of incisional wounds (177, 178). Due to the same mechanisms, however, TGF-β is also intimately related to scar formation. Thus the elimination of TGF-β from incisional wounds in rats (by neutralizing antibody) is able to prevent scar tissue formation (179, 620–622). Furthermore, it has been shown that the effect of TGF-β can be potentiated by the presence of PDGF and epidermal growth factor (EGF) (180). In experimental skin wounds in *animals*, an acceleration of both connective tissue and epithelial healing was found after topical application of EGF (181, 182). However, results after topical application of EGF to experimental wounds in *humans* have shown contradictory results on reepithelialization (178, 183–186). In the oral mucosa, salivary EGF has been shown to stimulate migration of oral epithelial cells (187).

An interesting observation in mice has been that saliva rinsing of skin wounds (by communal licking) both enhances coagulation and leads to acceleration of wound healing (182, 188–190). Due to the high concentration of EGF found in saliva (191) this effect has been suggested to be caused by EGF. Later experiments with induced tongue wounds in mice have shown that EGF (and possibly also TGF-β) is involved in healing of wounds of the oral mucosa (192, 193). Salivary EGF is suggested not only to accelerate wound healing in the oral cavity, but also to contribute to preserving integrity of the oral mucosa (194). Administration of IGF-I in skin wounds has no influence upon fibroblast proliferation or activity, or upon epithelialization (195–197). However, if IGF-I is administered together with PDGF or FGF, a marked fibroblast proliferation and collagen production can be observed as well as enhanced epithelialization (197).

## Periodontal healing

Experimental studies have suggested that PDGF-BB alone could have a regenerative effect on both formation of root cementum, periodontal ligament and alveolar bone (151, 198, 199, 200). PDGF has clinically, however, mainly been evaluated in combination with IGF-I where an increased bone fill could be observed both around periodontally compromised teeth and in periimplant defects (199, 201, 202). IGF used alone, TGF-β used alone, and the combination IGF-II/FGF-II/TGF-β has not been able to generate noteworthy periodontal regeneration in experimental studies (197, 203, 204). FGF-II has resulted in increased periodontal regeneration compared to control sites in experimentally created defects (205), used in a controlled release device in a sandwich membrane (206) but no clinical data are available. Experimental studies have reported regeneration of a periodontal ligament with Sharpey's fibers, inserted in the newly formed cementum and alveolar bone by using recombinant BMP-2, BMP-7 (OP-1) and recently also BMP-12. The treated periodontal defects have been either surgically created (207–209) or experimentally induced (210). This pronounced periodontal regeneration could not be obtained when BMP-12 was applied to extracted dog teeth before replantation. In contrast, ankylosis developed whether BMP-12 was applied or not (211).

## Bone healing

Information of the role of growth factors in bone healing mainly comes from preclinical studies of periodontal lesions and bone augmentation procedures before or in relation to implant placement. Numerous growth factors are deposited in bone matrix during bone formation (e.g. PDGF, TGF-β, FGF-II, and IGF-I). These are released during bone remodeling and in relation to trauma (256).

Contradictory results have been reported regarding the bone regenerative potential of PDGF. Both inhibition and stimulation of bone formation has been observed in rat calvarial defects (212, 213). PDGF alone has little impact on bone healing in vivo. However, a couple of studies have reported significant bone regeneration in periodontal and periimplant defects, when PDGF is combined with IGF (102, 201, 202, 214, 215). Likewise, IGF must be combined with other growth factors to promote bone healing. TGF-β has a strong impact on the healing of long-bone fractures (216). Only a few clinical data from the use of BMP in humans exist (217, 218). Experimental data, however, suggest an enhanced bone formation using BMP-2 and -7 for bone regeneration procedures (219–221).

## Pulp dentin complex

Attempts to regenerate the pulp dentin complex have mainly focused on the possibility of generating a hard tissue (dentin) closure to an exposed pulp in relation to pulp capping. The key question is how to induce uncommitted pulpal cells to differentiate into odontoblast-like cells secreting reparative dentin. TGF-βs, BMPs, FGFs and IGFs are harbored in dentin and are known to influence dentinogenesis during embryogenesis (222). BMP-2, BMP-4, and BMP-7 (OP-1) have all been shown to induce widespread dentin formation in the pulp, even leading to total occlusion of the pulp cavity when applied in high doses (223). Numerous studies have evaluated the revascularization of avulsed replanted teeth, but none have specifically studied the role of growth factors in this process.

## Platelet concentrate/platelet rich plasma

In the past few years, utilization of platelet concentrate (PC), also called 'platelet rich plasma' (PRP), has been increasingly recommended in patients undergoing osseous reconstruction and periodontal regeneration. PC has gained much attention since the presentation of very promising data for the resulting bone density by adding PC to iliac cancellous cellular bone marrow grafts in the reconstruction of mandibular continuity defects (224). An accelerated graft maturation rate and a denser trabecular bone configuration were observed in defects where PC had been added. It was speculated that the stimulating effect of PC was due to the accumulation of autogenous platelets, providing a high concentration of platelet growth factors with a well documented impact on bone regeneration (225, 226). The concept of using autogenous growth factors is attractive since there is no risk of disease transmission, and as it is relatively inexpensive compared to growth factors produced by recombinant techniques.

Additionally, one clinical study (227) and a series of clinical case reports and case series have presented the use of PC in different applications (228–236) leading to divergent recommendations. Data from experimental studies, evaluating addition of PC to bone graft materials have also been conflicting (237–247). In these studies a wide range of different animal models and PC preparation techniques have been used. Therefore, they are difficult to compare. Moreover, none of the studies have analyzed the growth factor content in the applied PC. Just one study analyzed the influence of PC platelet concentration in an in vivo model. The authors demonstrated a certain platelet concentration interval with the most positive biologic effect on bone regeneration, corresponding to a 3–5-fold increased concentration compared to whole blood. There was no effect using low concentrations (0–2 fold increased concentration), and there seemed to be an inhibitory effect on bone regeneration when higher concentrations were used (6–11-fold increased concentration compared to whole blood) (248).

In conclusion, no methods are currently available to produce standardized PC in which a certain whole blood platelet count will result in PC with a predictable amount of platelets and a predictable combination of growth factors. Use of autologous growth factors is simple and safe as compared with allogenic and xenogenic preparation methods. Consistent results, however, cannot be expected, until the ideal concentration of platelet growth factors has been identified and reliable PC preparation methods have been developed.

### Carriers/delivery systems for growth factors

Growth factors are in general volatile and need carriers to ensure continuance of the growth factor at the relevant site, and to provide sustained release of the growth factor in therapeutic doses. A carrier must be biocompatible. In addition, the carrier should be substituted concurrently with healing of the traumatized tissue, without causing an inflammatory reaction. Collagen can bind and release bioactive substances with some predictability (249, 250). Like other natural polymers, however, collagen has limitations in clinical use, due to difficulties in engineering its properties, handling problems, immunogenicity, and lack of resorption resistance (251, 252). Synthetic carriers for tissue promotive agents have therefore been extensively investigated. Traditionally copolymers such as lactic and glycolic acid have been utilized as vehicles for bioactive molecules due to their handling properties and biodegradability. They may, however, be associated with protein denaturation and inflammatory reactions along with the degradation process. More hydrophilic materials with controlled network properties thus offer an attractive alternative, but problems with loading the bioactive protein into the material is a common limitation related to these materials. A new polyethylene glycol (PEG) hydrogel may meet these demands. This hydrogels polymer network is synthesized around the bioactive molecules without modifying its action; it is highly water soluble, nontoxic, and nonimmunogenic (253).

In bone regeneration, a certain mechanical stability of the carrier is often required in order to avoid collapse of soft tissue into the defect and to protect against pressure from the overlying periosteum. *In vitro* investigations have shown that both adsorption of the bioactive substance and release kinetics exhibit pronounced variation when different carriers and growth factors are combined (254). In addition, the growth factor may be inactivated in relation to the release (254). PDGF-BB has, compared to IGF-I, been shown to adsorb better, be released more completely and keep its bioactivity in combination with an anorganic bovine bone substitute material (255).

In dental traumatology a carrier will probably be needed in case of pulp and PDL regeneration.

## Cells in wound healing

*F. Gottrup and S. Storgård Jensen*

### Platelets

Platelets (thrombocytes) are anucleate discoid fragments with a diameter of 2 μm (Fig. 1.8). They are formed in the bone marrow as fragments of cytoplasmatic buddings of megakaryocytes and have a life span of 7–10 days in the blood (260). Platelets contain various types of granules which, after release, have a number of effects upon hemostasis and initiation of wound healing processes (261–263) (Fig 1.4).

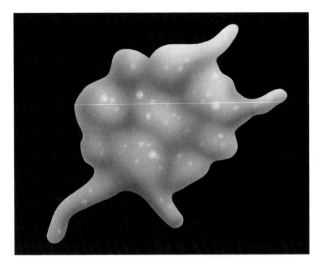

**Fig. 1.8** Activated platelet (thrombocyte).

The capacity of the platelets to adhere to exposed tissue surfaces as well as to each other after vessel injury is decisive for their hemostatic capacity (256–259). Adhesion and activation of platelets occurs when they contact collagen and microfibrils of the subendothelial matrix and locally generated factors such as thrombin, ADP, fibrinogen, fibronectin, thrombospondin and von Willebrand factor VIII.

Platelet activation results in degranulation and release of adenosine diphosphate (ADP), serotonin, thromboxane, prostaglandins and fibrinogen. The release of these substances initiates binding of other platelets to the first adherent platelets whereby blood loss is limited during formation of a hemostatic platelet plug (264). The blood loss is further reduced by the vasoconstrictor effect of thromboxane and serotonin.

The inflammatory response is initiated by activation of platelets due to liberation of serotonin, kinins and prostaglandins which leads to increased vessel permeability.

The platelet release of cytokines such as platelet derived growth factor (PDGF), platelet derived angiogenesis factor (PDAF), transforming growth factor α and β (TGF-α, TGF-β) and platelet factor 4 leads to an initiation of the wound-healing process (Fig. 1.9). Thus PDGF has been shown to have a chemotactic and activating effect upon neutrophils, monocytes and fibroblasts as well as a mitogenic effect upon fibroblasts and smooth muscle cells (263, 265). The release of TGF-β has been found to induce angiogenesis and collagen deposition (266, 267). Platelet derived angiogenesis factor (PDAF) has been shown to cause new capillary formation from the existing microvasculature (268–270). Finally, platelet factor 4 has been found to be a chemoattractant for neutrophils (271).

In summary, the platelets are the first cells brought to the site of injury. Apart from their role in hemostasis, they exert an effect upon the initiation of the vascular response and attraction and activation of neutrophils, macrophages, fibroblasts and endothelial cells. As wound healing progresses, the latter tasks are gradually assumed by macrophages.

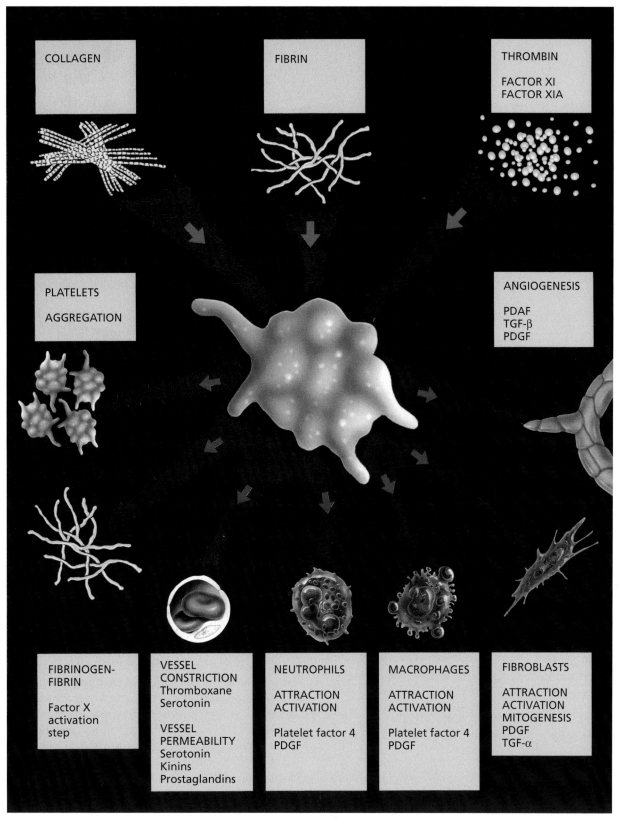

**Fig. 1.9** Role of platelets in wound healing. Exposure of platelets to collagen, fibrin, thrombin, factor XI and factor XI–A results in activation and degranulation. This then results in the release of a series of mediators influencing coagulation, vessel tone and permeability. Furthermore the initial cellular response of neutrophils, macrophages, fibroblasts and endothelial cells is established.

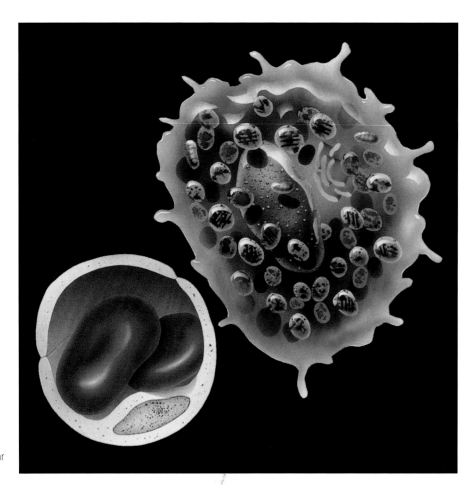

**Fig. 1.10** Mast cell in perivenular position.

## Erythrocytes

The influence of erythrocytes upon wound healing is not adequately documented except for the effect of carrying oxygen to healing tissue (40, 42, 48, 618). In one study it was found that neovascularization was stimulated in areas with erythrocyte debris (272). Another effect of the breakdown of erythrocytes is the liberation of hemoglobin, which has been found to enhance infection (273–276). In addition, the heme part of hemoglobin may contribute to the production of oxygen free radicals that can produce direct cell damage (277).

In summary, the role of erythrocytes in wound healing is doubtful, apart from being oxygen carriers.

## Mast cells

Masts cells, distinguished by their large cytoplasmatic granules, are located in a perivenular position at portals of entry of noxious substances and are especially prominent within the body surfaces that are subject to traumatic injury, such as mucosa and skin (278, 279) (Fig. 1.10).

The mast cell participates in the initial inflammatory response after injury via a series of chemical mediators such as histamine, heparin, serotonin, hyaluronic acid, prostaglandins and chemotactic mediators for neutrophils.

The release of mast cell mediators may occur as a direct result of trauma inflicted on the cell. Another means of acti-

vation after trauma appears to be when coagulation generates the mast cell activator bradykinin. An alternative means of mast cell activation appears to be the release of endotoxin during infection and the generation of C3a, C5a and cationic neutrophil protein during the inflammatory response (278).

The release of the mast cell mediators such as histamine, heparin, serotonin and slow reacting substance of anaphylaxis (SRS-A) results in active vasodilation of the small venules, which allows for the entrance of water, electrolyte and plasma proteins into the microenvironment. The maintenance of an open channel for this influx is promoted by the anticoagulant activity of heparin and by the proteolytic enzymes such as chymase. Histamine and heparin may also potentiate the angiogenesis when other angiogenic factors are present (280) (see p. 29).

The liberation of a neutrophil chemotactic factor and a lipid chemotactic factor from activated mast cells both result in attraction of neutrophils and the release of a platelet activating factor which results in degranulation and aggregation of platelets. Finally, hyaluronic acid promotes cell movement and may be crucial for cell division, which is essential in this phase of wound healing (9).

In summary the mast cell plays a role, together with platelets, in being the initiator of the inflammatory response. However, experiments with corneal wounds have shown that healing can proceed in the absence of mast cells (281).

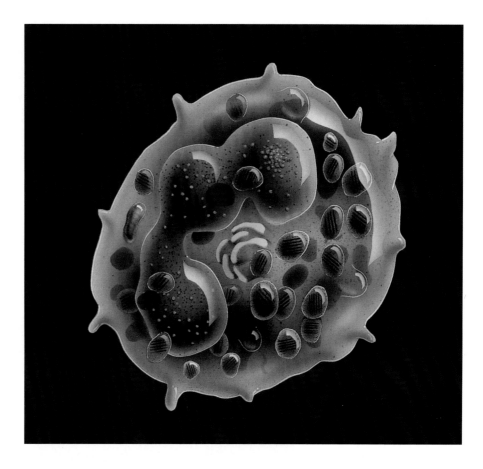

**Fig. 1.11** Neutrophil leukocyte.

## Neutrophils

The first wave of cells entering the wound site are neutrophil leukocytes which migrate from the microvasculature (Figs 1.11 and 1.12). The primary function of neutrophils is to phagocytize and kill microorganisms present within the wound (282, 283). They then degrade tissue macromolecules such as collagen, elastin, fibrin and fibronectin by liberation of digestive enzymes (Table 1.3). Finally, neutrophils release a series of inflammatory mediators which serve as chemotactic or chemokinetic agents (Fig. 1.4 and Table 1.4).

Upon exposure to chemoattractants from the clot, such as platelet factor 4, platelet derived growth factor (PDGF) kallekrein, C5a, leukotriene B4 (284, 285) and bacterial endotoxins (286–288), the granulocytes start to adhere locally to the endothelium of the venular part of the microvasculature next to the injury zone (289). Neutrophils begin to penetrate the endothelium between endothelial cells, possibly by active participation of the endothelium 2–3 hours after injury (290–293), and migrate into the wound area (291–293). Once a neutrophil has passed between endothelial cells, other leukocytes and erythrocytes follow the path (293, 294).

Once the neutrophil has passed between the endothelial cells it traverses the basement membrane by a degradation process and then moves into the interstitial tissue in the direction of the chemoattractant. This movement may be facilitated by proteolytic activity and enhanced by contact guidance. Thus neutrophils move preferentially along fiber

**Table 1.3** Neutrophil-produced degrading products.

| |
|---|
| **Primary granules (unspecific, azurophilic)** |
| Cathepsin A, G |
| Elastase |
| Collagenase (unspecific) |
| Myeloperoxidase |
| Lyzozyme |
| |
| **Secondary granules (specific)** |
| Lactoferrin |
| Collagenase (specific) |
| $B_{12}$-binding protein |
| Lyzozyme |
| |
| **Other products** |
| Gelatinase |
| Kininogenase |
| Oxygen radicals |

alignments, suggesting that tissue architecture may be a significant determinant of the efficacy of cellular mobilization.

At this point the wound contains a network of fibrin, leukocytes and a few fibroblasts. By the end of the second day most of the neutrophils have lost their ameboid properties and have released their granula into the surrounding tissue. This event apparently triggers a second migration where plasma, erythrocytes and neutrophils again leave the venules (295). In the case of uncomplicated non-infected healing, the numbers of neutrophils decrease after 3–5 days (Fig. 1.12).

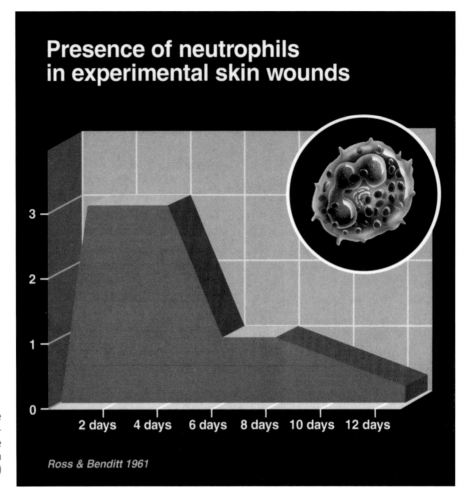

**Fig. 1.12** Schematic illustration of the presence of neutrophils in experimental skin wounds in guinea pigs. The scale is semiquantitative, graded from 0 to 3. From ROSS & BENDITT (73) 1961.

When the neutrophils have reached the site of injury they form a primary line of defense against infection by phagocytosis and intracellular killing of microorganisms (288). In this process each phagocyte may harbor as many as 30 or more bacteria (296).

Phagocytosis of bacteria by neutrophils induces a respiratory burst that produces toxic oxygen metabolites. These products include hypohalides, superoxide anion and hydroxyl radicals (288). Furthermore, they can generate chloramine formed by the reaction of hypochlorite with ammonia or amines (297). As a result of stimulation, phagocytosis or lysis, the neutrophils may release the content of their granules into the extracellular space. These granules contain oxygen radicals and neutral proteases, such as cathepsin G, elastase, collagenases, gelatinase and cationic proteins (288). All these products result in tissue damage and breakdown at an acid pH (298). A decrease or elimination of these products provided by experimental neutropenia has prevented the normally found decrease in wound strength in early intestinal anastomosis (299).

Despite these effects upon the wound the presence of neutrophils is not essential for the wound healing process itself. Thus wound healing has been found to proceed normally as scheduled in uncontaminated wounds in the absence of neutrophils (283, 300). A recent study, however,

**Table 1.4** Some chemotactic and chemokinetic agents. Modified from VENGE (136) 1985.

| **Humoral** | |
| --- | --- |
| Chemotactic | C3 and C5 fragments<br>Fibrin degradation products<br>Kallikrein<br>Plasminogen activator<br>Fibronectin<br>Casein |
| Chemokinetic | C3 and C5 fragments<br>Acute phase proteins (Orosomucoid, $\alpha_1$-antitrypsin,<br>$\alpha_2$-macroglobulin)<br>Hyaluronic acid |
| **Cellular** | |
| Chemotactic | Leukotriene $B_4$ (precursors and derivatives)<br>Platelet activating factor (PAF)<br>Transforming growth factor-$\beta$ (TGF-$\beta$)<br>Lymphokines<br>NCFs (neutrophil chemotactic factors)<br>ECFs (eosinophil chemotactic factors)<br>MCFs (monocyte chemotactic factors)<br>Formylated tripeptides (e.g. FMLP) |
| Chemokinetic | Cathepsin G |

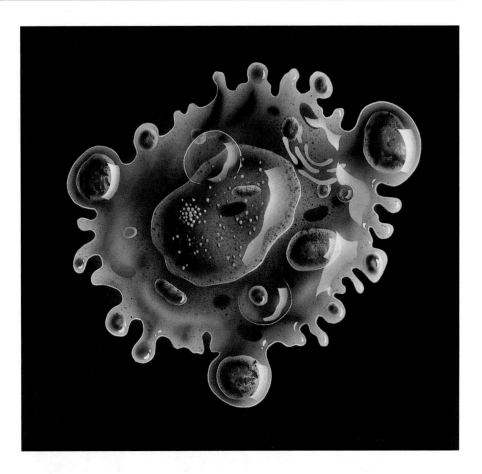

**Fig. 1.13** Macrophage.

demonstrating neutrophil expression of cytokines and TGF-β may indicate a positive influence on wound healing (301).

Recent research has elucidated a role of neutrophils in healing of chronic wounds (302–308). A consistent feature of chronic wounds is chronic inflammation associated with increased neutrophil infiltration (302). Once initiated, the inflammatory response is perpetuated and gradually converted into a chronic inflammatory state. Morphologically, the chronic inflammatory infiltrate is predominantly composed of macrophages and lymphocytes (304, 305). Mast cells may also contribute to the fibrotic response (304). It is likely that different polypeptidic cytokines and growth factors mediate some of these processes. One candidate is the profibrotic and proinflammatory TGF-β1, which is also increased at the mRNA and protein levels in the lower leg skin of class 4 patients (305, 306).

It is thought that excessive local proteolytic activity results in the breakdown of the matrix components of the skin with the end result of an ulcer.

Proteinases in skin homeostasis have multiple biological functions. Proteinases not only remodel extracellular matrix proteins but they also modulate the bioactivity of cytokines and growth factors by several different mechanisms (307, 308). In chronic wounds neutrophils are strong protease producers, delaying the wound healing process.

In summary, the main role of neutrophils in wound healing appears to be limited to elimination of bacteria within the wound area.

## Macrophages

Following the initial trauma and neutrophil accumulation, monocytes become evident in the wound area (Fig. 1.13). These cells arise from the bone marrow and circulate in blood (309, 310). In response to release of chemoattractants monocytes leave the bloodstream in the same way as neutrophils. These cells are a heterogeneous group of cells which can express an almost infinite variability of phenotypes in response to changes (311–313).

Monocytes appear in the wound after 24 hours, reach a peak after 2–4 days, and remain in the wound until healing is complete (73) (Fig. 1.14). When monocytes invade the wound area, they undergo a phenotypic metamorphosis to macrophages (314, 315). It should be mentioned that tissue macrophages can proliferate locally (314–317) and possibly play a significant role in the initial inflammatory response.

The arrival of macrophages in the wound area is a response to various chemoattractants released from injured tissue, platelets, neutrophils, lymphocytes and bacteria (Fig. 1.4). In Table 1.4 series of chemotactic factors are listed which have been shown to be chemotactic for macrophages. In this context, it should be mentioned that monocytes express multiple receptors for different chemotactic factors (317). As shown in Table 1.4, connective tissue fragments appear to be *chemotactic* for macrophages, i.e. forming gradients enabling directional movements, and *chemokinetic*, i.e. alter the rate of cell movements. These tissue fragments

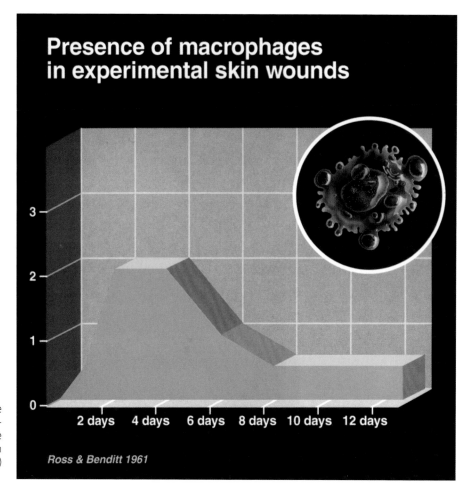

**Fig. 1.14** Schematic illustration of the presence of macrophages in experimental skin wounds in guinea pigs. The scale is semiquantitative, graded from 0 to 3. From ROSS & BENDITT (73) 1961.

are possibly generated by neutrophils which precede the appearance of monocytes (see p. 22). It has been shown that neutrophils contain enzymes such as elastase, collagenase and cathepsin which may degrade collagen and elastin, and fibronectin (Table 1.3) and thereby attract monocytes (317).

In contrast to neutrophils, depletion of circulating blood monocytes and tissue macrophages results in a severe retardation of tissue debridement and a marked delay in fibroblast proliferation and subsequent wound fibrosis (309). Macrophages therefore seem to have an important regulatory role in the repair process.

After migration from the vasculature into the tissue, the monocyte rapidly differentiates to an inflammatory macrophage, the mechanism of which is largely unknown. However, the binding of monocytes to connective tissue fibronectin has been found to drive the differentiation of monocytes into inflammatory macrophages (318, 319).

The regulatory and secretory properties of macrophages seem to vary depending on the state of activity: at rest, intermediate or in an activated state. Macrophage activation can be achieved by the already mentioned chemoattractants in higher concentrations. Further activation can be achieved through the products released from the phagocytotic processes described. These various stimuli induce macrophages to release a number of biologically active molecules with potential as chemical messengers for inflammation and wound repair (320) (Tables 1.1 and 1.2).

At the inflammatory site macrophages undertake functions similar to neutrophils, i.e. bacterial phagocytosis and killing and secretion of lysozomal enzymes and oxygen radicals $O_2$, $H_2O_2$, OH (62). Activated inflammatory macrophages have been found to be responsible for the degradation and removal of damaged tissue structures such as elastin, collagen, proteoglycans and glycoproteins by the use of secreted enzymes such as elastase, collagenase, plasminogen activator and cathepsin B and D. Both extra- and intracellular tissue debridement can occur (317).

Macrophages have been shown to release growth factors such as PDGF, TNF and TGF-β which stimulate cell proliferation in wound healing (321–323) (Fig. 1.4). These growth factors are collectively known as macrophage derived growth factors (MDGF). The level of MDGF can be significantly increased following stimulation of macrophages with agents such as fibronectin and bacterial endotoxin (324, 325).

Activation of macrophages has been found to lead to fibroblast proliferation (321, 326), increased collagen synthesis (322) and neovascularization (327–336).

Macrophages release their angiogenic mediator only in the presence of low oxygen tension in the injured tissue (i.e. 2–30 mm Hg) (268, 269). However, as macrophages have been found to release lactate even while they are well oxygenated, the stimulus to collagen synthesis remains even during hyperoxygenation (331, 332), a finding which is of importance in the use of hyperbaric oxygen therapy.

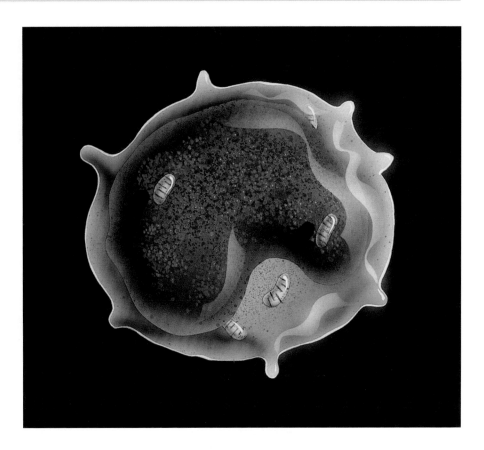

**Fig. 1.15** Lymphocyte.

Finally, macrophages can release a polypeptide, inter-leukin-1, that can function as a messenger for lymphocytes.

In summary, the macrophage seems to be the key cell in the inflammatory and proliferative phase of wound healing by secreting factors which stimulate proliferation of fibroblasts and secretion of collagen, as well as stimulation of neovascularization (Fig. 1.4). The macrophages also act as scavengers in the wound area and remove traumatized tissue and bacteria and neutralize foreign bodies by forming giant cells which engulf or surround the foreign matter. Moreover, signals released by traumatized bone or tooth substances cause some monocytes to fuse and form osteoclasts which will subsequently resorb damaged hard tissue (see Chapter 2, p. 78). Macrophages play a important role in the immune response to infection (Chapter 2, p. 78).

## Lymphocytes

Lymphocytes emigrating from the bloodstream into the injury site become apparent after one day and reach a maximum after six days (Figs 1.15 and 1.16). The role of these lymphocytes in the wound healing process has for many years been questioned as earlier investigations have pointed out that lymphocytes, like neutrophils, were not necessary for normal progression of healing in non-infected wounds (300). However, recent research has demonstrated that lymphocytes together with macrophages may modulate the wound healing process (333–335) (Fig. 1.17).

Lymphocytes can be divided into *T lymphocytes* (thymus derived lymphocytes) and *B lymphocytes* (bone marrow derived lymphocytes). Both types are attracted to the wound area, probably by activated complement on the surface of macrophages and neutrophils.

Lymphocyte infiltration in wounds is a dynamic process where both T-helper/effector and T-suppressor/cytotoxic lymphocytes are present in the wound after one week (336). These activated lymphocytes produce a variety of lymphokines of which interferon (IFN-$\alpha$) and TGF-$\beta$ have been shown to have a significant effect on endothelial cells and thereby may have an effect on angiogenesis. This effect may be secondary to other effects such as macrophage stimulation and activation (337). TGF-$\beta$ is also a potent fibroblast chemotactic molecule and, in addition, induces monocyte chemotaxis and secretion of fibroblast growth factor and activating factors (338).

Recent studies have indicated that there are at least two populations of T cells involved in wound healing. One population bearing the T cell marker appears to be required for successful healing, as shown by the impairment in healing caused by their depletion. The T-suppressor/cytotoxic subset appears to have a counterregulatory effect on wound healing, as their depletion enhances wound rupture strength and collagen synthesis (333–335, 337).

Based on present evidence, Barbul has postulated the following theory: macrophages exert a direct stimulatory effect on endothelial cells and fibroblasts (Fig. 1.17). A T cell marker positive subset (T$^+$), which is not yet fully characterized, has a direct action on endothelial cells and fibroblasts and acts indirectly by stimulating macrophages.

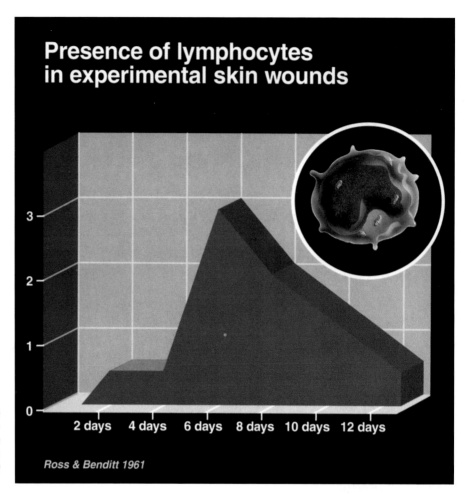

**Fig. 1.16** Schematic illustration of the presence of lymphocytes in experimental skin wounds in guinea pigs. The scale is semiquantitative, graded from 0 to 3. From ROSS & BENDITT (73) 1961.

T suppresser/cytotoxic cells (Ts/c) downregulate wound healing by direct action on macrophages and T cells (337, 338) (Fig. 1.17).

There is presently no evidence to suggest that the humoral immune system (B lymphocytes) participates in the wound healing process. The influence of lymphocytes therefore seems primarily to be through T lymphocytes.

In summary, lymphocytes appear indirectly to influence the balance between the stimulatory and inhibitory signals to fibroblasts and endothelial cells via the macrophages.

## Fibroblasts

The fibroblast is a pleomorphic cell. In the resting, non-functional state it is called a *fibrocyte*. The cytoplasm is scanty and often difficult to identify in ordinary histologic sections. In the activated, mature form the cell becomes stellate or spindle-shaped and is now termed a *fibroblast*. The most characteristic feature is now the extensive development of a dilated endoplasmic reticulum, the site of protein synthesis (339) (Fig. 1.18).

In the wound the fibroblast will produce collagen, elastin and proteoglycans (340). After injury, fibroblasts start to invade the area after three days stimulated by platelets and macrophage products and they become the dominating cell six to seven days after injury, being present in considerable

concentration until the maturation phase of the healing process (73) (Fig. 1.19).

Several studies have suggested that new fibroblasts arise from the connective tissue adjacent to the wound, principally from the perivascular undifferentiated mesenchymal cells (stem cells) (341–346) (see p. 30) and not from hematogenous precursors (346).

Once fibroblast precursors receive the proper signal they begin to reproduce and a mitotic burst is seen between the 2nd and 5th day after injury (347). Proliferating fibroblasts develop through cell divisions every 18 to 20 hours and remain in the mitotic phase for 30 minutes to 1 hour. The primary function of the activated fibroblast in the wound area is to produce collagen, elastin and proteoglycans. However, during the mitotic phase, the fibroblast does not synthesize or excrete external components. Progression factors are necessary to stimulate the fibroblast to undergo replication. Before this can happen the fibroblast must be made competent. Factors which induce this competence are platelet derived growth factor (PDGF), fibroblast growth factor (FGF) and calcium phosphate precipitates (26). PDGF-induced competence requires only transient exposure of cells to the factor. When competent, the fibroblast can replicate after stimulation by progression factors such as insulin-like growth factor-1 (IGF-1), epidermal growth factor (EGF) and other plasma factors (26). This dual

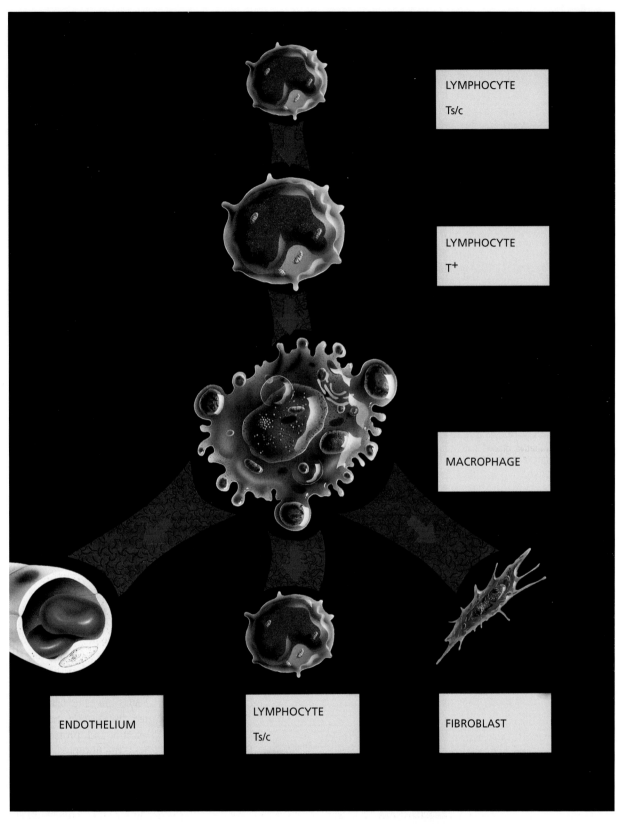

**Fig. 1.17** Role of lymphocytes in wound healing. Macrophages exert a direct stimulatory effect on endothelial cells and fibroblasts. A T-cell marker positive subset (T+), which is not fully characterized, has direct action on endothelial cells and fibroblasts and acts indirectly by stimulating macrophages. T-suppressor/cytotoxic cells (Ts/c) downregulate wound healing by direct action on macrophages and T cells. From BARBUL (337) 1992.

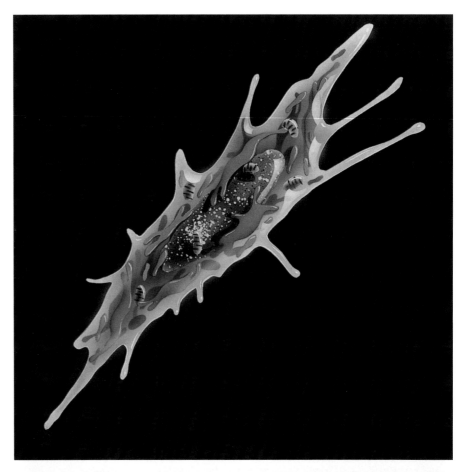

**Fig. 1.18** Active fibroblast.

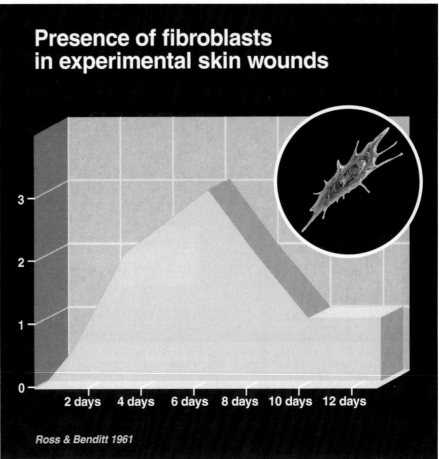

**Fig. 1.19** Schematic illustration of the presence of fibroblasts in experimental skin wounds in guinea pigs. The scale is semiquantitative, graded from 0 to 3. From ROSS & BENDITT (73) 1961.

control of fibroblast proliferation explains why fibroblasts can remain in a reversible quiescent state in the presence of progression factor. The transition to a proliferative stage then awaits the release of competence factors by activated cells, such as platelets, macrophages and lymphocytes.

PDGF is released in response to injury by platelets and production is continued by activated macrophages, which can induce migration into the wound and proliferation of fibroblasts over an extended period of time (Fig. 1.4).

TGF-β is a growth stimulator for mesenchymal cells and has been found to accelerate wound healing in rats (348, 349) by direct stimulation of connective tissue synthesis by fibroblasts and indirect stimulation of fibroblast proliferation by PDGF (350, 351). Other factors which may be involved in fibroblast proliferation include tumor necrosis factors (TNF-α and TNF-β) (26).

The best characterized inhibitor of fibroblast proliferation is β-fibroblast interferon (IFN-β). It has been suggested that IFN-β inhibits events involved in fibroblast competence and induction of competence of fibroblasts and by PDGF inhibition (352, 353).

Regulatory systems of fibroblast activity may operate through activation of macrophages, which generate an endogenous stimulus to fibroblast proliferation. Alternatively, fibroblast proliferation might be slowed by either inhibition of the release and activation of PDGF and TGF-β or by stimulation of inhibitory substances, such as IFN-β. Clinically this may suggest a specific stimulation of fibroblast proliferation by treatment with exogenous growth factors such as PDGF and TGF-β or by their activation (26).

Once fibroblasts have migrated into the wound, they produce and deposit large quantities of fibronectin, types I and III collagen and hyaluronidate. TGF-β is considered to be the most important stimulator of extracellular matrix production (354, 355).

Multiplication and differentiation of fibroblasts and synthesis of collagen fibers require oxygen as well as amino acids, carbohydrates, lipids, minerals and water. Collagen cannot be made in the mature fibroblast layer without oxygen (356–359). Consequently the nutritional demands of the wound are greater than that of non-wounded connective tissue (315) and the demand is greatest at a time when the local circulation is least capable of complying with that demand (316).

After collagen molecules are secreted into the extracellular space, they are polymerized in a series of steps in which the hydroxylysine groups of adjacent molecules are condensed to form covalent crosslinks. This step is rate-dependent on oxygen tension and gives collagen its strength (356, 361).

Fibroblasts have been shown to have chemotactic attraction to types I, II, and III collagen as well as collagen-derived peptides, with binding of these peptides directly to fibroblasts (362, 363).

Fibroblasts have been known for many years to be involved in wound contraction. In relation to this phenomenon, a specific type of fibroblast has been identified which has the characteristics of both fibroblasts and smooth muscle cells for which reason they have been termed myofi-broblasts. These cells are richly supplied with microfilament bundles that are arranged along the long axis of the cells and are associated with dense bodies for attachment to the surrounding extracellular matrix (364, 365). Besides numerous cytoplasmic microfilaments, large amounts of endoplasmic reticulum are also seen. In this respect these cells have characteristics of fibroblasts.

The myofibroblast has contractive properties and has been demonstrated in many tissues that form contracted and/or nodular scars (366). Myofibroblasts are present throughout granulation tissue and along wound edges at the time when active contraction occurs (367). For this reason the most generally accepted theory of wound contraction has involved the contribution by myofibroblasts (366).

Ehrlich and co-workers have presented a new theory for the phenomenon of wound contraction (368). In this fibroblast theory it is suggested that fibroblast locomotion is the mechanism that generates the contractive forces in wound contraction and that the connective tissue matrix is important in controlling these forces. It is suggested that the histological existence of myofibroblasts is a transitional state of the fibroblast in granulation tissue.

In summary, the fibroblasts are latecomers in the inflammation phase of wound healing. Their main function is to synthesize and excrete the major components of connective tissue: collagen, elastin and proteoglycans. The fibroblast is also involved in wound-contraction through a specific cell called the myofibroblast which has characteristics of both fibroblasts and smooth muscle cells.

## Endothelial cells and pericytes

The capillaries play an essential role in wound healing. The caliper of capillaries averages 9–12 μm which is just enough to permit unimpeded passage of cellular elements. In cross-section the capillary wall consists of 1–3 endothelial cells. (Fig. 1.20). Capillaries converge to form post capillary venules of slightly larger size (15–20 μm). The endothelial cells are surrounded by a network of pericytes. (Fig. 1.20). These cells appear to represent a pool of undifferentiated mesenchymal cells which have been found to participate in wound healing, and this applies also to the pulp and periodontium (see Chapter 3).

## Angiogenesis

Between 2 and 4 days after wounding, proliferation of capillaries and fibroblasts begins at the border of the lesion. However, studies have shown that blood cells and plasma perfuse the wound tissue several hours before the space is invaded by sprouting capillaries (295, 369). At first the blood cells move around randomly in the meshes of the fibrinous network but gradually preferential channels are formed in the wound through which cells pass more or less regularly. This phenomenon has been termed open circulation and it is suggested that the blood cells at this time are transported in a simple tube system which has not yet acquired an endothelial lining (295, 369, 370).

Angiogenesis is the process of formation of new blood vessels by directed endothelial migration, proliferation and lumen formation (262, 371–376) (Fig. 1.21). In wound healing, angiogenesis is crucial for oxygen delivery to ischemic or newly formed tissue. New vessels arise in most cases as capillaries from existing vessels and only from venules (376, 377) (Fig. 1.21). In early granulation tissue, after the wound healing module is assembled, capillary sprouts move just behind the advancing front of macrophages. Collagen secreting fibroblasts are placed between these sprouts and are nourished by the new capillaries (see Fig. 1.26).

Variants in healing of the vascular network are found according to the type of tissue involved and the extent of the

injury. In skin or mucosal lacerations, primarily closed, existing vessels may anastomose spontaneously and thereby re-establish circulation. In wounds with tissue defects or in non-closed wounds, a new vascular network has to be created via granulation tissue. The third variant in vascular healing is the revascularization of ischemic tissue as seen after skin grafting, tooth luxation, tooth replantation and transplantation. In these situations angiogenesis takes place in existing ischemic or necrotic tissue. The healing in these cases usually occurs as a mixture of gradual ingrowth of new vasculature combined with occasional end-to-end anastomosis between existing and ingrowing vessels (see Chapter 2, p. 90).

Angiogenesis in wounds has been examined in different *in vivo* assays such as the rabbit ear chamber (269, 378), the Algire chamber where a transparent plastic window is placed in the dorsal subcutaneous tissue of a mouse (379) or the hamster cheek pouch (380, 381). Furthermore, angiogenesis has been tested in corneal pockets (379, 382, 383), and chicken chorioallantoic membrane (384). These assays have been used to describe the dynamic process of angiogenesis together with the influence of different types of external factors on vascular proliferation.

Our current knowledge of the biochemical nature of the signals that induce angiogenesis has been derived primarily from *in vitro* observations using cultured vascular endothelial cells. *In vitro* assays have been used extensively in the identification and the purification of angiogenetic factors. In this context, as angiogenesis is considered to be a process of capillary growth, cultured capillary endothelial cells seem to be optimal for testing angiogenesis (385).

## Cellular events in angiogenesis

New capillaries usually start as outgrowths of endothelial cells lining existing venules. After exposure to an angiogenic stimulus, endothelial cells of the venules begin to produce enzymes that degrade the vascular basement membrane on the side facing the stimulus (376). After 24 hours the endothelial cells migrate through the degraded membrane in the direction of the angiogenic stimulus (Fig. 1.21).

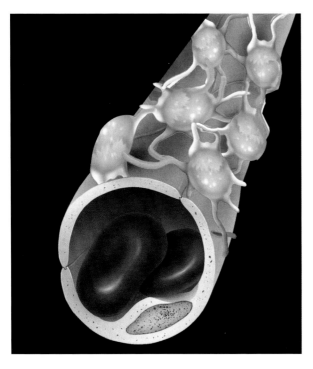

**Fig. 1.20** Endothelial cells and pericytes.

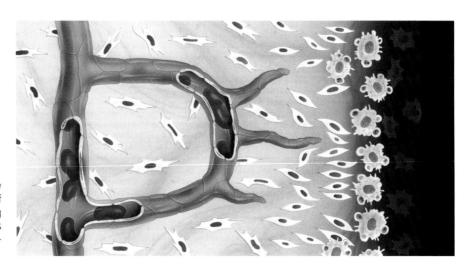

**Fig. 1.21** Neovascularization. New capillaries start as outgrowths of endothelial cells lining existing venules. Subsequent arcading sprouts unite and tubulization allows circulation to be established.

Behind the tip of the migrating wound edges, trailing endothelial cells divide and differentiate to form a lumen. The sprouts or buds can either connect with other sprouts to form vascular loops or can continue migrating. Capillary bud formation is found after 48 hours and these buds arise solely from venules (377).

When endothelial migration tips join to form capillary loops or join across a wound edge, blood flow begins within the formed lumen. As vessels mature, extracellular matrix components are laid down to form a new basement membrane (371, 376). Recent studies have shown that angiogenesis is closely related to fibroblast activity. Thus it appears that new vessels cannot grow beyond their collagenous support (356, 386).

The speed of neovascularization has been investigated in ear chambers and been found to range from 0.12 to 0.24 mm per day (272, 295, 387, 388). In dental pulps which become revascularized after replantation or transplantation, the speed is approximately twice this rate (see Chapter 2, p. 90).

In raised and repositioned skin flaps, angiogenesis along the cut margins is rapid and capillary sprouts advance across the wound space from the host bed. In rats, new vascular channels across the wound margin can be demonstrated within 3 days; and in pigs, normal blood flow has been observed within 2 to 3 days (389–391). After tissue grafting, specific vascular healing processes take place. Thus it has been shown in skin transplants that after an initial contraction of the vessels a so-called plasmatic circulation takes place in the zone next to the graft bed (392–400). This supply of fluids serves to prevent drying of the graft before blood supply has been restored (398). The role of the plasmatic circulation as a source of nourishment is, however, debatable (398).

Vascularization of skin transplants, although initially sluggish, takes place after 3 to 5 days (401–410). The role of already existing graft vessels is unsettled. Thus, in some studies, it has been shown that the original vessels act only as non-viable conduits for ingrowth of new vessels (388), and that revascularization takes place primarily from invading new vessels (408, 411). In other experiments, however, it has been shown that, depending upon the degree of damage to the grafted tissues and on local hemodynamic factors, the original graft vessels may be incorporated in the established new vascular network (409–413).

Teeth have a vascular system which in some situations is dissimilar to skin. In replantation and transplantation procedures of immature incisors, the severed periodontal ligament and the pulp can be expected to become revascularized. The process of revascularization of the periodontal ligament seems to follow the pattern of skin grafts (see Chapter 2, p. 90). There is limited diffusion of nutrients from the graft bed to the dental pulp due to its hard tissue confinement and extended length, which again leads to specific vascular healing events (see Chapter 2, p. 90).

In a closed skin wound, circulation bridging the wound edges can be established as early as the 2nd or the 3rd day and appears to be at a maximum after 8 days (73) (Fig. 1.22). The new vascular network is then remodeled. Some vessels differentiate into arteries and veins while others recede. The mechanism regulating this process is largely unknown. Active blood flow within the lumen may be a factor, as capillaries with decreased blood flow typically recede while those with active flow are usually maintained or expand into larger vessels (378, 414).

Factors determining angiogenesis represent a series of cellular and humoral events which lead to the initiation, progression and termination of angiogenesis (Figs 1.4 and 1.23). Initiation of angiogenesis appears to be related to signals released from activated platelets and fibrin at the site of vascular rupture (86, 285, 415, 416). During platelet activation, enzymes are released that degrade heparin and heparan sulfate components from the vascular basement membranes, whereby stored bFGF is liberated (417–421). This liberation of FGF has been shown to induce angiogenetic activity (422). Other bFGF signals are released from injured cells and matrix (376). This growth factor is partly responsible for angiogenesis through initiating a cascade of events (423). Thus bFGF stimulates endothelial cells to secrete procollagenase, plasmin and plasminogen. Plasmin, as well as plasminogen, activates procollagenase to collagenase. Together, these enzymes can digest the blood vessel basement membrane. Subsequently endothelial chemoattractants, such as fibronectin fragments generated from extracellular matrix degradation and heparin released from mast cells, draw endothelial cells through the disrupted basement membrane to form a nascent capillary bud (132).

Recruited and activated macrophages soon also promote angiogenesis (424) by liberating potent direct acting angiogenic factors such as tumor necrosis factor alpha (TNF-α), wound angiogenesis factor (WAF) and fibroblast growth factor (FGF). The macrophage signal seems to diminish as angiogenesis proceeds (268, 269, 356, 361, 425–428). Recent studies indicate that the effect of hypoxia within the wound upon angiogenesis is possibly mediated via stimulated macrophages (268, 429, 430) (see p. 39).

## Other factors controlling angiogenesis

Recently, a number of angiogenetic factors have been isolated which either have a direct effect on endothelial cell migration/proliferation or have an indirect effect via other cells. The exact mechanisms behind indirect angiogenetic activity are not yet known; but it is possible that they cause accumulation of other types of cells, e.g. platelets or macrophages, that release direct acting factors (126, 376, 431).

Once new blood vessels form, they acquire a layer of pericytes and the composition of their basement membrane changes. Pericytes inhibit the growth of adjacent endothelial cells and thereby direct growth toward the site of attraction (432).

Finally, it should be mentioned that angiogenesis is dependent upon the composition of the extracellular matrix (433, 623, 624). Thus, fibrin appears to promote angiogenesis (64) and the fibrin–fibronectin extravascular clot serves as a provisional stroma providing a matrix for macrophages, fibroblasts and new capillary migration. In this way, the

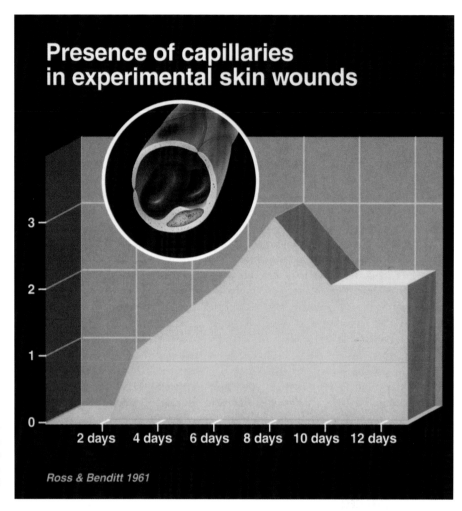

**Presence of capillaries in experimental skin wounds**

Ross & Benditt 1961

2 days  4 days  6 days  8 days  10 days  12 days

**Fig. 1.22** Schematic illustration of the presence of new capillaries in experimental skin wounds in guinea pigs. The scale is semiquantitative graded from 0 to 3. From ROSS & BENDITT (73) 1961.

fibrin–fibronectin gel is transformed to granulation tissue.

## Wound strength development

Wound strength, from a functional point of view, is the most important property for a healing wound. In surgical practice this is critical for the outcome of surgery. The time interval from injury to a healed wound is strong enough to resist mechanical stress in tissue. It is essential that an early return to normal life is facilitated with the development of significant wound strength. For ethical reasons this has to be based on investigations of tensile strength of experimental wounds.

In early wounds the tensile strength is low and insufficient to keep the tissue edges together without sutures. The strength of the wound is in this stage mainly based on fibrin in the wound cavity. Later, in the proliferation phase, the strength increases rapidly as granulation tissue is formed. The strength of the wound is in the collagen fibers, and is directly related to the collagen content of the tissue (Fig. 1.24) (434, 435). Some collagenous elements can be seen already after 2 to 3 days of injury, but the maximum period

of collagen synthesis most often starts the 5th to 6th days of healing. The collagen fibers are laid down in a random pattern and in the beginning possess little mechanical strength. Gradually a more systematic pattern of collagen fibrils develops, leading to stabilization by cross-linking and assembly of fibers into a more correct anatomical pattern. Experimental studies have shown that the 'biochemical active zone' encompasses tissue 5 to 7 mm from the incisional line.

The resulting tensile strength of a wound is the combined strength of old collagen (present in the wound area before injury) and diminishing by lyses of collagenases, and the increasing strength of new build collagen. The lowest tensile strength of a healing wound for this reason is after some days of healing (20) (Fig. 1.25).

Wound strength can in a functional way be described as the relative tensile strength of the wound. This is the actual tensile strength of the wound in relation to strength of intact tissue and is expressed as a percentage. Fig. 1.25 shows the relative tensile strength of healing incisional wounds in different types of tissues. In tissues with a low collagen content in intact tissue (gastrointestinal tract, muscle) (436, 437) the relative tensile strength increases rapidly and reaches intact level after 10–20 days. In tissues with high collagen content (fascia, skin, tendon) the relative strength increases slowly

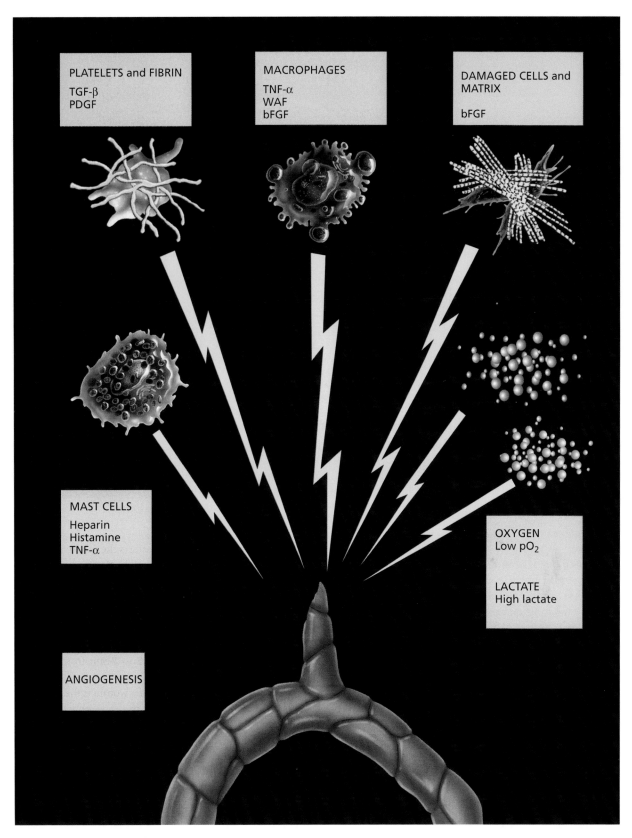

**Fig. 1.23** Cellular and humoral events leading to angiogenesis. Platelets, fibrin, mast cells, macrophages, injured cells and matrix all release angiogenic signals. Low oxygen tension and a high lactate concentration in the wound space represent also an important stimulation to angiogenesis.

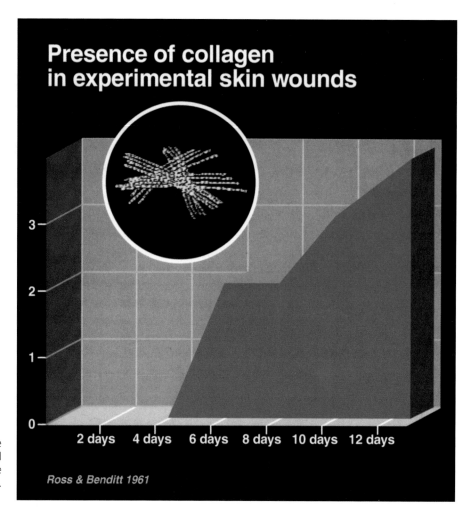

**Fig. 1.24** Schematic illustration of the presence of collagen in experimental skin wounds in guinea pigs. The scale is semiquantitative graded from 0 to 3. From ROSS & BENDITT (73) 1961.

and in skin and tendon the strength has after 60 days only reached 60% of intact level (Fig. 1.25) (435).

Collagen constitutes the principal structural protein of the body and is the main constituent of extracellular matrix in all species. At least 13 types of collagen have been identified. Despite their differences, all collagen molecules consist of a triple helix matrix protein which gives the tissues their strength (15, 437–442). Literature on wound healing and collagen contains only sparse information about the different types of collagens (437).

Type I collagen is the major structural components of skin, mucosa, tendons and bone (440).

Type II collagen is located almost exclusively in hyaline cartilage.

Type III collagen, also called reticular fibers (443), is found in association with Type I collagen although the ratio varies in different tissues (440). In a rat model, type III collagen could be demonstrated 10 hours after the start of wound healing in skin (444), and after 3 days in healing periodontal ligament (PDL) wounds (445, 446). The early appearance of type III collagen has been found associated with the deposition of fibronectin (see p. 11), indicating that type III collagen together with fibronectin may provide the initial scaffolding for subsequent healing events (447, 448).

In children, type III collagen can be detected between 24 and 48 hours in skin wounds, whereas no type I collagen is found in this type of wound (449). From 72 hours and onwards a substantial increase in type I collagen is found, together with the appearance of mature fibroblasts (449).

Type IV collagen together with other components, including heparan sulfate, proteoglycans and laminin, makes up the basement membranes in both epidermis and endothelium.

In dermal wound healing, type IV collagen synthesis by epidermis is connected with the reformation of the basement membrane and is a relatively late event in the wound healing process (450–452).

Type V collagen is found in almost all types of tissue and has been proposed to be involved in migration of capillary endothelial cells during angiogenesis (441). Type V collagen is synthesized while epidermal cells migrate; however, the regeneration of the basement membrane is delayed until the wound defect is covered and the epidermal cells are no longer in a migrating phase (451).

Type VII collagen has been found to be an anchoring fibril that attaches the basement membrane to underlying connective tissue (454–456).

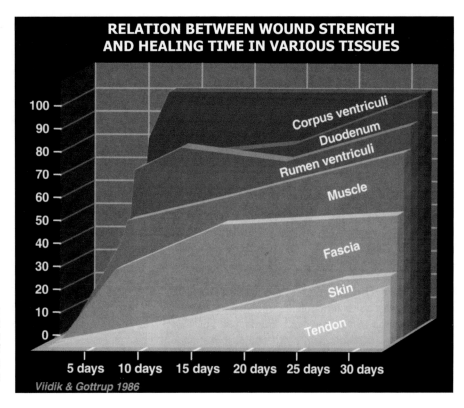

**RELATION BETWEEN WOUND STRENGTH AND HEALING TIME IN VARIOUS TISSUES**

Corpus ventriculi
Duodenum
Rumen ventriculi
Muscle
Fascia
Skin
Tendon

5 days   10 days   15 days   20 days   25 days   30 days

Viidik & Gottrup 1986

**Fig. 1.25** Relative healing rates for linear incisional wounds in different tissues in rats and rabbits; the tensile strength being calculated as percent of that of the respective intact tissues (taken as 100%). From VIIDIK & GOTTRUP (457) 1986.

The remaining types of collagen are less known in relation to the wound healing process and are therefore not discussed.

Collagen represents a key component in wound healing. Thus, immediately after injury the exposure of collagen fibers to blood results in platelet aggregation and activation with resultant coagulation and the release of chemotactic factors from platelets that initiate healing (e.g. PDGF, platelet factor IV, IGF-1 TGF-β and an unidentified chemoattractant to endothelial cells) (see p. 36). Collagen fragments are then degraded by the attracted neutrophils and leukocytes, which leads to attraction of fibroblasts.

Synthesis of new collagen in a wound starts with fibroblast proliferation and invasion and the deposition of a collagen based extracellular matrix. This event takes place after 3–5 days and persists for 10–12 days. During this period of time, there is a rapid synthesis primarily of type III and later of type I collagen, resulting in an increase in the tensile strength of the wound which is primarily dependent on the build-up of type I collagen (449, 458–460).

## Remodeling phase

Remodeling of the extracellular matrix is a continuous process which starts early in the wound healing process. Thus most fibronectin is eliminated within one or two weeks after granulation tissue is established. Hyaluronidate is replaced or supplemented with heparan sulfate proteoglycans in basement membrane regions and with dermatan chondroitin sulfate proteoglycans in the interstitium (61).

Type III collagen fibers are gradually replaced by type I collagen which becomes arranged in large, partly irregular, collagen bundles. These fiber bundles become oriented according to lines of stress and provide a slower increase in the tensile strength of the healing wound than found during the proliferation phase (460). In most tissues, this remodeling phase ultimately leads to formation of a scar (see p. 36).

The functional properties of the scar tissue vary considerably depending on the content of collagen in the intact original tissue. The healing rate, measured as the mechanical strength of the wound compared to adjacent intact tissue, therefore varies from one tissue type to another. In tissue with a low collagen content before injury (e.g. gastrointestinal tract (461) and other intra-abdominal organ systems), the primarily closed wound shows a rapid increase in relative strength (strength of wounded tissue compared to intact tissue) (457). As shown in Fig. 1.25 tensile strength close to the level of intact tissue levels of tensile strength is reached after 10 to 20 days of healing in tissues with a low collagen content before injury. In tissues with a high collagen content (e.g. tendon and skin) the increase in relative strength is much slower; and more than 100 days of healing are needed to achieve half the strength of intact tissue. In the wounded PDL, a very rapid increase in tensile strength has been found after severance of Sharpey's fibers (see Chapter 2, p. 80) Investigations of wounds closed 3 to 6 days after injury (delayed primary closure) has shown that this type of wound was significantly stronger than primarily closed wounds after 20 days of healing. After 60 days of healing, delayed primarily closed wounds were almost twice as strong as primarily closed wounds; and this difference persisted after 120 days (59, 60, 462). The mechanisms behind the different wound strength in primarily and delayed primarily closed wounds are probably related to an increase in tissue perfusion and oxygenation due to increased angiogenesis and oxygen delivery to the tissues (463).

## Hypertrophic scar and keloid

Excessive deposition of scar tissue is a clinical problem that has been difficult to resolve because of the lack of reliable animal models. Hypertrophic scar and keloid are both characterized by excessive accumulation of extracellular matrix especially collagen. The etiology is not known but abnormalities in cell migration and proliferation, inflammation, syntheses and secretion of extracellular matrix proteins and cytokines, and remodeling of wound matrix have been described. Also increased activity of fibrogenic cytokines (e.g. TGF-$\beta_1$, interleukin-1), abnormal epidermal–mesenchymal interaction and mutations in regulatory genes has been proposed (464). In healed burns the development of hypertrophic scars seems not to be the result of a continued proliferation phase, rather than an alteration of the remodeling phase (465).

The hypertrophic scar results from a full thickness injury and is characterized by a thick, raised scar that stays within the boundaries of the original injury. Keloids can develop from superficial injuries and exceed the boundaries of the initial injury. Histologically hypertrophic scars contain nodules and keloid does not. The collagen bundles on the surfaces of the nodule are arranged in parallel sheets, while randomly arranged fibrils within the centre (466). The collagen bundles of keloid are arranged in braided sheets running parallel to each other.

Hypertrophic scars most often regress over time and can be corrected by surgical intervention (620). Keloid scars as a rule do not regress over time and frequently recur after removal. Treatment of keloid scars is difficult, but pressure dressings and local application of glucocorticoids have been used with limited success. Silicone dressings and local use of calcium channel blockers have recently shown promising results.

## Epithelial cells

Epithelium covers all surfaces of the body, including the internal surfaces of the gastrointestinal, respiratory and genitourinary tract. The major function of epithelium is to provide a selective barrier between the body and the environment. The epithelial barrier is the primary defense against threats from the environment and is also a major factor in maintaining internal homeostasis. Physical and chemical injury of the epithelial layer must therefore be repaired quickly by cell proliferation.

After injury to the epidermis, wound protection is provided in two steps: within minutes there is a temporary coverage of the wound by coagulated blood which serves as a barrier to arrest the loss of body fluids. The second step is the movement of adjacent epithelium beneath the clot and over the underlying dermis to complete wound closure. Re-epithelialization of an injured surface is achieved either by movement or growth of epithelial cells over the wound area (467–469). In early phases of wound healing the most important process is cell migration which is independent of cell division (470–472).

In deep wounds the new epithelial cover arises from the wound periphery, whereas shallow wounds usually heal from residual pilosebaceous or eccrine structures (405, 473–475).

The cellular response of epithelial cells to an injury can be divided into four basic steps: *mobilization* (freeing of cells from their attachment; *migration* (movement of cells); *proliferation* (replacement of cells by mitosis of preexisting cells) and *differentiation* (restoration of cellular function, e.g. keratinization).

The first response of the epithelium after injury is *mobilization*, which starts after 12 to 24 hours. This involves detachment of the individual cells in preparation for migration. Epithelial cells lose hemidesmosomal junctions; the tonofilaments withdraw from the cell periphery; and the basal membrane becomes less well defined (15, 467, 476, 477). In addition, the cells of the leading edge become phagocytic, engulfing tissue debris and erythrocytes. Epithelialization occurs most rapidly in superficial wounds where the basal membrane is intact. Short tongues of epithelial cells grow out from the residual epithelial structures. By the 2nd or 3rd day, most of the wound base is covered with a thin epithelial layer; and, by the 4th day, by layered keratinocytes (453, 478, 479).

*Migration* of epithelial cells occurs as movement of clusters or sheets of cells. This movement of epithelial cells has been proposed to take place in a 'leapfrog' fashion of epidermal sheet movement (480). Fibronectin in connection with fibrin seems to make a provisional matrix for cellular anchorage and self-propelling traction of the epithelial cell for migration. A speculative mechanism has been that fibronectin is produced in front of the wound edge by epidermal cells and these then slide over the deposited fibronectin matrix and finally break down this matrix at a distance of some cell diameters behind the wound edge (481, 482). It seems that the motile cells use secreted fibronectin as a temporary basal membrane and use collagenase and plasminogen activators to facilitate passage through reparative connective tissue (483).

The specific signals or stimuli for epithelialization are unknown. Migration of epithelial cells takes place in a random fashion; however, orientation of the substrate on which the cells move, as well as the presence of other cells of the same type are determinants of the extent and direction of cell movement. Furthermore, cell migration appears to be at least in part initiated by a negative feedback mechanism from other epithelial cells in the free edge of the wound (5). Substances in the substrate which are important for direction of the migration seem to be collagen fibers, fibrin and fibronectin, as earlier described. Fibronectin appears to be a substrate for cell movement and to have a binding capacity for epithelial cells as well as monocytes, fibroblasts, and endothelial cells (101, 482–484).

Proliferation of epidermal cells starts after 1 to 2 days in the cells immediately behind the migrating edge, thereby generating a new pool of cells to cover the wound (472, 485). Mitosis in epidermal epithelium has a diurnal rhythm, being greatest during rest and inactivity. In normal epidermis, very few basal cells are in mitosis at any given time. Epidermal wounds, however, result in a change of the diurnal mitotic rhythm in cells adjacent to the wound, resulting in an absolute increase in mitotic activity and an increase in the size of epidermal cells (453). The maximal mitotic activity is found on the 3rd day and continues until epithelialization is complete and epithelial cells have reverted to their normal phenotype and reassumed their intercellular and basement membrane contacts by differentiation (486).

A number of stimuli for epidermal cell growth and thereby wound closure have been indentified, such as calcium in low concentration, interleukin-1, basic fibroblast growth factor (bFGF), epidermal growth factor (EGF), platelet derived growth factor (PDGF) and transforming growth factor-alpha (TGF-$\alpha$) (467, 482). The only factor known to block epithelial growth is TFG-$\beta$ (478, 487). Most of these molecules are released from cells within the wound environment such as platelets, inflammatory cells, endothelial cells and smooth muscle cells (Fig. 1.4).

Another factor which influences epithelialization is oxygen tension. Thus a high $pO_2$ has been found to increase epithelialization (488, 489).

Epithelial repair differs temporally in different types of wound. In incisional wounds, mobilization and migration of epithelial cells is a rapid response compared to other events of the wound healing process. Already after 24 to 48 hours the epithelial cells have bridged the gap in clean incisional and sutured wounds (142). In small excised and non-sutured wounds which heal by secondary intention the surface is initially covered by a blood clot. Migrating epithelium does not move through the clot, but rather beneath it in direct contact with the original wound bed. Epithelial cells appear to secrete a proteolytic enzyme that dissolves the base of the clot and permits unimpeded cell migration.

In large excised wounds, all stages of epithelial repair may be seen simultaneously. In such wounds epithelialization will not be complete before granulation tissue has developed. Epithelial cells will use this bed for subsequent migration. Depending upon the size of wound the surface will subsequently be covered by a scar epithelium which is thin, and lacks strong attachment to the underlying dermis as well as lacking Langerhans cells and melanocytes.

One factor which has a strong influence upon epithelial healing is the depth of the wound. In superficial wounds the regeneration from hair follicles coincides with epithelializa-

tion from the wound edges. In deeper wounds, all epidermal regrowth occurs from the wound edge.

Finally, it should be mentioned that reepithelialization is significantly enhanced if the wound is kept moist (481).

In the oral cavity the morphological changes seen during epithelialization of the rat molar extraction socket appear to be similar to wounds that involve oral mucosa (74, 490–494). Thus the epithelium migrates down into and across the wound with either fibrin–fibronectin or granulation tissue–fibronectin below it and the superficial wound contents (i.e. neutrophil leukocytes, tissue debris, food elements and bacteria) above it. This layer is subsequently lost in the form of a scab following reepithelialization (492).

## Microenvironnent in wounds

Microenvironments in wounds are the sum of the single processes mentioned earlier. Of particular interest for the wound healing process is the influence of the wound microenvironment as an initiator, supporter and terminator of the wound healing processes (495).

Cellular activity in the wound has already been discussed in detail, but can be described as three waves of cells invading the wound area. Apart from their role in hemostasis, platelets serve as the initiators of wound healing by their release of substances such as growth factors (e.g. PDGF, platelet factor IV, IGF-1, TGF-$\beta$ and an uncharacterized chemoattractant of endothelial cells at the moment of injury (Fig. 1.4). As the access of platelets to the wound area is limited by the coagulation process the supply of these factors is limited.

The second set of cells, polymorphonuclear leukocytes, migrate into the wound after a few hours largely under the direction of complement factors. Their role in the wound healing process appears mainly to be the control of infection.

The third type of cell invading the wound area are the monocytes, which are attracted to the injury site by platelet factors, complement and fibrinopeptides. After entering the wound, these cells are transformed to macrophages and take over the control of healing processes. It would appear that macrophages have the capacity to detect and interpret changes in the wound environment and thereby initiate appropriate healing responses.

In the early wound, cells float around in the tissue fluid of the wound and their function and movement are directed by different growth factors (e.g. TGF-$\beta$, IL-6, IGF-1 and insulin produced by platelets and/or macrophages).

The amino acid content of wound fluids reflects to some extent the metabolic events. Amino acid concentrations are initially close to those of serum. Later, they approach that of inflammatory cells. After some time particularly glutamine and glutamate rise well over that of serum, whereas arginine concentration falls to low levels due to conversion to ornithin and citrullin (495). Arginine has been shown to be active in influencing the wound healing process and seems to activate macrophages (496, 497).

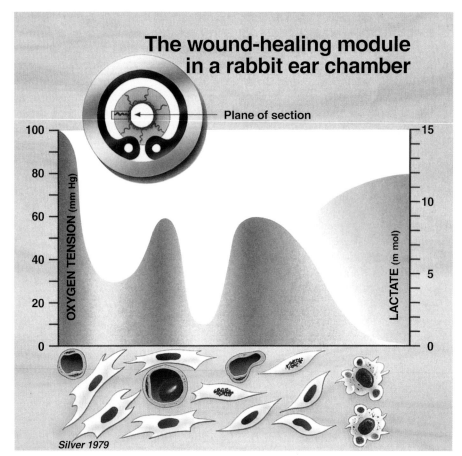

**Fig. 1.26** Cellular build-up, oxygen tension and lactate concentration in a rabbit ear chamber The center of the wound is to the right on the drawing. At this location where macrophages operate there is very low oxygen tension and a high lactate concentration. It appears that oxygen tension is closely related to the location of the vasculature. Replication of fibroblasts takes place ahead of the regenerating vessels, whereas fibroblasts begin collagen production when the neovascular front reaches the proliferating fibroblasts. From HUNT & VAN WINKLE (499) 1976.

It would seem that the wound fluid, with its mixture of growth factors, amino acids and other components, is conducive to cell proliferation. Thus, it has been found experimentally that cell growth was optimized in the presence of wound fluid compared to cell growth in serum (327).

Wound microenvironments have been studied in rabbit ear chambers in which healing tissues can be visualized between closely approximated, optically clear membranes mounted under a microscope (Fig. 1.26). This narrow space, as thin as 50 μm, forces healing cells to travel in coherent order, so that one or two cells pass at a time (49). In this model, influence of oxygen tension and lactate concentration could be measured by microprobes and has been characterized (49). An oxygen gradient from the central wound space in the chamber to the peripheral normal tissue has been described. While oxygen tension along the edges of the wound is very low, with hypoxia close to 0 mmHg, the oxygen tension at the periphery of the wound is up to 100 mmHg. This oxygen tension gradient seems to be important in the initiation of the wound healing process. Concurrently, lactate concentration in the wound space is 10–20 times that of venous blood, resulting in a fall in pH to 7.25 (498).

## Wound healing module

After the first phase of the inflammatory process occurs, a characteristic cell build-up is found after 3 to 4 days (Fig. 1.26). At the edge of a wound is a vanguard of scavenging cells, the majority of which in the non-infected wound are macrophages. If the wound is infected, these macrophages are accompanied by large numbers of neutrophilic leukocytes.

Beneath the phagocytes is a layer of immature fibroblasts, floating in a gelatinous, non-fibrillar matrix, which are unable to divide because of local hypoxia. Beneath this layer of fibroblasts is a group of dividing fibroblasts which are associated with the most distal perfused arcaded capillaries, and behind the first perfused capillary loops are more dividing fibroblasts which provide cells to form the new tissue.

Distal to this zone, blood vessels increase in size and become less dense, probably as a result of enlargement or coalescence of a few vessels, as the other channels recede from the pattern of vascular flow. Between these vessels lie mature fibroblasts and new fibrillar collagen. This arrangement of cells creates an environment that is favorable to angiogenesis and collagen deposition and has been termed the *wound healing module* (Fig. 1.4).

Fibroblasts in mitosis are always found just ahead of the regenerating vessels, where the tissue oxygen tension is optimal for replication (i.e. about 40 mmHg). It is assumed that these fibroblasts behave as growth centers and that new fibroblasts remain at this location until reached by the neovascular zone, whereafter they initiate collagen production (499). The hyperemic neovascular front has a higher $pO_2$ (Fig. 1.26) which is optimal for collagen synthesis. Thus the fibroblasts replicate and produce collagen in different wound environments.

It has been found that hypoxia or exposure to a high lactate concentration increases the capacity of fibroblasts to synthesize collagen when they are subsequently placed in an oxygenated environment (500, 501). It has been suggested that lactate stimulates collagen synthesis (495). Thus lactate has been shown to induce an increase in procollagen mRNA. Lactate concentration in test wounds is greatest in the central space and persists well into the zone of collagen synthesis (Fig. 1.26). It is therefore suggested that new vessels overtake the immature fibroblasts and change their environment from high lactate and low oxygen tension to high lactate and high oxygen tension and thereby increase both their collagen synthesis and their deposition. When the wound cavity is totally filled with granulation tissue, the hypoxia and high lactate concentration gradually diminish as does macrophage stimulation, whereupon the wound healing process will stop.

Oxygen tension in the wound has been shown to be important for collagen deposition and the development of the tensile strength of the wound (488, 502), for regulation of angiogenesis (369) and for the epithelialization of wounds (472). Oxygen in the wound's extracellular environment also has an important role in the intracellular killing of bacteria by granulocytes (503).

Neutrophil migration, attachment and ingestion of bacteria apparently are independent of oxygen; however, the killing of the most important wound pathogens is achieved by mechanisms that require molecular oxygen (504). These mechanisms are introduced through reducing extracellular molecular oxygen to superoxide which is then inserted into phagosomes. Here the superoxide is converted to high-energy bactericidal oxygen radicals for optimal bacterial killing (505).

Several studies in normal volemic animals have shown that they clear bacteria from wounds in proportion to the fraction of oxygen in the inspired gas. Infection was less invasive or failed to develop in hyperoxygenated guinea pigs when bacteria were injected into skin (505). Furthermore, infected skin lesions in dogs became invasive in tissues with extracellular fluid oxygen tension under 60 mmHg; however, they remained localized if the tissue was better oxygenated, as in the case of higher inspiratory oxygen concentration (506). Experience in human subjects tends to support these findings; but no trial has yet been performed supporting these observations.

## Factors affecting the wound healing process

External factors have an influence on the wound healing process. The categorization is often generally done as local or systematic. In acute surgical wounds a classification base on patient- and surgical-related factors is most convenient (Table 1.2). Patient-related factors are associated to the single patient and can alone or together with other factors inhibit or prevent wound healing. Surgical-related factors can be separated in pre-, peri- and postoperative influencing factors.

## Blood circulation and oxygenation of the wound

Continuous supply of oxygen to the tissue through a sufficient tissue perfusion is vital for the healing process as well as resistance to infection (488, 502, 507–509). Collagen production and development of strength of the wound is directly correlated to the partial pressure $PO_2$ of the tissue ($P_tO_2$). Epithelialization is also dependent on oxygen, but the humidity of the wound healing environment seems of more importance. Moist wound healing increases the epithelialization by a factor 2–3 while the optimal growth of epidermal cells is found at an oxygen concentration between 10 and 50%.

Anemia with hematocrite values of 15–20 has in experimental animal studies in cases of normal function of the heart and normal tissue perfusion been of minor importance for the $PO_2$ in the wound area and consequently for the healing. Evaluation of tissue perfusion and oxygenation is important in all types of wound. Monitoring systems should measure the hemodynamic situation and the ability of the cardiovascular system to deliver an adequate volume of oxygen to meet the metabolic demands of the peripheral tissue.

Tissue perfusion is determined by a variety of general and local factors. Peripheral tissue perfusion is influenced by multiple cardiovascular regulatory mechanisms. In response to hemorrhage, these mechanisms maintain blood flow to vital organs, such as the heart and brain, while blood flow to other tissues is decreased (510, 511). Circulatory adjustments are effected by local as well as systemic mechanisms that change the caliber of the arterioles and alter hydrostatic pressure in the capillaries. Detection of poor tissue perfusion, and especially tissue oxygenation, is crucial in the post-injury and care periods.

If wound edges show signs of ischemia, there is a risk of impaired wound healing with development of wound leakage and infection. From the knowledge of healing wounds of the oral cavity and the anus, it is obvious that perfusion is the major factor in resistance to infection. Despite contamination of both types of wound with bacteria, they almost always heal without infection if patients have a normally functioning immune system. The difference between these and other wounds (e.g. extremities) is not related to local immunity, but to differences in perfusion and oxygenation.

Increased oxygen tension improves resistance to infection through local leukocyte function (512). Thus, experimental data have shown that the killing capacity of granulocytes is normal only to the extent to which molecular oxygen is available (503, 513–519). Bacteria killing involves two major components. The first is degranulation of neutrophils in which bacteria located within the phagosome are exposed to various antimicrobial compounds from the granules. The effect of this system is unrelated to the environment of the leukocytes. The second system is the so-called oxidative killing and depends upon molecular oxygen absorbed by the leukocytes and converted to high energy radicals such as superoxide, hydroxyl radical, peroxides, aldehydes, hypochlorite, and hypoiodite, all substances which to varying degrees are toxic to bacteria. In this regard it is important to consider that the efficacy of oxidative bacteria killing is directly proportional to local oxygen tension (539).

The clinical relevance of blood flow and oxygen supply to healing and infection has been shown experimentally in skin flaps in dogs (32, 392, 395). In flaps with a high perfusion and tissue oxygen tension, no infection was found after injection of bacteria; whereas invasive, necrotizing infections were found in flap areas in which oxygen tension was less than 40 mmHg. When oxygen tension in inspired gas and arterial blood was raised or lowered, the infection rate corresponded to tissue oxygen tension, but not to oxygen carrying capacity.

With respect to healing of dental tissues, the oxygen tension may have a significant effect. Thus, several *in vivo* tissue culture studies have shown that low oxygen tension (e.g. a 5% oxygen atmosphere) results in reduced collagen and bone formation. A concentration of 35% $O_2$ was found to be optimal for collagen and bone formation, while a high oxygen concentration (95%) resulted in depression of collagen and bone formation as well as osteoclastic resorption of bone and cartilage (520–522). This *in vitro* relation between high oxygen concentration and osteoclastic activity may have an *in vivo* counterpart in vanishing bone disease (Gorhams disease or vanishing facial bone) (523, 524) as well as the internal surface resorption phenomenon seen in revascularization of the pulps of luxated or root-fractured teeth (525). In both instances active local hyperemia and increased oxygen supply may be related to osteoclastic activity.

Among local factors which can control blood supply and tissue perfusion to the injured tissue, tension caused by splints or sutures may seriously jeopardize local circulation. Thus, splinting types exerting pressure on the periodontium may disturb or prevent uneventful PDL or pulp healing and lead to disturbances, such as root resorption, ankylosis and pulp necrosis (see Chapter 2, p. 76). Furthermore, tension of sutured soft tissue wounds may lead to ischemia with subsequent risk of wound infection (see Chapter 21, p. 592).

## Hyperbaric oxygenation

Hyperbaric oxygen (HBO) has been introduced in the treatment of various oral conditions such as problem wounds subsequent to irradiation as well as in cases of grafting procedures where vascularization appears compromised, as well as in other types of chronic wounds (526, 617, 618).

HBO is administered in pressurized tanks where the patients inhale 100% oxygen at a pressure of 2 atmospheres. The interaction of HBO to hypoxic tissue has a range of effects (7). The most significant effect of HBO is that it aug-

ments the oxygen gradient within the wound healing site, thus leading to increased fibroblast and endothelial activity (269, 527–530) as well as increased epithelialization (489). HBO may also suppress growth of certain bacteria (512).

In experimental gingival wounds in rats, it has been found that HBO augments gingival connective tissue healing during the first 2 weeks, whereafter no difference was seen in comparison to wounds healed at normal atmosphere (531). In more extensive wounds in rats, where mandibular ramus osteotomy wounds severed the neurovascular supply in the mandibular canal, it was found that HBO reduced or prevented the ischemic damage to pulp cells, ameloblastema and adjacent bone on a short-term basis (i.e. after 10 days). With an observation period of 30 days, HBO was found to stimulate osteodentin and bone formation in the zones of injury (532).

This beneficial effect of HBO on bone healing after injury is supported by a human study where acceleration of bone healing after osteotomy could be demonstrated after the use of hyperbaric oxygen (533, 619).

## Smoking and alcohol

Smoking influences the healing process by different mechanisms. Nicotine is quickly absorbed and starts a release of catecolamines resulting in a peripheral vascular constriction followed by decrease in perfusion rate of 42% (534). Furthermore the CO in the cigarette smoke will reduce the oxygen content of the blood. These combined effects have been shown to decrease the tissue perfusion by more than 30% in more than 45 minutes in specific areas of the body (535). In such areas the production of collagen is 1.8 times higher in non-smokers compared to smokers (536). Leukocytes in smokers have also shown a decreased ability to kill bacteria resulting in a higher risk of wound infections in smokers. In surgical patients an increased risk of necrosis of the wound edge, diminished cosmetic result, increased risk of anastomic leakage after bowel surgery, and increased recurrence rate after hernia surgery have been described (49).

A recent study has found that healthy smokers have a higher incidence of wound infections and wound ruptures than never-smokers, and 4 weeks of abstinence from smoking reduces wound infections to a level similar to never-smokers (537).

Alcohol has also shown an increased risk of postoperative infection, bleeding, exudation and wound/anastomoses rupture. The specific influence on the wound healing process is not known, but alcohol consumption decreases total protein but not collagen in artificial wounds. These changes are reversible after stopping alcohol intake (538).

## Infection

Infection is the most common complication which can disturb wound healing (342). Development of infection is determined by the number and type of contaminating organisms, host defense capability and local environment (540).

When bacteria invade a wound, the final outcome of this event is related to the success of the initial phase of the inflammatory response in establishing an antibacterial defense (Fig. 1.27). Timing is critical and the fate of the contaminating bacteria appears to be determined within the first 3 to 4 hours after injury. During this period, the early inflammatory process is established and will usually result in the elimination of bacteria (539, 541, 542).

The risk of infection appears to be directly related to the number of bacteria initially present in the wound (540). If the bacteria are not eliminated during these first critical hours, a series of events which will effect wound healing will occur. Thus the formation of fibroblasts will be disturbed in several ways and fibroblast proliferation is generally inhibited; but stimulation may occur in certain circumstances (541–547). Liberation of toxins, enzymes and waste products from bacteria decrease or inhibit collagen synthesis (548) and increase the synthesis of collagenase, resulting in lysis of collagen (549). Furthermore, some bacteria decrease the amount of oxygen available in the infected tissue (550, 551) whereby healing processes suffer. Collagen formation is reduced, cell migration is delayed or arrested, cellular necrosis and microvascular thrombosis may result (552). Wounds have been classified as:

- *Clean wounds*, which are uninfected operative wounds in which no inflammation is encountered.
- *Potentially contaminated wounds*, in which the respiratory, alimentary or genitourinary tracts are entered under controlled conditions during surgery.
- *Contaminated wounds* where acute inflammation (without pus) is encountered or where there is a gross spillage from a hollow viscus during surgery.
- *Dirty wounds and infected wounds* which are old traumatic wounds and operating wounds in the presence of pus or those involving clinical infection of perforated viscera (552).

The level of aerobic and anaerobic contamination expressed as bacteria in the wound (i.e. colony forming units per unit area) is for clean wounds 2.2, for potentially contaminated wounds $2.4 \times 10^1$, for contaminated wounds $1.1 \times 10^3$, and for dirty wounds $3.7 \times 10^3$ (553).

Oral wounds are associated with a high risk of contamination as saliva contains $10^{8-9}$ bacteria per milliliter (554).

The infective dose of bacteria which results in a microscopic infection has been found to be $10^5$ bacteria per gram of tissue (555). A correlation has been found in different types of wounds between preclosure bacterial density of aerobic and anaerobic bacteria and post-surgical wound infections (553). It is recognized that both aerobic and

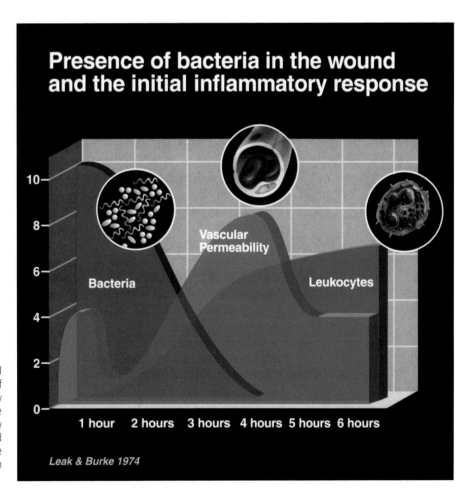

**Fig. 1.27** Bacteria and the initial inflammatory response. The period of active tissue antibacterial activity (decisive period) relates well to the establishing of the inflammatory response, as reflected by increased vascular permeability and leukocyte migration into the wound site. From LEAK & BURKE (539) 1974.

anaerobic organisms are implicated in most wound infections.

The use of antibiotics to supplement the natural host resistance (i.e. the early inflammatory response) has been found to be additive and sometimes even synergistic in bacteria killing. However, if antibiotics are given with more than a 3-hour delay, animal experiments have shown that the effect of antibiotics such as penicillin, erythromycin, chloramphenicol and tetracyclin was eliminated (556). The timing of antibiotics therefore seems to be of utmost importance.

Many factors are described as contributing to impaired wound healing as well as increased risk of infection. Some of these factors may have a direct influence on the healing process while other factors have an indirect influence by changing circulation and thereby oxygenation.

## Foreign bodies

The presence of foreign bodies can contribute to delayed healing, but is normally not by itself sufficient to prevent healing. Foreign bodies provide a focus for bacterial growth, and consequently a smaller amount of bacteria is needed to cause infection in the wound area. More than 50 years ago it was observed that just a single silk suture present in the wound area increased the susceptibility to bacteria (*Staphylococcus*) by a factor of × 10 000 (557, 558). Other types of foreign materials, such as soil, clothing and drains have also been shown to increase the risk of postoperative infection and impaired wound healing (559–561). Recently it has been found that bacteria may be camouflaged on artificial surfaces by producing an extracellular carbohydrate film (562). This film seriously affects the host response by inhibiting chemotaxis, bacterial engulfment and the oxidation response of the phagocytes.

Foreign bodies in oral and other soft tissue wounds consist mainly of soil and its contaminants (563), but also tooth fragments can be found. Soil has four major components: inorganic minerals, organic matter, water and air. The coarser components of soil are stone, gravel and sand. The smallest inorganic particle found in soil is clay. Not only does soil carry bacterial contamination into the wound, but the mere presence of inorganic and organic particles has been shown to lead to impairment of leukocyte ability to ingest and kill bacteria (559). Therefore very few bacteria are able to elicit purulent infections in the presence of foreign bodies. As there is no way of neutralizing the effect of soil, therapeutic efforts should be directed towards removing it from the wound area (see Chapter 21, p. 580).

In traumatic wounds, foreign bodies can usually be removed, improving wound healing and decreasing the risk of infection. In surgical wounds, however, this may not always be the case. The most common foreign bodies in surgical wounds are sutures, drains and biological materials such as hematomas.

## Sutures

The ideal suture can be described as free of infection, non-irritating to tissues, achieving its purpose and disappearing when the work is finished (435, 563). Such ideal sutures are still not available; but by choosing the best material, the complication rate provided by the suture material itself can be decreased. Bulky and braided suture materials are generally more likely to cause trouble than fine monofilament sutures (564, 565) (see Chapter 21, p. 592).

In non-infected multifilamentous sutures, fibroblasts and giant cells appear early and the suture strands remain tightly bound in comparison to infected sutures where bacteria are entrapped within the braids, leading to pus formation (566).

The reaction around a monofilament suture is minimal and a fibrous capsule appears after 10 days, even in the presence of infection. Apart from the knots, there is no space for bacteria to lodge (566). The ideal suture is therefore a monofilament type of suture with sufficient strength to hold the wound edges together until significant healing has occurred, even in delayed healing. The use of absorbable and non-absorbable sutures in relation to wound healing and infection is still controversial (567–569). The use of sutures in soft tissue wounds is further discussed in Chapter 21, p. 592.

## Distant wound response

For decades it has been known that a wound preceded by a previous injury heals faster than a primary wound. Thus from a mechanical point of view (wound strength) a second wound heals faster than the first (570). The explanation for this phenomenon is still uncertain. Another distant wound response is found when two wounds occur simultaneously in distant parts of the body. In these cases impaired blood circulation may be found in the wounds leading to impaired healing (571).

## Age

### Fetal wound healing

Healing of experimental oral wounds in a mammalian fetus differs greatly from similar wounds in adults (572–576). Thus accelerated healing without scarring is found in fetal wounds, even in defect wounds. The wound response appears to be without acute inflammation and with minimal fibroblast and endothelial cell proliferation (577). Furthermore the extracellular matrix appears collagen-poor and rich in hyaluronic acid.

Hyaluronic acid is laid down early in the matrix of both fetal and adult wounds; but sustained deposition of hyaluronic acid is unique to fetal wound healing (578). Hyaluronic acid is presently thought to play a decisive role in the regenerative process, as it provides a permissive environment for cell proliferation and mobility (572, 573, 577, 579) and suppresses macrophage-effected postnatal repair (579). It has been shown that the elimination of transforming growth factor β (TGF-β) from healing wounds in adult rats reversed the typical fibrous scar formation to a stage of fetal wound healing without scar tissue (580). This implies that the control of selected cytokines may be a future approach to control scarring.

### Adult wound healing

The relationship between age and healing of skin wounds in respect to speed of healing has been studied experimentally in rats (581–588), rabbits (589, 590) and in humans (591, 592). Experiments examining the role of the age factor upon wounding of oral mucosa and gingiva have been performed in rats (593–597) mice (598) and humans (599–601). In the most comprehensive studies using experimental skin wounds in rats and gingival wounds in humans, it was found that healing of gingival defects is slower and regeneration more incomplete in old than in young individuals. Furthermore, wound strength develops more slowly in old rats than in young rats, a finding which was related to the better functional arrangement of collagen fibers in the young animals (602). In the gastrointestinal tract, however, aging seems not to have an adverse influence on wound healing (603).

Wound infection is also strongly related to age (604, 605). Thus, in a prospective study on wound infection subsequent to surgical wounds, a wound infection rate of 0.6% was found in children aged 1–14 years and this rate rose to a maximum of 3.8% in patients over 66 years of age (604).

## Optimizing oral wound healing

An important principle to consider in this context is that the mode of action of both normal wound healing and the response to infection seems to follow a general pattern which is sometimes in conflict with the regeneration of injured organs. This is apparent in skin wounds where the need for rapid wound closure (in order to prevent infection from invading microorganisms) usually results in the formation of a scar. In the dental organ, an effective response against bacteria takes priority with activation of the neutrophils, lymphocytes, macrophages and osteoclasts leading to frequent bone and tooth loss due to hard tissue resorption (see Chapter 2, p. 80).

Presently, the most likely avenue whereby healing problems can be avoided appears to be careful tissue handling whereby tissue perfusion is re-established or stabilized and wound contaminants (e.g. foreign bodies and microbes) are reduced or eliminated.

To achieve this goal, various steps are necessary in the diffent phases of wound healing. In the coagulation phase, assistance in achieving hemostasis may be necessary. In performing this, it is important not to use excessive cautery, which results in tissue necrosis, or topical hemostatic agents (e.g. Surgicel®, Oxycel®, Gelfoam®) that may have a potentiating effect for infection (559). Instead, firm pressure exerted with a gauze sponge for several minutes usually results in hemostasis.

In handling oral wounds, a local anesthetic is usually necessary. In this regard it should be borne in mind that the vasoconstriction of the anesthetic solution increases the risk of infection of the wound due to interference with the inflammatory response in the critical first hours after injury (559, 606). Regional block anesthesia rather than local infiltration of the anesthetic solution is therefore to be recommended.

Wound debridement should be limited to removal of foreign bodies and obviously damaged tissue which cannot be anticipated to survive or become revascularized (see Chapter 21, p. 581).

The elimination and/or reduction in the size of the blood clot should be attempted in order to facilitate wound healing, including revascularization. This applies to soft tissues as well as tooth and bone repositioning.

The value of complete immobilization of the wound edges is presently under debate so only a few treatment principles can be suggested.

In soft tissue wounds any sutures used to immobilize the wound edges must be regarded as foreign bodies which increases the risk of infection (276, 559). Thus a minimal number of sutures should be used, and a suture type should be chosen which elicits minimal side effects (see Chapter 21, p. 593).

In regard to hard tissue healing, splinting should generally be performed. These splints should not augment the risk of infection, whereby the application and the design of the splints becomes crucial (see Chapter 32).

The value of antibiotics in oral wound healing is presently unsettled (see Chapters 17 and 21). If indicated, antibiotics should be administered as early as possible and preferably not later than in the first 3 to 4 hours after trauma and only maintained for a short period of time (540) (see Chapters 17, 18 and 21). Acceleration of oral wound healing by the use of growth factors is in its initial stage and has the potential to be an essential part of trauma treatment (Chapter 2). The fascinating perspective in the use of growth factors is the achievement of an orchestrated healing response whereby certain parts of the cellular response are promoted (e.g. angiogenesis, fibrillogenesis, dentinogenesis, osteogenesis and epithelialization). The initial attempts at such an approach to oral wound healing appear very promising (see Chapter 21).

## Essentials

Regeneration is a process whereby the original architecture and function of disrupted or lost tissue is completely restored.

Repair is a process whereby the continuity of disrupted or lost tissue is restored by new tissue, but which does not reproduce the original structure and function.

### The general steps in wound healing

- Control of bleeding by the combined action of vasoconstriction and coagulation
- Inflammatory response, whereby leukocytes migrate into the wound in order to protect the area against infection and perform cleansing of the wound site
- Connective and epithelial tissue migration and proliferation, which obturate the wound defect and add mechanical strength to the wound

- Reorganization of the tissue by a remodeling process which results in more functionally oriented collagen fibers which increase the strength of the wound.

## The main roles of the individual tissue cells

- *Platelets*, apart from their role in initial hemostasis and their activation of the coagulation cascade, serve as initiators of the wound healing process.
- *Polymorphonuclear leukocytes* prevent bacterial infection within the wound site.
- *Macrophages* are scavengers of tissue remnants and foreign bodies including bacteria and the key cells in coordinating the cellular events in wound healing.
- *Fibroblasts* produce collagen and ground substance which fills out the wound defect and adds mechanical strength to the wound.
- *Endothelial cells* in the venules are the key cells in angiogenesis. By coordinated endothelial cell proliferation and migration, a new vascular network is formed at the wound site.
- *Pericytes* represent a pool of undifferentiated mesenchymal cells.
- *Epithelial cells* close the gap against the external environment by cell migration and proliferation.

The coordinated action of the above-mentioned cells is found in the *wound healing module* created a few days after injury where leading macrophages clear damaged tissue, foreign bodies and bacteria with trailing fibroblasts and newly formed capillaries.

Significant stimuli for the invasive growth of new formed connective tissue and also termination of the wound healing module appear to be *growth factors* as well as *oxygen tension* and *lactate concentration* in the injury zone ahead of the wound healing module.

Of many factors known to disturb wound healing, the following are the most likely candidates affecting mucosa and skin, as well as the periodontium and the pulp of traumatized teeth:

- *Low oxygen* delivery to the wound site due to the initial trauma and/or improper tissue handling technique (e.g. suturing, splinting or lack of repositioning of tissues)
- *Infection* due to contamination of the injury site
- *Foreign bodies* including inappropriate use of sutures and drains.

## References

1. SUNDEL B. ed. Proceedings of a symposium on wound healing. Plastic surgical and dermatological aspects. Espoo, Finland, 1979.
2. HUNT TK. ed. *Wound healing and wound infection: theory and surgical practice.* New York: Appleton-Century-Crofts, 1980.
3. DINEEN P, HILDIC-SMITH G. eds. *The surgical wound.* Philadelphia: Lea & Febiger, 1981.
4. HUNT TK, HEPPENSTALL RB, PINES E, ROVEE D. eds. *Soft and hard tissue repair: biological and clinical aspects.* New York: Praeger, 1984.
5. PEACOCK EE Jr. *Wound repair.* 3rd edn. Philadelphia: WB Saunders, 1984.
6. WOO SLY, BUCKWALTER JA. eds. *Injury and repair of the musculoskeletal soft tissues.* Illinois: American Academy of Orthopedic Surgeons, 1988.
7. DAVIS JC, HUNT TK. eds. *Problem wounds: the role of oxygen.* New York: Elsevier, 1988.
8. CLOWES GHA Jr. ed. *Trauma, sepsis, and shock: the physiological basis of therapy.* New York: Mercel Dekker, 1988.
9. CLARK RAF, HENSON PM. eds. *The molecular and cellular biology of wound repair.* New York: Plenum Press, 1988.
10. LUNDBORG G. *Nerve injury and repair.* Edinburgh: Churchill Livingstone, 1988.
11. KLOTH LC, McCULLOCH JM, FEEDAR JA. eds. *Wound healing: alternatives in management.* Philadelphia: FA Davis Company, 1990.
12. JANSSEN H, ROOMAN R, ROBERTSON JIS. eds. *Wound healing.* Petersfield: Wrightson Biomedical Publishing, 1991.
13. COHEN IK, DIEGELMANN RF, LINDBLAD WJ. eds. *Wound healing: biochemical and clinical aspects.* Philadelphia: WB Saunders, 1992.
14. GILLMAN T. Tissue regeneration. In: Bourne GH. ed. *Structural aspects of ageing.* London: Pitman, 1961:144–76.
15. FEINBERG SE, LARSEN PE. Healing of traumatic injuries. In: Fonseca RJ, Walker RV. eds. *Oral and maxillofacial trauma.* Philadelphia: WB Saunders, 1991:13–56.
16. BARBUL A, CALDWELL MD, EAGLESTEIN WH. eds. *Clinical and experimental approaches to dermal and epidermal repair.* New York: Wiley-Liss, 1991.
17. BUCKNALL TE, ELLIS H. *Wound healing for surgeons.* London: Baillière Tindall, 1984.
18. HARTING G. ed. *Advanced wound healing resource theory.* Copenhagen: Coloplast, 1992.
19. GOTTRUP F. Advances in the biology of wound healing. In: Harding KG, Leaper DL, Turner TD. eds. *Advances in wound management.* London: Macmillan Magazines, 1992:7–11.
20. HUNT TK, DUNPHY JE. eds. *Fundamentals of wound management.* New York: Appleton-Century-Crofts, 1979.
21. IOCONCO JA, EHRLICH HP, GOTTRUP F, LEAPER DJ. The biology of healing. In: Leaper DJ, Harding KG. eds. *Wounds, biology and management.* Oxford: Oxford University Press, 1998:10–22.
22. FERGUSON MW, LEIGH IM. Wound healing. In: Champion RH, Burton JL, Burns DA, Breathnach SM. eds. *Textbook of dermatology.* 6th edn. Oxford: Blackwell Science, 1998:337–43.
23. SINGER AJ, CLARK RAF. Cutaneous wound healing. *N Engl J Med* 1999;**341**:738–46.
24. GOULD TRL. Ultrastructural characteristics of progenitor cell populations in the periodontal ligament. *J Dent Res* 1983;**62**:873–6.
25. BERNFIELD M, BANERJEE SD, KODA JE, RAPRAEGER AC. Remodeling of the basement membrane: morphogenesis

and maturation. *Ciba Foundation Symposium 108,* 1984:179–96.

26. MORGAN CJ, PLEDGER WJ. Fibroblast proliferation. In: Cohen IK, Diegelmann RF, Lindblad WJ. eds. *Wound healing: biochemical and clinical aspects.* Philadelphia: WB Saunders, 1992:63–78.

27. McCARTY JB, SAS DF, FURCHT LT. Mechanisms of parenchymal cell migration into wounds. In: Clark RAF, Henson PM. eds. *The molecular and cellular biology of wound repair.* New York: Plenum Press, 1988:281–319.

28. SINGER SJ, KUPFER A. The directed migration of eukaryotic cells. *Ann Rev Biol* 1986;**2**:337–65.

29. BRYANT WM. Wound healing. *Ciba Clin Symp* 1977;**29**:1–36.

30. REICH E, RIFKIN DB, SHAW E. eds. Proteases and biological control. Cold Spring Harbor: Cold Spring Harbor Conference on Cell Proliferation, 1976.

31. GOTTRUP F, ANDREASEN JO. Wound healing subsequent to injury. In. Andreasen JO, Andreasen FM. eds. *Textbook and color atlas of traumatic injuries to the teeth.* 3rd. edn. Copenhagen: Munksgaard, 1994:13–76.

32. GOTTRUP F, FIRMIN R, HUNT TK, MATHES S. The dynamic properties of tissue oxygen in healing flaps. *Surgery* 1984;**95**:527–37.

33. HUNT TK. Physiology of wound healing. In: Clowes GHA. ed. *Trauma, sepsis, and shock.* New York: Marcel Dekker, 1988:443–71.

34. TANDARA AA, MUSTOE TA. Oxygen in wound healing – more than a nutrient. *World J Surg* 2004;**28**:294–300.

35. SEN CK. The general case for redox control of wound repair. *Wound Rep Reg* 2003;**11**:431–8.

36. GORDILLO GM, CHEN CK. Revisiting the essential role of oxygen in wound healing. *Am J Surg* 2003;**186**:259–63.

37. SUNDARESAN M, YUZ X, FERRANS VJ, IRANI K, FINKEL T. Requirement for generation of $H_2O_2$ for platelet-derived growth factor signal transduction. *Science* 1995;**270**:296–9.

38. NIINIKOSKI J, GOTTRUP F, HUNT TK. The role of oxygen in wound repair. In: Janssen H, Rooman R, Robertson JIS. eds. *Wound healing.* Oxford: Blackwell Scientific, 1991:165–74.

39. JÖNSSON K, JENSEN JA, GOODSON WH, SCHEUENSTUHL H, WEST J, HOPF HW, HUNT TK. Tissue oxygenation, anemia and perfusion in relation to wound healing in surgical patients. *Ann Surg* 1991;**214**:605–13.

40. GOTTRUP F. Oxygen, wound healing and the development of infection, present status. *Eur J Surg* 2002;**168**:260–3.

41. HUNT TK, PAI MP. Effect of varying ambient oxygen tension on wound metabolism and collagen synthesis. *Surg Gynecol Obstet* 1972;**135**:257–60.

42. GOTTRUP F. Tissue perfusion and oxygenation related to wound healing and resistance to infection. In: Engemann R, Holzheimer R, Thiede A. eds. *Immunology and its impact on infections in surgery.* Berlin: Springer Verlag, 1995:117–26.

43. PROCKOP DJ, KIVIRIKKO KI, TUDERMAN L, GUZMAN NA. The biosynthesis of collagen and its disorders. *N Engl J Med* 1979;**301**:13–23.

44. ROY S, KHANNA S, BICKERSTAFF A, SUBRAMANIA SV, ATALAY M, BIERL M, PENDYALA S, LEVY D, SHAMA N,

VENOJARVI M, STRAUCH A, OROSZ CG, SEN CK. Oxygen sensing by primary cardiac fibroblasts: a key role of p21 (Waf1/Cip/Sdi 1). *Circ Res* 2003;**92**:264–71.

45. KNIGHTON D, SILVER I, HUNT TK. Regulation of wound healing and angiogenesis-effect of oxygen gradients and inspired oxygen concentrations. *Surgery* 1981;**90**:262–70.

46. SEMENZA GL. HIF-1 and human disease: one highly involved factor. *Genes Dev* 2000;**14**:1983–91.

47. YANG GP, LONGAKER MT. Abstinence from smoking reduces incisional infection: a randomised controlled trial (editorial). *Ann Surg* 2003;**238**:6–8.

48. GOTTRUP F. Oxygen in wound healing and infection. *World J Surg* 2004;**28**:312–15.

49. SILVER IA. The physiology of wound healing. In: Hunt TK. ed. *Wound healing and wound infection: theory and surgical practice.* New York: Appleton-Century-Crofts, 1980:11–31.

50. WINTER GD. Formation of the scab and the rate of epithelialization of superficial wounds in skin of the young domestic pig. *Nature* 1962;**193**:293–4.

51. WISEMAN DM, ROVEE DT, ALVAREZ OM. Wound dressing: design and use. In: Cohen K, Diegelman RF, Lindblad WJ. eds. *Wound healing: biochemical and clinical aspects.* Philadelphia: WB Saunders, 1992:562–80.

52. BULLOUGH WS, JOHNSON M. Epidermal mitotic activity and oxygen tension. *Nature* 1951;**167**:488.

53. KARASEK MA. *In vitro* culture of human skin epithelial cells. *J Invest Dermatol* 1966;**47**:533–40.

54. HORIKOSHI T, BALIN AK, CARTER DM. Effect of oxygen on the growth of human epidermal keratinocytes. *J Invest Dermatol* 1986;**86**:424–7.

55. DESMOLIERE A, REDARD M, DARBY I, GABBIANI G. Apoptosis mediated the decrease in cellularity during the transition between granulation tissue and scar. *Am J Pathol* 1995;**146**:56–66.

56. GOTTRUP F. Acute wound healing – aspects of wound closure. In: Leaper DJ. ed. *International symposium on wound management.* Bussum, the Netherlands: Medicom Europe, 1991:11–18.

57. GOTTRRUP F. Advances in the biology of wound healing. In: Harding KG, Leaper DL, Turner TD. eds. *Proceedings of 1st European Conference on Advances in Wound Management.* London: Macmillan, 1992:7–10.

58. GOTTRUP F. Surgical wounds – healing types and physiology. In: Harting K. ed. *Advanced wound healing resource theory.* Copenhagen: Coloplast, 1992, Chapter X:1–17.

59. GOTTRUP F, FOGDESTAM I, HUNT TK. Delayed primary closure: an experimental and clinical review. *J Clin Surg* 1982;**1**:113–24.

60. GOTTRUP F. Delayed primary closure of wounds. *Infect Surg* 1985;**4**:171–8.

61. CLARK RAF. Cutaneous wound repair: a review with emphasis on integrin receptor expression. In: Janssen H, Rooman R, Robertson JIS. eds. *Wound healing.* Petersfield: Wrightson Biomedical Publishing, 1991:7–17.

62. WAHL LM, WAHL SM. Inflammation. In: Cohen IK, Diegelmann RF, Lindblad WJ. eds. *Wound healing: biochemical and clinical aspects.* Philadelphia: WB Saunders, 1992:40–62.

63. DVORAK HF, KAPLAN AP, CLARK RAF. Potential functions of the clotting system in wound repair. In:

Clark RAF, Henson PM. eds. *The molecular and cellular biology of wound repair.* New York: Plenum Press, 1988:57–85.

64. DVORAK HF, HARVEY VS, ESTRELLA P, et al. Fibrin containing gels induce angiogenesis. Implications for tumor stroma generation and wound healing. *Lab Invest* 1987;**57**:673–86.

65. CHEN LB, BUCHANAN JM. Mitogenic activity of blood components. I. Thrombin and prothrombin. *Proc Natl Acad Sci USA* 1975;**72**:131–5.

66. WESLER BB, LEY CW, JAFFE EA. Stimulation of endothelial cell prostacycline production by thrombin, trypsin, and ionophore A23187. *J Clin Invest* 1978;**62**:923–30.

67. BAR-SHIVAT R, WILNER GD. Biologic activities of nonenzymatic thrombin: elucidation of a macrophage interactive domain. *Sem Throm Hem* 1986;**12**:244–9.

68. BAR-SHIVAT R, KAHN AJ, MANN KG, et al. Identification of a thrombin sequence with growth factor activity on macrophages. *Proc Natl Acad Sci* USA 1986;**83**:976–80.

69. CARNEY DH, CUNNINGHAM DD. Role of specific cell surface receptors in thrombin-stimulated cell division. *Cell* 1978;**15**:1341–9.

70. GRAY AJ, REEVES JT, HARRISON NK, et al. Growth factors for human fibroblasts in the solute remaining after clot formation. *J Cell Sci* 1990;**96**:271–4.

71. MAJNO G, BOUVIER CA, GABBIANI G, RYAN GB, STAIKOV P. Kymographic recording of clot retraction: Effects of papaverine, theophylline and cytochalasin B. *Thromb Diath Haemorrh* 1972;**28**:49–53.

72. ORDMAN LN, GILLMAN T. Studies in the healing of cutaneous wounds. Part III. A critical comparison in the pig of the healing of surgical incisions closed with sutures or adhesive tape based on tensile strength and clinical and histologic criteria. *Arch Surg* 1966;**93**:911–28.

73. ROSS R, BENDITT EP. Wound healing and collagen formation. I. Sequential changes in components of guinea pig skin wounds observed in the electron microscope. *J Biophys Biochem Cytol* 1961;**11**:677–700.

74. MCMILLAN MD. An ultrastructural study of the relationship of oral bacteria to the epithelium of healing tooth extraction wounds. *Arch Oral Biol* 1975;**20**:815–22.

75. MCMILLAN MD. The healing of oral wounds. *N Zealand Dent J* 1986;**82**:112–16.

76. POLK HC Jr, MILES AA. Enhancement of bacterial infection by ferric ion: kinetics, mechanisms and surgical significance. *Surgery* 1971;**70**:71–7.

77. POLK HC Jr, FRY DE, FLINT LM. Dissemination and causes of infection. *Surg Clin North Am* 1976;**56**:817–29.

78. WIKESJÖ UME, CLAFFEY N, EGELBERG J. Periodontal repair in dogs: effect of heparin treatment of the root surface. *J Clin Periodontol* 1991;**18**:60–4.

79. GRINNELL F, BENNETT MH. Fibroblast adhesion on collagen substrata in the presence and absence of plasma fibronectin. *J Cell Sci* 1981;**48**:19–34.

80. MOSHER DF, JOHNSON RB. Specificity of fibronectin–fibrin cross-linking. *Ann NY Acad Sci* 1983;**408**:583–94.

81. KITTLICK PD. Fibrin in fibroblast cultures: a metabolic study as a contribution of inflammation and tissue repair. *Exp Pathol (Jena)* 1979;**17**:312–26.

82. KNOX P, CROOKS S, RIMMER CS. Role of fibrinectin in the migration of fibroblasts into plasma clots. *J Cell Biol* 1986;**102**:2318–23.

83. WEIGEL PH, FULLER GM, LEBOEUF RD. A model for the role of hyaluronic acid and fibrin in the early events during the inflammatory response and wound healing. *J Theor Biol* 1986;**119**:219–34.

84. CIANO P, COLVIN R, DVORAK A, et al. Macrophage migration in fibrin gel matrices. *Lab Invest* 1986;**54**:62–70.

85. RICHARDSON DL, PEPPER DS, KAY AB. Chemotaxis for human monocytes by fibrinogen-derived peptides. *Br J Haematol* 1976;**32**:507–13.

86. KNIGHTON DR, HUNT TK, THAKRAL KK, et al. Role of platelets and fibrin and the healing sequence: an *in vivo* study of angiogenesis and collagen synthesis. *Ann Surg* 1782;**196**:379–88.

87. CLARK RAF, LANIGAN JM, DELLAPELLE P, et al. Fibronectin and fibrin provide a provisional matrix for epidermal cell migration during wound re-epithelialization. *J Invest Dermatol* 1982;**79**:264–9.

88. KURKINEN M, VAHERI A, ROBERTS PJ, et al. Sequential appearance of fibronectin and collagen in experimental granulation tissue. *Lab Invest* 1980;**43**:47–51.

89. ALLEN RA, PEPPER DC. Isolation and properties of human vascular plasminogen activator. *Thromb Haemost* 1981;**45**:43–50.

90. POLSON AM, PROYE MP. Fibrin linkage: a precursor for new attachment. *J Periodont* 1983;**54**:141–7.

91. MCDONALD JA. Fibronectin. A primitive matrix. In: Clark RAF, Henson PM. eds. *The molecular and cellular biology of wound repair.* New York: Plenum Press, 1988:405–35.

92. BROWN LF, DUBIN D, LAVIGNE L, DVORAK, HF, VAN DE WAER L. Macrophages and fibroblasts express embryonic fribronectins during cutaneous wound healing. *Amer J Pathol* 1993;**142**:793–801.

93. WILLIAMS IF, MCCULLAGH KG, SILVER IA. The distribution of types I and III collagen and fibronectin in the healing equine tendon. *Connect Tissue Res* 1984;**12**:211–27.

94. MCAUSLAN B, HANNAN G, REILLY W, STEWART F. Variant endothelial cells: fibronectin as a transducer of signals for migration and neovascularization. *J Cell Physiol* 1980;**104**:177–86.

95. MCAUSLAN B, HANNAN G, REILLY W. Signals causing change in morphological phenotype, growth mode, and gene expression of vascular endothelial cells. *J Cell Physiol* 1982;**112**:96–106.

96. KUBO M, NORRIS DA, HOWELL SE, RYAN SR, CLARK RA. Human keratinocytes synthesize, secrete, and deposit fibronectin in the pericellular matrix. *J Dermatol* 1984;**82**:580–6.

97. LIVINGSTON A, VAN DE WAER L, CONSTANT C, BROWN L. Fibronectin expression during cutaneous wound healing. In: Adzick NS, Longaker MT. eds. *Fetal wound healing.* New York: Elsevier, 1992:281–301.

98. KLEINMAN HK. Interactions between connective tissue matrix macromolecules. *Connective Tissue Res* 1982;**10**:61–72.

99. REPESH LA, FITZGERALD TJ, FURCHT LT. Fibronectin involvement in granulation tissue and wound healing in rabbits. *J Histochem Cytochem* 1982;**30**:351–8.

100. CLARK RA, WINN HJ, DVORAK HF, COLVIN RB. Fibronectin beneath reepithelializing epidermis *in vivo*: sources and significance. *J Invest Dermatol* 1982;**77**:26–30.

101. GRINNELL F, FELD MK. Initial adhesion of human fibroblasts in serum free medium: possible role of secreted fibronectin. *Cell* 1979;**17**:117–29.

102. LYNCH SE, BUSER D, HERNANDEZ RA, WEBER HP, STICH H, FOX CH, WILLIAMS RC. Effects of the platelet-derived growth factor/insulin-like growth factor-I combination on bone regeneration around titanium dental implants. Results of a pilot study in beagle dogs. *J Periodontol* 1991;**62**:710–16.

103. GUSTAFSON GT. Ecology of wound healing in the oral cavity. *Scand J Haematol* 1984;**33**:(Suppl 40):393–409.

104. IRISH PS, HASTY DL. Immunocytochemical localization of fibronectin in human cultures using a cell surface replica technique. *J Histochem Cytochem* 1983;**31**: 69–77.

105. POSTLETHWAITE A, KESKI-OJA J, BALIAN G, et al. Induction of fibroblast chemotaxis by fibronectin. Localization of the chemotactic region to a 14 000 molecular weight non-gelatin-binding fragment. *J Exp Med* 1981;**153**:494–9.

106. MCDONALD JA, KELLEY DG, BROEKELMANN TJ. Role of fibronectin in collagen deposition: Fab to the gelatin-binding domain of fibronectin inhibits both fibronectin and collagen organization in fibroblast extracellular matrix. *J Cell Biol* 1982;**92**:485–92.

107. GRINNEL F, BILLINGHAM RE, BURGES L. Distribution of fibronectin during wound healing *in vivo*. *J Invest Dermatol* 1981;**76**:181–9.

108. HÖLUND B, CLEMMENSEN I, JUNKER P, LYON H. Fibronectin in experimental granulation tissue. *Acta Pathol Microbiol Immunol Scand (A)* 1982;**90**:159–65.

109. DVORAK HF, FORM DM, MANSEAU EJ, SMITH BD. Pathogenesis of desmoplasia. I. Immunofluorescence identification and localization of some structural proteins of line 1 and line 10 guinea pig tumors and of healing wounds. *J Natl Cancer Inst* 1984;**73**:1195–205.

110. CARTER WG. The role of intermolecular disulfide bonding in deposition of GP 140 in the extracellular matrix. *J Cell Biol* 1984;**99**:105–14.

111. BAUR PS Jr, PARKS DH. The myofibroblast anchoring strand: the fibronectin connection in wound healing and the possible loci of collagen fibril assembly. *J Trauma* 1983;**23**:853–62.

112. CLARK RAF, DELLAPELLA P, MANSEAU E, LANIGAN JM, DVORAK HF, COLVIN RB. Blood vessel fibronectin increases in conjunction with endothelial cell proliferation and capillary ingrowth during wound healing. *J Invest Dermatol* 1982;**79**:269–76.

113. TAKASHIMA A, GRINNELL F. Human keratinocyte adhesion and phagocytosis promoted by fibroblast. *J Invest Dermatol* 1984;**83**:352–8.

114. TAKASHIMA A, GRINNELL F. Fibronectin-mediated keratinocyte migration and initiation of fibronectin receptor function *in vitro*. *J Invest Dermatol* 1985;**85**:304–8.

115. CLARK RAF, FOLKVORD JM, WERTZ RL. Fibronectin as well as other extracellular matrix proteins, mediate human keratinocyte adherance. *J Invest Dermatol* 1985;**84**:378–83.

116. O'KEEFE EJ, PAYNE RE Jr, RUSSELL N, WOODLEY DT. Spreading and enhanced motility of human keratinocytes on fibronectin. *J Invest Dermatol* 1985;**85**:125–30.

117. FERNYHOUGH W, PAGE RC. Attachment, growth and synthesis by human gingival fibroblasts on demineralized or fibronectin-treated normal and diseased tooth roots. *J Periodontol* 1983;**54**:133–40.

118. RIPAMONTI U, PETIT J-C, LEMMER J, AUSTIN JC. Regeneration of the connective tissue attachment on surgically exposed roots using a fibrin–fibronectin adhesive system. An experimental study on the baboon (*Papio ursinus*). *J Periodont Res* 1987;**22**:320–6.

119. CATON JG, POLSON AM, PINI PG, BARTOLUCCI EG, CLAUSER C. Healing after application of tissue-adhesive material to denuded and citric-treated root surfaces. *J Periodontol* 1986;**157**:385–90.

120. NASJLETI C, CAFFESSE RG. Effect of fibronectin on healing of replanted teeth in monkeys: a histological and autoradiographic study. *Oral Surg Oral Med Oral Pathol* 1987;**63**:291–9.

121. CAFFESSE RG, HOLDEN MJ, KON S, et al. The effect of citric acid and fibronectin application on healing following surgical treatment of naturally occurring periodontal disease in beagle dogs. *J Clin Periodont* 1985;**12**:578–90.

122. RYAN PC, WARING GJ, SEYMOUR GJ. Periodontal healing with citric acid and fibronectin treatment in cats. *Aust Dent J* 1987;**32**:99–103.

123. THOMPSON EW, SEYMOUR GJ, WHYTE GJ. The preparation of autologous fibronectin for use in periodontal surgery. *Aust Dent J* 1987;**32**:34–8.

124. FERNANDEZ HN, HENSON PM, OTANI A, HUGLI TE. Chemotactic response to human C3a and C5a anaphylatoxins. I. Evaluation of C3a and C5a leukotaxis *in vitro* and under stimulated *in vivo* conditions. *J Immunol* 1978;**120**:109–15.

125. FERNANDEZ HN, HUGLI TE. Primary structural analysis of the polypeptide portion of human C5a anaphylatoxin. *J Biol Chem* 1978;**253**:6955–64.

126. FOLKMAN J, KLAGSBRUN M. Angiogenesic factors. *Science* 1987;**235**:442–47.

127. WEITZHANDLER M, BERNFIELD MR. Proteoglycan glycoconjungates. In: Cohen K, Diegelmann RF, Lindblad WJ. eds. *Wound healing: biochemical and clinical aspects*. Philadelphia: WB Saunders, 1992:195–208.

128. STERN MG, LONGAKER MT, STERN R. Hyaluronic acid and its modulation in fetal and adult wounds. In: Adzick NS, Longaker MT. eds. *Fetal wound healing*. New York: Elsevier, 1992:189–98.

129. COUCHMAN JR, HOOK M. Proteoglycans and wound repair. In: Clark RAF, Henson PM. eds. *The molecular and cellular biology of wound repair*. New York: Plenum Press, 1988:437–70.

130. LATERRA J, ANSBACHER R, CULP LA. Glycosaminoglycans that bind cold–insoluble globulin in cell-substratum adhesion sites of murine fibroblasts. *Proc Natl Acad Sci USA* 1980;**77**:6662–6.

131. TOOLE BP, GROSS J. The extracellular matrix of the regenerating newt limb: synthesis and removal of hyaluronate prior to differentiation. *Dev Biol* 1971;**25**:57–77.

132. ALEXANDER SA, DONOFF RB. The glycosaminoglycans of open wounds. *J Surg Res* 1980;**29**:422–9.

133. GRIMES LN. The role of hyaluronate and hyaluronidase in cell migration during the rabbit ear regenerative healing response. *Anat Rec* 1981;**199**:100.

134. AZIZKHAN RG, AZIZKHAN JC, ZETTER BR, FOLKMAN J. Mast cell heparin stimulates migration of capillary endothelial cells *in vitro. J Exp Med* 1980;**152**:931–44.

135. ROSS R, GLOMSET JA. The pathogenesis of atherosclerosis. *N Engl J Med* 1976;**295**:369–77.

136. VENGE P. What is inflammation? In: Venge P, Lindblom A. eds. *Inflammation*. Stockholm: Almquist & Wiksell International, 1985:1–8.

137. MAJNO G, GILMORE V, LEVENTHAL M. On the mechanism of vascular leakage caused by histamine-type mediators. *Circ Res* 1967;**21**:833–47

138. KAHLSON G, NILSSON K, ROSENGREN E, ZEDERFELDT B. Histamine: Wound healing as dependent on rate of histamine formation. *Lancet* 1960;**2**:230–4.

139. MAJNO G, PALADE GE. Studies on inflammation. I. The effect of histamine and serotonin on vascular permeability: An electron microscopic study. *J Biol Phys Biochem Cytol* 1961;**11**:571–605.

140. MAJNO G, SCHOEFL GI, PALADE G. Studies on inflammation. II. The site of action of histamine and serotonin on the vascular tree: A topographic study. *J Biophys Biochem Cytol* 1961;**11**:607–26.

141. MAJNO G, SHEA SM, LEVENTHAL M. Endothelial contraction induced by histamine-type mediators. An electron microscopic study. *J Cell Biol* 1969;**42**:647–72.

142. PARRAT JR, WEST GB. Release of 5-hydroxytryptamine and histamine from tissues of the rat. *J Physiol* 1957;**137**:179–92.

143. ROBSON MC, HEGGERS JP. Eicosanoids, cytokines, and free radicals. In: Cohen IK, Diegelmann RF, Lindblad WJ. eds. *Wound healing: biochemical and clinical aspects*. Philadelphia: WB Saunders, 1992:292–304.

144. HEGGERS JP, ROBSON MC. Eicosanoids in wound healing. In: Watkins WD. ed. *Prostaglandins in clinical practice*. New York: Raven Press, 1989:183–94.

145. PENNEY NS. *Prostaglandins in skin*. Kalamazoo: Current Concept/Scope Publications, 1980.

146. FRANK MM. *Complement*. Kalamazoo: Current Concept/Scope Publications, 1975.

147. HELDIN CH, ERIKSSON U, ÖSTMAN A. New members of the platelet-derived growth factor family of mitogens. *Arch Biochem Biophys* 2002;**398**:284–90.

148. HELDIN CH, WESTERMARK B. Mechanism of action and *in vivo* role of platelet derived growth factor. *Physiol Rev* 1999;**79**:1283–316.

149. ANTONIADES HN, WILLIAMS LT. Human platelet derived growth factor: Structure and functions. *Fed Proc* 1983;**42**:2630–4.

150. ASSOIAN RK. The role of growth factors in tissue repair IV: Type beta-transforming growth factor and stimulation of fibrosis. In: Clark RAF, Henson PM. eds. *The molecular and cellular biology of wound repair*. New York: Plenum Press, 1988:273–80.

151. COHEN S. The epidermal growth factor (EGF). *Cancer* 1983;**51**:1787–91.

152. CHO M, LEE YL, GARANT PR. Radioautographic demonstration of receptors for epidermal growth factor in various cells of the oral cavity. *Anat Rec* 1988;**222**:191–200.

153. CHO MI, LIN WL, GENCO RJ. Platelet-derived growth factor-modulated guided tissue regenerative therapy. *J Periodontol* 1995;**66**:522–30.

154. GROVE RI, PRATT RM. Influence of epidermal growth factor and cyclic AMP on growth and differentiation of palatal epithelial cells in culture. *Dev Biol* 1984;**106**:427–37.

155. NAKAGAWA S, YOSHIDA S, HIRAO Y, et al. Biological effects of biosynthetic human EGF on the growth of mammalian cells *in vitro. Differentiation* 1985;**29**:284–8.

156. BLAY J, BROWN KD. Epidermal growth factor promotes the chemotactic migration of cultured rat intestinal cells. *J Cell Physiol* 1985;**124**:107–12.

157. CHUA CC, GEIMAN DE, KELLER GH, LADDA RL. Induction of collagenase secretion in human fibroblast cultures by growth promoting factors. *J Biol Chem* 1985;**260**:5213–16.

158. STEIDLER NE, READE PC. Epidermal growth factor and proliferation of odontogenic cells in culture. *J Dent Res* 1981;**60**:1977–82.

159. COHEN S. Isolation of a mouse submaxillary gland protein accelerating incisor eruption and eyelid opening on newborn animal. *J Biol Chem* 1962;**237**:1555–62.

160. CLEMMONS DR. Structural and functional analysis of insulin-like growth factors. *Br Med Bull* 1989;**45**:465–80.

161. BLOM S, HOLMSTRUP P, DABELSTEEN E. The effect of insulin-like growth factor-I and human growth hormone on periodontal ligament fibroblast morphology, growth pattern, DNA synthesis, and receptor binding. *J Periodontol* 1992;**63**:960–8.

162. LYNCH SE, COLVIN RB, ANTONIADES HN. Growth factors in wound healing: single and synergistic effects on partial thickness porcine skin wounds. *J Clin Invest* 1989;**84**:640–6.

163. FRANK S, HÜBNER G, BREIER G, LONGAKER MT, GREENHALGH DG, WERNER S. Regulation of vascular endothelial growth factor expression in cultured keratinocytes: implications for normal and impaired wound healing. *J Biol Chem* 1995;**270**:12607–13.

164. ROMANO di PEPPE S, MANGONI A, ZAMBRUNO G, SPINETTI G, MELILLO G, NAPOLITANO M, CAPOGROSSI MC. Adenovirus-mediated VEGF(165) gene transfer enhances wound healing by promoting angiogenesis in CD1 diabetic mice. *Gene Ther* 2002;**9**:1271–7.

165. KLEINHEINZ J, WIESMANN HP, STRATMANN U, JOOS U. Evaluating angiogenesis and osteogenesis modified by vascular endothelial growth factor (VEGF). *Mund Kiefer Gesichtschir* 2002;**6**:175–82.

166. BOSTROM MP. Expression of bone morphogenetic proteins in fracture healing. *Clin Orthop* 1998; S116–23.

167. URIST MR. Bone. Formation by autoinduction. *Science* 1965;**150**:893–9.

168. TOMPACH PC, LEW D, STOLL JL. Cell response to hyperbaric oxygen. *Int J Oral Maxillofac Surg* 1997;**26**:82–86.

169. GRANSTRÖM G. Radiotherapy, osseointegration and hyperbaric oxygen therapy. *J Periodontol* 2003;**33**:145–62.

170. KESSLER L, BILBAULT P, ORTEGA F, GRASSO C, PASSEMARD R, STEPHAN D, PINGET M, SCHNERIDER F. Hyperbaric oxygenation accelerates the healing rate of non-ischemic chronic diabetic foot ulcers: a prospective randomized study. *Diabetes Care* 2003;**26**:2378–82.

171. ROBERTS-CLARK DJ, SMITH AJ. Angiogenic growth factors in human dentine matrix. *Arch Oral Biol* 2000;**45**:1013–16.

172. STEED DL. Clinical evaluation of recombinant platelet-derived growth factor for the treatment of lower extremity diabetic ulcers. *J Vasc Surg* 1995;**21**:71–81.

173. EMBIL JM, NAGAI MK. Becaplermin: recombinant platelet-derived growth factor, a new treatment for healing diabetic foot ulcers. *Exp Opin Biol Ther* 2002;**2**:211–18.

174. COLLINS T, POBER JS, GIMBRONE MA Jr, HAMMACHER A, BETSCHOLTZ C, WESTERMARK B. Cultured human endothelial cells express platelet-derived growth factor A chain. *Am J Pathol* 1987;**126**:7–12.

175. ROBERTS AB, SPORN MB, ASSOIAN RK, et al. Transforming growth factor type beta: rapid induction of fibrosis and angiogenesis *in vivo* and stimulation of collagen formation *in vivo*. *Proc Natl Acad Sci USA* 1986;**83**:4167–71.

176. OGAWA Y, SAWAMURA SJ, KSANDER GA, et al. Transforming growth factors – b1 and b2 induce synthesis and accumulation of hyaluronate and chondroitin sulfate *in vivo*. *Growth Factors* 1990;**3**:53–62.

177. MUSTOE TA, PIERCE GF, THOMASON A, et al. Accelerated healing of incisional wounds in rats induced by transforming growth factor-beta. *Science* 1987;**237**:1333–6.

178. BROWN GL, CURTSINGER LJ, WHITE M, et al. Acceleration of tensile strength of incisions treated with EGF and TGF-β. *Ann Surg* 1988;**208**:788–94.

179. SHAH M, FOREMAN DM, FERGUSON MW. Control of scarring in adult wounds by neutralizing antibody to transforming growth factor beta. *Lancet* 1992;**339**:213–14.

180. LAWRENCE WT, NORTON JA, SPORN MB, GORSCHBOTH C, GROTENDORST GR. The reversal of an Adriamycin induced healing impairment with chemoattractants and growth factors. *Ann Surg* 1986;**203**:142–7.

181. FRANKLIN JD, LYNCH JB. Effects of topical applications of epidermal growth factor on wound healing: experimental study on rabbit ears. *Plast Reconst Surg* 1979;**64**:766–70

182. NIALL M, RYAN GB, O'BRIEN BM. The effect of epidermal growth factor on wound healing in mice. *J Surg Res* 1982;**33**:164–9.

183. BROWN GL, NANNEY LB, GRIFFEN L, et al. Enhancement of wound healing by topical treatment with epidermal growth factor. *N Engl J Med* 1989;**321**:76–7.

184. GREAVES MW. Lack of effect of topically applied epidermal growth factor (EGF) on epidermal growth in man *in vivo*. *Clin Exp Dermatol* 1980;**5**:101–3.

185. FALANGA V, EAGLSTEIN WH, BUCALO B, KATZ MH, HARRIS B, CARSON P. Topical use of human recombinant epidermal growth factor (h-EGF) in venous ulcers. *J Dermatol Surg Oncol* 1992;**18**:604–6.

186. COHEN IK, CROSSLAND MC, GARRETT A, DIEGELMANN RF. Topical application of epidermal growth factor onto partial thickness wounds in human volunteers does not enhance reepithelialization. *Plast Reconstr Surg* 1995;**96**:251–4.

187. ROYCE LS, BAUM BJ. Physiologic levels of salivary epidermal growth factor stimulate migration of an oral epithelium cell line. *Biochim Biophys Acta* 1991;**1092**:401–3.

188. HUTSON J, MALL M, EVANS D, FOWLER R. The effect of salivary glands on wound contraction in mice. *Nature* (London) 1979;**279**:793–5.

189. BODNER L, KNYSZYNSKI A, ADLER-KUNIN S, DANON D. The effect of selective desalivation on wound healing in mice. *Exp Gerontol* 1991;**26**:357–63.

190. LI AK, KOROLY MJ, SCHATTENKERK ME, MALT RA, YOUNG M. Nerve growth factor: acceleration of the rate of wound healing in mice. *Proc Natl Acad Sci USA* 1980;**77**:4379–81.

191. BYYNY RL, ORTH DN, DOYNE ES. Epidermal growth factor: effects of androgens and adrenergic agents. *Endocrinology* 1974;**95**:776–82.

192. NOGUCHI S, OHBA Y, OKA T. Effect of epidermal growth factor on wound healing of tongue in mice. *Am J Physiol* 1991;**260**:E620–5.

193. YEH YC, GUH JY, YEH J, YEH HW. Transforming growth factor type alpha in normal human adult saliva. *Mol Cell Endocrinol* 1989;**67**:247–54.

194. MANDEL ID. The functions of saliva. *J Dent Res* 1987;**66**:(Spec. No):623–7.

195. MAJNO G, GILMORE V, LEVENTHAL M. On the mechanism of vascular leakage caused by histamine-type mediators. *Circ Res* 1967;**21**:833–47.

196. LYNCH SE, NIXON JC, COLVIN RB, ANTONIADES HN. Role of platelet-derived growth factor in wound healing: synergistic effects with other growth factors. *Proc Natl Acad Sci USA* 1987;**84**:7696–700.

197. LYNCH SE, WILLIAMS RC, POLSON AM, REDDY MS, HOWELL TH, ANTONIADES HN. Effect of insulin-like growth factor-I on periodontal regeneration. *J Dent Res* 1989;**68**. Special issue 394 (abstract 1698).

198. WANG HL, PAPPERT TD, CASTELLI WA, CHIEGO JR, SHYR Y, SMITH BA. The effect of platelet-derived growth factor on cellular response of the periodontium: an autoradiographic study on dogs. *J Periodontol* 1994;**65**:429–36.

199. GIANNOBILE WV, HERNANDEZ RA, FINKELMANN RD, RYAN S, KIRITSY CP, D'ANDREA M, LYNCH SE. Comparative effects of platelet-derived growth factor-BB and insulin-like growth factor-I, individually and in combination on periodontal regeneration in *Macaca fascicularis*. *J Periodont Res* 1996;**31**:301–12.

200. CHO MI, LIN WL, GENCO RJ. Platelet-derived growth factor-modulated guided tissue regenerative therapy. *J Periodontol* 1995;**66**:522–30.

201. HOWELL TH, FIORELLINI JP, PAQUETTE DW, OFFENBACHER S, GIANNOBILE WV, LYNCH SE. A phase I/II clinical trial to evaluate a combination of recombinant human platelet-derived growth factor-BB and recombinant human insulin-like growth factor-I in patients with periodontal disease. *J Periodontol* 1997;**68**:1186–93.

202. Becker W, Lynch SE, Lekholm U, Caffesse R, Donath K, Sanchez R. A comparison of ePTFE membranes alone or in combination with platelet-derived growth factors and insulin-like growth factors-I or demineralised freeze-dried bone in promoting bone formation around immediate extraction socket implants. *J Periodontol* 1992;**63**:929–40.

203. Selvig KA, Wikesjö UM, Bogle GC, Finkelmann RD. Impaired early bone formation in periodontal fenestration defects in dogs following application of insulin-like growth factor (II). Basic fibroblast growth factor and transforming growth factor beta 1. *J Clin Periodontol* 1994;**21**:380–5.

204. Wikesjö UM, Razi SS, Sigurdsson TJ, Tatakis DN, Lee MB, Ongipipattanakul B, Nguyen T, Hardwick R. Periodontal repair in dogs: effect of recombinant human transforming growth factor-beta1 on guided tissue regeneration. *J Clin Periodontol* 1998;**25**:475–81.

205. Murakabi S, Takayama S, Kitamura M, Shimabukuru Y, Yanagi K, Ikezawa K, Saho T, Nozaki T, Okada H. Recombinant human basic fibroblast growth factor (bFGF) stimulates perodontal regeneration in class II furcation defects created in beagle dog. *J Clin Periodontol* 2003;**38**:97–103.

206. Nakahara T, Nakamura T, Kobayashi E, Inoue M, Shigeno K, Tabata Y, Eto K, Shimizu Y. Novel approach to regeneration of periodontal tissue based on in situ tissue engineering: effects of controlled release of basic fibroblast growth factor from a sandwich membrane. *Tissue Eng* 2003;**9**:153–62.

207. Ripamonti U, Duneas N. Tissue morphogenesis and regeneration by bone morphogenetic proteins. *Plast Reconstr Surg* 1998;**101**:227–39.

208. King GN, Hughes FJ. Bone morphogenetic protein-2 stimulates cell recruitment and cementogenesis during early wound healing. *J Clin Periodontol* 2001;**28**: 465–75.

209. Wikesjö UM, Sorensen RG, Kinoshita A, Li XJ, Wozney JM. Periodontal repair in dogs: effect of recombinant human bone morphogenetic protein-12 (rhBMP-12) on regeneration of alveolar bone and periodontal attachment. A pilot study. *J Clin Periodontol* 2004;**31**:662–70.

210. Sorensen RG, Wikesjö UM, Kinoshita A, Wozney JM. Periodontal repair in dogs: evaluation of a bioresorbable calcium phosphate cement (Ceredex) as a carrier for rhBMP-2. *J Clin Periodontol* 2004;**31**: 796–804.

211. Sorensen RG, Polimeni G, Kinoshita A, Wozney JM, Wikesjö UM. Effect of recombinant human bone morphogenetic protein-12 (rhBMP-12) on regeneration of periodontal attachment following tooth replantation. *J Clin Periodontol* 2004;**31**:654–61.

212. Chung CP, Kim DK, Pak YJ, Nam KH, Lee SJ. Biological effects of drug-loaded biodegradable membranes for guided bone regeneration. *J Periodont Res* 1997;**32**:304–11.

213. Marden LJ, Fan RS, Pierce GF, Reddi AH, Hollinger JO. Platelet-derived growth factor inhibits bone regeneration induced by osteogenin, a bone morphogenetic protein, in rat craniotomy defects. *J Clin Invest* 1993;**92**:2897–905.

214. Howell TH, Fiorellini JP, Paquette DW, Offenbacher S, Giannobile WV, Lynch SE. A phase I/II clinical trial to evaluate a combination of recombinant human platelet-derived growth factor-BB and recombinant human insulin-like growth factor-I in patients with periodontal disease. *J Periodontal* 1997;**68**:1186–93.

215. Stefani CM, Machado MA, Sallum EA, Sallum AW, Toledo S, Nociti FH Jr. Platelet-derived growth factor/insulin-like growth factor-1 combination and bone regeneration around implants placed into extraction sockets: a histometric study in dogs. *Implant Dent* 2000;**9**:126–31.

216. Lind M. Growth factor stimulation of bone healing. Effects on osteoblasts, osteotomies, and implant fixation. *Acta Orthop Scand Suppl* 1998;**283**:2–37.

217. Cochran DL, Jones AA, Lilly LC, Fiorellini JP, Howell H. Evaluation of recombinant human bone morphogenetic protein-2 in oral applications including the use of endosseous implants: 3-year results of a pilot study in humans. *J Periodont* 2000;**71**:1241–57.

218. van den Bergh JP, Ten Bruggenkate CM, Groenveld HH, Burger EH, Tuinzing DB. Recombinant human bone morphogenetic protein-7 in maxillary sinus floor elevation surgery in 3 patients compared to autogenous bone grafts. A clinical pilot study. *J Clin Periodontol* 2000;**27**:627–36.

219. Hanisch O, Tatakis DN, Rohrer MD, Wöhrle PS, Wozney JM, Wikesjö UM. Bone formation and osseointegration stimulated by rhBMP-2 following subantral augmentation procedures in nonhuman primates. *Int J Oral Maxillofac Surg* 1997;**12**: 785–92.

220. Nevins M, Kirker-Head C, Nevins M, Wozney JA, Palmer R, Graham D. Bone formation in goat maxillary sinus induced by absorbable collagen sponge implants impregnated with recombinant human bone morphogenetic protein-2. *Int J Periodontics Restorative Dent* 1996;**16**:8–19.

221. Terheyden H, Jepsen S, Möller B, Tucker MM, Rueger DC. Sinus floor augmentation with simultaneous placement of dental implants using a combination of deproteinized bone xenografts and recombinant osteogenic protein-1. *Clin Oral Impl Res* 1999;**10**:510–21.

222. Goldberg M, Smith AJ. Cells and extracellular matrices of dentin and pulp: a biological basis for repair and tissue engineering. *Crit Rev Oral Biol Med* 2004;**15**:13–27.

223. Rutherford RB. Regeneration of the pulp-dentin complex. In: Lynch SE, Genco RJ, Marx RE. eds. *Tissue engineering. applications in maxillofacial surgery and periodontics.* Illinois: Quintessence Publishing, 1999:185–99.

224. Marx RE, Carlson ER, Eichstaedt RM, Schimmele SR, Strauss JE, Georgeff KR. Platelet-rich plasma. Growth factor enhancement for bone grafts. *Oral Surg Oral Pathol Oral Med Oral Radiol Endod* 1998;**85**:638–46.

225. Slater M, Patava J, Kingham K, Mason RS. Involvement of platelets in stimulating osteogenic activity. *J Orthop Res* 1995;**13**:655–63.

226. Oprea WE, Karp JM, Hosseini MM, Davies JE. Effect of platelet releasate on bone cell migration and recruitment *in vitro*. *J Craniofac Surg* 2003;**14**:292–300.

227. Wiltfang J, Kloss FR, Zimmermann R, Schultze-Mosgau S, Neukam FW, Schlegel KA. Tierexperimentelle Studie zum Einsatz von Knochenersatzmaterialien und thrombozytenreichem Plasma in klinisch relevanten Defekten. *Dtsch Zahnärztl Z* 2002;**57**:307–11.

228. Kassolis JD, Rosen PS, Reynolds MA. Alveolar ridge and sinus augmentation utilizing platelet-rich plasma in combination with freeze-dried bone allograft: Case series. *J Periodontol* 2000;**71**:1654–61.

229. de Obarrio JJ, Arauz-Dutari JI, Chamberlain TM, Croston A. The use of autologous growth factors in periodontal surgical therapy: Platelet gel biotechnology – case reports. *Int J Periodont Restor Dent* 2000;**20**:487.

230. Anitua E. The use of plasmarich growth factors (PRGF) in oral surgery. *Pract Proced Aesthet Dent* 2001;**13**:437.

231. Danesh-Meyer MJ, Filstein MR, Shanaman R. Histological evaluation of sinus augmentation using platelet rich plasma (PRP): A case series. *J Int Acad Periodontol* 2001;**3**:48–56.

232. Petrungaro PS. Using platelet-rich plasma to accelerate soft tissue maturation in esthetic periodontal surgery. *Compend Contin Educ Dent* 2001;**22**:729–45.

233. Camargo PM, Lekovic V, Weinlaender M, Vasilic N, Madzarevic M, Kenney EB. Platelet-rich plasma and bovine porous bone mineral combined with guided tissue regeneration in the treatment of intrabony defects in humans. *J Periodont Res* 2002;**37**:300–6.

234. Froum SJ, Wallace SS, Tarnow DP, Cho S-C. Effect of platelet-rich plasma on bone growth and osseointegration in human maxillary sinus grafts: Three bilateral case reports. *Int J Periodont Restor Dent* 2002;**22**:45–53.

235. Rodriguez A, Anastassou GE, Lee H, Buchbinder D, Wettan H. Maxillary sinus augmentation with deproteinated bovine bone and platelet rich plasma with simultaneous insertion of endosseous implants. *J Oral Maxillofac Surg* 2003;**61**:157–63.

236. Thorn JJ, Sörensen H, Weis-Fogh U, Andersen M. Autologous fibrin glue with growth factors in reconstructive maxillofacial surgery. *Int J Oral Maxillofac Surg* 2004;**33**:95–100.

237. Kim E-S, Park E-J, Choung P-H. Platelet concentration and its effect on bone formation in calvarial defects: An experimental study in rabbits. *J Prosthet Dent* 2001;**86**:428–33.

238. Wiltfang J, Schlegel KA, Zimmermann R, Merten HA, Kloss FR, Neukam FW, Schultze-Mosgau S. Beurteilung der Knochenreparation nach kombinierter Anwendung von Platelet-rich-plasma und Knochenersatzmaterialien im Rahmen der Sinusbodenelevation. *Dtsch Zahnärztl Z* 2002; **57**:38–42.

239. Fennis JPM, Stoelinga PJW, Jansen JA. Mandibular reconstruction: A clinical and radiographic animal study on the use of autogenous scaffolds and platelet-rich plasma. *Int J Oral Maxillofac Surg* 2002;**31**:281–6.

240. Siebrecht MAN, de Rooij PP, Arm DM, Olsson ML, Aspenberg P. Platelet concentrate increases bone ingrowth into porous hydroxyapatite. *Orthopedics* 2002;**25**:169–72.

241. Schlegel KA, Kloss FR, Schultze-Mosgau S, Neukam FW, Wiltfang J. Implantat-Einheilvorgänge bei unterschiedlichen lokalen Knochenmassnahmen. *Dtsch Zahnärztl Z* 2002;**57**:194–9.

242. Aghaloo TL, Moy PK, Freymiller EG. Investigation of platelet-rich plasma in rabbit cranial defects: a pilot study. *J Oral Maxillofac Surg* 2002;**60**:1176–81.

243. Schlegel KA, Kloss FR, Schultze-Mosgau S, Neukam FW, Wiltfang J. Tierexperimentelle Untersuchung zum Einfluss verschiedener Thrombozytenkonzentrate auf die Defektregeneration mit autogenem Knochen und Kombinationen von autogenem Knochen und Knochenersatzmaterialien (Biogran® und Algipore®). Mikroradiographische Ergebungsbewertung. *Mund Kiefer Gesichtschir* 2003;**7**:112–18.

244. Fürst G, Gruber R, Tangl S, Zechner W, Haas R, Mailath G, Sanroman F, Watzek G. Sinus grafting with autogenous platelet-rich plasma and bovine hydroxyapatite. A histomorphometric study in minipigs. *Clin Oral Impl Res* 2003;**14**:500–8.

245. Jakse N, Tangl S, Gilli R, Berghold A, Lorenzoni M, Eskici A, Haas R, Pertl C. Influence of PRP on autogenous sinus grafts. An experimental study on sheep. *Clin Oral Impl Res* 2003;**14**:578–83.

246. Zechner W, Tangl S, Tepper G, Fürst G, Bernhart T, Haas R, Mailath G, Watzek G. Influence of platelet-rich plasma on osseous healing of dental implants: a histologic and histomorphometric study in minipigs. *Int J Oral Maxillofac Implants* 2003; **18**:15–22.

247. Terheyden H, Roldan J-C, Miller J, Jepsen S, Acil Y. Platelet-rich Plasma in der Knochenregeneration – Erste Ergebnisse zweier experimenteller Studien. *Implantologie* 2002;**10**:195–205.

248. Weibrich G, Hansen T, Buch R, Kleis W, Hitzler WE. Effect of platelet concentration in platelet-rich plasma on peri-implant bone regeneration. *Bone* 2004;**34**:665–71.

249. Boyne PJ. Animal studies of application of rhBMP-2 in maxillofacial reconstruction. *Bone* 1996;**19**:83–92.

250. Hollinger JO, et al. Recombinant human bone morphogenetic protein-2 and collagen for bone regeneration. *J Biomed Mater Res* 1998;**43**:356–64.

251. Ellingsworth LR, Delustro F, Brennan JE, Sawamura S, McPherson J. The immune response to reconstituted bovine collagen. *J Immunol* 1986;**136**:8877–82.

252. Delustro F, Dasch J, Keefe J, Ellingsworth L. Immune responses to allogeneic and xenogeneic implants of collagen and collagen derivatives. *Clin Orthop* 1990;**260**:263–79.

253. Elbert DL, Pratt AB, Lutolf MP, Halstenberg S, Hubbell JA. Protein delivery from materials formed by self-selective conjugate addition reactions. *J Control Release* 2001;**76**:11–25.

254. Ziegler J, Mayr-Wohlfart U, Kessler S, Breitig D, Gunther KP. Adsorption and release properties of growth factors from biodegradable implants. *J Biomed Mater Res* 2002;**59**:422–8.

255. JIANG D, DZIAK R, LYNCH SE, STEPHAN EB. Modification of an osteoconductive anorganic bovine bone mineral matrix with growth factors. *J Periodontol* 1999;**70**:834–9.

256. KHAN SN, BOSTROM MP, LANE JM. Bone growth factors. *Orthop Clin North Am* 2000;**31**:375–88.

257. MARX RE. Platelet-rich plasma (PRP): What is PRP and what is not PRP? *Implant Dentistry* 2001;**10**:225–8.

258. TERHEYDEN H, ROLDAN J-C, MILLER J, JEPSEN S, ACIL Y. Platelet-rich Plasma in der Knochenregeneration – Erste Ergebnisse zweier experimenteller Studien. *Implantologie* 2002;**10**:195–205.

259. TONNESEN MG, FENG X, CLARK RAF. Angiogenesis in wound healing. *J Invest Dermatol Symp Proc* 2000;**5**:40–6.

260. HARKER LA, FINCH CA. Thrombokinetics in man. *J Clin Invest* 1969;**48**:963–74.

261. HUANG JS, OLSEN TJ, HUANG SS. The role of growth factors in tissue repair I.:Platelet-derived growth factor. In: Clark RAF, Henson PM. eds. *The molecular and cellular biology of wound repair*. New York: Plenum Press, 1988:243–51.

262. JENNINGS RW, HUNT TK. Overview of postnatal wound healing. In: Adzick NS, Longaker MT. eds. *Fetal wound healing*. New York: Elsevier, 1992:25–52.

263. TERKELTAUB RA, GINSBERG MH. Platelets and response to injury. In: Clark RAF, Henson PM. eds. *The molecular and cellular biology of wound repair*. New York: Plenum Press, 1988:35–55.

264. MARK J, BARBORIAK JJ, JOHNSON SA. Relationship of appearance of adenosine diphosphate, fibrin formation, and platelet aggregation in the haemostatic plug *in vivo*. *Nature (London)* 1965;**205**:259–62.

265. DEUEL TF, HUANG JS. Platelet-derived growth factor: Structure, function, and roles in normal and transformed cells. *J Clin Invest* 1984;**74**:669–76.

266. ASSOIAN RK, SPORN MB. Type beta transforming growth factor in human pletelets: release during platelet degranulation and action on vascular smooth muscle cells. *J Cell Biol* 1986;**102**:1217–23.

267. ASSOIAN RK, SPORN MB. Anchorage-independent growth of primary rat embryo cells is induced by platelet-derived growth factor and inhibited by type-beta transforming growth factor. *J Cell Physiol* 1986;**126**:312–18.

268. KNIGHTON DR, HUNT TK, SCHEUENSTUHL H, HALLIDAY BJ, WERB Z, BANDA MJ. Oxygen tension regulates the expression of angiogenesis factor by macrophages. *Science* 1983;**221**:1283–5.

269. KNIGHTON DR, SILVER IA, HUNT TK. Regulation of wound healing angiogenesis: effect of oxygen gradients and inspired oxygen concentrations. *Surgery* 1981;**90**:262–70.

270. KNIGHTON DR, OREDSSON S, BANDA M, HUNT TK. Regulation of repair: hypoxic control of macrophage mediated angiogenesis. In: Hunt TK, Heppenstall RB, Pines E, Rovee D. eds. *Soft and hard tissue repair*. New York: Praeger, 1984:41–9.

271. HITI-HARPER J, WOHL H, HARPER E. Platelet factor 4: an inhibitor of collagenase. *Science* 1987;**199**:991–92.

272. ZAWICKI DF, JAIN RK, SCHMID-SHOENBEIN GW, CHIEN S. Dynamics of neovascularization in normal tissue. *Microvasc Res* 1981;**21**:27–47.

273. DAVIS JH, YULL AB. A toxic factor in abdominal injury. II. The role of the red cell component. *J Trauma* 1964;**4**:84–90.

274. KRIZEK TJ, DAVIS JH. The role of the red cell in subcutaneous infection. *J Trauma* 1965;**5**:85–95.

275. PRUETT TL, ROTSTEIN OD, FIEGEL VD, et al. Mechanism of the adjuvant effect of hemoglobin in experimental peritonitis. VIII. A leukotoxin is produced by *Escherichia coli* metabolism in hemoglobin. *Surgery* 1984;**96**:375–83.

276. EDLICH RF, RODEHEAVER GT, TRACKER JG. Surgical devices in wound healing management. In: Cohen IK, Diegelmann RF, Lindblad WJ. eds. *Wound healing: biochemical and clinical aspects*. Philadelphia: WB Saunders, 1992:581–600.

277. ANGEL MF, NARAYANAN K, SWARTZ WM, et al. The etiologic role of free radicals in hematoma-induced flap necrosis. *Plast Reconstr Surg* 1986;**77**:795–801.

278. YURT RW. Role of mast cells in trauma. In: Dineen P, Hildrick-Smith G. eds. *The surgical wound*. Philadelphia: Lea & Febiger, 1981:37–62.

279. ZACHRISSON BU. *Histochemical studies on the mast cell of the human gingiva in health and inflammation*. Oslo: Universitetsforlaget, 1968:135.

280. CLARK RAF. Cutaneous tissue repair: basic biologic considerations. *J Am Acad Dermatol* 1985;**13**:701–25.

281. HEROUX O. Mast cells in the skin of the ear of the rat exposed to cold. *Can J Biochem and Physiol* 1961;**39**:1871–8.

282. SIMPSON DM, ROSS R. Effects of heterologous antineutrophil serum in guinea pigs: hematologic and ultrastructural observations. *Am J Pathol* 1971;**65**:79–96.

283. SIMPSON DM, ROSS R. The neutrophilic leukocyte in wound repair: a study with antineutrophil serum. *J Clin Invest* 1972;**51**:2009–23.

284. DEUEL TF, SENIOR RM, CHANG D, et al. Platelet factor 4 is chemotactic for neutrophils and monocytes. *Proc Natl Acad Sci USA* 1981;**78**:4584–7.

285. DEUEL TF, SENIOR RM, HUANG JS, GRIFFIN GL. Chemotaxis of monocytes and neutrophils to platelet-derived growth factor. *J Clin Invest* 1982;**69**:1046–9.

286. BERGENHOLTZ G, WARFVINGE J. Migration of leucocytes in dental pulp in response to plaque bacteria. *Scand J Dent Res* 1982;**90**:354–62.

287. SAGLIE R, NEWMAN MG, CARRANZA FA Jr. A scanning electron microscopic study of leukocytes and their interaction with bacteria in human periodontitis. *J Periodont* 1982;**53**:752–61.

288. TONNESEN MG, WORTREN GS, JOHNSTON RB. Jr. Neutrophil emigration, activation, and tissue damage.In: Clark RAF, Henson PM. eds. *The molecular and cellular biology of wound repair*. New York: Plenum Press, 1988:149–83.

289. WILKINSON PC. *Chemotaxis and inflammation*. 2nd edn. New York: Churchill Livingstone, 1982.

290. SHAW JO. Leukocytes in chemotactic-fragment-induced lung inflammation. *Am J Pathol* 1980;**101**:283–91.

291. JANOFF A, SCHAEFER S, SHERER J, et al. Mediators in inflammation in leucocyte lysozymes. II Mechanisms of action of lysosomal cationic protein upon vascular permeability in the rat. *J Exp Med* 1965;**122**:841–51.

292. TEPLITZ C. The pathology and ultrastructure of cellular injury and inflammation in the progression and

outcome of trauma, sepsis, and shock. In: Clowes GHA Jr. ed. *Trauma, sepsis, and shock: the physiological basis of therapy.* New York: Marcek Dekker Inc, 1988.

293. MARCHESI VT. Some electron microscopic observations on interactions between leucocytes, platelets, and endothelial cells in acute inflammation. *Ann NY Acad Sci* 1964;**116**:774–88.

294. JOHNSTON DE. Wound healing in skin. *Vet Clin North Am* 1990;**20**:1–25.

295. LINDE J, BRÅNEMARK P-I. Observations on vascular proliferation in a granulation tissue. *J Periodont Res* 1970;**5**:276–92, 257.

296. BEASLEY JD, GROSS A, OUTRIGHT DE. Comparison of histological stained sections with culturing techniques in the evaluation of contaminated wounds. *J Dent Res* 1972;**51**:1624–31.

297. THOMAS EL. Myeloperoxydase, hydrogen peroxide, chloride antimicrobial system: nitrogen–chlorine derivatives of bactericidal action against *Escherichia coli. Infect Immun* 1979;**23**:522–31.

298. RAUSCHENBERGER CR, TURNER DW, KAMINSKI EJ, OSETEK EM. Human polymorphonuclear granule components: relative level detected by a modified enzyme-linked immunosorbent assay in normal and inflamed dental pulps. *J Endodont* 1991;**17**:531–6.

299. HÖGSTRÖM H, HAGLUND K. Neutropenia prevents decrease in strength of rat intestinal anastomoses: partial effect of oxygen free radicals scavengers and allopurinol. *Surgery* 1986;**99**:716–20.

300. STEIN JM, LEVENSON SM. Effect of the inflammatory reaction on subsequent wound healing. *Surg Forum* 1966;**17**:484–5.

301. GROTENDORST GR, SMALE G, PENCEV D. Production of transforming growth factor beta by human peripheral blood monocytes and neutrophils. *J Cell Physiol* 1989;**140**:396–402.

302. YAGER DR. The proteolytic environtment of chronic wounds. *Wound Repair Regen* 1999;**7**:433–41.

303. AGREN M, GOTTRUP F. Causation of venous leg ulcers. In: Morison MJ, Moffatt C, Franks P. eds. *Leg ulcers: a problem-based learning approach.* Edinburgh: Elsevier, 2006.

304. PAPPAS PJ, DEFOUW DO, VENEZIO LM, GORTI R, PADBERG FT Jr, SILVA MB Jr, GOLDBERG MC, DURAN WN, HOBSON RW 2nd. Morphometric assessment of the dermal microcirculation in patients with chronic venous insufficiency. *J Vasc Surg* 1997;**26**:784–95.

305. WILKINSON LS, BUNKER C. EDWARDS JC, SCURR JH, SMITH PD. Leukocytes: their role in the etiopathogenesis of skin damage in venous disease. *J Vasc Surg* 1993;**17**:669–75.

306. PAPPAS PJ, YOU R, RAMESHWAR P, GORTI R, DEFOUW DO, PHILLIPS CK, PADBERG FT Jr, SILVA MB Jr, SIMONIAN GT, HOBSON RW 2nd, DURAN WN. Dermal tissue fibrosis in patients with chronic venous insufficiency is associated with increased transforming growth factor–beta1 gene expression and protein production. *J Vasc Surg* 1999;**30**:1129–45.

307. ROGALSKI C, MEYER-HOFFERT U, PROKSCH E, WIEDOW O. Human leukocyte elastase induces keratinocyte proliferation *in vitro* and *in vivo. J Invest Dermatol* 2002;**118**:49–54.

308. STAMENKOVIC I. Extracellular matrix remodeling: the role of matrix metalloproteinases. *J Pathol* 2003;**200**:448–64.

309. LEIBOVICH SJ, ROSS R. The role of the macrophages in wound repair. A study with hydrocortisone and antimacrophage serum. *Am J Pathol* 1975;**78**:71–100.

310. STEWARD RJ, DULEY JA, DEWDNEY J, ALLARDYCE RA, BEARD MEJ, FIZGERALD PH. The wound fibroblast and macrophage. II. Their origin studied in a human after bone marrow transplantation. *Br J Surg* 1981;**68**:129–31.

311. COHN ZA. The activation of mononuclear phagocytes: fact, fancy, and future. *J Immunol* 1978;**121**:813–6.

312. VAN FURTH R. Current view of the mononuclear phagocyte system. *Immunobiol* 1982;**161**:178–85.

313. WERB Z. How the macrophage regulates its extracellular environment. *Am J Anat* 1983;**166**:237–56.

314. VAN FURTH R, COHEN ZA. The origin and kinetics of mononuclear phagocytes. *J Exp Med* 1968;**128**:415–35.

315. VAN FURTH R, DIESSELHOFFDEN DULK MMC, MATTIE H. Quantitative study on the production and kinetics of mononuclear phagocytes during an acute inflammatory reaction. *J Exp Med* 1973;**138**:1314–30.

316. VAN FURTH R, NIBBERIN PH, VAN DISSEL JT, DIESSELHOFFDEN DULK MMC. The characterization, origin and kinetics of skin machrophages during inflammation. *J Invest Dermatol* 1985;**85**:398–402.

317. RICHES DWH. The multiple roles of macrophages in wound repair. In: Clark RAF, Henson PM. eds. *Muscular and cellular biology of wound repair.* New York: Plenum Press, 1988:213–39.

318. HOSEIN B, BIANCO C. Monocyte receptors for fibronectin characterized by a monoclonal antibody that interferes with receptor activity. *J Exp Med* 1985;**162**:157–70.

319. HOSEIN B, MOSESSEN MW, BIANCO C. Monocyte receptors for fibronectin. In: van Furth R. ed. *Mononuclear phagocytes: characteristics, physiology, and function.* Dordrecht: Martinus Nijhoff, 1985:723–30.

320. BOUCEK RJ. Factors affecting wound healing. *Otolaryngol Clin North Amer* 1984;**17**:243–64.

321. LEIBOVICH S, ROSS R. A macrophage-dependent factor that stimulates the proliferation of fibroblasts *in vitro. Am J Pathol* 1976;**84**:501–14.

322. HUNT TK, KNIGHTON DR, THAKRAL KK, GOODSON WH, ANDREWS WS. Studies on inflammation and wound healing: angiogenesis and collagen synthesis stimulated *in vivo* by resident and activated wound macrophages. *Surgery* 1984;**96**:48–54.

323. MILLER B, MILLER H, PATTERSON R, RYAN SJ. Retinal wound healing. Cellular activity at the vitreoretinal interface. *Arch Ophthalmol* 1986;**104**:281–5.

324. GLENN KC. ROSS R. Human monocyte-derived growth factor(s) for mesenchymal cells: activation of secretion by endotoxin and concanavalin A. *Cell* 1981;**25**:603–15.

325. MARTIN BM, GIMBRONE MA, UNANUE ER, COTRAN RS. Stimulation of nonlymphoid mesenchymal cell proliferation by a macrophage-derived growth factor. *J Immunol* 1981;**126**:1510–15.

326. LEIBOVICH SJ. Production of macrophage-dependent fibroblast-stimulation activity (M-FSA) by murine macrophages. *Exp Cell Res* 1978;**113**:47–56.

327. GREENBERG GB, HUNT TK. The proliferative response *in*

*vitro* of vascular endothelial and smooth muscle cells exposed to wound fluid and macrophages. *J Cell Physiol* 1978;**97**:353–60.

328. THAKRAL KK, GOODSON WH, HUNT TK. Stimulation of wound blood vessel growth by wound macrophages. *J Surg Res* 1979;**26**:430–6.

329. POLVERINI PJ, COTRAN RS, GIMBRONE MA, UNANUE ER. Activated macrophages induce vascular proliferation. *Nature (London)* 1977;**269**:804–6.

330. POLVIRINI PJ, LEIBOVICH SJ. Induction of neovascularization *in vivo* and endothelial proliferation *in vitro* by tumor associated macrophages. *Lab Invest* 1984;**51**:635–42.

331. HUNT TK, ANDREWS WS, HALLIDAY B, et al. Coagulation and macrophage stimulation of angiogenesis and wound healing. In: Dineen P, Hildick-Smith G. eds. *The surgical wound*. Philadelphia: Lea & Febiger, 1981:1–18.

332. JENSEN JA, HUNT TK, SCHEUENSTUHL H, BANDA MJ. Effect of lactate, pyruvate and pH on secretion of angiogenesis and mitogenesis factors by macrophages. *Lab Invest* 1986;**54**:574–8.

333. PETERSON JM, BARBUL A, BRESLIN RJ, et al. Significance of T lymphocytes in wound healing. *Surgery* 1987;**102**:300–5.

334. BRESLIN RJ, BARBUL A, WOODYARD JP, et al. T-lymphocytes are required for wound healing. *Surg Forum* 1989;**40**:634–6.

335. BARBUL A, BRESLIN RJ, WOODYARD JP, et al. The effect of *in vivo* T helper and T suppressor lymphocyte depletion on wound healing. *Ann Surg* 1989;**209**:479–83.

336. FISHEL RS, BARBUL A, BESCHORNER WE, et al. Lymphocyte participation in wound healing. Morphological assesment using monoclonal antibodies. *Ann Surg* 1987;**206**:25–9.

337. BARBUL A. Role of immune system. In: Cohen IK, Diegel Mann RF, Lindblad WJ. eds. *Wound healing: biochemical and clinical aspects*. Philadelphia: WB Saunders, 1992:282–91.

338. REGAN MC, BARBUL A. Regulation of wound healing by the T cell-dependent immune system. In: Janssen H, Rooman R, Robertson JIS. eds. *Wound healing*. Petersfield, England: Wrightson Biomedical Publishing, 1991:21–31.

339. GABBIANI G, RUNGGER-BRÄNDLE E. The fibroblast. In: Glenn LE. ed. *Handbook of inflammation: tissue repair and regeneration*. Amsterdam: Elsevier/North Holland Biomedical Press, 1981:1–50.

340. ROSS R. The fibroblasts and wound repair. *Biol Rev* 1968;**43**:51–96.

341. MCDONALD RA. Origin of fibroblasts in experimental healing wounds: autoradiographic studies using tritiated thymidine. *Surgery* 1959;**46**:376–82.

342. GRILLO HC. Origin of fibroblasts in wound healing: an autoradiographic study of inhibition of cellular proliferation by local X-irradiation. *Ann Surg* 1963;**157**:453–67.

343. GLÜCKSMANN A. Cell turnover in the dermis. In: Montagna W, Billingham RE. eds. *Advances in biology of skin. Wound healing* Vol V. Oxford: Pergamon Press, 1964:76–94.

344. ROSS R, LILLYWHITE JW. The fate of buffy coat cells grown in subcutaneously implanted diffusion chambers.

A light and electron microscopic study. *Lab Invest* 1965;**14**:1568–85.

345. SPECTOR WG. Inflammation. In: Dunphy JE, VAN WINKLE HW. eds. *Repair and regeneration*. New York: McGraw-Hill Book Company, 1969:3–12.

346. ROSS R, EVERETT NB, TYLER R. Wound healing and collagen formation. VI. The origin of the wound fibroblast studied in parabiosis. *J Cell Biol* 1970;**44**:645–54.

347. HUNT TK. Disorders of repair and their management. In: Hunt TK, Dunphy JE. eds. *Fundamentals of wound management*. New York: Appleton-Century-Crofts, 1979:68–118.

348. SHIPLEY GD, TUCKER RF, MOSES HL. Type beta-transforming growth factor/growth inhibitor stimulate entry of monolayer culture of AKR-2B cells into S phase after prolonged prereplicative interval. *Proc Natl Acad Sci USA* 1985;**82**:4147–51.

349. SHIPLEY GD, TUCKER RF, MOSES HL. Type beta-transforming growth factor/growth inhibitor stimulate entry of monolayer culture of AKR-2B cells into S phase after prolonged prereplicative interval. *Proc Natl Acad Sci USA* 1985;**82**:4147–51.

350. PIERCE GF, MUSTOE TA, SENIOR RM, et al. *In vivo* incision wound healing augmented by platelet-derived growth factor and recombinant c-sis gene homodimeric proteins. *J Exp Med* 1988;**167**:974–87.

351. PIERCE GF, MUSTOE TA, LINGELBACH J, et al. Platelet-derived growth factor and transforming growth factor-beta enhance tissue repair activities by unique mechanisms. *J Cell Biol* 1989;**109**:429–40.

352. PLEDGER WJ, HART CA, LOCATELL KL, et al. Platelet derived growth factor-modulated proteins: constitutive synthesis by a transformed cell line. *Proc Natl Acad Sci USA* 1981;**78**:4358–62.

353. LIN SL, KIKUSKI T, PLEDGER WJ, et al. Interferon inhibits the establishment of competence in Go/S phase transition. *Science* 1986;**233**:356–9.

354. SPORN MB, ROBERTS AB, WAKEFIELD LM, DE CROMBRUGGHE B. Some recent advances in the chemistry and biology of transforming growth factor-beta. *J Cell Biol* 1987;**105**:1039–45.

355. WELCH MP, ODLAND GF, CLARK RAF. Temporal relationships of f-actin bundle formation, fibronectin and collagen assembly, fibronectin receptor expression to wound concentration. *J Cell Biol* 1990;**110**:133–45.

356. HUNT TK, PAI MP. Effect of varying ambient oxygen tension on wound metabolism and collagen synthesis. *Surg Gynecol Obstet* 1972;**135**:561–7.

357. HUNT TK. Disorders of repair and their management. In: Hunt TK, Dunphy JE. eds. *Fundamentals of wound management in surgery*. New York: Appleton-Century-Crofts, 1979:68–169.

358. NIINIKOSKI J, PENTTINEN R, KULONEN E. Effects of oxygen supply on the tensile strength healing wound and of granulation tissue. *Acta Physiol Scand* 1967;**70**:112–15.

359. LEVENSON S, SEIFTER E, VAN WINKLE E Jr. Nutrition. In: Hunt TK, Dunphy JE. eds. *Fundamentals of wound management*. New York: Appleton-Century-Crofts, 1979:286–363.

360. Douglas NJ, Twomey P, Hunt TK, Dunphy JE. Effects of exposure to 94% oxygen on the metabolism of wounds. *Bull Soc Int Chir* 1973;**32**:178–85.

361. Niinikoski J. Effect of oxygen supply on wound healing and formation of experimental granulation tissue. *Acta Physiol Scand* 1969;**334**:(Suppl 78): 1–72.

362. Postlethwaite AE, Seyer JM, Kang AH. Chemotactic attraction of human fibroblasts to type I, II and III collagens and collagen-derived peptides. *Proc Natl Acad Sci USA* 1978;**75**:871–5.

363. Chiang TM, Postlethwaite AE, Beachey EH, et al. Binding of chemotactic collagen-derived peptides to fibroblasts: the relationship to fibroblast chemotaxis. *J Clin Invest* 1978;**62**:916.

364. Gabbiani G, Hirschel BJ, Ryan GB, et al. Granulation tissue as a contractile organ. A study of structure and function. *J Exp Med* 1972;**135**:719–34.

365. Rudolph R, Gruber S, Suzuki M, et al. The life cycle of the myofibroblast. *Surg Gynecol Obstet* 1977;**145**:389–94.

366. Rudolph R, Berg JV, Ehrlich HP. Wound contraction and scar contracture. In: Cohen IK, Diegelmann RF, Lindblad WJ. eds. *Wound healing: biochemical and clinical aspects.* Philadelphia: WB Saunders, 1992:96–114.

367. Mango G, Gabbiani G, Hirschel BJ, et al. Contraction of granulation tissue *in vitro*: similarity to smooth muscle. *Science* 1971;**173**:548–50.

368. Ehrlich HP. The modulation of contraction of fibroblast populated collagen lattices by type I, II and III collagen. *Tiss Cell* 1988;**20**:47–50.

369. Brånemark P-I. Capillary form and function. The microcirculation of granulation tissue. *Bibl Anat* 1965;**7**:9–28.

370. Brånemark P-I, Breine U, Joshi M, et al. Microvascular pathophysiology of burned tissue. *Ann NY Acad Sci* 1968;**150**:474–94.

371. Ausprunk DH, Folkman J. Migration and proliferation of endothelial cells in performing and newly formed blood vessels during tumor angiogenesis. *Microvasc Res* 1977;**14**:53–63.

372. Clark ER, Clark EL. Observations on changes in blood vascular endothelium in the living animal. *Am J Anat* 1935;**57**:385–438.

373. Clark ER, Clark EL. Microscopic observations on the growth of blood capillaries in the living mammal. *Am J Anat* 1939;**64**:251–301.

374. Hunt TK, Conolly WB, Aronson SB. Anaerobic metabolism and wound healing. An hypothesis for the initiation and cessation of collagen synthesis in wounds. *Am J Surg* 1978;**135**:328–32.

375. Madri JA, Pratt BM. Angiogenesis. In: Clark RAF, Henson PM. eds. *The molecular and cellular biology of wound repair.* New York: Plenum Press, 1988:337–58.

376. Whalan GF, Zetter BR. Angiogenesis. In: Cohen IK, Diegelmann RF, Lindblad WJ. eds. *Wound healing: biochemical and clinical aspects.* Philadelphia: WB Saunders, 1992:77–95.

377. Phillips GD, Whitehead RA, Knighton DR. Initiation and pattern of angiogenesis in wound healing in rats. *Am J Anat* 1991;**192**:257–62.

378. Sandison JC. Observations on the growth of blood vessels as seen in the transparent chamber introduced in the rabbits ear. *Am J Anat* 1928;**41**:475–96.

379. Algire GH, Legallais FY. Recent developments in transparent-chamber technique as adapted to mouse. *J Natl Cancer Inst* 1949;**10**:225–53.

380. Sanders AG, Shubik P. A transparent window for use in the Syrian hamster. *Israel J Exp Med* 1964;**11**:118a.

381. Goodall CM, Sanders AG, Shubik P. Studies of vascular patterns in living tumors with a transparent chamber inserted in a hamster cheek pouch. *J Natl Cancer Inst* 1965;**35**:497–521.

382. Langham ME. Observations on the growth of blood vessels into the cornea. Application of a new experimental technique. *Br J Ophthalmol* 1953;**37**:210–22.

383. Gimbrone MA, Cotran RS, Leapman SB, et al. Tumor growth and neovascularization: an experimental model using the rabbit cornea. *J Natl Cancer Inst* 1974;**52**:413–27.

384. Auerbach R, Kubai L, Knighton D, et al. A simple procedure for the long term cultivation of chicken embryos. *Dev Biol* 1974;**41**:391–4.

385. Zetter BR. Endothelial heterogeneity: influence of vessel size, organ location and species specificity on the properties of cultured endothelial cell. In: Ryan U. ed. *Endothelial cells.* Orlando FL: CRC Press, 1988:63–80.

386. McGrath MH, Emery JM. The effect of inhibition of angiogenesis in granulation tissue on wound healing and the fibroblast. *Ann Plast Surg* 1985;**15**:105–22.

387. Cliff WJ. Kinetics of wound healing in rabbit ear chambers: a time lapse cinemicroscopic study. *Quart J Exp Physiol Cog Med Sci* 1965;**50**:79–89.

388. Zarem HA, Zweifach BW, McGehee JM. Development of microcirculation in full thickness autogeneous skin grafts in mice. *Am J Physiol* 1967;**212**:1081–5.

389. Tsur H, Danniler A, Strauch B. Neovascularization of the skin flap: route and timing. *Plast Reconstr Surg* 1980;**66**:85–93.

390. Nakanma T. How soon do venous drainage channels develop at the periphery of a free flap? A study on rats. *Br J Plast Surg* 1978;**31**:300–8.

391. Gatti JE, Larossa D, Brousseau DA, et al. Assessment of neovascularization and timing of flap division. *Plast Reconstr Surg* 1984;**73**:396–402.

392. Gottrup F, Oredson S, Price DC, Mathes SJ, Hohn D. A comparative study of skin blood flow in musculocutaneous and random pattern flaps. *J Surg Res* 1984;**37**:443–7.

393. Mir Y, Mir L. Biology of the skin graft. *Plast Reconstr Surg* 1951;**8**:378–89.

394. Hynes W. The early circulation in skin grafts with a consideration of methods to encourage their survival. *Br J Plast Surg* 1954;**6**:257–63.

395. Converse JM, Baliantyne DL, Rogers BO, Raisbeck AP. 'Plasmatic circulation' in skin grafts. *Transplant Bull* 1957;**4**:154.

396. Clemmesen T. The early circulation in split skin grafts. *Acta Chir Scand* 1962;**124**:11–18.

397. Clemmesen T. The early circulation in split-skin grafts. Restoration of blood supply to split-skin autografts. *Acta Chir Scand* 1964;**127**:1–8.

398. Clemmesen T. Experimental studies on the healing of free skin autografts. *Dan Med Bull* 1967;**14**:(Suppl.2):1–74.

399. Psillakis JM, de Jorge FB, Villardo R, de Malbano A, Martins M, Spina V. Water and electrolyte changes in autogeneus skin grafts. Discussion of the so–called 'plasmatic circulation'. *Plast Reconstr Surg* 1969;**43**:500–3.

400. Teich-Alasia S, Masera N, Massaioli N, Masse C. The disulphine blue colouration in the study of humoral exchanges in skin grafts. *Br J Plast Surg* 1961;**14**:308–14.

401. Scothorne RJ, McGregor IA. The vascularisation of autografts and homografts of rabbit skin. *J Anat* 1953;**87**:379–86.

402. Markmann A. Autologous skin grafts in the rat: vital microscopic studies of the microcirculation. *Angiology* 1966;**17**:475–82.

403. Ohmori S, Kurata K. Experimental studies on the blood supply to various types of skin grafts in rabbit using isotope P$^{32}$. *Plast Reconstr Surg* 1960;**25**:547–55.

404. Pihl B, Weiber A. Studies of the vascularization of free full–thickness skin grafts with radioisotope technique. *Acta Chir Scand* 1963;**125**:19–31.

405. Hinshaw JR, Miller ER. Histology of healing split-thickness, full thickness autogenous skin grafts and donor site. *Arch Surg* 1965;**91**:658–70.

406. Henry L, David C, Marshall C, Friedman A, Goldstein DP, Damhin GJ. A histologic study of the human skin autograft. *Am J Pathol* 1961;**39**:317–32.

407. Converse JM, Rapaport FT. The vascularization of skin autografts and homografts. An experimental study in man. *Ann Surg* 1956;**143**:306–15.

408. Converse JM, Filler M, Ballantyne DL. Vascularization of split-thickness skin autografts in the rat. *Transplantation* 1965;**3**:22–7.

409. Haller JA, Billingham RE. Studies of the origin of the vasculature in free skin grafts. *Ann Surg* 1967;**166**:896–901.

410. Smahel J, Ganzoni N. Contribution to the origin of the vasculature in free skin autografts. *Br J Plast Surg* 1970;**23**:322–5.

411. Converse JM, Ballantyne DL, Rogers BO, Raisbeck AP. A study of viable and non-viable skin grafts transplanted to the chorio-allantoic membrane of the chick embryo. *Transplantation* 1958;**5**:108–20.

412. Merwin RM, Algire GH. The role of graft and host vessel in the vascularization of grafts of normal and neoplastic tissue. *J Natl Cancer Inst* 1956;**17**:23–33.

413. Lambert PM. Vascularization of skin grafts. *Nature* 1971;**232**:279–80.

414. Schoefl GT. Electron microscopic obsrvations on the reactions of blood vessels after injury. *Ann N Y Acad Sci* 1964;**116**:789–802.

415. Ross R, Raines EW, Brwen-Pope DF. The biology of platelet-derived growth factor. *Cell* 1986;**46**:155–69.

416. Knighton DR, Ciresi KF, Fiegel VD, et al. Classification and treatment of chronic non-healing wounds. Successful treatment with autologous platelet derived wound healing factors. *Ann Surg* 1986;**104**:322–30.

417. Vlodasky I, Folkman J, Sullivan R, et al. Endothelial cell-derived basic fibroblast growth factor synthesis and deposition into subendothelial extracellular matrix. *Proc Natl Acad Sci USA* 1987;**84**:2292–6.

418. Oosta GM, Favreau LV, Beeler DL, et al. Purification and properties of human platelet heparitinase. *J Biol Chem* 1982;**257**:11249–55.

419. Buntrock P, Jentzsch KD, Heder G. Stimulation of wound healing, using brain extract with fibroblast growth (FGF) activity. I. Quantitative and biochemical studies into formation of granulation tissue. *Exp Pathol* 1982;**21**:46–53.

420. Broadley KN, Aquino AM, Woodward SC, et al. Monospecific antibodies implicate basic fibroblast growth factor in normal wound repair. *Lab Invest* 1989;**61**:571–5.

421. Baird A, Ling N. Fibroblast growth factors are present in the extracellular matrix produced by endothelial cells *in vitro*: implications for a role of heparinase-like enzymes in the neovascular response. *Biochem Biophys Res Commun* 1987;**142**:428–35.

422. Shing Y, Folkmann J, Sullivan R, Butterfeld C, Murray J, Klagsbrun M. Heparin affinity: purification of a tumor-derived capillary endothelial cell growth factor. *Science* 1984;**223**:1296–9.

423. Mignatti P, Tsuboi R, Robbins E, Rifkin DB. *In vitro* angiogenesis on the human amniotic membrane: requirement for basic fibroblast growth factor-induced proteinases. *J Cell Biol* 1989;**108**:671–82.

424. Polverini PJ, Cotran RS, Gimbrone MA, et al. Activated macrophages induce vascular proliferation. *Nature* 1977;**269**:804–6.

425. Hockel M, Beck T, Wissler JH. Neomorphogenesis of blood vessels in rabbit skin produced by a highly purified monocyte-derived polypeptide (monocyto-angiotropin) and associated tissue reactions. *Intl J Tiss Reac* 1984;**6**:323–31.

426. Meltzer T, Meyers B. The effect of hyperbaric oxygen on the bursting strength and rate of vascularization of skin wounds in the rat. *Am J Surg* 1986;**52**:659–62.

427. Silver IA. The measurement of oxygen tension in healing tissue. *Prog Resp Res* 1969;**3**:124–35.

428. Hunt TK, Conolly WB, Aronson SB, et al. Anaerobic metabolism and wound healing: an hypothesis for the initiation and cessation of collagen synthesis in wounds. *Am J Surg* 1978;**135**:328–32.

429. Banda MJ, Knighton DR, Hunt TK, et al. Isolation of a non-mitogenic angiogenesis factor from wound fluid. *Proc Natl Acad Sci USA* 1982;**79**:7773–7.

430. Hunt TK, Halliday B, Knighton DR, et al. Impairment of microbicidal function in wounds: correction with oxygen. In: Hunt TK, Heppenstall RB, Pines E, et al. eds. *Soft tissue repair. biological and clinical aspects*. Surgical Science Series Vol II. New York: Praeger, 1984:455–68.

431. D'Amore P, Braunhut SJ. Stimulatory and inhibitory factors in vascular growth control. In: Ryan U. ed. *The endothelial cell*. Boca Raton, FL: CRC Press, 1988:13–36.

432. Orlidge A, D'Amore P. Inhibition of capillary-endothelial cell growth by pericytes and smooth muscle cells. *J Cell Biol* 1987;**105**:1455–61.

433. Hay ED. *Cell biology of the extracellular matrix*. New York: Plenum Press, 1981.

434. Viidik A, Gottrup F. Mechanisms of healing soft tissue wounds. In: Schmid-Schonbein GW, Woo SLY, Zweifach BW. eds. *Frontiers in biomechanics*. New York: Springer, 1986:263–70.

435. Leaper DJ, Gottrup F. Surgical wounds. In: Leaper DJ, Harding KG. eds. *Wounds: biology and management*. Oxford: Oxford University Press, 1998:23–40.

436. GOTTRUP F. Models for studying physiology and pathophysiology of wound healing and granulation tissue formation in surgical research. In: Jeppsson B. ed. Animal modeling in surgical research. Philadelphia: Harwood Academic, 1998:29–35.

437. McPHERSON JM, PIEZ KA. Collagen in dermal wound repair. In: Clark RAF, Henson PM. eds. *The molecular and cellular biology of wound repair*. New York: Plenum Press, 1988:471–96.

438. PHILLIPS C, WENSTRUP RJ. Biosynthetic and genetic disorders of collagen. In: Cohen IK, Diegelmann RF, Lindblad WJ. eds. *Wound healing: biochemical and clinical aspects*. Philadelphia: WB Saunders, 1992:152–76.

439. MILLER EJ. Chemistry of collagens and their distribution. In: Piez KA, Reddi AH. eds. *Extracellular matrix biochemistry*. New York: Elsevier, 1984:41–78.

440. MARTIN GR, TIMPL R, MULLER PK, KUHN K. The genetically distinct collagens. *Trans Int Biol Soc* 1985;**115**:285–7.

441. MILLER EJ, GAY S. Collagen structure and function. In: Cohen IK, Diegelmann RF, Lindblad WJ. eds. *Wound healing: biochemical and clinical aspects*. Philadelphia: WB Saunders, 1992:130–51.

442. VIIDIK A, VUUST J. eds. *Biology of collagen*. London: Academic Press, 1980.

443. KANG AH. Connective tissue: collagen and elastin. In: Kelley WN, Harris ED Jr, Ruddy S, Sledge CB. eds. *Textbook of rheumatology*. Philadelphia: W B Saunders, 1981:221–38.

444. CLORE JN, COHEN IK, DIEGELMANN RF. Quantitation of collagen types I and III during wound healing in rat skin. *Proc Soc Exp Biol Med* 1979;**161**:337–40.

445. ANDREASEN JO. Histometric study of healing of periodontal tissues in rats after surgical injury. *Odont Rev* 1976;**27**:115–30.

446. ANDREASEN JO. Histometric study of healing of periodontal tissues in rats after surgical injury. *Odont Rev* 1976;**27**:131–44.

447. KURKINEN M, VAHERI A, ROBERTS PJ, et al. Sequential appearance of fibronectin and collagen in experimental granulation tissue. *Lab Invest* 1980;**43**:43–7.

448. GRINNELL F, BILLINGHAM RE, BURGESS L. Distribution of fibronectin during wound healing *in vivo*. *J Invest Dermatol* 1981;**76**:181.

449. GAY S, VILJANTO J, RAEKALLIO J, PETTINEN R. Collagen types in early phase of wound healing in children. *Acta Chir Scand* 1978;**144**:205–11.

450. FINE JD. Antigenic features and structural correlates of basement membranes. *Arch Dermatol* 1988;**124**:713.

451. STENN KS, MADRI JA, ROLL JF. Migrating epidermis produces AB2 collagen and requires continued collagen synthesis for movement. *Nature (London)* 1979;**277**:229–32.

452. STANLEY JR, ALVAREZ OM, BERE EW Jr, et al. Detection of basement membrane zone antigens during epidermal wound healing in pigs. *J Invest Dermatol* 1981;**77**:240.

453. ODLAND G, ROSS R. Human wound repair. I. Epidermal regeneration. *J Cell Biol* 1968;**39**:135–51.

454. SAKAI LY, KEENE DR, MORRIS NP, et al. Type VII collagen is a major structural component of anchoring fibrils. *J Cell Biol* 1986;**103**:2499–509.

455. BENTZ H, MORRIS NP, MURRAY LW, SAKAI LY, HOLLISTER DW, BURGESON RE. Isolation and partial characterization of a new human collagen with an extended triple-helical structural domain. *Proc Natl Acad Sci USA* 1983;**80**:3168–72.

456. GIPSON IK, SPURR-MICHAUD SJ, TISDALE SJ. Hemidesmosomes and anchoring fibril collagen appear synchronous during development and wound healing. *Develop Biol* 1988;**126**:253–62.

457. VIIDIK A, GOTTRUP F. Mechanics of healing soft tissue wounds. In: Schmid-Schonbein GW, Woo SLY, Zweifach BW. eds. *Frontiers in biomechanics*. New York: Springer, 1986:263–79.

458. ROSS R, BENDITT EP. Wound healing and collagen formation. I. Sequental changes in components of guinea pig skin wounds observed in the electron microscope. *J Biophys Biochem Cytol* 1961;**11**:677–700.

459. MADDEN JW, PEACOCK EE. Studies on the biology of collagen during wound healing. I. Rate of collagen synthesis and deposition in cutaneous wounds of the rat. *Surgery* 1968;**64**:288–94.

460. HEUGHAN C, HUNT T. Some aspects of wound healing research: a review. *Can J Surg* 1975;**18**:118–26.

461. GOTTRUP F. Healing of intestinal wounds in the stomach and duodenum. An experimental study. *Danish Med Bull* 1984;**31**:31–48.

462. FOGDESTAM I. A biomechanical study of healing rat skin incisions after delayed primary closure. *Surg Gynecol Obstet* 1981;**153**:191–9.

463. FOGDESTAM I. Delayed primary closure. An experimental study on the healing of skin incisions. Doctoral Thesis, University of Gothenburg, Sweden, 1980.

464. SINGER AJ, CLARK RAF. Cutaneous wound healing. *N Engl J Med* 1999;**341**:738–46.

465. IOCONO JA, EHRLICH HP, GOTTRUP F, LEAPER DJ. The biology of healing. In: Leaper DJ, Harding KG. eds. *Wounds: biology and management*. Oxford: Oxford University Press, 1998:10–22.

466. ERHLICH HP, DESMOULIERE A, DIEGELMANN RF, COHEN IK, COMPTON CC, GARNER WL, KAPANCI Y, GABBIANI G. Morphologial and immunochemical differences between keloids and hypertonic scar. *Am J Pathol* 1994;**145**:105–13.

467. STENN KS, MALHOTRA R. Epithelialization. In: Cohen IK, Diegelmann RF, Lindblad WJ. eds. *Wound healing: biochemical and clinical aspects*. Philadelphia: WB Saunders, 1992:115–27.

468. STENN KS, DEPALMA L. Re-epithelialization. In: Clark RAF, Henson PM. eds. *The molecular and cellular biology of wound repair*. New York: Plenum Press, 1988: 321–35.

469. KRAWCZYKW S. A pattern of epidermal cell migration during wound healing. *J Cell Biol* 1971;**49**:247–63.

470. AREY LB. Wound healing. *Physiol Rev* 1936;**16**:327–406.

471. KUWABARA T, PERKINS DG, COGAN DG. Sliding of the epithelium in experimental corneal wounds. *Invest Ophthalmol* 1976;**15**:4–14.

472. WINTER GD. Epidermal regeneration studied in the domestic pig. In: Maibach HI, Rovee DT. eds. *Epidermal wound healing*. Chicago: Year Book Med Publ. Inc., 1972:71–112.

473. PANG SC, DANIELS WH, BUCK RC. Epidermal migration during the healing of suction blisters in rat skin: a scanning and transmission electron microscopic study. *Am J Anat* 1978;**153**:177–91.

474. Gillman T, Penn J, Brooks D, et al. Reactions of healing wounds and granulation tissue in man to autothiersch, autodermal and homodermal grafts. *Br J Plast Surg* 1963;**6**:153–223.

475. Miller TA. The healing of partial thickness skin injuries. In: Hunt TK, ed. *Wound healing and wound infection*. New York: Appleton-Century-Crofts, 1980:81–96.

476. Andersen L, Fejerskov O. Ultrastructure of initial epithelial cell migration in palatal wounds of guinea pigs. *J Ultrastruc Res* 1974;**48**:313–24.

477. Gabbiani G, Ryan GB. Developments of contractile apparatus in epithelial cells during epidermal and liver regeneration. *J Submicr Cytol* 1974;**6**:143–57.

478. Mansbridge JN, Hanawalt PC. Role of transforming growth factor beta in maturation of human epidermal keratinocytes. *J Invest Dermatol* 1988;**90**:336–41.

479. Fejerskov O. Excision wounds in palatal epithelium in guinea pigs. *Scand J Dent Res* 1972;**80**:139–54.

480. Winter GD. Movement of epidermal cells over the wound surface. In: Montagna W, Billingham RE, eds *Advances in biology of skin*. New York: Pergamon Press, 1964:113–127.

481. Jonkman MF. Epidermal wound healing between moist and dry. Thesis, Groningen, 1990.

482. Clark RAF. Fibronectin matrix deposition and fibronectin receptor expression in healing and normal skin. *J Invest Dermatol* 1990;**94**:128–34.

483. Grøndahl-Hansen J, Lund LR, Ralfkier E, et al. Urokinase and tissue-type plasmin activators in keratinocytes during wound re-epithelization *in vivo*. *J Invest Dermatol* 1988;**90**:790–5.

484. Clark RAF, Folkvord JM, Wertz RL. Fibronectin as well as other extracellular matrix proteins, mediates keratinocytes adherence. *J Invest Dermatol* 1985;**84**:378–83.

485. Horsburg CR, Clark RAF, Kirkpatrick CH. Lymphokines and platelets promote human monocytes adherence to fibrinogen and fibronectin *in vitro*. *J Leuk Biol* 1987;**4**:14–24.

486. Laato M, Niinikoski J, Gerdin B, et al. Stimulation of wounds healing by epidermal growth factor: a dose dependent effect. *Ann Surg* 1986;**203**:379–81.

487. Moses HL, Coffey RJ, Leof EB, et al. Transforming growth factor beta regulation of cell proliferation. *J Cell Physiol* 1987;*(Suppl)***5**:1–7.

488. Pai MP, Hunt TK. Effect of varying ambient oxygen tensions on wound metabolism and collagen synthesis. *Surg Gynecol Obst* 1972;**135**:561–7.

489. Winter GD, Perrins JD. Effects of hyperbaric oxygen treatment on epidermal regeneration. In: Wada J, Iwa T. eds. *Proceedings of the Fourth International Congress on Hyperbaric Medicine*. Tokyo: Igaku Shoin, 1970:363–8.

490. McMillan MD. Oral changes following tooth extraction in normal and alloxan diabetic rats. Part II, microscopic observations. *N Z Dent J* 1971;**67**:23–31.

491. McMillan MD. Effects of histamine-releasing agent (compound 48–80) on extraction healing in rats. *N Z Dent J* 1973;**69**:101–8.

492. McMillan MD. The healing tooth socket and normal oral mucosa of the rat. PhD Thesis, University of Otago, 1978.

493. McMillan MD. Transmission and scanning electron microscope studies on the surface coat of oral mucosa in the rat. *J Periodont Res* 1980;**15**:288–96.

494. McMillan MD. Intracellular desmosome-like structures in differentiating wound epithelium of the healing tooth socket in the rat. *Arch Oral Biol* 1981;**26**:259–61.

495. Hunt TK, Hussain Z. Wound microenvironment. In: Cohen IK, Diegelmann RF, Lindblad WJ. eds. *Wound healing: biochemical and clinical aspects*. Philadelphia: WB Saunders, 1992:274–81.

496. Barbul A, Lazarou SA, Efron DT, et al. Arginine enhances wound healing and lymphocyte immune responses in humans. *Surgery* 1990;**108**:331–7.

497. Albina JE, Caldwell MD, Henry WL, et al. Regulation of macrophage functions by L-arginine. *J Trauma* 1989;**29**:842–6.

498. Hunt TK, Banda MJ, Silver IA. Cell interactions in posttraumatic fibrosis. In: Evered D, Weland J. eds. *Fibrosis*. Ciba Foundation Symposium 114. London: Pitman, 1985:127–9.

499. Hunt TK, van Winkle WJR. Wound healing: disorders of repair. In: Dunphy JE. ed. *Fundamentals of wound management in surgery*. South Plainfield: Chirurgecom, 1976:1–68.

500. Green H, Goldberg B. Collagen and cell protein synthesis by an established mammalian fibroblast line. *Nature* 1964;**204**:347–9.

501. Comstock JP, Udenfriend S. Effect of lactate on collagen proline hydroxylase activity in cultured L-929 fibroblasts. *Proc Natl Acad Sci USA* 1970;**66**:552–7.

502. Stephens FO, Hunt TK. Effects of changes in inspired oxygen and carbon dioxide tensions on wound tensile strength. *Ann Surg* 1971;**173**:515–19.

503. Hohn DC, Mackay RD, Halliday B, Hunt TK. The effect of $O_2$ tension on the microbicidal function of leucocytes in wounds and *in vitro*. *Surg Forum* 1976;**27**:18.

504. Ausprunk DH, Falterman K, Folkman J. The sequence of events in the regression of corneal capillaries. *Lab Invest* 1978;**38**:284–94.

505. Knighton DR, Halliday B, Hunt TK. Oxygen as an antibiotic: the effect of inspired oxygen on infection. *Arch Surg* 1984;**119**:199–204.

506. Johnson K, Hunt TK, Mathes SJ. Effect of environmental oxygen on bacterial induced tissue necrosis in flaps. *Surg Forum* 1984;**35**:589–91.

507. Niinikoski J, Gottrup F, Hunt TK. The role of oxygen in wound repair. In: Janssen H, Rooman R, Robertson JIS. eds. *Wound healing*. Petersfield, England: Wrightson Biomedical Publishing, 1991:165–74.

508. Johnson K, Hunt TK, Mathes SJ. Oxygen as an isolated variable influences resistance to infection. *Ann Surg* 1988;**208**:783–7.

509. Schandall A, Lowder R, Young HL. Colonic anastomotic healing and oxygen tension. *Br J Surg* 1986;**72**:606–9.

510. Gottrup F. Measurement and evaluation of tissue perfusion in surgery (to optimize wound healing and resistance to infection). In: Leaper DJ, Branicki FJ. eds. *International surgical practice*. Oxford: Oxford University Press, 1992:15–39.

511. Gottrup F, Niinikoski J, Hunt TK. Measurements of tissue oxygen tension in wound repair. In: Janssen H,

Rooman R, Robertson JIS. eds. *Wound healing.* Petersfield, England: Wrightson Biomedical Publishing, 1991:155–64.

512. Rabkin JM, Hunt TK. Infection and oxygen. In: Davis JC. ed. *Problem wounds: the role of oxygen.* New York: Elsevier, 1988:9–16.

513. Beaman L, Beaman BL. The role of oxygen and its derivatives in microbial pathogenesis and host defence. *Ann Rev Microbiol* 1984;**38**:27–48.

514. Hohn DC. Host resistance of infection: established and emerging concepts. In: Hunt TK. ed. *Wound healing and wound infection: theory and surgical practice.* New York: Appleton-Century-Crofts, 1980:264–80.

515. Hohn DC. Oxygen and leucocyte microbial killing. In: Davis JC, Hunt TK. eds. *Hyperbaric oxygen therapy.* Bethesda: Undersea Medical Society, 1977:101–10.

516. Hunt TK, Halliday B, Knighton DR, et al. Oxygen in prevention and treatment of infection. In: Root RK, Trunkey DD, Sande MA. eds. *Contemporary issues in infectious diseases* Vol VI. New York: Churchill Livingstone, 1986.

517. Klebanoff S. Oxygen metabolism and the toxic properties of phagocytes. *Ann Intern Med* 1980;**93**:480–9.

518. Mandell G. Bactericidal activity of aerobic and anaerobic polymorphonuclear neutrophils. *Infect Immun* 1974;**9**:337–41.

519. Johnson K, Hunt TK, Mathes SJ. Effect of environmental oxygen on bacterial induced tissue necrosis in flaps. *Surg Forum* 1984;**35**:589–91.

520. Goldhaber P. The effect of hyperoxia on bone resorption in tissue culture. *Arch Pathol* 1958;**66**:635–41.

521. Shaw JL, Bassett CAL. The effects of varying oxygen concentrations on osteogenesis and embryonic cartilage in vitro. *J Bone Joint Surg* 1967;**49**:73–80.

522. Bassett CAL, Herrmann I. Histology: influence of oxygen concentration and mechanical factors on differentiation of connective tissues in vitro. *Nature* 1961;**190**:460–1.

523. Gorham LW, Stout AP. Massive osteolysis (acute spontaneous absorption of bone, phantome bone, disappearing bone). Its relation to hemangiomatosis. *J Bone Joint Surg* 1955;**37–A**:985–1004.

524. Frederiksen NL, Wesley RK, Sciubba JJ, Helfrick J. Massive osteolysis of the maxillofacial skeleton: a clinical, radiographic, histologic, and ultrastructural study. *Oral Surg Oral Med Oral Pathol* 1983;**55**:470–80.

525. Andreasen JO, Andreasen FM. Root resorption following traumatic dental injuries. *Proc Finn Dent Soc* 1992;**88**:*(Suppl 1)*:95–114.

526. Marx RE, Johnson RP. Problem wounds in oral and maxillofacial surgery: the role of hyperbaric oxygen. In: Davis JC, Hunt TK. eds. *Problem wounds: the role of oxygen.* New York: Elsevier, 1988:123.

527. Udenfriend S. Formation of hydroxyproline in collagen. *Science* 1966;**152**:1335–40.

528. Niinikoski PB, Rajamaki A, Kulonen E. Healing of open wounds: effects of oxgen, distributed blood supply and hyperemia by infrared radiation. *Acta Chir Scand* 1971;**137**:399–401.

529. Ketchum SA, Thomas AN, Hall AD. Angiographic studies of the effect of hyperbaric oxygen on burn wound revascularization. In: Wada J, Iwa T. eds.

*Proceedings of the Fourth International Congress on Hyperbaric Medicine.* Baltimore: Williams and Wilkins, 1970:383–394.

530. Silver IA. Oxygen and tissue repair, an environment for healing: the role of occlusion. *Int Cong Symp Ser/Roy Soc Med* 1987;**88**:15–19.

531. Shannon MD, Hallmon WW, Mills MP, Newell DH. Periodontal wound healing responses to varying oxygen concentrations and atmospheric pressures. *J Clin Periodontol* 1988;**15**:222–6.

532. Nilsson LP, Granström G, Röckert HOE. Effects of dextrans, heparin and hyperbaric oxygen on mandibular tissue damage after osteotomy in an experimental system. *Int J Oral Maxillofacial Surg* 1987;**16**:77–89.

533. Wilcox JW, Kolodny SC. Acceleration of healing of maxillary and mandibular osteotomies by use of hyperbaric oxygen (a preliminary report). *Oral Surg Oral Med Oral Pathol* 1976;**11**:423–9.

534. Jörgensen LN. Collagen deposition in the subcutaneous tissue during wound healing in humans: a model evaluation. *APMIS* 2003;**111**:*(Suppl 115)*:1–56.

535. Jensen JA, Goodson WH, Hopf HW, Hunt TK. Cigarette smoking decreases tissue oxygen. *Arch Surg* 1991;**126**:1131–4.

536. Jörgensen LN, Kallehave F, Christensen E, Siana JE, Gottrup F. Less collagen production in smokers. *Surgery* 1998;**123**:450–5.

537. Sörensen LT, Karlsmark T, Gottrup F. Abstinence from smoking reduces incisional wound infection: a randomized controlled trial. *Ann Surg* 2003;**238**:1–5.

538. Jörgensen LN, Tønnesen H, Pedersen S, Lavrsen M, Tuxøe J, Gottrup F, Thomsen CE. Reduced amount of total protein in artificial wounds of alcohol abusers. *Br J Surg* 1998;**85**:*(Suppl)*:152–3.

539. Leak LV, Burke JF. In: Zweifach BW, Grant L, McCluskey RR. eds. *The inflammatory process* Vol. III. 2nd edn. New York: Academic Press, 1974:207.

540. Burke JF. Infection. In: Hunt TK, Dunphy JE. eds. *Fundamentals of wound management.* New York: Appleton-Century-Crofts, 1979:170–240.

541. Burke JF. Effects of inflammation on wound repair. *J Dent Res* 1971;**50**:296–303.

542. Burke JF. Infection. In: Hunt TK, Dunphy JE. eds. *Fundamentals of wound management.* New York: Appleton-Century-Crofts, 1979:170–241.

543. Kan-Gruber D, Gruber C, Seifter E, et al. Acceleration of wound healing by *Staphylococcus aureus.* II. *Surg Forum* 1981;**32**:76–9.

544. Tenorio A, Jindrak K, Weiner M, et al. Accelerated healing in infected wounds. *Surg Gynecol Obstet* 1976;**142**:537–44.

545. Oloumi M, Jindrak K, Weiner M, et al. The time at which infected postoperative wounds demonstrate increased strength. *Surg Gynecol Obstet* 1977;**145**:702–4.

546. Raju R, Jindrak K, Weiner M, et al. A study of the critical bacterial inoculum to cause a stimulus to wound healing. *Surg Gynecol Obstet* 1977;347–50.

547. Levenson SM, Gruber DK, Gruber C, et al. Wound healing accelerated by *Staphylococcus aureus.* *Arch Surg* 1983;**118**:310–19.

548. Niinikoski J. *Oxygen and trauma: studies on pulmonary oxygen poisoning and the role of oxygen in repair processes.* London: European Research Office United States Army, 1973:59.

549. Larjava H. Fibroblasts: bacteria interactions. *Proc Finn Dent Soc* 1987;**83**:85–93.

550. Smith IM, Wilson AP, Hazard EG, et al. Death from staphylococci in mice. *Infect Dis* 1960;**107**:369–78.

551. Bullen JJ, Cushnie GH, Stoner HB. Oxygen uptake by *Clostridium welchi* type A: its possible role in experimental infections in passively immunized animals. *Br J Exp Pathol* 1966;**47**:488.

552. Irvin TT. Wound infection. In: Irvin TT. ed. *Wound healing: principles and practice.* London: Chapman and Hall, 1981:64.

553. Raahave D. Wound contamination and post-operative infection. In: Taylor EW. ed. *Infection in surgical practice.* Oxford: Oxford University Press, 1992:49–55.

554. Becker GD. Identification and management of the patient at high risk for wound infection. *Head Neck Surg* 1986;**8**:205–10.

555. Robson MC, Heggers JP. Delayed wound closure based on bacterial counts. *J Surg Oncol* 1970;**2**:379–83.

556. Burke JF. The effective period of preventive antibiotic action in experimental incisions and dermal lesions. *Surgery* 1961;**50**:161–8.

557. Elek SD. Experimental staphylococcal infections in skin of man. *Ann NY Acad Sci* 1956;**65**:85–90.

558. Elek SD, Conen PE. The virulence of *Staphylococcus pyogenes* for man. A study of the problems of wound infection. *Br J Exp Pathol* 1957;**38**:573–86.

559. Edlich RF, Rodeheaver G, Thacker JG. Edgerton MT. Technical factors in wound management. In: Hunt TK, Dunphy JE. eds. *Fundamentals of wound management.* New York: Appleton-Century-Crofts, 1979:364–454.

560. Dougherty SH, Simmons RL. Infections in bionic man: the pathobiology of infections in prosthetic devices – Part II. *Curr Prob Surg* 1982;**19**:265–312.

561. Taylor EW. General principles of antibiotic prophylaxis. In: Taylor EW. ed. *Infection in surgical practice.* Oxford: Oxford University Press, 1992:76–81.

562. Costerton JW, Cheng KJ, Geesey GG, et al. Bacterial biofilms in nature and disease. *Ann Rev Microbiol* 1987;**41**:435–464.

563. Moyniham BJA. The ritual of surgical operations. *Br J Surg* 1920;**8**:27–35.

564. Bucknall TE. Factors affecting healing. In: Bucknall TE, Ellis H. eds. *Wound healing.* London: Baillière Tindall, 1984:42–74.

565. Osther PJ, Gjöde P, Mortensen BB, Bartholin J, Gottrup F. Randomized comparision of polyglycolic and polyglyconate sutures for abdominal fascia closure after laparotomy in patients with suspected impaired wound healing. *Br J Surg* 1995;**82**:1698–99.

566. Capperauld I, Bucknall TE. Sutures and dressings. In: Bucknall TE, Ellis H. eds. *Wound healing for surgeons.* London: Baillière Tindall, 1984:73–93.

567. Bucknall TE, Ellis H. Abdominal wound closure, a comparison of monofilament nylon and polyglycolic acid. *Surgery* 1981;**89**:672–7.

568. Savolainen H, Ristkari S, Mokka R. Early laparotomy wound dehiscence: a randomized comparison of three suture materials and two methods of fascial closure. *Ann Chir Gynecol* 1988;**77**:111–13.

569. Larsen PN, Nielsen K, Schultz A, Mejdahl S, Larsen T, Moesgaard F. Closure of the abdominal fascia after clean and clean-contaminated laparotomy. *Acta Chir Scand* 1989;**155**:461–4.

570. Viidik A, Holm-Pedersen P, Rundgren A. Some observations on the distant collagen response to wound healing. *J Plast Reconstr Surg* 1972;**6**:114–22.

571. Zederfeld TB. Factors influencing wound healing. In: Viidik A, Vuust S. eds. *Biology of collagen.* London: Academic Press, 1980:347–52.

572. Adzick NS, Longaker MT. Characteristics of fetal tissue repair. In: Adzick NS, Longaker MT. eds. *Fetal wound healing.* New York: Elsevier, 1992:53–70.

573. Adzick NS, Longaker MT. Scarless fetal healing: therapeutic implications. In: Adzick NS, Longaker MT. eds. *Fetal wound healing.* New York: Elsevier, 1992:317–24.

574. Longaker MT, Kaban LB. Fetal models for craniofacial surgery: cleft lip/palate and craniosynostosis. In: Adzick NS, Longaker MT. eds. *Fetal wound healing.* New York: Elsevier, 1992:83–94.

575. Ferguson MWJ, Howarth GF. Marsupial models of scarless fetal wound healing. In: Adzick NS, Longaker MT. eds. *Fetal wound healing.* New York: Elsevier, 1992:95–124.

576. Adzick NS. Fetal animal and wound implant models. In: Adzick NS, Longaker MT. eds. *Fetal wound healing.* New York: Elsevier, 1992:71–82.

577. Mast BA, Krummel TM. Acute inflammation in fetal wound healing. In: Adzick NS, Longaker MT. eds. *Fetal wound healing.* New York: Elsevier, 1992:227–40.

578. Chiu E, Longaker MT, Adzick NS, et al. Hyaluronic acid patterns in fetal and adult wound fluid. *Surg Forum* 1990;**41**:636–9.

579. Burd DAR, Siebert J, Garg H. Hyaluronan-protein interactions. In: Adzick NS, Longaker MT. eds. *Fetal wound healing.* New York: Elsevier, 1992:199–214.

580. Shah M, Foreman DM, Ferguson MWJ. Control of scarring in adult wounds by neutralising antibody to transforming growth factor. *Lancet* 1992;**339**:213–14.

581. Paul HE, Paul MF, Taylor JD, Marsters RW. Biochemistry of wound healing. II. Water and protein content of healing tissue of skin wounds. *Arch Biochem* 1948;**17**:269–74.

582. Bourlière F, Gourévitch M. Age et vitesse de réparation des plaies expérimentales chez le rat. *C R Soc Biol (Paris)* 1950;**144**:377–9.

583. Cuthbertson AM. Concentration of full thickness skin wounds in the rat. *Surg Gynec Obstet* 1959;**108**:421–32.

584. Engelhardt GH, Struck H. Effect of aging on wound healing. *Scand J Clin Lab Invest* 1972;**29**:(Suppl 123).

585. Holm-Pedersen P, Zederfeldt B. Strength development of skin incisions in young and old rats. *Scand J Plast Reconstr Surg* 1971;**5**:7–12.

586. Holm-Pedersen P, Viidik A. Maturation of collagen in healing wounds in young and old rats. *Scand J Plast Reconstr Surg* 1972;**6**:16–23.

587. Holm-Pedersen P, Nilsson K, Brånemark P-I. The microvascular system of healing wounds in young and old rats. *Advanc Microcirc* 1973;**5**:80–106.

588. Holm-Pedersen P, Viidik A. Tensile properties and morphology of healing wounds in young and old rats. *Scand J Plast Reconstr Surg* 1972;**6**:24–35.

589. Billingham RE, Russel PS. Studies on wound healing, with special reference to the phenomenon of contracture in experimental wounds in rabbits' skin. *Ann Surg* 1956;**144**:961–81.

590. Löfström B, Zederfeldt B. Wound healing after induced hypothermia. III. Effect of age. *Acta Chir Scand* 1957;**114**:245–51.

591. Sandblom P, Petersen P, Muren A. Determination of the tensile strength of the healing wound as a clinical test. *Acta Chir Scand* 1953;**105**:252–7.

592. Olsson A. Sårläkning hos homo. *Nord Med* 1955;**53**:128.

593. Forscher BK, Cecil HC. Some effect of age on the biochemistry of acute inflammation. *Gerontologia (Basel)* 1958;**2**:174–82.

594. Stahl SS. The healing of gingival wounds in male rats of various ages. *J Dent Med* 1961;**16**:100–3.

595. Stahl SS. Soft tissue healing following experimental gingival wounding in female rats of various ages. *Periodontics* 1963;**1**:142–6.

596. Butcher EO, Klingsberg J. Age, gonadectomy, and wound healing in the palatal mucosa of the rat. *Oral Surg Oral Med Oral Pathol* 1963;**16**:484–93.

597. Butcher EO, Klingsberg J. Age changes and wound healing in the oral tissues. *Ann Dent (Baltimore)* 1964;**23**:84–95.

598. Rovin S, Gordon HA. The influence of aging on wound healing in germfree and conventional mice. *Gerontologia (Basel)* 1968;**14**:87–96.

599. Holm-Pedersen P, Löe H. Wound healing in the gingiva of young and old individuals. *Scand J Dent Res* 1971;**79**:40–53.

600. Stahl SS, Witkin GJ, Cantor M, Brown R. Gingival healing. II. Clinical and histologic repair sequences following gingivectomy. *J Periodont* 1968;**39**:109–18.

601. Grove GL. Age-related differences in healing of superficial skin wounds in humans. *Arch Dermatol Res* 1982;**272**:381–5.

602. Holm-Pedersen P. *Studies on healing capacity in young and old individuals. Clinical, biophysical and microvascular aspects of connective tissue repair with special reference to tissue function in man and rat.* Copenhagen: Munksgaard, 1973.

603. Gottrup F. Healing of incisional wounds in stomach and duodenum. The influence of aging. *Acta Chir Scand* 1981;**147**:363–9.

604. Cruse PJE, Foord R. A five-year prospective study of 23,649 surgical wounds. *Arch Surg* 1973;**107**:206–10.

605. Davidson AIG, Clark C, Smith G. Postoperative wound infection: a computer analysis. *Br J Surg* 1971;**58**:333–7.

606. Stevenson TR, Rodeheaver GT, Golden GT, et al. Damage to tissue defenses by vasoconstrictors. *J Am Coll Emerg Phys* 1975;**4**:532.

607. Tomlinson A, Ferguson HW. Wound healing: a model of dermal wound repair. *Methods Mol Biol* 2003;**225**:249–60.

608. Diegelmann RF, Evans MC. Wound healing: an overview of acute, fibrotic and delayed healing. *Front Biosci* 2004;**9**:283–9.

609. Williams RL, Armstrong DG. Wound healing: new modalities for a new millennium. *Clin Podiatr Med Surg* 1998;**15**:117–28.

610. Hunt TK, Hopf H, Hussain Z. Physiology of wound healing. *Adv Skin Wound Care* 2000;**13**:6–11.

611. Ramasastry SS. Acute wounds. *Clin Plast Surg* 2005;**32**:195–208.

612. Bowler PG. Wound pathophysiology, infection and therapeutic options. *Ann Med* 2002;**34**:419–27.

613. Gottrup F. Wound closure techniques (update article). *J Wound Care* 1999;**8**:397–400.

614. Gottrup F. Prevention of surgical wound infections (editorial). *N Eng J Med* 2000;**342**:202–4.

615. Teot L, Banwell PE, Ziegler UE. *Surgery in wounds.* Springer Verlag, Berlin 2004.

616. Mustoe TA, Cooter R, Gold M, Hobbs R, Ramelet AA, Shakespeare P, Stella M, Teot L, Wood F, Ziegler U. International clinical guidelines for scar management. *Plast Reconstr Surg* 2002;**110**:560.

617. Kranke P, Bennett M, Roeckl-Wiedmann I, Delnis S. Hyperbaric oxygen therapy for chronic wounds. The Cochrane Database of Systemic Reviews 2004;(1) Art.No. CD004123,Pub2; DOI:10.1002/14651858. CD 004123, Pub 2.

618. Wang C, Schwaitzberg S, Berliner E, Zarin DA, Lau J. Hyperbaric oxygen treatment of wounds. *Arch Surg* 2003;**138**:272–9.

619. Thorn JJ, Kallehave F, Westergaard P, Hjørting Hansen E, Gottrup F. The effect of hyperbaric oxygen on irradiated oral tissue: transmucosal oxygen tension measurements. *J Oral Maxillofac Surg* 1997;**55**:1103–7.

620. Bayat A, McGrouther DA, Ferguson MW. Skin scarring. *BMJ* 2003;**326**:88–92.

621. Bayat A, Arscott G, Ollier WE, McGrouther DA, Ferguson MW. Keloid disease: clinical relevance of single versus multiple site scars. *Br J Plast Surg* 2005;**58**:28–37.

622. Gorvy DA, Herrick SE, Shah M, Ferguson MW. Experimental manipulation of transforming growth factor-beta isoforms significantly affects adhesion formation in a murine surgical model. *Am J Pathol* 2005;**167**:1005–19.

623. Tonnesen MG, Feng X, Clark RA. Angiogenesis in wound healing. *J Investig Dermatol Symp Proc* 2000;**5**:40–6.

624. Li J, Zhang YP, Kirsner RS. Angiogenesis in wound repair: angiogenic growth factors and the extracellular matrix. *Micros Res Tech* 2003;**60**:107–14.

625. Johnston RB Jr. Clinical aspects of chronic granulomatous disease. *Curr Opin Hematol* 2001;**8**:17–22.

# 2

# Response of Oral Tissues to Trauma

J. O. Andreasen & H. Løvschall

## Repair and regeneration of oral tissues

An injury can be defined as an interruption in the continuity of tissues, and healing as the reestablishment of that continuity. The result of this process can either be *tissue repair*, where the continuity is restored but the healed tissue differs in anatomy and function, or *tissue regeneration*, where both anatomy and function are restored.

In lower vertebrates, the regeneration of appendages such as limbs, tails and fins is common. In mammals, this healing capacity has generally been lost, although it has been reported that, in humans, digits amputated distal to the distal interphalangeal joint can regenerate in children (1). The explanation for this general loss of healing capacity in mammals is presently under investigation. However, the rapid epidermal healing response in mammals, which optimizes wound closure in skin and thereby limits the risk of infection, is currently believed to present an obstacle to tissue regeneration (2).

Healing of most wounds in humans, whether caused by trauma or surgery, includes repair with more or less fibrous scar tissue formation which subsequently leads to problems in function of the particular organ affected. In the oral region, skin wounds and to a lesser degree the oral mucosa are repaired with scar formation (see Chapter 21).

Dental tissues are unique in comparison to most other tissues in the body due to their marked capacity for regeneration. Thus tooth germs split by trauma or surgery may to a certain extent regenerate and the same applies to injured dentin, cementum, bone, and gingiva (see later).

Injuries to the pulp and the periodontal ligament (PDL) may sometimes regenerate or alternatively show repair with fibrous scar tissue or bone.

Understanding the circumstances leading to repair and regeneration in oral tissues has been a formidable challenge (3). In this regard, wounding releases a variety of signals that induce neighboring cell populations to respond by proliferation, migration, or differentiation.

The first prerequisite for tissue regeneration is that a tissue-specific cell population is present after wounding (e.g. pulp or PDL progenitor cells). If these cells are not present, repair rather than regeneration will take place. A typical example of this concept is the healing by ankylosis of teeth in which the PDL has been injured (see p. 81).

A second prerequisite for regeneration is that conditions exist that are conducive to migration of tissue-specific cells into the wound site. Thus, incomplete repositioning of a luxated tooth may lead to damage to the epithelial root sheath and thereby forcing ingrowth of PDL-derived cells and bone into the pulp canal. Another situation in which the topographic conditions of the wound may determine whether repair or regeneration take place is related to loss of periodontal attachment on a root or an implant. In this situation the insertion of a membrane may guide bone cells and/or PDL into the wound site (see Chapter 28, p. 779).

A third factor that may determine tissue repair or regeneration in oral wounds is the presence of contaminating foreign bodies and/or bacteria. Inflammation related to a contaminated wound has been found to lead to repair rather than regeneration, possibly because contamination leads to formation of a non-tissue-specific, inflamed granulation tissue at the expense of the proliferation and migration of tissue specific cells.

When assessing wound healing after trauma, it is not enough to understand the healing capacity of individual cell types; one must also consider the various tissue compartments, each consisting of different cellular systems. Differences in healing capacity and rates of healing can lead to competitive situations and thereby to variations in wound healing. Ischemia or the total destruction of cell layers may occur (2) (Fig. 2.1).

This chapter will present a brief description of the anatomy and function of cell compartments typically involved following a traumatic event. In the description of these compartments, anatomical borders have been chosen which are typically the result of separation lines or contusion locations subsequent to trauma. Using this approach, the following anatomical zones evolve in relation to teeth

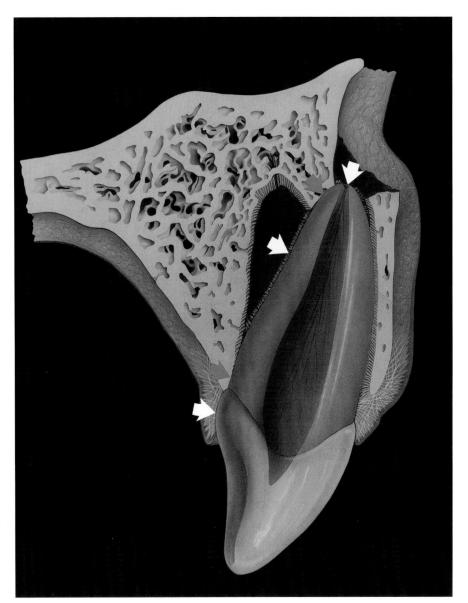

**Fig. 2.1** Injury zones after tooth luxation. A lateral luxation implies trauma to multiple cell systems in the periodontium and the pulp, as rupture (white arrows) or compression (blue arrows) or ischemia damage these cellular compartments. The outcome of the healing processes is entirely dependent upon the healing capacity of the different cellular systems involved. From ANDREASEN & ANDREASEN (3) 1989.

with completed root development: *gingival- and periosteal complex*; *cemento-periodontal ligament complex*; *alveolar bone complex* and *dentino pulpal complex*. In developing teeth, the following structures should be added: *dental follicle*, *enamel forming organ*; and *Hertwig's epithelial root sheath*.

For each tissue compartment, a description will be given of its anatomy and healing responses to trauma and infection.

## Developing teeth

### Dental follicle

The dental follicle (dental sac) has traditionally been considered the formative organ of the periodontium (Fig. 2.2). This concept has been supported by experimental studies of transplanted tooth germs which show that the innermost layer (dental follicle proper, which is in contact with the

tooth germ) give rise to all of the components of the periodontium (4–6). Based on these findings, it has been suggested that the term dental follicle should be reserved for the innermost layer of connective tissue separating the tooth germ from its crypt (7). The remaining peripheral tissue would therefore be designated as the perifollicular mesenchyme (5, 8). However, until further research has definitely ruled out the possibility of perifollicular mesenchymal participation in the formation of the periodontal attachment, it appears justified to use the term dental follicle for all the mesenchymal tissue interposed between the tooth germ and alveolar bone.

In addition to the role of the dental follicle in the formation of cementum and periodontal ligament fibers, it also has a significant osteogenic capacity. Thus, in several experiments it has been shown that heterotopic transplantation of tooth germs, including their follicles, to soft tissue sites results in formation of a complete periodontium including cementum, periodontal ligament fibers and an adjacent shell of bone (alveolar bone proper) (3, 5, 8–15).

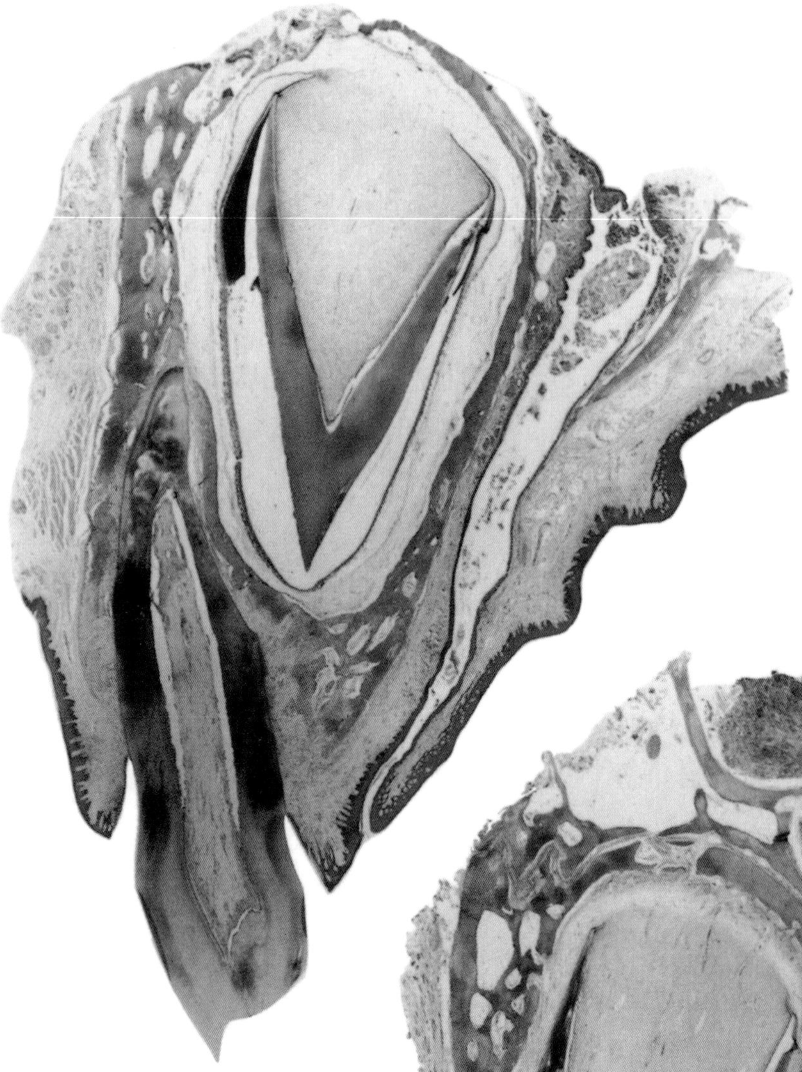

Fig. 2.2 Anatomy of a dental follicle of a monkey maxillary central tooth germ. Note the close proximity between the primary tooth and the permanent successor as well as the loose structure of the follicle. ×12.

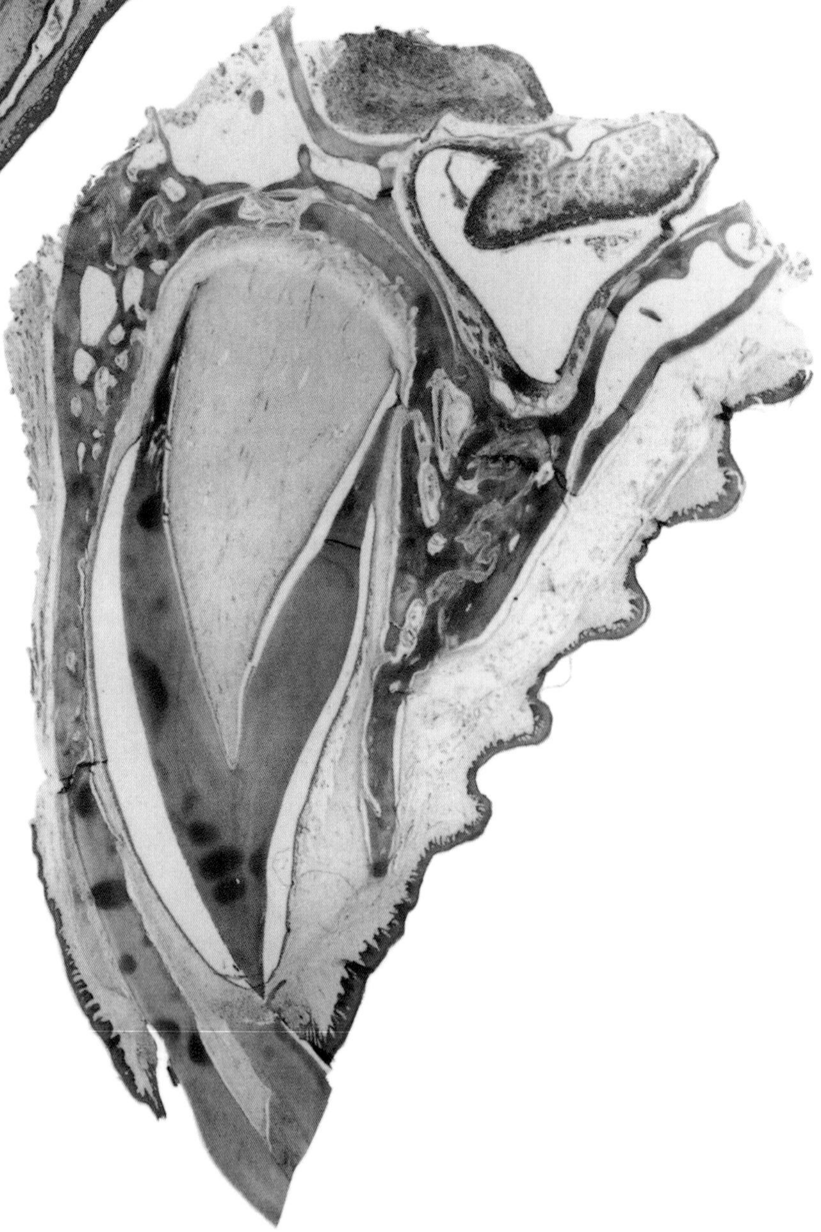

Fig. 2.3 Eruption of a permanent maxillary central monkey incisor. Note bone apposition apically, while active bone and tooth resorption takes place coronally. ×12.

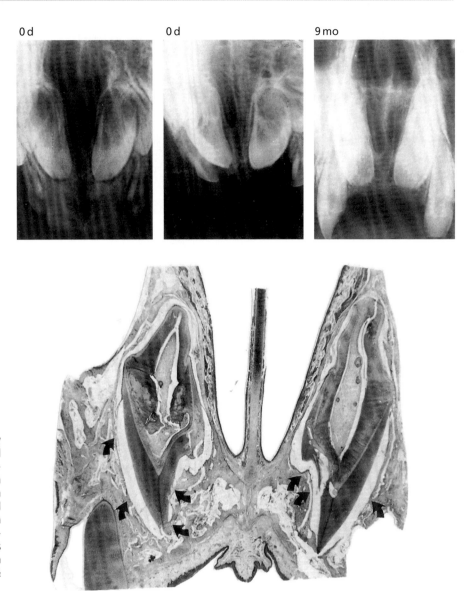

0 d          0 d          9 mo

**Fig. 2.4** Replantation of maxillary monkey tooth germs with damaged follicles. Preoperative and postoperative radiographs and the condition after 9 months. No eruption has taken place. Low power view of both central incisors. Note the lack of eruption despite almost complete root formation. Furthermore note the ankylosis sites affecting the crowns of both teeth (arrows). From KRISTERSON & ANDREASEN (25) 1984.

A number of events have been suggested to be responsible for tooth eruption, including root growth, dentin formation, pulp growth and changes in the dental follicle and the periodontal ligament (16–22). Recent experiments in dogs and monkeys have demonstrated that changes in the dental follicle (including the reduced enamel epithelium) are possibly responsible for the coordinated enlargement of the eruption pathway and movement of the tooth germ along this pathway in the initial phases of eruption (23–26). These findings, together with the established relationship between the dental follicle and distinct areas of bone resorption and bone formation, suggest that the dental follicle and/or the reduced enamel epithelium coordinate these processes during eruption (21, 22–30) (Fig. 2.3) (see Chapter 20). Consequently, severe disturbances in eruption can be anticipated if there is damage to the follicle

due to trauma or infection (see also Chapters 19 and 20).

### Response to trauma

Histologic studies have revealed a very close relationship between the primary teeth and the permanent dentition, especially in the initial phases of development (31, 32) (Figs 2.2 and 2.3). Traumatic injuries can therefore easily be transmitted from the primary to the permanent dentition (34).

While there is abundant clinical evidence to show that the dental follicle has a remarkable healing capacity after injury, certain limitations do exist. Thus, it has been shown that, when larger parts of the dental follicle are removed, an ankylosis is formed between the tooth surface and the crypt and eruption is arrested (23, 25) (Fig. 2.4). The extent to which

**Fig. 2.5 Follicular changes after pulp necrosis of a maxillary monkey central primary incisor**
Late stages of tooth development of permanent tooth germs. Low power view of control tooth (A) and experimental tooth (C). ×7.

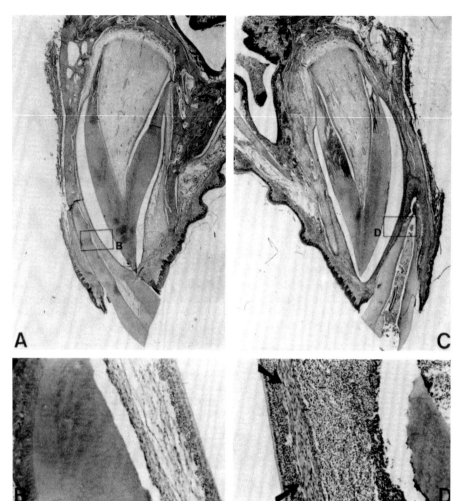

**Changes in the follicle**
B. Normal reduced enamel epithelium in control tooth. In the experimental tooth (D) there is intense periapical inflammation demarcated from reduced enamel epithelium by a thin layer of fibrous tissue (arrows). ×75. From ANDREASEN & RIIS (33) 1978.

a follicle can be damaged without leading to this complication is not known.

### Response to infection

Very little information exists on the reaction of the dental follicle to infection. In monkeys, it was found that follicles of permanent incisor tooth germs were resistant to short-term chronic periapical infection (i.e. 6 months exposure) originating from the root canals of primary incisors (Fig. 2.5), and no influence could be demonstrated on the permanent successors with respect to enamel mineralization (33). In rare instances, acute infection has been found to spread to the entire follicle and to lead to sequestration of the tooth germ. Such events have been reported after traumatic injuries to the primary dentition, in jaw fractures where the line of fracture involves a tooth germ, or in cases of osteomyelitis which affect the bony regions containing dental follicles (34). Apart from these rare occur-

rences, the dental follicle appears to be rather resistant to infection.

### Enamel-forming organ

The formation and maturation of enamel in the permanent dentition is often disturbed or arrested by trauma transmitted from primary teeth after displacement and/or periapical inflammation resulting from infection. The outcome of such events depends primarily upon the stage of enamel formation at the time of the injury.

The usual stage at which primary tooth injuries interfere with odontogenesis of the permanent dentition is the beginning of mineralization of the incisal portion of the crown. At this stage of development, the enamel-forming organ consists of the cervical loop placed apically to the site of active enamel and dentin formation. Coronally, the enamel epithelium is divided into the inner and outer enamel

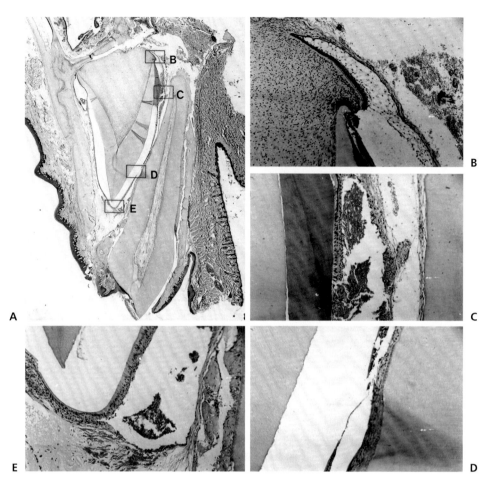

**Fig. 2.6** Immediate changes after intrusion of a primary monkey incisor. A. Low power view of specimen. ×8. B. Dislocation between mineralized tissues and cervical loop. ×75. C. Rupture and bleeding in stellate reticulum. ×75. D. Destruction of reduced enamel epithelium. ×75. E. Separation of reduced enamel epithelium from connective tissue. ×75. From ANDREASEN (37) 1976.

epithelium with an intervening stratum intermedium and stellate reticulum between them. The reduced enamel epithelium is found more coronally, where the full enamel thickness has been formed and mineralization completed. In the following, a synopsis of the anatomy and function of these structures will be presented, as well their response to trauma and infection.

## Cervical loop

At the free border of the enamel organ, the inner and outer enamel epithelial layers are continuous and form the cervical loop (35, 36). Progression of tooth development is entirely dependent upon the growth and action of this structure.

### Response to trauma

The cervical loop is highly resistant to trauma. Simple separation of the cervical enamel and dentin matrix does not prevent further enamel or dentin formation (37, 38) (Figs 2.6 and 2.7). However, profound contusion of this structure, as after intrusion of a primary incisor into the developing successor, may result in total arrest of further odontogenesis.

### Response to infection

The response of the cervical loop to infection has not yet been studied.

## Inner enamel epithelium

According to function, the inner enamel epithelium (ameloblasts) evolves through a number of functional stages (39–41) (Fig. 2.8). The first is the *morphogenetic stage* whereby the future outline of the crown is determined. This stage is followed by an *organizing stage*, with initiation of dentin formation. The *formative stage* is then reached, where enamel matrix formation as well as initial mineralization take place. The *maturation stage* follows enamel matrix formation. During this stage, there is partial removal of the organic enamel matrix accompanied by a complex mineralization process proceeding from the region immediately adjacent to dentin and progressing outward (42). These are followed by the *protective* and *desmolytic* stages, which will be described later. During these two stages, the tissue layer is now designated the *reduced enamel epithelium*.

**Fig. 2.7 Late changes after intrusion of primary incisors in a monkey**
Low power view of specimen (A), where the intruded tooth is preserved and the contralateral side where the intruded tooth was extracted (D). ×8.

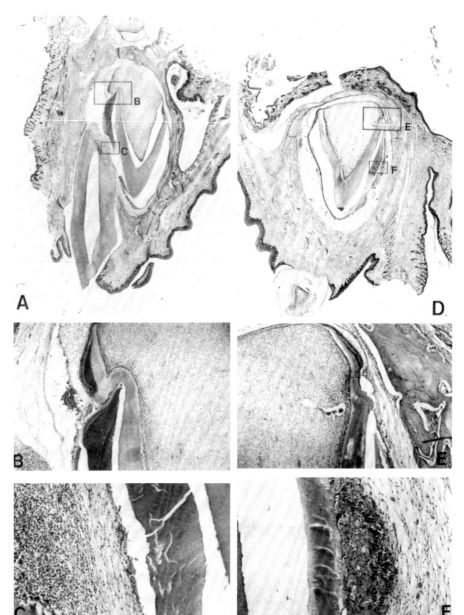

**Changes in enamel and dentin**
Morphologic changes in enamel matrix and dentin (B). Destruction of enamel epithelium and abnormal matrix formation (C). Partial arrest of enamel matrix formation (E). ×30. Metaplasia of enamel epithelium and abnormal matrix formation (F). ×75. From ANDREASEN (37) 1976.

### Response to trauma

To date, only limited knowledge exists concerning the response of the inner enamel epithelium to trauma (37, 38, 43–46). In the case of total loss of ameloblasts in the secretory phase, no regenerative potential exists (44). In the case of partial damage, the ameloblasts in the *secretory* stage may survive and continue enamel matrix formation, and later maturation may occur (42, 45–47) (Figs 2.6 and 2.7).

If there is total loss of the ameloblasts during the *maturation* stage, a hypomineralized area of enamel will develop. If partial damage occurs, the ameloblasts may recover and the result may be only a limited zone of hypomineralization (42).

### Response to infection

When chronic periapical inflammation develops due to the necrosis of an infected pulp in primary teeth, the effect upon permanent successors is very limited, at least over a short time (i.e. months) (33) (Fig. 2.5). When infection persists over longer periods (i.e. years), experimental and clinical studies have shown that enamel formation and maturation may be affected (48–50).

The response to acute infection is similar to the response to trauma and may lead to localized arrest of enamel formation (51–58). At the site of injury, a cementum-like tissue may later be deposited (59, 60). In this situation, the cementoblasts are most probably recruited from the follicle, shown to have cementogenic potential (61).

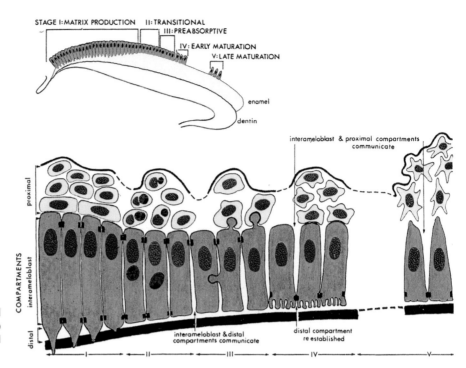

**Fig. 2.8** Changes in the enamel epithelial compartment related to enamel matrix production. From REITH (39) 1970.

## Reduced enamel epithelium

When enamel matrix formation is complete and enamel maturation begun, the ameloblasts become compact and the stellate reticulum disappears, and a multilayered epithelium is formed of cuboidal or flattened cells. The following functions are currently linked to the reduced enamel epithelium: protection of the enamel against the follicle until the tooth erupts (62), regulation of osteoclastic activity in the follicle preparatory to eruption (62), and participation in the breakdown of the connective tissue overlying the crown (63–66). In addition, the reduced enamel epithelium may play an active part in fusion with the oral epithelium as the tooth emerges into the oral cavity (64).

### Response to trauma

Minor injury to the reduced enamel epithelium is repaired with a thin squamous epithelium (37) (Fig. 2.9). The influence of this event upon eruption is presently unknown, but with larger areas of destruction of the reduced enamel epithelium, ankylosis and tooth retention have been demonstrated (67) (Fig. 2.4).

### Response to infection

The short-term effect (i.e. months) of chronic inflammation on primary teeth appears to be negligible (33) (Fig. 2.5), while the long-term effect appears to be ectopic or accelerated eruption (50).

## Enamel and enamel matrix

Mature enamel has the highest mineral content of any tissue in the body (i.e. 96–98%), whereas enamel matrix is con-siderably less mineralized. Thus, if maturation is interrupted due to infection or trauma, enamel hypomineralization will result. One may see problems clinically with increased caries or perhaps with difficulties regarding acid-etch restorative techniques. This problem is further discussed in Chapter 20.

### Response to trauma

Trauma to a primary tooth may cause contusion of the permanent enamel matrix (37, 38). The ameloblasts will also be destroyed, thereby arresting enamel maturation and resulting in a permanent hypomineralized enamel defect (see Chapter 20). In mature enamel, the result of a direct impact will be enamel infraction, i.e. a split along the enamel rods usually ending at the dentino-enamel junction (see Chapter 10), or a fracture, whereby part of the crown is lost.

### Response to infection

The response of enamel matrix or enamel to infection has been discussed earlier.

## Hertwig's epithelial root sheath

Hertwig's epithelial root sheath (HERS) is a continuous sleeve of epithelial cells which separates the pulp from the dental follicle. In all primates it consists of an inner layer of cuboidal cells and an outer layer of more flattened cells (68). (Fig. 2.10). Occasionally, there is an intermediate layer of elongated cells (69).

**Fig. 2.9 Late changes after intrusion in monkey**
Low power view of specimen (A) where the intruded primary tooth was preserved and the contralateral side where the intruded tooth was extracted (D). Arrows indicate length of disturbed reduced enamel epithelium. ×8.

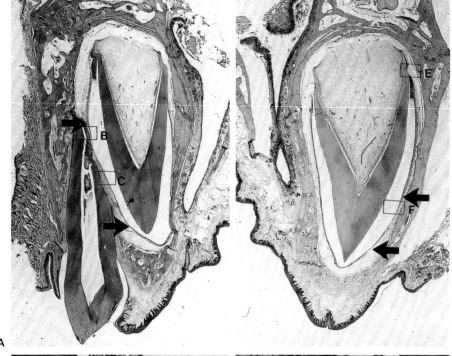

**Changes in follicle and hard tissues**
B. Periapical inflammation and disturbed enamel epithelium C. Amorphous eosinophilic substance deposited upon enamel. E. Area with temporary arrest of enamel matrix formation. ×75. F. Metaplastic reduced enamel epithelium. From ANDREASEN (37) 1976.

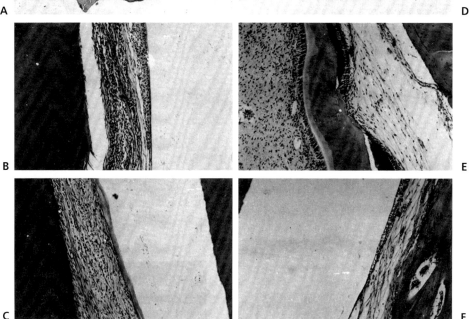

HERS completely encloses the dental papilla except for an opening in its base, the *primary apical foramen*, through which the pulp receives its neurovascular supply. Root formation is determined by the activity of HERS (70–74), and root growth is dependent upon a continuous proliferation of epithelium (75, 76). More incisally, dentin and cementum develop synchronously, ensuring a relatively constant sheath length throughout root formation up to the final phases of root development, when the root sheath becomes considerably shorter.

The width of the primary apical foramen as well as the number of vessels entering it appears to be relatively constant until final root length has been achieved (74). Thus, in a luxation, replantation or transplantation situation the

chances of revascularization through the primary apical foramen should theoretically be the same throughout the early stages of root development, until apical constriction starts. Such a relationship has in fact been found for luxated (75, 607) and replanted incisors (76, 608) as well as for autotransplanted human premolars (77).

In the following, a closer look will be taken at the role of HERS in *dentin* and *cementum formation*. Odontoblastic differentiation takes place adjacent to the basal aspect of HERS, after which the first dentin matrix is deposited (*mantle dentin*). At this time, the innermost layer of cells in the root sheath secrete a material which combines with the mantle dentin to form the so-called *intermediate cementum layer*. This layer has been found to contain enamel matrix protein

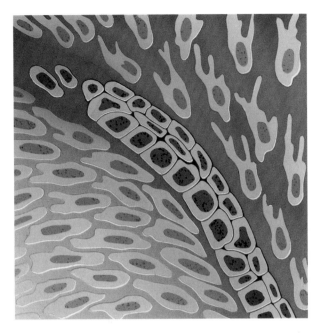

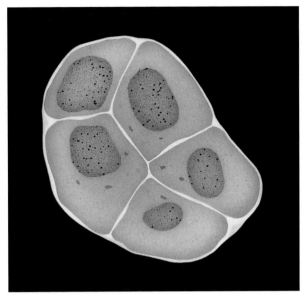

**Fig. 2.11** Epithelial island of Mallassez.

**Fig. 2.10** Hertwig's epithelial root sheath. The root sheath consists of 2 to 3 layers of epithelial cells.

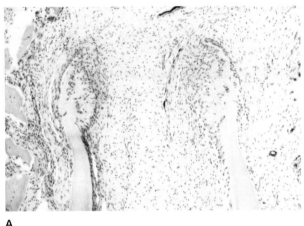

A

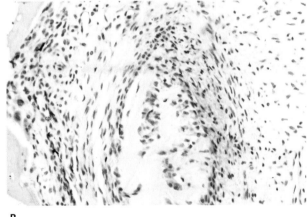

B

**Fig. 2.12** Hyperactivity of HERS with excessive production of dentin after replantation of a permanent maxillary lateral incisor. A. ×25. B. ×75. Observation period: 1 week.

and later becomes hypercalcified (78–80). The intermediate cementum layer has recently attracted interest (81). It has been found to be an effective barrier against the penetration of noxious elements placed in the root canal to the periodontal ligament via the dentinal tubules and possibly also to toxins produced by bacteria within the root canal (82).

After odontoblast induction and formation of intermediate cementum, the root sheath degenerates and the epithelial cells migrate away from the root surface to form the epithelial rests of Mallassez (Fig. 2.11). At the same time, cells from the periodontal ligament migrate towards the root surface and become cementoblasts. These cells then synthesize collagen and other organic constituents of cementum. The role of the epithelial root sheath in the induction of cementoblasts, however, has recently been questioned (75, 83–85).

## Response to trauma

*Chronic* trauma to the Hertwig's epithelial root sheath, such as orthodontic intrusion of immature teeth, often leads to its fragmentation. In these cases the epithelial fragments displaced into the pulp canal can induce true denticle formation (i.e. dentin-containing pulp stones) (86–90).

An injury close to the root sheath (e.g. a laceration in the PDL) may result in temporary hyperactivity of the root sheath which can initiate rapid production of both dentin and cementum in the apical area (Fig. 2.12). However, activity of the root sheath will later return to normal.

*Acute* trauma to the epithelial root sheath is transmitted indirectly, for example by the intrusion of a primary tooth, or directly by forceful displacement of immature permanent teeth, can damage HERS and lead to partial or complete arrest of root development (91–94) (Fig. 2.13).

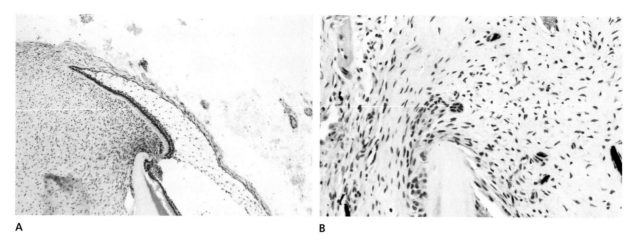

A                                                              B

**Fig. 2.13** Damage to the cervical diaphragm or the HERS subsequent to replantation of permanent lateral monkey incisors. Observation period: 1 week. A. Displacement of cervical diaphragm. ×25. B. Fragmentation of the root sheath. ×75.

During replantation, the root sheath may be injured either during avulsion, during extraoral storage, or by the repositioning procedure. Following such injury, further root growth will be partially or totally arrested; and bone and PDL-derived tissue from the base of the socket may invade the root canal to form intraradicular bone which is separated from the canal wall by an *internal periodontal ligament* (95) (Fig. 2.14) (see also Chapters 13 and 17). A similar bony invasion into the pulp of immature teeth is found when the epithelial root sheath is resected *in situ* (96–98), or when the root sheath is injured chemically, as with devitalization procedures that employ formaldehyde (99, 100).

### Response to infection

Hertwig's epithelial root sheath is rather resistant to inflammation in connection with partial pulp necrosis. Although sometimes restricted, root formation has been found to occur in most cases of partial pulp necrosis irrespective of whether endodontic therapy has been instituted or not (see also Chapter 22). This would seem to imply that HERS can continue to function despite inflammation (96, 101–108). In this context, there appears to be a critical distance between the root sheath and pathological changes in the pulp. If that distance is too short, inflammation will destroy the root sheath and root formation will be arrested (96) (Fig. 2.15). The fact that the epithelial root sheath can continue to function despite inflammation elicited by a partial pulp necrosis demonstrates that continued root development and apical closure as such cannot be taken as criteria for pulpal vitality (see Chapter 22).

### Teeth with developed roots

#### Gingival and periosteal complex

The gingiva is usually involved during crown-root and root fractures, luxation injuries and always during tooth avul-

sion. In addition, the periosteum is always involved during lateral luxation and alveolar bone fractures. In the following, the anatomy and function of the gingiva and periosteum will be described, as well as their response to trauma and infection.

#### GINGIVA

Gingiva is defined from an anatomic point of view as either *free* or *attached*. The *free gingiva* comprises the vestibular and oral gingival tissue as well as the interdental papilla. Clinically, the apical border of the free gingiva is usually circumscribed by the free gingival groove (Fig. 2.16).

The *attached gingiva* is circumscribed coronally by the free gingival groove and apically by the mucogingival junction. The attached gingiva is firmly bound to the periosteum by collagenous fibers and is resistant to elevation.

The *alveolar mucosa* borders the attached gingiva and is loosely bound to periosteum, thereby offering minimal resistance to the formation of a subperiosteal hematoma which can develop after lateral luxation, alveolar fracture, or rupture from traction due to an impact parallel to the labial surface of the mandible or maxilla.

The function of the *free gingiva* is to seal, maintain and defend the critical area where the tooth penetrates its connective tissue bed and enters the oral cavity.

The gingival epithelium immediately adjacent to the tooth and *junctional epithelium* is designed to seal the periodontium from the oral cavity (Fig. 2.16).

Gingival epithelium displays a specific anatomy, being narrow and consisting of a few cell layers without rete pegs. The development of the junctional epithelium is closely related to tooth eruption. Thus, the junctional epithelium shows cell division originating in the basal layers, with cells being ultimately exfoliated into the gingival sulcus. Two zones can be recognized by transmission electron microscopy between the superficial cells of the junctional epithelium and the enamel; namely, the *lamina densa* and the *lamina lucida*, together called the *internal basement*

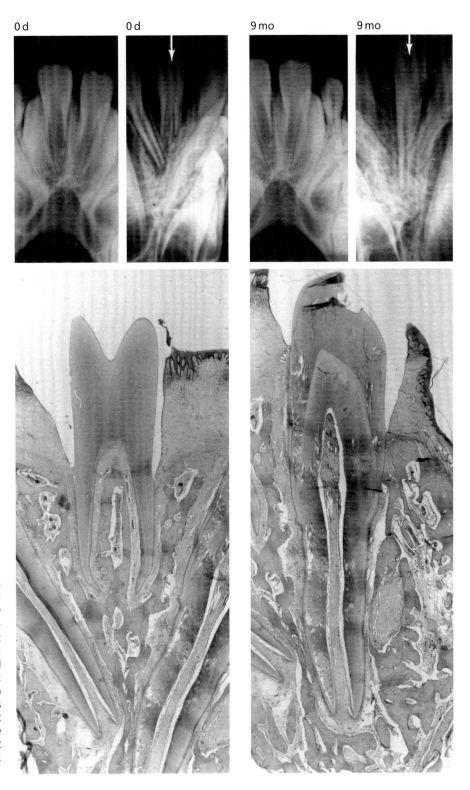

0 d    0 d    9 mo    9 mo

**Fig. 2.14** Effect of trauma to HERS upon root growth. Left: the right permanent central incisor in a monkey was extracted and the HERS was traumatized by pressing the apex against the socket wall before repositioning. The left central incisor was extracted and repositioned as a control. Right: condition 9 months after surgery in a monkey Root development has stopped and bone has entered the root canal in the right central incisor. The left central incisor shows normal root development. From ANDREASEN et al. (96) 1988.

*lamina*. Hemidesmosomes are formed by the epithelium adjacent to the lamina lucida, and these create an interphase with the enamel analogous to that with the subepithelial connective tissue (109).

Dental cuticle and sometimes a layer of fibrillar cementum can be seen interposed between this epithelium and the enamel. The *sulcular epithelium* faces the tooth without being in direct contact with it (Fig. 2.16). This epithelium is

thicker than the junctional epithelium and has abundant rete pegs.

The *fibrillar system* of the gingiva is complex, comprising groups of collagen fibers with different sites of insertion (110–116) (Fig. 2.16).

The *dentinogingival fibers* originate in cementum and insert in the free gingiva. The *dentoperiosteal fibers* start at the same site, but insert into the attached gingiva. The

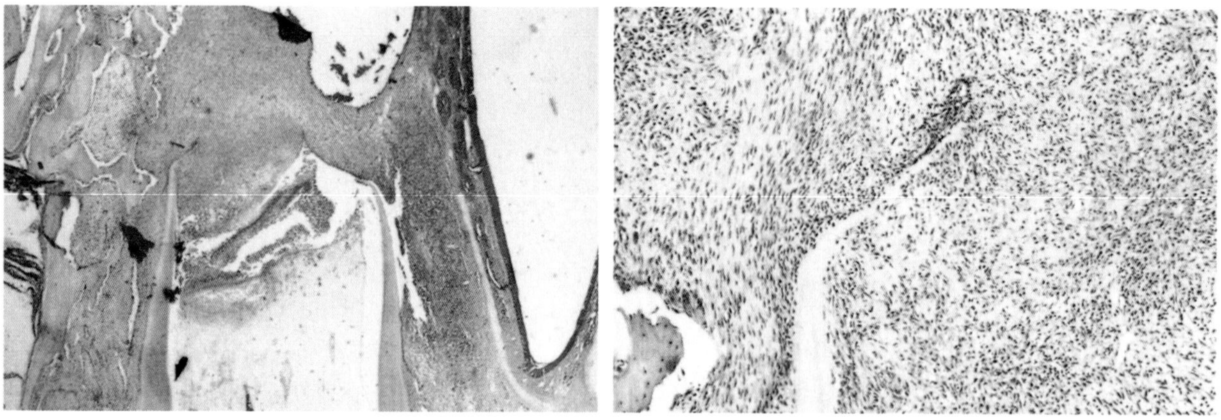

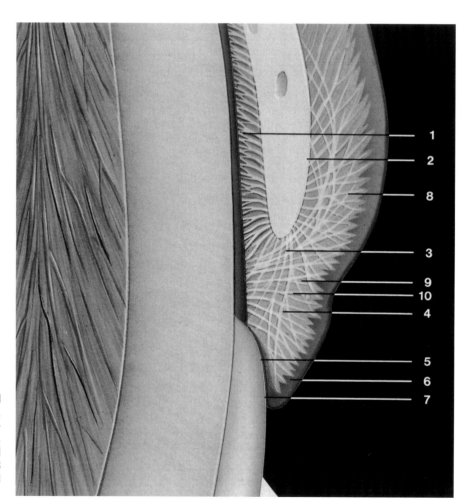

**A**                                                    **B**

**Fig. 2.15** Critical distance between pulp necrosis and survival of HERS. A. The permanent central maxillary incisor was autotransplanted to the contralateral side in a monkey 1 week previously. ×25. B. Pulp necrosis extending to the apex mesially whereas the pulp necrosis zone is 1 mm short of the distal aspect of the apex. The HERS has survived and some root formation has occurred. ×75. From ANDREASEN et al. (96) 1988.

**Fig. 2.16** Anatomy of the gingiva and periosteal complex. 1 Sharpey's fibers, 2 dentoperiosteal fibers, 3 alveolo-gingival fibers, 4 dentogingival fibers, 5 junctional epithelium, 6 gingival epithelium, 7 sulcular epithelium, 8 periosteogingival fibers, 9 intergingival fibers, 10 circular fibers.

*transseptal fibers* extend from cementum in the supra-alveolar region and insert into the supra-alveolar cementum of the adjacent tooth. The *circular fibers* encircle the tooth in a ring-like, supra-alveolar course. These fibers are responsible for the very rapid initial closure of an extraction wound (see p. 83), as well as the rapid adaptation of the gingiva around luxated or replanted teeth (see p. 75). Finally, *alveologingival*

*fibers* emanate from the top of the alveolar crest and fan out into the attached gingiva.

The blood supply to the gingiva originates from three sources: the periodontal ligament, the crestal bone and the supraperiosteal blood vessels (see p. 78). This ensures survival of the marginal gingiva even after severe laceration or contusion (see Chapter 21).

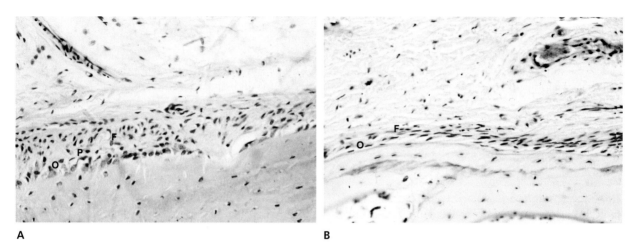

**Fig. 2.17** Differences in periosteum related to age. A. Cellular alveolar periosteum in a young monkey (root development of permanent incisors incomplete). O = osteoblasts, P = precursor cells, F = fibroblasts. ×75. B. Periosteum in an old monkey. Note the difference in the configuration of periosteum. ×75.

## PERIOSTEUM

The alveolar periosteum covers the alveolar process. In young individuals, at the time of active bone growth, it consists of an inner layer of angular osteoblasts followed by spindle-shaped precursor cells supported by loosely arranged collagen fibers (Fig. 2.17). In older individuals, where growth has ceased, the inner layer consists of flattened bone lining cells followed by an outer fibrous layer of inactive osteoprogenitor cells which, however, still maintain their potential for cell division (117–119) (Fig. 2.17).

The periosteum serves an important function in appositional growth, remodelling and bone repair after injury. Furthermore, it anchors muscles and carries blood vessels, lymphatic vessels and nerves.

### Response to trauma

The gingival attachment is often torn during luxation injuries and always during avulsions. In an experimental replantation study in monkeys, the junctional epithelium showed increased autoradiographic labelling of cells as early as after 1 day, and reached a peak after 3 days. After 7 days, a new junctional epithelium was formed (120). In the connective tissue, the ruptured gingival and transseptal collagen fibers were united in the majority of cases after 1 week (121–123).

The response of periosteum to trauma is not very well described. Displacement of the attached gingiva or the alveolar mucosa involves injury to the periosteum and the underlying bone (124–161). Thus, the surface of bone is affected in several ways. Firstly, the cortical bone plate loses an important part of its vascular supply. Secondly, the cellular cover of bone provided by the innermost layer of periosteum is partially or totally removed. These two events invite an initial resorption of the bony surface which, however, is then followed by bony deposition to repair the initial loss.

In addition to bone loss due to displacement of gingiva or alveolar mucosa, bone may also be lost directly due to trauma. In such cases, an important factor related to healing is the osteogenic potential of the periosteum, which is strongly influenced by age (152–154). Thus, when a periosteal flap is raised in *adult* animals, the osteogenic layer is usually disrupted and periosteal osteogenesis can only take place from the periphery of the wound where progenitor cells have not been disturbed (155–158), implying that bony repair will be limited and fibrous scar tissue will often form in its place (162, 163).

Conversely, in young animals, cells in the cambium layer of elevated flaps exhibit osteogenic potential and the bone contour is often fully repaired. In humans, surgical removal of large portions of the mandible, but with intentional preservation of the periosteum, has been seen to result in extensive new bone formation (160, 161).

### Response to infection

The general response of gingiva to infection has been the subject of numerous studies related to plaque-induced gingivitis and is beyond the scope of this text. The significance of infection will be discussed only as it relates to the gingival attachment after traumatic or surgical injury. In monkeys, it has been shown that incisional wounds from the gingival sulcus to the alveolar crest lead to epithelial growth through most of the supracrestal area when gingival inflammation was induced (164).

The role of bacteria in gingival healing after surgical injury has been assessed only indirectly through the effect of antibiotic therapy. The use of antibiotics (tetracycline) in rats after injuries to pulpal, gingival and root tissues was shown to promote gingival and periodontal reattachment (165–167). In humans, it was demonstrated that the administration of erythromycin for 4 days after gingivectomy led to completed epithelialization after 1 week, in contrast to only two-thirds of the specimens when no antibiotic coverage was given (167). In conclusion, there is some evidence that bacteria-induced gingival inflammation has a negative influence upon wound healing after trauma and surgical injury.

If an odontogenic infection spreads from bone marrow to the periosteal layer and an abscess is formed between periosteum and cortical bone, the blood supply to the immediately underlying cortical bone can be compromised. The cortical bone can then undergo ischemic necrosis, resulting in an undermining resorption (168).

## Periodontal ligament-cementum complex

The anatomical border for the PDL is the most cervically located of the principal fibers (Sharpey's fibers) that insert into both cementum and alveolar bone (Fig. 2.18). In this context, only the anatomy and function of the more important cellular and fibrillar structures of the periodontal ligament will be considered.

### CEMENTOBLASTS

Cementoblasts are spindle or polyhedral shaped cells whose long axes are usually oriented parallel to the root surface. The cytoplasm is basophilic and the nuclei are round or ovoid (Fig. 2.18). These cells are said to be active or resting according to the relative amount of cytoplasm. Resting cells contain less cytoplasm than active cementoblasts (169). Cementoblasts produce the organic matrix of cementum (i.e. intrinsic collagen fibers and ground substance), while the extrinsic fibers (i.e. Sharpey's fibers) are formed by fibroblasts from the PDL (170). If the cementoblast becomes incorporated into the mineralizing front, cellular cementum is formed. The deposition of cementum appears to occur rhythmically throughout life, at a speed of approximately 3 μm per year (171). Periods of activity alternate with periods of quiescence, thereby giving rise to incremental lines (172).

### PERIODONTAL FIBROBLASTS

These cells are spindle-shaped, with several points of contact with adjacent cells. The nuclei are oval, containing one or more prominent nucleoli (Fig. 2.18). In sections parallel to Sharpey's fibers, fibroblasts appear as spindle-shaped cells with only occasional contact with other fibroblasts (Fig. 2.18). In transverse sections, however, they are seen as stellate cells whose processes envelope the principal periodontal fiber bundles and connect with many other fibroblasts to form a cellular network (173). This intricate relationship between fibroblasts and Sharpey's fibers after injury may be important in the rapid degradation or reformation of Sharpey's fibers (175, 176). Anatomical (174) and *in vitro* studies (173) suggest that different fibroblast populations exist in the PDL (174).

Fibroblasts are responsible for the formation, maintenance and remodelling of PDL fibers and their associated ground substance. By using tritiated thymidine labelling, it has been found that fibroblasts comprise a very active cell renewal system. In mice, for example, a cell turnover rate of 30% was seen when continuous labelling was used over a period of 25 days (178, 179). Furthermore, cell renewal took place as a clonal paravascular proliferation of cells. Together

with programmed cell death (apoptosis) in the PDL, a steady state was created in the cellular content of the periodontal ligament (179–181).

As already stated, an important function of fibroblasts in the PDL is the maintenance of periodontal fibers. This function is manifested by very rapid collagen synthesis and degradation (turnover) (182–186), occurring primarily in the middle zone of the PDL (187). Thus, it has been shown that the half-life of collagen in the PDL of rats is about 6–9 days (188, 189). Moreover, collagen turnover is considerably more rapid in PDL collagen than in that of gingiva, pulp or other connective tissues in the body (190, 191). This very rapid turnover in the PDL is in agreement with findings from studies in PDL wound healing, where very rapid healing of the periodontium has been demonstrated after surgical injury (see p. 79).

Finally, for the sake of completeness, it should be mentioned that periodontal fibroblasts are also responsible for synthesis and maintenance of other fibers, such as elastin and oxytalan.

### OSTEOBLASTS

The osteoblast is slightly larger than the cementoblast and has a circular or ovoid nucleus which is usually located eccentrically. The cytoplasm is abundant and very basophilic during osteogenesis (Fig. 2.18). Like the cementoblast, the osteoblast is found in an active or resting form, as revealed by less cytoplasm in the latter form.

### EPITHELIAL RESTS OF MALLASSEZ

A network of epithelial cells is found in the PDL positioned close to the root surface (Fig. 2.18). These cells originate from the successive breakdown of the Hertwig's epithelial root sheath during root formation (see p. 69).

These epithelial cells have been proposed as playing a role in the homeostasis of the PDL (193–195, 659). However, other studies do not support this theory (196–200). On the other hand, these cells represent an important part of the defense system of the PDL against invading bacteria from the root canal. Bacterial invasion of both the main and lateral canals leads to proliferation and adherence of the epithelial cells to the root canal openings at the PDL to form an epithelial barrier against the invaders (201).

### PERIODONTAL LIGAMENT FIBERS

The vast majority of collagen fibers in the PDL are arranged in bundles, the so-called principal fibers (Sharpey's fibers) (Fig. 2.18). These fibers are embedded in both cementum and bone. In their course from cementum to alveolar bone, they are often wavy at their midpoint, giving the impression of an intermediate plexus, with interdigitation of fibers. However, recent scanning electron microscopic studies seem to indicate that the majority of the principal fibers span the entire PDL space, although they usually branch and join adjacent fibers to create a ladder-like architecture in the PDL (202–216) (Fig. 2.18). The principal fibers extending from

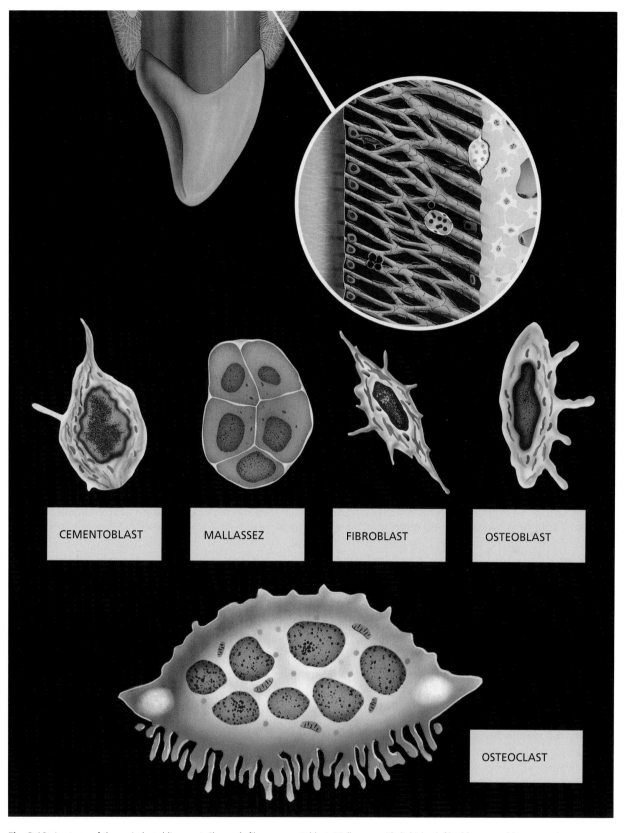

**Fig. 2.18** Anatomy of the periodontal ligament. Sharpey's fibers, cementoblast, Mallassez epithelial island, fibroblast, osteoblast, osteoclast.

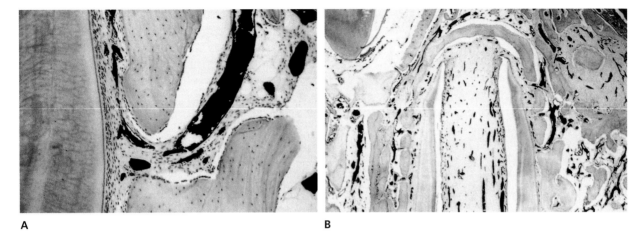

**Fig. 2.19** Vascular supply to the periodontium. A. Vascular supply to the PDL in a longitudinally sectioned permanent maxillary central incisor in a monkey shown by indian ink perfusion. ×10. B. The interdental arteries give off multiple branches to the midportion of the PDL. ×100.

cementum to bone can be classified according to their direction and location into horizontal, oblique and apical fibers. In the gingiva, the supra-alveolar (gingival) fibers can be classified into dentogingival fibers, dentoperiosteal fibers, interdental fibers and circular fibers (Fig. 2.16) (see p. 74).

The main function of the PDL is to support the tooth in its alveolus during function. Whenever functional demands are changed, corresponding adjustments take place in the architecture of the PDL, such that the orientation, amount and insertion pattern of the principal fibers are altered.

## PERIODONTAL VASCULATURE

The blood supply to the PDL at the midportion of the root appears to arise from branches of the superior or inferior alveolar arteries. Before these arteries enter the apical foramen, they give off branches to the interdental bone. On their way to the alveolar crest, they give off multiple branches which perforate the socket wall and form a plexus which surrounds the root surface (217–222). This plexus is located in the interstitial spaces between Sharpey's fibers. In primates, the majority of these vessels are located close to the bone surface (221). *Apically*, the blood supply to the PDL originates from branches of the dental arteries which are released as they cross the PDL and enter the pulp. *Cervically*, however, anastomoses are formed with gingival vessels (Fig. 2.19).

The blood supply to the gingiva appears to arise primarily from the supraperiosteal blood vessels, which anastomose in the gingiva with vessels from the PDL and branches of the interdental arteries and which perforate the crestal bone margin or the labial or lingual bone plate.

## PERIODONTAL INNERVATION

The PDL has receptors for pain, touch, pressure and proprioception, which all belong to the somatic nervous system. Autonomic nerves are also present, which innervate the blood vessels. In general, periodontal innervation follows the same pathways as the blood supply. In a recent experimental study it has also been found that sensory fibers promote root resorption after pulpo-periodontal injury (223).

## HOMEOSTATIC MECHANISM OF PDL

PDL appears to exist throughout life with minimal variations in width (224, 225). This dimension is primarily controlled by age and function, but it is also affected by pathology (226) (see Chapter 5).

The homeostasis against resorption in the periodontal ligament space (and the pulp) has always been an enigma. Previously, it has been hypothesized that the periodontal (227, 228, 255) and pulpal cells (229, 230) act as a barrier that prevents resorption of the roots by inhibiting the resorbing cells from gaining access to cementum and dentin (224, 229, 231–235).

Apparently, these cells on the root surfaces normally give protection against an osteogenic cell invasion. New molecular signals have recently been identified in various cell types (229, 230) such as periodontal ligament cells (PDL-cells), odontoblasts, osteoblasts, and cementoblasts (227), which may explain the homeostasis phenomenon.

Different cell types, including preosteoblasts, express active signal molecules in a membrane bound (RANKL) and a soluble (sRANKL) form. The RANKL (receptor activator of NFkappa-B-ligand) molecules are ligands with the capacity to activate mononuclear osteclast progenitor cells with receptor (RANK) attached to their surface. If these two molecules – the ligand and the receptor – meet, the osteoclast progenitor cells become differentiated and merge with other progenitor cells to form osteoclasts (236–241), which potentially may attack the root surface or the root canal.

A third molecule called osteoprotegerin (OPG) is a soluble molecule, i.e. a decoy receptor. The OPG is able to bind and cover both the RANKL molecules on adjacent cells and the soluble sRANKL, and OPG is thereby able to give protection to the root surface (236, 241) (Fig. 2.20).

When the OPG/RANK/RANKL signaling pathway is in action it is able to both protect against or activate osteoclastic activity, and recent studies suggest this as a possible explanation for the protective action of the hard tissue covering cells, i.e. odontoblasts, cementoblasts, and PDL-cells (Fig. 2.21). Furthermore, the OPG/RANKL ratio level can be upregulated or downregulated by growth factors, hormones

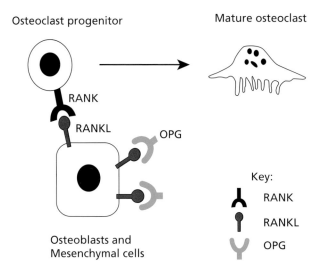

**Fig. 2.20** RANK, RANKL and OPG system monitoring osteoclast activity.

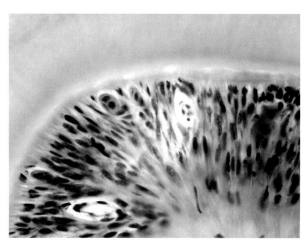

**Fig. 2.21** Intraradicular root surface of rat molar where migration of osteoclasts is arrested in the periodontal ligament.

and inflammatory factors (e.g. interleukins) which may explain a number of resorption phenomena such as osteoporosis and inflammatory root or bone resorption (238) (see Chapters 3 and 5).

The experience on periodontal homeostasis is supported with this new molecular evidence. The new knowledge about the OPG/RANK/RANKL system appear to explain central aspects of tooth eruption and shedding of primary teeth (241–244), progression of ankylosis (245–249), orthodontic tooth movement (250–253), periodontitis, periimplantitis and rheumatoid arthritis (253, 254).

Thus the molecules RANKL/OPG have been found involved in physiologic primary tooth resorption (240) and in the follicles of erupting teeth (243, 244), and primary tooth shedding appears to be regulated by the RANKL/OPG signaling system (241).

In conclusion the observations on the OPG/RANK/RANKL system in the PDL seem to agree and support the previous hypothesis that the PDL cells act as a barrier that prevents resorption of the roots by inhibiting the resorbing cells (617). For a further discussion of the OPG/RANK/RANKL system the reader is referred to Chapter 3.

## *Response to trauma*

Following a severe dental injury (e.g. lateral luxation or intrusion) the PDL must respond to a variety of insults. These can include temporary compressive, tensile or shearing stresses, which result in hemorrhage and edema, rupture or contusion of the PDL. Each of these injuries can induce varying wound-healing signals.

The cellular kinetics of healing in the PDL associated with a surgical wound have been examined using tritiated thymidine labelling of proliferating cells. Thus, in mice, paravascular cells were labelled within 100 μm of the margin of the injured PDL. Some of these cells moved into the injury zone 3–5 days after injury and divided (256). It would appear that in the PDL there is a population of paravascular stem cells which exhibits a high nuclear/cytoplasmic ratio and which

remains stable throughout wound healing, but provides a front of new cells that migrate towards the wound and then divide (256–259) (Fig. 2.22). The identity of these progenitor cells is only partially known at present (260–262). It is possible that progenitor cells placed in the middle of the PDL supply the fibroblast population (256, 259), while progenitor cells close to the alveolar bone develop into osteoblasts (256–259, 263, 264). Cementoblasts precursors have not yet been identified; however, there is some indication that the progenitors for this cell population are located away from blood vessels (259, 264) (see Chapter 3).

### Bleeding and edema

Very little is known about healing events after bleeding or edema in the PDL subsequent to minor trauma (e.g. concussion or subluxation). However, in a clinical luxation study, a higher frequency of surface resorption was seen following concussion injury than after subluxation (265), suggesting that pressure from bleeding into the PDL after a mild injury might elicit minor areas of damage to the root surface. In the case of subluxations, where the impact is great enough to cause tooth loosening, this pressure can be relieved; however when no loosening results (i.e. concussion), pressure will be reflected in subsequent surface resorption.

### Rupture of the PDL

There has been little investigation into the healing of a ruptured PDL. The few available studies are either of extrusive luxation (263, 266–268) or of extraction and subsequent replantation (120–122, 192, 269).

In monkeys, it appears that rupture of the fibers after extrusion or extraction usually occurs midway between the alveolar bone and the root surface. However, rupture can also be seen close to either the alveolar wall or the root surface. After 4 days the cervical and apical part of the PDL appears revascularized (270). After 1 week, the split in the periodontal ligament is occupied by proliferating fibroblasts and blood vessels. In isolated areas, union of the principal

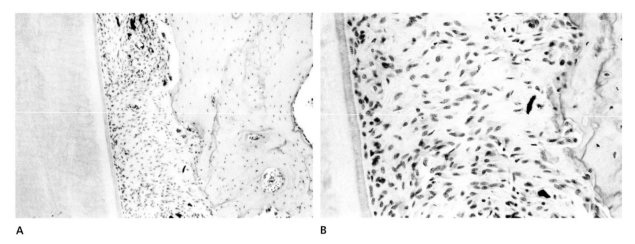

A                                                                              B

**Fig. 2.22** Healing of ruptured PDL. A. Healing of the periodontal ligament after replantation of a permanent monkey incisor. The monkey was perfused with India ink at sacrifice 1 week after replantation. ×25. B. The PDL is very cellular and has lost its typical parallel arrangement of the fibroblasts. In a few places Sharpey's fibers appear united. ×100.

fibers has already taken place (Fig. 2.22). After 2 weeks, a substantial number of principal fibers have healed. At that time, the mechanical properties of the injured PDL are about 50–60% of that of an uninjured PDL (266). With longer observation periods, an increased number of healed principal fibers can be seen. After 8 weeks, the injured PDL cannot be distinguished histologically from an uninjured control (266). If the alveolar bone is lost and there is an intact PDL covering the root, animal experiments have shown that the PDL will induce new bone (271, 272). In autotransplantation of teeth in humans the same phenomenon has been noted (see Chapter 27).

### Contusion injuries of the PDL

During intrusion, lateral luxation or avulsion with subsequent replantation, contusion of the PDL is a common occurrence (197). Wound healing is subsequently initiated when damaged tissue is removed by macrophage or osteoclast activity. During these events, not only are necrotic PDL tissue remnants removed, but sometimes also bone and cementum (273). The latter can lead to either **surface** or **inflammatory resorption** (repair- or infection-related resorption), depending upon the age of the patient, the stage of root development and pulp status (Figs 2.23 and 2.24) (224, 274). When large areas of the PDL are traumatized, competitive wound healing processes begin between bone marrow-derived stem cells destined to form bone and PDL-derived cells which are programmed to form PDL fibers and cementum (224, 274, 275) resulting in **replacement resorption** (ankylosis resorption) (Fig. 2.25).

### *Response to infection*

Progression of gingival infection or spread of infection from the root canal through the apical foramen, accessory canals or dentinal tubules are the most common routes of infection of the PDL. Accordingly, the following discussion will emphasize PDL reactions due to infection in the root canal, based on several studies in humans and animals (278–285).

Cellular kinetics of the PDL due to pulpal infection have been examined in rats using tritiated thymidine. It was shown that after 1 hour there was increased labelling of fibroblasts, osteoblasts and cementoblasts which reached a peak after 2 to 3 days. The increase in cellular activity continued in osteoblasts and fibroblasts for 30 days (the end of the experiment) while the cementoblast layer returned to its normal level after 25 days (276, 277).

Moderate or intense periapical inflammation has been found to lead to a breakdown of PDL fibers and resorption of the root apex and bone, resulting in an expansion of the PDL space or a periapical rarefaction (226–233) (Fig. 2.24). This resorption response has been found to be related to the presence of bacteria and their toxins in the root canal (286–295). This is supported by experiments in germ-free or conventional rats (617). The stimulus for osteoclastic activity affecting the root surface and alveolar bone appears to be a combination of a direct influence of bacteria and their toxins and an indirect influence on the osteoclast in response to inflammatory changes (224, 274, 296, 297) (Fig. 2.26). The cell population in the PDL, however, appears to be rather resistant to infection in the sense that, when infection has been eliminated, the PDL usually returns to normal. This phenomenon has been found in the marginal periodontium (298, 299), in the apical periodontium (300, 301) and in situations involving the entire PDL, such as after osteomyelitis (302). However, if the infection is not completely eradicated, chronic inflammation will develop and allow only minimal cementum and PDL repair (277, 303).

PDL healing after initial root resorption or surgical injury to the root surface is influenced by a number of factors including age, size of lesion, functional stimuli, but usually leads to healing with new formation of cementum and new inserting fibres (304). The process of healing is under control of a series of extracellular matrix, glycoproteins, growth factors and cytochines in a very complex process (for a survey see Amar 1996 (305)).

The presence of bacteria in the root canal and dentinal tubules has been shown experimentally to interfere with the

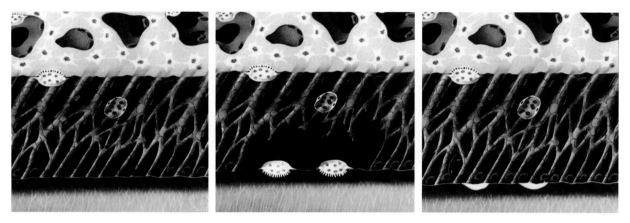

**Fig. 2.23** Pathogenesis of surface resorption (repair-related resorption): healing with minor injury to the periodontal ligament. The injury site is resorbed by macrophages and osteoclasts. The osteoclasts have exposed factors and other soluble molecules in dentin such as IGF-1, TGF-β, PDGF, BMPs, FGF-2 and A4 (amelogenin gene splice products). These molecules may serve as stimulators for cementoblasts (489). Subsequent repair takes place by the formation of new cementum and Sharpey's fibers.

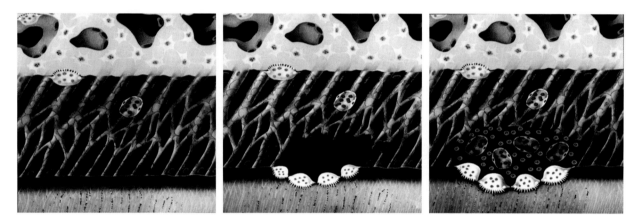

**Fig. 2.24** Pathogenesis of inflammatory resorption (infection-related resorption): healing with moderate or extensive injury to the periodontal ligament and associated infection in the pulp and/or dentinal tubules. The initial injury to the root surface triggers a macrophage and osteoclast attack on the root surface. Osteoclasts have exposed toxins from bacteria located in the root canal and dentinal tubules such as LPS (lipopolysaccharide), MDP (muramyl dipeptide) and LTA (lipoteichoic acid). These toxins serve as direct activators for osteoclastic activity. The resorption process is accelerated and granulation tissue ultimately invades the root canal.

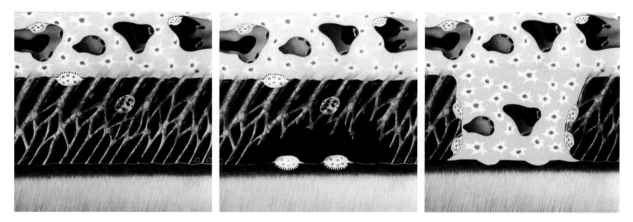

**Fig. 2.25** Pathogenesis of replacement resorption (ankylosis-related resorption): healing after extensive injury to the periodontal ligament. The osteoclasts have exposed factors and other soluble molecules in dentin such as IGF-1, TGF-β, PDGF, BMPs, FGF-2 and A4 (amelogenin gene splice products). These molecules may serve as stimulators for osteoclasts and/or bone formation (532). Ankylosis is formed because healing occurs almost exclusively by cells from the alveolar wall.

expected normal healing process with new deposition of cementum and reformation of PDL fibres. Instead a chronic inflammation occurs with osteoclastic activity and cementum repair becomes restricted (306, 307). The presence of

an intact cementum layer apparently prevents toxins and bacteria from interfering with healing.

With regard to periodontal apical healing, after endodontic treatment of an infected root canal a large study in

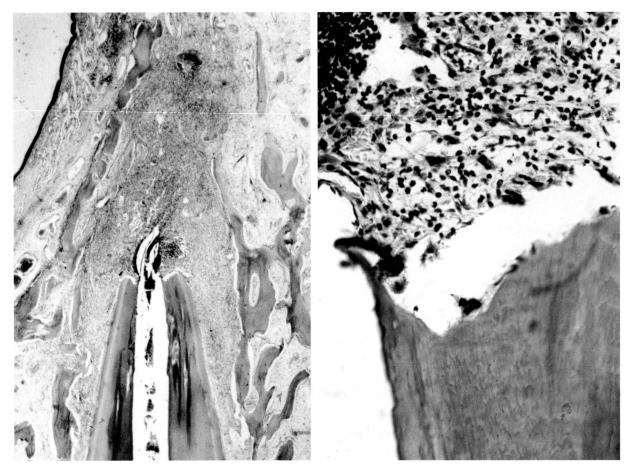

**Fig. 2.26** Periapical inflammation and apical root resorption subsequent to pulp necrosis in a replanted permanent monkey incisor. ×10 and ×100.

monkeys has shown that presence of bacteria in the canal after root filling results in significantly lower healing frequency (21% versus 72%) (618).

## Alveolar bone and marrow complex

The alveolar process may be defined as the tooth-supporting region of the mandible or maxilla (Fig. 2.27). It is made up of three components: (1) the *alveolar bone proper*, consisting of a thin plate of bone which provides attachment for either the dental follicle or the principal fibers of the PDL (308), (2) the *cortical bone plates* which form the outer and inner plates of the alveolar process, and (3) the *cancellous bone* and *bone marrow* which occupy the area between the cortical bone plates and the alveolar bone proper.

The *alveolar bone proper* consists of a thin, perforated bone plate which appears radiographically as a radiopaque lining around the radiolucent PDL space (i.e. lamina dura). The perforations in the socket wall function as gateways for vascular channels that supply the periodontal ligament (309) (see p. 83).

The *cortical bone plates* form the lateral borders of the alveolar process and are usually much thinner in the maxilla than in the mandible. In the incisor and canine regions, there is usually no cancellous bone or bone marrow to sep-

arate the lamina dura from the cortical plates, and this results in a fusion of these structures. For this reason, lateral luxation of maxillary incisors produces a combined fracture of the lamina dura and the cortical bone plate.

The *cancellous bone* consists of thin bone trabeculae which encircle the bone marrow. These trabeculae are lined with a delicate layer of connective tissue cells, the endosteum. The bone marrow consists of a reticulate tissue in which cells representing different stages of hematogenesis occupy the mesh (*red bone marrow*). If the hematopoietic cells disappear, the reticulate tissue is replaced either by adipose tissue (*yellow bone marrow*) or, as in some areas in the alveolar process, by fibrous tissue (*fibrous bone marrow*) (310). The exact topographical distribution of the various types of bone marrow in humans has not yet been documented.

As previously mentioned, the primary function of the *alveolar process* is to protect and support the dentition. More specifically, the alveolar bone proper protects the developing tooth and later provides an anchorage for the fibers of the PDL (311). Apart from its hemopoietic function, the *bone marrow* plays an important role in osteogenesis. Thus, the stromal cells of the bone marrow stroma can manifest osteogenic activity when stimulated by trauma (312). Furthermore, bone marrow plays an important role in the defense against infection (295).

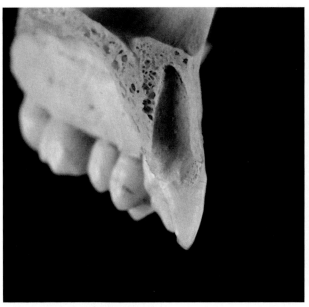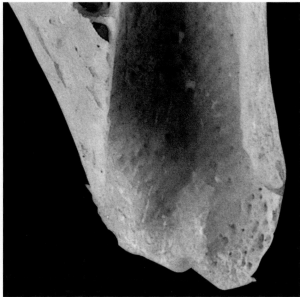

**Fig. 2.27** Anatomy of the alveolar bone. Section through the central incisor region in a human jaw. Note the fused alveolar bone proper and cortical bone plate labially whereas both structures can be recognized palatally. Furthermore, multiple vascular canals perforate the lamina dura.

## Response to trauma

The most common traumatic injury to the alveolar bone complex is the extraction/avulsion or luxation wound with displacement. Furthermore, the bone becomes involved after alveolar and bone fractures (see Chapter 18).

Extensive studies have been conducted regarding socket healing after extraction whereas none has yet been performed relating to tooth luxation. The following is a synopsis of what is presently known about human extraction wounds.

### Histologic evidence of socket healing

The following overlapping stages have been found histologically, based on biopsies from healing of normal extraction wounds in human patients (313–326).

*Stage I.* A *coagulum* is formed once hemostasis has been established. It consists of erythrocytes and leukocytes, in the same ratio as in circulating blood, entrapped in a mesh of precipitated fibrin.

*Stage II. Granulation tissue* is formed along the socket walls 2–3 days postoperatively and is characterized by proliferating endothelial cells, capillaries and many leukocytes. PDL ligament fibroblast appears to immigrate into the coagulum and differentiate into osteoblasts (327). Within 7 days, granulation tissue has usually replaced the coagulum.

*Stage III. Connective tissue* formation begins peripherally and, within 20 days postoperatively, replaces granulation tissue. This newly-formed connective tissue comprises cells, collagen and reticular fibers dispersed in a metachromatic ground substance.

*Stage IV. Bone development* begins 7 days postoperatively. It starts peripherally, at the base of the alveolus. The major contributors to alveolar healing appear to be cancellous bone and bone marrow while the remaining PDL apparently

plays an insignificant role (327, 328). By 38 days, the socket is almost completely occupied by immature bone. Within 2–3 months, this bone is mature and forms trabeculae; after 3–4 months maturation is complete (324).

*Stage V. Epithelial repair* begins closing the wound 4 days after extraction and is usually complete after 24 days.

Finally, it should be mentioned that socket healing has been found to be significantly influenced by the age of the individual (315, 325). Thus, histological alveolar socket repair is more active 10 days postoperatively in individuals in the 2nd decade of life, while the same stage of activity is seen about 20 days postoperatively in individuals in the 6th decade or more. However, after 30 days, the healing sequence levels out and becomes identical in the two age groups (325).

Finally, a significant amount of bone remodeling, especially of the labial bone, will take place in the following months (329), a phenomenon which has a significant influence upon timing of implant insertion (see Chapter 28, p. 764).

## Response to infection

The most common situations in which the alveolar bone becomes involved in infection are during marginal or periapical periodontitis (330, 331). As the most frequent complication after replantation procedures and certain luxation types is infection of necrotic pulp tissue, emphasis will be placed on the reaction of the alveolar bone to periapical infection.

Infected necrotic pulp tissue can elicit chronic or acute periapical inflammation. Acute inflammation in the form of a periapical abscess is the response to invasion by virulent bacteria or immune complexes in the periapex (287, 332). Histologically, there is an accumulation periapically of polymorphonuclear leukocytes and disintegration of the PDL. More peripherally, there is intense osteoclastic activity to remove periapical bone in order to provide space for the granulation tissue required to combat infection (333).

The result of a low-grade periapical infection is *chronic inflammation* in the formation of a periapical granuloma. In this situation, the bacterial front is either in the root canal or just outside the apical foramen (334–337). Lymphocytes appear to be the dominant cells in the immediate periapical region, accompanied by polymorphonuclear leukocytes, macrophages and fibroblasts (338–344). This cell population is identical to that of the infiltrate found in advanced marginal periodontitis (331, 345–347). In the capsule surrounding the periapical inflammatory zone, the dominant cell is the PDL fibroblast. Thus the capsule can be regarded as an extension of the PDL (344).

The osteoclastic activity responsible for resorption of periapical bone and subsequent expansion of the developing granuloma is most likely the result of the combined action of breakdown products of arachidonic acids (i.e. prostaglandins, thromboxanes, leukotrines and lipoxines) from phospholipids of cell membranes from leukocytes, macrophages and platelets (340, 348–359). Cytokines released by activated lymphocytes and plasma cells (352–362) include immunecomplexes released by B lymphocytes (349), and bacterial toxins (e.g. lipopolysaccaride (LPS), muramyl dipeptide (MDP) and, lipoteichoic acid (LTA) (363–371). These events are described in detail in Chapter 4.

Periapically, the long-term effect of chronic infection is a change in the bone marrow from predominantly fatty to predominantly fibrous (372, 373). An occasional finding is periapical osteosclerosis, whereby bone marrow is replaced by thickened spongiosa, resulting in a radiodense area (374, 375). The latter reaction is assumed to be the response to a low-grade irritant (infection) in the area. Supporting this hypothesis is the finding that osteosclerotic lesions often disappear when proper endodontic therapy is instituted (376, 377).

In jaw fractures, acute infection in the line of the fracture has been found to be related to a number of different factors, which are described in Chapter 18.

## Dentin-pulp complex

The functions of the dentin-pulp complex are multiple. After tooth development is accomplished the pulp-dentin organ is able to preserve a vital and rigid structure with flexibility which resists the challenge of repeated mechanical forces. At the same time it maintains an important neural sensitivity, and it preserves the ability to produce reparative dentin against noxious stimuli, such as trauma, attrition, abrasion, the progression of caries, and preparation.

Site-specific changes of pulp-dentin are seen with age. The number of odontoblasts decreases, leading to uncovered gaps on the dentin wall. However, continued dentin formation indirectly causes a tendency of crowding and accumu-lation of collagen fibers (31). Dentin continues to be laid down in vital teeth as secondary dentin and tertiary dentin in response to the physical impacts with a consequent obliteration of the pulp chamber, especially in the crown, and it proceeds apically.

## Dentin

Dentin consists of a mineralized organic matrix dominated by a collagen lattice skeleton traversed by dentinal tubules. Dentin contains numerous polypeptides and signalling molecules placed in a mineralized matrix (378–381). The exposure and release of these factors by a direct trauma to the tooth (e.g. intrusion or lateral luxation) or a root resorption process penetrating into dentin may have a potential effect of influencing the activity of a number of cells (e.g. cementoblasts, periodontal fibroblasts and osteoblasts).

### Response to trauma and infection

Any deviation in the composition of the organic structure of dentin may lead to fracture. Thus, teeth in patients suffering from dentinogenesis imperfecta, with its inherent defects in the collagen matrix, have a high risk of tooth fracture (382–384). Furthermore, exposure of dentinal tubules during trauma leads to bacterial invasion with a resultant permanent or transitory inflammatory reaction in the pulp (385, 386, 619). Finally, a weakening of the dentin under physical loads may occur due to early pulpectomy in immature teeth (387, 388). This may be intensified if inflammatory resorption weakens the root structure, especially in the cervical region (388).

In an *in vitro* study using extracted human teeth it has been found that enamel-dentin cracks induced experimentally allowed bacteria propagation to the pulp cavity (389). Based on these findings it was suggested to cover the enamel with unfilled resin in a replantation situation. However, experimental studies in dogs did not favour this approach and the chance of pulp revascularization (390).

## Pulp

The pulp is a highly specialized loose connective tissue with a specific response to traumatic injuries, as well as to bacterial insults (Fig. 2.28). The predominant cells in the pulp are the fibroblasts, which appear as spindle-shaped or stellate cells with oval nuclei and are dispersed uniformly throughout the pulp, except in the subodontoblastic layer. Undifferentiated mesenchymal cells are located paravascularly and can be recognized by their stunted or rounded form and their few, short processes. These cells probably play an important role in pulp repair (391) (see p. 86), and they probably include resident and migrating pericytes (Fig. 2.28, Chapter 3, p. 126).

Odontoblasts are elongated cells subjacent to the dentin. They have a polarized nucleus and processes which extend some distance into the dentinal tubules (392, 393) (Fig. 2.28). Their appearance varies from the coronal to the apical

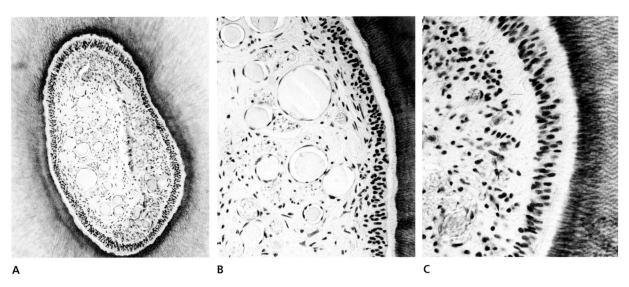

**A**                                   **B**                                   **C**

**Fig. 2.28** Anatomy of the pulp. A. Horizontal section of a pulp from a maxillary permanent monkey incisor. Root development is complete. Note the distribution of the larger vessels and nerves. B and C. The odontoblast layer and the subodontoblastic cell free zone. ×40 and ×100.

aspect of the pulp, being columnar coronally and flattened on the furcal wall and apically. Moreover, their appearance is also related to their functional stage i.e. preodontoblasts, secretory, transitional or aged (394). Odontoblasts have many adhesion molecules, e.g. for attachment, phenotype specification, gap-junctions used for intercellular communication between cells (395), and extracellular contacts with unmyelinated nerve fibres (396).

In the crown, a cell-free layer (i.e. the subodontoblastic layer or zone of Weil) exists that contains a network of nerve endings and vessels which, to a lesser degree, is also found in other parts of the pulp.

The cellular activities of odontoblasts are very complex. Beyond secretion of the organic matrix of predentin and control of calcium and phosphate ion transfer (395), the odontoblast also may release proteinases and degrade organic matrix. The average production of primary human dentin appears to be 3 μm per day during tooth formation and eruption (397). When eruption is complete, dentin formation decreases in the pulp chamber. In the root, production continues unchanged until root formation is complete, at which time dentin production is decreased to an extent that is not measurable over a 3-week period. Dentinogenesis, however, can be reactivated by external stimuli, such as dental caries, attrition and dentin fracture and luxation injuries. The production of new dentin can then rise to a level of that of primary dentin (397, 398).

## Pulpal vasculature

The vascular supply to the immature human dental pulp consists of multiple thin-walled arterioles, venules and veins passing through the apical foramen (399–340). In the mature tooth, vessels can also enter the tooth through lateral canals. The arterioles and venules run parallel to the canal walls up to the pulp horns (Fig. 2.28). En route, they give off branches to form a dense peripheral capillary plexus in the

subodontoblastic layer. A few loops are also found between the odontoblasts (399–403) (Fig. 2.29).

Within the pulp, especially apically, there are many arteriovenous connections (shunts) which facilitate and regulate blood flow (404–405). These shunts are important in the control of tissue pressure. When, during the initial inflammatory reaction, several vasoactive agents are released (see Chapters 1 and 4), these agents cause edema and an increase in tissue pressure. When this pressure exceeds that of the venules, a decrease in blood flow results. The arteriovenous anastomoses in the apical part of the pulp dilate in this situation and carry the blood away from the injury zone (403).

The number of vessels entering the apical foramen appears to a certain degree to be related to the maturity of the tooth. However, the density of the vessels is not in direct proportion to the constriction of the pulpo-periodontal interphase (406).

## Pulpal nerves

The pulpal nerves generally follow the course of the blood vessels (Fig. 2.28). The nerve fibers enter the pulp in multiple bundles that contain both mylinated and unmyelinated axons (407). The majority of the axons (70–80%) are unmyelinated. Both types terminate as free nerve endings. These endings are receptors which respond to various external stimuli, environmental changes, or inflammatory mediators under inflammatory conditions. They respond e.g. as nociceptors to mechanical forces and thermal changes (407). The number of myelinated fibers increases with tooth maturity and, at the same time, the threshold for electrometric pulp stimulation is lowered (408–411).

The innervation of the pulp–dentin border is extensive. A dense network of fine nerve filaments, known as the plexus of Raschkow, is formed close to the odontoblasts. A number of nerve terminals also enter the odontoblast layer and many of them extend into the dentinal tubules. A part of the

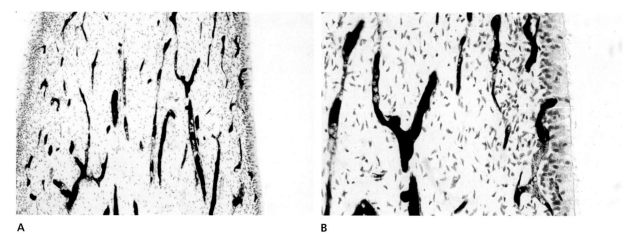

**Fig. 2.29** A. Vascular pattern in the pulp of a permanent monkey incisor as revealed by indian ink perfusion. B. Note the dense network of capillaries next to the odontoblastic layer. ×100.

axons also terminate in the deeper parts of the pulp, and they may have a significant role in sympathetic regulation of blood flow response to trauma, as well as in regulation of inflammation and repair (412, 413). Unmyelinated sympathetic nerves from the autonomic nervous system are associated with vasocontrol, and sympathetic impulses lead to constriction of arterioles (412).

## Tertiary dentin: reactionary or reparative

Extensive physical trauma may result in the formation of mineralized tissue. There is a strong relationship between traumas with their lesion environments, and different corresponding formations of *tertiary* dentine. After injury to the mature tooth, the fate of the odontoblast varies according to the intensity of the injury.

Milder injury can result in a stimulation of the involved odontoblastic cells leading to *reactionary* dentine formation. Upregulation of functional activity in primary surviving odontoblast cells leads to focal secretion of a reactionary dentin matrix in the dentinal tubules and predentin (414). Obturation of dentinal tubules are biologic responses that compensate for the loss of tissue.

Greater injury can lead to odontoblast cell death. Induction of differentiation of a new generation of odontoblast-like cells can then lead to *reparative* dentinogenesis. Secretion of matrix from a new generation of cells implies a discontinuity in tubular structure with subsequent reduction in dentin permeability. The initial repair response often represents a bonelike tissue, i.e. osteodentin, in the pulp chamber. The non-specific response leads to deposition of atubular dentinal matrix covered by cuboidal or polygonal preodontoblast-like cells, and inclusions of osteocyte-like cells are observed in a dense mineralizing matrix called osteodentin. Deep to the pulp injury surviving post-mitotic odontoblasts respond with deposition of reactionary dentin along the walls. In such situations we observe a reactionary dentin matrix with less tubular density than in the primary dentin. The dentinal tubules in tertiary dentin represent

often a mixture between reactionary and reparative dentinogenesis (415).

### *Response to trauma*

#### Repair after pulp exposure

The pulp-dentin organ must respond to a spectrum of traumatic events, such as exposed dentin due to fracture with subsequent bacterial invasion into the tubules (415). The pulp can be directly exposed to bacterial contamination from saliva following a complicated enamel-dentin fracture. Another, and usually sterile exposure occurs during root fracture, when the pulp is exposed to the periodontal ligament via the fracture line. Finally, the pulp may become partly or totally severed and sometimes crushed at the apical foramen or at the level of a root fracture during luxation injuries. These different traumatic insults, all of which interfere with the neurovascular supply to the pulp, give rise to various healing and defense responses ranging from localized or generalized tertiary dentin formation to pulpal inflammation, internal resorption, and bone metaplasia, as well as pulp necrosis with and without infection (416).

The general feature of the pulpal wound healing response is replacement of damaged tissue with newly formed pulp tissue. This can occur along the pulpo-dentin border if localized damage has been inflicted on the odontoblast layer (e.g. after dentin exposure), along an amputation zone in the coronal part of the pulp, or as a replacement of the major parts of the pulp if it has become necrotic because of ischemia (e.g. after a luxation injury). A common denominator of these different events is *replacement of pulp tissue* by the invasion of macrophages, new vessels, and pulp progenitor cells in the injury zone, whereby the traumatized pulp tissue is gradually replaced by new pulp tissue. The exact nature of this process is only partly understood at present (416, 417).

The character of the pulpal wound healing response varies according to the origin of the progenitor cells involved (also see Chapter 1). Thus, in the case of PDL-derived progenitor cells, PDL tissue will be formed with associated cementum deposition along the root canal walls. Moreover, if there is a patent apical foramen, periodontal stem cell progenitors may invade the root canal accompanied by bone formation and inserting Sharpey's fibers.

It has been found that if an accidental exposure of the pulp is left untreated, even over a period of 1 week, inflammation is superficial and limited to a depth of 2 mm. It can be seen at that time that the pulp tissue has proliferated through the exposure site (418, 419) (see also Chapter 22, p. 600). In cases where the entrance to the exposure site is covered with a suitable capping material (i.e. which limits or prevents bacterial contamination), a hard tissue barrier is normally established (420, 421). The cells responsible for the formation of this dentin bridge are apparently not odontoblasts, but most probably include mesenchymal cells located paravascularly that subsequently differentiate into odontoblasts (392, 422–426). This has been shown very convincingly in a study where the odontoblast population was eliminated in rats by colchicine administration. After 3–5 days, revascularization and cell proliferation into the necrotic cell layer adjacent to the predentin were observed. New odontoblasts seemed to develop from paravascular cells and, after initial formation of a non-mineralized collagenous matrix, tubular dentin was formed (427).

The wound healing response to pulp capping has recently been discussed in several survey articles (429–430). The ability to form a hard tissue bridge has been found to take place with a wide range of materials (428).

In the stimulation for a hard tissue bridge the formation of a necrosis and degenerative zone by the capping material appears to of importance (431–434). It has been speculated that this zone may mimic a basement membrane and serve as an attachment surface for components that induce odontoblasts and extracellular matrix production (e.g. fibronectin and TGF-β1) (428, 435, 436).

## Pulp healing after coronal exposure and capping

The events taking place after pulp wounding can be divided into the phases of hemostasis, inflammation, proliferation, and remodeling. Wound healing is, however, a continuous process where the beginning and the end of each phase cannot be clearly determined and phases overlap (440). The observed sequence of initial pulp reactions is that which is expected when connective tissue is wounded.

Fibrinogen exudation takes place under the capping material in the pulp tissue for up to 4 days (441). After approximately 3–6 days the inflammatory infiltration is replaced by a migration of granulation tissue originating from central pulp sites. The granulation tissue is arranged along the wound surface and consists primarily of newly-formed fibroblasts and capillary blood vessels which proliferate and grow into the damaged tissue. Layers of fibroblasts increase in thickness around the lesion. Synthesis of new collagen fibres along the tissue necrosis is detected from 4 days after application of pure calcium hydroxide. Cells sur-

rounded by new matrix including calcifying nodules are found after 7 days (442). The initial precipitation of minerals is associated with detection of matrix vesicles indicating close similarity to mineralization in bone (443). The minerals are found to originate from the blood supply (444). After 11 days the new matrix is associated with cuboidal cells, and some cells with odontoblast-like differentiation. After 14 days a clear odontoblast-like arrangement is observed (445). After one month dentin bridges can be seen around the trauma, which represents a defensive interface between the potential necrotic remnants and the new odontoblast layer (446). Microscopic evaluation, however, revealed 89% of all dentin bridges contained tunnel defects (447).

The pulp healing response replaces injured tissue with newly formed tissue. This can occur along the pulp-dentin border if localized damage has been inflicted on the odontoblast layer (e.g. after dentin exposure), along the wound surface in the coronal part of the pulp, or as a replacement of the major parts of the pulp if it has become necrotic because of ischemia (e.g. after a luxation injury) (416) (see p. 90).

## Biologic effects of calcium hydroxide

Calcium hydroxide containing agents have been widely used for vital pulp capping (442, 448, 449) and the wound healing response to pulp capping has recently been described in several survey articles (428–430).

The effect of calcium hydroxide materials on exposed connective pulp tissue has for decades been studied in experimental animals (450–453) as well as in man (442, 454–456). As experimental animals, the rat has been commonly used (453, 457–462), but also dogs (458, 459, 463, 464), pigs (452, 458) and primates (450, 451, 457) have been used. In comparative studies the conclusion has been that there is no significant differences in the reparative pulp response to calcium hydroxide between the different animal models (458–460). The ability to form hard tissue has been found to take place with a wide range of materials (428) irrespective of their pH (431).

The strong alkaline pH of $Ca(OH)_2$ contributes to its action. In the stimulation for a hard tissue bridge the formation of a necrosis and degenerative zone by the capping material appears to be of importance (432–434). Pulp capping using calcium hydroxide induces also apoptosis in the underlying pulp. Apoptosis is a non-inflammatory controlled cell death mechanism whereas necrosis induces a pro-inflammatory response (466, 467). The balance of apoptosis and necrosis after pulp capping, therefore, may influence the subsequent inflammatory response.

The high pH of calcium hydroxide appears to cause local necrosis of the pulp tissue. $Ca(OH)_2$ may thereby due to its pH effect prevent bacterial infection, and provide a bactericidal environment in which subsequent repair can occur. A few hours after application of calcium hydroxide on exposed pulp tissue an initial necrosis is created and inflammatory cells migrate towards the lesions and the inflammation lasts for a few days (468).

The signaling processes responsible for Ca(OH)$_2$-induced odontoblast-like cell differentiation remains to be clarified (468). It has been suggested that Ca(OH)$_2$ is able to solubilize bioactive molecules with appropriate signaling functions from the dentin matrix (469).

Much speculation has been made concerning identification of factors of importance for a successful outcome of calcium hydroxide treatment of pulp tissue (470). Efforts have been made to find a formula which minimizes the pro-inflammatory actions, and at the same time stimulate dentin bridge formation (468, 471, 472).

Apparently, the rather abnormal appearance of the initial matrix of the dentin bridge, which is usually of the osteo-dentin type, is followed with formation of tubular dentin. During later bridge formation, the matrix structure often becomes more regular, resembling true tubular orthodentin (68).

It has been claimed that the size of the defect, the degree of inflammatory reaction, the control of bleeding following surgical treatment, the amount of clotting, the amount of dentinal chips formed during preparation, the degree of immediate contact between tissue and agent, as well as the formulation of the calcium hydroxide material may play a key role (447, 472–474). Within the last decades several new capping materials have been introduced.

## Biologic effects of new pulp capping or pulpotomy materials

Calcium hydroxide compounds have throughout the years been the golden standard of a capping material but several other materials have also been suggested (437).

*Resin adhesive materials* used for pulp capping have had supporters based on experiments (439, 475, 482). The aim of using adhesive materials has been to minimize microleakage and thereby stimulate bridging. Recently criticism has been raised concerning their use, based on an analysis of human teeth treated with various resin adhesive systems showing poor results (438, 477, 478) (Fig. 2.30). Studies *in vitro* suggest components of the resin may inhibit odontoblast differentiation (614).

*MTA®* (mineral trioxide aggregate) has recently been shown in animal experiments to be a pulp capping material which consistently produces a hard tissue barrier (480, 481). The composition of MTA® is very similar to Portland cement and as such the material sets in a moist environment. During the setting reaction calcium hydroxide ions are released and a high alkalinity is present in the exposed area. Histological studies in animals have shown high sealing ability and hard tissue inducing capacity (482–486). MTA® used as a capping material was found to result in significantly less inflammation than calcium hydroxide (Dycal®). This material has furthermore been recommended for repair of root perforations and as a retrofill material (487–488). At present, MTA® appears to be a promising candidate as an alternative to calcium hydroxide. The clinical use of this material is described in Chapter 23.

Dentin contains numerous polypeptides and signaling molecules which may be released following a trauma. Among the growth factors isolated the following should be mentioned: IGF, TGF, PDGF and FGF, EGF and BMP (489). This is of importance as all of these substances have also been found to be involved in bone and PDL healing processes in animals (see Chapter 1).

*Bioactive substances* appear to represent a new way to stimulate formation of dentin bridges (489–497). Tissue injury leads to alterations in gene expression and release of a range of cytokines including growth factors. Cytokines play a determinant role in regulation of cell proliferation, migration and differentiation during pulp healing. In particular, members of the transforming growth factor beta (TGF-β) family have been implicated in dentin matrix formation (489–500). Nearly half of the TGF-β1 in dentin matrix has been reported to be present in active form (506). However, TGF-β activity decreases with a short half-life (2–3 min) (503) due to binding of active TGF-β to extracellular matrix (504).

A number of growth factors such as (BMP, TGF-β1, IGF, FGF, PDGF and EGF) have been tested in animal models for their capacity to stimulate dentin bridge formation (489–497). Among these TGF-β enhances dentinal matrix formation (497, 504–506). BMP 7 has been found to stimulate reparative dentin formation in rats (507), pigs (508), dogs (615) and monkeys (509, 516). BMP-7 failed to work in pulps with induced inflammation (511). The mechanism whereby ongoing inflammation inhibits dentin bridging remains to be elucidated (451, 512). IGF1 (493) and BSP (513) in rats, and GDF11 in dogs (514) have also been found to stimulate dentin bridge formation. Recently it has been shown experimentally in pigs that Emdogain® resulted in more complete bridges than calcium hydroxide induced bridges (515–517).

A matter of concern in evaluating the many experimental studies performed in rats, dogs, pigs and monkeys is that animal models do not always correlate very well with human studies (430, 437, 438). This implies that material only tested in animals should be considered with a certain skepticism until clinical studies in humans have been performed.

## Anatomy of dentin bridges

The cellular mechanisms in formation of a dentinal bridge have been reported in several studies (518–521). Almost all dentin bridges formed after calcium hydroxide application show multiple tunnel defects (522–524) and these tunnels may lead to microleakage (522, 523). The tunnel defects have been found not to decrease or be obliterated over time (523). The consequence of this should be that a bacteria-tight seal is established over the bridge (see Chapter 22). Furthermore, one of the requirements for potential new capping materials should be that they create a fast and thick dentin bridge with a minimum of tunnel defects.

Exposure of the dental pulp at the fracture site through a tooth fracture requires formation of another type of dentin

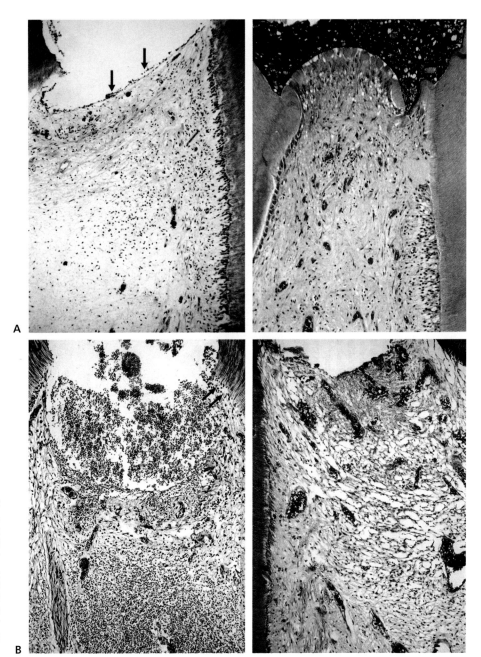

**Fig. 2.30** Pulp response to resin adhesive and calcium hydroxide. A. Human pulp capped with calcium hydroxide. Pulp response after 10 and 70 days. Note calcified barrier and the lack of inflammation. B. Pulp capping with a dentin bond adhesive. No hard tissue barrier is formed and the pulp tissue is necrotic next to the adhesive. After HÖRSTED-BINDSLEV et al. (479) 2003.

bridge. The formation of such a dentin bridge is usually favorable, provided that the pulp is not infected or inflamed.

The prognosis for healing of pulp capping is poor in locations with an inflamed pulp. Pulpotomy should be considered in order to create a wound in an uninflamed location (525).

## Extent of pulpal inflammation related to time of pulp exposure

It has often been cited that the time since exposure of the pulp should dictate the choice of treatment procedure i.e.

pulp capping, pulpotomy or pulp extirpation. However, clinical studies in humans do not confirm these statements (526). This may be explained by the nature of the inflammatory process occurring after pulp exposure. Thus it has been found in monkeys that there was only a moderate inflammatory invasion in the pulp after 1 week (527, 528). In a recent study in dogs the mean depths of inflammation were found to be 4.6 and 3.9 mm after 2 and 3 days, respectively (529) and based on these findings an easy treatment was indicated for humans. Again this statement is not supported by clinical evidence in humans (526, 530) and may represent specific experimental circumstances in pulp healing in the dog model.

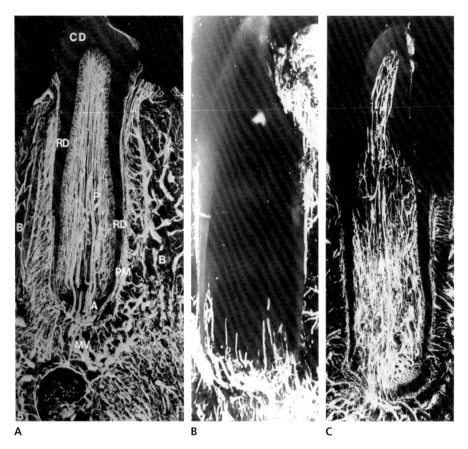

**Fig. 2.31** Ingrowth of vessels in the pulp after immediate replantation of an immature tooth in a dog demonstrated by a microangiographic technique. A. Control tooth. B. After 4 days, revascularization has begun in the apical portion of the pulp. C. After 3 weeks, revascularization is complete. From SKOGLUND et al. (531) 1978.

A                                    B                                    C

## Repair or regeneration of pulp due to luxation injuries or avulsion and replantation

Several clinical studies have shown that a pulp may heal after injuries where a complete severance of the neurovascular supply has taken place (see Chapters 13 and 17). The histological events during revascularization are also described in these chapters.

Luxation injuries usually imply total or complete severance of the neurovascular supply. The ensuing ischemia affects all cells in the pulp. The healing processes begin apically, move coronally and are highly dependent upon the size of the pulpo-periodontal interface (i.e. stage of root development) (607, 608). The outcome of pulpal severance will be either total pulpal revascularization (Fig. 2.31) or the development of partial or total pulp necrosis, usually determined by the presence or absence of bacteria in the injury zone. Revascularization of the pulp appears to have started after 4 days (270, 531) but no experiments have been done to examine exactly when it starts (Fig. 2.31). In some cases of successful revascularization, an intact odontoblast layer will be found with an apparent continuity of the odontoblastic processes (Fig. 2.32). The mechanism of this is speculative, but end-to-end anastomoses in the ruptured apical vascular supply is a possibility (531, 532) (Fig. 2.33).

Vascular alterations and inflammatory cell infiltration are activated in order to eliminate the irritating molecules.

Adhesion molecule interactions between blood leukocytes and endothelium enables transmigration of inflammatory cells from inside to outside the vessel wall (533). Failure to resolve inflammation after wounding leads to chronic non-healing wounds (534), and pulp tissue responds similarly with absence of hard tissue healing. The mechanism whereby foregoing inflammation may inhibit tissue repair (512) and potentially influence gene activity necessary for stem cell recruitment remains to be elucidated.

In the case of an invasion of PDL-derived progenitor cells into the root canal, connective tissue will form in association with cementum deposition along the root canal walls. Dependent on a patent apical foramen, bone may invade the root canal accompanied by inserting Sharpey's fibers.

The character of the pulpal wound healing response varies according to the origin of the progenitor cells involved (see Chapter 1). Thus, in the case of PDL-derived progenitor cells, PDL tissue will be formed with associated cementum deposition along the root canal walls. Moreover, if there is a patent apical foramen, periodontal stem cell progenitors may invade the root canal accompanied by bone formation and inserting Sharpey's fibers.

The source of the repopulating endothelial cells is variable (535). In most cases, osteo-dentin, bone or cementum-like tissue is formed on the canal walls as a response to the pulpal injury. The reasons for these varying responses have not yet been clarified.

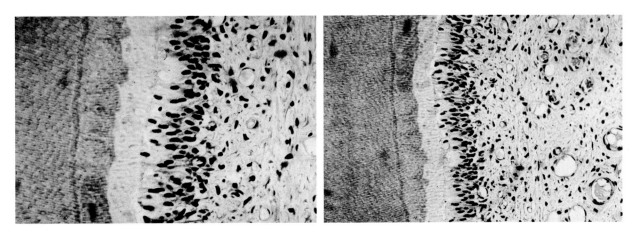

**Fig. 2.32** Continued dentin formation in a replanted permanent maxillary central incisor in a monkey. Observation period 8 weeks. Note continued dentinogenesis after replantation. Only a slight change in the direction of the dentinal tubules indicates the time of replantation. An average daily production of 2 µm of dentin was formed in the observation period. ×25 and ×50.

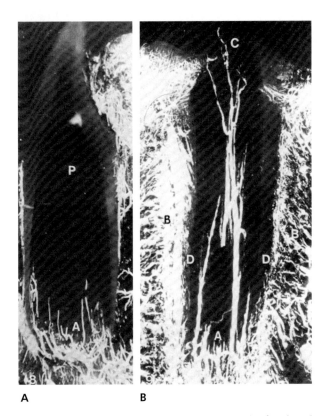

A                B

**Fig. 2.33** End-to-end anastomosis. A. Microangiograph of replanted mandibular third incisor in a dog, 4 days postoperatively. A few tiny vessels are seen in the apical region (A) of the pulp (P). B. Microangiograph of replanted first maxillary premolar, 4 days postoperatively. Some slender vessels are visible in the apical region of the pulp, but, in addition, a few larger vessels are seen running all the way to the coronal pulp. From SKOGLUND et al. (531) 1978.

Dentin formation after revascularization is usually very extensive and may soon lead to total pulp canal obliteration. In replanted or transplanted monkey incisors observed for 9 months, it was found that the average daily dentin production was 4 µm (25) (Fig. 2.34). The explanation for this accelerated dentin production is presumably a loss of autonomic and/or sensory nervous control of the pulp tissue (536–549).

## Response to infection

An untreated dentin fracture is a possible pathway for pulpal infection following bacterial invasion of the dentinal tubules. Pulpal reactions to crown fracture will be further described in Chapters 10 and 22. If the vascular supply to the pulp is intact and the bacterial insult moderate, the event will result in tertiary dentin formation and the pulp will survive (385, 386). However, if bacteria gain access to the pulp via dentin tubules, as in the case of dental caries or a crown fracture, where pulpal vascularity is in any way compromised (e.g. a luxation injury) pulpal healing will not take place (550, 551). This is probably due to impaired defense reactions and/or a loss of the pulpal hydrostatic pressure that presents a powerful barrier to bacterial invasion through the dental tubules (552, 553). An alternative route is through the apical foramen via a severed PDL (550, 551). Finally, a hematogenous route (anachoresis) cannot be excluded (554–562). The explanation for this transmission of bacteria appears to be an increased vascular leakage in the tissue bordering the traumatized pulp tissue (563, 564).

An interesting clinical study in humans has shown that the speed of invasion of bacteria in exposed dental tubules is dependent upon the pulp status. Thus in endodontically treated teeth bacteria invasion of up to 2.1 mm was found. In vital teeth bacteria invasion was significantly less pronounced (565). It was assumed that the dentinal fluid in a vital pulp or the pressure of intact odontoblastic processes may be the explanatory factor (565).

An interesting finding is that necrotic but sterile pulpal tissue can persist over a prolonged period (years) without becoming infected (332, 566–568). If the pulp becomes infected in its ischemic state, revascularization is apparently permanently arrested and a leukocyte zone is formed which

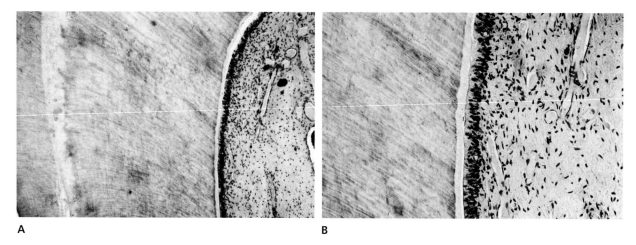

**Fig. 2.34.** Rapid dentinogenesis after pulp revascularization. A. Extensive dentin production after autotransplantation of a permanent maxillary central incisor in a monkey. Observation period: 9 months. ×10. B. An intact odontoblast layer is seen forming tubular dentin. The dentin formed immediately after transplantation is acellular. The average dentin production after transplantation is 4 μm daily. ×40.

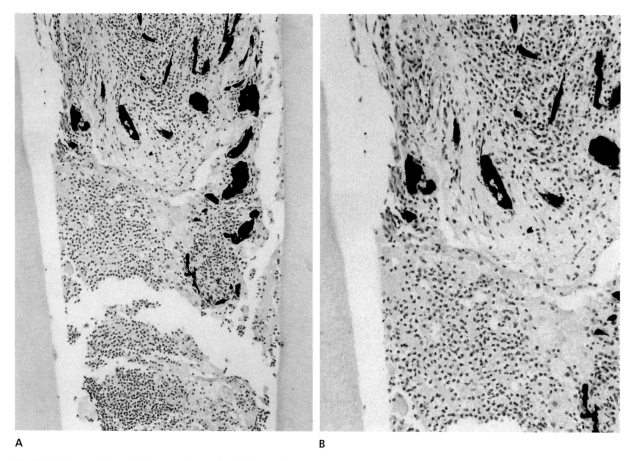

**Fig. 2.35** Infection in the pulp has caused arrest of pulpal revascularization. Status of a replanted permanent lateral incisor in a monkey. A. Low power view. There is autolysis and infection in the coronal part of the pulp. ×40. B. A leukocyte zone separating the infected part of the pulp from the revascularized part. ×100.

separates infected necrotic tissue from the ingrowing apical connective tissue (82) (Fig. 2.35). In these cases, bacteria are found in the necrotic pulp as well as in the leukocyte zone, but seldom in the adjacent vital connective tissue.

The pulpal response to infection differs from the general response to infection by the end-organ character of the pulp tissue, implying limitations in the initial inflammatory response to infection (i.e. swelling) and a restricted access of the defense system to privileged sites for bacteria, such as the dentinal tubules, lateral canals and vascular inclusions in dentin. These anatomical obstructions usually make complete microbial kill impossible. The best compromise is

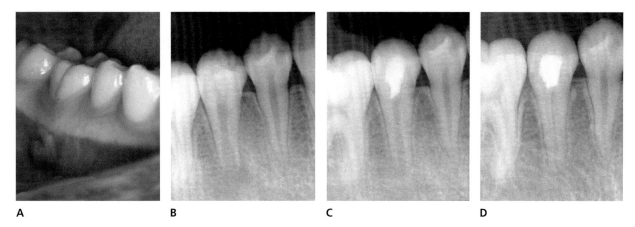

**Fig. 2.36** Revascularization of an immature premolar with apical periodontitis. A and B. Preoperative condition showing a fistula and an apical radio-lucency. C. The root canal was opened and the superficial part of the canal cleaned. The tooth was left open. At the following visits the upper part of the root canal was irrigated using 5% sodium hypoclorite and 3% hydrogen peroxide. Antimicrobial agents (metronidazole and ciprofloxacin) were placed into the root canal. The root canal was not mechanically cleaned during the treatment period (B). At the fifth visit, the existence of vital tissue approx-imately 5 mm apical to the canal orifice was confirmed by visual inspection. A radiograph taken 5 months after permanent closure of the access cavity revealed the first signs of apical closure. A slight increase in thickness of the root canal wall was also observed (C). D. 30 months after the intial treat-ment confirmed complete closure of the apex and thickening of the root wall due to a diminished pulp space. After IWAYA et al. (576) 2001.

usually the creation of a barrier against microorganisms, either by granulation tissue, hard tissue such as secondary dentin or cementum or proliferation of epithelium (282, 569–571). Obviously, this type of defense system is not absolute and with a change in the number of bacteria, their virulence, or the level of resistance of the patient, an exac-erbation of the infection may occur.

A specific response may be encountered during revascu-larization of an ischemic pulp if bacteria have invaded denti-nal tubules, as with an untreated dentin fracture. Resorption may then occur in relation to infected dentinal tubules (see Chapter 13, p. 393).

One factor found to arrest the revascularization process is infection whereby bacteria get access to the ischemic part of the pulp. This has so far been considered a definitive step preventing further advancement of the revascularization process. In the late 1960s and the 1970s attempts were made to examine whether removal of an ischemic pulp, steriliza-tion of the pulp canal and inserting or provoking a blood clot in the root canal would result in pulp revascularization, but these attempts were not successful apparently due to contamination of the root canal with bacteria (572–574). In a later study (575) it was found that extirpation of pulps from the apical end of root open dog incisors and subse-quent autotransplantation to another socket in three out of four teeth led to an almost complete revascularization. The character of the new tissue in the root canal was unfortu-nately not reported in detail (574).

A very interesting clinical human case has recently been reported where an immature premolar with an apical gran-uloma was treated with pulp extirpation and treatment of the root canal with antimicrobial solutions and this tooth showed gradual revascularization up to the coronal level and subsequently included gradual canal obliteration (576) (Fig. 2.36). If this technique can be shown to be reliable a com-pletely new treatment modality for teeth with immature root development can become a reality.

In immature teeth the response of Hertwig's epithelial root sheath to infection is also a part of the pulpal response. This response has already been described (see p. 72).

## Oral mucosa and skin

The lips comprise a complex unit of highly vascularized connective tissue, musculature, salivary glands and hair fol-licles (Fig. 2.37). Therefore, injury to this area can affect a number of different anatomical structures in which healing disturbances might arise.

### Response to injury

The main injuries affecting alveolar mucosa and lips are abrasions and lacerations. A combination of laceration and contusion is seen in the penetrating lip wound, where teeth have been forced through the tissues. In this type of lesion, tissue is lacerated and contused and contaminated by foreign bodies and bacteria.

The wound healing response in both oral mucosa and skin has been researched after incision injury (577–580, 609–612) or excision injury (581–595, 613). An excellent review on the healing events in oral mucoperiosteal wound healing has been published by Harrison 1991 (596).

Within 4 to 24 hours after injury, epithelial cells begin their migration from the basal cell layer peripherally to the base of the coagulum. A thin epithelial cover is thereby able to close a simple wound within 24 hours (582, 583). This event is seen earlier in mucosa than in cutis and is possibly related to the moist environment found in the oral cavity (611). By mitotic activity this epithelium will eventually achieve normal thickness.

In the connective tissue, a number of wound-healing processes are initiated. Thus after 2 days, proliferation of endothelium can be observed. A wound-healing module is created whereby macrophages, fibroblasts and capillaries,

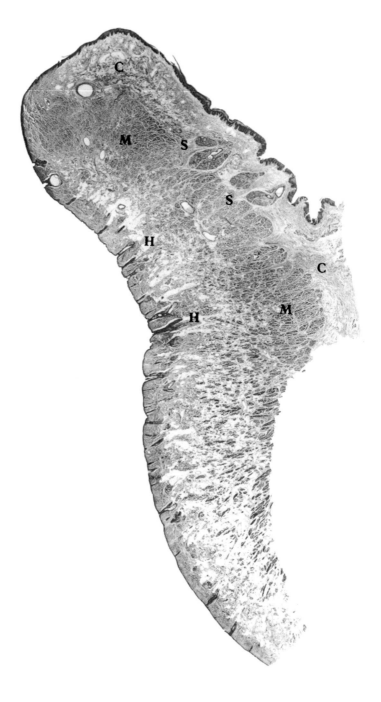

**Fig. 2.37** Anatomy of human lip. H, Hair follicles; S, sebaceous glands; M, musculature; C, connective tissue.

originating from existing venules, invade the injury zone (590). This process will close the wound with young mature connective tissue within 5–10 days. These events are described in detail in Chapter 1.

In general, wound healing processes are facilitated by a good vascular supply, as is seen in the lips; a fact which may explain the relatively rare occurrence of serious complications such as tissue necrosis in this region.

In an experimental study in monkeys, it was found that a penetration wound caused by an impact forcing the incisors through the lower lip resulted in crushing of musculature and salivary gland tissue, as well as occasional entrapment of foreign bodies (plaque, calculus, tooth fragments and remnants from the impacting object) (597). These events imply a complex pattern of healing in the oral mucosa, salivary gland tissue, muscular tissue and skin, simultaneously. The regenerative potential of each of these tissue components, as well as their response to infection, varies significantly. For example, oral mucosa lesions – in contrast to skin lesions – generally heal without scarring, an

**Fig. 2.38 Healing complications after a penetrating lip lesion**
Scarring in a lower lip due to persistence of foreign bodies. The patient has suffered a penetrating lip lesion 6 months previously. Induration is felt in the lower lip and a radiographic examination shows foreign bodies.

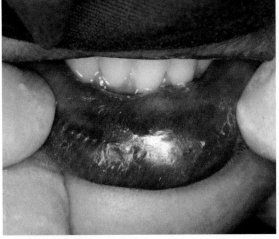 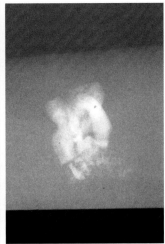

**Removed tissue**
The indurated tissue was removed and a histologic examination showed that it consisted of fibrous tissue and multiple foreign bodies, most likely enamel and dentin fragments. ×10 and ×40.

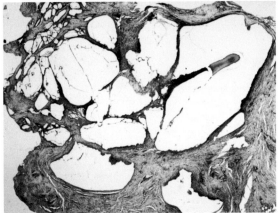 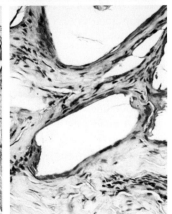

observation which is presently based only on clinical documentation.

Healing of damaged salivary gland tissue is presently not very well researched. However, considering that these cells are highly differentiated, only limited or no regenerative potential can be expected.

Muscle can regenerate (598–606), but this process is often complicated by competition from connective tissue, frequently leading to formation of scar tissue in the lips.

### Response to infection

The incorporation of foreign bodies during wound healing implies a risk of infection by their mere presence, as well as possible bacterial contamination. Furthermore, even sterile foreign bodies usually invoke a foreign body reaction and formation of fibrous scar tissue (see Chapter 1, p. 42). A longstanding chronic foreign body reaction and/or infection may lead to fibrosis which encapsulates the foreign body by a concentration of macrophages or giant cells (Fig. 2.38).

A common foreign body in the lips appears to be enamel fragments. The reaction to these appears to be fibrous encapsulation and a macrophage/giant cell response, whereas resorption by osteoclasts (recruited from the bloodstream) is sometimes found.

## Essentials

### Dental follicle

The dental follicle has some regenerative potential. Severe damage leads to ankylosis and/or disturbances in tooth eruption.

### Cervical loop

This structure has a great regenerative potential after trauma whereby crown and later root formation can usually be completed.

### Ameloblasts

These cells are very sensitive to trauma and infection. Both events usually lead to partial or total arrest of enamel formation and secondary mineralization.

### Reduced enamel epithelium

It has limited, if any, regenerative potential. Trauma and infection may therefore lead to defects in secondary mineralization.

## Enamel organ

The enamel organ is sensitive to trauma and infection; injuries lead to disturbances in mineralization and enamel matrix formation. Short-term chronic inflammation (i.e. months) has very little or no effect whereas persisting inflammation (years) results in disturbances in enamel matrix formation and mineralization.

## Hertwig's epithelial root sheath

This structure can be damaged directly during a luxation injury or indirectly by delayed revascularization due to incomplete repositioning. It has a certain regenerative potential and, depending on the extent of injury partial or total arrest of root development may occur. It appears to be rather resistant to even prolonged pulpal infection.

## Gingiva and periosteal complex

Regeneration of gingival anatomy usually takes place 1 week after wounding.

## Periodontal ligament-cementum complex

Traumatic injury to the periodontal ligament can lead to various types of resorption (i.e. surface resorption, inflammatory resorption and replacement resorption), depending upon the extent of the PDL injury, pulpal condition and the age of the patient. The periodontal ligament-cementum complex is resistant to chronic infection. However, acute infection leads to degradation of PDL fibers. Resorption of the root surface can occur subsequent to chronic or acute infection.

## Alveolar bone and marrow complex

The response to fracture or contusion is resorption of necrotic bone and subsequent osteogenesis. The reaction of bone to chronic infection is bone resorption and formation of granulation tissue which delimits the focus of infection. In acute infection, bacteria spread to the bone and bone marrow where they elicit severe inflammatory changes.

## Dentin pulp complex

The pulp exhibits a repair potential after traumatic injury as long as infection is avoided. This applies to accidental exposure of the coronal part of the pulp, where a hard tissue barrier usually walls off the exposure. In case of severance of the vascular supply to the pulp due to luxation or root fracture, the width of the pulp-periodontal interface is decisive for successful revascularization. If infection occurs in the pulp in its ischemic phase after luxation or replantation, the revascularization process becomes permanently arrested.

## Oral mucosa and skin

The lips have, due to their vascularity, an excellent healing capacity. Scar tissue formation is frequent in skin but rare in mucosa. Acute or chronic infection usually results from penetrating lip wounds due to contamination with foreign bodies.

# References

1. ILLINGWORTH CM. Trapped fingers and amputated fingertips in children. *J Pediatr Surg* 1974;**9**:853–8.
2. GOSS RJ. Regeneration versus repair. In: Cohen IK, Diegelmann RF, Lindblad JW. eds. *Wound healing: biochemical and clinical aspects.* Philadelphia: W.B. Saunders Company, 1992:20–39.
3. ANDREASEN JO, ANDREASEN FM. Biology of traumatic dental injuries. *Tandlaegebladet* 1989;**93**:385–92.
4. TEN CATE AR. Formation of supporting bone in association with periodontal ligament. *Arch Oral Biol* 1975;**20**:137–8.
5. TEN CATE AR, MILLS C, SOLOMON G. The development of the periodontium. A transplantation and autoradiographic study. *Anat Rec* 1971;**170**:365–80.
6. PALMER RM, LUMSDEN AGS. Development of periodontal ligament and alveolar bone in homografted recombinations of enamel organs and papillary, pulpal and follicular mesenchyme in the mouse. *Arch Oral Biol* 1987;**32**:281–9.
7. SCHROEDER HE. *The periodontium.* Berlin Heidelberg: Springer-Verlag, 1986:12–22.
8. FREEMAN E, TEN CATE AR, Development of the periodontium: an electron microscopic study. *J Periodont* 1971;**42**:387–95.
9. HOFFMAN RL. Formation of periodontal tissues around subcutaneously transplanted hamster molars. *J Dent Res* 1960;**39**:781–98.
10. HOFFMAN RL. Bone formation and resorption around developing teeth transplanted into the femur. *Am J Anat* 1960;**118**:91–102.
11. HOFFMAN RL. Tissue alterations in intramuscularly transplanted developing molars. *Arch Oral Biol* 1967;**12**:713–20.
12. BARTON JM, KEENAN RM. The formation of Sharpeys fibres in the hamster under nonfunctional conditions. *Arch Oral Biol* 1967;**12**:1331–6.
13. FREEMAN E, TEN CATE AR, DICKINSON J. Development of a gomphosis by tooth germ implants in the parietal bone of the mouse. *Arch Oral Biol* 1975;**20**:139–40.
14. YOSHIKAWA DK, KOLLAR EJ. Recombination experiments on the odontogenic roles of mouse dental papilla and dental sac tissues in ocular grafts. *Arch Oral Biol* 1981;**26**:303–7.
15. BARRETT P, READE PC. The relationship between degree of development of tooth isografts and the subsequent formation of bone and periodontal ligament. *J Periodont Res* 1981;**16**:456–65.
16. FREUND G. Über die Zahnleisten Kanäle und ihre Bedeutung für die Ätiologie der Follikularzysten und der Zahnretention. *Acta Anat* 1954;**21**:141–54.

17. CAROLLO DA, HOFFMAN RL, BRODIE AG. Histology and function of the dental gubernacular cord. *Angle Orthod* 1971;**41**:300–407.

18. MAGNUSSON B. Tissue changes during molar tooth eruption. Histologic and autoradiographic studies in monkeys and rats with special reference to dental epithelium, oral mucosa, periodontium, apical pulp and periapical tissue. *Trans Royal Dent Sch Stockholm, Umeâ* 1968:13.

19. BERKOVITZ BKB. Theories of tooth eruption. In: Poole DFG, Stack MV. eds. *The eruption and occlusion of teeth.* London: Butterworths, 1976:193–204.

20. JENKINS GN. Eruption and resorption. In: Jenkins GN. ed. *The physiology and biochemistry of the mouth.* 4th edn. Oxford: Blackwell Scientific Publications, 1978:197–214.

21. CAHILL DR, MARKS SC, WISE GE, GORSKI JP. A review and comparison of tooth eruption systems used in experimentation – a new proposal on tooth eruption. In: Davidovitch Z. ed. *The biological mechanisms of tooth eruption and root resorption.* Birmingham: EBSCO Media, 1988:1–7.

22. MARKS SC, GORSKI JP, CAHILL DR, WISE GE. Tooth eruption – a synthesis of experimental observations. In: Davidovitch Z. ed. *The biological mechanisms of tooth eruption and root resorption.* Birmingham: EBSCO Media, 1988:161–9.

23. CAHILL DR, MARKS SC Jr. Tooth eruption: evidence for the central role of the dental follicle. *J Oral Pathol* 1980;**9**:189–200.

24. CAHILL DR, MARKS SC Jr. Chronology and histology of exfoliation and eruption of mandibular premolars in dogs. *J Morphol* 1982;**171**:213–8.

25. KRISTERSON L, ANDREASEN JO. Autotransplantation and replantation of tooth germs in monkeys. Effect of damage to the dental follicle and position of transplant in the alveolus. *Int J Oral Surg* 1984;**13**:324–33.

26. BARFOED CO, NIELSEN LH, ANDREASEN JO. Injury to developing canines as a complication of intranasal antrostomy. *Int J Oral Surg* 1984;**13**:445–7.

27. CAHILL DR. Histological changes in the bony crypt and gubernacular canal of erupting permanent premolars during deciduous premolar exfoliation in beagles. *J Dent Res* 1974;**53**:786–91.

28. MARKS SC Jr, CAHILL DR, WISE GE. The cytology of the dental follicle and adjacent alveolar bone during tooth eruption in the dog. *Am J Anat* 1983;**168**:277–89.

29. MARKS SC Jr, CAHILL DR. Experimental study in the dog of the non-active role of the tooth in the eruptive process. *Arch Oral Biol* 1984;**29**:311–22.

30. WISE GE, MARKS SC Jr, CAHILL DR. Ultrastructural features of the dental follicle associated with formation of the tooth eruption pathway in the dog. *J Oral Pathol* 1985;**14**:15–26.

31. OOË T. On the early development on human dental lamina. *Folia Anat Jap* 1957;**30**:198–210.

32. OOË T. Changes of position and development of human anterior tooth germs after birth. *Folia Anat Jap* 1968;**45**:71–81.

33. ANDREASEN JO, RIIS I. Influence of pulp necrosis and periapical inflammation of primary teeth on their permanent successors. Combined macroscopic and histological study in monkeys. *Int J Oral Surg* 1978;**7**:178–87.

34. ANDREASEN JO. *Traumatic injuries of the teeth.* 2nd edn. Copenhagen: Munksgaard, 1981:304.

35. DIAMOND M, APPLEBAUM E. The epithelial sheath: histogenesis and function. *J Dent Res* 1942;**21**:403–11.

36. SCHOUR I. *Noyes' oral histology and embryology.* 8th edn. Philadelphia: Lea & Febiger, 1962.

37. ANDREASEN JO. The influence of traumatic intrusion of primary teeth on their permanent successors. A radiographic and histologic study in monkeys. *Int J Oral Surg* 1976;**5**:207–19.

38. THYLSTRUP A, ANDREASEN JO. The influence of traumatic intrusion of primary teeth on their permanent successors in monkeys. A macroscopic, polarized light and scanning electron microscopic study. *J Oral Pathol* 1977;**6**:296–306.

39. REITH EJ. The stages of amelogenesis as observed in molar teeth of young rats. *J Ultrastruct Res* 1970;**30**:111–51.

40. REITH EJ, COTTY VF. The absorptive activity of ameloblasts during maturation of enamel. *Anat Rec* 1967;**157**:577–88.

41. YEAGER JA. Enamel. In: Bhaskar N. ed. *Orban's oral histology and embryology.* Saint Louis: The CV Mosby Company, 1976:45.

42. SUGA S. Enamel hypomineralization viewed from the pattern of progressive mineralization of human and monkey developing enamel. *Adv Dent Res* 1989;**3**:188–98.

43. SUCKLING GW, CUTRESS TW. Traumatically induced defects of enamel in permanent teeth in sheep. *J Dent Res* 1977;**56**:14–29.

44. McKEE MD, WARSHAWSKY H. Response of the rat incisor dental tissues to penetration of the labial alveolar bone in preparation of a surgical window. *J Biol Buccale* 1986;**14**:39–51.

45. SUCKLING GW, PURDELL-LEWIS DJ. The pattern of mineralization of traumatically-induced developmental defects of sheep enamel assessed by microhardness and microradiography. *J Dent Res* 1982;**61**:1211–6.

46. SUCKLING GW. Developmental defects of enamel – historical and present-day perspectives of their pathogenesis. *Adv Dent Res* 1989;**3**:87–94.

47. SUCKLING GW, NELSON DGA, PATEL MJ. Macroscopic and scanning electron microscopic appearance and hardness values of developmental defects in human permanent tooth enamel. *Adv Dent Res* 1989;**3**:219–33.

48. VALDERHAUG J. Periapical inflammation in primary teeth and its effect on the permanent successors. *Int J Oral Surg* 1974;**3**:171–82.

49. ANDO S, SAKKO Y, NAKASHIMA T, et al. Studies on the consecutive survey of succedaneous and permanent dentition in Japanese children. Part III. Effects of periapical osteitis in the deciduous predecessors on the surface malformation of their permanent successors. *J Nihon Univ Sch Dent* 1966;**8**:233–41.

50. McCORMICK J, FILOSTRAT PJ. Injury to the teeth of succession by abscess of the temporary teeth. *ASDC J Dent Child* 1967;**34**:501–4.

51. RADKOVEC F. Les dents de Turner. *8 Congrés Dentaire International.* Paris 1931: 210–21.

52. Morningstar CH. Effect of infection of the deciduous molar on the permanent tooth germ. *J Am Dent Assoc* 1937;**24**:786–91.

53. Bauer W. Effect of periapical processes of deciduous teeth on the buds of permanent teeth. Pathological-clinical study. *Am J Orthod* 1946;**32**:232–41.

54. Taatz H, Taatz H. Feingewebliche Studien an permanenten Frontzähnen nach traumatischer Schädigung während der Keimentwicklung. *Dtsch Zahnärztl Z* 1961;**16**:995–1002.

55. Hitchin AD, Naylor MN. Acute maxillitis of infancy. Late sequelae of three cases, including a rhinolith containing a tooth and a compound composite odontome. *Oral Surg Oral Med Oral Pathol* 1964;**18**:423–31.

56. Binns WH, Escobar A. Defect in permanent teeth following pulp exposure of primary teeth. *ASDC J Dent Child* 1967;**34**:4–14.

57. Kaplan NL, Zach L, Goldsmith ED. Effects of pulpal exposure in the primary dentition of the succedaneous teeth. *ASDC J Dent Child* 1967;**34**:237–42.

58. Matsumiya S. Experimental pathological study on the effect of treatment of infected root canals in the deciduous tooth on growth of the permanent tooth germ. *Int Dent J* 1968;**18**:546–59.

59. Turner JG. Two cases of hypoplasia of enamel. *Br Dent Sci* 1912;**55**:227–8.

60. Hals E, Orlow M. Turner teeth. *Odont T* 1958;**66**:199–212.

61. Silness J, Gustavsen F, Fejerskov O, Karring T, Löe H. Cellular, afibrillar coronal cementum in human teeth. *J Periodontal Res* 1976;**11**:331–8.

62. Weinmann JP, Svoboda JF, Woods RW. Hereditary disturbances of enamel formation and calcification. *J Am Dent Assoc* 1945;**32**:397–418.

63. McHugh WD. The development of the gingival epithelium in the monkey. *Dent Pract Dent Rec* 1961;**11**:314–24.

64. Toto PD, Sicher H. Eruption of teeth through the oral mucosa. *Periodontics* 1966;**4**:29–32.

65. Melcher AH. Changes in connective tissue covering erupting teeth. In: Anderson DJ, Eastoe JE, Melcher AH, Picton DCA. eds. *The mechanism of tooth support.* Bristol: Wright, 1967:94–7.

66. Ten Cate AR. Physiological resorption of connective tissue associated with tooth eruption. *J Periodont Res* 1971;**6**:168–81.

67. Kristerson L, Andreasen JO. Autotransplantation and replantation of tooth germs in monkeys. Effect of damage to the dental follicle and position of transplant in the alveolus. *Int J Oral Surg* 1984;**13**:324–33.

68. Noble HW, Carmichael AF, Rankine DM. Electron microscopy of human developing dentine. *Arch Oral Biol* 1962;**7**:395–9.

69. Ooë T. *Human tooth and dental arch development.* Tokyo: Ishiyaku Publishers, 1981:86–94.

70. Diamond M, Applebaum E. The epithelial sheath: histogenesis and function. *J Dent Res* 1942;**21**:403–11.

71. Grant D, Bernick S. Morphodifferentiation and structure of Hertwig's root sheath in the cat. *J Dent Res* 1971;**50**:1580–8.

72. Owens PDA. A light microscopic study of the development of the roots of premolar teeth in dogs. *Arch Oral Biol* 1974;**20**:525–38.

73. Owens PDA. Ultrastructure of Hertwig's epithelial root sheath during early root development in premolar teeth in dogs. *Arch Oral Biol* 1978;**23**:91–104.

74. Andreasen FM, Andreasen JO. The relationship in monkeys between the functional, histological and radiographic diameter of the apical foramen and blood supply to the pulp. In preparation, 2006.

75. Diab MA, Stallard RE. A study of the relationship between epithelial root sheath and root development. *Periodontics* 1965;**3**:10–17.

76. Shibata F, Stern IB. Hertwig's sheath in the rat incisors. II. Autoradiographic study. *J Periodont Res* 1968;**2**:111–20.

77. Andreasen JO, Paulsen HU, Yu Z, Bayer T, Schwartz O. A long-term study of 370 autotransplanted premolars. Part II. Tooth survival and pulp healing subsequent to transplantation. *Eur J Orthod* 1990;**12**:14–24.

78. Lindskog S. Formation of intermediate cementum I: early mineralization of aprismatic enamel and intermediate cementum in monkey. *J Craniofac Genet Dev Biol* 1982;**7**:142–60.

79. Lindskog S. Formation of intermediate cementum II: a scanning electron microscopic study of the epithelial root sheath of Hertwig in monkey. *J Craniofac Genet Dev Biol* 1982;**2**:161–9.

80. Lindskog S, Hammarström L. Formation of intermediate cementum III: 3 H-tryptophan and 3 H-proline uptake into the epithelial root sheath of Hertwig *in vitro. J Craniofac Genet Dev Biol* 1982;**2**:171–7.

81. Harrison JW, Roda RS. Intermediate cementum. Development, structure, composition, and potential functions. *Oral Surg Oral Med Oral Pathol Oral Radiol Oral Endod* 1995;**79**:624–33.

82. Andreasen JO. Relationship between surface and inflammatory resorption and changes in the pulp after replantation of permanent incisors in monkeys. *J Endod* 1981;**7**:294–301.

83. Kenney EB, Ramfjord SP. Cellular dynamics in root formation of teeth in rhesus monkeys. *J Dent Res* 1969;**48**:114–19.

84. Lester KS. The unusual nature of formation in molar teeth of the laboratory rat. *J Ultrastruct Res* 1968;**28**:481–506.

85. Thomas HF, Kollar EJ. Tissue interactions in normal murine root development. In: Davidovitch Z. ed. *The biological mechanisms of tooth eruption and root resorption.* Birmingham: EBSCO Media, 1988: 145–51.

86. Stenvik A. Pulp and dentine reactions to experimental tooth intrusion (a histologic study – long-term effects). *Trans Eur Orthod Soc* 1970;**45**:449–64.

87. Stenvik A. The effect of extrusive orthodontic forces on human pulp and dentin. *Scand J Dent Res* 1971;**79**:430–5.

88. Stenvik A, Mjör IA. Epithelial remnants and denticle formation in the human dental pulp. *Acta Odontol Scand* 1970;**28**:721–8.

89. Stenvik A, Mjör IA. Pulp and dentine reactions to experimental tooth intrusion. A histologic study of the initial changes. *Am J Orthod* 1970;**57**:370–85.

90. Stenvik A, Mjör IA. The effect of experimental tooth intrusion on pulp and dentine. *Oral Surg Oral Med Oral Pathol* 1971;**32**:639–48.

91. Andreasen JO, Sundström B, Ravn JJ. The effect of traumatic injuries to primary teeth on their permanent successors. I. A clinical and histologic study of 117 injured permanent teeth. *Scand J Dent Res* 1971;**79**:219–83.

92. Andreasen JO, Ravn JJ. The effect of tramatic injuries to primary teeth on their permanent successors. II. A clinical and radiographic follow-up study of 213 teeth. *Scand J Dent Res* 1971;**79**:284–94.

93. Andreasen JO. The influence of traumatic intrusion of primary teeth on their permanent successors. A radiographic and histologic study in monkeys. *Int J Oral Surg* 1976;**5**:207–19.

94. Andreasen JO. *Traumatic injuries of the teeth.* 2nd edn. Copenhagen: Munksgaard, 1981:302–4.

95. Anderson AW, Massler M. Periapical tissue reactions following root amputation in immediate tooth replants. *Isr J Dent Med* 1970;**19**:1–8.

96. Andreasen JO, Kristerson L, Andreasen FM. Damage to the Hertwig's epithelial root sheath: effect upon growth after autotransplantation of teeth in monkeys. *Endod Dent Traumatol* 1988;**44**:145–51.

97. Waldhart E, Linares HA. Ist die Zahnpulpa zur Knochenbildung befähigt? *Dtsch Zahnärztl Z* 1972;**27**:52–55.

98. Andreasen JO, Borum M, Andreasen FM. Replantation of 400 avulsed permanent incisors. III. Factors related to root growth. *Endod Dent Traumatol* 1995;**11**:69–75.

99. Cvek M, Rüdhmer M, Granath L-E, Hollender L. First permanent molars subjected to mortal amputation before maturation of roots. I. Roentgenographic periradicular changes and peripheral root resorption after four years' observation. *Odont Rev J* 1969;**20**:119–22.

100. Granath L-E, Hollender L, Cvek M, Rüdhmer M. First permanent molars subjected to mortal amputation before maturation of roots. II. Roentgenologic and histologic study of ingrowth of vital tissue into devitalized, fixed pulp tissue. *Odont Rev J* 1970;**21**:319–30.

101. Stewart DJ. Traumatised incisors. An unusual type of response. *Br Dent J* 1960;**108**:396–9.

102. Rule DC, Winter GB. Root growth and apical repair subsequent to pulpal necrosis in children. *Br Dent J* 1966;**120**:586–90.

103. Barker BCW, Mayne JR. Some unusual cases of apexification subsequent to trauma. *Oral Surg Oral Med Oral Pathol* 1975;**39**:144–50.

104. Torneck CD, Smith J. Biologic effects of endodontic procedures on developing incisor teeth. I. Effect of partial and total pulp removal. *Oral Surg Oral Med Oral Pathol* 1970;**30**:258–66.

105. Tornech CD. Effects and clinical significance of trauma to the developing permanent dentition. *Dent Clin North Am* 1982;**26**:481–504.

106. Lieberman J, Trowbridge H. Apical closure of nonvital permanent incisor teeth where no treatment was performed: case report. *J Endod* 1983;**9**:257–60.

107. Holland R, de Souza V. Ability of a new calcium hydroxide root canal filling material to induce hard tissue formation. *J Endod* 1985;**11**:535–43.

108. Das S, Das AK, Murphy RA. Experimental apexigenesis in baboons. *Endod Dent Traumatol* 199;**13**:31–5.

109. Schroeder HE, Listgarten MA. Fine structure of the developing epithelial attachment of human teeth. *Monographs Develop Biol* 1971;**2**:1–134.

110. Goldman HM. The topography and role of the gingival fibers. *J Dent Res* 1951;**30**:331–6.

111. Arnim SS, Hagerman DA. The connective tissue fibers of the marginal gingiva. *J Am Dent Assoc* 1953;**47**:271–81.

112. Melcher AH. The interpapillary ligament. *Dent Practit* 1962;**12**:461–2.

113. Smukler H, Dreyer CJ. Principal fibres of the periodontium. *J Periodont Res* 1969;**4**:19–25.

114. Page RC, Ammons WF, Schectman LR, Dillingham A. Collagen fibre bundles of the normal marginal gingiva in the marmoset. *Arch Oral Biol* 1974;**19**:1039–43.

115. Atkinson ME. The development of transalveolar ligament fibres in the mouse. *J Dent Res* 1978;**57**:151 (abstract).

116. Garnick JJ, Walton RE. Fiber system of the facial gingiva. *J Periodont Res* 1984;**19**:419–23.

117. Tonna EA, Cronkite EP. The periosteum: autoradiographic studies of cellular proliferation and tranformation utilizing tritiated thymidine. *Clin Orthop* 1963;**30**:218–33.

118. Tonna EA. Electron microscopy of aging skeletal cells. III. The periosteum. *Lab Invest* 1974;**31**:609–32.

119. Tonna EA. Response of the cellular phase of the skeleton to trauma. *Periodontics* 1966;**4**:105–14.

120. Nasjleti CE, Cafesse RG, Castelli WA, Hoke JA. Healing after tooth reimplantation in monkeys. A radioautographic study. *Oral Surg Oral Med Oral Pathol* 1975;**39**:361–75.

121. Hurst RW. Regeneration of periodontal and transseptal fibres after autografts in Rhesus monkeys. A qualitative approach. *J Dent Res* 1972;**51**:1183–92.

122. Andreasen JO. A time-related study of periodontal healing and root resorption activity after replantation of mature permanent incisors in monkeys. *Swed Dent J* 1980;**4**:101–10.

123. Prove MP, Polson AM. Repair in different zones of the periodontium after tooth reimplantation. *J Periodontol* 1982;**53**:379–89.

124. Borden SM. Histological study of healing following detachment of tissue as is commonly carried out in the vertical incision for the surgical removal of teeth. *Can Dent Assoc* 1948;**14**:510–5.

125. Dedolph TH, Clark HB. A histological study of mucoperiosteal flap healing. *J Oral Surg* 1958;**16**:367–76.

126. Kohler CA, Ramfjord SP. Healing of gingival mucoperiosteal flaps. *Oral Surg Oral Med Oral Pathol* 1960;**13**:89–103.

127. Tayler AS, Cambell MM. Reattachment of gingival epithelium to the tooth. *J Periodontol* 1972;**43**:281–94.

128. GRUNG B. Healing of gingival mucoperiosteal flaps after marginal incision in apicoectomy procedures. *Int J Oral Surg* 1973;**2**:20–5.

129. TONNA EA, STAHL SS, ASIEDU S. A study of the reformation of severed gingival fibers in aging mice using 3H-proline autoradiography. *J Periodont Res* 1980;**15**:43–52.

130. ENGLER WD, RAMFJORD SP, HINIKER JJ. Healing following simple gingivectomy. A tritiated thymidine radioautographic study. I. Epithelialization. *J Periodontol* 1966;**37**:298–308.

131. RAMFJORD SP, ENGLER WO, HINIKER JJ. A radiographic study of healing following simple gingivectomy. II. The connective tissue. *J Periodontol* 1966;**37**:179–89.

132. LISTGARTEN MA. Electron microscopic features of the newly formed epithelial attachment after gingival surgery. *J Periodontol* 1966;**2**:46–52.

133. HENNING FR. Healing of gingivectomy wounds in the rat: reestablishment of the epithelial seal. *J Periodontol* 1968;**39**:265–9.

134. STAHL SS, WITKIN GJ, DICEASARE A, BROWN R. Gingival healing I. Description of the gingivectomy sample. *J Periodontol* 1968;**39**:106–8.

135. STAHL SS, WITKIN GJ, CANTOR M, BROWN R. Gingival healing II. Clinical and histologic repair sequences following gingivectomy. *J Periodontol* 1968;**39**:109–18.

136. STAHL SS, TONNA EA. Comparison of gingival repair following chemical or surgical injury. *Periodontics* 1968;**6**:26–9.

137. STAHL SS, TONNA EA, WEISS R. Autoradiographic evaluation of gingival response to injury – I. Surgical trauma in young adult rats. *Arch Oral Biol* 1968;**31**:71–86.

138. TONNA EA, STAHL SS, WEISS R. Autoradiographic evaluation of gingival response to injury – II. Surgical trauma in young rats. *Arch Oral Biol* 1969;**14**:19–34.

139. INNES PB. An electron microscopy study of the regeneration of gingival epithelium following gingivectomy in the dog. *J Periodont Res* 1970;**5**:196–204.

140. HOLM-PEDERSEN P, LÖE H. Wound healing in the gingiva of young and old individuals. *Scand J Dent Res* 1970;**79**:4053.

141. LISTGARTEN MA. Normal development, structure, physiology and repair of gingival epithelium. *Oral Sci Rev* 1972;**1**:63–8.

142. TONNA EA. A routine mouse gingivectomy procedure for periodontal research in aging. *J Periodontol* 1972;**7**:261–5.

143. TONNA EA, STAHL SS. A (3H)-thymidine autoradiographic study of cell proliferative activity of injured parodontal tissues of 5-week-old mice. *Arch Oral Biol* 1973;**18**:617–27.

144. BRAGAAM, SQUIER CA. Ultractructure of regenerating functional epithelium in the monkey. *J Periodontol* 1980;**51**:386–92.

145. WIRTHLIN MR, YEAGER JE, HANCOCK EB, GAUGLER RW. The healing of gingival wounds in miniature swine. *J Periodontol* 1980;**51**:318–27.

146. WIRTHLIN MR, HANCOCK EB, GAUGLER RW. The healing of atraumatic and traumatic incisions in the gingivae of monkeys. *J Periodontol* 1984;**55**:103–13.

147. LISTGARTEN MA, ROSENBERG S, LERNER S. Progressive replacement of epithelial attachment by a connective tissue junction after experimental periodontal surgery in rats. *J Periodontol* 1982;**53**:659–79.

148. WENNSTRÖM J. Regeneration of gingiva following surgical excision. A clinical study. *J Clin Periodontol* 1983;**10**:287–97.

149. SABAG N, MERY C, GARCIA M, VASQUEZ V, CUETO V. Epithelial reattachment after gingivectomy in the rat. *J Periodontol* 1984;**55**:135–40.

150. HENNING FR. Epithelial mitotic activity after gingivectomy – relationship to reattachment. *J Periodontol* 1969;**4**:319–24.

151. MONEFELDT I, ZACHRISSON BU. Adjustment of clinical crown height by gingivectomy following orthodontic space closure. *Angle Orthod* 1977;**47**:256–64.

152. HOLM-PEDERSEN P, LÖE H. Wound healing in the gingiva of young and old individuals. *Scand J Dent Res* 1971;**79**:40–53.

153. HOLM-PEDERSEN P. Studies on healing capacity in young and old individuals. Clinical, biophysical and microvascular aspects of connective tissue repair with special reference to tissue function in man and the rat (thesis). Copenhagen: Munksgaard, 1973.

154. LINDHE J, SOCRANSKY S, NYMAN S, WESTFELT E, HAFFAJEE A. Effect of age on healing following periodontal therapy. *J Clin Periodontol* 1985;**12**:774–87.

155. MELCHER AH. Role of the periosteum in repair of wounds of the parietal bone of the rat. *Arch Oral Biol* 1969;**14**:1101–9.

156. MELCHER AH. Wound healing in monkey (*Macaca irus*) mandible: effect of elevating periosteum on formation of subperiosteal callus. *Arch Oral Biol* 1971;**16**:461–4.

157. MELCHER AH, ACCURSI GE. Osteogenic capacity of periosteal and osteoperiosteal flaps elevated from the parietal bone of the rat. *Arch Oral Biol* 1971;**16**:573–80.

158. HJÖRTING-HANSEN E, ANDREASEN JO. Incomplete bone healing of experimental cavities in dog mandibles. *Br J Oral Surg* 1971;**9**:33–40.

159. MASCRÈS C, MARCHAND JF. Experimental apical scars in rats. *Oral Surg Oral Med Oral Pathol* 1980;**50**:164–74.

160. NWOKU AL. Unusually rapid bone regeneration following mandibular resection. *J Maxillofac Surg* 1980;**8**:309–15.

161. SHUKER S. Spontaneous regeneration of the mandible in a child. A sequel to partial avulsion as a result of a war injury. *J Maxillofac Surg* 1985;**13**:70–3.

162. DAHLIN C, LINDE A, GOTTLOW J, NYMAN S. Healing of bone defects by guided tissue regeneration. *Plast Reconstr Surg* 1988;**81**:672–76.

163. DAHLIN C, GOTTLOW J, LINDE A, NYMAN S. Healing of maxillary and mandibular bone defects using a membrane technique. *Scand J Plast Reconstr Hand Surg* 1990;**24**:13–19.

164. YUMET JA, POLSON AM. Gingival wound healing in the presence of plaque-induced inflammation. *J Periodontol* 1985;**56**:107–19.

165. STAHL SS. The influence of antibiotics on the healing of gingival wounds in rats. II. Reattachment potential of soft and calcified tissues. *J Periodontol* 1963;**34**:166–74.

166. STAHL SS. The influence of antibiotics on the healing of gingival wounds in rats. III. The influence of pulpal

necrosis on gingival reattachment potential. *J Periodontol* 1963;**34**:371–4.

167. STAHL SS, SOBERMAN A, de CESARE A. Gingiva healing. V. The effects of antibiotics administered during the early stages of repair. *J Periodontol* 1969;**40**:521–3.

168. KILLEY HC, KAY LW, WRIGHT HC. Subperiosteal osteomyelitis of the mandible. *Oral Surg Oral Med Oral Pathol* 1970;**29**:576–89.

169. YAMASAKI A, ROSE GG, PINERO GJ, MAHAN CJ. Ultrastructural and morphometric analyses of human cementoblasts and periodontal fibroblasts. *J Periodontol* 1987;**58**:192–201.

170. SELVIG KA. The fine structure of human cementum. *Acta Odontol Scand* 1965;**23**:423–41.

171. ZANDER HA, HÜRZELER B. Continuous cementum apposition. *J Dent Res* 1958;**37**:1035–44.

172. STOOT GG, SIS RF, LEVY BM. Cemental annulation as an age criterion in forensic dentistry. *J Dent Res* 1982;**61**:814–7.

173. ROBERTS WE, CHAMBERLAIN JG. Scanning electron microscopy of the cellular elements of rat periodontal ligament. *Arch Oral Biol* 1978;**23**:587–9.

174. BEERTSEN W, EVERTS V. Junction between fibroblasts in mouse periodontal ligament. *J Periodont Res* 1980;**15**:655–68.

175. GARANT PR. Collagen resorption by fibroblasts. A theory of fibroblastic maintenance of the periodontal ligament. *J Periodontol* 1976;**47**:380–90.

176. DEPORTER DA, TEN CATE AR. Collagen resorption by periodontal ligament fibroblasts at the hard tissue-ligament interfaces of the mouse periodontum. *J Periodontol* 1980;**51**:429–32.

177. BORDIN S, NARAYANAN AS, REDDY J, CLEVELAND D, PAGE RC. Fibroblast subtypes in the periodontium. A possible role in connective tissue regeneration and periodontal reattachment. *J Periodont Res* 1984;**19**:642–44.

178. MCCULLOCH CAG, BORDIN S. Role of fibroblast subpopulations in periodontal physiology and pathology. *J Periodont Res* 1991;**26**:144–54.

179. GOULD TRL, BRUNETTE DM, DOREY J. Cell turnover in the periodontium in health and periodontal disease. *J Periodont Res* 1983;**18**:353–61.

180. MCCULLOCH CAG, MELCHER AH. Continuous labelling of the periodontal ligament of mice. *J Periodont Res* 1983;**18**:231–41.

181. MCCULLOCH CAG, MELCHER AH. Cell density and cell generation in the periodontal ligament of mice. *Am J Anat* 1983;**167**:43–58.

182. LISTGARTEN MA. Intracellular collagen fibrils in the periodontal ligament of the mouse, rat, hamster, guinea pig and rabbit. *J Periodont Res* 1973;**8**:335–42.

183. TEN CATE AR, DEPORTER DA. The degradative role of the fibroblast in the remodelling and turnover of collagen in soft connective tissues. *Anat Rec* 1974;**182**:1–14.

184. CRUMLEY PJ. Collagen formation in the normal and stressed periodontium. *Periodontics* 1964;**2**:53–61.

185. GARANT PR. Collagen resorption by fibroblasts. A theory of fibroblastic maintenance of the periodontal ligament. *J Periodontol* 1976;**47**:380–90.

186. IMBERMAN M, RAMAMURTHY N, GOLUB L, SCHNEIR M. A reassessment of collagen half-life in rat periodontal tissues: application of the pool-expansion approach. *J Periodont Res* 1986;**21**:396–402.

187. BEERTSEN W, EVERTS V. The site of remodelling of collagen in the periodontal ligament of the mouse incisor. *Anat Rec* 1977;**189**:479–98.

188. RIPPIN JW. Collagen turnover in the periodontal ligament under normal and altered functional forces. I. Young rat molars. *J Periodont Res* 1976;**11**:101–07.

189. ORLOWSKI WA. Biochemical study of collagen turnover in rat incisor periodontal ligament. *Arch Oral Biol* 1978;**23**:1163–5.

190. SKOUGAARD MR, LEVY BM, SIMPSON J. Collagen metabolism in skin and periodontal membrane of the marmoset. *Scand J Dent Res* 1970;**78**:256–62.

191. KAMEYAM AY. Autoradiographic study of H 3-proline incorporation by rat periodontal ligament, gingival connective tissue and dental pulp. *J Periodont Res* 1975;**10**:98–102.

192. LÖE H, WAERHAUG J. Experimental replantation of teeth in dogs and monkeys. *Arch Oral Biol* 1961;**3**:176–83.

193. LINDSKOG S, BLOMLÖF L, HAMMARSTRÖM L. Evidence for a role of odontogenic epithelium in maintaining the periodontal space. *J Clin Periodontol* 1988;**15**:371–3.

194. HASEGAWA N, KAWAGUCHI H, OGAWA T, UCHIDA T, KURIHARA H. Immunohistochemical characteristics of epithelial cell rests of Malassez during cementum repair. *J Periodontol Res* 2003;**38**:51–6.

195. SCULEAN A, LIOUBAVINA N, THEILADE J, KARRING T. Absence of malassez epithelial rests in the regenerated periodontal ligament. A pilot study in the monkey. *J Periodont Res* 1998;**33**:310–14.

196. WESSELINK PR. *Disturbances in the homeostasis of the periodontal ligament: dento-alveolar ankylosis and root resorption.* Amsterdam: Joko Offset, 1992:100.

197. ANDREASEN JO. Review of root resorption systems and models. Etiology of root resorption and the homeostatic mechanisms of the periodontal ligament. In: Davidovitch Z. ed. *The biological mechanisms of tooth eruption and root resorption.* Birmingham: EBSCO Media, 1988:9–21.

198. ANDREASEN JO. Summary of root resorption. In: Davidovitch Z. ed. *Proceedings of the International Conference on the Biological Mechanisms of Tooth Eruption and Tooth Resorption.* Birmingham: EBSCO Media, 1988:399–400.

199. ANDREASEN JO, ANDREASEN FM. Root resorption following traumatic dental injuries. *Proc Finn Dent Soc* 1992; **88**:95–114.

200. WESSELINK PR, BEERTSEN W. The prevalence and distribution of rests of malassez in the mouse molar and their possible role in repair and maintenance of the periodontal ligament. *Arch Oral Biol* 1993;**38**:399–403.

201. NAIR PNR, SCHROEDER HE. Epithelial attachment at diseased human tooth-apex. *J Periodont Res* 1985;**20**:293–300.

202. BOYDE A, JONES SJ. Scanning electron microscopy of cementum and Sharpey's fibres. *Z Zellforsch* 1968;**92**:536–48.

203. SHACKLEFORD JM, ZUNIGA MA. Scanning electron microscopic studies of calcified and noncalcified dental

tissues. *Proc Cambridge Sterioscan Colloquium* 1970:113–19.

204. SHACKLEFORD JM. Scanning electron microscopy of the dog periodontium. *J Periodont Res* 1971;**6**:45–54.

205. SHACKLEFORD JM. The indifferent fiber plexus and its relationship to principal fibers of the periodontium. *Am J Anat* 1971;**131**:427–42.

206. SVEJDA J, KREJSA O. Die Oberflächenstruktur des Alveolarknochens, des extrahierten Zahnes and des Periodontiums im Rastereelektronenmikroskop (REM). *Schweiz Monatsschr Zahnheilk* 1972;**82**:763–76.

207. SVEJDA J, SKACH M. The periodontium of the human tooth in the scanning electron microscope (Stereoscan). *J Periodontol* 1973;**44**:478–84.

208. KVAM E. Scanning electron microscopy of organic structures on the root surface of human teeth. *Scand J Dent Res* 1972;**80**:297–306.

209. BERKOWITZ BKB, MOXHAM BJ. The development of the periodontal ligament with special reference to collagen fibre ontogeny. *J Biol Buccale* 1990;**18**:227–36.

210. YAMAMOTO T, WAKITA M. The development and structure of principal fibers and cellular cementum in rat molars. *J Periodont Res* 1991;**26**:129–37.

211. KVAM E. Topography of principal fibers. *Scand J Dent Res* 1973;**81**:553–7.

212. SHACKLEFORD JM. Ultrastructural and microradiographic characteristics of Sharpey's fibers in dog alveolar bone. *Ala J Med Sci* 1973;**10**:11–20.

213. SLOAN P, SHELLIS RP, BEKOWITZ BKB. Effect of specimen preparation on the appearance of the rat periodontal ligament in the scanning electron microscope. *Arch Oral Biol* 1976;**21**:633–5.

214. BERKOWITZ BKB, HOLLAND GR, MOXHAM BJ. *A colour atlas and textbook of oral anatomy, histology and embryology*. London: Wolfe Medical Publications, 1992.

215. SLOAN P. Scanning electron microscopy of the collagen fibre architecture of the rabbit incisor periodontium. *Arch Oral Biol* 1978;**23**:567–72.

216. SLOAN P. Collagen fibre architecture in the periodontal ligament. *J Roy Soc Med* 1979;**72**:188–91.

217. KINDLOVA M. The blood supply of the marginal periodontium in *Macacus rhesus. Arch Oral Biol* 1965;**10**:869.

218. FOLKE LEA, STALLARD RE. Periodontal microcirculation as revealed by plastic microspheres. *J Periodont Res* 1967;**2**:53–63.

219. LENZ P. Zur Gefässstruktur des Parodontiums. Untersuchungen an Korrosionspräparaten von Affenkiefern. *Dtsch Zahnärztl Z* 1968;**23**:357–61.

220. EDWALL LGA. The vasculature of the periodontal ligament. In: Berkowitz BKB, Moxham BJ, Newman HN. eds. *The periodontal ligament in health and disease*. Oxford: Pergamon Press, 1982:151–71.

221. LINDHE J, KARRING T. The anatomy of the periodontium. In: Lindhe J. *Textbook of clinical periodontology*. Copenhagen: Munksgaard, 1983: 19–66.

222. KVAM E. Topography of principal fibers. *Scand J Dent Res* 1973;**81**:553–7.

223. BERGGREN E, SAE-LIM V, BLETSA A, HEYERAAS KJ. Effect of denervation on healing after tooth replantation in the ferret. *Acta Odontol Scand* 2001;**59**:379–85.

224. ANDREASEN JO. Review of root resorption systems and models. Etiology of root resorption and the homeostatic mechanisms of the periodontal ligament. In: Davidovitch D. ed. *The biological mechanisms of tooth eruption and root resorption*. Birmingham: EBSCO Media, 1988:9–21.

225. McCULLOCH CAG. Origins and functions of cells essential for periodontal repair: the role of fibroblasts in tissue homeostasis. *Oral Diseases* 1995;**1**:271–8.

226. COOLIDGE ED. The thickness of the human periodontal membrane. *Am Dent Cosmos* 1937;**24**:1260–70.

227. BOABAID F, BERRY JE, KOH AJ, SOMERMAN MJ, McCAULEY LK. The role of parathyroid hormone-related protein in the regulation of osteoclastogenesis by cementoblasts. *J Periodontol* 2004;**75**:1247–4.

228. OGASAWARA T, YOSHIMINE Y, KIYOSHIMA T, KOBAYASHI I, MATSUO K, AKAMINE A, et al. *In situ* expression of RANKL, RANK, osteoprotegerin and cytokines in osteoclasts of rat periodontal tissue. *J Periodontal Res* 2004;**39**:42–9.

229. RANI CS, MacDOUGALL M. Dental cells express factors that regulate bone resorption. *Mol Cell Biol Res Commun* 2000;**3**:145–52.

230. HAMMARSTRÖM L, LINDSKOG S. Factors regulating and modifying dental root resorption. [Review]. *Proc Finn Dent Soc* 1992;**88**:*(Suppl 1)*:115–23.

231. BRUDVIK P, RYGH P. The repair of orthodontic root resorption: an ultrastructural study. *Eur J Orthod* 1995;**17**:189–98.

232. RYGH P. Orthodontic root resorption studied by electron microscopy. *Angle Orthod* 1977;**47**:1–16.

233. SASAKI T. Differentiation and functions of osteoclasts and odontoclasts in mineralized tissue resorption. *Microsc Res Tech* 2003;**61**:483–95.

234. ZHANG D, YANG YQ, LI XT, FU MK. The expression of osteoprotegerin and the receptor activator of nuclear factor kappa B ligand in human periodontal ligament cells cultured with and without 1 alpha, 25-dihydroxyvitamin D3. *Arch Oral Biol* 2004;**49**:71–6.

235. McCULLOCH CAG, MELCHER AH. Cell density and cell generation in the periodontal ligament of mice. *Amer J Anat* 1983;**167**:43–58.

236. KANZAKI H, CHIBA M, SHIMIZU Y, MITANI H. Dual regulation of osteoclast differentiation by periodontal ligament cells through RANKL stimulation and OPG inhibition. *J Dent Res* 2001;**80**:887–91.

237. TENG YT, NGUYEN H, GAO X, KONG YY, GORCZYNSKI RM, SINGH B, et al. Functional human T-cell immunity and osteoprotegerin ligand control alveolar bone destruction in periodontal infection. *J Clin Invest* 2000;**106**:R59–67.

238. HOFBAUER LC, HEUFELDER AE. Clinical review 114: hot topic. The role of receptor activator of nuclear factor-kappaB ligand and osteoprotegerin in the pathogenesis and treatment of metabolic bone diseases. *J Clin Endocrinol Metab* 2000;**85**:2355–63.

239. BUCAY N, SAROSI I, DUNSTAN CR, MORONY S, TARPLEY J, CAPPARELLI C, et al. Osteoprotegerin-deficient mice develop early onset osteoporosis and arterial calcification. *Genes Dev* 1998;**12**:1260–8.

240. HASEGAWA T, KIKUIRI T, TAKEYAMA S, YOSHIMURA Y, MITOME M, OGUCHI H, et al. Human periodontal

ligament cells derived from deciduous teeth induce osteoclastogenesis *in vitro. Tissue Cell* 2002;**34**: 44–51.

241. FUKUSHIMA H, KAJIYA H, TAKADA K, OKAMOTO F, OKABE K. Expression and role of RANKL in periodontal ligament cells during physiological root-resorption in human deciduous teeth. *Eur J Oral Sci* 2003;**111**: 346–52.

242. YAO S, RING S, HENK WG, WISE GE. *In vivo* expression of RANKL in the rat dental follicle as determined by laser capture microdissection. *Arch Oral Biol* 2004;**49**:451–6.

243. WISE GE, DING D, YAO S. Regulation of secretion of osteoprotegerin in rat dental follicle cells. *Eur J Oral Sci* 2004;**112**:439–44.

244. WISE GE, FRAZIER-BOWERS S, D'SOUZA RN. Cellular, molecular, and genetic determinants of tooth eruption. *Crit Rev Oral Biol Med* 2002;**13**:323–34.

245. HAMMARSTRÖM L, LINDSKOG S. Factors regulating and modifying dental root resorption. *Proc Finn Dent Soc* 1992;**88**:*(Suppl 1)*:115–23.

246. ANDREASEN JO, ANDREASEN FM. Root resorption following traumatic dental injuries. *Proc Finn Dent Soc* 1992;**88**:*(Suppl 1)*:95–114.

247. SCHWARTZ O, ANDREASEN FM, ANDREASEN JO. Effects of temperature, storage time and media on periodontal and pulpal healing after replantation of incisors in monkeys. *Dent Traumatol* 2002;**18**:190–5.

248. ANDREASEN JO. Effect of extra-alveolar period and storage media upon periodontal and pulpal healing after replantation of mature permanent incisors in monkeys. *Int J Oral Surg* 1981;**10**:43–53.

249. ANDREASEN JO. Analysis of pathogenesis and topography of replacement root resorption (ankylosis) after replantation of mature permanent incisors in monkeys. *Swed Dent J* 1980;**4**:231–40.

250. OSHIRO T, SHIOTANI A, SHIBASAKI Y, SASAKI T. Osteoclast induction in periodontal tissue during experimental movement of incisors in osteoprotegerin-deficient mice. *Anat Rec* 2002;**266**:218–25.

251. KANZAKI H, CHIBA M, SHIMIZU Y, MITANI H. Periodontal ligament cells under mechanical stress induce osteoclastogenesis by receptor activator of nuclear factor kappaB ligand up-regulation via prostaglandin E2 synthesis. *J Bone Miner Res* 2002;**17**:210–20.

252. KANZAKI H, CHIBA M, TAKAHASHI I, HARUYAMA N, NISHIMURA M, MITANI H. Local OPG gene transfer to periodontal tissue inhibits orthodontic tooth movement. *J Dent Res* 2004;**83**:920–5.

253. THEOLEYRE S, WITTRANT Y, TAT SK, FORTUN Y, REDINI F, HEYMANN D. The molecular triad OPG/RANK/RANKL: involvement in the orchestration of pathophysiological bone remodeling. *Cytokine Growth Factor Rev* 2004;**15**:457–5.

254. HAYNES DR, CROTTI TN. Regulation of bone lysis in inflammatory diseases. *Inflammopharmacology* 2003;**11**:323–31.

255. ANDREASEN JO. Relationship between cell damage in the periodontal ligament after replantation and subsequent development of root resorption. A time-related study in monkeys. *Acta Odontol Scand* 1981;**39**:15–25.

256. GOULD TRL, MELCHER AH, BRUNETTE DM. Location of progenitor cells in periodontal ligament of mouse molar stimulated by wounding. *Anat Rec* 1977;**188**:133–42.

257. YEE JA, KIMMEL DB, JEE WSS. Periodontal ligament cell kinetics following orthodontic tooth movement. *Cell Tissue Kinet* 1976;**9**:293–302.

258. ROBERT WE, CHASE DC. Kinetics of cell proliferation and migration associated with orthodontically induced osteogenesis. *J Dent Res* 1982;**60**:174–81.

259. GOULD TRL. Ultrastructural characteristics of progenitor cell population in the periodontal ligament. *J Dent Res* 1983;**62**:873–6.

260. MCCULLOCH CAG. Basic considerations in periodontal wound healing to achieve regeneration. *Periodontol 2000* 1993;**1**:16–25.

261. PITARU S, MCCULLOCH CAG, NARAYANAN SA. Cellular origins and differentiation control mechanisms during periodontal development and wound healing. *J Periodont Res* 1994;**29**:81–94.

262. SCHÜPBACH P, GABERTHÜEL T, LUTZ F, GUGGENHEIM B. Periodontal repair or regeneration: structures of different types of new attachment. *J Periodont Res* 1993;**28**:281–93.

263. BURKLAND GA, HEELEY JD, IRVING JT. A histological study of regeneration of the completely disrupted periodontal ligament in the rat. *Arch Oral Biol* 1967;**21**:349–54.

264. MCCULLOCH CAG, BORDIN S. Role of fibroblast subpopulations in periodontal physiology and pathology. *J Periodont Res* 1991;**26**:144–54.

265. ANDREASEN FM, VESTERGAARD PEDERSEN B. Prognosis of luxated permanent teeth – the development of pulp necrosis. *Endod Dent Traumatol* 1985;**1**: 207–20.

266. MANDEL U, VIIDIK A. Effect of splinting on the mechanical and histological properties of the healing periodontal ligament after experimental extrusive luxation in the monkey. *Arch Oral Biol* 1989;**34**: 209–17.

267. MIYASHIN M, KATO J, TAKAGI Y. Experimental luxation injuries in immature rat teeth. *Endod Dent Traumatol* 1990;**6**:121–8.

268. MIYASHIN M, KATO J, TAKAGI Y. Tissue reactions after experimental luxation injuries in immature rat teeth. *Endod Dent Traumatol* 1991;**7**:26–35.

269. ACETOZE PA, L SABBAG YS, RAMALHO AC. Luxacao dental. Estudo das alteracoes teciduais em dentes de crescimento continuo. *Rev Fac Farm Odont Araraquara* 1970;**4**:125–45.

270. CASTELLI WA, NASJLETI CE, CAFFESSE RG, DIAZ-PEREZ R. Vascular response of the periodontal membrane after replantation of teeth. *Oral Surg Oral Med Oral Pathol* 1980;**50**:390–7.

271. ISAKA J, OHAZAMA A, KOBAYASHI M, NAGASHIMA C, TAKIGUCHI T, KAWASAKI H, TACHIKAWA T, HASEGAWA K. Participation of periodontal ligament cells with regeneration of alveolar bone. *J Periodontol* 2001;**72**:314–23.

272. ANDREASEN JO. Interrelation between alveolar bone and periodontal ligament repair after replantation of mature permanent incisors in monkeys. *J Perio Dent Res* 1981;**16**:228–35.

273. EHNEVID H, LINDSKOG S, JANSSON L, BLOMLÖF L. Tissue formation on cementum surfaces *in vivo*. *Swed Dent J* 1993;**17**:1–8.

274. ANDREASEN JO, ANDREASEN FM. Root resorption following traumatic dental injuries. *Proc Finn Dent Soc* 1991;**88**:95–114.

275. BLOMLÖF L, LINDSKOG S. Quality of periodontal healing II. Dynamics of reparative cementum formation. *Swed Dent J* 1994;**18**:131–38.

276. STAHL SS, WEISS R, TONNA EA. Autoradiographic evaluation of periapical responses to pulpal injury. I. Young rats. *Oral Surg Oral Med Oral Pathol* 1969;**28**:249–58.

277. STAHL SS, TONNA EA, WEISS R. Autoradiographic evaluation of periapical responses to pulpal injury. II. Mature rats. *Oral Surg Oral Med Oral Pathol* 1970;**29**:270–4.

278. COOLIDGE ED. The reaction of cementum in the presence of injury and infection. *J Am Dent Assoc* 1931;**18**:499–525.

279. TAGGER M. Behaviour of cementum of rat molars in experimental lesions. *J Dent Res* 1964;**43**:777–8.

280. SINAI I, SELTZER S, SOLTANOFF W, GOLDENBERG A, BENDER IB. Biologic aspects of endodontics. Part II. Periapical tissue reactions to pulp extirpation. *Oral Surg Oral Med Oral Pathol* 1967;**23**:664–79.

281. TORNECK CD, TULANANDAN. Reaction of alveolar bone and cementum to experimental abscess formation in the dog. *Oral Surg Oral Med Oral Pathol* 1969;**28**:404–16.

282. HAIR PNR, SCHROEDER HE. Pathogenese periapikaler Läsionen (eine Literaturübersicht). *Schweiz Monatsschr Zahnheilk* 1983;**93**:935–52.

283. BLOCK RM, BUSHELL A, RODRIGUES H, LANGELAND K. A histopathologic, histobacteriologic, and radiographic study of periapical endodontic surgical specimens. *Oral Surg Oral Med Oral Pathol* 1976;**42**:656–78.

284. WALTON RE, GARNICK JJ. The histology of periapical inflammatory lesions in permanent molars in monkeys. *J Endod* 1986;**12**:49–53.

285. TAGGER M, MASSLER M. Periapical tissue reactions after pulp exposure in rat molars. *Oral Surg Oral Med Oral Pathol* 1975;**39**:304–17.

286. VAN MULLEM PJ, SIMON M, LAMERS AC, DE JONGE J, DE KOK JJ, LAMERS BW. Hard-tissue resorption and deposition after endodontic instrumentation. *Oral Surg Oral Med Oral Pathol* 1980;**49**:544–8.

287. MÖLLER RJR, FABRICIUS L, DAHLÉN G, ÖHMAN AE, HEYDEN G. Influence on periapical tissues of indigenous oral bacteria and necrotic pulp tissue in monkeys. *Scand J Dent Res* 1981;**89**:475–84.

288. PITT FORD TR. The effects on the periapical tissues of bacterial contamination of the filled root canal. *Int Endod J* 1982;**15**:16–22.

289. SIMON M, VAN MULLEM PJ, LAMERS AC, et al. Hard tissue resorption and deposition after preparation and disinfection of the root canal. *Oral Surg Oral Med Oral Pathol* 1983;**56**:421–4.

290. DWYER TG, TORABINEJAD M. Radiographic and histologic evaluation of the effect of endotoxin of the periapical tissues of the cat. *J Endod* 1981; **7**:31–5.

291. PITTS DL, WILLIAMS BL, MORTON TH. Investigation of the role of endotoxin in periapical inflammation. *J Endod* 1982;**8**:10–18.

292. SCHONFELD SE, GREENING AB, GLICK DH, FRANK AL, SIMON JH, HERLES SM. Endotoxin activity in periapical lesions. *Oral Surg Oral Med Oral Pathol* 1982;**53**:82–7.

293. JOHNSON NW, LINO Y, HOPPS RM. Bone resorption in periodontal diseases: role of bacterial factors. *Int Endod J* 1985;**18**:152–7.

294. MATTISON GD, HADDIX JE, KEHOE JC, PROGULSKE-FOX A. The effect of *Eikenella corrodens* endotoxin on periapical bone. *J Endod* 1987;**13**:559–65.

295. WANNFORS K, HAMMARSTRÖM L. A proliferative inflammation in the mandible caused by implantation of an infected dental root. A possible experimental model for chronic osteomyelitis. *Int J Oral Maxillofac Surg* 1989;**18**:179–83.

296. PIERCE AM. Experimental basis for the management of dental resorption. *Endod Dent Traumatol* 1989;**5**:255–65.

297. STASHENKO P. The role of immune cytokines in the pathogenesis of periapical lesions. *Endod Dent Traumatol* 1990;**6**:89–96.

298. KANTOR M, POLSON AM, ZANDER HA. Alveolar bone regeneration after removal of inflammatory and traumatic factors. *J Periodontol* 1976; **47**:687–95.

299. POLSON AM, MEITNER SW, ZANDER HA. Trauma and progression of marginal periodontitis in squirrel monkeys. IV. Reversibility of bone loss due to trauma alone and trauma superimposed upon periodontitis. *J Periodont Res* 1976;**11**:290–8.

300. JORDAN RE, SUZUKI M, SKINNER DH. Indirect pulp-capping of carious teeth with periapical lesions. *J Am Dent Assoc* 1978;**97**:37–43.

301. MALOOLEY JR.J, PATTERSON SS, KAFRAWY A. Response of periapical pathosis to endodontic treatment in monkeys. *Oral Surg Oral Med Oral Pathol* 1979;**47**:545–54.

302. MOSKOW BS, WASSERMAN BH, HIRSCHFELD LS, MORRIS ML. Repair of periodontal tissues following acute localized osteomyelitis. *Periodontics* 1967;**5**:29–36.

303. MERTE K, GANGLER P, HOFFMAN T. Morphophysiologische Untersuchungen der Zahnbildungs- and funktionsabhängigen Variationsmünster der periodontalen Regeneration. *Zahn Mund Kieferheilk* 1983;**71**:566–74.

304. LINDSKOG S, BLOMLÖF L. Mineralized tissue-formation in periodontal wound healing. *J Clin Periodontol* 1992;**19**:741–8.

305. AMAR S. Implications of cellular and molecular biology advances in periodontal regeneration. *Anat Rec* 1996;**245**:361–73.

306. ANDREASEN JO. Effect of pulpal necrosis upon periodontal healing after surgical injury in rats. *Int J Oral Surg* 1973;**2**:62–8.

307. HOLLAND R, OTOBONI FILHO JA, BERNABE PFE, NERY MJ, SOUZA V, BERBERT A. Effect of root canal status on periodontal healing after surgical injury in dogs. *Endod Dent Traumatol* 1994;**10**:77–82.

308. BHASKAR SN. Maxilla and mandible (alveolar process). In: Bhaskar SN. ed. *Orban's oral histology and embryology*. St. Louis: The CV Mosby Company, 1976:234–53.

309. Birn H. The vascular supply of the periodontal membrane. An investigation of the number and size of perforations in the alveolar wall. *J Periodont Res* 1966;**1**:51–68.

310. Weinmann JP, Sicher H. *Bone and bones. Fundamentals of bone biology.* St Louis: The CV Mosby Company, 1955:51–2.

311. Scott J. The development, structure and function of alveolar bone. *Dent Practit* 1968;**19**:19–22.

312. McLean FC, Urist MR. *Bone. An introduction to the physiology of skeletal tissue.* 2nd edn. Chicago: University of Chicago Press, 1961.

313. Amler MH, Johnson PL, Salman 1. Histological and histochemical investigation of human alveolar socket healing in undisturbed extraction wounds. *J Am Dent Assoc* 1960;**61**:32–44.

314. Amler MH, Salman I, Bungener H. Reticular and collagen fiber characteristics in human bone healing. *Oral Surg Oral Med Oral Pathol* 1964;**17**:785–96.

315. Amler MH. The time sequence of tissue regeneration in human extraction wounds. *Oral Surg Oral Med Oral Pathol* 1969;**27**:309–18.

316. Amler MH. Pathogenesis of disturbed extraction wounds. *J Oral Surg* 1973;**31**:666–74.

317. Amler MH. The age factor in human extraction wound healing. *J Oral Surg* 1977;**35**:193–7.

318. Amler MH. The interrelationship of dry socket sequelae. *NY J Dent* 1980;**50**:211–17.

319. Syrjanen SM, Syrjanen KJ. Influence of Alvogyl on the healing of extraction wound in man. *Int J Oral Surg* 1979;**8**:22–30.

320. Boyne PJ. Osseous repair of the postextraction alveolus in man. *Oral Surg Oral Med Oral Pathol* 1966;**21**:805–13.

321. Yoshiki S, Langeland K. Alkaline phosphatase activity in the osteoid matrix of healing alveolar socket. *Oral Surg Oral Med Oral Pathol* 1968;**26**:381–9.

322. Syrjanen SM, Syrjänen KJ. Mast cells in the healing process of the extraction wound in man. *Proc Finn Dent Soc* 1977;**73**:220–4.

323. Syrjanen SM, Syrjanen KJ. Prevention and treatment of post-extraction complications. A comparison of the effects of Alvogyl and a new drug combination on wound healing. *Proc Finn Dent Soc* 1981;**77**:305–11.

324. Evian CI, Rosenberg ES, Coslet JG, Corn H. The osteogenic activity of bone removed from healing extraction sockets in humans. *J Periodontol* 1982;**53**:81–5.

325. Andreasen JO, Sindet-Petersen S. Wound healing after surgery. In: Andreasen JO, Kølsen Petersen J, Laskin DM. ed. *Texbook and color atlas of tooth impactions.* Copenhagen: Munksgaard, 1996:440–61.

326. Gergely E, Bartha N. Die Wirkung der in der Extractionswunde gebliebenen Wurzelhautreste auf den Heilungsverlauf. *Dtsch Stomatol* 1961;**11**:494–8.

327. Lin W-L, McCulloch CAG, Cho M-I. Differentiation of periodontal ligament fibroblasts into osteoblasts during socket healing after tooth extraction in the rat. *Anat Rec* 1994;**240**:492–506.

328. Simpson HE. The healing of extraction wounds. *Br Dent J* 1969;**126**:555–7.

329. Schropp L, Wenzel A, Kostopoulos L, Karring T. Bone healing and soft tissue contour changes following single-tooth extraction: a clinical and radiographic 12-months prospective study. *Int J Periodont Restor Dent* 2003;**4**:313–23.

330. Guggenheim B, Schroeder HE. Reactions in the periodontium to continuous antigenic stimulation in sensitized gnotobiotic rats. *Infect Immun* 1974;**10**:565–77.

331. Page RC, Schroeder HE. Pathogenesis of inflammatory periodontal disease. *Lab Invest* 1976;**33**:235–49.

332. Sundqvist G. Bacteriological studies of necrotic dental pulps. Thesis. Umeå: Umeå University-Odontological Faculty, 1976.

333. Fish EW. Bone Infection. *J Am Dent Assoc* 1939;**26**:691–712.

334. Möller AJR. Microbiological examination of root canals and periapical tissues of human teeth. Thesis. Odontologisk Tidsskrift (Special Issue) 1966;**74**:1–380.

335. Andreasen JO, Rud J. A histobacteriologic study of dental and periapical structures after endodontic surgery. *Int J Oral Surg* 1972;**1**:272–81.

336. Walton RE. Histological evaluation of the presence of bacteria in induced periapical lesions in monkeys. *J Endod* 1992;**18**:216–21.

337. Langeland K, Block RM, Grossman LI. A histopathologic and histobacteriologic study of 35 periapical endodontic surgical speciments. *J Endod* 1977;**3**:8–23.

338. Torabinejad M, Kiger RD. Experimentally induced alterations in periapical tissues of the cat. *J Dent Res* 1980;**59**:87–96.

339. Torabinejad M, Kettering JD. Identification and relative concentration B and T lymphocytes in human chronic periapical lesions. *J Endod* 1985;**11**:479–88.

340. Torabinejad M, Eby WC, Naidorf IJ. Inflammatory and immunological aspects of the pathogenesis of human periapical lesions. *J Endod* 1985;**11**:479–88.

341. Stern H, Mackler BF, Dreizen S. A quantitative analysis of cellular composition of human periapical granuloma. *J Endod* 1981;**7**:70–4.

342. Stern H, Dreizen S, Mackler BF, Selbst AG, Levy BM. Quantitative analysis of cellular composition of human periapical granuloma. *J Endod* 1981;**7**:117–22.

343. Stern H, Dreizen S, Mackler BF, Levy BM. Isolation and characterization of inflammatory cell from the human periapical granuloma. *J Dent Res* 1982;**61**:1408–12.

344. Bergenholtz G, Lekholm U, Liljenberg B, Lindhe J. Morphometric analysis of chronic inflammatory periapical lesions in root-filled teeth. *Oral Surg Oral Med Oral Pathol* 1983;**55**:295–301.

345. Lindhe J, Liljenberg B, Listgarten M. Some microbiological and histopathological features of periodontal disease in man. *J Periodontol* 1980;**51**:264–9.

346. Yanagisawa S. Pathologic study of periapical lesions. I. Periapical granulomas: clinical, histopathologic and immunohistopathologic studies. *J Oral Pathol* 1980;**9**:288–300.

347. Cymerman JJ, Cymerman DH, Walters J, Nevins AJ. Human T lymphocyte subpopulations in chronic periapical lesions. *J Endod* 1984;**10**:9–11.

348. Klein DC, Raisz LG. Prostaglandins: stimulation of bone resorption in tissue culture. *Endocrinology* 1970;**86**:1436–40.

349. Raisz LG, Sandberg AL, Goodson JM, Simmons HA, Mergenhagen SE. Complement-dependent stimulation of prostaglandin synthesis and bone resorption. *Science* 1974;**185**:789–91.

350. Torabinejad M, Clagett J, Engel D. A cat model for the evaluation of mechanisms of bone resorption: induction of bone loss by simulated immune complexes and inhibition by indomethacin. *Calcif Tissue Int* 1979;**29**:209–14.

351. Matejka M, Porteder H, Kleinert W, Ulrich W, War Zek G, Sinzinger H. Evidence that PGI-generation in human dental cysts is stimulated by leucotrienes C and D. *J Maxillofac Surg* 1985;**13**:93–6.

352. Horton JE, Raisz G, Simmons HA, Oppenheim JJ, Mergehagen SE. Bone resorbing activity in supernatant fluid from cultured human peripheral blood leucocytes. *Science* 1972;**177**:793–5.

353. Luben RA, Mundy GR, Trummel CL, Raisz LG. Partial purification of osteoclast-activating factor from phytohemagglutinin-stimulated human leukocytes. *J Clin Invest* 1974;**53**:1473–80.

354. Dietrich JW, Goodson JM, Raisz LG. Stimulation of bone resorption by various prostaglandins in organ culture. *Prostaglandins* 1975;**10**:231–40.

355. Horton JE, Wezeman FH, Kuettner KE. Regulation of osteoclast-activating factor (OAF)-stimulated bone resorption in vitro with an inhibitor of collagenase. In: Horton JE, Tarpley TM, Davis WF. eds. *Mechanisms of localized bone loss*. Arlington: Information Retrieval Inc, 1978:127–50.

356. Horton JE, Koopman WJ, Farrar JJ, Fuller-Bonar J, Mergenhagen SE. Partial purification of a bone-resorbing factor elaborated from human allogeneic cultures. *Cell Immunol* 1979;**43**:1–10.

357. Fitzgerald M. Cellular mechanics of dentinal bridge repair using 3H-thymidine. *J Dent Res* 1979;**58**:2198–206.

358. Holtrop ME, Raisz LG. Comparison of effects of 1, 25-dihydroxycholecalciferol, prostaglandin E, and osteoclast-activating factor with parathyroid hormone on the ultrastructure of osteoclasts in cultures of long bones of fetal rats. *Calcif Tissue Int* 1979;**29**:201–5.

359. Yoneda T, Mundy GR. Monocytes regulate osteoclast-activating factor production by releasing prostaglandins. *J Exp Med* 1979;**149**:338–50.

360. Luben RA, Mohler MA, Nedwin GE. Production of hybridomas secreting monclonal antibodies against the lymphokine osteoclast activating factor. *J Clin Invest* 1979;**64**:337–41.

361. Dewhirst FE, Moss DE, Offenbacher S, Goodson JM. Levels of prostaglandin E, thromboxane, and prostacyclin in periodontal tissues. *J Periodont Res* 1983;**18**:156–63.

362. Torabinejad M, Luben RA. Presence of osteoclast activating factor in human periapical lesions. *I Endod* 1985;**10**:145.

363. Hausmann E, Raisz LG, Miller WA. Endotoxin stimulation of bone resorption in tissue culture. *Science* 1970;**168**:862–4.

364. Raisz LG, Alander C, Eilon G, Whitehead SP, Nuki K. Effects of two bacterial products, muramyl dipeptide endotoxin on bone resorption in organ culture. *Calcif Tissue Int* 1982;**34**:365–9.

365. Chambers TJ. The cellular basis of bone resorption. *Clin Orthop* 1980;**151**:283–93.

366. Raisz LG, Nuki K, Alander CB, Craig RG. Interactions between bacterial endotoxin and other stimulators of bone resorption in organ culture. *J Periodont Res* 1981;**16**:1–7.

367. Nair BC, Mayberry WR, Dziak R, Chen PB, Levine MJ, Hausmann E. Biological effects of a purified lipopolysaccharide from *Bacteroides gingivalis*. *J Periodont Res* 1983;**18**:40–9.

368. Johnson NW, Iino Y, Hopes RM. Bone resorption in periodontal diseases: role of bacterial factors. *Int Endod J* 1985;**18**:152–7.

369. Miller SJ, Goldstein EG, Levine MJ, Hausmann E. Lipoprotein: a Gram-negative cell wall component that stimulates bone resorption. *J Periodont Res* 1986;**21**:256–9.

370. Yoneda T, Mundy GR. Prostaglandins are necessary for osteoclast-activating factor production by activated peripheral blood leukocytes. *J Exp Med* 1979;**149**:279–83.

371. Bockman RS, Repo MA. Lymphokine-mediated bone resorption requires endogenous prostaglandin synthesis. *J Exp Med* 1981;**154**:529–34.

372. Andreasen JO, Rud J. Modes of healing histologically after endodontic surgery in 70 cases. *Int J Oral Surg* 1972;**1**:148–60.

373. Brynolf I. A histological and roentgenological study of the periapical region of human upper incisors. *Odontologisk Revy* 1967;**18**:(Suppl 11):1–176.

374. Boyle PE. *Kronfeld's histopathology of the teeth and their surrounding structures*. 4th edn. Philadelphia: Lea & Fibiger, 1955:17–19.

375. Bender IB, Mori K. The radiopaque lesion: a diagnostic consideration. *Endod Dent Traumatol* 1985;**1**:2–12.

376. Moscow BS, Wasserman BH, Hirschfeld LS, Morris ML. Repair of periodontal tissues following acute localized osteomyelitis. *J Am Soc Periodont* 1967;**5**:29–36.

377. Hedin M, Polhagen L. Follow-up study of periradicular bone condensation. *Scand J Dent Res* 1971;**79**:436–40.

378. Silva TA, Rosa AL, Lara VS. Dentin matrix proteins and soluble factors: intrinsic regulatory signals for healing and resorption of dental and periodontal tissues? *Oral Dis* 2004;**10**:63–74.

379. Finkelman RD, Mohans, Jennings JC, et al. Quantification of growth factors IGF-I, SGF/IGFII and TGF-beta in human dentin. *J Bone Miner Res* 1990;**5**:717–23.

380. Roberts-Clark DJ, Smith AJ. Angiogenic growth factors in human dentine matrix. *Arch Oral Biol* 2000;**45**:1013–16.

381. Veis A, Sires B, Clohisy J. A search for the osteogenic factor in dentin. *Connect Tissue Res* 1989;**23**:137–44.

382. Wilson GW, Steinbrecher M. Heriditary hypoplasia of the dentin. *J Am Dent Ass* 1929;**16**:866–86.

383. Hodge HC. Correlated clinical and structural study of hereditary opalescent dentin. *J Dent Res* 1936;**15**:316–17.

384. OVERVAD H. Et tilfälde af osteogenesis imperfecta med dentinogenesis imperfecta. *Tandlaegebladet* 1969;**73**:840–50.

385. BRÄNNSTRÖM M. Observations on exposed dentine and the corresponding pulp tissue. A preliminary study with replica and routine histology. *Odont Rev J* 1962;**13**:235–45.

386. BRÄNNSTRÖM M, ÅSTRÖM A. A study on the mechanism of pain elicited from the dentin. *J Dent Res* 1964;**43**:619–25.

387. FUSAYAMA T, MAEDA T. Effect of pulpectomy on dentin hardness. *J Dent Res* 1969;**48**:452–60.

388. CVEK M. Prognosis of luxated non-vital maxillary incisors treated with calcium hydroxide and filled with guttapercha. A retrospective clinical study. *Endod Dent Traumatol* 1992;**8**:45–55.

389. LOVE RM. Bacterial penetration of the root canal of intact incisor teeth after a simulated traumatic injury. *Endod Dent Traumatol* 1996;**12**:289–93.

390. YANPISET K, TROPE M. Pulp revascularization of replanted immature dog teeth after different treatment methods. *Endod Dent Traumatol* 2000;**16**:221–7

391. BAUME LJ. The biology of pulp and dentine. A historic, terminologic-taxonomic, histologic-biochemical, embryonic and clinical survey. *Monographs Oral Science* 1980;**8**:1–220.

392. RUCH JV. Odontoblast differentiation and the formation of the odontoblast layer. *J Dent Res* 1945;**64**:489–98.

393. HOLLAND GR. The odontoblast process: form and function. *J Dent Res* 1985;**64**:499–514.

394. COUVE E. Ultrastructural changes during the life cycle of human odontoblasts. *Arch Oral Biol* 1986;**31**: 643–51.

395. FRANK RM, NALBANDIAN J. Development of dentine and pulp. In: Berkowitz BKB, Boyde A, Frank RM, et al. eds. *Teeth*. Berlin: Springer-Verlag, 1989:73–171.

396. KOLING A, RASK-ANDERSEN H. Membrane junctions between odontoblasts and associated cells. A freeze-fracture study of the human odontoblastic cell layer with special reference to its nerve supply. *Acta Odontol Scand* 1984;**42**:13–22.

397. MELSEN B, MELSEN F, RÖLLING I. Dentin formation rate in human teeth. *Calcif Tissue Res* 1977;**24**:*(Suppl)*:Abstr no 62.

398. STANLEY HR, WHITE CL, McCRAY L. The rate of tertiary (reparative) dentine formation in the human tooth. *Oral Surg Oral Med Oral Pathol* 1966;**21**:180–9.

399. KRAMER IHR, RUSSELL LH. Observations on the vascular architecture of the dental pulp. *J Dent Res* 1956;**35**:957.

400. KRAMER IRH. The vascular architecture of the human dental pulp. *Arch Oral Biol* 1960;**2**:177–89.

401. SAUNDERS RL. X-ray microscopy of the periodontal and dental pulp vessels in the monkey and in man. *Oral Surg Oral Med Oral Pathol* 1966;**22**:503–18.

402. TAKAHASHI K, KISHI Y, KIM S. Scanning electron microscope study of the blood vessels of dog pulp using corrosion resin casts. *J Endod* 1982;**8**:131–5.

403. KIM S. Microcirculation of the dental pulp in health and disease. *J Endod* 1985;**11**:465–71.

404. KIM S. Regulation of pulpal blood flow. *J Dent Res* 1985;**64**:590–6.

405. HEYERAAS KJ. Pulpal, microvascular, and tissue pressure. *J Dent Res* 1985;**64**:585–9.

406. LÖVSCHALL H, FEJERSKOV O, JOSEPHSEN K. Age-related and site-specific changes of pulp histology in Wistar rat molar. *Arch Oral Biol* 2002;**47**:361–7.

407. DAHL E, MJÖR IA. The structure and distribution of nerves in the pulp-dentin organ. *Acta Odontol Scand* 1973;**31**:349–56.

408. BERNICK S. Differences in nerve distribution between erupted and non-erupted human teeth. *J Dent Res* 1964;**43**:406–11.

409. FULLING H-J, ANDREASEN JO. Influence of maturation status and tooth type of permanent teeth upon electrometric and thermal pulp testing. *Scand J Dent Res* 1976;**84**:286–90.

410. JOHNSEN DJ, HARSHBARGER J, RYMER HD. Quantitative assesment of neural development in human premolars. *Anat Rec* 1983;**205**:421–9.

411. JOHNSEN DJ. Innervation of teeth: qualitative, quantitative, and developmental assessment. *J Dent Res* 1985;**64**(*Spec. Issue*):555–63.

412. BYERS MR. Dental sensory receptors. *Int Rev Neurobiol* 1984;**25**:39–94.

413. BYERS MR, NARHI MV. Dental injury models: experimental tools for understanding neuroinflammatory interactions and polymodal nociceptor functions. *Crit Rev Oral Biol Med* 1999;**10**:4–39.

414. SMITH AJ, LESOT H. Induction and regulation of crown dentinogenesis: embryonic events as a template for dental tissue repair? *Crit Rev Oral Biol Med* 2001;**12**:425–37.

415. MJOR IA. Pulp-dentin biology in restorative dentistry. Part 5: Clinical management and tissue changes associated with wear and trauma. *Quintess Int* 2001;**32**:771–88.

416. ANDREASEN JO, KRISTERSON L, ANDREASEN FM. Relation between damage to the Hertwig's epithelial root sheath and type of pulp repair after autotransplantation of teeth in monkeys. *Endod Dent Traumatol*1988;**4**:145–51.

417. SKOGLUND A, TROWSTAD K, WALLENIUS K. A microradiographic study of vascular changes in replanted and autotransplanted teeth of young dogs. *Oral Surg Oral Med Oral Pathol* 1978;**45**: 17–28.

418. CVEK M, CLEATON-JONES PE, AUSTIN JC, ANDREASEN JO. Pulp reactions to exposure after experimental crown fractures of grinding in adult monkeys. *J Endod* 1982;**9**:391–7.

419. HEIDE S, MJÖR IA. Pulp reactions to experimental exposures in young permanent monkey teeth. *Int Endod J* 1983;**16**:11–9.

420. WATTS A, PATERSON RC. Cellular responses in the dental pulp: a review. *Int Endod J* 1981;**14**:10–21.

421. CVEK M. Endodontic treatment of traumatized teeth. In: Andreasen JO. *Traumatic injures of the teeth*. Copenhagen: Munksgaard, 1981:321–83.

422. SVEEN OB, HAWES RR. Differentiation of new odontoblasts and dentine bridge formation in rat molar teeth after tooth grinding. *Arch Oral Biol* 1968;**13**:1399–412.

423. ZACH L, TOPAL R, COHEN G. Pulpal repair following operative procedures. Radioautographic demonstration with tritiated thymidine. *Oral Surg Oral Med Oral Pathol* 1969;**28**:587–97.

424. FEIT J, METELOVA M, SINDELKA Z. Incorporation of 3H-thymidine into damaged pulp of rat incisors. *J Dent Res* 1970;**49**:783–6.

425. LUOSTARINEN V. Dental pulp response to trauma. An experimental study in the rat. *Proc Finn Dent Soc* 1971;**67**:1–51.

426. YAMAMURA T. Differentation of pulpal cells and inductive influences of various matrices. *J Dent Res* 1985;**64**:530–40.

427. SENZAKI H. A histological study of reparative dentinogenesis in the rat incisor after colchicine administration. *Arch Oral Biol* 1980;**25**:737–43.

428. TJÄDERHANE L. The mechanism of pulpal wound healing. *Aust Endod J* 2002;**28**:68–74.

429. TZIAFAS D, BELIBASAKIS G, VEIS A, PAPADIMITRIOU S. Dentin regeneration in vital pulp therapy: design principles. *Adv Dent Res* 2001;**15**:96–100.

430. DE SOUZA COSTA CA, HEBLING J, HANKS CT. Current status of pulp capping with dentin adhesive system: a review. *Dent Mater* 2000;**16**:188–97.

431. SNUGGS HM, COX CF, POWELL CS, WHITE KC. Pulpal healing and dentinal bridge formation in an acidic environment. *Quintessence Int* 1993;**24**: 501–10.

432. SCHRÖDER U, GRANATH L-E. Early reaction of intact human teeth to calcium hydroxide following experimental pulpotomy and its significance to the development of hard tissue barrier. *Odont Revy* 1971;**22**:379–96.

433. HOLLAND R, PINHEIRO CR, MELLO W, NERY MJ, SOUZA V. Histochemical analysis of the dogs' dental pulp after pulp capping with calcium barium and strontium hydroxides. *J Endodon* 1982;**8**:444–7.

434. HIGASHI T, OKAMOTO H. Characteristics and effect of calcified degenerative zones on the formation of hard tissue barriers in amputated canine dental pulp. *J Endod* 1996;**22**:168–72.

435. TZIAFAS D, PANAGIOTAKOPOULOS N, KOMNENOU A. Immunolocalization of fibronectin during early response of dog dental pulp demineralized dentine or calcium hydroxide-containing cement. *Arch Oral Biol* 1995;**40**:23–31.

436. YOSHIBA K, YOSHIBA N, NAKAMURA H, IWAKU M, OZAWA H. Immunolocalization of fibronectin during reparative dentinogenesis in human teeth after pulp capping with calcium hydroxide. *J Dent Res* 1996;**75**:1590–7.

437. OLSBURGH S, JACOBY T, KREJCI I. Crown fractures in the permanent dentition: pulpal and restorative considerations. *Dent Traumatol* 2002;**18**:103–15.

438. HEBLING J, GIRO EMA, COSTA CAS. Biocompatibility of an adhesive system applied to exposed human dental pulp. *J Endodontics* 1999;**25**:676–82.

439. COX CF, HAFEZ AA. Biocomposition and reaction of pulp tissues to restorative treatments. *Dent Clin North Am* 2001;**45**:31–48.

440. GOTTRUP F, ANDREASEN JO. Wound healing subsequent to injury. In: Andreasen JO, Andreasen FM. eds. *Textbook and color atlas of traumatic injuries to the teeth.* Copenhagen: Munksgaard, 1994:13–76.

441. FITZGERALD M. Cellular mechanics of dentinal bridge repair using 3H-thymidine. *J Dent Res* 1979;**58**:2198–206.

442. SCHRÖDER U, GRANATH LE. Early reaction of intact human teeth to calcium hydroxide following experimental pulpotomy and its significance to the development of hard tissue barrier. *Odontol Revy* 1971;**22**:379–95.

443. HAYASHI Y. Ultrastructure of initial calcification in wound healing following pulpotomy. *J Oral Pathol* 1982;**11**:174–80.

444. PISANTI S, SCIAKY I. Origin of calcium in the repair wall after pulp exposure in the dog. *J Dent Res* 1964;**43**:641.

445. MJÖR IA, DAHL E, COX CF. Healing of pulp exposures: an ultrastructural study. *J Oral Pathol Med* 1991;**20**:496–501.

446. BAUME LJ. The biology of pulp and dentine. A historic, terminologic-taxonomic, histologic-biochemical, embryonic and clinical survey. *Monogr Oral Sci* 1980;**8**:1–220.

447. COX CF, SUBAY RK, OSTRO E, SUZUKI S, SUZUKI SH. Tunnel defects in dentin bridges: their formation following direct pulp capping. *Oper Dent* 1996;**21**:4–11.

448. STANLEY HR. Pulp capping: conserving the dental pulp – can it be done? Is it worth it? *Oral Surg Oral Med Oral Pathol* 1989;**68**:628–39.

449. CHRISTENSEN GJ. Pulp capping 1998. *J Am Dent Assoc* 1998;**129**:1297–9.

450. HÖRSTED P, EL ATTAR K, LANGELAND K. Capping of monkey pulps with Dycal and a Ca-eugenol cement. *Oral Surg Oral Med Oral Pathol* 1981;**52**:531–53.

451. COX CF, BERGENHOLTZ G, HEYS DR, SYED SA, FITZGERALD M, HEYS RJ. Pulp capping of dental pulp mechanically exposed to oral microflora: a 1–2 year observation of wound healing in the monkey. *J Oral Pathol* 1985;**14**:156–68.

452. OGUNTEBI BR, HEAVEN T, CLARK AE, PINK FE. Quantitative assessment of dentin bridge formation following pulp-capping in miniature swine. *J Endod* 1995;**21**:79–82.

453. NEGM MM, COMBE EC, GRANT AA. Reaction of the exposed pulps to new cements containing calcium hydroxide. *Oral Surg Oral Med Oral Pathol* 1981;**51**:190–204.

454. HERMANN BW. Calciumhydroxyd als Mittel zum Behandeln und Fullen von Wurzelkanalen. Dissertation. Würtzburg: 1920.

455. FRANZ FE, HOLZ J, BAUME LJ. Ultrastructure (SEM) of dentine bridging in the human dental pulp. *J Biol Buccale* 1984;**12**:239–46.

456. SUBAY RK, SUZUKI S, KAYA H, COX CF. Human pulp response after partial pulpotomy with two calcium hydroxide products. *Oral Surg Oral Med Oral Pathol Oral Radiol Endod* 1995;**80**:330–7.

457. CHIEGO DJJ. An ultrastructural and autoradiographic analysis of primary and replacement odontoblasts following cavity preparation and wound healing in the rat molar. *Proc Finn Dent Soc* 1992;**88**:(Suppl 1):243–56.

458. JEAN AH, POUEZAT JA, DACULSI G. Pulpal response to calcium phosphate materials. *In vivo* study of calcium

phosphate materials in endodontics. *Cell Mater* 1993;**3**:193–200.

459. WATTS A, PATERSON RC. A comparison of pulp responses to two different materials in the dog and the rat. *Oral Surg Oral Med Oral Pathol* 1981;**52**:648–52.

460. HARRIS R, BULL AW. The healing of the traumatized dental pulp following capping. *Aust Dent J* 1966;**11**:236–47.

461. JABER L, MASCRES C, DONOHUE WB. Reaction of the dental pulp to hydroxyapatite. *Oral Surg Oral Med Oral Pathol* 1992;**73**:92–8.

462. SASAKI T, KAWAMATA-KIDO H. Providing an environment for reparative dentine induction in amputated rat molar pulp by high molecular-weight hyaluronic acid. *Arch Oral Biol* 1995;**40**:209–19.

463. PITT FORD TR. Pulpal response to a calcium hydroxide material for capping exposures. *Oral Surg Oral Med Oral Pathol* 1985;**59**:194–7.

464. HIGASHI T, OKAMOTO H. Characteristics and effects of calcified degenerative zones on the formation of hard tissue barriers in amputated canine dental pulp. *J Endod* 1996;**22**:168–72.

465. BERGENHOLTZ G, REIT C. Reactions of the dental pulp to microbial provocation of calcium hydroxide treated dentin. *Scand J Dent Res* 1980;**88**:187–92.

466. LÖVSCHALL H, MOSEKILDE L. Apoptosis: cellular and clinical aspects. *Nord Med* 1997;**112**:133–7.

467. LÖVSCHALL H, KASSEM M, MOSEKILDE L. Apoptosis: molecular aspects. *Nord Med* 1997;**112**:271–5.

468. SCHROEDER HE. *Pathologie oraler Strukturen*. 3rd edn. Basel: Karger, 1997.

469. TZIAFAS D, SMITH AJ, LESOT H. Designing new treatment strategies in vital pulp therapy. *J Dent* 2000;**28**:77–92.

470. MESSER HH. Calcium hydroxide: is there a biological basis for its use in dentistry? *Northwest Dent* 1983;**62**:13–17.

471. MCSHANE CJ, STIMSON PG, BUGG JL, JENNINGS RE. Tissue reactions to Dycal. *ASDC J Dent Child* 1970;**37**:466–74.

472. WATTS A, PATERSON RC. Pulp-capping studies with Analar calcium hydroxide and zinc oxide-eugenol. *Int Endod J* 1987;**20**:169–76.

473. STANLEY HR. Criteria for standardizing and increasing credibility of direct pulp capping studies. *Am J Dent* 1998;**11**: *(Spec No)*:S17–S34.

474. SCHRÖDER U. Effects of calcium-hydroxide-containing pulp-capping agents on pulp cell migration, proliferation, and differentiation. *J Dent Res* 1985;**64**:*(Spec Iss)*:541–8.

475. COX CF, HAFEZ AA, AKIMOTO N, OTSUKI M, SUZUKU S, TARIM B. Biocompatibility of primer, adhesive and resin composite systems on non-exposed pulps of non-human primate teeth. *Am J Dent* 1998;**10**:S55–63.

476. IWAYA S, IKAWA M, KUBOTA M. Revascularization of an immature permanent tooth with apical periodontitis and sinus tract. *Dent Traumatol* 2001;**17**:185–7.

477. BERGENHOLTZ G. Factors in pulpal repair after oral exposure. *Adv Dent Res* 2001;**15**:84.

478. BERGENHOLTZ G. Evidence for bacterial causation of adverse pulpal response in rein-based dental restoration. *Crit Rev Oral Biol Med* 2000;**11**:467–80.

479. HÖRSTED-BINDSLEV P, VILKINIS V, SIDLAUSKAS A. Direct capping of human pulps with a dentin bonding system or with calcium hydroxide cement. *Oral Surg Oral Med Oral Pathol Oral Radiol Oral Endod* 2003;**86**:591–600.

480. TZIAFAS D, PANTELIDOU O, ALVANOU A, BELIBASAKIS G, PAPADIMITRIOU S. The dentinogenic effect of mineral trioxide aggregate (MTA) in short-term capping experiments. *Int Endod J* 2002;**35**:245–54.

481. FARACO IM Jr, HOLLAND R. Response of the pulp of dogs to capping with mineral trioxide aggregate or a calcium hydroxide cement. *Dent Traumatol* 2001;**17**:163–6.

482. TORABINEJAD M, PITT FORD TR, MCKENDRY DJ, ABEDI HR, MILLER DA, KARIYAWASAM SP. Histologic assessment of mineral trioxide aggregate as a root-filling material in monkeys. *J Endod* 1997;**23**:225–8.

483. FARACO IM Jr, HOLLAND R. Response of the pulp of dogs to capping with mineral trioxide aggregate or a calcium hydroxide cement. *Dent Traumatol* 2001;**17**:163–6.

484. HOLLAND R, DE SOUZA V, MURATA SS, NERY MJ, BERNABE PFE, OTOBONI FILHO JA, et al. Healing process of dog dental pulp after pulpotomy and pulp covering with mineral trioxide aggregate or Portland cement. *Braz Dent* 2001;**12**:109–13.

485. HOLLAND R, DE SOUZA V, MURATA SS, NERY MJ, BERNABE PFE, OTOBONI FILHO JA, et al. Reaction of rat connective tissue to implanted dentin tube filled with mineral trioxide aggregate, Portland cement or calcium hydroxide. *Braz Dent* 2001;**12**:3–8.

486. TZIAFAS D, PANTELIDOU E, ALVANOU A, BELIBASAKIS G, PAPADIMITRIOU S. The dentinogenic effect of mineral trioxide aggregate (MTA) in short-term capping experiments. *Int Endod J* 2002;**35**:245–54.

487. TORABINEKAD M, CHIVIAN N. Clinical applications of mineral trioxide aggregate. *J Endod* 1999;**25**:197–205.

488. SHABAHANG S, TORABINEJAD M, BOYNE PP, ABEDI H, MCMILLAN P. A comparative study of root-end induction using osteogenic protein-1, calcium hydroxide, and mineral trioxide aggregate in dogs. *J Endod* 1999;**25**:1–5.

489. SILVA TA, ROSA AL, LARA VS. Dentin matrix proteins and soluble factors: intrinsic regulatory signals for healing and resorption of dental and periodontal tissues. *Oral Dis* 2004;**10**:63–74.

490. RUTHERFORD RB. Regeneration of the dentin-pulp complex. In: Lynch SE, Genco RJ, Marx RE. eds. *Tissue engineering, applications in maxillofacial surgery and periodontics*. Chicago: Quintessence Int., 1999: 185–99.

491. RUTHERFORD RB, GU K. Treatment of inflamed ferret dental pulps with recombinant bone morphogenetic protein-7. *Eur J Oral Sci* 2000;**108**:202–6.

492. NAKASHIMA M, REDDI AH. The application of bone morphogenetic proteins to dental tissue engineering. *Nat Biotechnol* 2003;**21**:1025–32.

493. LOVSCHALL H, FEJERSKOV O, FLYVBJERG A. Pulp capping with recombinant human insulin-like growth factor I (rhIGF-I) in rat molars. *Adv Dentl Res* 2001;**35**: 108–12.

494. TZIAFAS D. *Reparative dentinogenesis*. University of Thessaloniki, Greece, 1997.

495. TZIAFAS D, SMITH AJ, LESOT H. Designing new treatment strategies in vital pulp therapy. *J Dent* 2000;**28**:77–92.

496. SMITH AJ, MURRAY PE, LUMLEY PJ. Preserving the vital pulp in operative dentistry: I. A biological approach. *Dent Update* 2002;**29**:64–9.

497. HU CC, ZHANG C, QIAN Q, TATUM NB. Reparative dentin formation in rat molars after direct pulp capping with growth factors. *J Endod* 1998;**24**:744–51.

498. RUTHERFORD RB, WAHLE J, TUCKER M, RUEGER D, CHARETTE M. Induction of reparative dentine formation in monkeys by recombinant human osteogenic protein-1. *Arch Oral Biol* 1993;**38**:571–6.

499. NAKASHIMA M. Induction of dentin formation on canine amputated pulp by recombinant human bone morphogenetic proteins (BMP)-2 and -4. *J Dent Res* 1994;**73**:1515–22.

500. RUTHERFORD RB, SPANGBERG L, TUCKER M, RUEGER D, CHARETTE M. The time-course of the induction of reparative dentine formation in monkeys by recombinant human osteogenic protein-1. *Arch Oral Biol* 1994;**39**:833–8.

501. SMITH AJ, MATTHEWS JB, HALL RC. Transforming growth factor-beta1 (TGF-beta1) in dentine matrix. Ligand activation and receptor expression. *Eur J Oral Sci* 1998;**106**:(*Suppl 1*):179–84.

502. SMITH AJ, MURRAY PE, SLOAN AJ, MATTHEWS JB, ZHAO S. Trans-dentinal stimulation of tertiary dentinogenesis. *Adv Dent Res* 2001;**15**:51–4.

503. WAKEFIELD LM, WINOKUR TS, HOLLANDS RS, CHRISTOPHERSON K, LEVINSON AD, SPORN MB. Recombinant latent transforming growth factor beta 1 has a longer plasma half-life in rats than active transforming growth factor beta 1, and a different tissue distribution. *J Clin Invest* 1990;**86**:1976–84.

504. MELIN M, JOFFRE-ROMEAS A, FARGES JC, COUBLE ML, MAGLOIRE H, BLEICHER F. Effects of TGF beta1 on dental pulp cells in cultured human tooth slices. *J Dent Res* 2000;**79**:1689–96.

505. SLOAN AJ, SMITH AJ. Stimulation of the dentine-pulp complex of rat incisor teeth by transforming growth factor-beta isoforms 1–3 *in vitro*. *Arch Oral Biol* 1999;**44**:149–56.

506. TZIAFAS D, ALVANOU A, PAPADIMITRIOU S, GASIC J, KOMNENOU A. Effects of recombinant basic fibroblast growth factor, insulin-like growth factor-II and transforming growth factor-beta 1 on dog dental pulp cells *in vivo*. *Arch Oral Biol* 1998;**43**:431–44.

507. GOLBERG M, SIX N, DECUP F, NUCH D, MAJD ES, LASFARGUES J-J, SALIH E, STANISLAWSKI L. Application of bioactive molecules in pulp-capping situations. *Adv Dent Res* 2001;**15**:91–105.

508. JEPSEN S, ALBERS H-K, FLEINER B, TUCKER M, RUEGER D. Recombinant human osteogenic protein-1 induces dentin formation: an experimental study in miniature swine. *J Endod* 1997;**23**:378–82.

509. RUTHERFORD B, FITZGERALD M. A new biological approach to vital pulp therapy. *Crit Rev Oral Biol Med* 1995;**44**:361–71.

510. RUTHERFORD RB, WAHLE J, TUCKER M, RUEGER D, CHARETTE M. Induction of reparative dentine formation in monkeys by recombinant human osteogenic protein-1. *Arch Oral Biol* 1993;**38**:571–6.

511. RUTHERFORD RB. BMP-7 gene transfer to inflamed ferret dental pulps. *Eur J Oral Sci* 2001;**109**:422–4.

512. WATTS A, PATERSON RC. Bacterial contamination as a factor influencing the toxicity of materials to the exposed dental pulp. *Oral Surg Oral Med Oral Pathol* 1987;**64**:466–74.

513. DECUP F, SIX N, PALMIER B, BUCH D, LASFARGUES JJ, SALIH E, et al. Bone sialoprotein-induced reparative dentinogenesis in the pulp of rat's molar. *Clin Oral Investig* 2000;**4**:110–19.

514. NAKASHIMA M, MIZUNUMA K, MURAKAMI T, AKAMINE A. Induction of dental pulp stem cell differentiation into odontoblasts by electroporation-mediated gene delivery of growth/differentiation factor 11 (Gdf11). *Gene Ther* 2002;**9**:814–18.

515. NAKAMURA Y, SLABY I, MATSUMOTO K, RITCHIE HH, LYNGSTADAAS SP. Immunohistochemical characterization of rapid dentin formation induced by enamel matrix derivate. *Calcif Tissue Int* 2004;**75**:243–52.

516. NAKAMURA Y, HAMMARSTRÖM L, MATSUMOTO K, LYNGSTADAAS SP. The induction of reparative dentine by enamel proteins. *Int Endod J* 2002;**35**:407–17.

517. NAKAMURA Y, HAMMARSTRÖM L, LUNDBERG E, EKDAHL H, MATSUMOTO K, GESTRELIUS S, LYNGSTADAAS SP. Enamel matrix derivate promotes reparative processed in the dental pulp. *Adv Dent Res* 2001;**15**:105–7.

518. FITZGERALD M. Cellular mechanics of dental bridge using $^3$H-thymidine. *J Dent Res* 1979;**58**:198–206.

519. CLARKE NG. The morphology of the reparative dentin bridge. *Oral Surg Oral Med Oral Pathol* 1970;**29**:746–52.

520. MJÖR IA, DAHL E, COX CF. Healing of pulp exposures: an ultra-structural study. *J Oral Pathol Med* 1991;**20**:496–501.

521. KIRASAKO Y, SHIBATA S, ARAKAWA M, COX CF, TAGAMI J. A light and transmission microscopic study of mechanically exposed monkey pulps. *Oral Surg Oral Med Oral Pathol Oral Radiol Endod* 2000;**89**:224–30.

522. GOLDBERG F, MASSONE EJ, SPIELBERG C. Evaluation of the dentinal bridge after pulpotomy and calcium hydroxide dressing. *J Endo* 1984;**10**:318–20.

523. COX CF, BERGENHOLTZ G, HEYS DR, SYED SA, FITZGERALD M, HEYS RJ. Pulp capping of dental pulp mechanically exposed to oral microflora: a 1–2 year observation of wound healing in the monkey. *J Oral Pathol* 1985;**14**:165–8.

524. COX CF, SÜBAY RK, OSTRO E, SUZUKI S, SUZUKI SH. Tunnel defects in dentin bridges: their formation following direct pulp capping. *Oper Dent* 1996;**21**:4–11.

525. MJÖR IA. Pulp-dentin biology in restorative dentistry. Part 7: the exposed pulp. *Quintess Int* 2002;**33**:113–35.

526. CVEK M. Partial pulpotomy in crown-fractured incisors – results after 3 to 15 years after treatment. *Acta Stomatol Croatica* 1993;**97**:167–73.

527. CVEK M, CLEATON-JONES PEM, AUSTIN JC, ANDREASEN JO. Pulpal reactions to exposure after experimental

crown fractures or grinding in adult monkeys. *J Endod* 1982;**9**:391–7.

528. HEIDE S, KEREKES K. Delayed direct pulp capping in permanent incisors of monkeys. *Int Endod J* 1987;**20**:65–74.

529. HARRAN-PONCE E, HOLLAND R, BARREIRO-LOIS A, LOPEZ-BECEIRO AM, PEREIRA-ESPINEL JL. Consequences of crown fractures with pulpal exposure: histopathological evaluation in dogs. *Dent Traumatol* 2002;**18**:196–205.

530. ANDREASEN JO, ANDREASEN FM, SKEIE A, HJÖRTING-HANSEN E, SCHWARTZ O. Effect of treatment delay upon pulp and periodontal healing of traumatic dental injuries – a review article. *Dent Traumatol* 2002;**18**:1–13.

531. SKOGLUND A, TRONSTAD L, WALLENIUS K. A micorangiographic study of vascular changes in replanted and autotransplanted teeth of young dogs. *Oral Surg Oral Med Oral Pathol* 1978;**45**:17–28.

532. SKOGLUND A. Vascular changes in replanted and autotransplanted apicoectomized mature teeth of dogs. *Int J Oral Surg* 1981;**10**:100–10.

533. ALBELDA SM, SMITH CW, WARD PA. Adhesion molecules and inflammatory injury. *FASEB J* 1994;**8**:504–12.

534. SINGER AJ, CLARK RA. Cutaneous wound healing. *N Engl J Med* 1999;**341**:738–46.

535. BARRETT AP, READE PC. Revascularization of mouse tooth isografts and allografts using autoradiography and carbon perfusion. *Arch Oral Biol* 1981;**26**:541–5.

536. AVERY JK, STRACHAN DS, CORPRON RE, COX CF. Morphological studies of the altered pulps of the New Zealand white rabbit after resection of the inferior alveolar nerve and/or the superior cervical ganglion. *Anat Rec* 1971;**171**:495–508.

537. AVERY JK, COX CF, CORPRON RE. The effects of combined nerve resection and cavity preparation and restoration on response dentin formation in rabbit incisors. *Arch Oral Biol* 1974;**19**:539–48.

538. AVERY JK, COX CF, CHIEGO DJ JR. Presence and location of adrenergic nerve endings in the dental pulps of mouse molars. *Anat Rec* 1980;**198**:59–71.

539. CHIEGO DJ JR, SINGH IJ. Evaluation of the effects of sensory deveration on osteoblasts by 3H-proline autoradiography. *Cell Tissue Res* 1981;**217**:569–76.

540. CHIEGO DJ JR, KLEIN RM, AVERY JK. Tritiated thymidine autoradiographic study of the effect of inferior alveolar nerve resection of the proliferative compartments of the mouse incisor formative tissue. *Arch Oral Biol* 1981;**26**:83–9.

541. CHIEGO DJ JR, FISHER MA, AVERY JK, KLEIN RM. Effects of denervation of 3H-fucose incorporation by odontoblasts in the mouse incisor. *Cell Tissue Res* 1983;**230**:197–203.

542. CHIEGO DJ JR, KLEIN RM, AVERY JK, GRUHL IM. Denervation induced changes in cell proliferation in the rat molar after wounding. *Anat Rec* 1986;**214**:348–52.

543. CHIEGO DJ JR, AVERY JK, KLEIN RM. Neuroregulation of protein synthesis in odontoblasts of the first molar of the rat after wounding. *Cell Tissue Res* 1987;**248**:119–23.

544. KLEIN RM, CHIEGO DJ JR, AVERY JK. Effect of chemical sympathectomy on cell proliferation in the progenitive

compartments of the neonatal mouse incisor. *Arch Oral Biol* 1981;**26**:319–25.

545. KUBOTA K, YONAGA T, HOSAKA K, KATAYAMA T, NAGAE K, SHIBANAI S, SATO Y, TAKADA K. Experimental morphological studies on the functional role of pulpal nerves in denti nogenesis. *Anat Anz (Jena)* 1985;**158**:323–36.

546. ANDREASEN FM. Pulpal healing after luxation injuries and root fracture in the permanent dentition. *Endod Dent Traumatol* 1989;**5**:111–31.

547. ANDREASEN FM, JUHL M, ANDREASEN JO. Pulp reaction to replantation of teeth with incomplete root development. *Endod Dent Traumatol* 2006. To be submitted.

548. INOUE H, KUROSAKA Y, ABE K. Autonomic nerve endings in the odontoblast/predentin border and predentin of the canine teeth of dogs. *J Endod* 1992;**18**:149–51.

549. OLGART L, MATSUO M, LINDSKOG S, WALL L. Enhanced formation of secondary dentin in the absence of nerve supply to feline teeth. *Eur J Oral Sci* 1995;**103**:160–5.

550. CVEK M, CLEATON-JONES P, AUSTIN J, KLING M, LOWNIE J, FATTI P. Pulp revascularization in reimplanted immature monkey incisors – predictability and the effect of antibiotic systemic prophylaxis. *Endod Dent Traumatol* 1990;**6**:157–9.

551. CVEK M, CLEATON-JONES P, AUSTIN J, LOWNIE J, KLING M, FATTI P. Effect of topical application of doxycycline on pulp revascularization and periodontal healing in reimplanted monkey incisors. *Endod Dent Traumatol* 1990;**6**:170–6.

552. OLGART L, BRÄNNSTRÖM M, JOHNSON G. Invasion of bacteria into dentinal tubules. Experiments *in vivo* and *in vitro*. *Acta Odontol Scand* 1974;**32**:61–70.

553. VONGSAVAN N, MATTHEWS B. Fluid flow through cat dentine in vivo. *Arch Oral Biol* 1992;**37**:175–85.

554. GROSSMAN LI. Origin of migroorganisms in traumatized, pulpless, sound teeth. *J Dent Res* 1967;**46**:551–3.

555. ROBINSON HBG, BOLING LR. The anachoretic effect in pulpitis. I. Bacteriologic studies. *J Am Dent Assoc* 1941;**28**:268–82.

556. BOLING LR, ROBINSON HBG. Anachoretic effect in pulpitis. II. Histologic studies. *Arch Pathol* 1942;**33**:477–86.

557. BURKE GW, KNIGHTON HT. The localization of microorganisms in inflamed dental pulps of rats following bacteremia. *J Dent Res* 1960;**39**:205–14.

558. GIER RE, MITCHELL DF. Anachoretic effect of pulpitis. *J Dent Res* 1968;**47**:564–70.

559. SMITH LS, TAPPE GD. Experimental pulpitis in rats. *J Dent Res* 1962;**41**:17–22.

560. CSERNYEI J. Anachoresis and anachoric effect of chronic periapical inflammations. *J Dent Res* 1939;**18**:527–31.

561. TZIAFAS D. Experimental bacterial anachoresis in dog dental pulps capped with calcium hydroxide. *J Endod* 1989;**15**:591–5.

562. TZIAFAS D, KOLOKURIS J, ZAGAKIS P. Experimentally induced pulpal anachoresis. A histologic study in dogs. *Hell Stom Rev* 1985;**29**:121–7.

563. ALLARD U, STRÖMBERG T. Inflammatory reaction in the apical area of pulpectomized and sterile root canals in

dogs. *Oral Surg Oral Med Oral Pathol* 1979;**48**: 463–6.

564. ALLARD U, NORD C-E, SJÖBERG L, STRÖMBERG T. Experimental infections with staphylococcus aureus, streptococcus sanguis, pseudomonas aeruginosa, and bacteroides fragilis in the jaws of dogs. *Oral Surg Oral Med Oral Pathol* 1979;**48**:454–62.

565. NAGAOKA S, MIYAZAKI Y, LUI H-J, IWAMOTO Y, KITANO M, KAWAGOE M. Bacterial invasion into dentinal tubules of human vital and nonvital teeth. *J Endo* 1995;**21**: 70–73.

566. BERGENHOLTZ G. Microorganisms from necrotic pulp of traumatized teeth. *Odont Rev J* 1974;**25**:347–58.

567. MÖLLER AJR, FABRICIUS L, DAHLÉN G, ÖHMAN AE, HEYDEN G. Influence on periapical tissues of indigenous oral bacteria and necrotic pulp tissue in monkeys. *Scand J Dent Res* 1981;**89**:475–84.

568. DELIVANIS PD, SNOWDEN RB, DOYLE RJ. Localization of blood-borne bacteria in instrumented unfilled root canals. *Oral Surg Oral Med Oral Pathol* 1981;**52**:430–2.

569. SONNABEND E, ÖH C-S. Zur Frage des Epithels im apikalen Granulationsgewebe (Granulom) menschlicher Zähne. *Dtsch Zahnärztl Z* 1966;**21**:627–43.

570. NAIR PNR. Light and electron microscopic studies of root canal flora and periapical lesions. *J Endod* 1987;**13**:29–39.

571. NAIR PNR, SCHROEDER HE. Epithelial attachment at diseased human tooth-apex. *J Periodont Res* 1985;**20**:293–300.

572. ÖSTBY B. The role of the blood clot in endodontic therapy. *Acta Odontol Scand* 1961;**19**:323–53.

573. ÖSTBY B, HJORTDAL O. Tissue formation in the root canal following pulp removal. *Scand J Dent Res* 1971;**79**:333–49.

574. MEYERS WC, FOUNTAIN SB. Dental pulp regeneration aided by blood and blood substitutes after experimentally induced periapical infection. *Oral Surg Oral Med Oral Pathol* 1974;**37**:441–50.

575. CLAUS I, LAUREYS W, CORNELISSEN R, DERMAUT LR. Histologic analysis of pulpal revascularization of autotransplanted immature teeth after removal of the original pulp tissue. *Am J Orthod Dentofacial Orthop* 2004;**125**:93–9.

576. IWAYA S, IKAWA M, KUBOTA M. Revascularization of an immature permanent tooth with apical periodontis and sinus tract. *Dent Traumatol* 2001;**17**:185–7.

577. LUOMANEN M. A comparative study of healing of laser and scalpel incision wounds in rat oral mucosa. *Scand J Dent Res* 1987;**95**:65–73.

578. LUOMANEN M, VIRTANEN I. Healing of laser and scalpel incision wounds of rat tongue mucosa as studied with cytokeratin antibodies. *J Oral Pathol* 1987;**16**:139–44.

579. LUOMANEN M, MEURMAN JH, LEHTO V-P. Extracellular matrix in healing $CO_2$ laser incision wound. *J Oral Pathol* 1987;**16**:322–31.

580. LUOMANEN M, LEHTO V-P, MEURMAN JH. Myofibroblasts in healing laser wounds of rat tongue mucosa. *Arch Oral Biol* 1988;**33**:17–23.

581. ROVIN S, COSTICH ER, FLEMING JE, GORDON HA. Healing of tongue wounds in germfree and conventional mice. *Arch Pathol* 1965;**79**:641–3.

582. FEJERSKOV O. Excision wounds in palatal epithelium in guinea pigs. *Scand J Dent Res* 1972;**80**:139–54.

583. FEJERSKOV O, PHIILIPSEN HP. Incisional wounds in palatal epithelium in guinea pigs. *Scand J Dent Res* 1972;**80**:47–62.

584. DABELSTEEN E, MACKENZIE I. Selective loss of blood group antigens during wound healing. *Acta Pathol Microbiol Scand* 1974;**84**:445–50. Sect A.

585. ANDERSEN L, FEJERSKOV O. Ultrastructure of initial epithelial cell migration in palatal wounds of guinea pigs. *J Ultrastruct Res* 1974;**48**:113–24.

586. ANDERSEN L, FEJERSKOV O. Ultrastructural localisation of acid phosphatase in oral mucosal wounds. In: Bierring E. ed. *Proc 9th Congress Nord Soc Cell Biol.* Odense: Odense University Press, 1976:89–99.

587. ANDERSEN L. Quantitative analysis of epithelial changes during wound healing in palatal mucosa of guinea pigs. *Cell Tissue Res* 1978;**193**:231–46.

588. ANDERSEN L. Cell junctions in squamous epithelium during wound healing in palatal mucosa of guinea pigs. *Scand J Dent Res* 1980;**88**:328–39.

589. ANDERSEN L. Ultrastructure of squamous epithelium during wound healing in palatal mucosa of guinea pigs. *Scand J Dent Res* 1980;**88**:418–29.

590. NOBUTO T, TOKIOKA T, IMAI H, SUWA F, OHTA Y, YAMAOKA A. Microvascularization of gingival wound healing using corrosion casts. *J Periodontol* 1987;**58**:240–6.

591. WIJDEVELD MGMM, GRUPPING EM, KUIJPERS-JAGTMAN AM, MALTHA JC. Wound healing of the palatal mucoperiosteum in beagle dogs after surgery at different ages. *J Cranio Maxillofac Surg* 1987;**15**:51–7.

592. KAHNBERG K-E, THILANDER H. Healing of experimental excisional wounds in the rat palate. I. Histological study of the interphase in wound healing after sharp dissection. *Int J Oral Surg* 1982;**11**:44–51.

593. HEDNER E, VAHLNE A, HIRSCH J-M. Herpes simplex virus (type 1) delays healing of oral excisional and extraction wounds in the rat. *J Oral Pathol Med* 1990;**19**:471–6.

594. HARRISON JW, JUROSKY KA. Wound healing in the tissues of the periodontium following periradicular surgery. I. The incisional wound. *J Endod* 1991;**17**:425–35.

595. HARRISON JW, JUROSKY KA. Wound healing in the tissues of the periodontium following periradicular surgery. II. The dissectional wound. *J Endod* 1991;**17**:544–52.

596. HARRISON JW. Healing of surgical wounds in oral mucoperiosteal tissue. *J Endod* 1991;**17**:401–8.

597. ANDREASEN JO. Histologic aspects of penetrating lip wounds. 2006. In preparation.

598. ALLBROOK D, BAKER W DE C, KIRKALDY-WILLIS WH. Muscle regeneration in experimental animals and in man. The cycle of tissue change that follows trauma in the injured limb syndrome. *J Bone Joint Surg* 1966;**48**:153–69.

599. BETZEH, FIRKET H, REZNIK M. Some aspects of muscle regeneration. In: Bourne GH, Danielli JF. eds. *International review of cytology.* New York, London: Academic Press, 1966:203–25.

600. CHURCH JCT, NORONHA RFX, ALLBROOK DB. Satellite cells and skeletal muscle regeneration. *Br J Surg* 1966;**53**:638–42.

601. JÄRVINEN M, SORVARI T. Healing of a crush injury in rat striated muscle. I. Description and testing of a new method of inducing a standard injury to the calf muscles. *Acta Pathol Microbiol Scand* 1975;**83**:259–65.

602. JÄRVINEN M. Healing of a crush injury in rat striated muscle. II. A histological study of the effect of early mobilization and immobilization of the repair processes. *Acta Pathol Microbiol Scand* 1975;**83**:269–82.

603. ROWSELL AR. The intra-uterine healing of foetal muscle wounds: experimental study in the rat. *Br J Plast Surg* 1984;**37**:635–42.

604. GARRETT WE Jr, SEABER AV, BOSWICK J, URBANIAK JR, GOLDNER JL. Recovery of skeletal muscle after laceration and repair. *J Hand Surg* 1984;**9**:683–92.

605. LEHTO M, ALANEN A. Healing of a muscle trauma. Correlation of sonographical and histological findings in an experimental study in rats. *J Ultrasound Med* 1987;**6**:425–9.

606. HURME, T KALIMO H, LEHTO M, JÄRVINEN M. Healing of skeletal muscle injury: an ultrastructural and immunohistochemical study. *Med Sci Sports Exerc* 1991;**23**:801–10.

607. ANDREASEN FM, YU Z, THOMSEN BL. The relationship between pulpal dimensions and the development of pulp necrosis after luxation injuries in the permanent dentition. *Endod Dent Traumatol* 1986;**2**:90–8.

608. ANDREASEN JO, BORUM M, JACOBSEN HL, ANDREASEN FM. Replantation of 400 avulsed permanent incisors. II. Factors related to pulp healing. *Endod Dent Traumatol* 1995;**11**:59–68.

609. ROSS R. Wound healing. *Sci Am* 1969;**220**:40–8.

610. ROSS R, ODLAND G. Human wound repair. II. Inflammatory cells. Epithelial-menechymal interrelations, and fibrinogenesis. *J Cell Biol* 1968;**39**:152–68.

611. SCIUBBA JJ, WATERHOUSE JP, MEYER J. A fine structural comparison of the healing of incisional wounds of mucosa and skin. *J Oral Pathol* 1978;**7**:214–27.

612. FEJERSKOV O, PHILIPSEN HP. Incisional wounds in palatal epithelium in guinea pigs. *Scand J Dent Res* 1972;**80**:47–62.

613. FEJERSKOV O. Excision wounds in palatal epithelium in guinea pigs. *Scand J Dent Res* 1972;**80**:139–54.

614. ABOUT I, CAMPS J, MITSIADIS TA, BOTTERO MJ, BUTLER W, FRANQUIN JC. Influence of resinous monomers on the differentiation *in vitro* of human pulp cells into odontoblasts. *J Biomed Mater Res* 2002;**63**(**4**): 418–23.

615. NAKASHIMA M. Induction of dentine in amputated pulp of dogs by recombinant human bone morphogenetic proteins-2 and -4 with collagen matrix. *Arch Oral Biol* 1994;**39**:1085–9.

616. FUJIYAMA K, YAMASHIREO T, FUKUNAGA T, BALAM TA, ZHENG L, TAKANO-YAMAMATO T. Denervation resulting in dento-alveolar ankylosis associated with decreased Malassez epithelium. *J Dent Res* 2004;**83**:625–9.

617. NISHIOKA M, SHIIYA T, UEMO K, SUDA H. Tooth replantation in germ-free and conventional rats. *Endod Dent Traumatol* 1998;**14**:163–73.

618. FABRICIUS L, DAHLÉN G, SUNDQVIST G, HAPPONEN R-P, MÖLLER ÅJR. Influence of residual bacteria on periapical tissue healing after chemomechanical treatment and root filling of experimentally infected monkey teeth. *Eur J Oral Sci* 2006;**114**:278–85.

619. ROBERTSON A, ANDREASEN FM, BERGENHOLTZ G, ANDREASEN JO, MUNKSGAARD C. Pulp reactions to restoration of experimentally induced crown fractures. *J Dent* 1998;**26**:409–16.

# 3

# Stem Cells and Regeneration of Injured Dental Tissue

H. Løvschall, W. V. Giannobile, M. J. Somerman, Q. Jin & J. O. Andreasen

*H. Løvschall and J. O. Andreasen*

## Introduction

The integrity of the tooth organ is, among other factors, dependent on stem cells located in the pulp and the periodontium. After tooth trauma adult stem cells are the reservoir of reparative cells. They proliferate and migrate to the wound site, where, in cooperation with local cells, they participate in repair. Adult stem cells have the capacity to grow into many types of tissue. Their capacity for regeneration is being studied in transplantation models. In this section we focus on the evidence in the field of tooth and periodontal regeneration with focus on stem cells.

Advances in regeneration of oro-facial tissues are based on contributions from molecular biology, stem cell biology, developmental biology, the human genome project, and development of new biomaterials. These disciplines have merged in a discipline called **tissue engineering**. This field provides new dental tissue engineering modalities, including generation of teeth (1–3).

Recent studies in a variety of systems have highlighted new perspectives for stem cell-based treatments. Here are a few examples: one group in Washington isolated pulpal stem cells capable of making dentin after transplantation (4); Another group claimed they were able to develop tooth crowns with dentin and enamel using cells cultivated from tooth buds in rats (5); In London another group was capable of making new teeth *ex situ* by transplantation of embryonic stem cells (6). Therefore, the recent studies indicate new avenues for dental tissue engineering, and they suggest that knowledge about cells may become relevant in future traumatology.

## The stem cell

### What is a stem cell?

The stem cell is a cell from the embryo, or adult organism, that has, under certain conditions, the ability to reproduce itself. It can give rise to specialized cells that make up the tissues and organs of the body (7).

Stem cells initially undergo asymmetric cell division where one daughter cell is a duplicate of the original stem cell. However, the other stem cells undergo further cell divisions and produce progenitor cells (Fig. 3.1) (8). Progenitor cells, also called precursor cells, can divide further as a transit amplifying cell pool and eventually give rise to a pool of differentiated cells.

Progenitor/precursor cells can replace cells that are damaged or dead, and thereby repair a defect. After terminal differentiation the cells are able to maintain their integrity and functions and thus achieve tissue regeneration.

Stem cells are capable of making copies. We have stem cells, not only in the embryo, but also in adults throughout life. They have been found in dental pulp, periodontal ligament, bone marrow, blood, the cornea and the retina of the

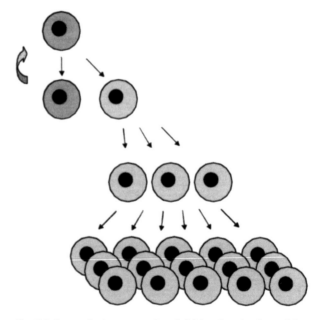

**Fig. 3.1** Stem cells show asymetric cell division. One daughter cell is a duplicate of the stem cell. The others continue division and thereby represent an amplifying cell pool.

eye, brain, skeletal muscle, liver, skin, the lining of the gastrointestinal tract, and pancreas (4, 9, 10).

## Embryonic stem cells

The fertilized egg cell is capable of developing into all types of tissue, and it is therefore totipotent. After cell division in four days it develops into a blastocyst where the cells have divided into an outer and an inner cell mass. The inner cell mass is pluripotent and develops into all tissue in the body. By adding specific growth and differentiation factors to a culture medium, stem cells are induced to differentiate into certain specialized cell types (Fig. 3.2).

Once removed from their environment the inner cell mass lacks signals regulating the cell fate, and they can proliferate indefinitely as embryonic stem cells in the laboratory while retaining the ability to differentiate into all somatic cells, a property that is not shared by adult stem cells (Fig. 3.2) (9).

The mechanism by which embryonic stem cells are determined for differentiation is dependent on a network of developmental signaling molecules. The local environment of stem cells plays an important role.

Embryonic stem cells have tremendous potential in development. Embryonic stem cells can now be cultured and even produced from adult cells by the nuclear transfer method (11). It has been claimed that cells may be added to injured regions, develop *in situ*, and restore function in a part of the body (2). They can also make small segments of tissue which are usable for developing into regular tissue transplants (6). However, there are not only scientific and biotechnical problems when using embryonic stem cells: ethical and legal aspects need to be clarified (12).

## Adult stem cells

In the mature tissue of adults, stem cells play a major role in homeostasis and tissue repair. Stem cells have been isolated from many tissues, including bone, periosteum, synovium, and teeth (10, 13–15). In contrast to embryonic stem cells, the adult stem cells do not replicate indefinitely in culture (9).

Evidence suggests that adult stem cells have more developmental potential than previously thought. They may adopt different cell types after differentiation (3). Given the right environment adult stem cells from bone marrow (16), skin (17) and dental pulp (18) can differentiate into neurons and adipocytes.

Differentiation is the process by which an unspecialized cell, such as a stem cell, becomes specialized into one of the cell types that make up the tissues. During differentiation, certain genes become activated and other genes become inactivated in a regulated fashion. As a result, a differentiated cell develops specific structures and certain functions.

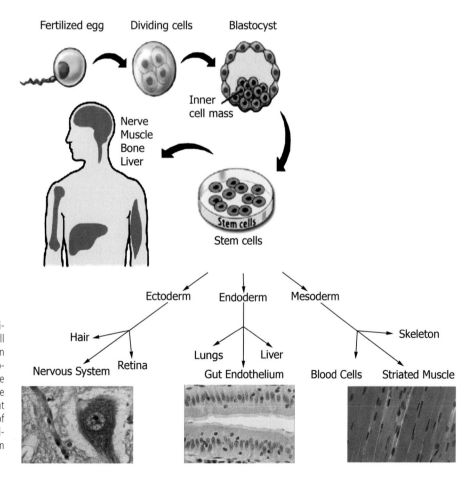

**Fig. 3.2** The fertilized ovum is totipotent. First, it develops the inner cell mass and subsequently the three main types of embryonal stem cells in ectoderm, mesoderm and endoderm. These stem cells can *in vitro* develop a wide range of specific cell types dependent on the culture conditions. Segments of tissue can be developed for experimental implantation. Modified from KREBSBACH & ROBEY (12) 2002.

Apparently, differentiated cells from one germ layer may be 'genetically re-programmed' to generate new specialized cells that are characteristic of tissues originating from another, a phenomenon called 'plasticity' (19). The evidence of stem cell plasticity is controversial and more studies are anticipated (20, 21). Much work has to be done in order to map the tree of stem cell lineages.

## Detection of stem cells

There is a lack of data on the fate of stem cells and their progenitors in the environment of dental trauma. They work in an environment that has a crucial, but not necessarily irreversible, influence on the differentiation of genes in a particular direction (22).

Adult stem cells are rare, and they are therefore often difficult to identify, isolate, and purify. Stem cells are often interspersed between differentiated cells.

In light of previous discoveries of adult stem cells in tissues where they were not expected, it was hypothesized that they could also be present in hard tissues of the oral cavity. By using techniques previously established for isolation of stem cells and progenitors from bone and its marrow, it is now possible to isolate fractions of dental cells enriched in stem cells (see later). By using cell sorting technology it is possible to label individual cell types with specific antibodies and isolate the cell fractions. It is thereby possible to isolate cell groups with an extensive clonogenic capacity, and also an ability to regenerate hard tissue after transplantation (23).

Today, a new interpretation of stem cells is developing. We know that stem cells are not necessarily typical undifferentiated cells. On the contrary they may, to some extent, express a selection of molecules which are characteristic for differentiated cells (19). Stem cells may apparently adopt some reversible changes in direction of changes seen after irreversible terminal differention.

It can be difficult to ascertain scientifically whether a single cell is capable of developing an array of cell types, or whether multiple cell types, when grown together, are capable of forming the same cell type. Development in the detection of specific stem cell markers, including production of specific antibodies, is anticipated with great interest.

## Origin of dental stem cells

The origin of stem cells is important in the understanding of their competence and fate. The embryo is developed from three layers of multipotent stem cells called ectoderm, mesoderm, and endoderm. In the primitive oral cavity two cell types are juxtaposed, ectoderm in the epithelial surface and ecto-mesenchyme (including mesoderm) below. They interact to control the process of tooth initiation (24). Tooth organs have to develop at precisely determined sites and time-points. The first fundamental patterning in jaw morphogenesis is controlled by the early separation of specific areas of ectoderm that are regulated specifically by ectoderm-endoderm interactions (25).

The branchial arches are derived when ecto-mesenchymal stem cells migrate under the ectoderm into the cranial mesoderm. The ecto-mesenchyme has been called the fourth germ layer. This important tissue is derived from the cranial neural crest at the junction between the neuroectoderm of the closing neural tube and the surface ectoderm. The neural crest tissue, which is filled with pluripotential stem cells, migrates from the dorsal side around the primitive brain into the branchial arches on the ventral side (26). The mammalian jaw apparatus including teeth is derived from the first branchial arch in the embryo (27).

## Tooth initiation

In tooth development the epithelium covering the inside of the developing oral cavity secretes the first instructive signals. Signaling molecules thereby position the sites of subsequent tooth development (28) (Fig. 3.3).

The patterning of the dentition is based on a nested pattern of homeobox genes that are expressed in the mesenchyme (29). These genes include Msx1, -2, Dlx1, -2, -3, -5, -6, -7, Barx1, Otlx2, Lhx6, -7, in specific spatial patterns before any morphological manifestation of tooth development (13, 30–34).

From anterior to posterior, the dentition is divided into regions of incisor, canine, premolar and molar tooth types. The teeth are initiated as discrete organs (35). Manipulation of homeobox code causes transformations in tooth type, for example, from incisor to molar (36).

## Tooth development

The shape of the tooth crown results from growth and folding of inner enamel epithelium. The cusp patterning is regulated by transient signaling centers, the enamel knots (37).

The development of individual teeth involves epithelial-mesenchymal interactions that are mediated by molecular signals shared with other organs, particularly in the four major groups of signaling molecules, and they regulate the early steps of organ development: Hh (hedgehog), wnt (went), FGF (fibroblast growth factor) and TGF super family (transforming growth factors) which include the BMP (bone morphogenetic proteins).

Recent evidence suggests that largely the same signaling cascade is used reiteratively throughout tooth development. Tooth type appears to be determined by epithelial signals and to involve differential activation of homeobox genes in the mesenchyme (35). Tooth initiations involve interaction between Sonic hedgehog (Shh) and wnt signalling molecules in the oral epithelium (29).

Today we are beginning to understand the molecular networks regulating tissue interactions unfolding in time and space during tooth development (38). Hundreds of genes involved in tooth formation have been described (see http://bite-it.helsinki.fi).

The dental mesenchyme, including the dental papilla and follicle, is derived from the cranial neural crest primarily and

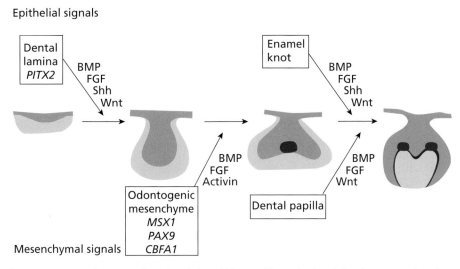

**Fig. 3.3** Tooth development. During tooth initiation the oral epithelium thickens and forms the dental placode. Most ectodermal organs start their development with an epithelial thickening. The epithelium then buds into or protrudes out from the mesenchyme with mesenchyme condensing around the epithelium. From that moment on the development of different organs take on different shapes and quite different functions. The tooth development is characterized by molecular signalling with reciprocal dynamic interaction between epithelium and mesenchyme during all stages. The instructive competence switches between these tissues. From THESLEFF (38) 2003.

few mesodermal cells (26, 39, 40). It is conceivable that stem cells in the dental papilla acquire commitment to differentiate into odontoblasts during their development (41). Dental follicle cells develop commitment to form cementoblasts, PDL-fibroblasts and osteoblasts (42).

The epithelial FGFs and BMPs initially regulate mesenchymal transcription factors including Msx1 and Pax9 (43). These and other signaling molecules are used for temporo-spatial regulation of interaction between adjacent epithelium and underlying mesenchyme (29, 38, 44).

It is well established that odontogenic competence, with information for identity and shape of the teeth, is induced by the epithelium, and subsequently resides in the tooth mesenchyme (45).

Study of the cell signaling ectodysplasin (Eda) gene showed that with increasing expression levels, the number of cusps increases, cusp shapes and positions change, and number of teeth increases (46). The shape of the resulting tooth is coordinated by the enamel-knot signaling centre (29).

Human dental disorders have been shown to involve many of the genes that have important roles in early tooth development (47).

## Cross-talk of genes

Interaction between the local environment of a tissue injury and adult stem cells is a dynamic, complex, ongoing set of interactions. The genes that regulate tooth development (35) are, at least to some extent, reactivated following injury. Members of the Notch signaling pathway operate through local cell–cell interactions and regulate the fate of stem cells. Results suggest activation of Notch signaling is also involved in regulation of adult stem cells during pulp regeneration (48).

Proinflammatory molecules, such as those redistributed from immune responsive cells, root canal microbiota, and necrotic pulp tissue, in the hostile environment created by the injury, influence genes and factors that are involved in regulation of the stem cells and their progenitors during wound healing. When the treatment is successful the inflammatory phase is followed by a reparative phase with proliferation, and eventually a regeneration phase (49).

The progression of the inflammatory phase leads to dampening of complex and potentially aggressive defense reactions. The modifications in the inflammatory signaling network allow for upregulation of the upcoming proliferation phase. Some inflammatory cytokines may be growth stimulatory, but in the fetus wound healing reactions may occur successfully without inflammation (50). Studies on reparative dentinogenesis in germ free animals have shown that pulp cells express the odontoblast phenotype much more early when inflammatory factors are not present (51).

Insight into some of the environmental influences on stem cells in wound healing, such as interaction between stem cells and inflammatory cytokine networks, seems relevant for optimal development of tissue engineering.

## Bone marrow cells

The bone marrow harbors stem cells capable of differentiating between hematopoietic and stromal cell lineages. Both stem cell types are capable of contributing to multiple cell lineages (52, 53). The bone marrow stromal cells (BMSCs) include a group of mesenchymal stem cells capable of forming e.g. cartilage and bone (54). BMSCs can be expanded *in vitro*, but they only form bone after implantation with a 3-dimensional matrix, such as that based on hydroxyapatite. Addition of bone morphogenetic protein7

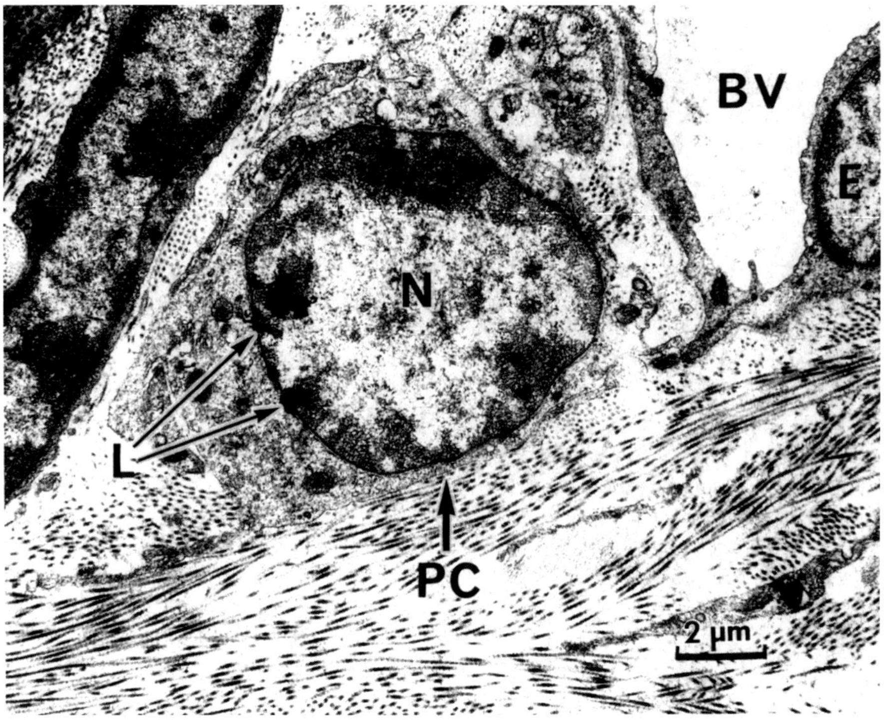

**Fig. 3.4** PDL stem cell. Electron microscope radio-autograph of an undifferentiated paravascular progenitor cell labeled with $H^3$-TdR 29 hours after wounding. BV = lumen of blood vessel; E = endothelial cell; L = radioactive label; N = nucleus; PC = progenitor cell. From GOULD (183) 1983.

(BMP7) stimulates the cells' bone formation in defects which are not capable of repair by themselves (54).

When bone marrow stromal cells with a reporter gene coding for green fluorescent protein (GFP) are transplanted into mice without bone marrow, several organs with experimental injury, including liver, heart and muscle, regenerate with the help of GFP-labeled bone marrow cells (20, 55, 56). It has been proposed that circulating skeletal stem cells can adhere to local cell adhesion molecules (CAMs) in damaged tissue and migrate out and subsequently contribute to tissue regeneration (53).

## Stem cell plasticity, fusions and confusion

Postnatal cells have been suggested to possess some degree of plasticity with de-differentiation of differentiated cells as the basis for recruitment of new stem cells (20).

After pulp exposure it has been suggested that endothelial cells and pericytes may become undifferentiated mesenchymal cells, and that they hypothetically re-differentiate into odontoblasts (57). Cells in the fibroblast cell family may transdifferentiate. However, terminal differentiation is normally irreversible, and conclusions on reversible de-differentiation, with plasticity of mature somatic cells changing to stem cells, need more evidence. Existing evidence suggests that *in vivo* such unexpected transformations are exceedingly rare (21).

The scale of cell recruitment, such as (1) through a transit amplifying cell pool, (2) the potential dedifferentiation due to cell plasticity, or (3) the migration of already determined precursor cells, remains to be clarified (20).

Our concept of stem cells during tissue regeneration has been radically changed, and unfortunately more compli-

cated, by discovery of stem cell fusion and plasticity with potential de-differentiation of differentiated cells as the source of new stem cells.

New discoveries on the Twist-1 gene expression indicate it can be responsible for epithelial-mesenchymal transitions during development (EMT) (58, 59).

*In vitro* coculture of embryonic stem cells and somatic cells can result in spontaneous cell fusion (60, 61). Liver cells are known to form heterokaryons, but only in severe pathological conditions (62, 63). *In vivo* bone marrow stem cells may derive hepatocytes, cardiomyocytes, and Purkinje cells due, at least in part, to fusion with these cell types (60, 61, 64–67). Apparently, stem cells may under specific circumstances fuse with local differentiated cells.

## Stem cells in the periodontium

The periodontium consists of soft and mineralized tissues, and together they provide an attachment for the tooth to the bone while allowing the tooth to withstand physical forces. The periodontal tissues are arranged in cellular domains of remarkable coherence and preserved dimensions (68).

The periodontal ligament is a specialized connective tissue that connects the cementum and the inner wall of the alveolar socket to maintain and support teeth *in situ* and preserve tissue homoeostasis (10). The cementum is a thin layer of mineralized tissue on the surface of the roots (69).

The adult periodontium contains stem cell progenitors, which are involved in tooth maintenance and repair after injury (Fig. 3.4). *In situ*, these cells often have a low cycling rate and locate in specific regions or niches (70, 71).

Adult stem cells and their progenitors proliferate and migrate before arrival at sites of periodontal injury. The advent of new cells has been followed in several studies in rodents by using a marker of DNA synthesis prior to cell division.

An increased number of labeled cell populations are seen to be associated with bone surfaces and ligaments after injury (72). They proliferate in adjacent and unwounded tissues from where they migrate as labeled cells into the wound defect (73, 74). They migrate and differentiate into fibroblasts, osteoblasts or cementoblasts forming new bone and cement (70, 72).

The number of labeled cells in wounded ligaments increased from days 1 to 7 suggesting a prolonged repopulation response after wounding (73).

Studies in mouse molars suggest there is a slowly dividing cell population within 10 microns of blood vessels which may represent stem cells (74, 75). They divide several times before day 3 (74). From day 3 to day 7 after wounding the majority of cells were found to be paravascular. The majority of the dividing cells appeared to belong to two populations, one adjacent to bone, the other in the body of the ligament. A third and minor population, not paravascular, lay adjacent to cementum (72).

Endosteal spaces of alveolar bone apparently also contribute with progenitors (70). Data also from mouse molars with ligament wounding indicate that endosteal spaces are enriched with labeled progenitor cells whose progeny rapidly migrate out of the compartment, and there they subsequently express the phenotype for osteoblasts or cementoblasts (70).

Periodontal ligament contiguous with the endosteal spaces exhibited 5 times as many mitosis-labeled cells as other sites in this tissue. Thickened cementum was coincident with the openings of endosteal spaces in most of the observations (70). Taken together, the data sugggest that periodontal tissues respond with site-specific recruitment of stem cell progenitors.

## Stem cells in the pulp

The dentin provides a structural basis for the function of the tooth which allows the tooth to withstand physical forces while protecting the pulp. The pulp-dentinal organ consists of soft and mineralized tissues, and together they interact in order to maintain the function of the tooth.

The pulp-dentin tissues are integrally connected in the sense that pathologic reactions in one of the tissues will also affect the other (69).

The peripheral part of the pulp comprises a single layer of polarized cells, the odontoblasts, which separate the dentin from the pulp stroma. Each odontoblast secretes predentin and makes an extension into a dentinal tubule, the odontoblast process. After odontoblasts have formed they secrete *primary dentin*, after eruption they continue to form *secondary dentin* at a slow rate, and *tertiary dentin* is formed in response to localized irritation (Fig. 3.5).

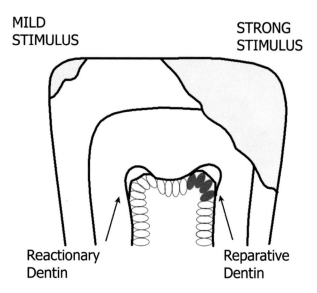

**Fig. 3.5** Reactionary and reparative dentin. The range of confusing terms used to describe physiological and pathological dentin, secreted after primary dentin formation, has led to redefinition of 'tertiary dentin', which is subdivided into reactionary and reparative dentin. The localized tertiary dentin formed by surviving primary odontoblasts following mild impacts, has been referred to as reactionay dentin, whereas that formed by a new odontoblasts has been called reparative dentin (76, 77).

The range of confusing terms used to describe physiological and pathological dentin, secreted after primary dentin formation, has led to redefinition of 'tertiary dentin', which is subdivided into reactionary and reparative dentin (76).

The localized tertiary dentin formed by surviving primary odontoblasts following mild impacts, has been referred to as *reactionary dentin*, whereas that formed by a new odontoblasts has been called *reparative dentin* (77) (Fig. 3.5).

The pulp stroma is a specialized loose connective tissue including blood and lymph vessels, nerves, and interstitial fluid (69). The adult pulp contains immature stem cell-like cells, which are involved in pulp-dentin repair after injury. They have the potential to develop into specialized odontoblast-like cells, and they are duplicated in the stromal pulp after greater injuries, where they migrate to the injured site as described in the following.

## Pericytes, the primary stem cell candidate

Earlier studies suggest the dentinogenic stem cells are associated with the blood vessel walls (2).

Studies in rodents suggest that progenitor cells located around the blood vessels (78), and especially endothelial cells and pericytes, are involved in repair (57).

The *pericytes* in human dental pulp are abluminal perivascular cells located around the endothelial cells in capillaries and blood vessels. They are enclosed in basement membrane matrix, and they can be recognized by their stunted or rounded form and their few, short processes (Fig. 3.6). The pericytes represent undifferentiated mesenchymal cells.

*Transitional cells* are partly surrounded by basement membrane. *Fibroblast-like cells* are outside, but adjacent to the basement membrane. Some pericytes may migrate away

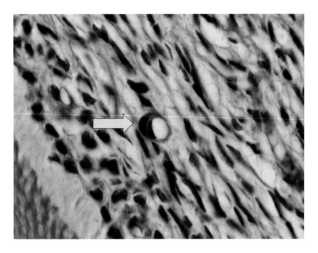

**Fig. 3.6** Pericyte. The pericyte is seen close to cuboidal odontoblasts on the dentin wall of a mouse molar. Dental pulp stem cells are expected to include pericytes. Pericytes are located around endothelial cells embedded in the basal lamina. They are abluminal and small with big nuclei, and a plump and rounded morphology with only few lamellipodia. The PAS staining labels glycoproteins in the perivascular basal lamina.

from the vessel wall to undergo transition to another phenotype (28).

Recent evidence supports that dentinogenic progenitor cells are of perivascular origin with pericytes as the primary dentinogenic stem cell candidate (28).

Stem cells have been found in human dental pulp in permanent (79) and exfoliated deciduous teeth (18). It has been shown that it is possible to isolate a fraction of pulp cells enriched in stem cells by using STRO-1, CD-146, and 3G5 antigens for selection of cells and fluorescence activated cell sorting (FACS). The Gronthos & Shi group confirmed the stem-cell-like properties as two-thirds of the single-colony-derived cell populations generated abundant ectopic dentin *in vivo* after transplantation (80). STRO-1 and CD-146 antigens colocalized *in vivo* on the outer walls of large blood vessels in human adult pulp (80), whereas 3G5 is a general pericyte-associated cell surface antigen (81, 82). Therefore, it is suggested that dental pulp stem cells reside in the microvasculature of the pulp, and that pulpal pericytes, which fulfil a role in angiogenesis and blood vessel homeostasis, may also contribute as adult dentinogenic stem cells (26).

## Stem cells and pulp injury

Experimental animal studies have demonstrated that repair of the pulp-dentin organ occurs with recruitment of new odontoblast-like cells (83) (Fig. 3.7). Studies using tritiated thymidine described an increased number of labeled cells 3–4 days after pulp capping, and the progenitor cells migrated toward the wound clot and adjacent dentin walls where odontoblasts had been lost. No label incorporation was observed in surviving odontoblasts close to the injury (84). Accordingly, new pre-odontoblasts replacing lost odontoblasts were labeled and recruited by multiplication and not only migration (85).

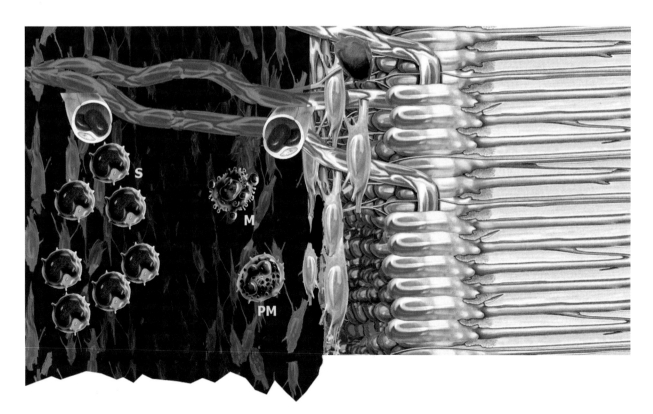

**Fig. 3.7** Pulp healing after crown fracture. Stem cells participate in healing after a crown fracture with deep dentin exposure or direct pulp exposure. The offspring of paravascular stem cells (S) migrate together with polymorphonuclear leukocytes (PM) and macrophages (M) to the injury site.

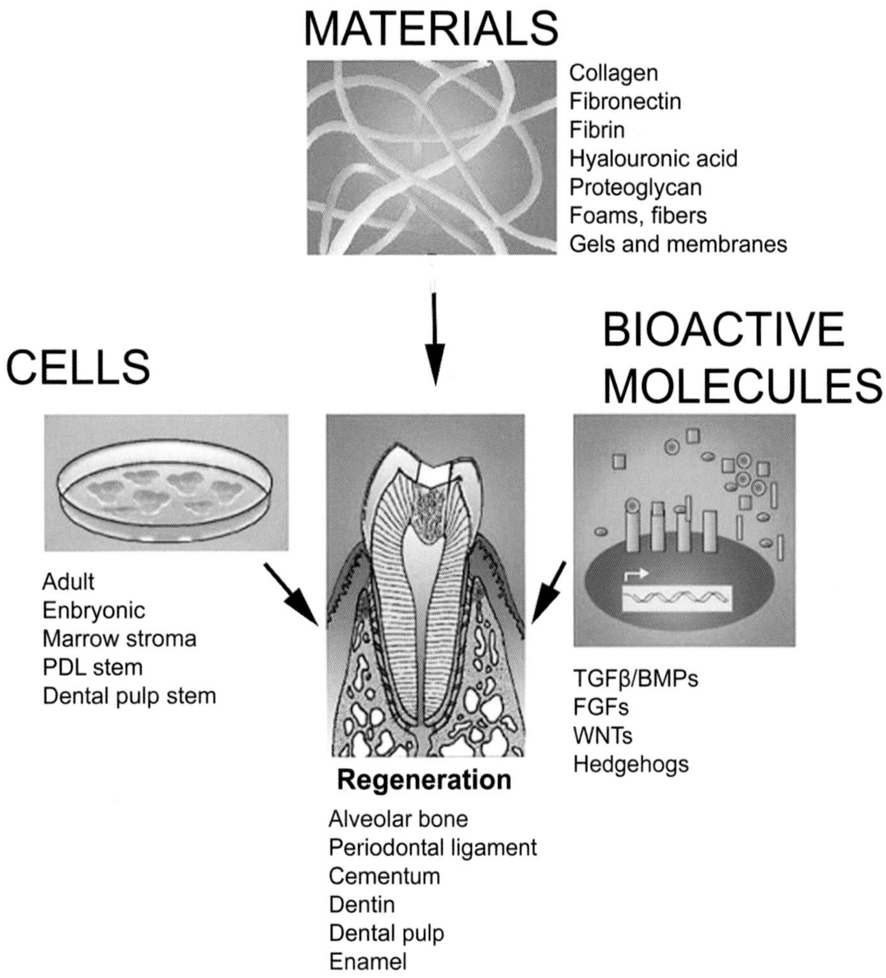

## MATERIALS

Collagen
Fibronectin
Fibrin
Hyalouronic acid
Proteoglycan
Foams, fibers
Gels and membranes

## CELLS

## BIOACTIVE MOLECULES

**Fig. 3.8** Tissue engineering. The triad: *bioactive molecules, cells* and *materials* (scaffolds/carriers) can be used for regeneration of bone, PDL, cementum and dentin. The key bioactive molecules are the morphogenetic signaling families: BMPs, FGFs, Shh and Wnts. The cells include progenitor/stem cells derived from marrow, dental pulp and PDL-derived cells. The materials consist of extracellular matrix scaffold, hydroxy apatite, collagens, fibronectin, proteoglycans including hyaluronic acid, synthetic foams, fibers, gels and membranes, which can be incorporated with biomimetic biomaterials. From NAKASHIMA & REDDI (92) 2003.

Adult
Enbryonic
Marrow stroma
PDL stem
Dental pulp stem

TGFβ/BMPs
FGFs
WNTs
Hedgehogs

**Regeneration**
Alveolar bone
Periodontal ligament
Cementum
Dentin
Dental pulp
Enamel

Different labeling responses have been described after superficial and deep pulp injuries. In superficial injuries increased labeling of fibroblasts and perivascular cells were described early and close to the lesion and decreasing by time, whereas under deep exposures similar labeling changed from low to high over time (86). Continuous influx of newly differentiating odontoblast-like cells at the material–pulp interface was observed to be cells originating from the deeper pulp. At least two replications of DNA are required after pulp capping before cell migration and expression of the new odontoblast-like phenotype (86, 87). Transplantation of pulp tissue from transgenic mice carrying a GFP-reporter gene confirmed that the stromal dental pulp contains progenitors that can differentiate into odontoblast- or osteocyte-like cells giving rise to tubular reparative dentin or atubular bone-like dentin, dependent on the conditions (7).

## Tissue engineering

### A triade of biomolecules, biomaterials and cells

Tissue engineering is the manipulation and development of molecules, cells, tissues and organs, to replace or support the function of defective or injured body parts.

Tissue engineering is based on the research triade of cells, biomolecules and biomaterials (Fig. 3.8). The list of tissues with the potential to be engineered is growing steadily (3).

Progress in understanding tooth development, the role of stem cells, carriers, scaffolds, and bioactive molecules, have set the stage for engineering of traumatized dental tissue.

The designs and approaches are endless, and range from conductive membranes to using stem cells *ex vivo* for construction of whole teeth. This section briefly reviews the role of biomaterials, biomolecules, and cells, in dental tissue engineering.

### Biomaterials: the third generation

Biomaterials for conductive, inductive, and also cell-based tissue replacement strategies, are in development (88). Biodegradable or nondegradable scaffolds can be used as space-filling matrices for tissue development and barriers to migration of epithelial cells in tissue conductive approaches (88). The biomaterials may also include matrix and vehicle for cell adhesion and distribution of bioactive molecules.

Inductive approaches involve sustained delivery of bioactive factors, such as protein growth factors and plasmid DNA, to alter cell function in localized regions. Factors can be released from highly porous polymer scaffolds to allow factor delivery and tissue development to occur in concert (88).

Recent bone research described the response of osteoblasts to the ionic solution products of bioactive glasses, which have proven to be effective tools with osteo-productive properties. The activated genes express numerous proteins that influence all aspects of proliferation and differentiation of osteoblasts:

- Transcription factors and cell cycle regulators
- Signal transduction molecules
- Proteins involved in DNA synthesis, repair, and recombination
- Growth factors and cytokines that influence the inflammatory response to the material
- Cell-surface antigens and receptors
- Extracellular matrix components and enzymes
- Apoptosis regulators (89).

Where the second generation biomaterials were designed to be either resorbable or bioactive the third generation of biomaterials is combining these two properties, with the aim of developing materials that, once implanted, will help the body heal itself (90). The separate concepts of using bio-resorbable and bioactive materials have converged.

Two alternative routes of repair with the use of bioactive biomaterials are available (90).

In one approach, tissue engineering is performed before implantation. Progenitor cells are seeded onto modified resorbable scaffolds. The cells grow outside the body and become differentiated and mimic naturally occurring tissues.

In another approach, tissue engineering is performed after implantation *in situ*. This approach involves the use of bio-materials in the form of powders, solutions, or micropartices to stimulate local stem cell recruitment. Extracellular matrix molecules can also mimic the extracellular environment and provide a multifunctial cell-adhesive surface (90).

The new third-generation implants, as mentioned above, include both resorbable biomaterials and a molecular tailoring of immobilized proteins, peptides, and other bioactive substances seems to show great promise.

## Biomolecules: growth and differentiation factors

Although numerous molecules can be used to stimulate tissue formation including mitogenic signals and differentiation factors, only a small number are yet being pursued clinically (91–95).

As reviewed by Silva, et al. 2004 several growth factors and other soluble molecules have been identified in human dentin including IGF-I, IGF-II, TGF-β1, TGF-β2, TGF-β3, MMP gelatinase A, PDGF-AB, VEGF, PlGF, FGF2, and EGF (96).

Classic receptor-mediated peptide signaling supported with extracellular matrix molecules for stimulation of tissue formation cascades lead to cellular events such as chemotaxis, angiogenesis, proliferation, differentiation, and eventually formation of soft or hard tissue (91).

The application of polypeptides such as PDGF, TGFβ and IGF has apparently led to successful enough outcomes to facilitate clinical regulatory approval (91–95).

Another therapeutic candidate is enamel matrix derivative, a set of matrix proteins. Enamel matrix derivative appears to stimulate first acellular cementum formation, which may, in a limited extent, support functional periodontal ligament formation (91).

It is evident that the BMPs are excellent molecules and candidates for stimulation of oral mineralizing tissues and periodontal ligament (91). BMPs have been introduced for pulp capping showing marked stimulation of reparative dentinogenesis (97, 98); however, blood vessel invasion into the pulp implant appears to be a side-effect which has to be conquered. The recent approval by the US Food and Drug Administration of rhBMPs for accelerating bone fusion in slow-healing fractures indicates that this protein family may prove useful in designing regenerative dental treatments both in endodontics and periodontics (92).

## Biomolecules: gene therapy

Gene therapy represents a promising approach for local delivery of bioactive molecules to specific tissues. Advances in the techniques to genetically modify the gene activity of stem cells during their *ex vivo* expansion may offer a unique opportunity to influence a patient's own stem cells even better. It is actually possible to replace a gene activity which is missing, and it is also possible to silence a gene activity that is defective and unwanted (12).

Several laboratories have shown that virus-based expression vectors can stimulate for example BMP expression and osteoblast differentiation leading to increased bone formation *in vivo*. Both *in vivo* and *ex vivo* transduction of cells can induce bone formation at ectopic and orthotopic sites. Bone regeneration may also be achieved through the use of inducible promoters and, in so doing, be able to precisely control both the amount and type of bone regenerated (99).

## Cell implantation

The isolation of adult stem cell populations that reproducibly can form bone and its marrow, dentin, cementum, and periodontal ligament, support an envision of complete restoration of complex oro-facial structures by using the patients own cells and, thereby, avoid the issues of histo-compatibility.

The molecular techniques for expansion and induction of specific stem cell progenitors, and also the biomaterials used as carrier, are developing. Recent approaches have been based on seeding of cells, for example onto polymeric scaffolds *in vitro* and subsequent transplantation of the scaffold. New scaffold materials are being developed that address specific tissue engineering design requirements, and in some cases attempt to mimic natural extracellular matrices (88).

These strategies together offer the possibility of forming specific tissue structures, and may provide answers to problems with exposed pulps, injured periodontal ligaments, furcation defects, bone and root resorptions, and ankylosis (88).

Stem cells from teeth have been isolated from teeth by using activated cell sorting. It was possible to transplant a mix of human stem cells with hydroxyl apatite carrier into immunocompromized mice and develop PDL/cementum from isolated fractions of PDL stem cells (10), dentin from subpopulations of pulp stem cells, and bone from stromal marrow cells (23), respectively.

There are several aspects that need to be addressed as we attempt to explore the mechanisms underlying the potentials of stem cell therapy. These questions include at present the host immune response to implanted cells, the homing mechanisms that guide delivered cells to a site of injury, and differentiation of implanted cells under the influence of local signals (40).

## Periodontal tissue regeneration

### Stem cells and periodontal regeneration

Successful regeneration of tooth and bone fractures requires repair and regeneration with the tissues in the right place. Several tissues can be involved in dental traumas: ligament, cement, bone, dentin, pulp, vessels, and neurons. Regeneration of tooth injuries can therefore be a complex process requiring recruitment of specific adult stem cells in specific locations. Evidence to date suggests that future treatment of periodontal traumas may benefit from studies focusing on stem cells.

### Traumatized or lost periodontal ligament

The periodontal ligament is a specialized connective tissue that connects cementum and alveolar bone to maintain and support teeth *in situ* and preserve tissue homeostasis. The prognosis of tooth regeneration depends on the extent and nature of the trauma. When periodontal tissues are lost it is important that PDL-derived progenitor cells are formed and regenerate the PDL with associated cementum deposition along the root in order to save the tooth.

Cases of acute injury to the PDL are represented by luxation injuries, root fracture, alveolar bone fractures and avulsions. It has been found that the healing of most of these traumas is uneventful leading to regeneration of the PDL within approximately two weeks (see Chapter 2).

In some instances where a significant part of the PDL has been destroyed, root resorption may become a significant problem. This relates especially to intrusive luxation and avulsion with subsequent replantation.

Improved regeneration of lost periodontal tissue is a major goal in traumatology. Animal experiments have shown that the decisive factor in these cases is the survival, or destruction, of the innermost layer of the PDL (cementoblasts and possibly also the PDL cells next to the cementoblast) (see Chapter 2). Although a number of treatment approaches have been made using various chemical and antibiotic procedures, these have so far not been able to prevent establishment and progression of root resorption. Strategies used to treat loss of periodontal support include those that arrest the progression of periodontitis (100) and reconstruct lost support with surgical approaches (101–103). In the following a number of new assays will be presented to cope with this problem.

## Bone engineering

Several previous studies have focused on alveolar bone regeneration. The formation of bone can be achieved by several approaches. Many materials have been used: several graft, derivatives and substitutes (104).

The biological bone reaction cascade during integration of transplanted teeth or artificial implants *in situ*, can be deconvoluted into three phases. First, *osteoconduction* relies on the migration of differentiating osteogenic cells to defect. Second, *bone formation*, results in a mineralized matrix equivalent to that seen in cement lines in natural bone tissue. Third, *bone remodeling* will follow. Stimulation of bone formation rather than just bone replacement is dependent on several factors. Stem cells which will form the bone are needed, as well as for a scaffold for them, a bony bed, or they will resorb, and a blood supply, stability, continual micro-mechanical forces, and freedom from infection (105).

Transplantation of bone marrow stromal cells (BMSC) including osteogenic stem cells has been suggested as an approach for reconstruction of craniofacial bone defects by circumventing many of the limitations of auto- and allografting (3).

It is evident that, in order to make bone by using the adherent stromal cells from bone marrow aspirates, it is necessary to transplant the stem cells together with an organized framework to which they can adhere and proliferate long enough to ensure differentiation and bone formation (12). Skeletal stem cells can be isolated from a limited volume of bone marrow and expanded *in vitro* and loaded onto an appropriate carrier, and locally transplanted for bone reconstruction. Successful bone engineering by using stem cells has been shown in calvarial and long bones models (1, 106–109). This procedure can result in effective repair of critical size defects, which are larger than what can be repaired by resident cells guided by an osteoconductive device in the local environment (3).

Gene transfer may offer new possibilities by transducing into cells from the host *ex vivo* before they are seeded onto carriers and implanted in the host again. When the BMP-7 gene is transferred to dermal fibroblasts it has been shown it is possible to stimulate healing of alveolar bone defects in rats (110). The use of stem cells for regenerative therapy is in development; however it has primarily been demonstrated in animal models.

## PDL engineering

Regeneration of periodontal defects requires recruitment of stem cell progenitors, which originally are developed from the dental follicle (68). It has been proposed that, for new cementum and attachment during periodontal regeneration, the local environment must be conducive for the recruitment and function of cementum-forming cells (111). Studies have described that clonogenic cells isolated from human periodontal ligament cementum can be expanded *in vitro*. Furthermore, these cells are capable of forming a cementum-like tissue, in contrast to bone stem cells which, for example, make trabecular structures and hematopoietic compartments when transplanted into immunocompromized mice (14, 15).

Preliminary cell transplantation studies suggest transplanted PDL-derived stem cells (10) and cementoblasts (14, 15) can be used for cementum formation when transplanted into immunocompromized mice with a carrier (10, 184). It was shown cementoblasts can be used for repairing root injuries (112).

Periodontal ligament stem cells were isolated by using the stem and cell markers STRO-1 and CD146/MUC18 for activated cell sorting. The Gronthos group thereby demonstrated stem-cell-like properties and the cells' capacity to generate a cementum/PDL-like structure after transplantation into immunocompromized mice (10).

Whether organization of bone, cementum and ligament are also formed by stem cells from distinct tissues, or only by pluripotent cells responding with plasticity to local environmental cues, has not been verified. Distinguishing between these possibilities has been difficult as cell specific markers for labeling and distinction of cementoblast and osteoblast precursors are lacking (12).

Developing and wounded periodontal tissues exhibit fundamental differences. The developing periodontium is governed by epithelial-mesenchymal signal interactions which regulate specific cell populations in time and space. During wound healing the cell fates are regulated by a vast array of extracellular molecules that induce responses in the different cell lineages and their precursors (68).

According to the concept of *in situ* tissue engineering the use of a third generation resorbable and bioactive membrane has been demonstrated in dogs. To regenerate periodontal tissues, a sandwich membrane has been developed that is composed of a collagen sponge scaffold and gelatin microspheres containing basic fibroblast growth factor (bFGF) in a controlled-release system.

New cementum was formed on the exposed root surface at 4 weeks, and functional recovery of the periodontal ligament was indicated in part by the perpendicular orientation of regenerated collagen fibers. In the control group, epithelial downgrowth and root resorption occurred and the defects were filled with connective tissue (113). Thus, sandwich membrane with bioactive molecules may induce regeneration of the periodontal tissues. Other studies have shown that new bone formation is apparently affected by rapid-release kinetics of bone morphogenetic proteins (BMPs). In contrast, new cementum formation is promoted by slow release of BMP (114).

*W. V. Giannobile, M. J. Somerman and Q. Jin*

## Cementum engineering

### Influence of amelogenins on cementogenesis

Periodontal regenerative therapies have focused traditionally on regeneration of alveolar bone, with a paucity of approaches targeted on cementum regeneration. Evidence to date suggests that cementum regeneration is a key consideration for designing predictable approaches to restore tooth-supporting tissues (115). One strategy for promoting periodontal tissue regeneration is to mimic the specific events that occur during development of these tissues. In this regard, some investigators have reported that epithelial cells deposit enamel matrix-related proteins onto the root surface prior to cementum formation, and that these proteins trigger follicle cell differentiation toward a cementoblast phenotype and subsequently cementogenesis (116) (Fig. 3.9). These findings, suggesting that epithelial-mesenchymal interactions are required for cementum formation, prompted the formation of a company to develop an enamel matrix derivative (EMD) product for regenerating periodontal tissues (Straumann, Switzerland) (117–119). Enamel matrix derivative (EMD) is predominately composed of amelogenin (90%), suggesting that the role of enamel matrix derivative is realized mainly through amelogenin. The results of amelogenin knock-out mice show that without amelogenin, cementum will be resorbed. However, caution must be used in interpreting the data, since the weak enamel structure itself may activate osteoclasts during mastication (120). In addition, amelogenins have been reported to regulate hard tissue forming markers: osteocalcin and bone sialoprotein expression, as well as osteoprotegerin, in cementoblasts (121). However, there are differences between EMD and amelogenin responsiveness (e.g. EMD promotes proliferation of mesenchymal cells, but amelogenins do not), and thus, some of the clinical effects of EMD may not be related to amelogenin. At the clinical level, application of EMD improves periodontal tissue regeneration (122).

In order to confirm that amelogenins have a direct effect on mesenchymal cells, additional investigations are needed, including identification of specific cell surface receptors associated with amelogenin.

### BMP and noggin

Bone morphogenetic proteins (BMP) are multifunctional signaling molecules belonging to the transforming growth factor-superfamily, which are involved in embryonic development and bone formation and turnover in post-natal life (122, 123).

The effects of BMPs represent both stimulation and inhibition of dental tissue formation. Most BMP members have the ability to induce ectopic bone formation (92). BMPs are

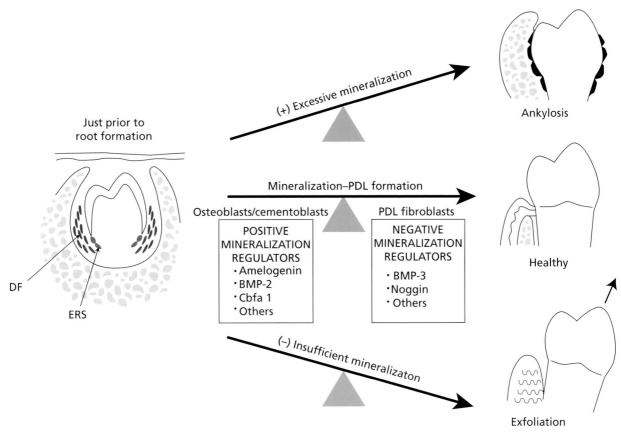

**Fig. 3.9** Potential factors and cells regulating formation and regeneration of the periodontium. Appropriate development of the periodontium requires a balance between formation of soft connective tissues, i.e. PDL, and hard connective tissues, i.e. bone and cementum. Periodontal tissue development includes formation of the root/cementogenesis, supporting alveolar bone and PDL. Molecules suggested as keys for promoting formation/regeneration of periodontal tissues include: a) *amelogenin* and/or amelogenin-like molecules secreted by surrounding epithelial cells that may promote follicle cells to express genes linked with the cementoblast/osteoblast phenotype; b) *BMPs*: BMP-3, found in high concentrations within the follicle cell region, functions as a negative regulator of mineralization, while BMP-2, -4 and -7 function as a positive regulator of mineralization promoting follicle cells to differentiate along the cementoblast/osteoblast pathway; c) *noggin*, a negative regulator of BMP-2, -4 and -7 activity; d) *Runx2*, a putative master switch, may be important for promoting differentiation of follicle cells along a cementoblast/osteoblast pathway (Abbreviations: DF = dental follicle; ERS = epithelial root sheath).

differentially expressed during tooth development and periodontal repair (124–126). BMP-2 triggers the differentiation of dental follicle cells into cementoblasts or osteoblasts *in vitro* (42). The expression of BMP-3 is seen in particular in the dental follicle cells which give rise to cementoblasts (124), especially cementoblasts close to epithelial cell rests of Malassez continuing to express Msx2 (127). Moreover, BMPs potently stimulate alveolar bone regeneration around teeth, as well as initiate cementogenesis in periodontal wounds (110, 128). Noggin is a BMP antagonist that binds specific BMPs and prevents them docking to cognate receptors (129). The BMP binding proteins including Noggin regulate the bioavailability of BMPs, and they may thereby influence the development and regeneration of ligaments and joints (130). Noggin plays an important role in tooth development. For example, local application of noggin to embryonic tooth bud explants transforms tooth type from incisor teeth to molar teeth (36).

BMP-7 induces noggin expression in cementoblasts, PDL fibroblasts, and osteoblasts, which suggests that there is a feedback regulatory mechanism between BMP and its antagonist (110, 131). Furthermore, sustained delivery of noggin reduces cementogenesis *in vivo* (110, 131). The complex BMP signaling pathways and feedback loops, and also the threshold dependent action of BMPs, emphasize the need for a balance between multiple factors for application of BMPs in tissue engineering with a successful regeneration of both soft or hard tissues.

## Cell transplantation for cemental repair

In order to better understand the potential of cementum-derived cells in the restoration of lost cemental support, cell populations of dental follicle cells and cementoblasts have been evaluated in a model of cementum and periodontal regeneration (112, 133–134).

Using a periodontal defect model in rodents, periodontal traumas were treated with transplanted cell lines of dental follicle cells and cementoblasts (112) to determine the ability to promote periodontal wound healing (Fig. 3.10). The extent of bone and cementum regeneration and the gene expression of mineral-associated bone sialoprotein and

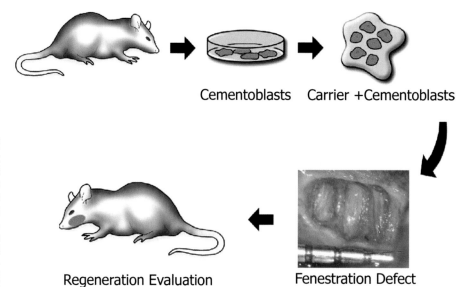

Cementoblasts　　　Carrier +Cementoblasts

Regeneration Evaluation

Fenestration Defect
Cell transplantation

**Fig. 3.10** Cementum engineering of cementum *in vivo*. This schematic representation demonstrates a method for delivery of cells/scaffolds to sites of periodontal wound healing in a rodent model. First, cells such as cementoblasts are expanded *in vitro*, followed by seeding in bioresorbable polymer carriers and then transplanted to alveolar bone wounds for quantitative assessment of periodontal regeneration. Adapted from ZHAO et al. (112) 2004.

osteocalcin were observed at early time points after the cell therapy (112). The results showed that follicle cells failed to restore periodontal bone and cementum support, while cementoblast transplantation promoted both bone and early cementum-like tissue formation (Fig. 3.11). Interestingly, follicle cells negatively regulated healing versus sites with no cells added, supporting the concept that cells within the local periodontal environment secrete factors that inhibit mineral formation. These findings suggest that mature cementoblast populations can promote periodontal repair, while less differentiated cells (i.e. dental follicle cells) require additional triggers in order to promote mineral formation (135).

A variety of approaches have been undertaken to regenerate tooth root cementum with the goal that cementogenesis will promote further periodontal regeneration, i.e. restoration of the cementum, alveolar bone and a functional PDL. Continued studies focused on defining the key regulators of cementogenesis will assist in designing predictable regenerative therapies.

*H. Løvschall and J. O. Andreasen*

## Pulp-dentin regeneration after trauma

The pulp must respond to a spectrum of traumatic events. The character of the pulp-dentin healing response varies according to the origin of the progenitor cells involved.

The early reparative responses include proliferation of mesenchymal stem cells and formation of new blood vessels. The formation of a granulation tissue provides a niche with many vascular cells which allows for self-renewal of stem cells and progenitors, an environment which putatively is instructive in generation of the dental progeny (49).

During pulp-dentin repair, the tooth development processes are somehow mimicked leading to focal deposition of reactionary and reparative dentin at injury sites. The nature of these responses is determined in part by the extent of tissue injury (136).

The mildest traumatic entity is represented by an *uncomplicated crown* or *crown-root fracture* which exposes dentin, leading to various external stimuli through the dentinal tubules (e.g. thermal, chemical). After some time bacteria invasion into the dentinal tubules may increase the pulp inflammation (see Chapter 2).

Deep to the pulp injury surviving odontoblasts respond with deposition of reactionary dentin along the walls. In such a situation we observe formation of a reactionary dentin matrix with less tubular density than in the primary dentin (Fig. 3.6).

If the odontoblast layer is damaged new secondary odontoblast-like cells are recruited from the bank of dentinogenic stem cells precursors. The differentiation of odontoblasts is characterized by a sequence of cytological and functional changes which occur at each site in the pulp chamber according to a specific pattern (137–139).

The new odontoblast-like cells secrete reparative dentine and the prognosis of pulp vitality is influenced by the residual dentin thickness and the choice of restorative materials (140). Secretion of matrix from the new generation of cells implies a discontinuity in tubular structure with subsequent reduction in dentin permeability.

In case of a *complicated crown fracture*, the pulp is exposed and thereby directly exposed to the same stimuli as described above. In these cases the optimal healing sequence is to ensure a hard tissue closure of the exposure (see Chapter 2).

The cells responsible for the formation of this dentin bridge have been described as mesenchymal cells located

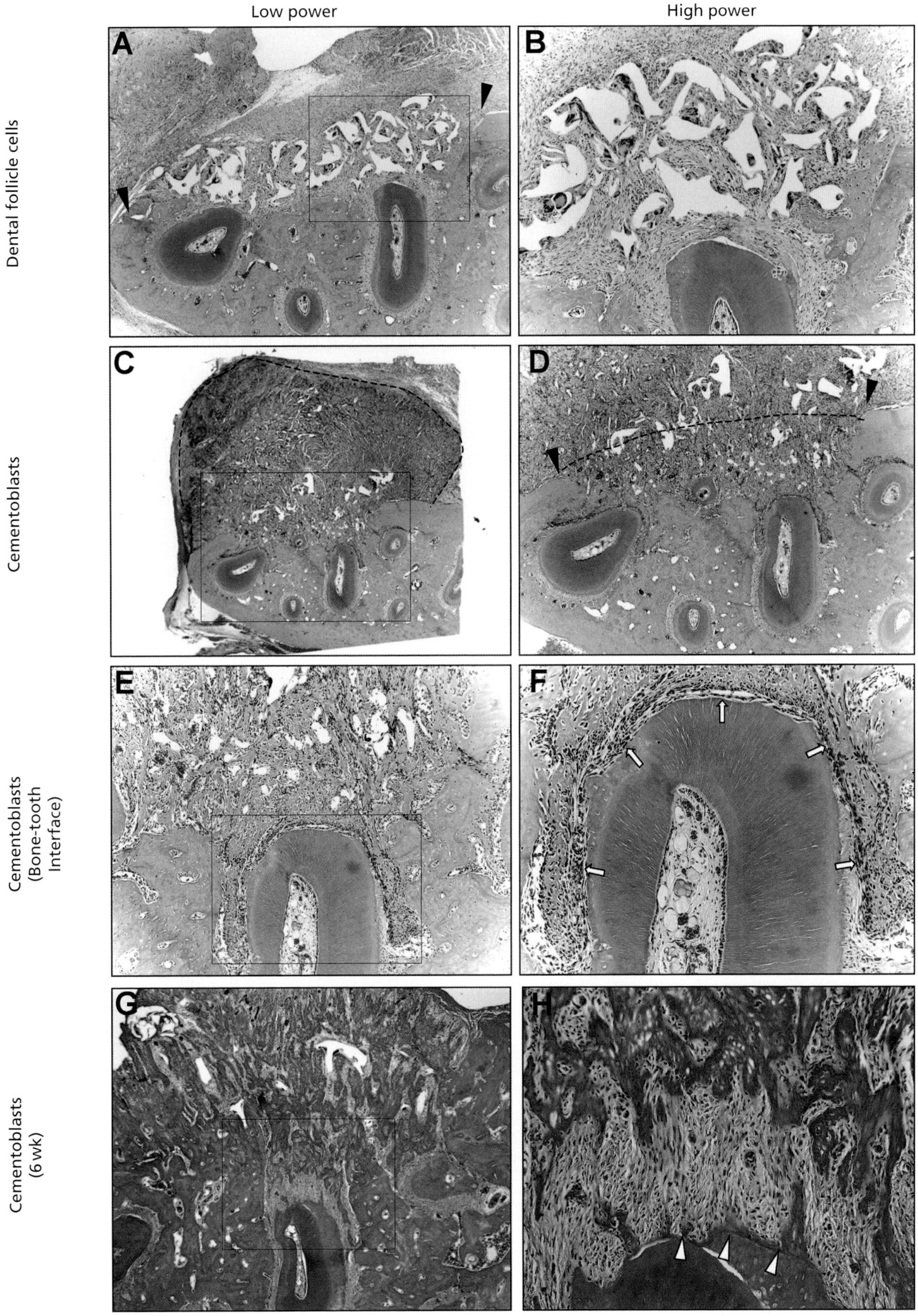

**Fig. 3.11** Transplantation of cementoblasts promotes regeneration of cementum and bone, while dental follicle cell transplantation fails to restore periodontal support. A and B. Polymer carrier (polylactic co-glycolide polymer) + dental follicle cells at 3 weeks. The defect contains polymer particles and fibrous tissue interspersed with numerous spindle-shaped and multinucleated cells. There is minimal evidence of new bone formation, except at the surgical margin (original magnification A: ×4, B: ×10). C–F. Cementoblasts at 3 weeks. Newly formed mineralized tissue with numerous blood vessels is observed filling the defect region and laterally beyond the envelope of the buccal plate of bone (dotted line in D). The newly formed mineralized tissue merges with surrounding bone in some areas, but is separated from the root surface by a layer of connective tissue (white arrows in F) containing spindle-shaped cells and small blood vessels (original magnification C: ×2, D: ×4, E: ×10, F: ×20). G and H: cementoblasts at 6 weeks. Newly formed mineralized tissues fill the defect in a similar fashion to the 3-week specimens. A well-organized PDL region is now seen, with organized fibers connecting the root surface and mineralized tissue. A thin layer of cementum-like tissue on the root surface is also seen (arrowheads in H). From ZHAO et al. (112) 2004.

paravascularly that subsequently differentiate into odonto-blasts (57, 141) (Fig. 3.7).

The first stem cell progenitors deposit an atubular denti-nal matrix covered by cuboidal or polygonal preodonto-blast-like cells. Some of the cells are embedded, as osteocyte-like cells, in a dense mineralizing matrix called osteodentin. Subsequently, a layer of tubular dentin is deposited on top the osteodentin.

The tissue reactions to experimental pulp capping in dogs' teeth with calcium hydroxide have been summarized in 4 stages: the exudative stage (1–5 days), the proliferative stage (3–7 days), osteodentin formative stage (5–14 days), and the tubular dentin formative stage (14 days and more) (142).

Several studies using a number of organ, explant, and cell-culture methods have noted the ability of such cultures to mineralize (143–146). The reason for the varying responses has not yet been clarified.

In cases where the entrance to the exposure site is covered with a suitable capping material (i.e. which limits or pre-vents bacterial contamination), a hard tissue barrier is nor-mally established (147–150).

It has been found that if an accidental exposure of the pulp is left untreated over a period of 1 week the pulp tissue can proliferate through the exposure site (151, 152).

In the case of a *root fracture*, the coronal part will suffer a partial or total severance of the neurovascular supply which leads to ischemia and cell death in this region (see Chapter 12).

The healing process moves coronally with vascular stem cell progenitors, and eventually revascularization. If the pulp becomes infected in its ischemic state, reparative angiogen-esis is apparently permanently arrested and an inflammatory cell infiltration separates infected tissue from ingrowing apical tissue.

Finally in *luxation injuries* (eg. extrusion, lateral luxation and intrusion), the neuro-vascular supply to the pulp is totally severed and most of the populations in the pulp will die after a few days. The ensuing ischemia affects all cells in the pulp (see Chapter 12).

The outcome will be either pulpal revascularization or the development of partial or total pulp necrosis, usually deter-mined by the presence or bacteria in the injury zone. Both trauma and bacterial infection stimulate release of pro-inflammatory cytokines and activate inflammatory cell infil-tration. Failure to resolve inflammation after wounding leads to chronic nonhealing wounds (153), and the pulp tissue responds with absence of hard tissue healing (see Chapter 22).

The general feature of the pulp healing response is replacement of damaged tissue with newly formed pulp tissue. This can occur *along the dentin wall* if localized pulp damage has been inflicted on the odontoblast layer, along an *amputation zone* in the coronal part of the pulp, or as a *replacement of the major parts* of the pulp tissue if it has become necrotic because of ischemia (154).

During pulp repair, cells are able to proliferate, migrate, and differentiate into pre-odontoblasts and odontoblasts outside the specific temporo-spatial pattern of tooth devel-opment, and in the absence of a developing epithelial appendage from the oral ectoderm (49, 136). Local activa-tion after pulp capping of stem cell regulating molecules belonging to the Notch signaling pathway, indicate more cell populations are involved (48, 155).

Further characterization of reparative angiogenesis and dentinogenesis with clarification on the role of stem cell populations during pulp healing, may help in utilization of their potentials.

## Experimental pulp cell transplantation

In recent studies adult stem cells have been isolated from dental pulp (157) and expanded *in vitro* in order to examine their behaviour after transplantation.

Transplantation of dental papilla from rodent or bovine tissue may lead to ectopic dentin formation (52, 160). It was observed that transplantation of developing human dental papilla into immuncompromised mice failed to generate mineralized dentin matrix or odontoblast-like cells (161, 162). However, when the human papillae (158) and also FACS-isolated (STRO-1 and CD-146) (80) and cultured adult dental pulp cells (79) were transplanted with a suitable conductive carrier, such as hydroxyapatite/tricalcium phos-phate particles, dentin formation was observed *in vivo*.

The dentin formation was characterized by a well-defined layer of aligned odontoblast-like cells expressing the dentin-specific protein dentin sialophosphoprotein (DSPP) with their processes oriented in the same direction and extend-ing into tubular structures within newly generated dentin (79).

The data demonstrate that postnatal dental pulp contains dentinogenic cells that are clonogenic, highly proliferative, and capable of regenerating a tissue, properties that effec-tively define them as stem cells (23).

The future research directions for designing regenerative therapies include studies on stem cells in the pulp and their associated signals which are instrumental in regulating their behavior.

## Bioactive molecules and pulpal stem cells

The identification of bio-active molecules, including growth factors sequestered in the dentin matrix (163, 164), has given new insight and opportunities for their exploitation in dental treatments (77, 92, 163).

Trans-dentinal stimulation of tertiary dentinogenesis has long been recognized. Release of bio-active components from dentin matrix may arise during injury to the tissue, and also during subsequent surgical intervention and restoration of the tooth. Identification of bioactive components, includ-ing TGF-beta, sequestered within dentin matrix provides a new explanation for cellular signaling during tertiary dentinogenesis (165).

The understanding of the regulation of cell proliferation and differentiation has increased, but we are far from being able to apply specific cocktails of factors and stimulate cell differentiation into specific pathways *in vivo* (166).

Tissue injury leads to alterations in gene expression and release of a range of cytokines including growth factors. The cytokines are released as a signal network and they play determinant and complex roles in regulation of cell proliferation, migration and differentiation. In particular, members of the FGF and TGFβ superfamily including BMPs have been implicated in repair of dental hard tissues (92, 167–169). However, many growth factors and receptors specific for individual cell types are involved (170–172).

BMPs are growth and differentiation factors that can stimulate the differentiation of stromal bone marrow stem cells into osteoblasts, pulp cells into odontoblasts, and dental follicle cells into cementoblasts (92).

Several studies have shown that growth factor rBMP-7 implantation markedly stimulates reparative dentin with vascular inclusions (168, 169, 173), but fails in inflamed pulps with pulpitis (174).

The mechanism whereby foregoing inflammation may inhibit tissue repair (175, 176) and potentially influence gene activity necessary for stem cell recruitment remains to be elucidated.

Application of exogenous signaling molecules offers opportunities for development of new therapies (136). Stimulation of odontoblast differentiation and enhanced reparative dentinogenesis has been observed after basic fibroblast growth factor (bFGF) and TGFβ-1 implantation (177), and insulin-like growth factor I (IGF-I) application (178) (see Chapter 2).

Further studies are needed and a number of delivery considerations must be addressed before implantation of pulp cells or bioactive molecules can be introduced into clinical endodontic practice (136).

Small agarose beads that release bioactive molecules have been used for stimulation of dental cells *in vitro*. Could they be used for pulp capping *in vivo*, or triggering of the epithelium to induce a new tooth?

## *H. Løvschall and J.O. Andreasen*

## Growing teeth

The challenge of restoring tissue lost through disease or trauma will be with us for many years to come. Dental scientists in the field of developmental biology throughout the world provide the foundation upon which it is possible to build future strategies for engineering human teeth. New interesting advances have been made toward tissue engineering of teeth (12, 179, 180, 181; Fig. 3.12).

Whole teeth are often found in ectopic teratomas, and it is noteworthy that they may have a normal shape and structure (180).

Teeth were lost in birds 70–80 million years ago. However, it has been shown that avian oral epithelium is able to initiate evidence of tooth formation in mouse mesenchymal cells from the neural crest (181).

One tissue engineering group seeded cultured tooth germ cells from pigs (182) or rats (5) on biodegradable scaffolds.

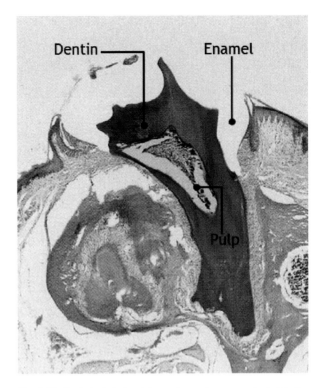

**Fig. 3.12** Tooth buds isolated from mice embryos transplanted to the mandible of adult mice has resulted in formation and eruption of a molar-like tooth. From SHARPE et al. (188) 2005.

They were then implanted in the abdomen of rats in order to generate tooth tissue (5). The cultured tooth bud cells were seeded on PGA or PLGA scaffolds where they generated dental-like tissues. Recognizable tooth structures formed that contained dentin, odontoblasts, a pulp chamber, putative Hertwig's root sheath epithelia, putative cementoblasts, and a morphologically correct enamel organ containing fully formed enamel. It was concluded that tooth-tissue-engineering methods can be used to generate porcine (182) and rat tooth tissues (5). The method was suggested to have a potential for regeneration of human dental tissues (5).

Another group has also been able to generate tooth-like structures. Their approach was based on the ability of oral epithelium to provide instructive information for initiation of tooth development. They transplanted embryonic oral epithelium to an ectopic site and in contact with non-dental mesenchymal cells. Oral epithelium, in association with uncommitted mesenchymal stem cells, thereby mimicked developmental events leading to initiation of a tooth structure comprising enamel, dentin, and pulp, with a morphology resembling that of a natural tooth (6).

Recombinations between non-dental cell-derived mesenchyme and embryonic oral epithelium stimulate an odontogenic response in different stem cells. Embryonic stem cells, neural stem cells, and adult bone-marrow-derived cells all responded by expressing odontogenic genes. Transfer of the tissue recombinations into adult renal capsules resulted in the development of tooth structures and associated bone. Moreover, transfer of embryonic tooth primordia into the

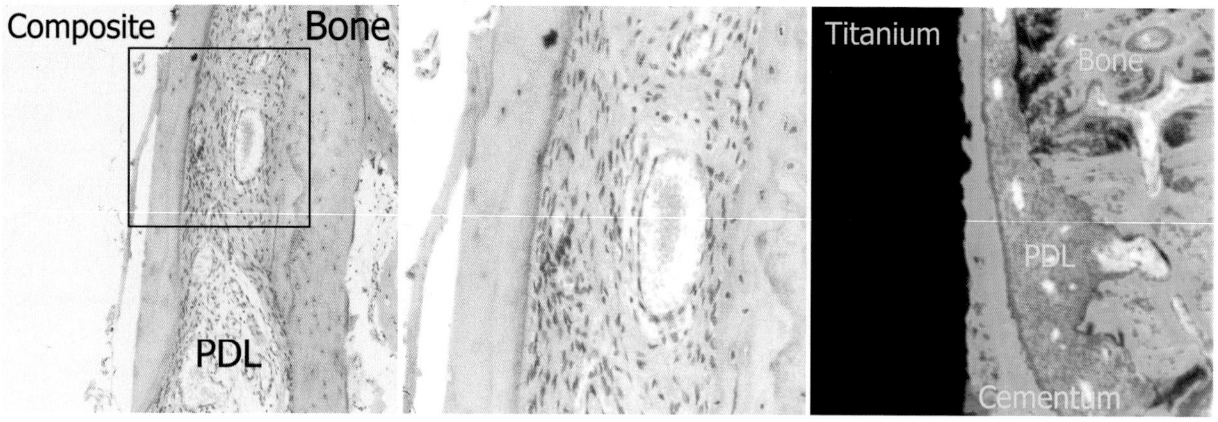

**Fig. 3.13** A. Human incisor with an apex covered with composite 3 years after surgery. The empty space represents the lumen after composite loss during tissue preparation. Higher magnification shows deposition of cementum upon the composite and reformation of PDL fibers. From ANDREASEN et al. (184) 1993. B. Implant placed next to a root in a monkey. The portion of the implant next to the root became covered with new cementum and a new periodontal ligament. From BUSER et al. (186) 1990.

adult jaw resulted in development of tooth structures. This study shows that an embryonic primordium can develop in its adult environment (6). Lately, transplanted stem cells from mouse embryos that have been implanted into the jaws of adult mice have resulted in the development of mature teeth (188) (Fig. 3.12).

*J. O. Andreasen and H. Løvschall*

## Implant/transplant teeth

In spite of the above mentioned promising animal experiments, the prospects for the use of such techniques to create a tooth graft to replace missing or lost teeth in children or young adults seems far away due to a number of major obstacles:

(1) How to recruit odontogenic stem cells that are acceptable to the recipient.
(2) How to develop methods to control the composition (enamel/dentin/cementum/pulp and PDL), shape and color of the graft to fit the potential new recipient site.
(3) How to develop reliable transplantation procedures to ensure optimal PDL and pulp healing.
(4) How to prevent the graft-versus-host response if stem cells do not originate from the patient.

These considerations mean the whole idea of growing new teeth needs to be rethought. Do we need enamel dentin and pulp in those grafts? Can artificial materials such as porcelain, composite, hydroxyapatite or titanium be used to replace these tissues? This would imply that only a PDL has to be created and anchored on top of tooth replicas, i.e. a hybrid tooth.

Experiments have shown that a new functioning PDL can be regenerated on top of materials such as composite, hydroxyapatite (185) and titanium (186) (Fig. 3.13). This would simplify the tooth replacement procedure significantly as tooth replicas can be made and then implanted after PDL cells are attached to their surface. This naturally raises the problem of where to get recipient-acceptable PDL cells. Right now four approaches seem possible:

(1) Auto- or allografted adult stem cells altered to become differentiated into PDL cells.
(2) PDL cells recruited from third molars.
(3) PDL cells from extracted persistent primary teeth (canines or molars).
(4) Gingival PDL-programed cells removed with a biopsy (187).

Future research may clarify which of these solutions has a future for use in hybrid grafts used in growing individuals.

## Essentials

New evidence from experimental animal studies focusing on stem cells introduces a range of new possibilities for dental tissue engineering. Tissue engineering is the manipulation and development of molecules, cells, tissues and organs, to replace or support the function of defective or injured body parts. Tissue engineering is based on a triade of stem cells, materials (carriers/scaffolds), and bioactive molecules. The tissue engineering designs and approaches are endless, and range from using conductive membranes to *ex vivo* construction of root analogs or whole teeth.

When a stem cell divides, one 'daughter' cell has the potential to remain a stem cell, while the other 'daughter' cell divides repeatedly giving a cell group which develops a specialized function, such as a muscle cell, a red blood cell, or a brain cell.

*Embryonic stem cells* are derived from the fertilized egg. Embryonic stem cells can divide almost indefinitely and can give rise to every cell type in the body. They divide continuously in tissue culture dishes in an incubator, but at the same time they maintain the ability to generate any cell type when placed into the correct environment to cause their differentiation.

Embryonic stem cells have great potential, but they are more difficult to obtain. The use of embryonic stem cells transplanted across natural boundaries of embryos, developing organs, age, and individuals, at the expense of the donor, give important information from animal studies. However, the application in humans raises ethical and legal problems.

The organs contain stem cells that persist throughout adult life and contribute to the maintenance and repair of the organs. The *adult stem cells* have restricted developmental potential, in that their capacity for proliferation is limited and they can give rise only to a few cell types. Regeneration therapies targeting bioactivation of adult stem cells in the organ and the neigboring tissue seem at present closer to clinical implementation.

Adult stem cells are more available, but they have a limited range of cell doublings and fates, and they may be affected by aging. The risk of rejection is lowered when adult stem cells are derived from the same patient. Adult stem cells have been used with a carrier for dental tissue engineering in transplantation animal models. Adult human stem cells from bone marrow are quite easily obtained by aspiration, and stem cells can also be collected from teeth pulp, PDL, and bone samples. They can putatively be isolated and expanded *in vitro*, or stimulated *in situ*. *Stem cell therapy* based on transplantation is currently in its infancy.

Targeting stem cells *in situ* is closer to clinical implementation. *Regeneration therapies* targeting bioactivation of stem cells *in situ*, rather than transplantation of stem cells *ex vivo*, seem at present closer to being implemented in the clinic.

*Bioactive molecules* have had limited success due to problems of dosage, lack of full activity of recombinant factors, and inability to sustain a factor's presence for an appropriate time.

*Local gene-therapy* is a new strategy. Development of local gene transfer techniques, for example using 'gene-activating matrices' may provide a second-generation of transcription, growth, and differentiation factor therapy for long-term stimulation of tissue regeneration.

# References

1. LANZA RP, LANGER R, CHICK WL (eds). *Principles of tissue engineering.* Austin: AP, 1997.
2. MURRAY PE, GARCIA-GODOY F. Stem cell responses in tooth regeneration. *Stem Cells Dev* 2004;**13**:255–62.
3. BIANCO P, ROBEY PG. Stem cells in tissue engineering. *Nature* 2001;**414**:118–121.
4. GRONTHOS S, CHERMAN N, ROBEY PG, SHI S. Human dental pulp stem cells – characterization and developmental potential. In: Turkun M. ed. *Adult Stem Cells.* Totowa, New Jersey: Humana Press, 2004:67–81.
5. DUAILIBI MT, DUAILIBI SE, YOUNG CS, BARTLETT JD, VACANTI JP, YELICK PC. Bioengineered teeth from cultured rat tooth bud cells. *J Dent Res* 2004;**83**:523–8.
6. OHAZAMA A, MODINO SA, MILETICH I, SHARPE PT. Stem-cell-based tissue engineering of murine teeth. *J Dent Res* 2004;**83**:518–22.
7. BRAUT A, KOLLAR EJ, MINA M. Analysis of the odontogenic and osteogenic potentials of dental pulp *in vivo* using a Col1a1-2.3-GFP transgene. *Int J Dev Biol* 2003;**47**:281–92.
8. FUCHS E, RAGHAVAN S. Getting under the skin of epidermal morphogenesis. *Nat Rev Genet* 2002;**3**:199–209.
9. NIH. *Stem cells: scientific progress and future research directions.* Washington: National Institute of Health, 2001.
10. SEO BM, MIURA M, GRONTHOS S, BARTOLD PM, BATOULI S, BRAHIM J, et al. Investigation of multipotent postnatal stem cells from human periodontal ligament. *Lancet* 2004;**364**:149–55.
11. DO JT, SCHOLER HR. Nuclei of embryonic stem cells reprogram somatic cells. *Stem Cells* 2004;**22**:941–9.
12. KREBSBACH PH, ROBEY PG. Dental and skeletal stem cells: potential cellular therapeutics for craniofacial regeneration. *J Dent Educ* 2002;**66**:766–73.
13. BARRY FP, MURPHY JM. Mesenchymal stem cells: clinical applications and biological characterization. *Int J Biochem Cell Biol* 2004;**36**:568–84.
14. GRZESIK WJ, KUZNETSOV SA, UZAWA K, MANKANI M, ROBEY PG, YAMAUCHI M. Normal human cementum-derived cells: isolation, clonal expansion, and *in vitro* and *in vivo* characterization. *J Bone Miner Res* 1998;**13**:1547–54.
15. GRZESIK WJ, CHENG H, OH JS, KUZNETSOV SA, MANKANI MH, UZAWA K, et al. Cementum-forming cells are phenotypically distinct from bone-forming cells. *J Bone Miner Res* 2000;**15**:52–59.
16. BIANCO P, RIMINUCCI M, GRONTHOS S, ROBEY PG. Bone marrow stromal stem cells: nature, biology, and potential applications. *Stem Cells* 2001;**19**:180–92.
17. TOMA JG, AKHAVAN M, FERNANDES KJ, BARNABE-HEIDER F, SADIKOT A, KAPLAN DR, et al. Isolation of multipotent adult stem cells from the dermis of mammalian skin. *Nat Cell Biol* 2001;**3**:778–84.
18. MIURA M, GRONTHOS S, ZHAO M, LU B, FISHER LW, ROBEY PG, et al. Stem cells from human exfoliated deciduous teeth. *Proc Natl Acad Sci USA* 2003;**100**:5807–12.
19. HUYSSEUNE A, THESLEFF I. Continuous tooth replacement: the possible involvement of epithelial stem cells. *Bioessays* 2004;**26**:665–71.
20. WEISSMAN IL, ANDERSON DJ, GAGE F. Stem and progenitor cells: origins, phenotypes, lineage commitments, and transdifferentiations. *Annu Rev Cell Dev Biol* 2001;**17**:387–403.
21. WAGERS AJ, WEISSMAN IL. Plasticity of adult stem cells. *Cell* 2004;**116**:639–48.
22. FUCHS E, SEGRE JA. Stem cells: a new lease on life. *Cell* 2000;**100**:143–55.
23. GRONTHOS S, MANKANI M, BRAHIM J, ROBEY PG, SHI S. Postnatal human dental pulp stem cells (DPSCs) *in*

*vitro* and *in vivo*. *Proc Natl Acad Sci U S A* 2000;**97**: 13625–30.

24. Sharpe PT. Neural crest and tooth morphogenesis. *Adv Dent Res* 2001;**15**:4–7.

25. Haworth KE, Healy C, Morgan P, Sharpe PT. Regionalisation of early head ectoderm is regulated by endoderm and prepatterns the orofacial epithelium. *Development* 2004;**131**:4797–806.

26. Miletich I, Sharpe PT. Neural crest contribution to mammalian tooth formation. *Birth Defects Res Part C Embryo Today* 2004;**72**:200–12.

27. Cobourne MT, Sharpe PT. Tooth and jaw: molecular mechanisms of patterning in the first branchial arch. *Arch Oral Biol* 2003;**48**:1–14.

28. Carlile MJ, Sturrock MG, Chisholm DM, Ogden GR, Schor AM. The presence of pericytes and transitional cells in the vasculature of the human dental pulp: an ultrastructural study. *Histochem J* 2000;**32**:239–245.

29. Tucker A, Sharpe P. The cutting-edge of mammalian development; how the embryo makes teeth. *Nat Rev Genet* 2004;**5**:499–508.

30. Froum S, Lemler J, Horowitz R, Davidson B. The use of enamel matrix derivative in the treatment of periodontal osseous defects: a clinical decision tree based on biologic principles of regeneration. *Int J Periodontics Restorative Dent* 2001;**21**:437–49.

31. Berry JE, Zhao M, Jin Q, Foster BL, Viswanathan H, Somerman MJ. Exploring the origins of cementoblasts and their trigger factors. *Connect Tissue Res* 2003;**44**:(Suppl 1):97–102.

32. Mitsiadis TA, Cheraud Y, Sharpe P, Fontaine-Perus J. Development of teeth in chick embryos after mouse neural crest transplantations. *Proc Natl Acad Sci USA* 2003;**100**:6541–45.

33. Duailibi MT, Duailibi SE, Young CS, Bartlett JD, Vacanti JP, Yelick PC. Bioengineered teeth from cultured rat tooth bud cells. *J Dent Res* 2004;**83**:523–8.

34. Ohazama A, Modino SA, Miletich I, Sharpe PT. Stem-cell-based tissue engineering of murine teeth. *J Dent Res* 2004;**83**:518–22.

35. Jernvall J, Thesleff I. Reiterative signaling and patterning during mammalian tooth morphogenesis. *Mech Dev* 2000;**92**:19–29.

36. Tucker AS, Matthews KL, Sharpe PT. Transformation of tooth type induced by inhibition of BMP signaling. *Science* 1998;**282**:1136–8.

37. Wang XP, Suomalainen M, Jorgez CJ, Matzuk MM, Wankell M, Werner S, et al. Modulation of activin/bone morphogenetic protein signaling by follistatin is required for the morphogenesis of mouse molar teeth. *Dev Dyn* 2004;**231**:98–108.

38. Thesleff I. Epithelial-mesenchymal signalling regulating tooth morphogenesis. *J Cell Sci* 2003;**116**:1647–8.

39. Chai Y, Jiang X, Ito Y, Bringas P, Jr., Han J, Rowitch DH, et al. Fate of the mammalian cranial neural crest during tooth and mandibular morphogenesis. *Development* 2000;**127**:1671–9.

40. Barry FP, Murphy JM. Mesenchymal stem cells: clinical applications and biological characterization. *Int J Biochem Cell Biol* 2004;**36**:568–84.

41. Thesleff I, Vaahtokari A. The role of growth factors in determination and differentiation of the odontoblastic cell lineage. *Proc Finn Dent Soc* 1992;**88**:(Suppl 1):357–68.

42. Zhao M, Xiao G, Berry JE, Franceschi RT, Reddi A, Somerman MJ. Bone morphogenetic protein 2 induces dental follicle cells to differentiate toward a cementoblast/osteoblast phenotype. *J Bone Miner Res* 2002;**17**:1441–51.

43. Peters H, Balling R. Teeth. Where and how to make them. *Trends Genet* 1999;**15**:59–65.

44. Thesleff I, Sharpe P. Signalling networks regulating dental development. *Mech Dev* 1997;**67**:111–23.

45. Kollar EJ, Baird GR. The influence of the dental papilla on the development of tooth shape in embryonic mouse tooth germs. *J Embryol Exp Morphol* 1969;**21**:131–48.

46. Kangas AT, Evans AR, Thesleff I, Jernvall J. Nonindependence of mammalian dental characters. *Nature* 2004;**432**:211–14.

47. Thesleff I. The genetic basis of normal and abnormal craniofacial development. *Acta Odontol Scand* 1998;**56**:321–5.

48. Lövschall H, Tummers M, Thesleff I, Fuchtbauer EM, Poulsen K. Activation of notch signaling pathway in response to capping of rat molars. *Eur J Oral Sci* 2005;**113**:1–23.

49. Hörsted-Bindslev P, Lövschall H. Treatment outcome of vital pulp treatment. *Endodontic Topics* 2002;**2**:24–34.

50. Martin P, Parkhurst SM. Parallels between tissue repair and embryo morphogenesis. *Development* 2004;**131**:3021–34.

51. Inoue T, Shimono M. Repair dentinogenesis following transplantation into normal and germ-free animals. *Proc Finn Dent Soc* 1992;**88**:(Suppl 1):183–94.

52. Lyaruu DM, van Croonenburg EJ, van Duin MA, Bervoets TJ, Woltgens JH, Blieck-Hogervorst JM. Development of transplanted pulp tissue containing epithelial sheath into a tooth-like structure. *J Oral Pathol Med* 1999;**28**:293–6.

53. Kuznetsov SA, Mankani MH, Gronthos S, Satomura K, Bianco P, Robey PG. Circulating skeletal stem cells. *J Cell Biol* 2001;**153**:1133–40.

54. Krebsbach PH, Kuznetsov SA, Bianco P, Robey PG. Bone marrow stromal cells: characterization and clinical application. *Crit Rev Oral Biol Med* 1999;**10**:165–81.

55. Corti S, Locatelli F, Donadoni C, Guglieri M, Papadimitriou D, Strazzer S, et al. Wild-type bone marrow cells ameliorate the phenotype of SOD1-G93A ALS mice and contribute to CNS, heart and skeletal muscle tissues. *Brain* 2004;**127**:2518–32.

56. Poulsom R, Alison MR, Forbes SJ, Wright NA. Adult stem cell plasticity. *J Pathol* 2002;**197**:441–56.

57. Yamamura T. Differentiation of pulpal cells and inductive influences of various matrices with reference to pulpal wound healing. *J Dent Res* 1985;**64**(Spec. Issue):530–40.

58. Kang Y, Massague J. Epithelial-mesenchymal transitions: twist in development and metastasis. *Cell* 2004;**118**:277–9.

59. BLOCH-ZUPAN A, PARDAL, HUNTER N, MANTHEY A, GIBBINS J. R-twist gene expression during rat palatogenesis. *Int J Dev Biol* 2001;**45**:397–404.

60. TERADA N, HAMAZAKI T, OKA M, HOKI M, MASTALERZ DM, NAKANO Y, et al. Bone marrow cells adopt the phenotype of other cells by spontaneous cell fusion. *Nature* 2002;**416**:542–45.

61. YING QL, NICHOLS J, EVANS EP, SMITH AG. Changing potency by spontaneous fusion. *Nature* 2002;**416**:545–8.

62. LERUT JP, CLAEYS N, CICCARELLI O, PISA R, GALANT C, LATERRE PF, et al. Recurrent postinfantile syncytial giant cell hepatitis after orthotopic liver transplantation. *Transpl Int* 1998;**11**:320–2.

63. HICKS J, BARRISH J, ZHU SH. Neonatal syncytial giant cell hepatitis with paramyxoviral-like inclusions. *Ultrastruct Pathol* 2001;**25**:65–71.

64. VASSILOPOULOS G, WANG PR, RUSSELL DW. Transplanted bone marrow regenerates liver by cell fusion. *Nature* 2003;**422**:901–4.

65. WANG X, WILLENBRING H, AKKARI Y, TORIMARU Y, FOSTER M, AL DHALIMY M, et al. Cell fusion is the principal source of bone-marrow-derived hepatocytes. *Nature* 2003;**422**:897–901.

66. WEIMANN JM, JOHANSSON CB, TREJO A, BLAU HM. Stable reprogrammed heterokaryons form spontaneously in Purkinje neurons after bone marrow transplant. *Nat Cell Biol* 2003;**5**:959–66.

67. ALVAREZ-DOLADO M, R, GARCIA-VERDUGO JM, FIKE JR, LEE HO, PFEFFER K, et al. Fusion of bone-marrow-derived cells with Purkinje neurons, cardiomyocytes and hepatocytes. *Nature* 2003;**425**:968–73.

68. PITARU S, MCCULLOCH CA, NARAYANAN SA. Cellular origins and differentiation control mechanisms during periodontal development and wound healing. *J Periodontal Res* 1994;**29**:81–94.

69. MJÖR IA, SVEEN OB, HEYERAAS KJ. Pulp-dentin biology in restorative dentistry. Part 1: normal structure and physiology. *Quintess Int* 2001;**32**:427–46.

70. MCCULLOCH CA, NEMETH E, LOWENBERG B, MELCHER AH. Paravascular cells in endosteal spaces of alveolar bone contribute to periodontal ligament cell populations. *Anat Rec* 1987;**219**:233–42.

71. MCCULLOCH CA. Progenitor cell populations in the periodontal ligament of mice. *Anat Rec* 1985;**211**:258–62.

72. GOULD TR, MELCHER AH, BRUNETTE DM. Location of progenitor cells in periodontal ligament of mouse molar stimulated by wounding. *Anat Rec* 1977;**188**:133–41.

73. LEKIC P, SODEK J, MCCULLOCH CA. Relationship of cellular proliferation to expression of osteopontin and bone sialoprotein in regenerating rat periodontium. *Cell Tissue Res* 1996;**285**:491–500.

74. GOULD TR, MELCHER AH, BRUNETTE DM. Migration and division of progenitor cell populations in periodontal ligament after wounding. *J Periodontal Res* 1980;**15**:20–42.

75. MCCULLOCH CA. Progenitor cell populations in the periodontal ligament of mice. *Anat Rec* 1985;**211**:258–62.

76. SMITH AJ, CASSIDY N, PERRY H, BEGUE KIRN C, RUCH JV, LESOT H. Reactionary dentinogenesis. *Int J Dev Biol* 1995;**39**:273–80.

77. SMITH AJ, LESOT H. Induction and regulation of crown dentinogenesis: embryonic events as a template for dental tissue repair? *Crit Rev Oral Biol Med* 2001;**12**:425–37.

78. SVEEN OB, HAWES RR. Differentiation of new odontoblasts and dentine bridge formation in rat molar teeth after tooth grinding. *Arch Oral Biol* 1968;**13**:1399–1409.

79. GRONTHOS S, BRAHIM J, LI W, FISHER LW, CHERMAN N, BOYDE A, et al. Stem cell properties of human dental pulp stem cells. *J Dent Res* 2002;**81**:531–5.

80. SHI S, GRONTHOS S. Perivascular niche of postnatal mesenchymal stem cells in human bone marrow and dental pulp. *J Bone Miner Res* 2003;**18**:696–704.

81. ANDREEVA ER, PUGACH IM, GORDON D, OREKHOV AN. Continuous subendothelial network formed by pericyte-like cells in human vascular bed. *Tissue Cell* 1998;**30**:127–35.

82. NAYAK RC, BERMAN AB, GEORGE KL, EISENBARTH GS, KING GL. A monoclonal antibody (3G5)-defined ganglioside antigen is expressed on the cell surface of microvascular pericytes. *J Exp Med* 1988;**167**:1003–15.

83. MJÖR IA. *Pulp-dentin biology in restorative dentistry.* Carol Stream: Quintessence Publishing Co, 2002.

84. FEIT J, METELOVA M, SINDELKA Z. Incorporation of 3H thymidine into damaged pulp of rat incisors. *J Dent Res* 1970;**49**:783–6.

85. DAHL JE. Proliferation and migration of rat incisor mesenchymal cells. *Scand J Dent Res* 1983;**91**:335–40.

86. CHIEGO DJ Jr. An ultrastructural and autoradiographic analysis of primary and replacement odontoblasts following cavity preparation and wound healing in the rat molar. *Proc Finn Dent Soc* 1992;**88**:(*Suppl*):243–56.

87. FITZGERALD M, CHIEGO DJJ, HEYS DR. Autoradiographic analysis of odontoblast replacement following pulp exposure in primate teeth. *Arch Oral Biol* 1990;**35**:707–15.

88. MURPHY WL, MOONEY DJ. Controlled delivery of inductive proteins, plasmid DNA and cells from tissue engineering matrices. *J Periodontal Res* 1999;**34**:413–19.

89. XYNOS ID. EDGAR AJ, BUTTERY LD, HENCH LL, POLAK JM. Gene-expression profiling of human osteoblasts following treatment with the ionic products of Bioglass45S5 dissolution. *J Biomed Mater Res* 2001;**55**:151–7.

90. HENCH LL, POLAK JM. Third-generation biomedical materials. *Science* 2002;**295**:1014–17.

91. COCHRAN DL, WOZNEY JM. Biological mediators for periodontal regeneration. *Periodontol 2000* 1999;**19**:40–58.

92. NAKASHIMA M, REDDI AH. The application of bone morphogenetic proteins to dental tissue engineering. *Nat Biotechnol* 2003;**21**:1025–32.

93. REDDI AH. Cartilage morphogenetic proteins: role in joint development, homoeostasis, and regeneration. *Ann Rheum Dis* 2003;**62**:(*Suppl 2*):ii73–8.

94. SONG Q, LAVIN MF. Calyculin A, a potent inhibitor of phosphatases-1 and -2A, prevents apoptosis. *Biochem Biophys Res Commun* 1993;**190**:47–55.

95. RAMOSHEBI LN, MATSABA TN, TEARE J, RENTON L, PATTON J, RIPAMONTI U. Tissue engineering: TGF-beta

superfamily members and delivery systems in bone regeneration. *Expert Rev Mol Med* 2002;**2002**:1–11.

96. SILVA TA, ROSA AL, LARA VS. Dentin matrix proteins and soluble factors: intrinsic regulatory signals for healing and resorption of dental and periodontal tissues? *Oral Dis* 2004;**10**:63–74.

97. RUTHERFORD B, FITZGERALD M. A new biological approach to vital pulp therapy. *Crit Rev Oral Biol Med* 1995;**6**:218–29.

98. RUTHERFORD RB, GU K. Treatment of inflamed ferret dental pulps with recombinant bone morphogenetic protein-7. *Eur J Oral Sci* 2000;**108**:202–6.

99. FRANCESCHI RT, YANG S, RUTHERFORD RB, KREBSBACH PH, ZHAO M, WANG D. Gene therapy approaches for bone regeneration. *Cells Tissues Organs* 2004;**176**:95–108.

100. HAFFAJEE AD, SOCRANSKY SS, GUNSOLLEY JC. Systemic anti-infective periodontal therapy. A systematic review. *Ann Periodontol* 2003;**8**:115–81.

101. ANUSAKSATHIEN O, GIANNOBILE WV. Growth factor delivery to re-engineer periodontal tissues. *Curr Pharm Biotechnol* 2002;**3**:129–39.

102. MURPHY KG, GUNSOLLEY JC. Guided tissue regeneration for the treatment of periodontal intrabony and furcation defects. A systematic review. *Ann Periodontol* 2003;**8**:266–302.

103. REYNOLDS MA, AICHELMANN-REIDY ME, BRANCH-MAYS GL, GUNSOLLEY JC. The efficacy of bone replacement grafts in the treatment of periodontal osseous defects. A systematic review. *Ann Periodontol* 2003;**8**:227–65.

104. URIST MR, O'CONNOR BT, BURWELL RG. *Bone grafts, derivatives and substitutes.* Oxford: Butterworth-Heinemann, 1994.

105. ROBINSON C, SHORE RC, WOOD SR, BROOKES SJ, SMITH DA, KIRKHAM J. Critical issues in endosseous peri-implant wound healing. In: Ellingsen JE, Lyngstadaas JP. eds. *Bio-implant interface. Improving biomaterials and tissue reactions.* Boca Raton: CRC Press, 2003:219–28.

106. MANKANI MH, KREBSBACH PH, SATOMURA K, KUZNETSOV SA, HOYT R, ROBEY PG. Pedicled bone flap formation using transplanted bone marrow stromal cells. *Arch Surg* 2001;**136**:263–70.

107. KREBSBACH PH, MANKANI MH, SATOMURA K, KUZNETSOV SA, ROBEY PG. Repair of craniotomy defects using bone marrow stromal cells. *Transplantation* 1998;**66**:1272–8.

108. QUARTO R, MASTROGIACOMO M, CANCEDDA R, KUTEPOV SM, MUKHACHEV V, LAVROUKOV A, et al. Repair of large bone defects with the use of autologous bone marrow stromal cells. *N Engl J Med* 2001;**344**:385–6.

109. BRUDER SP, KRAUS KH, GOLDBERG VM, KADIYALA S. The effect of implants loaded with autologous mesenchymal stem cells on the healing of canine segmental bone defects. *J Bone Joint Surg Am* 1998;**80**:985–96.

110. JIN QM, ANUSAKSATHIEN O, WEBB SA, RUTHERFORD RB, GIANNOBILE WV. Gene therapy of bone morphogenetic protein for periodontal tissue engineering. *J Periodontol* 2003;**74**:202–13.

111. GRZESIK WJ, NARAYANAN AS. Cementum and periodontal wound healing and regeneration. *Crit Rev Oral Biol Med* 2002;**13**:474–84.

112. ZHAO M, JIN Q, BERRY JE, NOCITI FH, JR., GIANNOBILE WV, SOMERMAN MJ. Cementoblast delivery for periodontal tissue engineering. *J Periodontol* 2004;**75**:54–161.

113. NAKAHARA T, NAKAMURA T, KOBAYASHI E, INOUE M, SHIGENO K, TABATA Y, et al. Novel approach to regeneration of periodontal tissues based on *in situ* tissue engineering: effects of controlled release of basic fibroblast growth factor from a sandwich membrane. *Tissue Eng* 2003;**9**:153–62.

114. TALWAR R, DI SILVIO L, HUGHES FJ, KING GN. Effects of carrier release kinetics on bone morphogenetic protein-2-induced periodontal regeneration *in vivo*. *J Clin Periodontol* 2001;**28**:340–7.

115. SAYGIN NE, GIANNOBILE WV, SOMERMAN MJ. Molecular and cell biology of cementum. *Periodontol 2000* 2000;**24**:73–98.

116. GESTRELIUS S, LYNGSTADAAS SP, HAMMARSTROM L. Emdogain-periodontal regeneration based on biomimicry. *Clin Oral Investig* 2000;**4**:120–5.

117. LINDSKOG S. Formation of intermediate cementum. I: early mineralization of aprismatic enamel and intermediate cementum in monkey. *J Craniofac Genet Dev Biol* 1982;**2**:147–60.

118. LINDSKOG S. Formation of intermediate cementum. II: a scanning electron microscopic study of the epithelial root sheath of Hertwig in monkey. *J Craniofac Genet Dev Biol* 1982;**2**:161–9.

119. SLAVKIN HC, BRINGAS P, JR., BESSEM C, SANTOS V, NAKAMURA M, HSU MY, et al. Hertwig's epithelial root sheath differentiation and initial cementum and bone formation during long-term organ culture of mouse mandibular first molars using serumless, chemically-defined medium. *J Periodontal Res* 1989;**24**:28–40.

120. HATAKEYAMA J, SREENATH T, HATAKEYAMA Y, THYAGARAJAN T, SHUM L, GIBSON CW, et al. The receptor activator of nuclear factor-kappa B ligand-mediated osteoclastogenic pathway is elevated in amelogenin-null mice. *J Biol Chem* 2003;**278**: 35743–8.

121. VISWANATHAN HL, BERRY JE, FOSTER BL, GIBSON CW, LI Y, KULKARNI AB, et al. Amelogenin: a potential regulator of cementum-associated genes. *J Periodontol* 2003;**74**:1423–31.

122. GIANNOBILE WV, SOMERMAN MJ. Growth and amelogenin-like factors in periodontal wound healing. A systematic review. *Ann Periodontol* 2003;**8**:193–204.

123. REDDI AH. BMPs: actions in flesh and bone. *Nat Med* 1997;**3**:837–9.

124. ABERG T, WOZNEY J, THESLEFF I. Expression patterns of bone morphogenetic proteins (BMPs) in the developing mouse tooth suggest roles in morphogenesis and cell differentiation. *Dev Dyn* 1997;**210**:383–96.

125. AMAR S, CHUNG KM, NAM SH, KARATZAS S, MYOKAI F, VAN DYKE TE. Markers of bone and cementum formation accumulate in tissues regenerated in periodontal defects treated with expanded polytetrafluoroethylene membranes. *J Periodontal Res* 1997;**32**:148–58.

126. THOMADAKIS G, RAMOSHEBI LN, CROOKS J, RUEGER DC, RIPAMONTI U. Immunolocalization of bone morphogenetic protein-2 and -3 and osteogenic protein-

1 during murine tooth root morphogenesis and in other craniofacial structures. *Eur J Oral Sci* 1999;**107**:368–77.

127. YAMASHIRO T, TUMMERS M, THESLEFF I. Expression of bone morphogenetic proteins and MSX genes during root formation. *J Dent Res* 2003;**82**:172–6.

128. GIANNOBILE WV, RYAN S, SHIH MS, SU DL, KAPLAN PL, CHAN TC. Recombinant human osteogenic protein-1 (OP-1) stimulates periodontal wound healing in class III furcation defects. *J Periodontol* 1998;**69**:129–37.

129. ZIMMERMAN LB, JESUS-ESCOBAR JM, HARLAND RM. The Spemann organizer signal noggin binds and inactivates bone morphogenetic protein 4. *Cell* 1996;**86**:599–606.

130. REDDI AH. Interplay between bone morphogenetic proteins and cognate binding proteins in bone and cartilage development: noggin, chordin and DAN. *Arthritis Res* 2001;**3**:1–5.

131. JIN QM, ZHAO M, ECONOMIDES AN, SOMERMAN MJ, GIANNOBILE WV. Noggin gene delivery inhibits cementoblast-induced mineralization. *Connect Tissue Res* 2004;**45**:50–9.

132. KING GN, KING N, CRUCHLEY AT, WOZNEY JM, HUGHES FJ. Recombinant human bone morphogenetic protein-2 promotes wound healing in rat periodontal fenestration defects. *J Dent Res* 1997;**76**:1460–70.

133. ANDREASEN JO. Histometric study of healing of periodontal tissues in rats after surgical injury. I. Design of a standardized surgical procedure. *Odontol Rev* 1976;**27**:115–30.

134. ANDREASEN JO. Histometric study of healing of periodontal tissues in rats after surgical injury. II. Healing events of alveolar bone, periodontal ligaments and cementum. *Odontol Rev* 1976;**27**:131–44.

135. NOCITI FH, JR., BERRY JE, FOSTER BL, GURLEY KA, KINGSLEY DM, TAKATA T, et al. Cementum: a phosphate-sensitive tissue. *J Dent Res* 2002;**81**: 817–21.

136. TZIAFAS D, SMITH AJ, LESOT H. Designing new treatment strategies in vital pulp therapy. *J Dent* 2000;**28**:77–92.

137. JERNVALL J, KERANEN SV, THESLEFF I. From the cover: evolutionary modification of development in mammalian teeth: quantifying gene expression patterns and topography. *Proc Natl Acad Sci U S A* 2000;**97**:14444–8.

138. RUCH JV. Odontoblast differentiation and the formation of the odontoblast layer. *J Dent Res* 1985;**64**:(*Spec No.*):489–98.

139. LÖVSCHALL H, FEJERSKOV O, JOSEPHSEN K. Age-related and site-specific changes of pulp histology in Wistar rat molars. *Arch Oral Biol* 2002;**47**:1–7.

140. MURRAY PE, SMITH AJ, WINDSOR LJ, MJÖR IA. Remaining dentine thickness and human pulp responses. *Int Endod J* 2003;**36**:33–43.

141. FITZGERALD M. Cellular mechanics of dentinal bridge repair using 3H-thymidine. *J Dent Res* 1979;**58**:2198–206.

142. YAMAMURA T. Differentiation of pulpal cells and inductive influences of various matrices with reference to pulpal wound healing. *J Dent Res* 1985;**64**:(*Spec No.*):530–40.

143. COUBLE ML, FARGES JC, BLEICHER F, PERRAT-MABILLON B, BOUDEULLE M, MAGLOIRE H. Odontoblast

144. KUO MY, LAN WH, LIN SK, TSAI KS, HAHN LJ. Collagen gene expression in human dental pulp cell cultures. *Arch Oral Biol* 1992;**37**:945–52.

145. TSUKAMOTO Y, FUKUTANI S, SHIN-IKE T, KUBOTA T, SATO S, SUZUKI Y, et al. Mineralized nodule formation by cultures of human dental pulp-derived fibroblasts. *Arch Oral Biol* 1992;**37**:1045–55.

146. SHIBA H, NAKAMURA S, SHIRAKAWA M, NAKANISHI K, OKAMOTO H, SATAKEDA H, et al. Effects of basic fibroblast growth factor on proliferation, the expression of osteonectin (SPARC) and alkaline phosphatase, and calcification in cultures of human pulp cells. *Dev Biol* 1995;**170**:457–66.

147. BAKLAND LK. Management of traumatically injured pulps in immature teeth using MTA. *J Calif Dent Assoc* 2000;**28**:855–8.

148. FARACO IM, JR, HOLLAND R. Response of the pulp of dogs to capping with mineral trioxide aggregate or a calcium hydroxide cement. *Dent Traumatol* 2001;**17**:163–6.

149. SAIDON J, HE J, ZHU Q, SAFAVI K, SPANGBERG LS. Cell and tissue reactions to mineral trioxide aggregate and Portland cement. *Oral Surg Oral Med Oral Pathol Oral Radiol Endod* 2003;**95**:483–9.

150. HÖRSTED P, SANDERGAARD B, THYLSTRUP A, EL ATTAR K, FEJERSKOV O. A retrospective study of direct pulp capping with calcium hydroxide compounds. *Endod Dent Traumatol* 1985;**1**:29–34.

151. HEIDE S, MJÖR IA. Pulp reactions to experimental exposures in young permanent monkey teeth. *Int Endod J* 1983;**16**:11–19.

152. CVEK M, CLEATON JONES PE, AUSTIN JC, ANDREASEN JO. Pulp reactions to exposure after experimental crown fractures or grinding in adult monkeys. *J Endod* 1982;**8**:391–7.

153. SINGER AJ, CLARK RA. Cutaneous wound healing. *N Engl J Med* 1999;**341**:738–46.

154. ANDREASEN JO, KRISTERSON L, ANDREASEN FM. Damage of the Hertwig's epithelial root sheath: effect upon root growth after autotransplantation of teeth in monkeys. *Endod Dent Traumatol* 1988;**4**: 145–51.

155. MITSIADIS TA, RAHIOTIS C. Parallels between tooth development and repair: conserved molecular mechanisms following carious and dental injury. *J Dent Res* 2004;**83**:896–902.

156. SHORT B, BROUARD N, OCCHIODORO-SCOTT T, RAMAKRISHNAN A, SIMMONS PJ. Mesenchymal stem cells. *Arch Med Res* 2003;**34**:565–71.

157. BATOULI S, MIURA M, BRAHIM J, TSUTSUI TW, FISHER LW, GRONTHOS S, et al. Comparison of stem-cell-mediated osteogenesis and dentinogenesis. *J Dent Res* 2003;**82**:976–81.

158. HOLTGRAVE EA, DONATH K. Response of odontoblast-like cells to hydroxyapatite ceramic granules. *Biomaterials* 1995;**16**:155–9.

159. ISHIZEKI K, NAWA T, SUGAWARA M. Calcification capacity of dental papilla mesenchymal cells transplanted in the isogenic mouse spleen. *Anat Rec* 1990;**226**:279–87.

160. PRIME SS, READE PC. Xenografts of recombined bovine odontogenic tissues and cultured cells to hypothymic mice. *Transplantation* 1980;**30**:149–52.

161. PRIME SS, SIM FR, READE PC. Xenografts of human ameloblastoma tissue and odontogenic mesenchyme to hypothymic mice. *Transplantation* 1982;**33**:561–2.

162. BUURMA B, GU K, RUTHERFORD RB. Transplantation of human pulpal and gingival fibroblasts attached to synthetic scaffolds. *Eur J Oral Sci* 1999;**107**: 282–9.

163. TZIAFAS D, SMITH AJ, LESOT H. Designing new treatment strategies in vital pulp therapy. *J Dent* 2000;**28**:77–92.

164. SMITH AJ, MATTHEWS JB, HALL RC. Transforming growth factor-beta1 (TGF-beta1) in dentine matrix. Ligand activation and receptor expression. *Eur J Oral Sci* 1998;**106**:(*Suppl 1*):179–84.

165. SMITH AJ, MURRAY PE, SLOAN AJ, MATTHEWS JB, ZHAO S. Trans-dentinal stimulation of tertiary dentinogenesis. *Adv Dent Res* 2001;**15**:51–4.

166. THESLEFF I, TUMMERS M. Possibilities to improve implants and regenerate dento-alveolar tissue engineering using stem cells and growth factors. In: Ellingsen JE, Lyngstadaas JP. eds. *Bio-implant interface. improving biomaterials and tissue reactions.* Boca Raton: CRC Press, 2003:205–17.

167. RUTHERFORD RB, SPANGBERG L, TUCKER M, RUEGER D, CHARETTE M. The time-course of the induction of reparative dentine formation in monkeys by recombinant human osteogenic protein-1. *Arch Oral Biol* 1994;**39**:833–38.

168. RUTHERFORD RB, WAHLE J, TUCKER M, RUEGER D, CHARETTE M. Induction of reparative dentine formation in monkeys by recombinant human osteogenic protein-1. *Arch Oral Biol* 1993;**38**:571–6.

169. NAKASHIMA M. Induction of dentin formation on canine amputated pulp by recombinant human bone morphogenetic proteins (BMP)-2 and -4. *J Dent Res* 1994;**73**:1515–22.

170. HU CC, ZHANG C, QIAN Q, TATUM NB. Reparative dentin formation in rat molars after direct pulp capping with growth factors. *J Endod* 1998;**24**:744–51.

171. TZIAFAS D, ALVANOU A, PAPADIMITRIOU S, GASIC J, KOMNENOU A. Effects of recombinant basic fibroblast growth factor, insulin-like growth factor-II and transforming growth factor-beta1on dog dental pulp cells *in vivo*. *Arch Oral Biol* 1998;**43**:431–44.

172. RUTHERFORD RB. Regeneration of the dentin-pulp complex. In: Lynch SE, Genco RJ, Marx RE. eds. *Tissue engineering, applications in maxillofacial surgery and periodontics.* Chicago: Quintessence Int., 1999: 185–99.

173. JEPSEN S, ALBERS HK, FLEINER B, TUCKER M, RUEGER D. Recombinant human osteogenic protein-1 induces dentin formation: an experimental study in miniature swine. *J Endod* 1997;**23**:378–82.

174. RUTHERFORD RB. BMP-7 gene transfer to inflamed ferret dental pulps. *Eur J Oral Sci* 2001;**109**:422–4.

175. COX CF, BERGENHOLTZ G, HEYS DR, SYED SA, FITZGERALD M, HEYS RJ. Pulp capping of dental pulp mechanically exposed to oral microflora: a 1–2 year observation of wound healing in the monkey. *J Oral Pathol* 1985;**14**:156–68.

176. WATTS A, PATERSON RC. Bacterial contamination as a factor influencing the toxicity of materials to the exposed dental pulp. *Oral Surg Oral Med Oral Pathol* 1987;**64**:466–74.

177. TZIAFAS D. *Reparative dentinogenesis.* University of Thessaloniki, Greece, 1997.

178. LOVSCHALL H, FEJERSKOV O, FLYVBJERG A. Pulp capping with recombinant human insulin-like growth factor I (rhIGF-I) in rat molars. *Adv Dent Res* 2001;**35**:108–12.

179. SMITH AJ. Tooth tissue engineering and regeneration – a translational vision! *J Dent Res* 2004;**83**:517.

180. THESLEFF I, TUMMERS M. Stem cells and tissue engineering: prospects for regenerating tissues in dental practice. *Med Princ Pract* 2003;**12**:(*Suppl 1*):43–50.

181. MITSIADIS TA, CHERAUD Y, SHARPE P, FONTAINE-PERUS J. Development of teeth in chick embryos after mouse neural crest transplantations. *Proc Natl Acad Sci U S A* 2003;**100**:6541–5.

182. YOUNG CS, TERADA S, VACANTI JP, HONDA M, BARTLETT JD, YELICK PC. Tissue engineering of complex tooth structures on biodegradable polymer scaffolds. *J Dent Res* 2002;**81**:695–700.

183. GOULD TRL. Ultrastructural characteristics of progenior cell populations in the periodontal ligament. *J Dent Res* 1983;**62**:873–6.

184. ANDREASEN JO, MUNKSGAARD EC, FREDEBO L, RUD J. Periodontal tissue regeneration including cementogenesis adjacent to dentin-bonded retrograde composite fillings in humans. *J Endod* 1993;**19**:151–3.

185. TAKATA, T, KATAUCHI K, AKAGAWA Y, NIKAI H. New periodontal ligament formation on a synthetic hydroxyapatite surface. *Clin Oral Impl Res* 1993;**4**:130–6.

186. BUSER D, WARRER K, KARRING T, STICH H. Titanium implants with a true periodontal ligament: an alternative to osseointegrated implants. *Int J Oral Maxillofac Impl* 1990;**5**:113–16.

187. GROISMAN M, SCHWARZ O, ANDREASEN JO, ATTSTRÖM R. Supra-alveolar periodontal healing of auto- and allotransplanted teeth in monkeys. *Endod Dent Traum* 1989;**5**:229–33.

188. SHARPE P, YOUNG CS. Test tube teeth. *Sci Am* 2005;**293**(2):34–41.

# 4

# Osteoclastic Activity

S. F. Lindskog, C. W. Dreyer, A. M. Pierce, M. Torabinejad & S. Shabahang

*S. F. Lindskog, C. W. Dreyer and A. M. Pierce*

## Osteoclast histogenesis

Roodman in 1996 (1) described bone resorption as a life-long physiological process, initially involved with the processes of growth and modelling and continuing as remodelling of the mature skeleton. The main cellular agent involved in the removal of bone has been identified as the osteoclast, and extensive reviews, as well as entire books, have been written on this unique cell (1–20). The osteoclast is described as a large multinucleated cell usually containing between 10 and 20 nuclei (21, 22) (Fig. 4.1).

## The origin of osteoclasts

Kölliker, in 1873, is credited as the first to identify an association between the osteoclast and bone (23). It is currently believed that this multinucleated cell is derived from the pluripotential hemopoietic stem cell and remains the principal cell involved in bone resorption (24).

Early reports suggested that osteoblasts possess the dual capabilities of osteogenesis and bone resorption (2). This impression was based on histological evidence of the close relationship between osteoblasts and osteoclasts and it was suggested that osteoblasts were mononuclear precursors that coalesced to form the multinucleated osteoclasts (2). Subsequent parabiotic research indicated that osteoclasts are of haemopoietic origin (25–27). Additional experiments again using parabiotic rats, one of which was exposed and the other shielded from irradiation, demonstrated that osteoclasts form in and are derived from bone marrow tissue in the protected animal (28). This important finding has been utilized in the management of infantile and juvenile osteopetrosis by bone marrow transplantation (29). Further transplantation studies using quail-chick chimeras revealed that osteoclasts are host derived and clearly indicated that osteoclast precursors are present in marrow, spleen and also detectable in circulating peripheral blood (30).

While there is general agreement that osteoclasts form from mononuclear cells of extraskeletal origin, debate exists as to whether this originating stem cell is part of the mononuclear phagocyte system (31). Circulating blood monocytes have been shown to fuse and form osteoclasts in tissue culture (32) and osteoclasts have differentiated from proliferating bone marrow mononuclear phagocytes *in vitro* (33). Whereas monocytes have been shown to be capable of causing bone resorption (34), transplantation studies have revealed a bone marrow (35) and/or a splenic origin for the osteoclast precursor (36). Surface antigens of osteoclasts have been found to share certain determinants with multinucleated giant cells and monocyte derived macrophages (38).

Under experimental conditions using incubated mouse and rat monocytes, macrophages, spleen and marrow

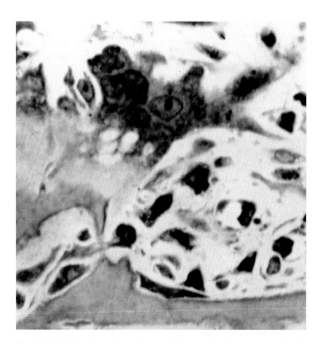

**Fig. 4.1** Multinucleated osteoclast actively resorbing bone as seen by the fuzzy bone-cell interface.

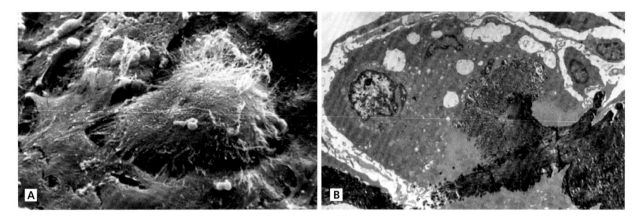

**Fig. 4.2** A. Scanning electron microscopy of an actively resorbing osteoclast attached to a bone surface and surrounded by osteoblasts. The periphery of the osteoclast consists of a fringe of filopodia. B. The TEM image was taken of undecalcified bone and shows the actively resorbing *ruffled border* as at dark tree-like structure (dissolved hydroxyapatite crystallites) connecting the cell with the bone surface. It is surrounded by the *sealing zone* void of cell organelles.

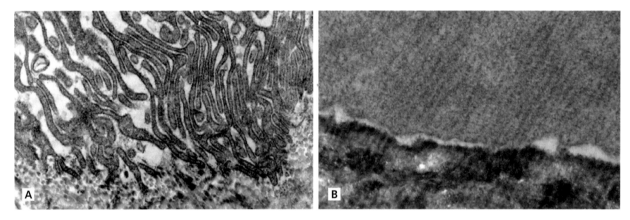

**Fig. 4.3** A. Detail from the ruffled border in a decalcified TEM-section showing plasma membrane foldings stretching towards the resorbed bone. B. Detail demonstrating that the sealing zone is free of cell organelles and that it is microphilamentous. It attaches to the bone surface in focal points.

hemopoietic cells as well as foreign body macrophages and macrophage polykaryons, with UMR 106 osteoblast-like cells on bone slices in the presence of 1,25-dihydroxyvitamin D₃ it was noted that numerous tartrate-resistant acid phosphatase-positive cells formed in these co-cultures and extensive lacunar resorption was observed on bone surfaces (37). It was further reported that a bone-derived stromal cell element was necessary for the differentiation of monocytes and macrophages into osteoclast-like cells capable of bone resorption and based on these findings it was suggested that osteoclasts are members of the mononuclear phagocyte system (38).

## Osteoclast morphology

Bone biologists have described osteoclasts as large, multinucleated cells found in resorption bays (Howship's lacunae) on the surface of bone (2, 23, 39, 40, 41). Under high-power light microscopy, infoldings of the plasma membrane termed *ruffled borders* are observed in close contact with the hard tissue surface (Figs 4.2B, 4.3A). The dramatic and revealing ultrastructural appearance of the ruffled border was first described by Scott and Pease in 1956 (42) as a complex series of finger-like cytoplasmic folds and projections. The ruffled border appears to be the true resorptive organ of the active osteoclast (43) and has been further reported to be an ultrastructural feature not seen in other giant cells (21, 43, 44). It is suggested that the ruffled area is formed by the fusion of intracellular vesicles with membranous proteins, matching those present in the osteoclast's plasma membrane (43, 44). Furthermore it is suggested that the ruffled border is a specialized form of lysosomal membrane based on the localization of a mannose-6-phosphate receptor and a lysosomal proton pump (46). Another view has been that the ruffled border proteins are more consistent with endosomal rather than lysosomal membranes (46). Bone resorption and degradation of bone matrix has been found to occur in a resorptive compartment beneath the ruffled border, as a result of the cellular release of proteolytic enzymes and hydrogen ions (45).

On either side of the ruffled border an organelle-free area of cytoplasm (*sealing zone*) associated with a portion of cell membrane is seen in intimate contact with the hard tissue surface (Fig. 4.3B) (21, 22). It has been suggested that this intimate contact creates a sealing zone which anchors the

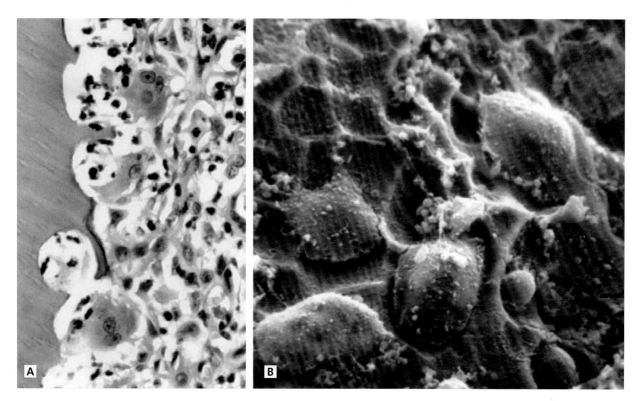

**Fig. 4.4** Odontoclasts in varying stages of resorbing activity on a dentine surface. A. Multinucleated odontoclasts surrounded by a mixed infiltrate of inflammatory cells. B. Odontoclasts in an area of inflammatory root resorption.

osteoclast to bone via specific adhesion molecules collectively termed integrins (47). This adhesion zone effectively isolates the resorptive compartment from the extracellular environment and in doing so creates a resorptive microenvironment. The adjacent intracellular cytoplasmic clear zone has been shown to contain actin-like filaments (β-actinin, talin, vinculin) but is void of organelles (48).

The remaining cytoplasm of the osteoclast contains the necessary intracellular organelles to fulfil its digestive functions. An extensive endoplasmic reticulum involved in protein (enzyme) synthesis in company with ribosomes, occurring singly or as polyribosomes has been described (22). Perinuclear Golgi bodies were identified for vesicle production and numerous mitochondria provided the cell's energy requirements. Osteoclast mitochondria have been found associated with adenosine triphosphatase (ATPase) release as a by-product of the conversion of water and intracellular carbon dioxide to $H^+$ and $HCO_3^-$ ions under the catalytic action of carbonic anhydrase II (47, 49). Numerous intracellular vesicles have also been identified carrying secretory products towards the ruffled border and in the transcytotic process of moving bone dissolution products through the cell towards the basolateral membrane for excretion into the extracellular space (45, 46, 95). Apart from a role in cell adhesion, the clear zone filaments are supposed to act as intracellular guides for the vacuolar transcytotic process (51). The multiple nuclei seen are not considered a unique features of the osteoclast but the ruffled border and intracellular organelles are what distinguish this cell from other polykaryons.

Scanning electron microscopic studies have revealed the complexity of the osteoclast's plasma membrane (52, 53). Prominent microvilli or pseudopodia are located over the central portion of the cell and associated with excavation cavities (Figs 4.3, 4.4). The osteoclasts appear to be connected to adjacent cells and is suggested to be part of the formation of a functional syncytium (53). Because of their pseudopodia and observations using time-lapse video photography (54), osteoclasts have been reported to be highly motile cells that contract when exposed to calcitonin or prostaglandin $E_2$ (55).

## Odontoclast function

The process of bone resorption requires a series of events leading from the differentiation and recruitment of mononuclear osteoclast precursors, to their multinucleation and attachment to the hard tissue surface, before the removal of the inorganic and organic hard tissue components (4, 56, 57, 58). Many studies have identified the osteoblast as the principal regulator of resorption (3, 14, 59, 60).

Osteoclasts have the capacity to digest mineralized matrices such as bone, mineralized cartilage and dentine (61, 62) (Figs 4.4, 4.5). An initial step in the sequence of events leading to bone digestion is the formation of the osteoclast from mononuclear progenitor cells from the monocyte lineage (63). Fusion of the mononuclear precursors to form osteoclasts at the site of resorption is followed by attachment

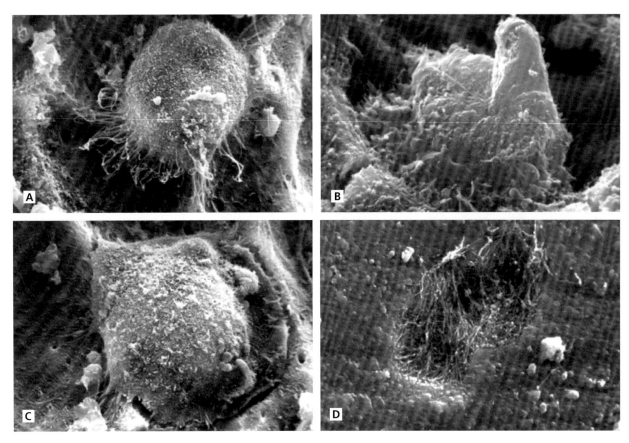

**Fig. 4.5** Odontoclasts in progressive stages of attachment. A and B show polarization including formation of a ruffled border. C shows formation of a sealing zone. D shows a resorption lacuna after an odontoclast has detached. The mineral has been dissolved exposing the collagenous matrix.

to the bony surface which is facilitated by membrane-bound integrins and bone-associated proteins (64–66). Osteoblast-derived collagenase (MMP-1) plays a prime role in facilitating osteoclast attachment by the degradation of surface osteoid (67). Pretreatment of bone with mammalian collagenase predisposes surface tissue to osteoclastic resorption which has led to the concept that the layer of osteoid acts as a protective barrier against osteoclastic contact with the underlying, resorption-stimulating bone mineral (67). In between episodes of resorption it has been shown that the surface of bone is largely covered by a layer of non-mineralized collagen fibrils which have the effect of making bone resistant to osteoclastic attack (68). In addition, it has been shown that cells isolated from the tissues in close apposition to bone and subsequently seeded on to bone slices possess the capacity to render the mineralized surface accessible to osteoclasts. It was concluded that bone needs to be cleared of non-mineralized collagen prior to osteoclastic attack (67, 69), and further, that bone-tissue derived osteoblast-like cells have the capacity to strip the surface of bone of its collagenous fringe (70). It has furthermore been suggested that osteoblasts are responsible for the removal of non-mineralized collagen and, further, indicated that collagen elimination depends on the activity of matrix metalloproteinases (MMP) which are manufactured and secreted by the osteoblast (71, 72).

Further evidence for implicating the involvement of osteoblasts in the initiation of bone resorption has been that the incubation of osteoblast-like cells with parathyroid hormone (PTH) results in a decreased amount of non-mineralized collagen (62, 73). It has been established that PTH stimulates the breakdown of the investing collagenous layer by increasing the activity of PTH-sensitive cells such as the osteoblast, and possibly the fibroblast.

Enzymes other than MMPs, of which collagenase is a member, are possibly also involved in bone resorption. The cysteine proteinases (cathepsins K, B and L) have been shown to play a crucial role in the digestion of phagocytosed fibrillar collagen (74). Both MMPs and cysteine proteinases have been found to mediate pathophysiological bone resorption, a phenomenon depending upon the environmental pH (75). Delaissé et al. (76) reviewed the various proteinases involved in bone resorption and indicated that they may be of importance in determining the site of bone resorption and possibly whether bone formation will eventuate.

## Osteoclast recruitment

The determining factors governing sites of resorption are largely unknown, as are the factors guiding osteoclast precursors to resorptive sites (43). It has been suggested that *complement* mediates the recruitment of mononuclear osteoclasts and also *macrophage inflammatory protein-1α* plays an attracting role (77, 78). Osteoclasts are seen in the vicinity of osteoblasts producing macrophage inflammatory protein-1α which has lead to the concept that this chemokine is involved in haemopoiesis as well as bone remodeling (78). Alternatively, it has been suggested that *human osteogenic protein-1*, in combination with *1,25-dihydroxyvitamin D₃* has a profound effect on osteoblastic growth as well as the recruitment of osteoclasts as judged by vitronectin receptor and carbonic anhydrase activity (79). Proteinase inhibitors have been used to show that MMPs play a major role in determining where and when osteoclasts attack bone (80). Importantly, *tumor necrosis factor receptors* types 1 and 2 are found to differentially regulate osteoclastogenesis (81) while *interleukin-1* and *tumor necrosis factor*, by stimulating the inflammatory process, lead to osteoclast recruitment and bone resorption (82). Osteoclast recruitment has also been found to occur at sites of periodontal ligament compression as a result of orthodontic tooth movement due to the likely release of *local mediators* (83). Osteoclast recruitment appears to be related to local factors (84) which are governed by *hormonal, cytokine, growth* and *colony-stimulating factor* interaction (11). Once at a site of resorption, a complex multistep series of events occurs, representing osteoclast attachment and polarization, the formation of a sealing zone followed by active bone resorption, and finally cell detachment and death (85).

## Osteoclast attachment

The physical intimacy between the osteoclast and bone is considered essential in order to create and isolate an acidic extracellular resorptive microenvironment (51). The most striking and unique feature of the osteoclast cytoskeleton is found at the site of cell contact with the substratum (12). These specialized sealing areas appear as a prominent peripheral ring of filaments containing F-actin, orientated parallel to the plane of the substrate (12). In addition, numerous punctate structures of F-actin filaments orientated perpendicular to the substratum have been described and termed *podosomes* (48). These podosomes occur in cells of monocytic origin and also in cells that have been transformed by *src, fps* and *abl* oncogenes (86). Furthermore, it has been indicated that podosomes contain other proteins which have been associated with sites of cell-substratum and cell-cell interaction. These were spatially described as *rosette structures* surrounding podosome cores (91). Also several tyrosine kinases and substrates localized to focal adhesions and to the sealing zone in osteoclasts have been identified (91).

A dynamic view of the attachment of osteoclasts to bone matrix was provided by Kanehisa et al. (87) who described highly motile cells with few podosomes located mainly at the cell's leading edge. Upon osteoclast attraction and attachment an increase in the number of podosomes has been found arranged in a peripheral ring (64, 87). The establishment of this seal results in the replacement of the punctate podosomes by two concentric protein rings of vinculin and talin that surround a central zone of F-actin. It is suggested that these observations provided a distinction in time and in specific cell-matrix interactions between a motile cell and one that stops at a prospective bone-resorbing site (12).

The mediation of cell-substratum interaction at the interface between the osteoclast and bone is facilitated by proteins of the integrin family (12). Integrins have been described as heterodimeric molecules containing $\alpha$ and $\beta$ subunits which, when combined, have specific, receptor-like, extracellular binding sites that recognize the Arginyl-Glycyl-Aspartyl (RGD) sequence (88). It has been ascertained that the RGD sequence represents a core ligand for all members of the integrin family and, furthermore, found that the amino acid sequence surrounding this motif determined which integrin would recognize and bind to a specific matrix protein (89).

Osteoclasts appear to express multiple integrin proteins, some of which are involved in cell adhesion to bone matrix (88). Several RGD-bone matrix proteins have been identified, of which collagen type I, osteopontin, and bone sialoprotein are the most likely candidates to fill the integrin-binding role (90, 91). The important use of integrins in osteoclast attachment and function has been demonstrated in the way that several RGD-containing proteins inhibit bone resorption *in vitro* and *in vivo* (92).

## Osteoclast polarization

Osteoclasts show organization of their cytoplasmic elements during resorptive activation (85, 93). They become more highly polarized via changes in their plasma membrane morphology (43, 94) with the sealing area of cell attachment to bone separating the ruffled border and the basolateral membrane into distinct basal membrane specializations (Fig. 4.5). It appears that there are at least two functionally different basal membrane domains and the intervening central area is postulated to be involved with the transcytotic movement of degraded bone products (50). Both organic and inorganic bone degradation products are transported in vesicles through the osteoclast and liberated into the extracellular environment via the specialized and polarized basal membrane area (95). Transcytosis of proteins liberated from mineralized matrix to the basolateral membrane for extracellular release has been reported (96, 97). An intracellular polarization of organelles which accumulated adjacent to the basolateral region of the cell away from the ruffled border and sealing zone has also been found (98). These polarized organelles synthesized the lysosomal enzymes and vesicles for vectorial transport towards the resorptive compartment.

## Dissolution of bone mineral

The crystalline salts comprising the inorganic component of bone are calcium and phosphate in the form of hydroxyapatite (99) (Fig. 4.2B). It appears that osteoclasts degrade bone mineral and collagen with temporal asynchrony suggesting that the inorganic phase is removed prior to collagenolysis (100). Bone mineral dissolves in a low pH environment and the acidic nature of the resorptive lacunae has been demonstrated (101, 102). Furthermore, the ruffled border of actively resorbing osteoclasts contains a vacuolar-type of proton pump involved in the acidification of the resorptive compartment (103). Protons appears to be pumped across the ruffled border into the sealed extracellular microenvironment via a complex ionic-balance process requiring co-ordinated electrogenic ion pumps, ion channels and electroneutral ion exchangers to maintain cytoplasmic pH (12). In addition to protons, the ruffled border plasma membrane expresses chloride channels that are an essential requirement of the acidification process (50, 91).

A series of intracellular processes have been shown to produce the protons for exchange (51). Cytosolic hydration of carbon dioxide to carbonic acid is catalysed by mitochondrial carbonic anhydrase II (104, 105). This is followed by dissociation of carbonic acid to produce protons and bicarbonate ions. The protons are secreted into the resorption lacunae in an energy-dependent manner while at the basolateral surface opposite the resorbing zone, the bicarbonate ions are exchanged for chloride ions to maintain homeostasis (90, 91). In addition, intracellular pH recovery is assisted by a $Na^+$-$H^+$ exchange process (106).

The osteoclast appears to be similar to acid-secreting epithelial cells found in other areas of the body such as the gastrointestinal tract and the kidney (45). However, subtle differences in vacuolar-type ATPases in chicken osteoclasts compared with kidney intercalated epithelial cells have been found suggesting that the osteoclast proton pump is pharmacologically unique (107).

## Removal of organic matrix

The organic matrix of bone consists predominantly of type I collagen and non-collagenous matrix components comprising structural glycoproteins, proteoglycans and specific bone-related proteins (99, 108). The organic matrix has been found to contain numerous growth factors which provide bone with a remarkable ability to repair and regenerate itself (109). In contrast, dentine contains type I as well as a small percentage of type III collagen. Matrix components of dentin include glycoproteins and proteoglycans of a similar nature but not identical with those of bone (110). An odontoblast-produced phosphoprotein and dentine sialoprotein appear to be specific for dentine (111). Cementum also has a similar organic composition compared with bone but an adhesion molecule and a growth factor possibly remain unique to this material (112).

Removal of matrix proteins is presently far from clear but several major classes of lysosomal proteolytic enzymes are likely to be involved (43). These enzymes can be divided into four groups; namely, *matrix metalloproteinases* (MMPs) and *serine*, *cysteine* and *aspartic proteinases* (109). MMPs are qualitatively and quantitatively the most important, because they function at neutral pH and are apparently capable of digesting all of the bone matrix proteins (109). Biochemical and clonal studies where MMPs were subgrouped into collagenases, gelatinases and stromelysins, found all were active on matrix components working synergistically and with broad specificity (115).

The presence of *collagenase* in rat osteoclasts and in their resorption lacunae has been shown using immunohistochemistry (113) and it has been shown that odontoclasts are capable of expressing *m*RNA for collagenase (115). However, this finding was not supported in another study despite its presence in other bone cells (116). Furthermore, MMP-2 and MMP-3 are not found in osteoclasts, and MMP-9 is possibly expressed at *m*RNA and protein levels, but not in the resorption lacunae (117, 118). MMP-9 has been found to be as an enzyme localized exclusively in osteoclasts and perhaps involved in the degradation of bone collagen below the ruffled border in concert with cysteine proteinases (118). Multinucleated giant cells from osteoclastomas and osteoclasts from patients with Paget's disease have also been reported to have high levels of MMP-9 activity (119). MMP-9 has been found to be expressed early in osteoclastic differentiation (1).

*Cysteine proteinases* (cathepsins/caspases) appear to be able to degrade type I collagen in an acidic environment in the process of bone resorption (120). A number of cysteine proteinases have been found in intracellular lysosomes located in osteoclasts as well as in their resorption lacunae (122, 123, 131). Cathepsin B1 degrades collagen in solution at an optimal pH of 4.5–5.0 and also degrades insoluble collagen at a pH lower than 4 (124). In addition, collagen degradation by cathepsin L is five times faster at a pH of 3.5 compared with higher pH levels and its specific activity is five to ten times greater than that of cathepsin B (122). These enzymes participate directly and effectively in the degradation of bone matrix (125, 126). The cysteine protease inhibitors reduce resorption pit formation by osteoclasts in a concentration-dependent manner. The inhibition of resorption by other cysteine proteinase inhibitors provides direct evidence for the importance of these enzymes in bone resorption where they are able to function in the acidic microenvironment beneath the osteoclast where neutral collagenases (MMPs) cannot (109, 127, 128).

Cathepsin L has been suggested to be the main cysteine proteinase responsible for bone collagen degradation since the epoxysuccinyl peptide inhibitor, CA074, specific for the inactivation of cathepsin B, fails to inhibit bone resorption (129).

More recently, cloned human cysteine proteinase (cathepsin K) has been shown to be predominantly expressed in osteoclasts, although not exclusively (130, 131). Furthermore, cathepsins B, D, L and K appears important in the breakdown of extracellular matrix during osteoclastic bone resorption and therefore possible markers for resorptive activity (131).

## Removal of degradation products

Breakdown products from the resorptive process need to be continuously removed from the extracellular resorptive compartment (43). As there is no experimental evidence to support leakage of material through the sealing zone, it is suggested that vesicular transcytotic passage through the osteoclast is the most likely pathway. Confocal microscopic analysis has been used to show that released matrix proteins, including degraded type I collagen, are endocytosed along the ruffled border and transcytosed through the osteoclast to the basolateral membrane (96). Earlier ultrastructural studies suggested that bone mineral may be phagocytosed

**Table 4.1** Stimulatory and inhibitory factors associated with osteoclast activity.

| Substance | Stimulatory | Inhibitory | |
|---|---|---|---|
| **Hormones** | | | |
| Amylin | | + | Alam et al. (1993) (139) |
| Androgens | | + | Bellido et al. (1995) (140) |
| Calcitonin | | + | Zaidi et al. (1991) (141) |
| Calcitonin gene-related peptide | | + | Alam et al. (1991) (142) |
| Glucocorticoids | + | | Delany et al. (1994) (143) |
| Oestrogen | | + | Oursler et al. (1993) (141) |
| Parathyroid hormone | + | | Talmage (1967) (145) |
| PTHrP | + | | Moseley and Gillespie (1995) (146) |
| Thyroid hormone | + | | Mundy et al. (1979) (147) |
| 1,25(OH)$_2$ vitamin D3 | + | | Reichel et al. (1989) (148) |
| | | | |
| **Cytokines and growth factors** | | | |
| Bone morphogenic proteins, BMP | + | | Udagawa (2002) (149) |
| Colony stimulating factors, CSF-1 | + | | Hattersley et al. (1991) (150) |
| Endothelin-1 | + | | Tarquini et al. (1998) (151) |
| Epidermal growth factor, EGF | + | | Tashjian et al. (1986) (152) |
| Fibroblast growth factor, FGF | + | + | Shen et al. (1989) (153) |
| | | | Chikazu et al. (2001) (154) |
| Granulocyte macrophage colony stimulating factor, GM-CSF | + | | Kurihara et al. (1989) (155) |
| Insulin-like growth factor, IGF-1 | + | | Mochizuki et al. (1992) (156) |
| Interferon-$\gamma$, IF-$\gamma$ | | + | Gowen et al. (1986) (157) |
| Interleukin-1, IL-1 | + | | Lorenzo et al. (1987) (158) |
| Interleukin-4 | | + | Shioni et al. (1991) (159) |
| Interleukin-6 | + | | Peters et al. (1996) (160) |
| Interleukin-8 | | + | Fuller et al. (1995) (161) |
| Interleukin-10 | | + | Burger and Dayer (1995) (162) |
| Interleukin-11 | + | | Manolagas and Jilka (1995) (163) |
| Interleukin-18 | | + | Udagawa et al. (1997) (164) |
| Kinins | + | | Lerner et al. (1987) (165) |
| Macrophage inflammatory protein 1-$\alpha$, MIP-1$\alpha$ | + | | Choi et al. (2000) (166) |
| Nitric oxide | | + | MacIntyre et al. (1991) (167) |
| Platelet-derived growth factor, PDGF | + | | Canalis et al. (1989) (168) |
| Prostaglandins | + | | Akatsu et al. (1991) (169) |
| Transforming growth factor alpha, TGF-$\alpha$ | + | | Tashjian et al. (1986) (152) |
| Tissue inhibitors of metalloproteinases, TIMP | + | | Sobue et al. (2001) (170) |
| Transforming growth factor $\beta$, TGF-$\beta$ | + | | Udagawa (2002) (149) |
| Tumor necrosis factor $\alpha$, TNF-$\alpha$ | + | | Kobayashi et al. (2000) (171) |
| Tumor necrosis factor $\beta$, TNF-$\beta$ | + | | Bertolini et al. (1986) (172) |
| Substance P | + | | Lotz et al. (1988) (173) |
| Vasoactive intestinal peptide, VIP | + | | Hohmann et al. (1983) (174) |
| | | | |
| **Pharmaceuticals** | | | |
| Bisphosphonates | | + | Fleisch et al. (1969) (175) |
| Corticosteroids | | + | Pierce et al. (1987, 1988, 1989) (176, 177, 178) |

by osteoclasts and subsequently removed in the low pH of lysosomes as degradation products are transcytosed (184). Bone degradation products, both organic and inorganic, appear to be transported in vesicles through the cell to the middle of the basolateral membrane domain where they are released into the extracellular space (95). It is suggested that the osteoclast is *similar* to epithelial cells in this metabolite transport mechanism but that the process is significantly more complicated and the endocytic and exocytic processes are *dissimilar* to those previously encountered in other cell types and require a specialized area of the osteoclast basolateral membrane (97).

## The fate of osteoclasts

Osteoclasts appear to be are able to pass through more than one resorption cycle but their fate is uncertain once resorp-

tion had ceased (132). Apparently, a mechanism exists to remove or destroy multinucleated cells *in situ* (43). The effects of bisphosphonates *in vitro* and *in vivo* have revealed a 4- to 24-fold increase in the number of apoptotic osteoclasts (133). This has led to the suggestion that osteoclasts, formed by the aggregation of mononuclear cells rather than by mitosis, are removed by apoptosis.

## Regulation of osteoclast activity

The majority of regulatory factors operate via surface receptors located on *osteoblasts* whereas few act directly on *osteoclasts*. Extensive reviews have been written (6, 14, 20, 84, 134–138). A summary of regulatory factors involved in clast cell activity is presented in Table 4.1 (139–178). These

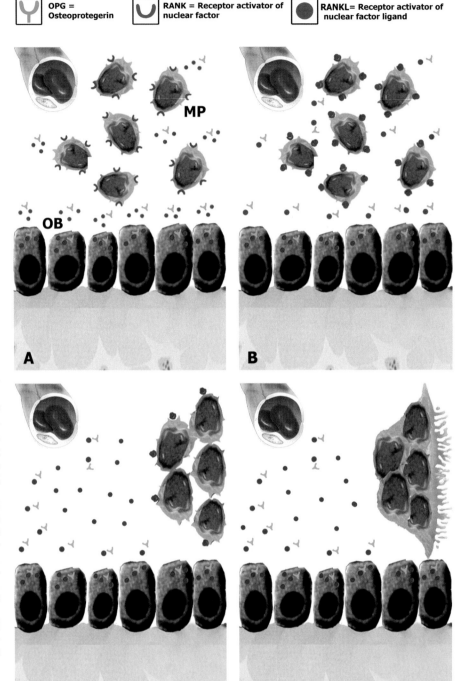

**OPG =**
**Osteoprotegerin**

**RANK = Receptor activator of**
**nuclear factor**

**RANKL= Receptor activator of**
**nuclear factor ligand**

**Fig. 4.6** Activation of the ODF/ OPGL/RANKL system. Osteoclastogenesis is the result of differentiation of mononuclear/macrophage progenitor cells (MP) and fusion of these cells to become osteoclasts. The commitment of these cells to become osteoclasts depends on the activation of the RANK receptors on the surface of RANKL, which is produced by stroma cells and osteoblasts (OB). A and B. RANKL is liberated into the tissue and attaches to the receptors of the mononuclear/macrophage progenitor cells. C. Mononuclear/macrophage cells aggregate, fuse and form osteoclasts (D). Proresorptive factors are hormones and cytokines such as PTH, $1,25(OH)_2D_3$, IL-1, IL-6, TNF, LIF and corticosteroids, which activate osteoblasts and stroma cells to produce RANKL and depress OPG.

include factors important in physiological bone resorption as well as those produced by an inflammatory reaction subsequent to mechanical injury or infection (see Effects on osteoclasts of chemical mediators of inflammation p. 148).

Of interest in a therapeutic context is that Pierce and Lindskog provided evidence for direct inhibition of inflammatory root resorption by the use of corticosteroids. The culture of isolated dentinoclasts with a steroid paste inhibited cell spreading which suggested that the intrapulpal *in vivo* application of a steriod paste could arrest inflammatory root resorption by the detachment of dentinoclasts from the root surface, provided the pathogenic bacteria are eliminated (176).

Recent literature has described a newly discovered regulator of clast cell activity termed *osteoclast differentiation factor/osteoprotegerin ligand* (ODF/OPGL/RANKL) and its antagonist *osteoprotegerin/osteoclast inhibitory factor* (OPG/OCIF). Hofbauer et al. (136, 179, 180) indicated that many of the above-listed regulatory factors operate via stimulation of the RANKL/OPG system. A schematic diagram of the RANKL/RANK/OPG interaction between osteoblasts/ stromal cells and osteoclasts appears in Figs 4.6–4.8. Its dis-

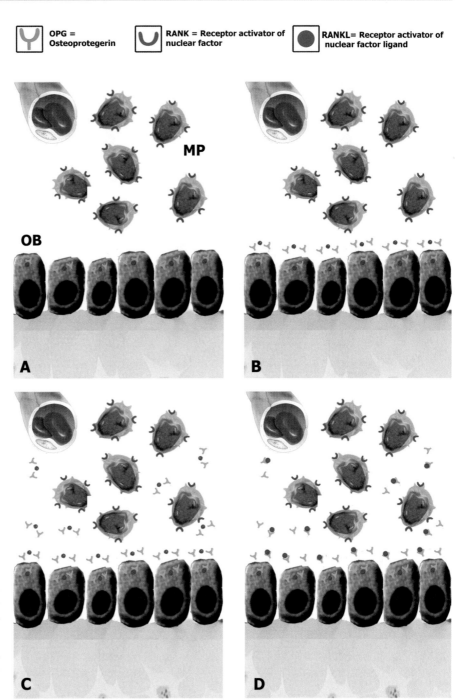

**OPG =**
**Osteoprotegerin**

**RANK = Receptor activator of**
**nuclear factor**

**RANKL= Receptor activator of**
**nuclear factor ligand**

**Fig. 4.7** Inactivation of the OPG/OCIF system. Anti-resorptive factors such as estrogens, calcitonin, BMP, TGF-β, IL-17, PDGF and calcium depress RANKL production by osteoblasts and stroma cells and activate their OPG production (A–C). OPG binds and neutralizes RANKL (D), leading to a block in osteoclastogenesis and decreased survival of osteoclasts.

covery and implications for other systems in the body such as the immune system is described below. In summary, it provides a link between the osteoblast/stromal cells in the bone marrow and the osteoclast precursor cells. The dependence of osteoclast formation on osteoblasts/stromal cells has been recognized for a long time but the details are largely unknown. Stimulation of osteoblasts/stromal cells with, for example, PTH results in release of M-CSF (macrophage-colony stimulation factor) thus increasing the locally available number of osteoclast precursor cells (MP) derived from hematopoetic stem cells (Fig. 4.6A). Concomitantly, RANKL is expressed on the surface of osteoblasts/stromal cells, a ligand which in turn activates the RANK receptor on the surface of the osteoclast precursor cells (Fig. 4.6B). This direct contact stimulates the cell to dif-

ferentiate into osteoclasts (Fig. 4.6C, D). OPG is a soluble receptor which is secreted by osteoblasts/stromal cells and is capable of inhibiting RANKL from interacting with RANK thus regulating osteoclast formation in an autocrine manner through the osteoblasts/stromal cells. Resorption stimulants such as PTH, vitamin D3 and IL-1 inhibit formation and release of OPG and stimulate expression of RANKL. In this context, IL-1 is one of the most important links between inflammation and resorption of bone and dental tissues as seen in traumatic injuries to the teeth.

Antiresorptive factors such as estrogen, calcitonin, IL-17, PGDF and calcium depress RANKL production and activate OPG leading to a block in osteoclastogenesis and decreased survival of osteoclasts (Fig. 4.7).

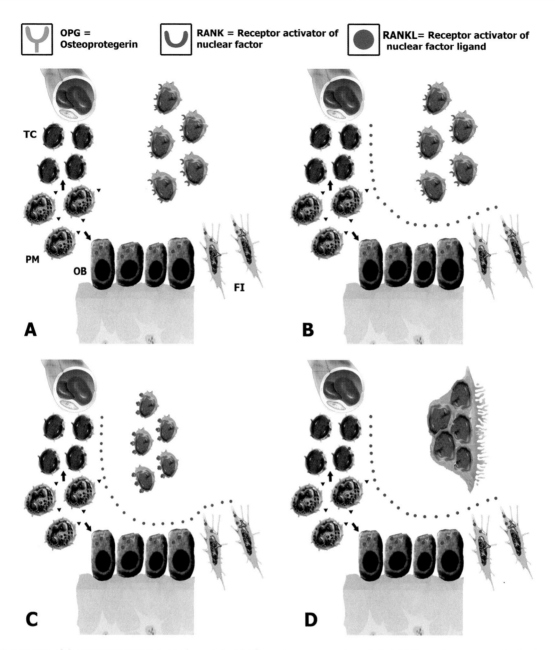

**Fig 4.8** Activation of the ODF/OPGL/RANKL system by periodontal inflammatory processes. In periodontal inflammatory processes leading to root and bone resorption RANKL is produced by T-cells (TC), gingival fibroblasts/PDL cells (FI) and osteoblasts (OB), whereby osteoclasts are induced and activated, attacking root or bone substances. Furthermore, polymorph nuclear leukocytes (PM) release pro-inflammatory substances (cytokines, kinins, thrombin and prostaglandins), illustrated as black triangles, which activate PDL cells and osteoblasts to produce RANKL (arrow). An activation also occurs on the T-cells (arrow).

In periodontal inflammatory processes (marginal or periapical) a number of activators are released (Figs 4.8A–C) which result in osteoclast induction and activation (Fig. 4.8D).

## Identification of osteoclasts and odontoclasts

Apart from the uniqueness of the calcitonin receptor (181), traditional methods of osteoclast identification have relied on enzyme histochemistry and immunolabelling to distinguish this cell from other multinucleated giant cells (13). Although possessing unique morphological differences, it

has been reported that osteoclasts contain a number of phenotypic features that enable their detection (206).

The cells implicated in root resorption have been identified as clastic in nature since they are large, multinucleated and possess properties similar to the osteoclast (182). Based on the identification of the osteoclast and odontoclast cell types as both resorptive, located in Howship's lacunae and possessing similar cytological features, Jones and Boyd (183) and Pierce (184) have stated that there is no reason to believe that the cell type differ except in their relative substrata (Figs 4.4 and 4.5). These authors reported that multinucleated odontoclasts are polarized with respect to dental tissues and possess a ruffled border within an annular clear zone that is closely adherent to mineralized tissues

(Fig. 4.5). It has been found that odontoclasts are capable of having two ruffled border areas that resorbed bone and tooth surfaces simultaneously (185). Accordingly, Jones and Boyd suggested that if an odontoclast was defined as an eukaryotic cell that is capable of resorbing mineralized dental tissues, 'osteoclasts became odontoclasts with alacrity' (183).

Odontoclasts have been isolated from rat molars and cultured successfully (186, 187). It has been shown that the odontoclastic tooth resorption *in vitro* may be controlled by the early administration of calcitonin and prednisolone or exacerbated by the introduction of hydrocortisone (176, 178). Scanning electron microscope evidence indicates that both substances inhibit odontoclast spreading and attachment and hence resorption. It is considered that the direct effect of steroids on resorption is one of inhibition but that local secondary effects might moderate a systemic *in vivo* effect (178).

Odontoclasts appear to spread and colonize surface dentine in a time-related fashion (Fig. 4.8). Scanning electronmicroscopy at predetermined time intervals has determined that dentinoclasts follow a general pattern of attachment and spreading on solid substrata (187).

In a comparative study by Addison (188) the enzyme histochemical characteristics of human and kitten odontoclasts and osteoclasts were studied. Enzyme profiles suggested that odontoclasts have similar properties and metabolic functions to those of osteoclasts and that species differences appear to be minor (188). In a later study, Addison (189) described the effects of low dose PTH on feline odontoclasts and, in particular, on the number of odontoclast nuclei. PTH administered intravenously was found to have a dramatic and almost instantaneous effect on increasing numbers of nuclei.

Earlier ultrastructural studies examined the effects of PTH on both the fine structure of odontoclasts and on their acid phosphatase activity (190). It has been found that active odontoclasts possess cytoplasmic processes that enter dentinal tubules, and that acid phosphatase is present both intra- and extra-cellularly (190). Subcutaneous administration of PTH has been found to increase the number of extracellular dense bodies showing acid phosphatase activity but did not appear to influence intracellular phosphatase activity (190). The identification of odontoclasts might therefore be possible by the localization of certain plasma proteins. By using immunofluorescent staining it has been possible to demonstrate albumin, α-antitrypsin, α$_2$-HS glycoprotein, transferrin and several immunoglobulins in the cytoplasm of odontoclasts and also within human dentine (115).

Odontoclast research has mainly utilized the physiological resorption of deciduous teeth as an experimental model. Matsuda (191) conducted an ultrastructural and cytochemical study of odontoclasts gathered from trypsin-treated dentine and cemental surfaces and showed extensive ruffled borders along with multiple phagosomes containing tannic-acid stainable amorphous inclusions (191). It was further noted that odontoclasts did not phagocytose collagen fibrils but they exhibited acid phosphatase activity. These observations have led to the conclusion that odontoclasts resorb the non-collagenous component of the dental organic matrix via the release of hydrolytic enzymes and have the capacity to demineralize hard tissue by H$^+$- K$^+$-ATPase activity (191).

Sahara et al. (192), employing a similar model, expanded Matsuda's study (191) and reported that odontoclasts are capable of resorbing the superficial non-mineralized layer of predentine. Light and electron microscopy indicated that, as root resorption was nearing completion, multinucleated cells were observed between degenerative osteoblasts on the predentine surface of the coronal dentine. These cells had the same ultrastructural characteristics as odontoclasts and excavated resorption lacunae in the non-mineralized dentine. In addition, histochemical demonstration of tartrate-resistant acid phosphatase activity revealed intense staining in intracellular lysosomes. It was concluded that multinucleated odontoclasts are capable of resorbing non-mineralized predentine matrix *in vivo*, probably in a similar fashion to the manner in which they resorb demineralized dentine matrix (192).

Collagenase *m*RNA expression has been identified in odontoclasts, macrophages, fibroblasts, odontoblasts and cementoblasts around bovine resorbing tooth roots. In addition, TRAP activity and interleukin-1 *m*RNA expression was also observed in odontoclasts, fibroblasts and macrophages indicating that odontoclasts might play a role in dentine collagen degradation and that interleukins could be an important factor in promoting root resorption (115).

Cathepsins B and G have been demonstrated in lysosomes, vacuoles and within the extracellular channels of the ruffled border in odontoclasts (193). The presence of these proteolytic enzymes suggest that they are of prime importance in the intra- or extra-cellular degradation of collagen and other non-collagenous matrix proteins in the resorption of deciduous teeth.

Histological and histochemical observations of deciduous teeth have demonstrated that odontoclastic resorption usually occurs at the pulpal surface of coronal dentine, and in a specific time-related pattern. During physiological root resorption, coronal pulpal tissue retains its normal structure until root loss is almost complete. Multinucleated odontoclastic resorption appears to proceed from predentine to dentine on the pulpal surface at the cervical areas of the crown before spreading towards the pulp horns (194).

The cytodifferentiation of odontoclasts during root resorption has been studied in a light and electron microscopic study. Odontoclasts differentiated from TRAP-positive mononuclear cells which were presumed to originate from circulating progenitors. Ruffled borders, clear cytoplasmic zones and multinucleation occurred only after contact with the substrate surface (195). Odontoclasts appear to resorb predentine before dentine and it is suggested that the processes are similar to those responsible for the resorption of bone. It was also noted that the end of the resorptive process was characterized by loss of the odontoclast ruffled border and detachment from the resorbed surface (195).

Resorption at the cemento-enamel junction in feline teeth has been examined using specific antibodies and immunohistochemical analyses to localize adhesion molecules associated with mineralized tissues. Osteoclast/odontoclast numbers were found to increase in resorptive lesions, bone sialoprotein (BSP) and osteopontin (OPN) were identified in tissues, and a complementary clast cell surface receptor (integrin $\alpha_v\beta_3$) was linked to these molecules (197). OPN was found localized to resorption fronts and reversal lines whereas BSP was localized to reversal lines only. Odontoclasts were found in juxtaposition to mineralized surfaces not associated with OPN and the cell surface integrin receptor, $\alpha_v\beta_3$, was localized to odontoclastic surfaces. It was concluded that this integrin receptor is involved in the resorptive process and facilitates the attachment of clastic cells to their substrate (197).

In conclusion, based on morphological and functional similarities between odontoclasts or dentinoclasts and osteoclasts there is every reason to believe that factors regulating osteoclast activity under normal physiological as well as pathological conditions also regulate resorption of teeth following traumatic injuries whether accompanied by infection and inflammation or not. Clinically a number of different types of resorptions following such injuries have been described ranging from self-limiting surface resorption to progressive inflammatory resorption and replacement resorption (see Chapter 2). An inflammatory root resorption is almost inevitably accompanied by an infection in the root canal and requires treatment. Ankylosis with subsequent bony replacement resorption is, from a prognostic point of view, a treatment sequela with a relatively poor prognosis when it affects a large surface area of the root. The rate at which the root is replaced by bone largely depends on systemic factors which normally regulate bone remodeling in addition to the age of the patient.

*M. Torabinejad and S. Shabahang*

## Osteoclast activity in general

Osteoblasts and osteoclasts are involved in bone formation and maintenance of bone. The osteoclast, the main bone-resorbing cell, plays also an important role in the healing events after trauma to bone and teeth as well as in the defense system established in response to infection (198–212). Consequently, marked osteoclastic activity may be the explanation for a number of radiographic phenomena including transient or permanent apical and marginal breakdown of the bony socket as well as root surface and root canal resorption (209, 210) (see Chapter 13, p. 392).

### GROWTH AND MAINTENANCE

Under normal physiologic conditions, osteoclast activity is regulated by a combination of direct and indirect osteoclast *activators* (e.g. parathyroid hormone (PTH), vitamin D metabolites, plasma calcium concentration, neurotransmitters, growth factors and cytokines (20, 209, 213), and osteoclast *inhibitors* (e.g. calcitonin and estrogen) (20, 209, 213) (Fig. 4.9). The sum of osteoblast/osteoclast activity (i.e. net bone balance) can be seen in normal tooth eruption, growth and maintenance of the jaws, as well as homeostasis of plasma calcium and phosphate.

### REPAIR

With respect to wound healing in hard tissues, the osteoclast can be considered analogous to the macrophage system operating in soft tissue wounds in its response to trauma and/or infection (205, 210, 212).

There are three hard tissues in the oral cavity that are subject to resorption subsequent to trauma, *alveolar bone*, *dentin* and *cementum*. Alveolar bone is itself highly vascular, while dentin and cementum are adjacent to the vascular tissues of the dental pulp and periodontal ligament (PDL), respectively. Thus, all three of these hard tissues are readily accessible to blood-derived inflammatory cells and serum proteins and can be resorbed as a result of inflammatory reactions.

Hard tissues may be injured following trauma either *directly* (e.g., crushing injuries) or *indirectly*, (e.g., ischemic injuries). In both instances, an inflammatory response is elicited which results in the liberation of cytokines and the promotion of hard tissue resorption (Figs 4.10 and 4.11). The purpose of this response is to remove the damaged hard tissue prior to healing. In this regard, the integrity of the cementoblast and odontoblast layers that cover cementum and dentin, respectively, is of paramount importance. If the traumatic event results in an irreparable injury to these cell layers, the hard tissue surface may succumb to resorption due to the intense osteoclastic activity that results from the liberation of a series of osteoclast-activating factors (210), (Figs 4.10 and 4.11). Resorption of dental tissues may be regulated similarly to that of osseous tissues. RANK-positive multinucleated odontoclasts have been immunohistochemically localized near the dentinal surface in resorption lacunae (213–215). Thus the RANK/RANKL/OPG-system may contribute to this process under both physiological and pathological conditions (215).

## Inflammation and mediators of hard tissue resorption

In the case of bacterial contamination of dentin and pulp, this response is a necessary step in the fight against invading bacteria (Fig. 4.11). Resorption of dentin serves to eliminate bacteria residing in dentinal tubules and the pulp canal while periradicular bone resorption and the development of an apical granuloma builds up an area of defense against the bacteria residing in the pulp canal (207). Bacterial by-products, i.e. lipopolysaccharide (LPS), can lead to inflammatory bone resorption. The mechanism involved differs from physiological bone resorption in that the pathway is independent of osteoblasts. LPS from *Porphyromonas gingivalis* and *Escherichia coli* induce differentiation of murine leukocytes into osteoclasts in the absence of osteoblasts (216).

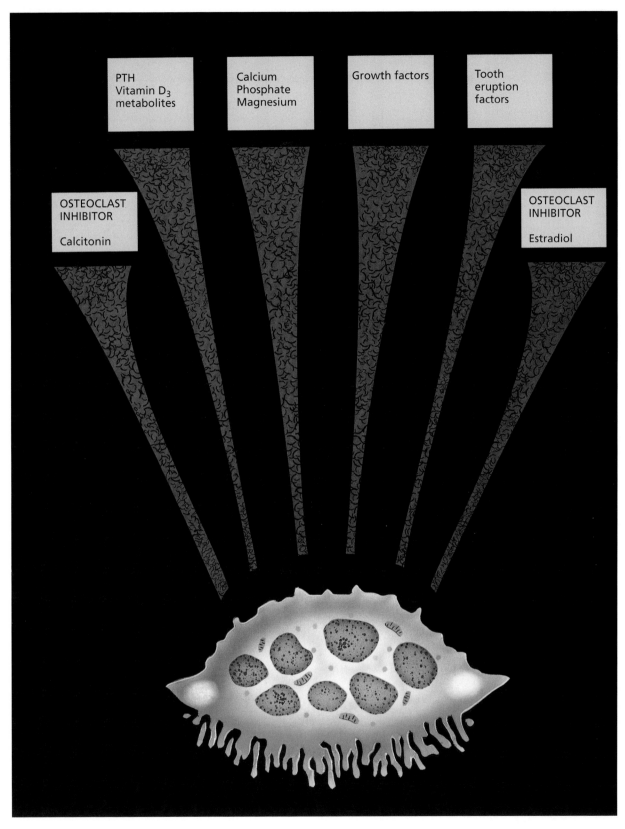

**Fig. 4.9** Activators and inhibitors regulating osteoclast activation during growth and maintenance of bone.

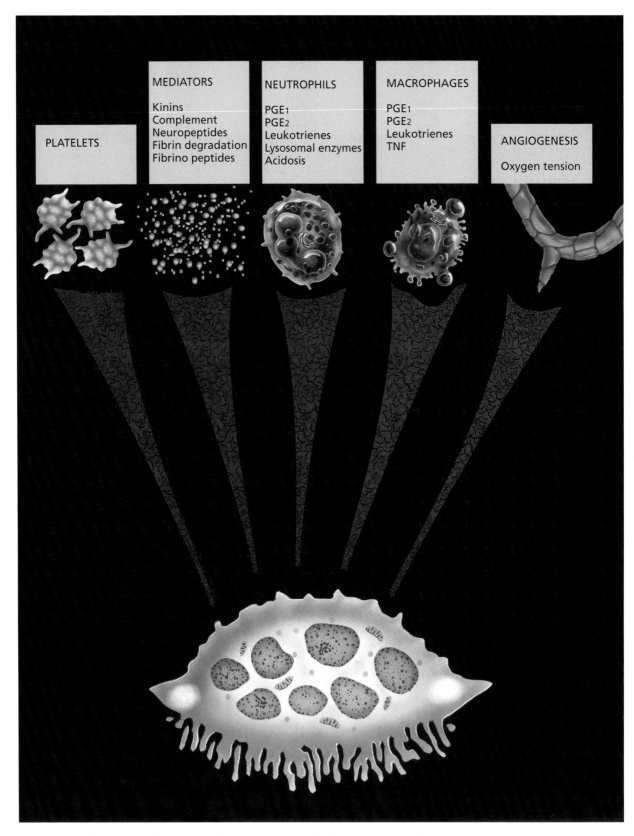

**Fig. 4.10** Osteoclast activators released during inflammatory response elicted by a traumatic dental injury.

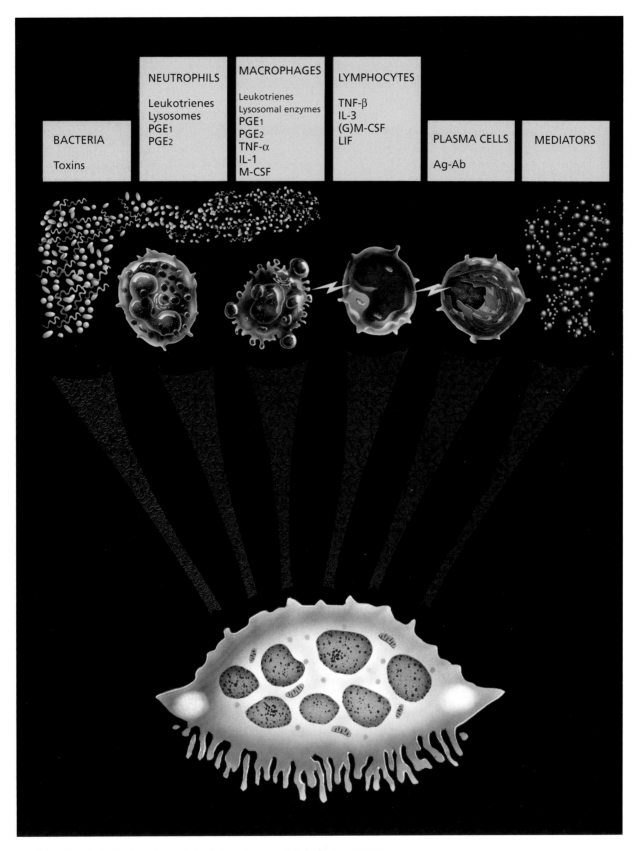

**Fig. 4.11** Osteoclast activators released by bacteria and the associated inflammatory response.

Regardless of whether the source of the injury is bacterial, mechanical or chemical, tissue injury leads to the host response of inflammation. The inflammatory reaction is characterized by the movement of fluid, proteins and white blood cells from the intravascular compartment into the extravascular space (see Chapter 1, p. 9). The inflammatory reaction can also initiate a resorptive process, the net result of which is a loss of hard tissue volume. In the following, the cells and chemical mediators involved in inflammation and hard tissue resorption will be described.

## Cells of inflammation

Although the inflammatory response is not completely understood, the precipitating event in any inflammatory process is tissue injury. Such injury is quickly followed by a vascular response that includes vasodilation, vascular stasis and increased vascular permeability, which then results in the extravasation of fluid and soluble components into the surrounding tissues (217–220; see Chapter 1). These vascular changes lead to the redness, heat, swelling and pain that are the cardinal signs of inflammation. The vascular response also includes margination of leukocytes, pavementing of these cells and, finally, their egress from the vascular space. The immune system consists of a number of inflammatory cell types that can control and direct the activities of other cells via secreted factors. Inflammatory cells involved in the various stages of tissue injury and repair include platelets, polymorphonuclear (PMN) leukocytes, mast cells, basophils, eosinophils, macrophages and lymphocytes (Figs 4.10, 4.11). The response of these cells to injury has already been described in detail in Chapter 1.

## Chemical mediators of inflammation

Immune cells, along with other cells associated with local tissue injury and inflammation, produce a number of soluble factors that further accentuate the inflammatory response and may elicit osteoclastic activity (Figs 4.11, 4.12, Table 4.2). These endogenous chemical mediators of inflammation include neuropeptides, fibrinolytic peptides, kinins, complement components, vasoactive amines, lysosomal enzymes, arachidonic acid metabolites and other mediators of immune reactions.

## Neuropeptides

Neuropeptides are proteins generated from somatosensory and autonomic nerve fibers following tissue injury. A number of neuropeptides have been characterized, including *substance P* (SP), *calcitonin gene-related peptide* (CGRP), *dopamine-β-hydrolase* (DβH), *neuropeptide Y* (NPY), originating from sympathetic nerve fibers, and *vasoactive intestinal polypeptides* (VIP), generated from parasympathetic nerve fibers (220). Physiological and pharmacological studies have shown that these substances have both vasodilatory and vasoconstrictive effects.

*Substance P* (SP) is a multifunctional neuropeptide present both in the peripheral and central nervous systems. The release of SP causes transmission of pain signals,

regulation of the immune system (vasodilation, increased vascular permeability and increased blood flow), and stimulation of bone resorptive activity of osteoclasts. Sensory denervation with capsaicin in rats reduces SP-IR fibers in numbers by 49%, with a corresponding reduction in bone resorption (221). This finding is directly correlated with a significant decrease in the number of actively resorbing osteoclasts. More current evidence suggests that Substance P can inhibit osteoblastic cell differentiation and this effect is potentiated in the presence of *P. gingivalis* LPS (222).

*Calcitonin gene-related peptide* (CGRP) is another neuropeptide, which has been localized in small to medium sensory nerve fibers of several organs of experimental animals. CGRP has an inhibitory effect on bone resorption (223). Both SP and CGRP have been identified in dental tissues (222). SP was the first neuropeptide to be detected in dental pulp (224), and the presence of CGRP in dental pulp was demonstrated almost ten years later (225–227). Sectioning of the inferior alveolar nerve results in complete disappearance of SP- and CGRP-containing granules from nerve fibers, suggesting that these substances originate from the sensory fibers of the trigeminal ganglion (225–230). Davidovitch and co-workers found intense staining for SP in PDL tension sites in cats one hour after orthodontic tooth movement (231). Intra-arterial infusion with SP and CGRP produces vasodilation in feline dental pulps as measured by laser Doppler flowmetry and $^{125}$I with clearance techniques (232).

*Vasoactive intestinal peptide* (VIP), a 28-amino acid residual peptide originally extracted from porcine duodenum, appears to be a stimulator of bone resorption. Hohmann and associates have shown that VIP stimulates bone resorption by a prostaglandin (PG)-E$_2$-independent mechanism (233). Furthermore, they showed the presence of functional receptors for VIP on human osteosarcoma cells (234). VIP is reportedly present in the dental pulp (220). Sectioning of the inferior alveolar nerve or sympathectomy do not abolish VIP-containing granules in nerve fibers, indicating that VIP is of parasympathetic origin (220).

**Table 4.2** Local factors that may affect osteoclasts; effect on osteoclasts.

| Factor | kDa | Osteoclast precursor growth or differentiation | Function of mature osteoclasts |
|---|---|---|---|
| IL-1 | 17.4 | ↑ | ↑ |
| IL-3 | 28 | ↑ | – |
| IL-6 | 23–30 | ↑ | – |
| TNFs | 17–18.8 | ↑ | ↑ |
| CSFs | 14–35 | ↑ | – |
| PGs | 0.35 | ↑ | ↓ |
| 1,25(OH)$_2$D$_3$ | 0.42 | – | ↑ |
| LIT | 45–58 | ↑ | ↑ |
| TGF-β* | 25 | ↓ | ↓ |

IL, interleukin; TNF, tumor necrosis factor; CSF, colony-stimulating factor; PG, prostaglandin; 1,25(OH)$_2$D$_3$, 1,25-dihydroxyvitamin D$_3$; LIF, leukemia inhibitory factor; TGF-β, transforming growth factor β.
Signatures: ↑ increases; ↓ decreases; – effects not shown.
*TGF-β stimulates PG production by mouse calvariae, causing increased bone resorption in the neonatal mouse calvarial assay.

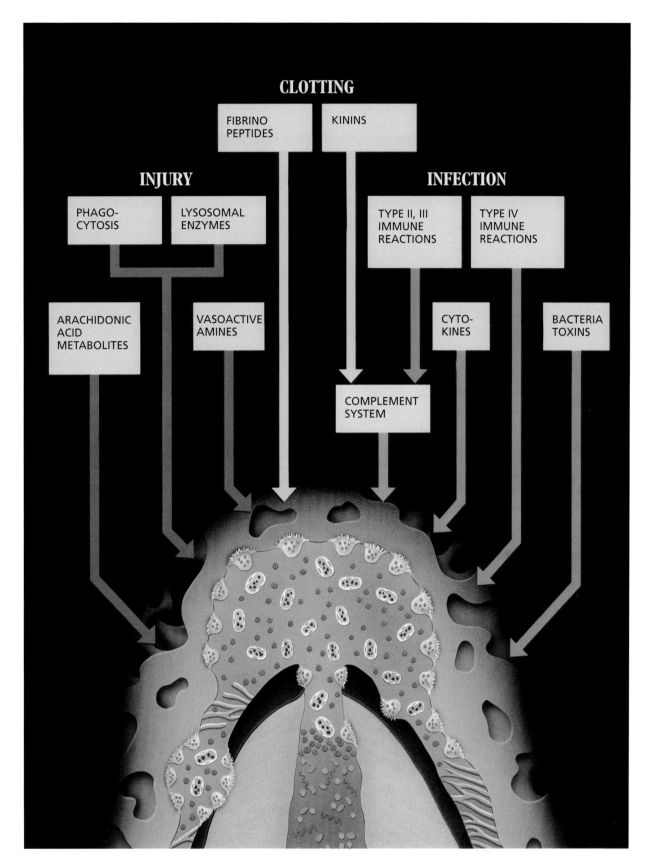

**Fig. 4.12** Mediators of inflammation and tooth and bone resorption released by a mechanical, chemical or bacterial injury to the pulp or periodontium.

Lastly, two other neuropeptides that have been only briefly characterized, DβH and NPY, have been localized in dental pulp (220). In this case, removal of the superior cervical ganglion results in the complete disappearance of NPY from nerve fibers, indicating that the origin of NPY in fibers is sympathetic in nature.

The presence of these neuropeptides has been clearly demonstrated in pulpal tissues; however, their role in the pathogenesis of periapical pathology following pulpal necrosis has not been completely elucidated. Recent studies suggest a possible role between sympathetic nerves and bone remodeling. In fact, sympathectomized rats demonstrate a near complete loss of NPY-immunoreactive fibers and a corresponding increase in the size of periapical lesions and the number of osteoclasts in the inflamed sites (235).

## Fibrinolytic peptides

Proper hemostasis depends on the coordinated activity of blood vessels, platelets and plasma proteins. Following tissue injury, circulating platelets immediately adhere to the subendothelial collagen and form a primary platelet plug. This initial hemostasis is followed by the coagulation cascade, which involves both an intrinsic pathway, and exposure of coagulation factor XII to negatively charged collagen and an extrinsic pathway and activation of factor VII. After a complex sequence of reactions, both pathways jointly convert prothrombin into thrombin, which in turn cleaves fibrinogen to fibrin (see Chapter 1, p. 9).

While hemostasis is taking place, however, a fibrinolytic system is activated which subsequently dissolves the newly formed blood clot. Circulating plasminogen is activated to plasmin (fibrinolysin) by the action of factor XIIa or by a tissue factor (236). Plasmin digests the clot and forms fibrin and fibrinogen degradation products. Fibrinopeptides and fibrin degradation products are themselves promoters of inflammation and cause increased vascular permeability and chemotaxis of leukocytes to the site of injury (236).

Severance of the blood vessels in the PDL or bone during root canal instrumentation can activate intrinsic and extrinsic coagulation pathways. Contact of Hageman factor with the collagen content of basement membranes, with enzymes such as kallikrein or plasmin or even with endotoxins from infected root canals can all activate the clotting cascade and the fibrinolytic system. Fibrinopeptides released from fibrinogen molecules and fibrin degradation products released during the proteolysis of fibrin by plasmin can also contribute to the inflammatory process.

## Kinins

Kinins are able to produce many of the characteristic signs of inflammation (237). They can cause chemotaxis of inflammatory cells, contraction of smooth muscles, dilation of peripheral arterioles and increased capillary permeability. They are also able to cause pain by direct action on the nerve fibers. The kinins are produced by proteolytic cleavage of kininogen by trypsin-like serine proteases, the kallikreins.

Kinins are subsequently inactivated by removal of the last one or two C-terminal amino acids by the action of peptidase (238). The kallikreins are also able to react with other systems, such as the complement and coagulation systems, to generate other trypsin-like serine proteases (239). Elevated levels of kinins have been detected in human periapical lesions (240), with acute periradicular lesions containing higher concentrations than chronic ones (Fig. 4.13).

## Complement system

The complement system consists of at least 26 distinct plasma proteins capable of interacting with each other and with other systems to produce a variety of effects (241). Complement is able to cause both cell lysis if activated on the cell membrane and to enhance phagocytosis through interaction with complement receptors on the surface of phagocytic cells. Complement can also increase vascular permeability and act as a chemotactic factor for granulocytes and macrophages. The complement system is a complex cascade that has two separate activation pathways that converge to a single protein (C3) and complete the cascade in a final, common sequence. Complement can be activated through the classical pathway by antigen-antibody complexes or through the alternate pathway by directly interacting with complex carbohydrates on bacterial and fungal cell walls or with substances such as plasmin (Figs 4.11 and 4.12).

Several investigators have found C3 complement components in human periradicular lesions (242–245). Activators of the classical and alternative pathways of the complement system include IgM, IgG, bacteria and their by-products, lysosomal enzymes from PMN leukocytes and clotting factors. Most of these activators are present in periradicular lesions. Activation of the complement system in these lesions can contribute to bone resorption either by destruction of already existing bone or by inhibition of new bone formation via the production of prostaglandins (PGs). Addition of complement to organ cultures of fetal rat long bones *in vitro* stimulates the release of previously incorporated $^{45}Ca$ to a greater extent than heat-inactivated complement (245, 246).

The activated complement system can stimulate phospholipid metabolism (247) and cause the release of lipids from cell membranes (248–250). Consequently, the activated complement system may provide a source for the precursor of PGs, arachidonic acid (see below).

## Vasoactive amines

The two major vasoactive amines involved in inflammatory reactions are histamine and serotonin (Fig. 4.12). Both exist preformed in a variety of cells, most notably in mast cells, basophils and platelets. These two factors lead to increased capillary permeability and dilation and can cause smooth muscle contraction. Histamine is present in preformed granules in mast cells and is released by a number of stimuli including physical and chemical injury (251), complement activation products (252), activated T lymphocytes (253)

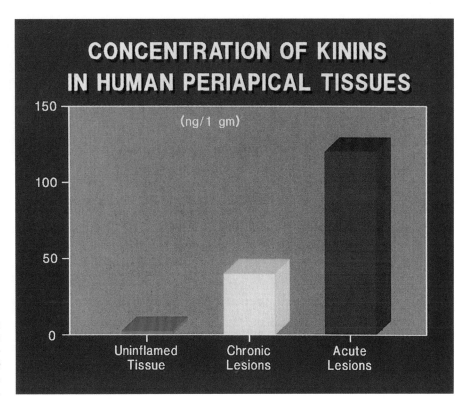

**Fig. 4.13** Concentration of kinins in chronic (yellow) and acute (red) human periapical lesions as well as uninflamed negative control connective tissue (green), ng/g of tissue weight. From TORABINEJAD et al. (240) 1968.

and bridging of membrane-bound IgE by allergens (254). Mast cells have been detected in human periradicular lesions (255, 256). Physical or chemical injury of periradicular tissues during cleaning, shaping or obturation of the root canal system with antigenic substances can cause mast cell degranulation. Mast cells discharging vasoactive amines into the periradicular tissues can in turn initiate an inflammatory response or aggravate an existing inflammatory process.

Recent studies have found a potential role of histamine as a mediator regulating estrogen deficiency induced bone resorption (257). H(2) blockers, such as cimetidine, attenuate trabecular bone volume reduction in ovariectomized rats by 50% (258). The mechanism involved may be through direct inhibition of osteoclastogenesis and indirect increase in calcitriol synthesis (259).

## Lysosomal enzymes

While dissolution of the inorganic fraction of the bone matrix is mediated by acidification of the bone surface in contact with the osteoclast, secreted lysosomal enzymes digest the organic components (260) (Fig. 4.12). Lysosomal enzymes are potent proteolytic enzymes that are stored in small, membrane-bound bodies termed lysosomes within the cytoplasm of inflammatory cells such as neutrophils, macrophages and platelets (261). These enzymes are released via two principal mechanisms: cytotoxic release during cell lysis (as in gout or silicosis) and secretory release, often during phagocytosis. Examples include acid and alkaline phosphatases, lysozyme, peroxidase, cathepsins and collagenase. Cathepsin K is responsible for degradation of collagen type I and other bone proteins. Osteoclasts deficient in this enzyme can demineralize bone but cannot

degrade the protein matrix. Patients with pycnodysostosis demonstrate mutations in the cathepsin K gene. Animal models of cathepsin K deficiency are available providing a tool to study osteoclast function and treatment for cathepsin K deficiency (262).

The effects of lysosomal enzyme release can be modulated by inhibitors of vacuolar-type H(+)-ATPase, such as bafilomycin A1, and E-64, a cysteine proteinase inhibitor (263). In cell cultures, bafilomycin A1 treatment prevents formation of ruffled borders associated with osteoclasts, and resorption lacuna formation is markedly diminished. This effect on osteoclast structure is reversible by removal of the compound. E-64 shows no effect on demineralization of dentin slices; however, it reduces resorption lacuna formation in a dose-dependent manner (263).

Depending on their physiological pH activities, the lysosomal enzymes have been subdivided into acid, basic and neutral proteases. Because the inflammatory site typically has an acidic pH, the acidic proteases may have the greatest activity in these locations. Factors that could help to determine the extent of tissue damage after the release of lysosomal enzymes might include the nature of the stimulus, the type of tissue or the absence of appropriate control mechanisms.

Release of lysosomal enzymes can also result in increased vascular permeability and further chemotaxis of leukocytes and macrophages. In addition, lysosomal enzymes can cause cleavage of C5 and generation of C5a, a potent chemotactic component, and liberate active bradykinin from plasma kininogen (261).

Lysosomal enzymes have been immunolocalized in odontoblasts suggesting a similar mechanism for root resorption compared to that of osteoclastic bone resorption (264).

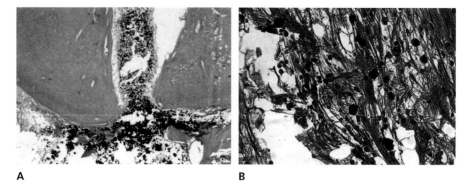

**Fig. 4.14** A. Egress of vitreous carbon particles from the root canal of a canine tooth into the periodontal ligament. ×20. B. Phagocytosis of carbon particles by macrophages present in the periodontal ligament. ×200.

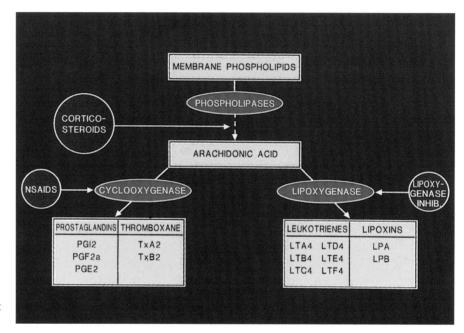

**Fig. 4.15** Pathways of arachidonic acid metabolism.

Lysosomal enzyme release can also occur following endodontic manipulation. Extrusion of filling materials into the periradicular tissues can result in phagocytosis and release of lysosomal enzymes (Fig. 4.14). Thus, root canal obturating materials themselves, if improperly used, can be potent sources of inflammation and resorption. In fact, cathepsin K has been identified in granulomatous lesions (265). Therefore, persistent foreign body reaction to extruded material can lead to the secretion of lysosomal enzymes.

## Arachidonic acid metabolites

Arachidonic acid is a naturally occurring acid that is incorporated into phospholipids of the cell membrane. Oxidation of arachidonic acid leads to the generation of a group of biologically important products including prostaglandins (PG), thromboxanes and leukotrienes. Products of the arachidonic acid cascade are not preformed and stored within intracellular granules, but instead are synthesized from cell membrane components as a result of cell membrane injury (266). There are several pathways by which arachidonic acid is metabolized (Fig. 4.15).

### Prostaglandins

PGs are produced from arachidonic acid via the cyclooxygenase pathway. The PGs, particularly PGE2 and PGI2, have been shown to be associated with vascular permeability and pain in conjunction with the action of other chemical mediators of acute inflammation, such as histamine and kinins (236).

PGs have been implicated in pathological changes associated with human pulpal and periradicular diseases (267). The role of PGs in periradicular bone resorption was investigated by Torabinejad et al. (268) who demonstrated that the formation of periradicular lesions in cats is inhibited by systemic administration of indomethacin (Fig. 4.16). In another study, McNicholas et al. (269) showed the presence of high levels of PGE2 in acute periradicular abscesses. The

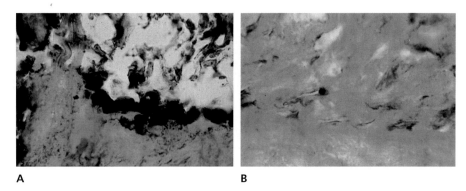

A B

**Fig. 4.16** A. Horizontal 5 μm section of periradicular tissue of a feline tooth after 6 weeks of exposure to the oral flora, stained histochemically for PGE$_2$. Note: dark staining for the presence of PGE$_2$ on the surface of alveolar bone. ×500. B. No staining is noted in the contralateral tooth not exposed to the oral flora. From TORABINEJAD et al. (68) 1979.

mechanisms by which PGs are involved in bone resorption will be discussed in greater detail later in this chapter.

### Leukotrienes

The leukotrienes are produced from arachidonic acid via the lipo-oxygenase pathway. The biological activities of leukotrienes include chemotactic effects for neutrophils, eosinophils and macrophages, increased vascular permeability, and release of lysosomal enzymes from PMN leukocytes and macrophages (270). High concentrations of leukotriene B4, a potent chemotactic agent, have been found in periradicular lesions (271) (Fig. 4.13). In addition, a positive correlation has been found between the concentration of this substance and the number of PMN leukocytes. The actions of these mediators can be further enhanced by vasoactive amines and kinins.

## Immunological reactions

Immunological reactions can be divided into antibody- and cell-mediated reactions. The role of IgE-mediated reactions in hard tissue resorption was described earlier under vasoactive amines (Fig. 4.12). In addition to immediate hypersensitivity reactions, immune complex reactions as well as cell-mediated reactions can also participate in inflammation and hard tissue reactions.

## Antigen-antibody complex reactions

Immune complexes in periradicular tissues can be formed when extrinsic antigens such as bacteria or their by-products interact with either IgG or IgM antibodies. The resultant complexes bind to platelets, leading to the release of vasoactive amines and to increased vascular permeability and PMN leukocyte chemotaxis. The binding of immune complexes in periradicular lesions has been demonstrated in experimental animals. Simulated immune complexes placed in feline root canals can lead to rapid formation of periradicular lesions, notably characterized by bone loss and the accumulation of numerous PMN leukocytes and osteoclasts (268) (Fig. 4.13). This finding has been confirmed by Tora-

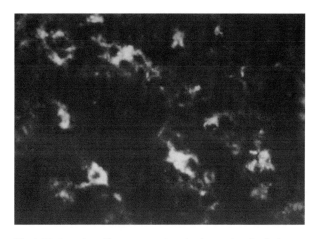

**Fig. 4.17** Detection of immune complexes in phagocytic cells of a human periapical lesion using anticomplement immunofluorescence technique. ×200. From TORABINEJAD & KETTERING (273) 1979.

binejad and Kiger (272) who immunized cats with subcutaneous injections of keyhole limpet hemocyanin until the presence of circulating antibody to this antigen was detected. Challenge doses of the same antigen were then administered via the root canals. Radiographic and histological observations showed the development of periradicular lesions consistent with characteristics of an Arthus-type reaction.

Immune complexes in periradicular tissues in humans have been studied as well. Torabinejad and Kettering (273), using the anticomplement immunofluorescence technique, presented evidence to support the localization of immune complexes in human periradicular specimens (Fig. 4.17). Furthermore, in two separate investigations, Torabinejad and associates quantitated the serum concentrations of circulating immune complexes, various classes of immunoglobulins and a C3 complement component in patients with chronic and acute periradicular lesions (274, 275). The results indicated that immune complexes formed in chronic periradicular lesions are either minimal or are confined within the lesions and do not enter into the systemic circulation. In contrast, when the serum concentrations of circulating immune complexes in patients with acute abscesses were compared with those of individuals

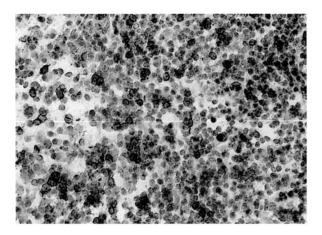

**Fig. 4.18** Presence of numerous T lymphocytes (red cell membrane) in a human periradicular lesion. From TORABINEJAD & KETTERING (276) 1985.

without these lesions, a significant difference was found between the two groups. Complexes were present in the circulation of patients with lesions, but they were undetectable in the blood of unaffected controls.

Although immune complex formation can often be considered a protective mechanism for the neutralization and elimination of antigens, the data from studies on experimental animals and from patients with periradicular lesions suggest that this complex formation in the periapical space can lead to periradicular lesions that can include hard tissue resorption.

## Cell-mediated immune reactions

The presence and relative concentration of B and T lymphocytes and their subpopulations were determined in human periradicular lesions by the indirect immunoperoxidase method (276). Many B cells, T suppressor (S) cells and T helper (H) cells were detected in these lesions; but the T cells outnumbered the B cells significantly (Fig. 4.18). Other investigators found approximately equal numbers of T-cell subsets in chronic lesions (TH/TS ratio) (277–280). Further immune cell specificity in developing lesions was shown by Stashenko and Yu (279), who demonstrated in rats that TH cells outnumber TS cells during the acute phase of lesion expansion, whereas TS cells predominate at later time periods when lesions are stabilized. Based on these results it appears that TH cells may participate in the development of periradicular lesions, whereas TS cells may decrease excessive immune reactivity, leading to cessation of lesion growth.

The specific role of T lymphocytes in the pathogenesis of periradicular lesions has been studied by a number of investigators. Wallström (281) exposed the pulps of mandibular molars of athymic and conventional rats and left them open to the oral flora for 2, 4 or 8 weeks. Tissue sections were quantified by percentages of surface areas of bone, connective tissue, bone marrow, intrabony spaces, periradicular lesions and numbers of osteoclasts. Statistical analysis

showed no significant difference between periradicular tissue responses of the two treated groups. Finally, Waterman (282) compared periradicular lesion formation in immunosuppressed rats with that in normal rats and found no significant histological differences between the two groups. These findings suggest that the pathogenesis of periradicular lesions is a multifactorial phenomenon and is not totally dependent on the presence of circulating lymphocytes.

### Interleukin-1 (IL-1)

The cytokine most widely studied for its effects on bone resorption is IL-1. IL-1 is produced primarily by monocytes and macrophages (260, 283), and human monocytes produce at least two IL-1 species, IL-1α and IL-1β (285). IL-1β is the major form secreted by human monocytes. The chief component of osteoclast activating factor (OAF) was purified and found to be identical to IL-1β (285). IL-1β is the most active of the cytokines in stimulating bone resorption *in vitro* (half-maximal activity at $4.5 \times 10^{-11}$ M), 15-fold more potent than IL-1α and 1,000-fold more potent than the tumor necrosis factors (TNFs) (286). The genes for IL-1 have been cloned, and IL-α, and IL-β are related molecules of nearly identical molecular weight (17.4 kDa), but sharing only 35% sequence homology (284).

The effects of IL-1 on bone resorption have been widely studied. IL-1 strongly stimulates bone resorption (287) and inhibits bone formation (288). IL-1 stimulates the growth of osteoclast precursor cells, the differentiation of committed osteoclast precursors and the activity of mature osteoclasts (289, 290). As is the case with other bone resorptive agents, the actions of IL-1 on osteoclasts are mediated through osteoblasts (25). IL-1β is also produced by osteoblasts and hence may serve as a messenger to communicate bone-resorptive signals to osteoclasts (291).

IL-1 has been associated with increased bone resorption *in vivo* in several disease conditions. For example, IL-1 is produced by tumor cells in several malignancies associated with increased bone resorption and hypercalcemia (292–295). In addition, since IL-1 may be produced by activated macrophages or inflammatory cells and has been identified in human dental pulp (296), IL-1 has been implicated in the bone resorption of several chronic inflammatory diseases including periodontal disease (297) and periradicular lesions (298–301).

### Interleukin-3 (IL-3)

IL-3 is a T lymphocyte-derived, 28 kDa glycoprotein which supports growth and differentiation of hematopoietic progenitor cells (302, 303). In bone marrow, IL-3 will induce the differentiation of precursors to osteoclast-like cells, an effect that was independent of $1,25(OH)_2D_3$ and inhibited by an anti-IL-3 inhibitory antibody (304, 305). IL-3 has also been implicated in the bone resorption that occurs in chronic inflammatory diseases, such as rheumatoid arthritis or periodontitis (306–308).

## Interleukin-6 (IL-6)

IL-6 is a glycoprotein produced by a large number of cells and with a wide range of cell targets (309). It is produced by osteoblasts, but in response to other bone resorptive agents including PTH, IL-1 and 1,25(OH)$_2$D$_3$ (310). IL-6 has been reported to be a potent stimulator of osteoclast-like cell formation in human bone marrow cultures (311), although it did not stimulate resorption in neonatal mouse calvariae (312). It does stimulate resorption, however, in an organ culture system that contains more primitive osteoclastic precursors (313).

IL-6 is produced during immune responses and may play a role in human disease. For example, IL-6 may be an important mediator of the increased number of osteoclasts in Paget's disease (314), implicating IL-6 in the pathogenesis of diseases of increased osteoclast formation. Nude mice carrying CHO tumors overexpressing IL-6 develop hypercalcemia (315), and IL-6 may be involved in the hypercalcemia and bone lesions associated with other malignancies. Lastly, IL-6 may play a role in the bone resorption observed with inflammatory diseases. Thus IL-6 has been isolated from diseased tissues associated with adult periodontitis (316) and rheumatoid arthritis (317).

## Tumor necrosis factors (TNFs)

The monocyte-macrophage-derived TNF-$\alpha$ and the lymphocyte-derived TNF-3 (previously called lymphotoxin) have effects on bone resorption that are similar to IL-1. Both stimulate resorption and inhibit formation of bone in organ culture (286). TNFs stimulate both the growth of osteoclast progenitor cells and the differentiation of committed precursors (289). Their effects on osteoclasts are also indirect and are mediated through osteoblasts (318). The ability of TNF-$\alpha$ to stimulate bone resorption is dependent on prostaglandin (PG) synthesis (319).

TNFs may be associated with bone resorption *in vivo* in a number of diseases. Although TNF has not been shown to be produced directly by solid tumor cells, many such tumors cause host defense cells to produce excess TNFs, leading to increased resorption and hypercalcemia of malignancy (320–322). Direct injections *in vivo* of TNF-$\alpha$ in intact mice cause hypercalcemia. TNF has been implicated in the hypercalcemia and bone resorption with multiple myeloma as well (323). Finally, the TNFs, produced by activated immune cells, may be associated with bone resorption resulting from chronic inflammatory disease. For example, TNFs were detected in all samples of gingival and periradicular tissues associated with disease but were scarcely detectable in sites associated with health (297, 301).

## Prostaglandins

PGs, products of arachidonic acid metabolism as described earlier, have long been implicated in bone resorption. PGE$_1$ and PGE$_2$ were first reported to stimulate $^{45}$Ca release from fetal rat bone *in vitro* in 1970 (324). The stimulatory effect of PGEs on bone resorption has been confirmed by many groups (325–330). Paradoxically, Chambers and co-workers reported that PGE$_2$ had a direct inhibitory effect on bone resorption by isolated osteoclasts (329) and inhibited osteoclast motility (330), suggesting that the stimulation of bone resorption by PGs in organ culture is due to indirect effects of PGs on cells other than osteoclasts. This suggestion was further strengthened by the finding that PGE$_2$ initially inhibited and then stimulated bone resorption in isolated rabbit osteoclast cultures, consistent with the idea that the stimulated resorption was due to late, indirect effects mediated by marrow stromal cells (331). It appears that PGs induce osteoclastic differentiation from precursor cells but inhibit the activity of mature osteoclasts (332).

PGs have been implicated in both the local bone resorption of chronic inflammation and in systemic resorption as well. PGE$_2$ is elevated in inflamed, periodontally diseased sites and in symptomatic pulpal tissue compared to control sites (333–336). The importance of PGs in periodontal disease progression was further suggested by the finding that an inhibitor of PGs, flurbiprofen, decreased naturally occurring periodontal disease destruction in beagle dogs (337). Synovial tissue from patients with rheumatoid arthritis produced PGE$_2$ and caused bone resorption *in vitro*, an effect inhibited by indomethacin (338). Tumor cells producing large amounts of PGE$_2$ lead to extensive bone resorption and hypercalcemia, effects also blocked by indomethacin (339, 340). Similarly to PTH, however, infusions of PGE$_2$ *in vivo* actually increase bone formation (341), and PG inhibitors decrease fracture repair in rats (342).

PGs may interact with other local cytokines. IL-I (343, 344) and TNF-$\alpha$ (319) increase PGE$_2$ production. PGE$_2$ has been reported to inhibit IL-1 production, perhaps acting as a negative feedback system (344). PTH-related protein will also stimulate PGE$_2$ from human osteoblast-like cells, suggesting that PGs also may communicate bone resorptive signals locally (345).

## Leukemia-inhibitory factor (LIF)

LIF, a glycoprotein derived from activated T lymphocytes which stimulates differentiation of myeloma cells to mature monocytes (346), is identical in activity to a glycoprotein shown to stimulate bone resorption *in vitro* called differentiation-inducing factor (DIF, 347). It also stimulates osteoclast-like cell formation in marrow cultures (348).

## Local inhibitors of resorption

Three local inhibitors of osteoclastic bone resorption have been described. *Transforming growth factor-$\beta$* (TGF-$\beta$) is one of several growth factors that are abundant in bone and known to stimulate bone cell growth. TGF-$\beta$ is a powerful stimulator of bone cell growth and function and has been shown to stimulate bone formation in a number of *in vivo* models (349–352). TGF-$\beta$ also affects bone resorption, but its effects vary depending on the model system studied. For example, in human marrow cultures, TGF-β inhibits the formation of osteoclast-like cells (353). In the neonatal mouse calvarial assay, however, TGF-β treatment leads to an increase in bone resorption secondarily due to an increased production of PGs (354).

Another agent shown to inhibit osteoclastic bone resorption is *γ-interferon*, which completely abolished the resorption stimulated by IL-1, TNF-α and TNF-β, but that stimulated by PTH and $1,25(OH)_2D_3$ was not significantly affected (355). In addition, γ-interferon also inhibited the bone resorption induced by bradykinin, only partially through a PG-mediated mechanism (356).

The most recently described local inhibitor of osteoclastic bone resorption is the *IL-1 receptor antagonist (IL-1ra)* (357–360). *IL-1ra* is a cytokine that is related to the IL-1 family and specifically inhibits the bone-resorptive effects of IL-1α and IL-1β, but not that of PTH or $1,25(OH)_2D_3$ (361, 362). It also inhibits the bone resorption and hypercalcemia caused by IL-1 injections *in vivo*.

As summarized in Fig. 4.12, present studies indicate that multiple mechanisms are involved in the pathological changes that are associated with hard tissue resorption. Mechanical injury to the periodontium or periradicular tissues is likely to initiate the release of nonspecific mediators of inflammation and activate several pathways of inflammation. Continuous egress of irritants, antigens or toxic bacterial materials, as from a pathologically involved root canal, can result in one or more immunological reactions. Present data indicate that a number of these reactions can lead to hard tissue resorption at both the periradicular and periodontal sites. Because of complex interactions between the various components of these systems, the dominance of any one pathway or substance may be difficult to establish. Much research is still needed to characterize the specific roles of mediators of inflammation in pathogenesis of hard tissue resorption.

## Essentials

### Origin of osteoclasts

- Mononuclear phagocyte system
- Bone marrow-derived mononuclear precursor cells

### Regulation of osteoclast activity

- RANKL
- RANK
- OPG
- Cytokines
- Hormones

### Osteoclast participation in root and bone resorption

- Growth
- Maintenance
- Repair
- Inflammation and mediation of hard tissue resorption

## References

1. Roodman GD. Advances in bone biology: the osteoclast. *Endocrine Rev* 1996;**13**:66–80.
2. Arey LB. The origin, growth and fate of osteoclasts and their relation to bone resorption. *Am J Anat* 1920;**26**:315–45.
3. Chambers TJ. The cellular basis of bone resorption. *Clin Orthop* 1980;**151**:283–93.
4. Chambers TJ. The pathobiology of the osteoclast. *J Clin Pathol* 1985;**38**:241–52.
5. Chambers TJ. The regulation of osteoclastic development and function. In: Evered D, Harnett S. eds. *Cell and molecular biology of vertebrate hard tissues*. New York: John Wiley and Sons, 1988:92–100.
6. Chambers TJ. Regulation of the differentiation and function of osteoclasts. *J Pathol* 2000;**192**:4–13.
7. Hall BK. The origin and fate of osteoclasts. *Anat Rec* 1975;**183**:1–12.
8. Hall BK. The osteoclast. In: Hall BK. ed. *Bone volume 2*. Boca Raton, FL: CRC Press, 1991.
9. Pierce AM, Lindskog S, Hammarström L. Osteoclasts: structure and function. *Electron Microscopy Review* 1991;**4**:1–45.
10. Rifkin BR, Gay CV. In: Rifkin BR, Gay CV. eds. *Biology and physiology of the osteoclast*. Boca Raton, FL: CRC Press, 1992.
11. Zaidi M, Towhidul Alam ASM, Shankar VS, Bax BE, Bax CMR, Moonga BS, Bevis PJR, Stevens C, Blake DR, Pazianas M, Huang CLH. Cellular biology of bone resorption. *Biology Reviews* 1993;**68**:197–264.
12. Baron R. Molecular mechanisms of bone resorption – an update. *Acta Orthop Scan* 1995;**66**:(*Suppl 266*):66–70.
13. Athanasou NA. Cellular biology of bone-resorbing cells. *J Bone Joint Surg* 1996;**78A**:1096–112.
14. Greenfield EM, Bi Y, Miyauchi, A. Regulation of osteoclast activity. *Life Sci* 1999;**65**:1087–102.
15. Lerner UH. Osteoclast formation and resorption. *Matrix Biology* 2000;**19**:107–20.
16. Väänänen HK, Zhao H, Mulari M, Halleen JM. The cell biology of osteoclast function. *J Cell Sci* 2000;**113**:377–81.
17. Suda T, Kobayashi K, Jimi E, Udagawa N, Takahashi N. The molecular basis of osteoclast differentiation and activation. *Novartis Foundation Symposium* 2001;**232**:235–50.
18. Marks SC Jr. Osteoclast biology: lessons from mammalian mutations. *Am J Med Genet* 1989;**34**:43–54.
19. Bucay N, Sarosi I, Dunstan CR, Morony S, Tarpley J, Capparelli C, Scully S, Tan HL, Xu W, Lacey DL, Boyle WJ, Simonet WS. Osteoprotegerin-deficient mice develop early onset osteoporosis and arterial calcification. *Genes Develop* 1998;**12**:1260–8.
20. Lerner UH. New molecules in the tumor necrosis factor ligand and receptor super-families with importance for physiological and pathological resorption. *Crit Rev Oral Biol* 2004;**15**:64–81.
21. Lucht U. Osteoclasts and their relationship to bone as studied by electron microscopy. *Z Zellforsch Mikrosk Anat* 1972;**135**:211–28.
22. Lucht U. Osteoclasts: ultrastructure and function. In: Carr I and Daems WT, eds. *The reticuloendothelial*

*system. A comprehensive treatise*. Vol. I Morphology. New York: Plenum Press, 1980:70–734.

23. KÖLLIKER A. *Die normale Resorption der Knochengewebes und ihre Bedeutung fur die Entstehung der typischen Knochenformen*. Leipzig, GDR: Vogel, 1873.

24. BURGER EH, NIJWEIDE PJ. Cellular origin and theories of osteoclast differentiation. In: Hall BK. ed. *Bone*. Boca Raton, FL: CRC Press, 1992:31–60.

25. WALKER DG. Congenital osteopetrosis in mice cured by parabiotic union with normal siblings. *Endocrinology* 1972;**91**:916–20.

26. WALKER DG. Osteopetrosis cured by temporary parabiosis. *Science* 1973;**180**:875.

27. GÖTHLIN G, ERICSSON JL. The osteoclast: review of ultrastructure, origin, and structure-function relationship. *Clin Orthop* 1976;**120**:201–31.

28. WALKER DG. Control of bone resorption by hemapoietic tissue. The induction and reversal of congenital osteopetrosis in mice through use of bone marrow and splenic transplants. *J Exper Med* 1975;**142**:651–63.

29. COCCIA PF, KRIVIT W, CERVENKA K, CLAWSON C, KERSEY JH, KIM TH, NESBIT ME, RAMSAY NK, WARKENTIN PI, TEITELBAUM SL, KAHN AJ, BROWN DM. Successful bone-marrow transplantation for infantile malignant osteopetrosis. *N Engl J Med* 1980;**302**:701–8.

30. KAHN AJ, SIMMONS DJ. Investigation of cell lineage in bone using a chimera of chick and quail embryonic tissue. *Nature* 1975;**258**:325–7.

31. MARKS SC. The origin of osteoclasts: evidence, clinical implications and investigative challenges of an extraskeletal source. *J Oral Pathol* 1983;**12**:226–56.

32. ZAMBONIN-ZALLONE A, TETI A, PRIMAVERA MV. Monocytes from circulating blood fuse *in vitro* with purified osteoclasts in primary culture. *J Cell Science* 1984;**66**:335–42.

33. BURGER EH, VAN DER MEER JWM, VAN DER GEVEL JS, GRIBNAN JC, THESINGH CW, VAN FURTH R. *In vitro* formation of osteoclasts from long term cultures of bone marrow mononuclear phagocytes. *J Experiment Med* 1982;**156**:1604–14.

34. MUNDY GR, ALTMAN AJ, GONDER MD, BANDELIN JG. Direct resorption of bone by human monocytes. *Sci* 1977;**196**:1109–11.

35. ASH P, LOUTIT JF, TOWNSEND KMS. Osteoclasts derived from haemopoietic stem cells. *Nature* 1980;**283**:669–70.

36. MARKS SC, WALKER DG. The hematogenous origin of osteoclasts: experimental evidence from osteoppetrotic (microphthalmic) mice treated with spleen cells from beige mouse donors. *Am J Anat* 1981;**161**:1–10.

37. OURSLER MJ, BELL LV, CLEVENGER B, OSDOBY P. Identification of osteoclast-specific monclonal antibodies. *J Cell Biol* 1985;**100**:1592–600.

38. QUINN JMW, SABOKBAR A, ATHANASOU NA. Cells of the mononuclear phagocyte series differentiate into osteoclastic lacunar bone resorbing cells. *J Pathol* 1996;**179**:106–11.

39. HANCOX NM. Osteoclastic bone resorption. In: Hancox NM. ed. *Biology of bone*. Cambridge, England: Cambridge University Press, 1972:113–35.

40. BARNES DM. Close Encounters with an osteoclast. *Science* 1987;**236**:914–16.

41. HOLTROP ME. Light and electronmicroscopic structure of osteoclasts. In: Hall BK. ed. *Bone* Vol. II. The Osteoclast. CRC Press, Boca Raton, FL: Florida 1992, p. 1–29.

42. SCOTT BL, PEASE DC. Electron microscopy of the epiphyseal apparatus. *Anat Rec* 1956;**125**:465–95.

43. VÄÄNÄNEN HK. Osteoclast function: biology and mechanisms. In: Bilezikian JP, Raisz LG, Rodan GA. eds. *Principles of bone biology*. San Diego: Academic Press, 1996:103–13.

44. HOLTROP ME, KING GJ. The ultrastructure of the osteoclast and its functional implications. *Clin Orthop* 1977;**123**:177–96.

45. BARON R, NEFF L, BROWN W, COURTOY PJ, LOUVARD D, FARQUHAR MG. Polarized secretion of lysosomal enzymes: co-distribution of cation-independent mannose-6-phosphate receptors and lysosomal enzymes along the osteoclast exocytic pathway. *J Cell Biol* 1988;**106**:1863–72.

46. LUCHT U. Cytoplasmic vacuoles and bodies of the osteoclast. An electron microscope study. *Z Zellforsch Mikrosk Anat* 1972;**135**:229–44.

47. GAY CV. Osteoclast ultrastructure and enzyme histochemistry: functional implications. In: Rifkin BR, Gay CV. eds. *Biology and physiology of the osteoclast*. Boca Raton, FL: CRC Press, 1992:129–50.

48. MARCHISIO PC, CIRILLO D, NALDINI L, PRIMAVERA MV, TETI A, ZAMBONIN-ZALLONE A. Cell-substratum interaction of cultured avian osteoclasts is mediated by specific adhesion structures. *J Cell Biology* 1984;**99**:1696–705.

49. BARON R, NEFF L, LOUVARD D, COURTOY PJ. Cell-mediated extracellular acidification and bone resorption: evidence for a low pH in resorbing lacunae and localization of a 100-kD lysosomal membrane protein at the osteoclast ruffled border. *J Cell Biol* 1985;**101**:2210–22.

50. SALO J, METSIKKO K, PALOKANGAS H, LEHENKARI P, VÄÄNÄNEN HK. Bone-resorbing osteoclasts reveal a dynamic division of basal plasma membrane into two different domains. *J Cell Sci* 1996;**109**:301–07.

51. TEITELBAUM SL, TONDRAVI MM, ROSS FP. Osteoclasts, macrophages, and the molecular mechanisms of bone resorption. *J Leucocyte Biology* 1997;**61**:381–8.

52. JONES SJ, BOYDE A. Some morphological observations on osteoclasts. *Cell Tissue Res* 1977;**185**:387–97.

53. de St GEORGES L, MILLER SC, BOWMAN BM, JEE WSS. Ultrastructural features of osteoclasts in situ. *Scan Micros* 1989;**3**:1201.

54. KURIHARA S. 16mm cinematographic observation on behavior of a multinucleated cell cultured with a dentine slice. In: Davidovitch, Z. ed. *The biological mechanisms of tooth eruption and root resorption*. Birmingham, Alabama: EBSCO Media, 1988:371–7.

55. CHAMBERS TJ, McSHEEHY PM, THOMSON BM, FULLER K. The effect of calcium-regulating hormones and prostaglandin on bone resorption by osteoclasts disaggregated from neonatal rabbit bones. *Endocrinology* 1985;**116**:234–9.

56. MARKS SC, POPOFF SN. Bone cell biology: the regulation of development, structure, and function in the skeleton. *Am J Anat* 1988;**183**:1–44.

57. Suda T, Tanaka S, Udagawa N, Tamura T, Takahashi N. The role of osteoblastic cells in osteoclast differentiation. In: Slavkin H, Price P. eds. *Chemistry and biology of mineralized tissues.* Elsevier Science Publishers, 1992:329–38.

58. Loutit JF, Nisbet NW. Resorption of bone. *Lancet* 1979;**2**:26–7.

59. Rodan GA, Martin TJ. Role of osteoblasts in hormonal control of bone resorption. A hypothesis. *Calcified Tissue Int* 1981;**33**:348–51.

60. McSheehy PM, Chambers TJ. Osteoblastic cells mediate osteoclastic responsiveness to parathyroid hormone. *Endocrinol* 1986;**118**:824–8.

61. Vaes G. Cellular biology and biochemical mechanism of bone resorption. A review of recent developments on the formation, activation, and mode of action of osteoclasts. *Clin Orthopaed Related Res* 1988;**231**:239–71.

62. Delaissé JM, Vaes LG. Mechanism of mineral solubilization and matrix degradation in osteoclastic bone resorption. In: Rifkin BR, Gay CV. eds. *Biology and physiology of the osteoclast.* Boca Raton, FL: CRC Press, 1992:289–314.

63. Burger EH, van der Meer JWM, Nijweide PJ. Osteoclast formation from mononuclear phagocytes, role of bone-forming cells. *J Cell Biol* 1984;**99**: 1901–6.

64. Lakkakorpi PT, Horton MA, Helfrich MH, Karhukorpi EK, Väänänen HK. Vitronectin receptor has a role in bone resorption but does not mediate tight sealing zone attachment of osteoclasts to the bone surface. *J Cell Biology* 1991;**115**:1179–86.

65. Horton MA, Taylor ML, Arnett TR, Helfrich MH. Arg-Gly-Asp (RGD) peptides and the anti-vitronectin receptor antibody 23C6 inhibit resorption and cell spreading by osteoclasts. *Exp Cell Res* 1992;**195**: 368–75.

66. Helfrich MH, Nesbitt SA, Dorey EL, Horton MA. Rat osteoclasts adhere to a wide range of RGD (Asp-Gly-Asp) peptide-containing proteins, including the bone sialoproteins and fibronectin, via a beta 3 integrin. *J Bone Miner Res* 1992;**7**:335–43.

67. Chambers TJ, Darby JA, Fuller K. Mammalian collagenase predisposes bone surfaces to osteoclastic resorption. *Cell Tissue Res* 1985;**241**:671–5.

68. Chow J, Chambers TJ. An assessment of the prevalence of organic matter on bone surfaces. *Calcified Tissue Int* 1992;**50**:118–22.

69. Chambers TJ, Revell PA, Fuller K, Athanasou NA. Resorption of bone by isolated rabbit osteoclasts. *J Cell Sci* 1984;**66**:383–99.

70. Chambers TJ, Fuller K. Bone cells predispose bone surfaces to resorption by exposure of mineral to osteoclastic contact. *J Cell Sci* 1985;**76**:155–65.

71. Meikle MC, McGarrity AM, Thomson BM, Reynolds JJ. Bone-derived growth factors modulate collagenase and TIMP (tissue inhibitor of metalloproteinases) activity and type 1 collagen degradation by mouse calvarial osteoblasts. *Bone Miner* 1991;**12**:41–55.

72. Meikle MC, Bord S, Hembry RM, Compston J, Croucher PI, Reynolds JJ. Human osteoblasts in culture synthesize collagenase and other matrix metalloproteinases in response to osteotropic hormones and cytokines. *J Cell Sci* 1992;**103**:1093–9.

73. Jilka RL. Stimulation of collagenolytic enzyme release from cultured bone cells of normal and osteopetrotic (mi/mi) mice by parathyroid hormone and lipopolysaccharide. *J Bone Miner* 1989;**6**:277–87.

74. Everts V, Delaissé JM, Korper W, Niehof A, Vaes G, Beertsen W. Degradation of collagen in the bone-resorbing compartment underlying the osteoclast involves both cysteine-proteinases and matrix metalloproteinases. *J Cell Physiol* 1992;**150**:221–31.

75. Reynolds JJ, Meikle MC. Mechanisms of connective tissue matrix destruction in periodontitis. *Periodont 2000* 1997;**14**:144–57.

76. Delaissé JM, Ensig MT, Everts V, del Carmen Overjero M, Ferreras M, Lund L, Vu TH, Werb Z, Winding B, Lochter A, Karsdal MA, Troen T, Kirkegaard T, Lenhard T, Heegaard AM, Neff L, Baron R, Foged NT. Proteinases in bone resorption: obvious and less obvious roles. *Clin Chim Acta* 2000;**291**:223–34.

77. Mangham DC, Scoones DJ, Drayson MT. Complement and the recruitment of mononuclear osteoclasts. *J Clin Pathol* 1993;**46**:517–21.

78. Kukita T, Nomiyama H, Ohmoto Y, Kukita A, Shuto A, Hotokebuchi T, Sugioka Y, Miura R, Iijima T. Macrophage inflammatory protein-1 alpha (LD78) expressed in human bone marrow: its role in regulation of hematopoiesis and osteoclast recruitment. *Laboratory Invest* 1997;**76**:399–406.

79. Hentunen TA, Lakkakorpi PT, Tuukkanen J, Lehenkari PP, Sampath TK, Väänänen HK. Effects of recombinant human osteogenic protein-1 on the differentiation of osteoclast-like cells and bone resorption. *Biochem Biophys Res Com* 1995;**209**:433–43.

80. Blavier L, Delaissé JM. Matrix metalloproteinases are obligatory for the migration of preosteoclasts to the developing marrow cavity of primitive long bones. *J Cell Science* 1995;**108**:3649–59.

81. Abu-Amer Y, Erdmann J, Alexopoulou L, Kollias G, Ross FP, Teitelbaum SL. Tumor necrosis factor receptors types 1 and 2 differentially regulate osteoclastogenesis. *J Bio Chem* 2000;**275**:27307–27.

82. Assuma R, Oates T, Cochran D, Amar S, Graves DT. IL-1 and TNF antagonists inhibit the inflammatory response and bone loss in experimental periodontitis. *J Immunol* 1998;**160**:403–9.

83. Rody WJJ, King GJ, Gu G. Osteoclast recruitment to sites of compression in orthodontic tooth movement. *Am J Orthodont Dentofacial Orthop* 2001;**120**:477–89.

84. Suda T, Udagawa N, Nakamura I, Miyaura C, Takahashi N. Modulation of osteoclast differentiation by local factors. *Bone* 1995;**17**:87S–91S.

85. Lakkakorpi PT, Väänänen HK. Cytoskeletal changes in osteoclasts during the resorption cycle. *Micro Res Technique* 1996;**33**:171–81.

86. Marchisio PC, Cirillo D, Teti A, Zambonin-Zallone A, Tarone G. Rous sarcoma virus-transformed fibroblasts and cells of monocyte origin display a peculiar dot-like organization of cytoskeletal proteins involved in microfilament-membrane interactions. *Experiment Cell Res* 1987;**169**:202–14.

87. Kanehisa J, Yamanaka T, Doi S, Turksen K, Heersche JNM, Aubin JE, Takeuchi H. A band of F-actin containing podosomes is involved in bone resorption by osteoclasts. *Bone* 1990;**11**:287–93.

88. Nesbitt SA, Nesbit A, Helfrich M, Horton M. Biochemical characterization of human osteoclast integrins: Osteoclasts express alpha v beta 3, alpha 2 beta 1 and alpha v beta 1 integrins. *J Biological Chemistry* 1993;**268**:16737–45.

89. Ruoslahti E, Pierschbacher MD. New perspectives in cell adhesion: RGD and integrins. *Sci* 1987;**238**:491–7.

90. Teti A, Blair HC, Schlesinger PH, Grano M, Zambonin-Zallone A, Kahn AJ, Teitelbaum SL, Hruska KA. Extracellular protons acidify osteoclasts, reduce cytosolic calcium, and promote expression of cell-matrix attachment structures. *J Clin Invest* 1989;**84**:773–80.

91. Teti A, Blair HC, Teitelbaum SL, Kahn AJ, Koziol C, Konsek J, Zambonin-Zallone A, Schlesinger PH. Cytoplasmic pH regulation and chloride/bicarbonate exchange in avian osteoclasts. *J Clin Invest* 1989;**83**:227–33.

92. Fisher JE, Caufield MP, Sato M, Quartuccio HA, Gould RJ, Garsky VM, Rodan GA, Rosenblatt M. Inhibition of osteoclastic bone resorption *in vivo* by echistatin, an 'arginyl-glycyl-aspartyl' (RGD)-containing protein. *Endocrinol* 1993;**132**:1411–13.

93. Lakkakorpi PT, Tuukkanen J, Hentunen T, Jarvelin K, Väänänen HK. Organization of osteoclast microfilaments during the attachment to bone surface *in vitro*. *J Bone Min Res* 1989;**4**:817–25.

94. Väänänen HK, Horton M. The osteoclast clear zone is a specialized cell-matrix adhesion structure. *J Cell Sci* 1995;**108**:2729–32.

95. Salo J, Lehenkari P, Mulari M, Metsikko K, Väänänen HK. Removal of osteoclast bone resorption products by transcytosis. *Sci* 1997;**276**:270–3.

96. Nesbitt SA, Horton MA. Trafficking of matrix collagens through bone-resorbing osteoclasts. *Sci* 1997;**276**:266–9.

97. Mostov K, Werb Z. Journey across the osteoclast. *Sci* 1997;**276**:219–20.

98. Baron R. Polarity and membrane transport in osteoclasts. *Con Tissue Res* 1989;**20**:109–20.

99. Buckwalter JA, Glimcher MJ, Cooper RR, Recker R. Bone biology. *J Bone Joint Surg* 1995; 77-A:1256–75.

100. Blair HC, Kahn AJ, Crouch EC, Jeffrey JJ, Teitelbaum SL. Isolated osteoclasts resorb the organic and inorganic components of bone. *J Cell Bio* 1986;**102**:1164–72.

101. Fallon MD. Bone resorbing fluid from osteoclasts is acidic. An *in vitro* micropuncture study. In: Cohn DV, Fujita T, Potts JT Jr, Talmage RV. eds. *Endocrine control of bone and calcium metabolism* Vol IV. Amsterdam: Elsevier Science, 1984:144–6.

102. Fallon MD. Alterations in the pH of osteoclast resorbing fluid reflects changes in bone degradative activity. *Cal Tissue Int* 1984;**36**:458.

103. Blair HC, Teitelbaum SL, Ghiselli R, Gluck S. Osteoclastic bone resorption by a polarized vacuolar proton pump. *Science* 1989;**245**:855–7.

104. Hall GE, Kenny AD. Carbonic anhydrase in bone resorption induced by prostaglandin $E_2$ *in vitro*. *Pharmacology* 1985;**30**:339–47.

105. Hall GE, Kenny AD. Role of carbonic anhydrase in bone resorption induced by 1,25 dihydroxyvitamin $D_3$ *in vitro*. *Calc Tissue Int* 1985;**37**:134–42.

106. Ravesloot JH, Eisen T, Baron R, Baron WF. Role of $Na^+$-$H^+$ exchangers and vacuolar $H^+$ pumps in entracellular pH regulation in neonatal rat osteoclasts. *J General Physiol* 1995;**105**:177–208.

107. Wang Z, Gluck S. Isolation and properties of bovine kidney brush border vacuolar $H^+$-ATPase. A proton pump with enzymatic and structural differences from kidney microsomal $H^+$-ATPase. *J Biological Chemistry* 1990;**265**:21957–65.

108. Robey PG. Bone Matrix Proteoglycans and Glycoproteins. In: Bilezikian JP, Raisz LG, Rodan GA. eds. *Principles of bone biology*. San Diego: Academic Press, 1996:155–65.

109. Meikle MC. Control mechanisms in bone resorption: 240 years after John Hunter. *Annals Royal Coll Surg of Engl* 1997;**79**:20–7.

110. Mjör IA. The morphology of dentin and dentinogenesis. In: Linde A. ed. *Dentin and dentinogenesis* Volume I. Boca Raton, FL: CRC Press, 1984:1–18.

111. Butler WT. Dentin matrix proteins. *Euro J Oral Sci* 1998;**106**:(*Suppl 1*):204–10.

112. Saygin NE, Giannobile WV, Somerman MJ. Molecular and cellular biology of cementum. *Periodontol 2000* 2000;**24**:73–98.

113. Delaissé JM, Eeckhout Y, Neff L, Francois-Gillet C, Henriet P, Su Y, Vaes G, Baron R. (Pro)collagenase (matrix metalloproteinase-1) is present in rodent osteoclasts and in the underlying bone-resorbing compartment. *J Cell Sci* 1993;**106**:1071–82.

114. Murphy G, Reynolds JJ. Extracellular matrix degradation. In: Royce PM, Steinmann B. eds. *Connective tissue and its heritable disorders*. New York: Wiley-Liss Inc., 1993:287–316.

115. Okamura T, Shimokawa H, Takagi Y, Ono H, Sasaki S. Detection of collagenase mRNA in odontoclasts of bovine root-resorbing tissue by *in situ* hybridization. *Calcified Tissue Int* 1993;**52**:325–30.

116. Fuller K, Chambers TJ. Localization of mRNA for collagenase in osteocytic, bone surface and chondrocytic cells but not in osteoclasts. *J Cell Sci* 1995;**108**: 2221–30.

117. Reponen P, Sahlberg C, Munaut C, Thesleff I, Tryggvason K. High expression of 92-kD type IV collagenase (gelatinase B) in the osteoclast lineage during mouse development. *J Cell Bio* 1994;**124**:1091–102.

118. Okada Y, Naka K, Kawamura K, Matsumoto, T. Localization of matrix metalloproteinase 9 (92-kilodalton gelatinase/type IV collagenase = gelatinase B) in osteoclasts: implications for bone resorption. *Lab Invest* 1995;**72**:311–22.

119. Wucherpfenning AL, Li Y, Stetler-Stevenson WG, Rosenberg AE, Stashenko P. Expression of 92 kD type IV collagenase/gelatinase B in human osteoclasts. *J Bone Min Res* 1994;**9**:549–56.

120. Etherington DJ. The nature of the collagenolytic cathepsin of rat liver and its distribution in other rat tissues. *Biochem J* 1972;**127**:685–92.

121. Sasaki T, Ueno-Matsuda E. Immunocytochemical localization of cathepsins B and G in odontoclasts of human deciduous teeth. *J Dent Res* 1992;**71**:1881–4.

122. Kirschke H, Kembhavi AA, Bohley P, Barrett AJ. Action of rat liver cathepsin L on collagen and other substrates. *Biochemical J* 1982;**201**:367–72.

123. Goto T, Tsukuba T, Kiyoshima T, Nishimura Y, Kato K, Yamamoto K, TANAKA, T. Immunohistochemical localization of cathepsins B, D and L in the rat osteoclast. *Histochem* 1993;**99**:411–14.

124. Burleigh MC, Barrett AJ, Lazarus GS. Cathepsin B1. A lysosomal enzyme that degrades native collagen. *Biochem J* 1974;**137**:387–98.

125. Debari K, Sasaki T, Udagawa N, Rifkin BR. An ultrastructural evaluation of the effects of cysteine-proteinase inhibitors on osteoclastic bone resorption. *Calcified Tissue Int* 1995;**56**:566–70.

126. Inui T, Ishibashi O, Inaoka T, Irigane Y, Kumegawa M, Kokubo T, Yamamura T. Cathepsin K Antisense oligodeoxynucleotide inhibits osteoclastic bone resorption. *J Biol Chem* 1997;**272**:8109–12.

127. Delaissé JM, Eeckhout Y, Vaes G. Inhibition of bone resorption in culture by inhibitors of thiol proteinases. *Biochem J* 1980;**192**:365–8.

128. Delaissé JM, Eeckhout Y, Vaes G. *In vivo* and *in vitro* evidence for the involvement of cysteine proteinases in bone resorption. *Biochem Biophys Res Com* 1984;**125**:441–7.

129. Murata M, Miyashita S, Yokoo C, Tamai M, Hanada K, Hatayama K, Towatari T, Nikawa T, Katunuma N. Novel epoxysuccinyl peptides: seletive inhibitors of cathepsin B. *FEBS Letters* 1991;**280**:307–10.

130. Inaoka T, Bilbe G, Ishibashi O, Tezuka K, Kumegawa M, Kokubo T. Molecular cloning of human cDNA for cathepsin K: Novel cysteine proteinase predominantly expressed in bone. *Biochem Biophysic Res Com* 1995;**206**:89–96.

131. Goto T, Kiyoshima T, Moroi R, Tsukuba T, Nishimura Y, Himeno M, Yamamoto K, Tanaka T. Localization of cathepsins B, D and L in the rat osteoclast by immuno-light and -electron microscopy. *Histochem* 1994;**101**:33–40.

132. Lakkakorpi PT, Väänänen HK. Kinetics of the osteoclast cytoskeleton during the resorption cycle *in vitro*. *J Bone Min Res* 1991;**6**:817–26.

133. Hughes DE, Wright HR, Uy HL, Sasaki A, Yoneda T, Roodman GD, Mundy GR, Boyce BF. Bisphosphonates promote apoptosis in murine osteoclasts *in vitro* and *in vivo*. *J Bone Min Res* 1995;**10**:1478–87.

134. Heymann D, Guicheux J, Gouin F, Passuti N, Daculsi G. Cytokines, growth factors and osteoclasts. *Cytokine* 1998;**10**:155–68.

135. Manolagas SC. Birth and death of bone cells: basic regulatory mechanisms and indications for the pathogenesis and treatment of osteoporosis. *Endocrine Rev* 2000;**21**:115–37.

136. Hofbauer LC, Khosla S, Dunstan CR, Lacey DL, Boyle WJ, Riggs BL. The roles of osteoprotegerin and osteoprotegerin ligand in the paracrine regulation of bone resorption. *J Bone Min Res* 2000;**15**:2–12.

137. Khosla S. Minireview: the OPG/RANKL/RANK system. *Endocrinol* 2001;**142**:5050–5.

138. Duong LT, Rodan GA. Regulation of osteoclast formation and function. *Rev Endocrin Metabolic Dis* 2001;**2**:95–104.

139. Alam AS, Moonga BS, Bevis PJ, Huang CL, Zaidi M. Amylin inhibits bone resorption by a direct effect on the motility of rat osteoclasts. *Exper Physiol* 1993;**78**:183–96.

140. Bellido T, Jilka RL, Boyce BF, Girasole G, Broxmeyer H, Dalrymple SA, Murray R, Manolagas SC. Regulation of interleukin-6, osteoclastogenesis, and bone mass by androgens. The role of the androgen receptor. *J Clin Invest* 1995;**95**:2886–95.

141. Zaidi M, Moonga B, Bevis PJR, Towhidul Alam ASM, Legon S, Wimalawansa S, MacIntyre I, Breimer LH. Expression and function of calcitonin gene products. *Vitamins and Hormones* 1991;**46**:87–164.

142. Alam AS, Moonga B, Bevis PJR, Huang CLH, Zaidi M. Selective antagonism of calcitonin-induced osteoclastic quiescence (Q effect) by human calcitonin gene-related peptide (Val8Phe37). *Biochem Biophys Res Com* 1991;**179**:134–9.

143. Delany AM, Dong Y, Canalis E. Mechanisms of glucocorticoid action on bone cells. *J Cell Biochem* 1994;**56**:295–302.

144. Oursler MJ, Landers JP, Riggs BL, Spelsberg TC. Oestrogen effects on osteoblasts and osteoclasts. *Ann Med* 1993;**25**:361–71.

145. Talmage RV. A study of the effect of parathyroid hormone on bone remodeling and on calcium homeostasis. *Clin Orthop* 1967;**54**:163–73.

146. Moseley JM, Gillespie MT. Parathyroid related protein. *Crit Rev Clin Lab Sci* 1995;**32**:299–343.

147. Mundy GR, Shapiro JL, Bandelin JG, Canalis EM, Raisz LG. Direct stimulation of bone resorption by thyroid hormones. *J Clin Invest* 1979;**58**:529–34.

148. Reichel H, Koeffler HP, Norman AW. The role of the vitamin D endocrine system in health and disease. *New England J Med* 1989;**320**:980–91.

149. Udagawa N. Mechanisms involved in bone resorption. *Biogerontology* 2002;**3**:79–83.

150. Hattersley G, Owens J, Flanagan AM, Chambers TJ. Macrophage colony stimulating factor (M-CSF) is essential for osteoclast formation *in vitro*. *Biochem Biophys Res Com* 1991;**177**:526–31.

151. Tarquini R, Perfetto F, Tarquini B. Endothelin-1 and Paget's bone disease: is there a link? *Calcified Tissue Int* 1998;**63**:118–20.

152. Tashjian AH, Voelkel EF, Lloyd W, Derynck L, Winkler ME, Levine L. Actions of growth factors on plasma calcium. Epidermal growth factor and transforming growth factor cause elevation of plasma calcium in mice. *J Clin Invest* 1986;**78**:1405–9.

153. Shen V, Kohler G, Huang J, Huang SS, Peck WA. An acidic fibroblast growth factor stimulates DNA synthesis, inhibits collagen and alkaline phosphatase synthesis and induces resorption in bone. *Bone Miner* 1989;**7**:205–19.

154. Chikazu D, Katagiri M, Ogasawara T, Ogata N, Shimoaka T, Takato T, Nakamura K, Kawaguchi H. Regulation of osteoclast differentiation by fibroblast

growth factor 2: stimulation of receptor activator kappa alpha ligand/osteoclast differentiation factor expression in osteoblasts and inhibition of macrophage colony-stimulating factor function in osteoclasts. *J Bone Miner Res* 2001;**16**:2074–81.

155. KURIHARA H, SUDA T, MIURA Y, NAKAUCHI H, KODAMA H, HIURA K, HAKEDA Y, KUMEGAWA M. Generation of osteoclasts from isolated hematopoietic progenitor cells. *Blood* 1989;**74**:1295–302.

156. MOCHIZUKI H, HAKEDA Y, WAKASUKI N, USUI N, AKASHI S, SATO T, TANAKA K, KUMEGAWA M. Insulin-like growth factor-1 supports formation and activation of osteoclasts. *Endocrinol* 1992;**131**:1075–80.

157. GOWEN M, NEDWIN GE, MUNDY GR. Preferential inhibition of cytokine-stimulated bone resorption by recombinant interferon gamma. *J Bone Miner Res* 1986;**1**:469–74.

158. LORENZO JA, SOUSA SL, ALANDER C, RAISZ LG. Comparison of the bone-resorbing activity in the supernatants from phyohemagglutin-stimulated human peripheral blood mononuclear cells with that of cytokines through the use of an antiserum to interleukin 1. *Endocrinology* 1987;**121**:1164–70.

159. SHIONI A, TEITELBAUM SL, ROSS FP, WELGUS HG, SUZUKI H, OHARA J, LACEY DL. Interleukin 4 inhibits murine osteoclast formation *in vitro*. *J Cell Biochem* 1991;**47**:272–7.

160. PETERS M, MEYER ZUM, BUSCHENFELDE KH, ROSE-JOHN S. The function of the soluble IL-6 receptor *in vivo*. *Immunology Letters* 1996;**54**:177–84.

161. FULLER K, OWENS J, CHAMBERS TJ. Macrophage inflammatory protein-1 alpha and IL-8 stimulate the motility but suppress the resorption of isolated rat osteoclasts. *J Immunol* 1995;**154**:6065–72.

162. BURGER D, DAYER JM. Inhibitory cytokines and cytokine inhibitors. *Neurology* 1995;**45**:S39–S43.

163. MANOLAGAS SC, JILKA RL. Bone marrow, cytokines and bone remodeling – emerging insights into the pathophysiology of osteoporosis. *New England J Med* 1995;**332**:305–11.

164. UDAGAWA N, HORWOOD NJ, ELLIOTT J, MACKAY A, OWENS J, OKAMURA H, KURIMOTO M, CHAMBERS TJ, MARTIN TJ, GILLESPIE MT. Interleukin (IL)-18 (interferon gamma inducing factor) is produced by osteoblasts and acts via granulocyte macrophage-colony stimulating factor and not via interferon-gamma to inhibit osteoclast formation. *J Experimental Med* 1997;**185**:1005–12.

165. LERNER UH, JONES IL, GUSTAFSON GT. Bradykinin, a new potential mediator of inflammatory-induced bone resorption. *Arthritis Rheumatol* 1987;**30**:530–40.

166. CHOI SJ, CRUZ JC, CRAIG F, CHUNG H, DEVLIN RD, ROODMAN GD, ALSINA M. Macrophage inflammatory protein 1-alpha is a potential osteoclast stimulating factor in multiple myeloma. *Blood* 2000;**96**:671–5.

167. MACKINTYRE I, ZAIDI M, TOWHIDU L, ALAM AS, DATTA HK, MOONGA BS, LIDBURY PS, HECKER M, VANE JM. Osteoclast inhibition: an action of nitric oxide not mediated by cGMP. *Proc Nat Acad Sci USA* 1991;**88**:2936–40.

168. CANALIS EM, MCCARTHY TL, CENTRELLA M. Effects of platelet-derived growth factor on bone formation in vitro. *J Cell Physiol* 1989;**140**:530–37.

169. AKATSU T, TAKAHASHI N, UDAGAWA N, IMAMURA K, YAMAGUCHI A, SATO K, NAGATA N, SUDA T. Role of prostaglandins in interleukin-1 induced bone resorption in mice *in vitro*. *J Bone Miner Res* 1991;**6**:183–90.

170. SOBUE T, HAKEDA Y, KOBAYASHI Y, HAYAKAWA H, YAMASHITA K, AOKI T, KUMEGAWA M, NOGUCHI T, HAYAKAWA T. Tissue inhibitor of metalloproteinases 1 and 2 directly stimulate the bone-resorbing activity of isolated mature osteoclasts. *J Bone Miner Res* 2001;**16**:2205–14.

171. KOBAYASHI K, TAKAHASHI N, JIMI E, UDAGAWA N, TAKAMI M, KOTAKE S, NAKAGAWA N, KINOSAKI M, YAMAGUCHI K, SHIMA N, YASUDA H, MORINAGA T, et al. Tumor necrosis factor α stimulates osteoclastic differentiation by a mechanism independent of the ODF/RANKL-RANK interaction. *J Experimental Med* 2000;**191**:275–86.

172. BERTOLINI D, NEDWIN G, BRINGMAN T, SMITH D, MUNDY G. Stimulation of bone resorption and inhibition of bone formation *in vitro* by human tumor necrosis factors. *Nature* 1986;**319**:516–18.

173. LOTZ E, VAUGHAN JH, CARSON DA. Effect of neuropeptides on production of inflammatory cytokines by human monocytes. *Science* 1988;**241**:1218–20.

174. HOHMANN EL, LEVINE L, TASHJIAN AH. Vasoactive intestinal peptide stimulates bone resorption via a cyclic adenosine 3′,5′-monophosphate-dependent mechanism. *Endocrinol* 1983;**112**:1233–9.

175. FLEISCH H, RUSSELL RGG, FRANCIS MD. Diphosphonates inhibit hydroxyapatite dissolution *in vitro* and bone resorption in tissue culture and *in vivo*. *Science* 1969;**165**:1262–4.

176. PIERCE AM, LINDSKOG S. The effect of an antibiotic/corticosteroid paste on inflammatory root resorption *in vivo*. *Oral Surg Oral Med Oral Pathol* 1987;**64**:216–20.

177. PIERCE AM, HEITHERSAY GS, LINDSKOG S. Evidence for direct inhibition of dentinoclasts by a corticosteroid/antibiotic paste. *Endodont Dent Traumatol* 1988;**4**:44–5.

178. PIERCE AM, LINDSKOG S. Early responses by osteoclasts *in vivo* and dentinoclasts *in vitro* to corticosteroids. *J Submicroscopic Cytology Pathol* 1989;**21**:501–8.

179. HOFBAUER LC, GORI F, RIGGS BL, LACEY DL, DUNSTAN CR, SPELSBERG TC, KHOSLA S. Stimulation of osteoprotegerin ligand and inhibition of osteoprotegerin production by glucocorticoids in human osteoblastic lineage cells: potential paracrine mechanisms of glucocorticoid-induced osteoporosis. *Endocrinology* 1999;**140**:4382–9.

180. HOFBAUER LC, LACEY DL, DUNSTAN CR, SPELSBERG TC, RIGGS BL, KHOSLA S. Interleukin-1-beta and tumor necrosis factor alpha, but not inrerleukin-6, stimulate osteoprotegerin ligand gene expression in human osteoblastic cells. *Bone* 1999;**25**:255–9.

181. HATTERSLEY G, CHAMBERS TJ. Calcitonin receptors as markers for osteoclastic differentiation: correlation between generation of bone-resorptive cells and cells that express calcitonin receptors in mouse bone marrow cultures. *Endocrinol* 1998;**125**:1606–12.

182. ADDISON WC. *Properties and functions of odontoclasts. A*

*comparative study.* PhD Thesis, University of Birmingham, 1976.

183. JONES SJ, BOYD A. The resorption of dentine and cementum *in vivo* and *in vitro*. In: Davidovitch Z. ed. *The biological mechanisms of tooth eruption and root resorption*. Birmingham, Alabama: EBSCO Media, 1988:335–54.

184. PIERCE AM. Experimental basis for the management of dental resorption. *Endod Dent Traumatol* 1989;**5**:255–65.

185. WESSELINK PR, BEERTSEN W, EVERTS V. Resorption of the mouse incisor after the application of cold to the periodontal attachment apparatus. *Calcified Tissue Int* 1986;**36**:11–21.

186. GILLES JA, CARNES DL, WINDELER AS. Development of an *in vitro* culture system for the study of osteoclast activity and function. *J Endodont* 1994;**20**:327–31.

187. LINDSKOG S, PIERCE AM. Spreading of dentinoclasts on various substrata *in vitro*. *Scan J Dent Res* 1988;**96**:310–16.

188. ADDISON WC. The distribution of nuclei in human odontoclasts in whole cell preparations. *Arch Oral Pathol* 1978;**23**:1167–71.

189. ADDISON WC. The effect of parathyroid hormone on the numbers of nuclei in feline odontoclasts *in vivo*. *J Periodont Res* 1980;**15**:536–43.

190. FREILICH LS. Ultrastructure and acid phosphatase cytochemistry of odontoclasts: effects of parathyroid extract. *J Dent Res*, 1971;**50**:(Suppl 5):1047–55.

191. MATSUDA E. Ultrastructural and cytochemical study of the odontoclasts in physiologic root resorption of human deciduous teeth. *J Electron Microscopy* 1992;**41**:131–40.

192. SAHARA N, OKAFUJI N, TOYOKI A, ASHIZAWA Y, DEGUCHI T, SUZUKI K. Odontoclastic resorption of the superficial nonmineralized layer of predentine in the shedding of human deciduous teeth. *Cell Tissue Res* 1994;**277**:19–26.

193. SASAKI T, UENO-MATSUDA E. Immunocytochemical localization of cathepsins B and G in odontoclasts of human deciduous teeth. *J Dent Res* 1992;**71**:1881–4.

194. SAHARA N, OKAFUJI N, TOYOKI A, SUZUKI I, DEGUCHI T, SUZUKI K. Odontoclastic resorption at the pulpal surface of coronal dentin prior to the shedding of human deciduous teeth. *Arch Histol Cytol* 1992;**55**:273–85.

195. SAHARA N, TOYOKI A, ASHIZAWA Y, DEGUCHI T, SUZUKI K. Cytodifferentiation of the odontoclast prior to the shedding of human deciduous teeth: an ultrastructural and cytochemical study. *Anat Rec* 1996;**244**:33–49.

196. SASAKI T. Differentiation and functions of osteoclasts and odontoclasts in mineralized tissue resorption. *Microsc Res Tech* 2003;**61**:483–95.

197. SHIGEYAMA Y, GROVE TK, STRAYHORN C, SOMERMAN MJ. Expression of adhesion molecules during tooth resorption in feline teeth: a model for aggressive osteoclast activity. *J Dent Res* 1996;**75**:1650–7.

198. TORABINEJAD M, BAKLAND LK. Prostaglandins: their possible role in the pathogenesis of pulpal and periapical diseases, part 1. *J Endodont* 1980;**6**:733–39.

199. TORABINEJAD M, BAKLAND LK. Prostaglandins: their possible role in the pathogenesis of pulpal and periapical diseases, part 2. *J Endodont* 1980;**6**:769–75.

200. TORABINEJAD M, EBY WC, NAIDORF IJ. Inflammatory and immunological aspects of the pathogenesis of human periapical lesions. *J Endodont* 1985;**11**:479–87.

201. STERRETT JD. The osteoclast and periodontitis. *J Clin Periodontol* 1986;**13**:258–69.

202. ANDREASEN JO. External root resorption: its implication in dental traumatology, paedodontics, periodontics, orthodontics and endodontics. *Int Endodont J* 1985;**18**:109–18.

203. HAMMARSTRÖM L, LINDSKOG S. General morphological aspects of resorption of teeth and alveolar bone. *Int Endodont J* 1985;**18**:93–8.

204. ANDREASEN JO. Experimental dental traumatology: development of a model for external root resorption. *Endodont Dent Traumatol* 1987;**3**:269–87.

205. ANDREASEN FM, ANDREASEN JO. Resorption and mineralization processes following root fracture of permanent incisors. *Endodont Dent Traumatol* 1988;**4**:202–14.

206. ATHANASOU NA, QUINN J. Immunophenotypic differences between osteoclasts and macrophage polykaryons: immunohistochemical distinction and implications for osteoclast ontogeny and function. *J Clin Pathol* 1990;**43**:997–1003.

207. STASHENKO P. The role of immune cytokines in the pathogenesis of periapical lesions. *Endodont Dent Traumatol* 1990;**6**:89–96.

208. TORABINEJAD M, COTTI E, LESSARD G. Leukotrienes: their possible role in pulpal and periapical diseases. *Endodont Dent Traumatol* 1991;**7**:233–41.

209. PIERCE AM, LINDSKOG S, HAMMARSTRÖM L. Osteoclasts: structure and function. *Electron Microsc Rev* 1991;**4**:1–45.

210. ANDREASEN JO, ANDREASEN FM. Root resorption following traumatic dental injuries. *Proc Finn Dent Soc* 1992;**88**(Suppl.1):95–14.

211. CAHILL DR, MARKS SC Jr, WISE GE, GORSKI JP. A review and comparison of tooth eruption systems used in experimentation – a new proposal on tooth eruption. In: Davidovitch Z. ed. *The biological mechanism of tooth eruption and root resorption*. Birmingham, Alabama: EBSCO media, 1988:1–7.

212. HEPPENSTALL RB. Fracture healing. In: Hunt TK, Heppenstall RB, Pines E, Rovee D. eds. *Soft and hard tissue repair*. New York: Praeger, 1984:101–42.

213. SASAKI T. Differentiation and functions of osteoclasts and odontoclasts in mineralized tissue resorption. *Microsc Res Tech* 2003;**61**:483–95.

214. LOSSDORFER S, GOTZ W, JAGER A. Immunohistochemical localization of receptor activator of nuclear factor kappaB (RANK) and its ligand (RANKL) in human deciduous teeth. *Calcif Tissue Int* 2002;**71**:45–52.

215. SAIDENBERG KERMANACH N, BESSIS N, COHEN-SOLAL M, de VERNEJOUL MC, BOISSIER MC. Osteoprotegerin and inflammation. *Eur Cytokine Netw* 2002;**13**:144–53.

216. JIANG Y, MEHTA CK, HSU TY, ALSULAIMANI FF. Bacteria induce osteoclastogenesis via an osteoblast-independent pathway. *Infect Immun* 2002;**70**:3143–8.

217. FANTONE JC, WARD PA. Inflammation. In: Rubine, Farber JL. eds. *Pathology*. Philadelphia: JB Lippincott, 1988:34–64.

218. TROWBRIDGE HO, EMLING RC. *Inflammation: a review of*

*the process.* 2nd edn. Bristol, Pennsylvania. Comsource Distribution Systems Inc, 1983.

219. Seltzer S. *Inflammation: an update.* The Research and Education Foundation of the American Association of Endodontists, 1990.

220. Wakisaka S. Neuropeptides in the dental pulps: distribution, origin, and correlation. *J Endodont* 1990:67–69.

221. Adam C, Llorens A, Baroukh B, Cherruau M, Saffar JL. Effects of capsaicin-induced sensory denervation on osteoclastic resorption in adult rats. *Exp Physiol* 2000;**85**:62–6.

222. Azuma H, Kido J, Ikedo D, Kataoka M, Nagata T. Substance P enhances the inhibition of osteoblastic cell differentiation induced by lipopolysaccharide from Porphyromonas gingivalis. *J Periodontol* 2004;**75**:974–81.

223. Akopian A, Demulder A, Ouriaghli F, Corazza F, Fondu P, Bergmann P. Effects of CGRP on human osteoclast-like cell formation: a possible connection with the bone loss in neurological disorders? *Peptides* 2000;**21**:559–64.

224. Olgart L, Hockfelt T, Nilsson G, Pernow B. Localization of substance P-like immunoreactivity in nerves of the tooth pulp. *Pain* 1977;**4**:153–9.

225. Uddman R, Grunditz T, Sundler F. Calcitonin gene-related peptide: a sensory transmitter in dental pulp. *Scand J Dent Res* 1986;**94**:219–24.

226. Wakisaka S, Ichikawa H, Nishikawa S, Matsuo S, Takano Y, Akai M. The distribution and origin of calcitonin gene-related peptide-containing nerve fibers in feline dental pulp: relationship with substance-P containing nerve fibers. *Histochemistry* 1987;**86**:585–89.

227. Silverman JD, Kruger L. An interpretation of dental innervation based upon the pattern of calcitonin gene-related (CGRP)-immunoreactive thin sensory axons. *Somatosens Res* 1987;**5**:157–75.

228. Wakisaka S, Ichikawa H, Nishimoto T, et al. Substance P-like immunoreactivity in the pulp-dentine zone of human molar teeth demonstrated by indirect immunofluorescence. *Arch Oral Biol* 1984;**29**:73–5.

229. Takahashi N, Yamana H, Yoshiki S, et al. Osteoclast-like cell formation and its regulation by osteotropic hormones in mouse bone marrow cultures. *Endocrinology* 1988;**122**:1373–82.

230. Wakisaka S, Nishikawa S, Ichikawa H, Matsuo S, Takano Y, Akai M. The distribution and origin of substance P-like immunoreactivity in rat molar pulp and periodontal tissues. *Arch Oral Biol* 1985;**30**:813–8.

231. Davidovitch Z, Nicolay OF, Ngan PW, Shanfeld JL. Neurotransmitters, cytokines, and the control of alveolar bone remodeling in orthodontics. *Dent Clin N Am* 1988;**31**:411–35.

232. Gazelius B. Edwall B, Olgart L, Lundberg JM, Hök Felt T, Fischer JA. Vasodilatory effects and coexistence of calcitonin gene-related peptide (CGRP) and substance P in sensory nerves of cat dental pulp. *Acta Physiol Scand* 1987;**130**:33–40.

233. Hohmann E, Levine L, Tashjian AH Jr. Vasoactive intestinal peptide stimulates bone resorption via a cyclic adenosine 3′,5′-monophosphate-dependent mechanism. *Endocrinology* 1983;**112**:1233–9.

234. Hohmann E, Tashjian AH Jr. Functional receptors for vasoactive intestinal peptide of human osteosarcoma cells. *Endocrinology* 1984;**114**:1321–7.

235. Haug SR, Heyeraas KJ. Effects of sympathectomy on experimentally induced pulpal inflammation and periapical lesions in rats. *Neuroscience* 2003;**120**:827–36.

236. Torabinejad M, Eby WC, Naidorf IJ. Inflammatory and immunological aspects of the pathogenesis of human periapical lesions. *J Endodont* 1985;**11**:479–88.

237. Marceau F, Lussier A, Regoli D, Giroud JP. Pharmacology of kinins: their relevance to tissue injury and inflammation. *Gen Pharmacol* 1983;**14**:209–29.

238. Plummer TH, Erodos EG. Human plasma carboxypeptidase. *Methods Enzymol* 1981;**80**(part c): 442–49.

239. Kaplan AP, Silverberg M, Dunn JT, Ghebrehiwet B. Interaction of the clotting, kinin-forming, complement and fibrinolytic pathways in inflammation. C-reactive protein and the plasma protein response to tissue injury. *Ann NY Acad Sci* 1982;**389**:23–38.

240. Torabinejad M, Midrou T, Bakland L. Detection of kinins in human periapical lesions. *J Dent Res* 1968;**68**:201 (Abs 156).

241. Muller-Eberhard HJ. Chemistry and reaction mechanisms of complement. *Adv Immunol* 1968;**8**:1–80.

242. Malmström M. Immunoglobulin classes of IgG, IgM, IgA, and complement components C3 in dental periapical lesions of patients with rheumatoid disease. *Scand J Rheumatol* 1975;**4**:57–64.

243. Kuntz DD, Genco RJ, Gutruso J, Natiella JR. Localization of immunoglobulins and the third component of complement in dental periapical lesions. *J Endodont* 1977;**3**:68–73.

244. Pulver WH, Taubman MA, Smith DJ. Immune components in human dental periapical lesions. *Arch Oral Biol* 1978;**23**:435–43.

245. Raisz LG, Sandberg AL, Goodson JM, Simmons HA, Mergenhagen SE. Complement dependent stimulation of prostaglandin synthesis and bone resorption. *Science* 1974;**185**:789–91.

246. Sandberg AL, Raisz LG, Goodson JM, Simmons HA, Mergenhagen SE. Initiation of bone resorption by the classical and alternative C pathways and its mediation by prostaglandins. *J Immunol* 1977;**119**:1378–81.

247. Kaliner M, Austen KF. Cyclic AMP, ATP, and reversed anaphylactic histamine release from rat mast cells. *J Immunol* 1974;**112**:664–74.

248. Guttler F. Phospholipid synthesis in HeLa cells exposed to immunoglobulin G and complement. *Biochem* 1972;**128**:953–60.

249. Inoue K, Kinoshitat, Okada M, Akiyama Y. Release of phospholipids from complement-mediated lesions on the surface structure of *Escherichia coli.* *J Immunol* 1977;**119**:65–72.

250. Schlager SI, Ohanian SH, Borsos T. Stimulation of the synthesis and release of lipids in tumor cells under attack of antibody and complement. *J Immunol* 1978;**120**:895–901.

251. Wilhelm DL. The mediation of increased vascular permeability in inflammation. *Pharmacol Rev* 1962;**14**:251–80.

252. Willouby DA, Dieppe P. Anti-inflammatory models in animals. *Agents Actions* 1976;**6**:306–12.

253. VANLOVEREN H, KRAEUTER-KOPS S, ASKEMASE PW. Different mechanisms of release of vasoactive amines by mast cells occur in T cell-dependent compared to IgE-dependent cutaneous hypersensitivity responses. *Eur J Immunol* 1984;**14**:40–7.

254. ISHIZAKA K, ISHIZAKA T. Immune mechanisms of reversed type reaginic hypersensitivity. *J Immunol* 1973;**103**:588–95.

255. MATHIESEN A. Preservation and demonstration of mast cells in human apical granulomas and radicular cysts. *Scand J Dent Res* 1973;**81**:218–29.

256. PERRINI N, FONZI L. Mast cells in human periapical lesions: ultrastructural aspects and their possible phys-iopathological implications. *J Endodont* 1985;**11**:197–202.

257. LESCLOUS P, GUEZ D, SAFFAR JL. Short-term prevention of osteoclastic resorption and osteopenia in ovariectomized rats treated with the H(2) receptor antagonist cimetidine. *Bone* 2002;**30**:131–6.

258. LESCLOUS P, GUEZ D, BAROUKH B, VIGNERY A, SAFFAR JL. Histamine participates in the early phase of trabecular bone loss in ovariectomized rats. *Bone* 2004;**34**:91–9.

259. FITZPATRICK LA, BUZAS E, GAGNE TJ, NAGY A, HORVATH C, FERENCZ V, MESTER A, KARI B, RUAN M, FALUS A, BARSONY J. Targeted deletion of histidine decarboxylase gene in mice increases bone formation and protects against ovariectomy-induced bone loss. *Proc Natl Acad Sci U S A* 2003;**100**:6027–32.

260. MIZEL SB. Interleukin 1 and T cell activation. *Immunol Rev* 1982;**63**:51–72.

261. RYAN GB, MAJNO G. *Inflammation.* Kalamazoo, MI: The Upjohn Company, 1980:52–5.

262. MOTYCKOVA G, FISHER DE. Pycnodysostosis: role and regulation of cathepsin K in osteoclast function and human disease. *Curr Mol Med* 2002;**2(5)**:407–21.

263. SAHARA T, ITOH K, DEBARI K, SASAKI T. Specific biological functions of vacuolar-type H(+)-ATPase and lysosomal cysteine proteinase, cathepsin K, in osteoclasts. *Anat Rec A Discov Mol Cell Evol Biol* 2003;**270**:152–61.

264. GOTZ W, QUONDAMATTEO F, RAGOTZKI S, AFFELDT J, JAGER A. Localization of cathepsin D in human odontoclasts. A light and electron microscopical immunocytochemical study. *Connect Tissue Res* 2000;**41**:185–94.

265. DIAZ A, WILLIS AC, SIM RB. Expression of the proteinase specialized in bone resorption, cathepsin K, in granulomatous inflammation. *Mol Med* 2000;**6**:648–59.

266. TORABINEJAD M, BAKLAND LK. Prostaglandins: their possible role in the pathogenesis of pulpal and periapical diseases. Part 1. *J Endodont* 1980;**6**:733–9.

267. TORABINEJAD M, BAKLAND LK. Prostaglandins: their possible role in the pathogenesis of pulpal and periapical diseases. Part 2. *J Endodont* 1980;**6**:769–76.

268. TORABINEJAD M, CLAGETT J, ENGEL D. A cat model for evaluation of mechanism of bone resorption: induction of bone loss by simulated immune complexes and inhibition by indomethacin. *Calcif Tissue Int* 1979;**29**:207–14.

269. MCNICHOLAS S, TORABINEJAD M, BLANKENSHIP J, BAKLAND LK. The concentration of prostaglandin E2 in human periradicular lesions. *J Endodont* 1991;**17**:97–100.

270. NACCACHE PH, SHAAM RI. Arachidonic acid, leukotriene B4, and neutrophil activation. *Ann NY Acad Sci* 1983;**514**:125–39.

271. TORABINEJAD M, COTTI E, JUNG T. The concentration of leukotriene B4 in symptomatic and asymptomatic lesions. *J Endodont* 1992;**18**:205–8.

272. TORABINEJAD M, KIGER RD. Experimentally induced alterations in periapical tissues of the cat. *J Dent Res* 1980;**59**:8796.

273. TORABINEJAD M, KETTERING JD. Detection of immune complexes in human periapical lesions by anticomplement immunofluorescence technique. *Oral Surg Oral Med Oral Pathol* 1979;**48**:256–61.

274. TORABINEJAD M, THEOFILOPOULOS AN, KETTERING JD, BAKLAND LK. Quantitation of circulating immune complexes, immunoglobulins G and M, and C3 complement in patients with large periapical lesions. *Oral Surg Oral Med Oral Pathol* 1983;**55**:186–90.

275. KETTERING JD, TORABINEJAD M. Concentration of immune complexes, IgG, IgM, IgE, and C3 in patients with acute apical abscesses. *J Endodont* 1984;**10**: 417–21.

276. TORABINEJAD M, KETTERING JD. Identification and relative concentration of B and T lymphocytes in human chronic periapical lesions. *J Endodont* 1985;**11**:122–25.

277. BABAL P, SOLER P, BROZMAN M, JAKUBOVSKY J, BEYLY M, BASSET F. *In situ* characterization of cells in periapical granulomas by monoclonal antibodies. *Oral Surg Oral Med Oral Pathol* 1987;**64**:548–52.

278. CYMERMAN JJ, CYMERMAN DH, WALTERS J, NEVINS AJ. Human T lymphocyte subpopulations in chronic periapical lesions. *J Endodont* 1984;**10**:9–11.

279. STASHENKO P, YU SM. T helper and T suppressor cells reversal during the development of induced rat periapical lesions. *J Dent Res* 1989;**68**:830–4.

280. BARKHORDAR RA, RESOUZA YG. Human T lymphocyte subpopulations in periapical lesions. *Oral Surg Oral Med Oral Pathol* 1988;**65**:763–6.

281. WALLSTRÖM J. *Surgical exposure of pulp tissues in conventional and nude rats.* Thesis, Loma Linda University, 1990.

282. WATERMAN PA. *Development of periapical lesions in immunosuppressed rats.* Thesis, Loma Linda University, 1992.

283. GERY I, LUPE-ZUNIGA JL. Interleukin 1: uniqueness of its production and spectrum of activities. *Lymphokines* 1984;**9**:109–25.

284. MARCH CJ, MOSLEY B, LARSEN A, et al. Cloning, sequence and expression of two distinct human interleukin-1 complementary DNAs. *Nature* 1985;**315**:641–7.

285. DEWHIRST FE, STASHENKO PP, MOLE JE, TSURUMACHI T. Purification and partial sequence of human osteoclast-activating factor: identity with interleukin 1 beta. *Immunol* 1985;**136**:2562–8.

286. BERTOLINI DR, NEDWIN GE, BRINGMAN TS, SMITH DD, MUNDY GR. Stimulation of bone resorption and inhibition of bone formation *in vitro* by human tumor necrosis factors. *Nature* 1986;**319**:516–18.

287. GOWEN M, WOOD DD, IHRIE EJ, MCGUIRE MKB, RUSSELL RGG. An interleukin 1 like factor stimulates bone resorption *in vitro*. *Nature* 1983;**306**:378–80.

288. Stashenko P, Dewhirst FE, Rooney ML, Desjardins LA, Heeley JD. Interleukin-1 β is a potent inhibitor of bone formation *in vitro*. *J Bone Miner Res* 1987;**2**:559–65.

289. Pfeilschifter J, Chenu C, Bird A, Mundy GR, Roodman GD. Interleukin-1 and tumor necrosis factor stimulate the formation of human osteoclastlike cells *in vitro*. *J Bone Miner Res* 1989;**4**:113–18.

290. Thomson BM, Saklatvala J, Chambers TJ. Osteoblasts mediate interleukin 1 stimulation of bone resorption by rat osteoclasts. *J Exp Med* 1986;**164**:104–12.

291. Keeting PE, Rifas L, Harris SA, et al. Evidence for interleukin-β production by cultured normal human osteoblast-like cells. *J Bone Miner Res* 1991;**6**:827–33.

292. Fried RM, Voelkel EF, Rice RH, Levine L, Gaffney EV, Tashjian AH Jr. Two squamous cell carcinomas not associated with humoral hypercalcemia produce a potent bone resorption-stimulating factor which is interleukin-1 alpha. *Endocrinology* 1989;**125**:742–51.

293. Sato K, Fuju Y, Kasono K, et al. Parathyroid hormone-related protein and interleukin-1 alpha synergistically stimulate bone resorption *in vitro* and increase the serum calcium concentration in mice *in vivo*. *Endocrinology* 1989;**124**:2172–8.

294. Kawano M, Tanaka H, Ishikawah, et al. Interleukin-1 accelerates autocrine growth of myeloma cells through interleukin-6 in human myeloma. *Blood* 1989;**73**: 2145–8.

295. Cozzolino F, Torcia M, Aldinucci D, et al. Production of interleukin-1 by bone marrow myeloma cells. *Blood* 1989;**74**:380–7.

296. D'Souza R, Brown LR, Newland JR, Levy BM, Lachman LB. Detection and characterization of IL-1 in human dental pulps. *Arch Oral Biol* 1989;**34**:307–13.

297. Stashenko P, Jandinski JJ, Fujiyoshi P, Rynar J, Socransky SS. Tissue levels of bone resorptive cytokines in periodontal disease. *J Periodontol* 1991;**62**:504–9.

298. Stashenko P, Yu SM, Wang C-Y. Kinetics of immune cell and bone resorptive responses to endodontic infections. *J Endodont* 1992;**18**:422–6.

299. Safavi KE, Rossomando EF. Tumor necrosis factor identified in periapical tissue exudates of teeth with apical periodontitis. *J Endodont* 1991;**17**:12–14.

300. Barkhordarr A, Hussain MZ, Hayashi C. Detection of IL-1β in human periapical lesions. *Oral Surg Oral Med Oral Pathol* 1992;**73**:334–6.

301. Lim G, Torabinejad M, Kettering J, Linkhart T, Finkelman R. Concentration of interleukin 1 β- in symptomatic and asymptomatic human periradicular lesions. *J Endodont* 1992;**18**:189 (Abs 10).

302. Schrader JW. The panspecific hemopoietin of activated T lymphocytes (interleukin-3). *Annu Rev Immunol* 1986;**4**:205–30.

303. Ihle JN, Weinstein Y. Immunological regulation of hematopoietic/lymphoid stem cell differentiation by interleukin 3. *Adv Immunol* 1986;**39**:1–50.

304. Barton BE, Mayer R. IL-3 induces differentiation of bone marrow precursor cells to osteoclast-like cells. *J Immunol* 1989;**143**:3211–16.

305. Hattersley G, Chambers TJ. Effects of interleukin 3 and of granulocyte-macrophage and macrophage colony stimulating factors on osteoclast differentiation from

mouse hemopoietic tissue. *J Cellular Physiol* 1990;**142**:201–9.

306. Yoshie H, Taubman MA, Olson CL, Ebersole JL, Smith DJ. Periodontal bone loss and immune characteristics after adoptive transfer of Actinobacillus-sensitized T cells to rats. *J Periodont Res* 1987;**22**:499–505.

307. Kennedy AC, Lindsay R. Bone involvement in rheumatoid arthritis. *Clin Rheum Dis* 1977;**3**:403–20.

308. Kennedy AC, Lindsay R, Buchanan WW, Allam BF. Bone resorbing activity in the sera of patients with rheumatoid arthritis. *Clin Sci Mol Med* 1976;**51**:205–7.

309. Billiau A, van Damme J, Ceuppens J, Baroja M. Interleukin 6, a ubiquitous cytokine with paracrine as well as endocrine functions. In: Fradelizi D, Bertoglio J. eds. *Lymphokine receptor interactions*. London: John Libby Eurotext, 1989:133–42.

310. Feyen JHM, Elford P, di Padova FE, Trechsel U. Interleukin-6 is produced by bone and modulated by parathyroid hormone. *J Bone Miner Res* 1989;**4**: 633–8.

311. Kurihara N, Bertolini D, Suda T, Akiyama Y, Roodman GD. IL-6 Stimulates osteoclast-like multinucleated cell formation in long term human marrow cultures by inducing IL-1 release. *J Immunol* 1990;**144**:4226–30.

312. Al-Humidan A, Ralston SH, Hughes DE et al. Interleukin-6 does not stimulate bone resorption in neonatal mouse calvariae. *J Bone Min Res* 1991;**6**:3–8.

313. Ishimi Y, Miyaura C, Jin CH, et al. IL-6 is produced by osteoblasts and induces bone resorption. *J Immunol* 1990;**145**:3297–03.

314. Roodman GD, Kurihara N, Ohsaki Y et al. Interleukin 6. A potential autocrine/paracrine factor in Paget's disease of bone. *J Clin Invest* 1992;**89**:46–52.

315. Black K, Garret IR, Mundy GR. Chinese hamster ovarian cells transfected with the murine interleukin-6 gene cause hypercalcemia as well as cachexia, leukocytosis and thrombocytosis in tumor-bearing nude mice. *Endocrinology* 1991;**128**:2657–59.

316. Kono Y, Beagley KW, Fujihashi K, et al. Cytokine regulation of localized inflammation. Induction of activated B cells and IL-6-mediated polyclonal IgG and IgA synthesis in inflamed human gingiva. *J Immunol* 1991;**146**:1812–21.

317. Al-Balaghi S, Strom H, Moller E. B cell differentiation factor in synovial fluid of patients with rheumatoid arthritis. *Immunol Rev* 1984;**78**:7–23.

318. Thomson BM, Mundy GR, Chambers TJ. Tumor necrosis factors α and β induce osteoblastic cells to stimulate osteoclastic bone resorption. *J Immunol* 1987;**138**:775–9.

319. Tashjian AH Jr, Voelkel EF, Lazzaro M, Goad D, Bosma T, Levine L. Tumor necrosis factor-a (cachectin) stimulates bone resorption in mouse calvaria via a prostaglandin-mediated mechanism. *Endocrinology* 1987;**120**:2029–36.

320. Sabatini M, Mates AJ, Garrett IR, et al. Increased production of tumor necrosis factor by normal immune cells in a model of the humoral hypercalcemia of malignancy. *Lab Invest* 1990;**63**:676–82.

321. Sabatini M, Chavez J, Mundy GR, Bonewald LF.

Stimulation of tumor necrosis factor release from monocytic cells by the A375 human melanoma via granulocyte-macrophage colony stimulating factor. *Cancer Res* 1990;**50**:2673–8.

322. YONEDA T, ALSINA MA, CHAVEZ JB, BONEWALD L, NISHIMURA R, MUNDY GR. Evidence that tumor necrosis factor plays a pathogenetic role in the paraneoplastic syndromes of cachexia, hypercalcemia, and leukocytosis in a human tumor in nude mice. *J Clin Invest* 1991;**87**:977–85.

323. GARRETT IR, DURIE BGM, NEDWIN GE et al. Production of lymphotoxin, a bone resorbing cytokine, by cultured human myeloma cells. *N Engl J Med* 1987;**317**:526–32.

324. KLEIN DC, RAISZ LG. Prostaglandins: stimulation of bone resorption in tissue culture. *Endocrinology* 1970;**86**:1436–40.

325. DIETRICH JW, GOODSON JM, RAISZ LG. Stimulation of bone resorption by various prostaglandins in organ culture. *Prostaglandins* 1975;**10**:231–40.

326. RAISZ LG, DIETRICH JW, SIMMONS HA, SEYBERTH HW, HUBBARD W, OATES JA. Effect of prostaglandin endoperoxides and metabolites on bone resorption *in vitro*. *Nature* 1977;**267**:532–4.

327. TASHJIAN AH Jr, TICE JE, SIDES K. Biological activities of prostaglandin analogues and metabolites on bone in organ culture. *Nature* 1977;**266**:645–7.

328. DEWHIRST FE. 6-Keto-prostaglandin E1-stimulated bone resorption in organ culture. *Calcif Tissue Int* 1984;**36**:380–3.

329. CHAMBERS TJ, MCSHEHY PMJ, THOMPSON BM, FULLER K. The effect of calcium-regulating hormones and prostaglandins on bone resorption by osteoclasts disaggregated from neonatal rabbit bones. *Endocrinology* 1985;**116**:234–9.

330. CHAMBERS TJ, ALI NN. Inhibition of osteoclastic motility by prostaglandins 12, E1, E2 and 6-oxo E1. *J Pathol* 1983;**139**:383–97.

331. OKUDA A, TAYLOR LM, HEERSCHE JNM. Prostaglandin E2 initially inhibits and then stimulates bone resorption in isolated rabbit osteoclast cultures. *Bone Min* 1989;**7**:255–66.

332. COLLINS DA, CHAMBERS TJ. Effect of prostaglandins E1, E2, and F2 alpha on osteoclast formation in mouse bone marrow cultures. *J Bone Min Res* 1991;**6**:157–64.

333. GOODSON JM, DEWHIRST FE, BRUNETTI A. Prostaglandin E2 levels and human periodontal disease. *Prostaglandins* 1974;**6**:81–5.

334. OFFENBACHER S, ODLE BM, VAN DYKE TE. The use of crevicular fluid prostaglandin E2 levels as a predictor of periodontal attachment loss. *J Periodont Res* 1986,**21**:101–12.

335. COHEN JS, READER A, FERTEL R, BECK M, MEYERS WJ. A radioimmunoassay determination of the concentrations of prostaglandins E2 and F2 alpha in painful and asymptomatic human dental pulps. *J Endodont* 1985;**11**:330–5.

336. LESSARD G, TORABINEJAD M, SWOPE D. Arachidonic acid metabolism in canine tooth pulps and the effects of non-steroidal anti-inflammatory drugs. *J Endodont* 1986;**12**:146–9.

337. JEFFCOAT MK, WILLIAMS RC, WECHTER WJ, et al.

Flurbiprofen treatment of periodontal disease in beagles. *J Periodont Res* 1986;**21**:624–33.

338. ROBINSON DR, TASHJIAN AH Jr, LEVINE L. Prostaglandin stimulated bone resorption by rheumatoid synovia. *J Clin Invest* 1975;**56**:1181–8.

339. VOELKEL EF, TASHJIAN AH Jr, FRANKLIN R, WASSERMAN E, LEVINE L. Hypercalcemia and tumor prostaglandins: The VX2 carcinoma model in the rabbit. *Metabolism* 1975;**24**:973–86.

340. SEYBERTH HW, SEGRE GV, MORGAN JL, SWEETMAN BJ, POTTS JT Jr, OATES JA. Prostaglandins as mediators of hypercalcemia associated with certain types of cancer. *N Engl J Med* 1975;**293**:1278–3.

341. CHYUN YS, RAISZ LG. Stimulation of bone formation by prostaglandin E2. *Prostaglandins* 1984;**27**:97–103.

342. RÖ S, SUDMANN E, MARTON PF. Effect of indomethacin on fracture healing in rats. *Acta Orthop Scand* 1976;**47**:558–99.

343. MIZEL SB, DAYER J-M, KRANE SM, MERGENHAGEN SE. Stimulation of rheumatoid synovial cell collagenase and prostaglandin production by partially purified lymphocyte activating factor (interleukin 1). *Proc Natl Acad Sci U S A* 1981;**78**:2474–7.

344. KNUDSEN PJ, DINARELLO CA, STROM TB. Prostaglandins posttranscriptionally inhibit monocyte expression of interleukin 1 activity by increasing intracellullar cyclic adenosine monophosphate. *J Immunol* 1986;**137**:3189–94.

345. MITNICK M, ISALES C, PALIWAL I, INSOGNA K. Parathyroid hormone-related protein stimulates prostaglandin E2 release from human osteoclast-like cells: modulating effect of peptide length. *J Bone Min Res* 1992;**7**:887–96.

346. METCALF D, GEARING DP. Fatal syndrome in mice engrafted with cells producing high levels of the leukemia inhibitory factor. *Proc Natl Acad Sci U S A* 1989;**86**:5948–52.

347. ABE E, TANAKA H, ISHIMI Y, et al. Differentiation-inducing factor purified from conditioned medium of mitogen-treated spleen cell cultures stimulates bone resorption. *Proc Natl Acad Sci U S A* 1986;**83**:5958–62.

348. ABE E, ISHIMI Y, TAKAHASHI N, et al. A differentiation-inducing factor produced by the osteoclastic cell line MC3T3El stimulates bone resorption by promoting osteoclast formation. *J Bone Min Res* 1988;**3**:635–45.

349. MACKIE EJ, TRECHSEL U. Stimulation of bone formation *in vivo* by transforming growth factor-β: remodeling of woven bone and lack of inhibition by indomethacin. *Bone* 1990;**11**:295–300.

350. NODA M, CAMILLIERE JJ. *In vivo* stimulation of bone formation by transforming growth factor-β. *Endocrinology* 1989;**124**:2991–4.

351. JOYCE ME, ROBERTS AB, SPORN MB, BOLANDER ME. Transforming growth factor-β and the initiation of chondrogenesis and osteogenesis in the rat femur. *J Cell Biol* 1990;**110**:2195–7.

352. BECK LS, DEGUZMAN L, LEE WP, XU Y, MCFATRIDGE LA, GILLETT NA, AMENTO EP. TGF-βl induces bone closure of skull defects. *Bone Min Res* 1991;**6**:1257–65.

353. CHENU C, PFEILSCHIFTER J, MUNDY GR, ROODMAN GD. Transforming growth factor β inhibits formation of

osteoclast-like cells in long-term human marrow cultures. *Proc Natl Acad Sci U S A* 1988;**85**:5683–7.

354. TASHJIAN AH Jr, VOELKEL EF, LLOYD W, DERYNCK R, WINKLER ME, LEVINE L. Actions of growth factors on plasma calcium. Epidermal growth factor and human transforming growth factor-alpha cause elevation of plasma calcium in mice. *J Clin Invest* 1986;**78**:1405–9.

355. GOWEN M, NEDWIN GE, MUNDY GR. Preferential inhibition of cytokine-stimulated bone resorption by recombinant interferon gamma. *J Bone Min Res* 1986;**1**:469–74.

356. LERNER UH, LJUNGGREN O, RANSJÖ M, KLAUSHOFER K, PETERLIK M. Inhibitory effects of γ-interferon on bradykinin induced bone resorption and prostaglandin formation in cultured mouse calvarial bones. *Agents Actions* 1991;**32**:305–11.

357. CARTER DB, DEIBEL MR, DUNN CJ, et al. Purification, cloning, expression and biological characterization of an interleukin-1 receptor antagonist protein. *Nature* 1990;**344**:633–8.

358. HANNUM CH, WILCOX CJ, AREND WP, et al. Interleukin-1 receptor antagonist activity of a human inerleukin-1 inhibitor. *Nature* 1990;**343**:336–40.

359. EISENBERG SP, EVANS RJ, AREND WP, et al. Primary structure and functional expression from complementary DNA of a human interleukin-1 receptor antagonist. *Nature* 1990;**343**:341–6.

360. AREND WP, JOSLIN FG, THOMPSON RC, HANNUM CH. An IL-1 inhibitor from human monocytes. Production and characterization of biologic properties. *J Immunol* 1989;**143**:1851–58.

361. GARRETT IR, BLACK KS, MUNDY GR. Interactions between interleukin-6 and interleukin-1 in osteoclastic bone resorption in neonatal mouse calvariae. *Calcif Tissue Int* 1990;**46**:(*Suppl 2*):140.

362. SECKINGER P, KLEIN-NULEND J, ALANDER C, THOMPSON RC, DAYER J-M, RAISZ LG. Natural and recombinant human IL-1 receptor antagonists block the effects of IL-1 on bone resorption and prostaglandin production. *J Immunol* 1990;**145**:4181–4.

# 5

# Physical and Chemical Methods to Optimize Pulpal and Periodontal Healing After Traumatic Injuries

M. Trope

When a tooth suffers a traumatic injury, a variable degree of damage will occur to the periodontal structures as well as the neurovascular bundle at the root apex (1). Under all circumstances the first reaction to a trauma will be an inflammatory process. If this process is minimal, healing of the PDL will take place without resorption (*normal healing*) which is considered a *favorable healing.*

If the root surface damage and subsequent inflammation are of sufficient intensity, root resorption will result through osteoclastic activity (2) (Fig. 5.1). Under most circumstances, this resorption will be transient with spontaneous healing resulting in *surface resorption with cemental repair (repair related resorption)*; this healing is also considered *favorable.*

If a continual stimulus is present e.g. if the pulp canal becomes infected or sulcular infection corresponds to an affected root surface, no healing takes place and the active inflammatory resorption will continue until the entire root is lost. This will be referred to as *infection-related resorption* (see Chapter 2, p. 80) (Fig. 5.2).

The type of healing that occurs after the initial inflammation subsides is also (apart from the pulp condition) dependent on the surface area of root that is damaged. If the surface area of damaged root is small, the surviving cementoblasts that surround the area will produce new cementum and periodontal ligament in time to cover the denuded area and result in the above mentioned surface resorption with cemental repair which can be considered a favorable healing. This type of healing is favorable or cemental healing (2) (see Chapter 2, p. 80) (Fig. 5.3).

If on the other hand, the damage to the root covers a large surface area, bone producing cells will attach directly onto the root before the area can be healed by new cementum. When the bone has attached directly to the root it undergoes physiologic turnover comprising resorption and apposition. The osteoclasts have little difficulty resorbing dentin;

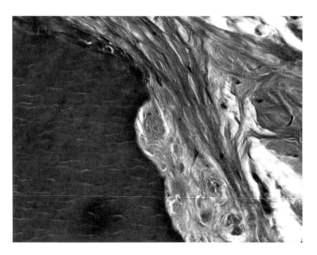

**Fig. 5.1** Multinucleated osteoclasts are formed in reaction to the damage to the root caused by the traumatic injury and are now resorbing the root.

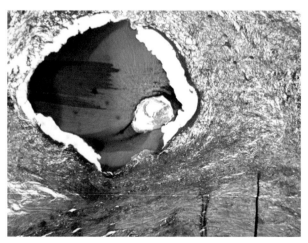

**Fig. 5.2** Infection related inflammatory root resorption that has destroyed almost the entire root.

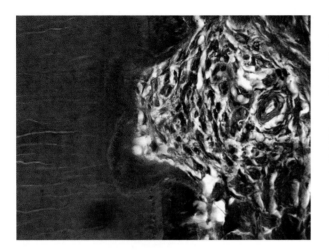

**Fig. 5.3** Favorable healing. The inflammatory root resorption has stopped and the denuded root surface is covered with cementoblasts and new cementum.

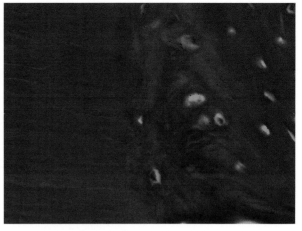

**Fig. 5.4** Unfavorable healing with osseous replacement. Bone has attached directly to the root surface. In time the osteoclasts will resorb the dentin and osteoblasts will lay down new bone. In this way the root dentin will be replaced by bone.

however in the apposition stage, bone (rather than dentin) is formed and thus the root is slowly replaced by bone. This osseous replacement is obviously an *unfavorable healing* outcome. It has been termed *osseous replacement resorption* in Chapter 2 (2) (Fig. 5.4) (see also Chapter 2, p. 80).

Therefore in order to optimize healing after a traumatic injury it is essential to ensure that the surface area of root damage is as small as possible. It is not possible to control the physical damage to the root surface due to the trauma itself. However, if the initial inflammatory response after the injury can be minimized, additional 'secondary' root damage will be limited thus promoting cemental (favorable) healing. Also it is essential to ensure that the pulp canal does not become infected and act as a continuous stimulus for inflammatory root resorption. Thus the treatment objective after a traumatic injury is to limit active inflammation immediately after the injury and to prevent or treat pulpal infection (2, 3). In addition attempts have been made to stimulate cemental healing so as to aid in favorable healing (4, 5). In this chapter a series of experiments will be shown demonstrating the effect of physical and chemical methods to optimize healing. In this regard the above mentioned distinction of healing types has been made. In a few studies an alternative classification has been used dividing healing into two groups:

- Favorable healing
  — Normal healing (without root resorption)
  — Suface resorption with cemental repair (repair-related resorption)
- Unfavorable healing
  — Osseous replacement resorption (ankylosis)
  — Infection related resorption.

When the experimental results are evaluated the major interest will naturally be the proportion of the root surface showing favorable healing. Osseous replacement resorption can be an acceptable healing in adults, especially if the extent of the ankylosis is rather limited. Inflammatory root

resorption cannot be regarded as a healing process but a pathologic infection related condition which will transfer either into favorable or unfavorable healing when the infection is treated.

## Treatment strategies

### Accident site

The best healing results are obtained if the traumatized tooth is returned to its original position as soon as possible. The sooner this is achieved the better the prognosis (6–8). Most luxated teeth require repositioning. This should be performed as gently as possible so as to limit additional trauma.

Avulsed teeth pose a unique challenge. The damage to the cemental layer/periodontal ligament when a tooth is avulsed is usually not extensive since in most cases the periodontal ligament tears leaving viable cells on the root surface that are capable of healing (Fig. 5.5).

In fact the damaged root surface usually covers a small surface area with a good potential for favorable healing. The potential danger for unfavorable healing in an avulsed tooth is if the periodontal ligament cells on the root surface dry out and die before replantation (2, 6, 8, 9). The dead cells will then act as potent inflammatory stimulators on replantation. Therefore dry time must be kept to a minimum.

Strategies at the accident site to limit the inflammatory potential of the root periodontal ligament are:

- **Physical**: Gently wash the root surface of gross debris with tap water (Fig. 5.6) or sterile saline if the tooth is to be replanted immediately (2, 10).
- **Chemical**: If the tooth cannot be replanted immediately it should be placed in an appropriate storage medium until it can be replanted. Dry time must be avoided. Acceptable media include physiological saline, milk or the patient's

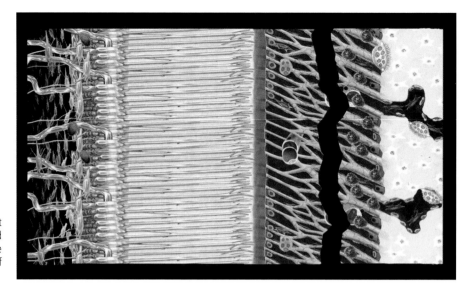

**Fig. 5.5** After an avulsion injury most of the external root surface is covered with periodontal ligament fibers since the avulsion occurs due to tearing of the periodontal ligament.

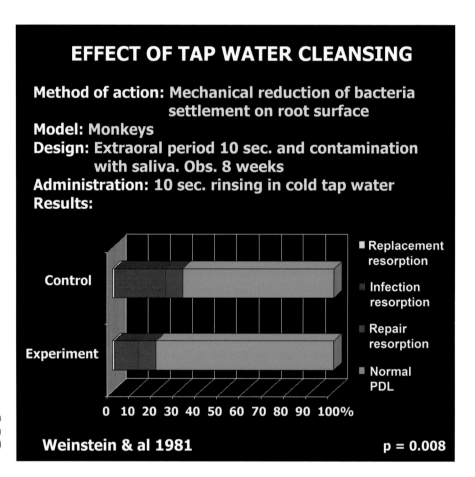

# EFFECT OF TAP WATER CLEANSING

**Method of action: Mechanical reduction of bacteria settlement on root surface**
**Model: Monkeys**
**Design: Extraoral period 10 sec. and contamination with saliva. Obs. 8 weeks**
**Administration: 10 sec. rinsing in cold tap water**
**Results:**

- Replacement resorption
- Infection resorption
- Repair resorption
- Normal PDL

Control

Experiment

0  10  20  30  40  50  60  70  80  90  100%

**Weinstein & al 1981**                                    p = 0.008

**Fig. 5.6** Effect of saline cleansing on PDL healing after replantation in monkeys. After WEINSTEIN et al. (10) 1981.

saliva (in cheek, under tongue or in a cup with patient's spit). These media can keep the periodontal ligament cells viable for healing for about 2 hours (6, 11, 12). Hanks Balanced Salt Solution (HBSS) if available at the accident site may extend the extra oral period to up to 8 hours (13, 14). In special circumstances, such as possible neurological damage or a life threatening accident, storage media e.g. Viaspan® can be used to retain a periodontal ligament viable for healing for longer periods (14) (see later). Since in the majority of cases the accident occurs near the home or school, milk appears to be the most appropriate and popular storage medium.

## Emergency dental visit

At this visit minimizing the external inflammatory root resorption due to the traumatic injury and promoting cemental regeneration is the focus. Pulp space infection is a slower process and is the focus of later visits.

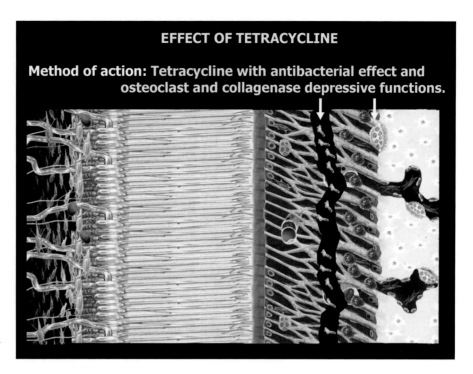

**EFFECT OF TETRACYCLINE**

**Method of action: Tetracycline with antibacterial effect and osteoclast and collagenase depressive functions.**

**Fig. 5.7** Possible ways that tetracycline may optimize PDL healing.

## General strategies

### Physical

If the tooth is in the socket (luxation injury or replanted at the accident site) its positioning should be checked. If repositioning is required it should be performed as atraumatically as possible.

In an intruded tooth the practitioner may chose to allow for spontaneous re-eruption depending on the stage of root development (15) (see Chapter 16).

If the tooth has been avulsed the root should be soaked in physiologic saline or HBSS while the history and examination are performed so as to flush debris and dead cells off the root surface (14, 16).

The tooth is retained in position using a physiologic splint. A physiologic rather than rigid splint has been shown to favor cemental healing (15, 17). The movement of the tooth is thought to break up ankylotic areas on the root surface which are then replaced by cementum and periodontal ligament.

### Chemical

There has been extensive research done in order to chemically prepare the root to promote favorable healing or in situations where favorable healing is not possible to slow down the osseous replacement of the root. The strategies employed are dependent upon the extent of the injury to the root surface and/or the potential for repair at the time of replantation and/or repositioning. Obviously a tooth that has undergone a luxation injury without avulsion cannot have the root surface treated. Therefore most of the strategies described will be relevant only for the avulsed tooth. After an avulsion injury deleterious effects occur to the peri-

odontal ligament very quickly. Recent clinical research has shown that after approximately 20 minutes dry time some degree of unfavorable healing is expected (7, 8). However, most of the research into the beneficial effects of anti-inflammatory or anti-resorptive procedures has been performed on roots that have been dry for 60 minutes or more. It is assumed (although not proven) that medicaments that are beneficial after 60 minutes dry time will be beneficial after shorter dry periods as well.

### Mature tooth – short (<20 minutes) extra-oral dry time

After the tooth has been soaked in physiologic saline or HBSS while the history and examination has taken place these teeth should be replanted and splinted as soon as possible.

### Mature tooth – intermediate (20 to 60 minutes) extra-oral dry time

A number of medicaments have been studied in order to minimize the initial inflammation after replantation by soaking the root surface.

#### Tetracycline

Tetracyclines are antibacterial and have proven anti-resorptive properties. It has been theorized that by soaking the tooth in the tetracycline antibiotic the reduction in bacteria on the root surface would decrease the potential for inflammation and in addition the anti-resorptive actions would limit the area of root surface damaged thus promoting favorable healing by the process already described (Figs 5.7, 5.9). Tetracyclines exert their antimicrobial activity by inhibiting protein synthesis, are broad-spectrum antibiotics

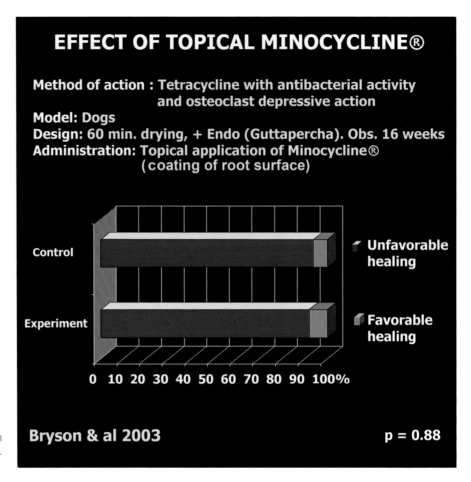

## EFFECT OF TOPICAL MINOCYCLINE®

**Method of action : Tetracycline with antibacterial activity
and osteoclast depressive action**

**Model: Dogs**
**Design: 60 min. drying, + Endo (Guttapercha). Obs. 16 weeks**
**Administration: Topical application of Minocycline®
(coating of root surface)**

Control

Experiment

0  10 20 30 40 50 60 70 80 90 100%

⏴ **Unfavorable
healing**

⏴ **Favorable
healing**

**Bryson & al 2003**                              **p = 0.88**

**Fig. 5.8** Effect of minocycline® upon
PDL healing after replantation in dogs.
After BRYSON et al. (22) 2003.

providing action against anaerobes and facultative organisms. They provide bactericidal action at the high concentration occurring with local delivery of the drug (18).

Tetracyclines are substantive due to their hard tissue binding capability and also have an innate anti-resorptive action. They have the ability to bind to the tooth surface and then be slowly released in active form (19). Tetracyclines also promote fibroblast and connective tissue attachment, enhancing regeneration of periodontal attachment lost to pathologic processes (20). Tetracyclines inhibit collagenase activity and osteoclast function (21), which could be beneficial to a replanted tooth. Their effects on the osteoclasts include diminished acid production, decreased ruffled border area, and decreased adhesive properties, all of which inhibit bone resorption. Despite these effects, Bryson et al. (2003) in endodontically treated dogs teeth dried for 60 minutes were not able to show a beneficial effect of soaking the tooth in minocycline for 60 minutes (22) (Fig. 5.8).

Ma and Sae-Lim (2003) in monkey teeth dried for 60 minutes showed an increase in normal periodontal healing after soaking the roots in minocycline (23) (Fig. 5.9). However, there was no decrease in osseous replacement in the experimental teeth. Thus, the favorable healing occurred by decreasing the inflammatory root resorption. Since the teeth were not endodontically treated as in the Bryson study it can be assumed that the effect was due to an inhibition of bacteria from the root canal space. Since in the clinical situation these teeth would be root treated, it is assumed that

the effect would be similar to the Bryson study, where root treatment was performed on the teeth. Here, too, little effect of enhancing favorable healing would be seen. *Thus, these studies were not able to validate the use of this method after an avulsion injury.* Further research needs to be performed in roots where the dry time is less than 60 minutes.

### Corticosteroids

Glucocorticosteroids have been widely used to reduce the deleterious effects of inflammatory responses. They have been reported to reduce and block the expression of macrophage activation, thus affecting IL-1, TNFα, IL-6 and prostaglandin production (24). These effects have been attributed to inhibition at the transcriptional level of processes leading to the complex events of macrophage activation (24). Long-term systemic administration of dexamethasone is known to reduce skeletal bone mass. Nevertheless, its local administration has been shown to reduce osteoclastic bone resorption. Several mechanisms have been reported for this effect, including reduction of the number of osteoclasts by direct receptor mediated and specific toxicity to these cells (25, 26) and enhancement of calcitonin receptors on these cells, making them more responsive to the existing systemic concentration of hormone whose main function is to reduce bone resorptive activity (Fig. 5.10). This up-regulation is also steroid-receptor mediated and is effective at the transcriptional level (27, 28).

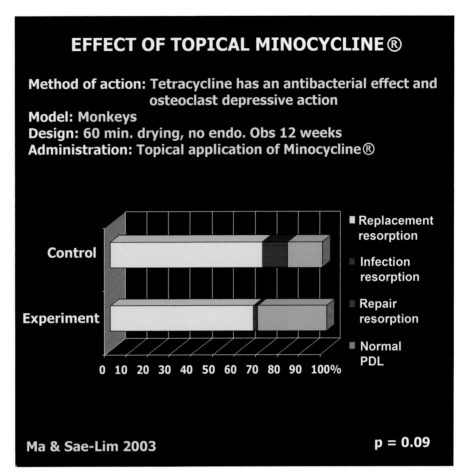

**Fig. 5.9** Effect of minocycline® upon PDL healing after replantation in monkeys. After MA & SAE-LIM (23) 2003.

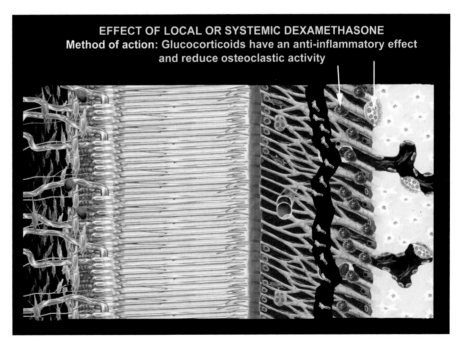

**Fig. 5.10** Possible effect of local or systemic dexamethasone.

Sae-Lim et al. (1998) found that in dogs the topical (and not systemic) application of corticosteroids had a beneficial effect on the production of favorable healing (29). In this experiment the teeth had been stored in a wet medium for 48 hours (Fig. 5.11). The beneficial effect of the corticos-teroid was presumably due to its ability to locally shut down the inflammatory response thus limiting the damage to the root surface. The reason that dexamethasone was ineffective systemically is subject to speculation. It may not have been adequately absorbed in time or may not have reached a

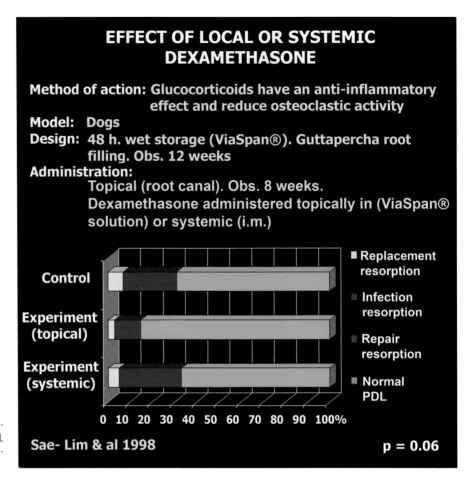

**Fig. 5.11** Effect of topical and systemic dexamethosone upon PDL healing after replantation. After SAE-LIM et al. (29) 1998.

concentration in the periodontal space that was adequate to shut down the inflammation.

### Alendronate

Alendronate (ALN) is currently being used to inhibit pathologic osteoclast-mediated hard tissue resorption in disease states such as osteoporosis, Paget's disease, and osteolytic malignancies of bone (57). The affinity of ALN for calcium phosphate and its tenacious binding to hydroxyapatite lead to a rapid uptake into the skeleton (30). Once incorporated into the skeleton, the terminal half-life of ALN activity has been determined to be as high as 1000 days in dogs (31). The mechanism of osteoclast inhibition has been attributed to a decrease in osteoclast activity with minimal effects on recruitment (58), the interference of receptors on the osteoclasts for specific bone matrix proteins (32), promoting the production of an osteoclast-inhibitor by osteoblasts which reduces the lifespan and/or the number of differentiated osteoclasts (59), and the obstruction of resorption by interfering with the ruffled border of the osteoclast (57) (Fig. 5.12). Most importantly, the inhibitory effect of ALN on osteoclasts is widely recognized and is currently used therapeutically in the osteoclast-mediated disease states previously mentioned (57). Dog roots soaked in HBSS followed by alendronate had statistically significantly more healing than the roots soaked in HBSS without alendronate (30% vs.11%) (33). This was true for roots dried for 40 or 60 minutes (Fig. 5.13). Soaking in alendronate also resulted in significantly less loss in root mass due to resorption compared to those teeth soaked in HBSS without alendronate.

### Calcitonin

Calcitonin is a hormone secreted by the parafollicular cells of the thyroid gland and is known to cause contraction of osteoclasts and inhibit their activity (see Chapter 4, p. 149) (Fig. 5.14). Topical use of calcitonin (placed in the root canal) has been found to be effective in controlling inflammation related to root resorption (Fig. 5.15) (70).

### Emdogain® (enamel matrix protein)

Emdogain® has been shown to promote periodontal ligament proliferation. Enamel matrix molecules are inductive for acellular cementum formation on traumatized root surfaces. The progenitor cell pool for repopulating the root surface is thought to be the remaining vital cells on the root surface, undifferentiated cells from the marrow and progenitor cells from the socket. Trope et al. have shown that the socket environment plays an important role in the healing of replanted teeth (34) suggesting that the periodontal

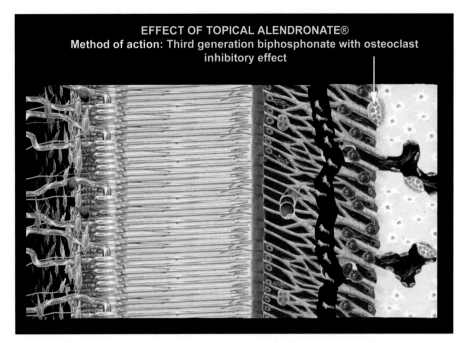

**Fig. 5.12** Possible ways that a biphosphonate may optimize PDL healing.

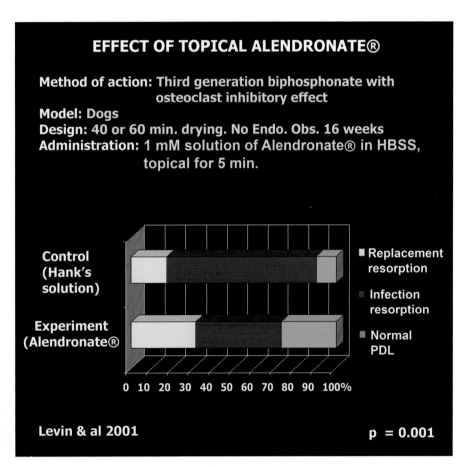

**Fig. 5.13** Effect of topical biphosphonate upon PDL healing after replantation in dogs. After LEVIN et al. (33) 2001.

ligament cells on the socket wall may be important progenitor cells for Emdogain® (Fig. 5.16).

Once the PDL has been destroyed due to avulsion, the cell surface can be repopulated by cementum derived cells or with osteogenic cells from the marrow.

It is optimal to repopulate the surface with PDL or cementum-derived cells. Guided tissue regeneration techniques are designed to facilitate cell-specific repopulation. Barrier techniques can inhibit competition between marrow-derived cells and cementum-derived cells to favor

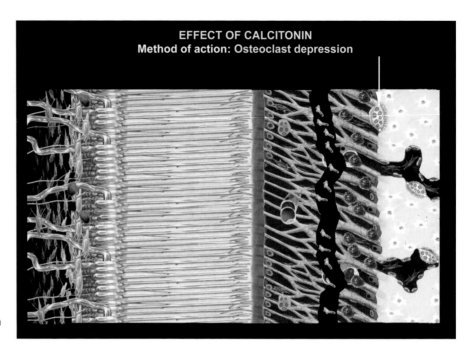

**Fig. 5.14** Possible ways calcitonin may optimize PDL healing.

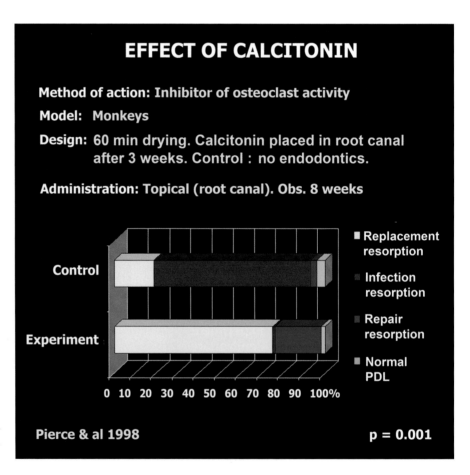

**Fig. 5.15** Effect of topical placed calcitonin (root canal) upon PDL healing. After PIERCE et al. (70) 1988.

the latter. Thus, a lower number of seeding cells would be required to repopulate the root surface. The prognosis may, therefore, be improved for teeth with longer extraoral times.

Emdogain® was shown in a study by Igbal and Bamaas (2001) to almost double the favorable healing in dogs teeth dried for 60 minutes (5) (Fig. 5.17).

Araujo et al. (2003) failed to show a benefit in healing after soaking roots in Emdogain® (35) (Fig. 5.18).

There have been numerous case reports in which Emdogain® was used after extended dry times. It is obvious from these reports that while the use of Emdogain® slowed down the osseous replacement it was not able to reconstitute the

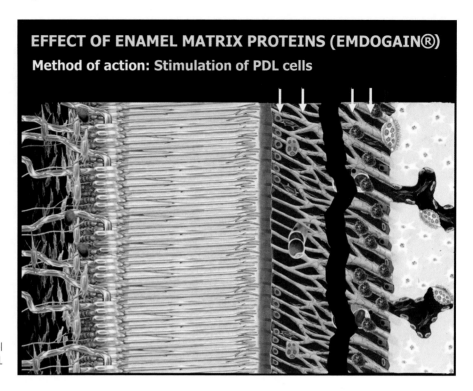

**Fig. 5.16** Possible ways that enamel matrix proteins may optimize PDL healing.

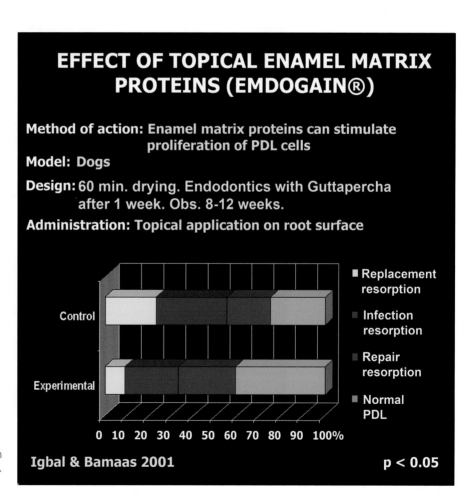

**Fig. 5.17** Effect of Emdogain® upon PDL healing in dogs after replantation. After IQBAL & BAMAAS (5) 2001.

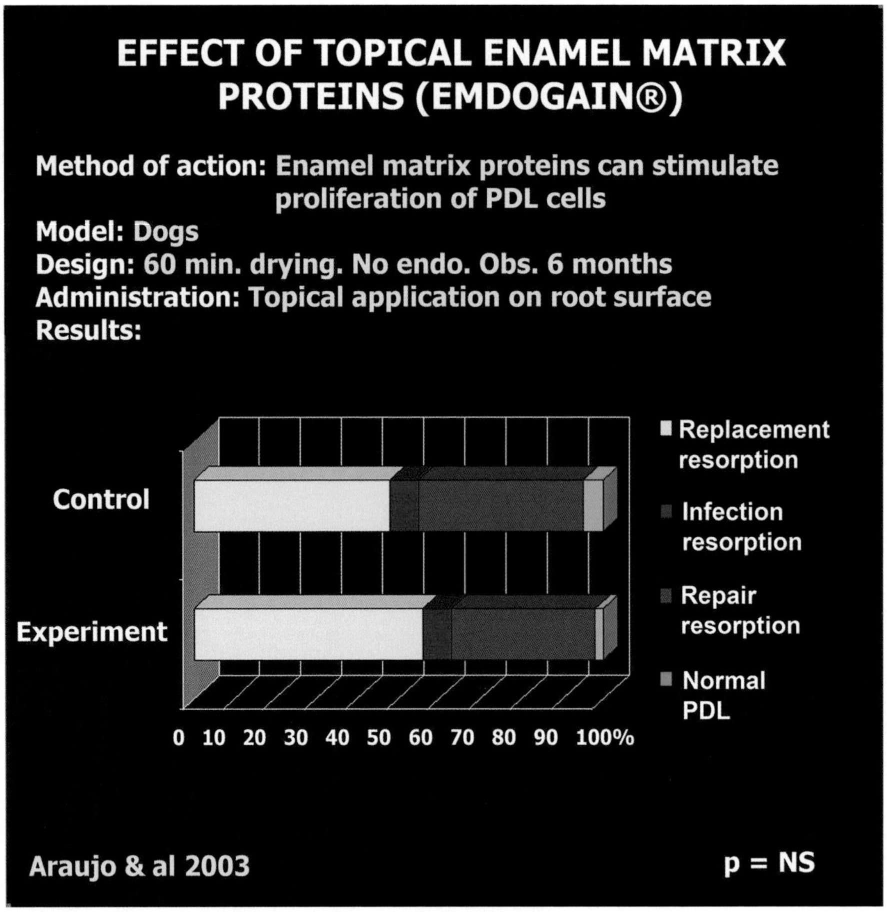

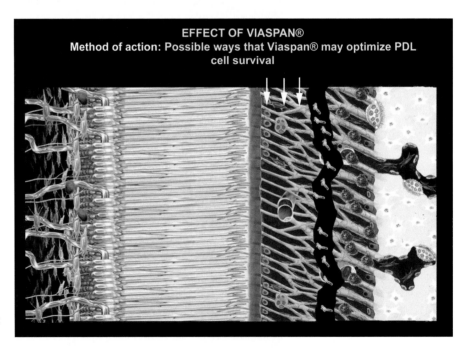

## EFFECT OF TOPICAL ENAMEL MATRIX PROTEINS (EMDOGAIN®)

**Method of action: Enamel matrix proteins can stimulate proliferation of PDL cells**

**Model: Dogs**
**Design: 60 min. drying. No endo. Obs. 6 months**
**Administration: Topical application on root surface**
**Results:**

Control

Experiment

0 10 20 30 40 50 60 70 80 90 100%

■ Replacement resorption

■ Infection resorption

■ Repair resorption

■ Normal PDL

**Araujo & al 2003**

**p = NS**

**Fig. 5.18** Effect of Emdogain® upon PDL healing after replantation in dogs. After ARAUJO et al. (35) 2003.

### EFFECT OF VIASPAN®
**Method of action: Possible ways that Viaspan® may optimize PDL cell survival**

**Fig. 5.19** Possible ways that ViaSpan® may optimize PDL healing.

periodontal ligament completely (35). Like the other medicaments discussed in this chapter most research has been performed on roots that have been left dry for 60 minutes. These medicaments should be tested at shorter dry times where there is more likelihood of remaining progenitor cells on the root surface.

### Specialized tissue storage medium

ViaSpan® is a storage medium used when transporting livers for transplantation (63) and this medium has been found also to be an excellent storage media for teeth (62) (Fig. 5.19). In a study on dog teeth extraction with varying drying periods, it was found that teeth dried for 45 to 60 minutes

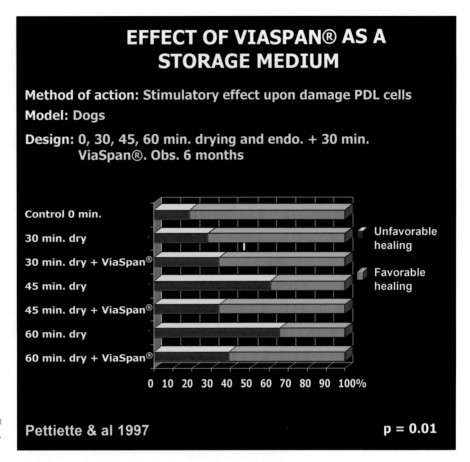

**Fig. 5.20** Effect of ViaSpan® upon PDL healing after replantation in dogs. After PETTIETTE et al. (64) 1997.

showed an improvement in periodontal healing after 30 minutes soaking in ViaSpan® compared to dried replantation after 45 to 60 min. dry storage (64) (Fig. 5.20).

### Slow release anti-inflammatory drugs using the root canal as a reservoir

Exciting experimental results have been obtained recently by placing anti-inflammatory agents inside the root canal so as to achieve a slow and continuous release of the medicaments through the dentinal tubules to the site of osteoclastic activity.

Ledermix® is a water soluble paste containing 1% triamcinolone and 3% demeclocycline. Triamcinolone is a highly active steroid providing potent anti-inflammatory action and demeclocycline is a broad-spectrum antibiotic effective against a large range of Gram positive and Gram negative bacteria. Studies have shown that the active agents in Ledermix® have a rapid initial release followed by a slow steady release. Ledermix® is able to diffuse through dentin and levels of triamcinolone sufficient for anti-inflammatory action have been recorded in the periradicular area. In addition, triamcinolone has been shown to directly inhibit the spreading of dentinoclasts *in vitro* (36–38). Ledermix® has been previously proposed as a medicament to control pulp infection. This procedure is usually delayed until the second visit. The hypothesis in this experiment was that the Ledermix® should be used at the emergency visit so as to use its

anti-inflammatory action when the initial active inflammation occurs (Fig. 5.21).

Bryson et al. (2002) tested the effect of the immediate placement of Ledermix® compared to calcium hydroxide in the pulp canal of dog teeth that had been dried for 60 minutes (39). The Ledermix® treated roots showed 59% favorable healing compared to 14% for the calcium hydroxide group which was not different from the control group (Fig. 5.22). In addition the remaining root structure was significantly more in the Ledermix® treated teeth.

In monkey teeth Wong and Sae-Lim (2002) also found a three-fold favorable healing compared to the control teeth (40) (Fig. 5.23). This high incidence of favorable healing is extremely promising under the conditions of these studies and may constitute a major step forward in the treatment of these types of traumatic injuries.

Pierce and Lindskog (1987) had previously used Ledermix® in the root canals of monkey teeth and did not show a beneficial effect in relation to normal PDL (41) (Fig. 5.24). However, they placed the medicament 3 weeks after the experimental injury when presumably the acute inflammation had subsided and already produced its deleterious effect.

The placement of an anti-inflammatory medicament at the emergency visit is a deviation from previous practice where the root canal was not considered until the second visit. In addition the tetracycline medicament in the Ledermix® has the potential to discolor the tooth. In order to

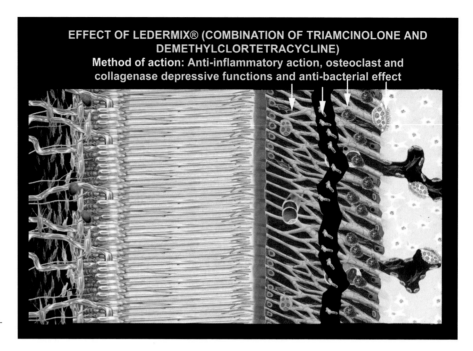

**Fig. 5.21** Possible ways that Ledermix® may optimize PDL healing.

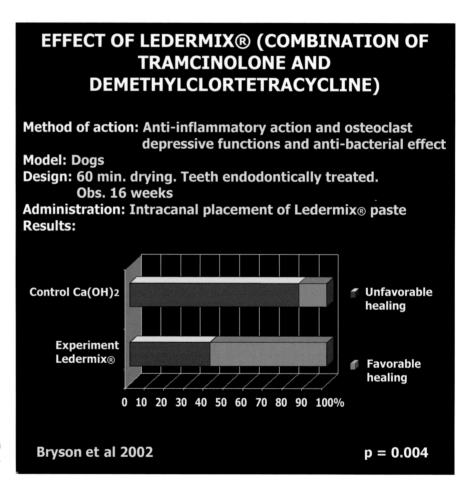

**Fig. 5.22** Effect of Ledermix® upon PDL healing in dogs after replantation. After BRYSON et al. (39) 2002.

address the discoloration potential of the medicament Chen et al. (61) examined the potential for favorable healing when tetracycline and the corticosteroid were placed alone compared to in combination in the Ledermix® medicament. The favorable effect of Ledermix® was confirmed in this experiment. In addition the corticosteroid was shown to have an equally positive effect (Fig. 5.25). Thus it appears that the corticosteroid may be used instead of the Ledermix® negating the discoloration problem when Ledermix® is used.

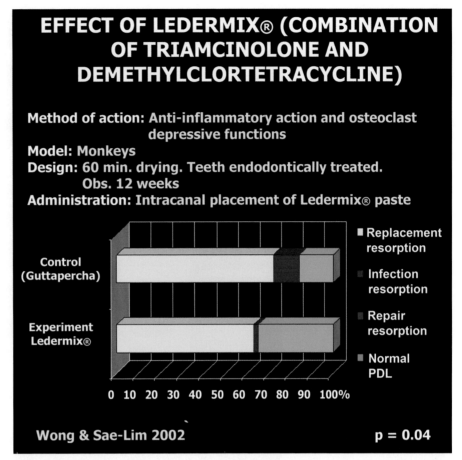

**Fig. 5.23** Effect of Ledermix® upon periodontal healing in monkeys after replantation. After WONG & SAE-LIM (40) 2002.

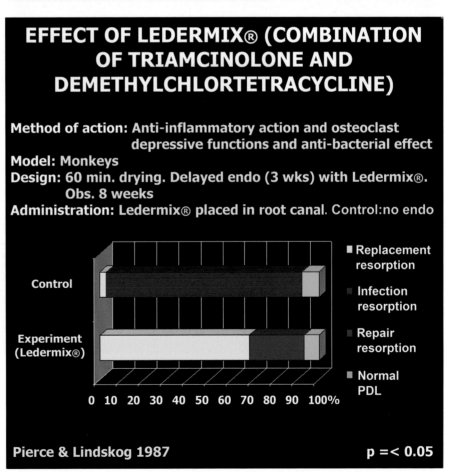

**Fig. 5.24** Effect of Ledermix® upon periodontal healing in monkeys after replantation. After PIERCE & LIND-SKOG (41) 1987.

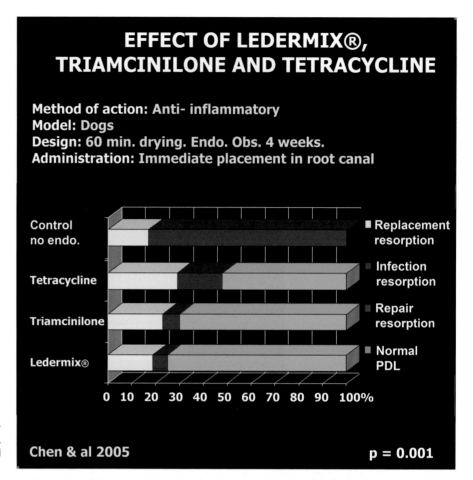

**Fig. 5.25** Effect of Ledermix®, triamcinilone and tetracycline upon PDL healing after replantation. After CHEN et al. (61) 2005.

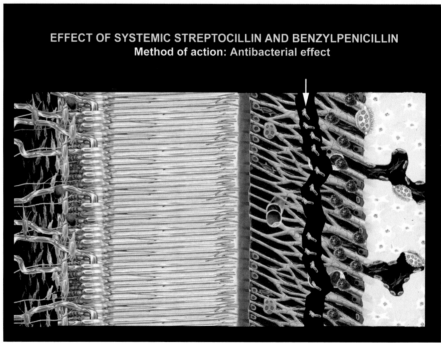

**Fig. 5.26** Effect of antibiotics upon PDL healing after replantation.

## Systemic methods to limit inflammation

As previously discussed the traumatic injury will predictably cause inflammation due to the physical damage on the root surface. In addition if bacteria are able to colonize the root surface an additional inflammatory stimulus is present. The most likely source of bacteria is the external environment at the site of the injury or bacteria from the mouth that migrate down the blood clot that forms in the periodontal ligament (Fig. 5.26).

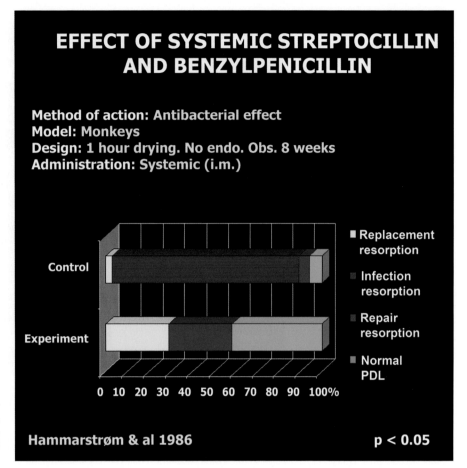

**Fig. 5.27** Effect of systemic streptocillin and benzylpenicillin upon PDL healing after replantation in monkeys. After HAMMARSTRÖM et al. (42) 1986.

Systemic antibiotics have been tested in order to remove socket bacteria that may act as inflammatory stimuli. These are started immediately at the time of repositioning at the emergency visit when the bacterial count and thus the resultant inflammatory response should be highest.

*Penicillin.* Penicillin is the traditional antibiotic used in oral infections and thus logically would appear to be the drug of choice to counteract bacteria within the periodontal space after a traumatic injury (Fig. 5.28).

Hammarström et al. (1986) tested penicillin under two experimental conditions. In the first experiment the root canals were infected in addition to an extra-oral dry time of 60 minutes. In this experiment the use of systemic antibiotic has a marked beneficial effect on healing by eliminating active inflammatory root resorption (42) (Fig. 5.27).

In the second experiment root canal therapy was performed and thus root canal bacteria did not play a role after the 60 minute dry time. Under these circumstances the antibiotic did not have an appreciable effect on the healing results (43) (Fig. 5.28).

Since at the emergency visit periodontal inflammation is unlikely to be present due to pulp space infection, the experiment where endodontic treatment was performed before replantation appears to be more relevant to the emergency visit and the use of systemic penicillin was not shown to be beneficial, a finding supported by a clinical study of avulsed and replanted teeth (7).

*Tetracycline.* As already described tetracyclines have anti-resorptive properties in addition to their anti-bacterial properties. Therefore they may be ideal as a drug to act systemically against bacteria on the root surface and also act against the resorbing osteoclasts.

Sae-Lim et al. (1998) (44, 45) tested systemic doxycycline in similar models to the previous studies performed by Hammarström et al. with penicillin.

When the root canals were infected in roots dried for 60 minutes both doxycycline and amoxicillin showed improved healing compared to the control. The healing with doxycycline was equal to that shown with the amoxicillin (Fig. 5.29). Thus it appears that the antibacterial effect of the tetracycline was similar to that of the penicillin drugs used by the Hammarström group (42, 45).

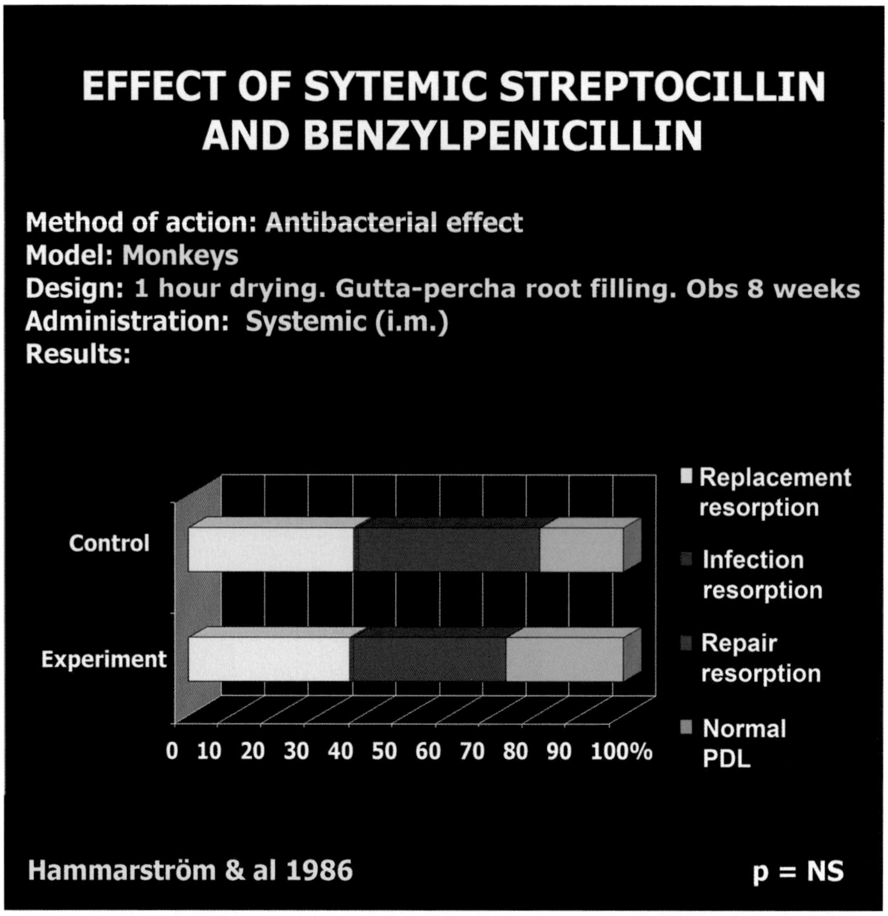

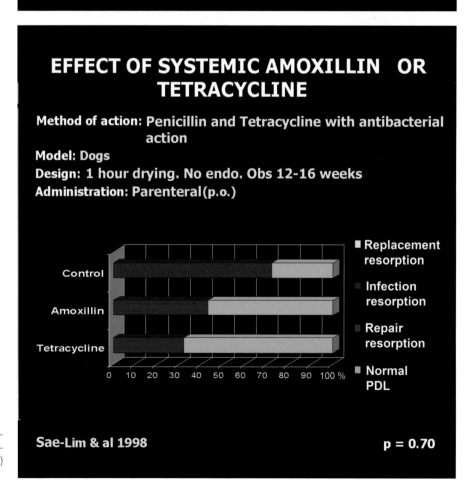

**Fig. 5.28** Effect of streptocillin and benzylpenicillin upon PDL healing after replantation in monkeys. After HAMMARSTRÖM et al. (42) 1986.

**Fig. 5.29** Effect of amoxillin or tetracycline upon PDL healing after replantation in dogs. After SAE-LIM et al. (45) 1998.

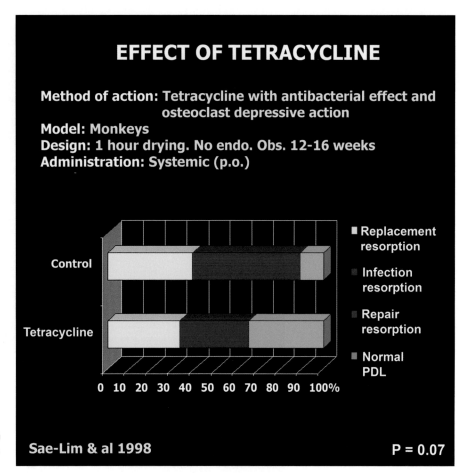

**EFFECT OF TETRACYCLINE**

**Method of action: Tetracycline with antibacterial effect and osteoclast depressive action**
**Model: Monkeys**
**Design: 1 hour drying. No endo. Obs. 12-16 weeks**
**Administration: Systemic (p.o.)**

Sae-Lim & al 1998                                    P = 0.07

**Fig. 5.30** Effect of tetracycline upon PDL healing after replantation in dogs. After SAE-LIM et al. (44) 1998.

However, when the tetracycline antibiotics were tested in the model where 60 minute dried dog teeth were endodontically treated before re-implantation, an almost significant improvement in normal healing was seen compared to the controls (44) (Fig. 5.30). This was presumably due to the anti-resorptive effect of the tetracycline which is not present for the penicillin drugs.

Thus it appears that systemic tetracycline rather than penicillin is the appropriate antibiotic for severe avulsion injuries and should be started at the emergency visit.

### Mature tooth – extra-oral dry time >60 minutes

If a root has been dry for more than 60 minutes the periodontal ligament is not expected to be viable. Thus eventual osseous replacement of the root is inevitable. However, with traumatic injuries particularly in young patients, a slow replacement of the tooth root can be an important benefit compared to a root that is replaced quickly. Therefore, when the practitioner deems that it is worthwhile to keep the tooth, the aim of treatment is to prepare the tooth for as slow a replacement process as possible.

### Fluoride pre-treatment of the root

Since 1968 it has been known that sodium fluoride treatment of the root surface before replantation may decrease the rate of osseous replacement in experimental replanted teeth in monkeys (65) (Fig. 5.31). A study in humans likewise demonstrated a 50% reduction in progression of root resorption after replantation (66). In later experimental studies it was found that a 1% stannous fluoride supplemented with tetracycline had an ankylosis depressing effect; however a long-standing inflammating reaction in the PDL was found (67, 68). In a subsequent study the concentration of stannous fluoride was lowered from 1 to 0.1% which resulted in a significant reduction of inflammation in the PDL (Fig. 5.32) and with a minimal amount of ankylosis. Although this study seems promising it should be considered that the observation period in this experiment was only 4 weeks, an observation period which in similar experiments has been found much too short to exclude later osseous replacement (66). This implies that the concept of sodium fluoride solution (2.4%) is the only tested and useful method to be recommended (66).

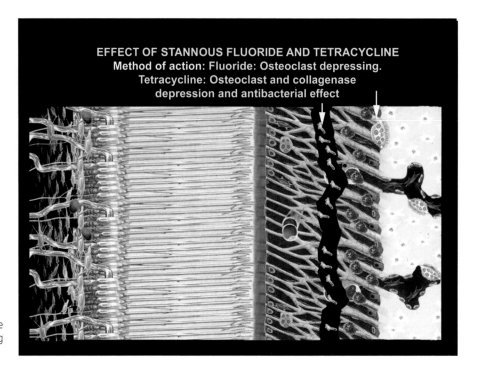

**Fig. 5.31** Effect of stannous fluoride and tetracycline upon PDL healing after replantation.

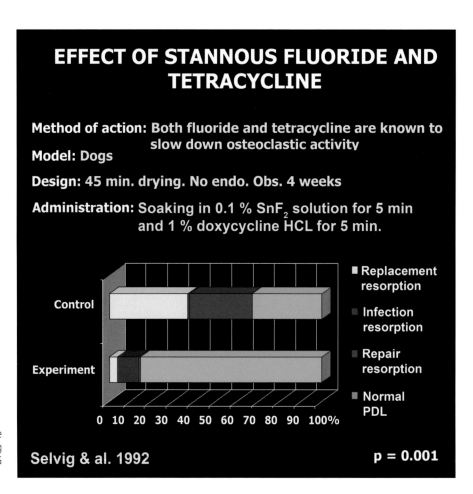

**Fig. 5.32** Effect of stannous fluoride and doxycycline upon PDL healing after replantation in dogs. After SELVIG et al. (60) 1992.

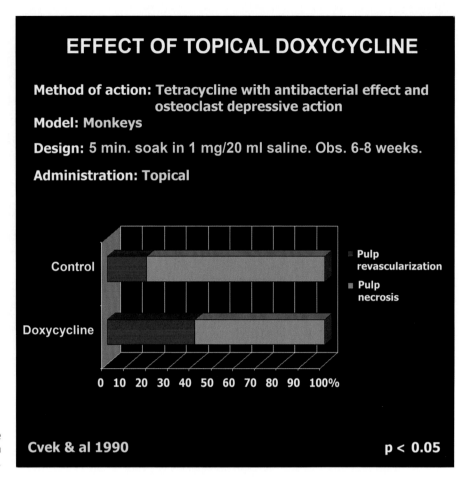

**EFFECT OF TOPICAL DOXYCYCLINE**

**Method of action: Tetracycline with antibacterial effect and osteoclast depressive action**

**Model: Monkeys**

**Design: 5 min. soak in 1 mg/20 ml saline. Obs. 6-8 weeks.**

**Administration: Topical**

Control

Doxycycline

0  10  20  30  40  50  60  70  80  90  100%

■ **Pulp revascularization**

■ **Pulp necrosis**

**Cvek & al 1990**                                                        **p < 0.05**

**Fig. 5.33** Effect of topical doxycycline upon pulp healing after replantation in monkeys. After CVEK et al. (47) 1990.

## Physical methods

Probably the most important action that should be taken in order to slow down the osseous replacement is to remove the dead periodontal ligament cells on the root surface (2, 8, 16). If these cells remain after replantation they will act as potent inflammatory stimulators. In order to remove the remaining cells the root can be soaked in sodium hypochlorite or a weak acid. Some authors have proposed using a periodontal curette to remove the cells. Logically this may not be as good since scraping off the cemental layer would probably allow the resorption to progress at a more rapid rate.

## Chemical methods

### Immature tooth – extra-oral dry time <60 minutes

The luxated or avulsed immature tooth is different from the mature tooth in that the pulp that is necrotic due to the traumatic injury has the possibility for revascularization. Revascularization of an immature tooth is of tremendous benefit in that the root canal walls continue to develop and strengthen and the apex closes, making future endodontic treatment if needed, a more predictable procedure. The less developed the root at the time of injury the greater the potential for revascularization (47–49).

It appears that bacteria on the root surface and particularly at the apical foramen are the reason for failure of revascularization (47). Thus it is essential to limit these bacteria from the accident site and those tracking down the blood clot in the socket.

Doxycycline as discussed has antibacterial and anti-resorptive properties. Cvek et al. (1990) tested the effect of soaking extracted immature monkey teeth in doxycycline before replantation (47). They found that the revascularization rate doubled (18–41%) after the doxycycline soak (Fig. 5.33).

They could not reproduce this effect with systemic doxycycline (Fig. 5.34) (71).

Yanpiset and Trope repeated the Cvek study in dogs and were able to replicate the doubling of healing rates with the use of the doxycycline (30–60%) compared to saline controls (48) (Fig. 5.35).

Recently Ritter et al. (2004) were able to further increase the revascularization rate in dogs with the use of minocycline (50) (Fig. 5.36).

Minocycline is a slow-release tetracycline that has been shown to decrease periodontal bone loss when administered topically. Its slow release action may keep bacteria from

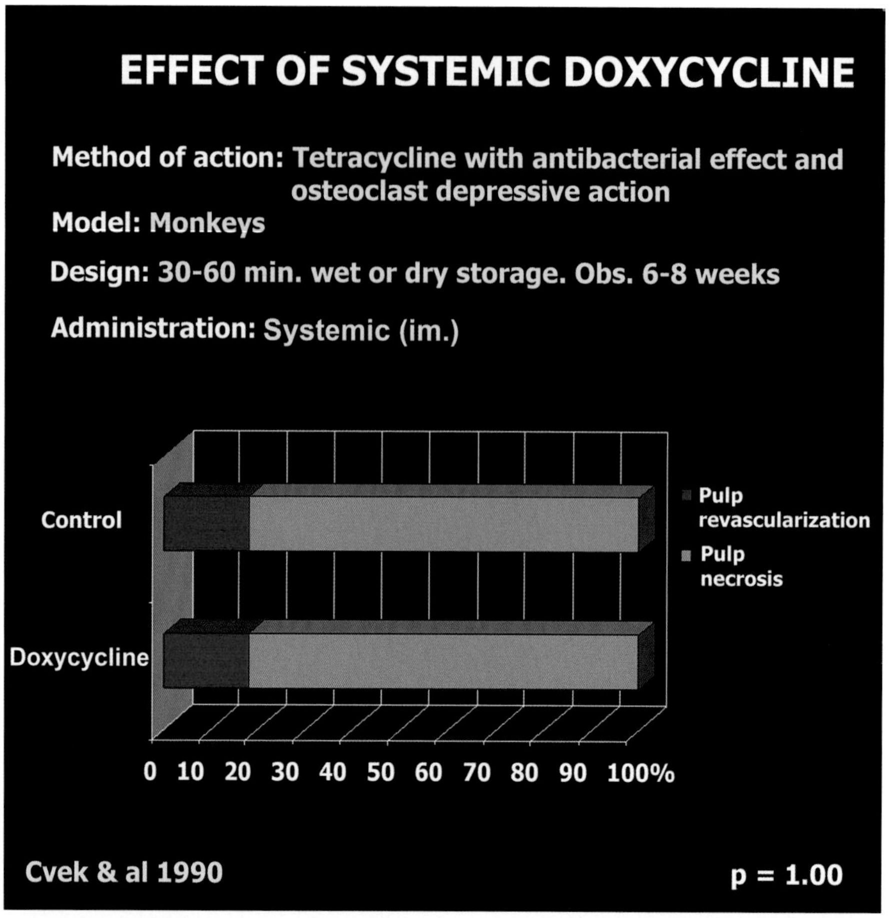

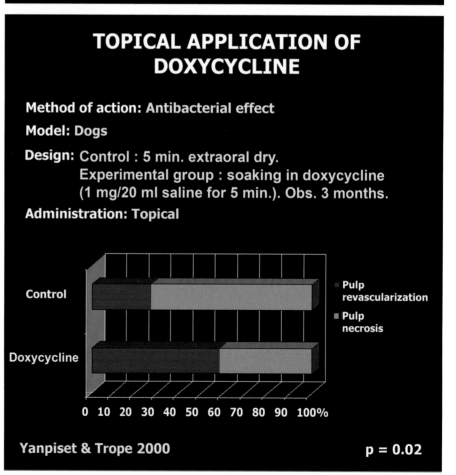

**Fig. 5.34** Effect of systemic doxycycline upon pulp healing after replantation in monkeys. After CVEK et al. (71) 1990.

**Fig. 5.35** Effect of topical application of doxycycline upon pulp healing after replantation in dogs. After YANPISET & TROPE (48) 2000.

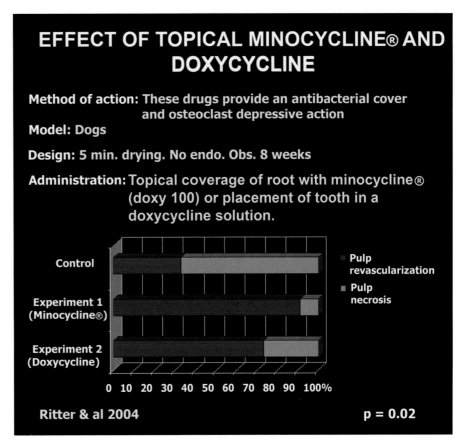

**Fig. 5.36** Effect of topical application of minocycline and tetracycline upon pulp healing in dogs. After RITTER et al. (50) 2004.

entering the pulp space long enough to allow a higher incidence of revascularization than doxycycline, which has a shorter period of action. A number of studies show that the local administration of a 2% minocycline gel is effective in the treatment of periodontitis (51–53).

Minocycline is available in the form of Arestin™ Microspheres (OraPharma, Inc.) which is a sustained release product containing minocycline hydrochloride into a bioabsorbable polymer (polyglycolide-co-DL lactide). The resulting microspheres combine the minocycline and bioabsorbable polymer in a powder form. Immediately upon contact with moisture, the polymer hydrolyzes releasing minocycline. Concentrations of 340 ug of minocycline per ml have been measured in human crevicular fluid after 14 days, exceeding the minimum inhibitory concentrations of many pathogens (54).

### Immature tooth – extra-oral dry time >60 minutes

The benefit of replanting an immature tooth that will definitely be lost due to osseous replacement has been debated; and some authors have concluded that such teeth should not be replanted (see Chapter 17).

In this author's opinion, such teeth can provide a benefit to the young patient while waiting for facial growth to be completed. If the tooth is replanted with the root condi-

tioned similar to the adult tooth with an extended dry time and then submerged it can help to maintain the height and width of the socket for an extended time period (see Chapter 24, p. 703). In some cases this will negate the need for complicated prosthetic reconstruction when facial growth is completed.

## Second visit

The attachment damage due to the traumatic injury and minimizing the subsequent inflammation was the focus of the emergency visit. The second visit should be scheduled 10 to 14 days after the emergency visit. At this visit the focus is on preventing pulp space infection which would sustain active inflammatory root resorption and result in loss of the root structure in a very short period of time (2, 7).

Root canal disinfection removes the stimulus to the periradicular inflammation and the active resorption will stop (55, 56). In most cases a new attachment will form; but if a large area of root is affected, osseous replacement can result by the mechanism already described. Again treatment principles include prevention of pulp space infection or elimination of the bacteria if they are present in the pulp space.

Details of how to achieve the aims described above for the second visit are described in detail in Chapters 22 and 23.

## Essentials

A series of physical and chemical methods have been used experimentally to optimize periodontal and/or pulpal healing after replantation of avulsed teeth. Most are experimental methods that have been validated in animals only and need to be verified in future clinical studies. For treatment guidelines of avulsion see also Chapter 17, Avulsions.

## Summary of experimental findings

### PDL healing

(1) Rinsing of the root surface with tap water for 10 sec before replantation appears to favor PDL healing.
(2) Minimizing dry time and appropriate storage is critical.
(3) 30 minutes extra storage in a tissue storage medium may improve PDL healing after 45 to 60 minutes dry storage.
(4) A combination of triamcinolone and tetracycline or triamcinolone alone placed in the root canal at time of replantation appears to favor PDL healing.
(5) Tetracycline hydrochloride systemically administered appears to favor PDL healing.
(6) Amoxillin systematically administered for 7 days (22 mg/kg) appears to favor PDL healing.
(7) Sodium fluoride, 2.4% used topically for 20 minutes appears to slow down progression of replacement resorption but should only be used in cases with extensive damage to the PDL.

### Pulpal healing

**Immature tooth**
Doxycycline (1 mg/20 ml saline) soaked for 5 minutes or minocyline topically appears to greatly improve the chance of pulp revascularization.

**Mature tooth**
Pulp healing is not possible. Endodontic treatment to prevent pulp space infection is critical.

## References

1. Trope M. Root resorption of dental and traumatic origin: classification based on etiology. *Pract Periodontics Aesthet Dent* 1998;**10**:515–22.
2. Trope M. Clinical management of the avulsed tooth: present strategies and future directions. *Dent Traumatol* 2002;**18**:1–11.
3. Trope M. Root resorption due to dental trauma. *Endodontic Topics* 2002;**1**:79–100.
4. Filippi A, Pohl Y, von Arx T. Treatment of replacement resorption with Emdogain – preliminary results after 10 months. *Dent Traumatol* 2001;**17**:134–8.
5. Iqbal MK, Bamaas N. Effect of enamel matrix derivative (EMDOGAIN) upon periodontal healing after replantation of permanent incisors in beagle dogs. *Dent Traumatol* 2001;**17**:36–45.
6. Andreasen JO. Effect of extra-alveolar period and storage media upon periodontal and pulpal healing after replantation of mature permanent incisors in monkeys. *Int J Oral Surg* 1981;**10**:43–53.
7. Andreasen JO, Borum MK, Jacobsen HL, Andreasen FM. Replantation of 400 avulsed permanent incisors. 4. Factors related to periodontal ligament healing. *Endod Dent Traumatol* 1995;**11**:76–89.
8. Barrett EJ, Kenny DJ. Avulsed permanent teeth: a review of the literature and treatment guidelines. *Endod Dent Traumatol* 1997;**13**:153–63.
9. Trope M. Luxation injuries and external root resorption – etiology, treatment, and prognosis. *J Calif Dent Assoc* 2000;**28**:860–6.
10. Weinstein FM, Worsaae N, Andreasen JO. The effect on the periodontal and pulpal tissues of various cleansing procedures prior to replantation of extracted teeth. An experimental study in monkeys. *Acta Odontol Scand* 1981;**39**:251–5.
11. Blomlöf L. Milk and saliva as possible storage media for traumatically exarticulated teeth prior to replantation. *Swed Dent J Suppl* 1981;**8**:1–26.
12. Blomlöf L, Lindskog S, Andersson L, Hedström KG, Hammarström L. Storage of experimentally avulsed teeth in milk prior to replantation. *J Dent Res* 1983;**62**:912–6.
13. Hiltz J, Trope M. Vitality of human lip fibroblasts in milk, Hanks balanced salt solution and Viaspan storage media. *Endod Dent Traumatol* 1991;**7**:69–72.
14. Trope M, Friedman S. Periodontal healing of replanted dog teeth stored in Viaspan, milk and Hank's balanced salt solution. *Endod Dent Traumatol* 1992;**8**:183–8.
15. Andreasen JO. The effect of splinting upon periodontal and pulpal healing after replantation of permanent incisors in monkeys. *Acta Odontol Scand* 1975;**33**:313–23.
16. Lindskog S, Pierce AM, Blomlöf L, Hammarström L. The role of the necrotic periodontal membrane in cementum resorption and ankylosis. *Endod Dent Traumatol* 1985;**1**:96–101.
17. Andersson L, Friskopp J, Blomlöf L. Fiber-glass splinting of traumatized teeth. *ASDC J Dent Child* 1983;**50**:21–4.
18. Greenstein G, Polson A. The role of local drug delivery in the management of periodontal diseases: a comprehensive review. *J Periodontol* 1998;**69**:507–20.
19. Baker PEA. Tetracycline and its derivatives strongly bind to and are released from the tooth surface in an active form. *J Periodontol* 1983;**54**:580–6.
20. Terranova VEA. A biochemical approach to periodontal regeneration: tetracycline treatment of dentin promotes fibroblast adhesion and growth. *J Periodont Res* 1986;**21**:330–7.
21. Golub LM, Ramamurthy NS, McNamara TF, Greenwald RA, Rifkin BR. Tetracyclines inhibit connective tissue breakdown: new therapeutic implications for an old family of drugs. *Crit Rev Oral Biol Med* 1991;**2**:297–321.

22. BRYSON EC, LEVIN L, BANCHS F, TROPE M. Effect of minocycline on healing of replanted dog teeth after extended dry times. *Dent Traumatol* 2003; **19**:90–5.

23. MA KM, SAE-LIM V. The effect of topical minocycline on replacement resorption of replanted monkeys' teeth. *Dent Traumatol* 2003;**19**:96–102.

24. LINDEN M, BRATTSAND R. Effects of a corticosteroid, budesonide, on alveolar macrophage and blood monocyte secretion of cytokines: differential sensitivity of GM-CSF, IL-1 beta, and IL-6. *Pulm Pharmacol* 1994;**7**:43–7.

25. TOBIAS J, CHAMBERS TJ. Glucocorticoids impair bone resorptive activity and viability of osteoclasts disaggregated from neonatal rat long bones. *Endocrinology* 1989;**125**:1290–5.

26. DEMPSTER DW, MOONGA BS, STEIN LS, HORBERT WR, ANTAKLY T. Glucocorticoids inhibit bone resorption by isolated rat osteoclasts by enhancing apoptosis. *J Endocrinol* 1997;**154**:397–406.

27. WADA S, UDAGAWA N, AKATSU T, NAGATA N, MARTIN TJ, FINDLAY DM. Regulation by calcitonin and glucocorticoids of calcitonin receptor gene expression in mouse osteoclasts. *Endocrinology* 1997;**138**:521–9.

28. WADA S, YASUDA S, NAGAI T, MAEDA T, KITAHAMA S, SUDA S, et al. Regulation of calcitonin receptor by glucocorticoid in human osteoclast-like cells prepared *in vitro* using receptor activator of nuclear factor-kappaB ligand and macrophage colony-stimulating factor. *Endocrinology* 2001;**142**:1471–8.

29. SAE-LIM V, METZGER Z, TROPE M. Local dexamethasone improves periodontal healing of replanted dogs' teeth. *Endod Dent Traumatol* 1998;**14**:232–6.

30. FLEISCH H. Bisphosphonates in osteoporosis: an introduction. *Osteoporos Int* 1993;**3**:(Suppl 3): S3–5.

31. LIN JH, DUGGAN DE, CHEN IW, ELLSWORTH RL. Physiologic disposition of alendronate, a potent anti-osteolytic bisphosphonate, in laboratory animals. *Drug Metab Dispos* 1991;**19**:926–32.

32. COLUCCI S EA. Alendronate reduces adhesion of human osteoclast-like cells to bone and bone protein-coated surfaces. *Calcif Tissue Int* 1998;**63**:230–5.

33. LEVIN L, BRYSON EC, CAPLAN D, TROPE M. Effect of topical alendronate on root resorption of dried replanted dog teeth. *Dent Traumatol* 2001;**17**:120–6.

34. TROPE M, HUPP JG, MESAROS SV. The role of the socket in the periodontal healing of replanted dogs' teeth stored in ViaSpan for extended periods. *Endod Dent Traumatol* 1997;**13**:171–5.

35. ARAUJO M, HAYACIBARA R, SONOHARA M, CARDAROPOLI G, LINDHE J. Effect of enamel matrix proteins (Emdogain') on healing after re-implantation of 'periodontally compromised' roots. An experimental study in the dog. *J Clin Periodontol* 2003;**30**: 855–61.

36. ABBOTT PV, HUME WR, HEITHERSAY GS. Barriers to diffusion of Ledermix paste in radicular dentine. *Endod Dent Traumatol* 1989;**5**:98–104.

37. ABBOTT PV, HUME WR, HEITHERSAY GS. The release and diffusion through human coronal dentine *in vitro* of triamcinolone and demeclocycline from Ledermix paste. *Endod Dent Traumatol* 1989;**5**:92–7.

38. PIERCE A, HEITHERSAY G, LINDSKOG S. Evidence for direct inhibition of dentinoclasts by a corticosteroid/antibiotic endodontic paste. *Endod Dent Traumatol* 1988;**4**:44–5.

39. BRYSON EC, LEVIN L, BANCHS F, ABBOTT PV, TROPE M. Effect of immediate intracanal placement of Ledermix Paste® on healing of replanted dog teeth after extended dry times. *Dent Traumatol* 2002;**18**:316–21.

40. WONG KS, SAE-LIM V. The effect of intracanal Ledermix on root resorption of delayed-replanted monkey teeth. *Dent Traumatol* 2002;**18**:309–15.

41. PIERCE A, LINDSKOG S. The effect of an antibiotic/corticosteroid paste on inflammatory root resorption *in vivo*. *Oral Surg Oral Med Oral Pathol* 1987;**64**:216–20.

42. HAMMARSTRÖM L, BLOMLÖF L, FEIGLIN B, ANDERSSON L, LINDSKOG S. Replantation of teeth and antibiotic treatment. *Endod Dent Traumatol* 1986;**2**:51–7.

43. HAMMARSTRÖM L, PIERCE A, BLOMLÖF L, FEIGLIN B, LINDSKOG S. Tooth avulsion and replantation – a review. *Endod Dent Traumatol* 1986;**2**:1–8.

44. SAE-LIM V, WANG CY, CHOI GW, TROPE M. The effect of systemic tetracycline on resorption of dried replanted dogs' teeth. *Endod Dent Traumatol* 1998;**14**:127–32.

45. SAE-LIM V, WANG CY, TROPE M. Effect of systemic tetracycline and amoxicillin on inflammatory root resorption of replanted dogs' teeth. *Endod Dent Traumatol* 1998;**14**:216–20.

46. ANDREASEN JO, KRISTERSON L. The effect of limited drying or removal of the periodontal ligament. Periodontal healing after replantation of mature permanent incisors in monkeys. *Acta Odontol Scand* 1981;**39**:1–13.

47. CVEK M, CLEATON-JONES P, AUSTIN J, LOWNIE J, KLING M, FATTI P. Effect of topical application of doxycycline on pulp revascularization and periodontal healing in reimplanted monkey incisors. *Endod Dent Traumatol* 1990;**6**:170–6.

48. YANPISET K, TROPE M. Pulp revascularization of replanted immature dog teeth after different treatment methods. *Endod Dent Traumatol* 2000;**16**:211–7.

49. KLING M, CVEK M, MEJARE I. Rate and predictability of pulp revascularization in therapeutically reimplanted permanent incisors. *Endod Dent Traumatol* 1986;**2**: 83–9.

50. RITTER AL, RITTER AV, MURRAH V, SIGURDSSON A, TROPE M. Pulp revascularization of replanted immature dog teeth after treatment with minocycline and doxycycline assessed by laser Doppler flowmetry, radiography, and histology. *Dent Traumatol* 2004;**20**:75–84.

51. HIRASAWA M, HAYASHI K, TAKADA K. Measurement of peptidase activity and evaluation of effectiveness of administration of minocycline for treatment of dogs with periodontitis. *Am J Vet Res* 2000;**61**:1349–52.

52. THOMAS BS, VARMA BR, BHAT KM. Efficacy of minocycline as a root conditioner in comparison to citric

acid and tetracycline. An *in vitro* evaluation. *Indian J Dent Res* 1999;**10**:69–75.

53. van Steenberghe D, Rosling B, Söder PO, Landry RG, van der Velden U, Timmerman MF, et al. A 15-month evaluation of the effects of repeated subgingival minocycline in chronic adult periodontitis. *J Periodontol* 1999;**70**:657–67.

54. Williams RC, Paquette DW, Offenbacher S, Adams DF, Armitage GC, Bray K, et al. Treatment of periodontitis by local administration of minocycline microspheres: a controlled trial. *J Periodontol* 2001;**72**:1535–44.

55. Trope M, Moshonov J, Nissan R, Buxt P, Yesilsoy C. Short vs. long-term calcium hydroxide treatment of established inflammatory root resorption in replanted dog teeth. *Endod Dent Traumatol* 1995;**11**:124–8.

56. Trope M, Yesilsoy C, Koren L, Moshonov J, Friedman S. Effect of different endodontic treatment protocols on periodontal repair and root resorption of replanted dog teeth. *J Endod* 1992;**18**:492–6.

57. Sato M, Grasser W, Endo N, Akins R, Simmons H, Thompson DD, et al. Bisphosphonate action: aledronate localization in rat bone and effects on osteoclast ultrastructure. *J Clin Invest* 1991;**88**:2095–105.

58. Breuil V, Cosman F, Stein L, et al. Human osteoclast formation and activity *in vitro*: effects of alendronate. *J Bone Min Res* 1998;**13**:1721–29.

59. Vitte C, Fleisch H, Guenther HL. Bisphosphonate induce osteoblast to secrete an inhibitor of osteoclast-mediated resorption. *Endocrinology* 1996;**137**:2324–33.

60. Selvig KA, Bjorvatn K, Bogle GC, Wikesjo UM. Effects of stannous fluoride and tetracycline on periodontal repair after delayed tooth replantation in dogs. *Scan J Dent Res* 1992;**100**:200–203.

61. Chen H, Teixira FB, Ritter AL, Levin L, Trope M. The effect of intracanal anti-inflammatory medicaments on external root resorption of replanted dog teeth after extended extra-oral dry time. Abstract AAE meeting, Dallas 2005.

62. Hiltz J, Trope M. Vitality of human lip fibroblasts in milk, Hank's balanced salt solution and ViaSpan storage media. *Endod Dent Traumatol* 1991;**7**:69–72.

63. Ploeg RJ, Goossens D, Vreugdenhil P, McNulty JF, Southard JH, Belzer FO. Successful 72-hour cold storage kidney preservation with UW solution. *Transplantation* 1988;**46**:196.

64. Pettiette M, Hupp J, Mesaros S, Trope M. Periodontal healing of extracted dog's teeth air-dried for extended periods and soaked in various media. *Endod Dent Traumatol* 1997;**13**:113–18.

65. Shulman LB, Kalis P, Goldhaber P. Fluoride inhibition of tooth-replant root resorption in cebus monkeys. *J Oral Ther Pharmacol* 1998;**4**:331–7.

66. Coccia CT. A clinical investigation of root resorption rates in reimplanted young permanent incisors: A five-year study. *J Endodont* 1980;**6**:413–20.

67. Bjorvatn K, Selvig KA, Klinge B. Effect of tetracycline and SnF$_2$ on root resorption in replanted incisors in dogs. *Scand J Dent Res* 1989;**97**:477–82.

68. Selvig KA, Bjorvatn K, Claffey N. Effect of stannous fluoride and tetracycline on repair after delayed replantation of root-planed teeth in dogs. *Acta Odontol Scand* 1990;**48**:107–12.

69. Barbakow FH, Austin JC, Cleaton-Jones PE. Histologic response of replanted teeth pre-treated with acidulated sodium fluoride. *Oral Surg Oral Med Oral Pathol* 1978;**45**:621–8.

70. Pierce A, Berg JO, Lindskog S. Calcitonin as an alternative therapy in the treatment of root resorption. *J Endodont* 1988;**14**:459–64.

71. Cvek M, Cleaton-Jones P, Austin J, Lownie J, Kling M, Fatti P. Pulp revascularization in reimplanted immature monkey incisors – predictability and the effect of antibiotic systemic prophylaxis. *Endod Dent Traumatol* 1990;**6**:157–69.

# 6

# Socio-Psychological Aspects of Traumatic Dental Injuries

W. Marcenes & U. Rydå

## Introduction

Facial esthetics play an important role in self-identification, self-image, self-presentation and interpersonal confidence (1). Furthermore, they affect social behavior (2). Therefore, in most cultures, the face is regarded as the most salient characteristic of one's identity (1). Facially unattractive people tend to be less liked, less preferred as friends and less desirable as 'dates' and marriage partners, less trustworthy, less intelligent, less successful, more aggressive, and more antisocial (3–6). The combined effect of these factors disrupts normal social role functioning and brings about a major impact on quality of daily life due to their cumulative effect. There is a clear chain of risk from being unattractive, which may lead to poor educational performance, which in turn may reduce job prospects later in life. Taken together, these factors will significantly reduce mating chances.

The mouth is of primary importance in determining overall facial attractiveness (Fig. 6.1). The features more commonly associated with facial attraction are the eyes and the mouth (7). An attractive dentition and smile is an essential feature, for both children and adults. People with a relatively normal dental appearance are judged to be better looking, more desirable as friends, more intelligent, and less likely to behave aggressively (8); and teachers have higher expectations of them (9). Any deviation from the 'norm,' such as a dentofacial disfigurement, will stigmatize a person and make them less acceptable socially (10). Thus, it is not

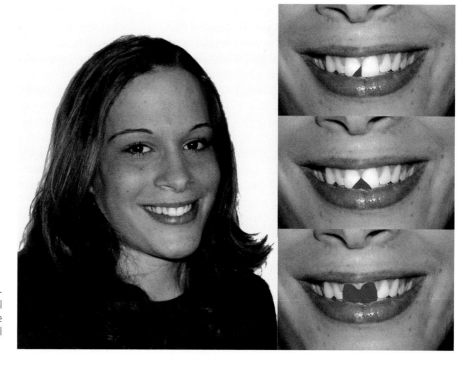

**Fig. 6.1** The fracture or loss of incisors may dramatically alter facial appearance. The photographs at the right simulate various types of dental trauma.

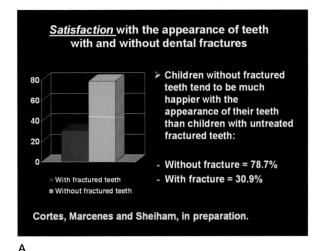
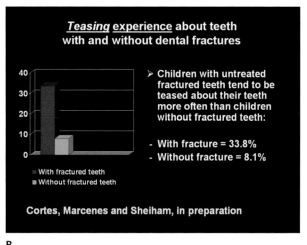

**Fig. 6.2** Patient satisfaction and teasing experience related to trauma experience. After CORTES et al. (80) 2006.

surprising that dental problems are linked to social and psychological well-being; and the contribution of dentofacial characteristics to dimensions of personality, self-esteem and body image is well documented (10–12).

Deviation from the 'norm' can be as simple as a dental anomaly or as complex as a craniofacial deformity (13). A traumatic dental injury (TDI), be it a fracture, discoloration of teeth, or avulsion of a tooth will alter facial appearance (14). What is more, the effects of TDIs on self-esteem and self-awareness are important because the majority of TDIs occur in the early years of life and adolescence (15, 16), which are periods of important psychological development when the growing person is particularly sensitive to impacts, however small (17–19). This may lead to long-term psychological effects, in particular if the TDI is associated with a physical as well as a psychological traumatic experience.

Psychologists define a traumatic experience as an intense and sudden event that overwhelms the child's capacity to cope with the memories and feelings that are triggered by it. Such traumatic experiences may lead to psychological symptoms such as depression and anxiety (20). Undoubtedly, a significant proportion of physical events, for example, traffic accidents, assaults, and physical abuse that cause TDIs, have strong psychological overlays (see also Chapter 3 and Chapter 7). Indeed, the actual treatment of a TDI may well be a source of psychological stress. So it is not surprising that a TDI may have social and psychological implications. There is a chain of risk from having a TDI to the development of adverse social and psychological outcomes; and, later in life, to experiencing poor educational performance which in turn affects job prospects and the chances of getting married (14).

Surprisingly, these important psychological issues have been neglected in dentistry and dental research. A review of the dental literature reveals that rarely has the social and psychological impact of TDI been studied (14), and although some research was carried out on the social and psychological aspects of maxillofacial injuries (21, 22), the majority of those studies had serious methodological shortcomings,

such as small sample sizes, low response rate and short-term follow-up.

This chapter will outline the social and psychological impacts of traumatic dental injuries on quality of life and set out how very basic procedures can be incorporated into dental practice to prevent or reduce the negative social and psychological outcomes of having a TDI.

## Socio-psychological impacts of traumatic dental injuries

Oral health influences people's quality of life: how people look, speak, smile, chew, taste and enjoy food and interpersonal relations (23). Thus it influences how people socialise, their self-esteem, self-image and their feelings of social well-being (24, 25). Cortes et al. (14) showed that children with untreated fractured teeth were very significantly more dissatisfied with the appearance of their teeth and experienced a significantly greater impact on their daily life than children without any traumatic dental injury. Children with fractured teeth were significantly more likely to report problems with 'eating and enjoying food', 'cleaning teeth', 'smiling, laughing and showing teeth without embarrassment', 'maintaining usual emotional state without being irritable' and 'enjoying contact with people' than children without any traumatic injury (Figs 6.2, 6.3). On average, children with an untreated traumatic dental injury were 20 times more likely to report an impact on quality of life due to the injury when compared with children without any traumatic dental injury (14). These findings suggest that untreated tooth fractures affect people's quality of life (80). In a study of 218 Australian children suffering a dental trauma, 66% felt worried or very worried after the injury. This applied especially to girls (79) (Fig. 6.2).

One important aspect of daily life that is affected by untreated TDI is unfavorable social responses. Children who sustain untreated TDI become targets for harassment and teasing by other schoolchildren and often have nicknames

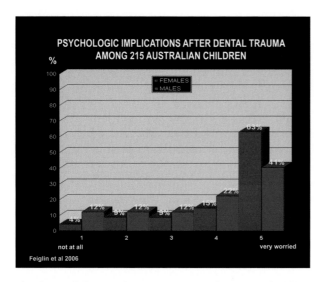

**Fig. 6.3** Psychologic implications in an Australian group of children affected by a dental trauma. After FEIGLIN et al. (79) 2006.

(26). Indeed, children with dentofacial deviations report negative socio-psychological impacts such as teasing, embarrassment and lack of social acceptance (8, 11, 27–29). Nicknames referring to physical features are usually disliked and individuals who have been teased and ridiculed tend to develop insecure behavior, limited social interaction and low self-esteem (10, 30, 80) (Fig. 6.3). The long-term effects of teasing due to dental features on the development of personality is unknown, but it is likely that some children who have been exposed to ridicule and insults may develop lower self-confidence and a sense of alienation (11).

The magnitude of the psychological impact of the TDI will depend on the type of event associated with the injury. For example, an injury event such as an assault causes significantly higher levels of stress than an accidental fall. An even more serious psychological impact is observed when the physical injuries are due to domestic abuse. This is not rare and includes child abuse, torture and domestic violence against children, older adults, women and men. A retrospective review of 236 patients treated for domestic violence injuries at an inner-city hospital over a 5-year period confirmed that 81% of victims presented with maxillofacial injuries at accident and emergency departments (31).

The psychological impact of traumatic injuries increases even further if associated with intense pain, loss of function and control, social isolation, as well as separation from parents and fear of death or future impairment (32). The child's immediate reaction to a traumatic experience will probably be dominated by tears, horror and shock. The physiological reaction to the incident will often be of the 'fight-flight-freeze' nature, a situation in which any person needs very good quality care. Afterwards, the child may be haunted by intense thoughts about the incident. Such thoughts could be particularly troublesome when the child is at rest. Later on, the person will experience a wide range of additional symptoms such as sleep disturbances and nightmares, different types of fears, difficulties in separat-

ing from parents, emotional distress and cognitive problems (33).

Experiences which have a strong sensory impact in terms of pain, fear, and fear of death could lead to serious and permanent psychological problems such as post-traumatic stress disorder (PTSD) (34). The diagnosis of PTSD was first conceptualized in Vietnam veterans, but later also applied to children who have experienced 'an event outside the range of usual human experience that would be markedly distressing to anyone'. A particular pattern of symptoms is described in children. This can be defined in three clusters (33): intrusive thoughts about a traumatic event; emotional numbing and avoidance of reminders of that event; and physiological hyperarousal.

Post-traumatic stress disorder is common after all traumatic events, including maxillofacial injury, and can become chronic unless recognized and treated (22). Glynn assessed a sample of 287 urban oral facial trauma survivors and found that approximately one in four reported experiencing symptoms consistent with a diagnosis of acute PTSD one month after the event of injury. This rate is similar to those observed after a car accident (35, 36). Another study including 40 patients showed that post-traumatic psychological symptoms were present in 54% of participants and that 41% met the diagnostic criteria for post-traumatic stress disorder 4–6 weeks later (22). Other psychiatric problems, such as anxiety and depression, were identified by the *General Health Questionnaire* and the *Hospital Anxiety and Depression Scale*. The long-term effects of lack of treatment include many psychological and social difficulties. Acute traumatic episodes in children, adolescents and adults can have long-term psychiatric consequences (20, 34, 37–39).

The psychosocial consequences of TDIs take on another dimension when one considers the dimension of the impacts at a population level. As the prevalence of TDI is relatively high (see Chapter 3) and the majority of damaged teeth remain untreated in both developing and developed countries, the cumulative impact of the consequences of experiencing a TDI is considerable (40–42). When one adds to this the financial cost of treating the TDIs, most of which are untreated or improperly treated (43), it is apparent that TDIs constitute an important dental public health problem and pose a significant challenge to dental professionals (40). To address that challenge, dental professionals need to be aware of basic psychological concepts. These are discussed next. We recommend reading textbooks on psychology for further understanding of children's psychology.

## Stages of psychological development

An understanding of the different stages of psychological development is crucial to the success of an intervention which will reduce the impact of TDI and associated events. Toddlers aged about one and a half to three years are developing a sense of doing things on their own. The child has a very strong drive to investigate the boundaries set by adults, to try out its own power and abilities, and to experience new, thrilling situations (44). Sometimes, toddlers exceed the limits of their capacity and expose themselves to a trauma. A traumatic experience such as intense pain puts limits on the child's expanding world (45). Furthermore, the experience of pain is imprinted on the mind of young children (46, 47).

During later childhood, aged 3–5 years, the child develops a clear concept of itself as a 'me', knowing it is a person in itself, and is no longer dependent on its parents in familiar situations. Development brings the child into a world of magic, oscillating between reality and fantasy. Intellectual growth is dominated by the increasing use of symbols, the most important of which is language. Words become loaded with feelings, ideas and associations and help the child to create an understanding of the world that is not strictly logical but holds a deep meaning for the child (48). The child internalizes the parent's guidelines for right and wrong and, during this process, the child gradually develops a conscience, and an inner representation of values and the rules that parents represent (17). Having a conscience means that one feels guilt when one does the 'wrong thing'. In addition, children may feel guilt even if they are not responsible for the TDI event. For example, a child may imagine he/she caused the painful incident by being angry with Mum that morning. A feeling of guilt may intensify the psychological impact. Furthermore, at this age, children perceive the body as a bag containing feelings and tears and food and heart and blood: it is frightening if there is a hole in the bag so it has to be mended as soon as possible. This is really the 'age of plaster'.

School age (6–12 years) is a period of life characterized by intensive development in social skills and cognitive growth. Intellectual development in the period has been described by Piaget as concrete, operational thinking, meaning that the child develops the ability to 'make up things in its head', starting from his/her own knowledge and experience (48). This is, however, limited and might lead the child to unrealistic conclusions. Logical ability increases, and therefore accuracy is needed when explaining something to the school age child. A very strong sense of justice is accompanied by a strong wish to punish the wrongdoer. This punishment could also be directed to the self, if he/she is the one to be blamed for the TDI event. At about the age of 9 years old, the child reaches an adult conception of life and death, namely a full understanding that everyone who lives will also die, including oneself. This leads to a deeper understanding of the transient nature of life and might cause an easily evoked fear of death and illness (49). Such a fear could easily be triggered off by a TDI event associated with intense pain.

Adolescence (13–20 years) is the final period of the child's development into adulthood. Intellectually, the young person is capable of formal operations (48). This means, for example, using double symbols (as in mathematics), handling hypothetical facts. Thus, an adolescent has adult intellectual concepts, but less experience than an adult. Teenagers often experience mood swings, as they are trying to achieve a stable inner identity and self-esteem. This is a process that goes on for years and takes great energy. Emotionally, the teenager will pass through different periods, the first of which is dominated by regression, as the wish to remain an innocent child clashes with the need to grow up. The next period is typically dominated by easily invoked aggression, when all earlier self-evident values and norms have to be questioned. The last period also represents the final emotional separation from parents and the security of childhood, in which there is loss and often some degree of depression until the young person finds a new sense of belonging (19). A traumatic experience with intense pain during this period of development may exaggerate any expression of regression, aggression or depression.

## Implications for treatment

Normative assessments of need for restoring enamel-dentine tooth fractures are commonly based on the premise, stated by Brännström (50), that bacterial invasion in the exposed dentinal tubules should determine inflammation that could lead to either repair or necrosis of the pulp, which neglects the role of facial esthetic. The assessment of treatment needs and the treatment plan must also reflect psychosocial factors in order to prevent an undesirable outcome to the treatment. This is because the ultimate goal of treatment is to restore the capacity of people to perform desired social roles and activities. Dentists should remember that oral health is defined as 'a standard of health of the oral and related tissues which enables an individual to eat, speak and socialize without active disease, discomfort or embarrassment and which contributes to general well-being'. Clearly the definition of oral health has evolved and expanded from a purely biological outlook to include a socio-psychological meaning.

The esthetic implications of TDI are perhaps the most important motivator in seeking treatment (14). The psychological impact of the TDI event and pain associated with the injury may be even more serious than the physical damage. Furthermore, the treatment and prognosis of a TDI may be an additional source of psychological stress.

A subjective assessment (51) of patients with traumatized teeth in a 15-year follow-up study identified that 39% of the patients reported dissatisfaction either with the color and/or anatomic form of the traumatized teeth or reconstruction. Twenty-one per cent of the patients remembered pain during treatment, and 25% remembered only the behavior and attitudes of the dental team. Most of the individuals did not remember having received any information about prognosis for the traumatized teeth. Thus, there is an urgent need to improve the quality of care of traumatic dental injuries.

### Assessments of need

Social functions such as communication and esthetics may be more important than biting and chewing and may be the main determinants of an individuals' subjective or perceived need for replacement of missing natural teeth and their feelings about the loss of teeth (52, 53). Keeping the front teeth is more important than keeping molars (54). Similarly, dentofacial esthetics and self-perceptions of dental appearance are important factors in deciding to seek orthodontic treatment (55–59). Dissatisfaction with esthetics has been consistently reported as the main reason for seeking orthodontic treatment and more important than the ability to chew (57). Hence, it is not surprising that children with fractured teeth tend to be more concerned with esthetics than with function (14). There is a strong case for the argument that dentistry should concentrate more on psychological and social functioning than on functional restoration (63). Research to date confirms the concern expressed by patients in relation to their appearance, with any shortfall between the individual's ideal and perceived expectations resulting in discontent and a possible desire for improvement (60). Both children and their parents alike believe that the cosmetic improvement of the mouth will enhance the social acceptance and self-esteem of an individual (61). In a self-assessment of their own appearance, children mentioned teeth as a feature which they would like to change first of all (62).

Despite the fact that demand for treatment of traumatic dental injuries may be mostly related to esthetic or psychosocial factors, assessments of treatment need due to a traumatic dental injury do not include a valid measurement of the psychosocial impact of these on quality of life (14). The assessment is based primarily on normative need judged by a dentist. Clinical measures used to define oral health status and needs in populations are subject to serious limitations as they do not take into account the World Health Organizations's (WHO) definition of oral health. For example, they tell us nothing about the functioning of the oral cavity or the person as a whole, or about subjectively perceived symptoms. Traditional normative assessment of treatment need does not inquire into people's capacity to carry out desired daily roles and activities and whether people could take advantage of important opportunities in life, if treatment is provided (63).

Clearly, the assessment of need for treatment should include the patient's perception of their need for treatment in order to restore the 'capacity of individuals to perform desired roles and activities' (64, 65). This led Cohen and Jago (66) to call for the development of socio-dental indicators, with the rationale of improving clinical indicators of oral health by adding a dimension of social impact, and their subsequent development (66). Socio-dental indicators are measures of oral health-related quality of life and range from survival, through impairment, to function and perceptions (63). Oral health-related quality of life is a multi-dimensional concept that incorporates survival, illness and impairment, social, psychological and physical function and disability, oral health perceptions, opportunity, as well as interactions between the aforementioned domains (67). They measure the extent to which dental and oral disorders disrupt normal social role functioning and bring about

major changes in daily life, such as an inability to work or attend school, or undertake parental or household duties (68, 69). They are subjective and their use should be complementary to the clinical measures of oral status and needs (23, 70). WHO policies state clearly that the enhancement of people's quality of life and extension of their life spans are the two central goals for health care since 1981 (71).

The assessment of treatment need, and treatment provided due to traumatic dental injuries must include an oral health-related quality of life measure because this condition has considerable psychosocial implications for patients. Several dental researchers have developed validated measures to assess the effects of oral disorders on the functional, social and psychological well-being and these are easily available in the dental literature (65). Slade et al. (72) reviewed the pertinent literature and concluded that there is not any single instrument that is better than the others or can be regarded as a gold-standard set of questions.

One socio-dental measure devised specifically for use with children, the Child OIDP, assesses socio-dental impacts in children and relates these impacts to the cause by asking the child what dental condition, including TDIs, provoked the impact (73). Another socio-dental indicator developed for children, the **Child Oral Health Quality of Life** questionnaire, was designed to assess the impact of oral and orofacial conditions on the quality of life of children and their families (74, 75).

## Treatment plan

In order to understand fully the psychological impact of TDI and the implications for treatment of this condition, it might be useful to consider first the sequence of events experienced by someone involved in a TDI event, including the potential negative impact of the treatment regimen. A typical scenario includes:

(1) *Injury event*: A TDI event is characterized by a collision that can generate enough mechanical energy to produce the injury and often releases immediate intense pain. This is the first psychological impact, and its magnitude will depend on the type of injury, intensity of pain released and type of event associated with the injury. Therefore, dental professionals must be prepared to deal with the physical and psychological impact of a TDI.

(2) *Emergency procedures*: The majority of traumatic dental injuries occur outside office hours. To visit an emergency room is an unpleasant experience that may increase the psychological impact of a TDI. Emergency rooms tend to be crowded and populated by people who are experiencing stressful circumstances. This atmosphere is not conducive to the reduction of the psychological impact caused by the injury event.

(3) *Treatment*: Immediate treatment of TDI may be frightening and painful, especially if adequate pain control is not administered and proper information about treatment procedures is not provided. In addition, lack of

postoperative information about future treatment and prognosis may cause further concern.

(4) *Post-treatment follow-up*: Studies have shown that treatment of traumatic dental trauma in emergency care services is often inadequate (43). Unsuccessful emergency care affects the outcome of treatment of TDI. For example, successful outcomes following avulsion injuries significantly depend on early treatment. This includes the need for further and more complex treatment (e.g. endodontic procedures) or loss of the tooth or teeth affected. Exposure to these further stressors may increase the psychological impact of a TDI event.

(5) *Economic consequences* for the family may be the final step in this series of unpleasant experiences in relation to the trauma.

## Suggested approaches to reduce the impact of a traumatic dental injury

There is a clear need for stopping or at least minimizing pain caused by acute damage as early as possible; and procedural pain should be avoided, to prevent or reduce the negative social and psychological outcomes of having a TDI. The most serious effect of experiencing strong pain is the potential development of permanent psychological problems such as post-traumatic stress disorder (34). There are also other reasons to consider stopping or at least minimizing pain:

* *Humanitarian reasons*, as stated in the UN Convention on the Rights of the Child.
* *Medical reasons*, since uncontrolled pain causes the release of local and general stress hormones, which will increase the tissue damage and make the healing of wounds more difficult (76). There is also some evidence that insufficient pain control from the outset can diminish the effect of subsequent efforts to control pain during surgery (76).
* *Practical reasons*: A child in pain will have much greater problems in co-operating with treatment (76).

Despite the importance of this, there is evidence that children are often given inadequate pain control when experiencing acute damage (76). The sequence of events experienced by someone involved in a TDI event was presented above. The implications for treatment from the injury event to post-treatment follow-up are discussed next.

### Injury event

The first people to help and transport the patient to an emergency service have the responsibility for relieving pain and calming the patient, and they are normally well trained to do this job. Food, shelter and medical care do not heal the psychological trauma but ensure survival and might give strength, will and mental readiness to confront the trauma and cope with the experience.

### Emergency treatment

In hospitals, the waiting rooms should have a friendly appearance; and children, as a rule, should have preferential treatment before adults to relieve their anxiety as fast as possible. It is also of great value to have a separate room for waiting children, so as to avoid them being exposed to frightening sights. The first step in the treatment of patients in an emergency setting is to tell them that you are going to help them and that you expect that there will be a successful outcome to the treatment. In those rare cases where it is obvious that nothing can be done, and that the teeth have to be extracted, this remark has naturally to be omitted. The next issue is to relieve pain. This is a precondition in order to be able to treat the patient and to reduce the psychological impact of the treatment situation. Pain can be treated pharmacologically and non-pharmacologically, and both means should be used in combination as they are complementary and reinforce each other. The non-pharmacological methods are mainly directed towards diminishing fear and anxiety. Only methods that can be used in acute situations will be mentioned here. Methods for decreasing anxiety in the acute situation can roughly be grouped into four: preparation, support, distraction and discussion of post-trauma treatment.

### Preparation

There is always time to prepare, and to give some information (unless there is an immediate threat to life). The principle of 'tell-show-do' will allow the child to learn something about what will happen during treatment which will diminish anxiety. In other words, it is not a waste of time to prepare for treatment but an 'investment'. Tell the child in an age appropriate manner what is going to happen. Ask the child questions and give him/her answers, with details according to the child's age. It is important to be honest about what may happen during treatment. Take care that the child does not use questions as a delaying technique just to postpone treatment. In a more developed form, these principles are used as modelling/role-playing and behavioral rehearsal (47). Allow the child to take control over details by giving a choice that is realistic (i.e. the child might decide on which side one should start preparation). This will make the child feel that he/she is participating and strengthen his co-operation, since it makes clear to the child that it is possible for him to influence the treatment.

### Support

The presence of the parents is important to provide support to the child. If this is not possible, an appropriate alternative adult will need to be identified. Include the parents in all that is going to happen, give sufficient explanation to reassure them, make them feel secure about the treatment and they will comfort the child. This holds true, even for a teenager, and not only for a small child. The behavior from the whole staff in the emergency room is important: adults who take time to listen to the child, who keep calm even if the situation is stressful, who know what to do and how to do it in an efficient and confident way, will give the child a sense of security. Also, the environment could make the child relax. An emergency treatment ward designed for children with toys and pictures feels friendly and more familiar than a common hospital environment, and it offers some distraction. Support also means that the staff explain everything, emphasize the aspect of mending and tell about the way to heal. Early treatment of pain is also supportive and will make things easier not only in the emergency room but also further on during long-term treatment. Short pauses are important to give the child an opportunity to relax for a while, maybe move around a little and ask questions before concentrating on another session.

### Distraction

The child could be distracted in the emergency room by listening to music (take care to have records that are popular among children of different ages), by watching videos or by telling a thrilling story. You could also distract the child from surgical procedures by making him/her concentrate upon something else, for example counting (i.e. number of lights in the room) or pressing a hand very firmly for a certain time. It might also be possible to involve the child in a detailed imaginative story, thus concentrating upon something that is going on outside the emergency room (46). It is recommended that children younger than five should preferably be distracted from the surgical procedure, whereas older children should have the choice whether they prefer to look or to be distracted.

### Discussion

Post-trauma treatment information is an essential part of the treatment and will decrease anxiety significantly if given in a proper way. This issue is further described in Chapter 35. Post-procedure discussion allows the child to ask questions about what happened and to clarify things that might have been misunderstood in the acute situation. It is important to give credence to the child's thoughts and to answer honestly. Some children will need active encouragement from the staff to start talking. This post procedure 'discussion' could be done as a play with the youngest children.

### Treatment

The same principles as those mentioned above regarding the emergency situation are relevant also during treatment and post-treatment and will not be repeated here. Remember that information given in a stressful situation might not be fully understood or remembered (51). Therefore it is necessary to repeat all that has been told, maybe several times, to check that it has been correctly interpreted. It is also important to give written information and to give opportunities for the patient and/or parents to ask questions more than once. It is important to handle the acute situation in a way that makes the person feel safe and protected so as to avoid or limit the psychological secondary effects of the physical trauma.

### Post-treatment follow-up

The same factors should be followed as mentioned for emergency treatment. It is very important that the patients are adequately informed about the reasons for follow-up (identifying healing complications) and the necessity to perform certain procedures, e.g. endodontics, extractions). See also Chapter 35.

### Economic consequences

In relation to this it is important to inform the patient about means to reduce the economic impact of the trauma (e.g. support from public or insurance companies; see also Chapter 34).

## Talking to children

Health professionals need to be aware of and able to control their own emotions in relation to the patient. Even if one is affected by what one sees, one must not express such feelings in front of the child or the parents. As far as verbal expression is concerned, most professionals are probably trained to control themselves. However, it is important to remember that body language expresses just as much as words; and for the youngest children it is even more important than words.

To communicate with an infant means that you mainly 'talk with the body' and the young child 'talks' to you in the same way. Words by themselves mean nothing: what counts is eye contact, mimicry, and pitch of the voice. The child answers by smiling, crying, yelling, moving away or showing interest and by imitating (78). All this is perceived by the young child, whereas the words you use will be directed to and understood by the parent(s). The toddler is very much dependent upon body language in its communication and, in particular, if words are contradictory they will rely upon the body signals rather than the words to understand the message.

Words will become more and more important as children get older, and they act as an important support for the child's memory. In a sense, words are regarded as something one collects, rather than concepts to describe a whole world of associations; as a description, rather than as a symbol of the thing concerned (48). During this period of life, children love to imitate, for example, animals, and to identify themselves with familiar persons. This offers a way for them to make contact. Children want certainty and regularity. They want things to be repeated and done the same way every time. You could ask their parents about the child's specific rituals, which animals or people or cartoon figures they prefer to imitate or with which they identify. This might be very helpful in establishing contact and making the child cooperate. Remember that the child is still very dependent upon the parents to understand and handle the environment around him.

In late childhood, there is still a great dependency upon parents, but the child has reached a concept of self as a 'me' (18). Their verbal capacity has increased, which adds to the child's self-assurance in new situations and with foreign people. It is important to remember that a child in crisis and pain will not be able to handle the situation as in normal circumstances (and this holds true for all ages). The child of this age likes to use new adult words, but does not always know the exact meaning. Thus it is crucial to ask the child: 'What do you mean exactly?' Praise the child for whatever he/she achieves. A 4-year-old will be happy to try to follow your instructions as long as he/she feels that you appreciate his/her efforts.

During school age, children gradually achieve an adult way of handling language: they talk correctly and are logical. Still there is a lack of experience and a certain rigidity in their thinking which might lead to false conclusions (48). Therefore it is preferable to ask questions to find out exactly how they think, what ideas they have about the outcome of treatment, and the procedures involved. Always answer their questions and answer honestly. The dentist must never be dishonest! It is important to make sure that the school age child has a correct explanation for anything they may ask. If the dentist is not honest, he/she will probably lose the child's confidence forever, or at least for a very long time. Listen carefully to understand the child's real worries, and attempt to try to understand and respond to the child's thoughts. Sometimes one might need to use adult technical terms. If so, take care to explain the new word very precisely. Making a 'contract' might be a way to solve a critical situation during treatment. This will usually be made between three parties: the child, the parent and the professional (45).

During adolescence, the teenager expects to be treated like an adult and also has the intellectual capacity to discuss and think like one (48). Still, as a professional, one must remember that mood swings are common and there is a lack of experience that might make things seem and feel worse. Thus, as a professional, one has to be patient and to show that you really want to understand the teenager's thoughts, ideas and feelings. The way you do this does not differ from the techniques you use in talking to adults. There will probably be a great deal of arguing, which is typical for the age group. You should be understanding, but also clear about what can and cannot be done.

## Essentials

- Dento-facial disfigurement may have social and psychological implications.
- In most cultures the face is regarded as the most precious characteristic of human identity and, therefore, it enjoys a privileged status in relation to the rest of the body. There is evidence that the oral region is of primary importance in determining overall facial attractiveness.
- Any deviation from the 'norm', such as a dento-facial disfigurement, will stigmatize a person and make that person less acceptable socially. Deviation from the 'norm' can be as simple as a dental anomaly or as complex as a cranio-facial deformity.
- A pretty dentition (smile) is an essential feature both for children and adults. A traumatic dental injury (TDI) may destroy that appearance due to a fracture, discoloration of teeth, and avulsion of teeth.
- Oral health influences how people look, speak, chew, taste and enjoy food. Thus it influences how people socialize, their self-esteem, self-image and their feelings of social well-being.
- People with a relatively normal dental appearance are judged as better looking, more desirable as friends, more intelligent, and less likely to behave aggressively, and teachers have higher expectations from them.
- There is some evidence to suggest that children who sustain untreated TDI can attract unfavorable social responses in becoming targets for nicknames, harassment and teasing from other schoolchildren.
- The magnitude of the psychological impact will depend on the type and severity of the injury, type of event associated with the injury, level of pain and fear, and quality of treatment provided.
- The trauma event in itself might have serious psychological effects. Further negative effects could be reduced by means of good emergency care, provision of shelter and support to the child both at the site of injury and during transport.
- Awaiting treatment is a stressful experience for children, especially if they are also exposed to the frightening sight of other emergency patients and are in unfriendly surroundings. Try to reduce stress by arranging a separate waiting room for children at the emergency ward and to give them priority over adult patients, if possible for medical reasons.
- Pain adds significantly to both physiological and psychological stress. This means that immediate and skilful pain control should be given very early at the emergency ward or if possible at the place of injury.
- Lack of postoperative information might add to emotional stress during emergency treatment as the child anticipates future problems. Give information, in as concise and positive a manner as possible, emphasise likelihood of recovery and also give written information.
- Post-traumatic follow-up gives an excellent opportunity to talk the whole treatment through: from the moment of the injury until the expected end result. This will reduce negative feelings about dental care.

## References

1. BERSCHEID E, GANGESTAD S. The social psychological implications of facial physical attractiveness. *Clin Plast Surg* 1982;**9**:289–96.
2. RUMSEY N, BULL R, GAHAGAN DA. A development study of children's stereotyping of facially deformed adults. *Brit J Psych* 1986;**77**:269–74.

3. WALSTER E, ARONSON V, ABRAHAMS D, ROTTMAN L. Importance of physical attractiveness in dating behavior. *J Pers Soc Psychol* 1966;**4**:508–16.

4. DION K, BERSCHEID E, WALSTER E. What is beautiful is good. *J Pers Soc Psychol* 1972;**24**:285–90.

5. MATHES EW, KAHN A. Physical attractiveness, happiness, neuroticism, and self-esteem. *J Psychol* 1975;**90**:27–30.

6. TAYLOR PA, GLENN ND. The utility of education and attractiveness for females status attainment through marriage. *Am Soc Rev* 1976;**61**:486–98.

7. BALDWIN DC. Appearance and esthetics in oral health. *Community Dent Oral Epidemiol* 1980;**8**:244–56.

8. SHAW WC. Factors influencing the desire for orthodontic treatment. *Eur J Orthod* 1981;**3**:151–62.

9. ADAMS GR. Physical attractiveness, personality, and social reactions to peer pressure. *J Psychol* 1977;**96**:287–96.

10. MACGREGOR FC. Social and psychological implications of dentofacial disfigurement. *Angle Orthod* 1970;**3**:231–3.

11. SHAW WC, MEEK SC, JONES DS. Nicknames, teasing, harassment and the salience of dental features among school children. *Br J Orthod* 1980;**7**:75–80.

12. STRICKER G. Psychological issues pertaining to malocclusion. *Am J Orthod* 1970;**58**:276–83.

13. CUNNINGHAM SJ. The psychology of facial appearance. *Dent Update* 1999;**26**:438–43.

14. CORTES MI, MARCENES W, SHEIHAM A. Impact of traumatic injuries to the permanent teeth on the oral health-related quality of life in 12–14-year-old children. *Community Dent Oral Epidemiol* 2002;**30**:193–8.

15. GLENDOR U, HALLING A, ANDERSSON L, EILERT-PETERSSON E. Incidence of traumatic tooth injuries in children and adolescents in the county of Vastmanland, Sweden. *Swed Dent J* 1996;**20**:15–28.

16. EILERT-PETERSSON E, SCHELP L. An epidemiological study of bicycle-related injuries. *Accid Anal Prev* 1997;**29**:363–72.

17. ERIKSON EH. *Childhood and society.* New York: WW Norton & Company, 1963.

18. MAHLER MS, McDEVITT JB. Thoughts on the emergence of the sense of self, with particular emphasis on the body self. *J Am Psychoanal Assoc* 1982;**30**:827–48.

19. KAPLAN LJ. *Adolescence: The farewell to childhood.* New York: Simon & Schuster, 1984.

20. PINE CM, COHEN LK. Trauma in children and adolescence. *Biol Psychiatry* 2002;**51**:519–31.

21. LASKIN DM. The psychological consequences of maxillofacial injury. *J Oral Maxillofac Surg* 1999;**57**: 1281.

22. HULL AM, LOWE T, DEVLIN M, FINLAY P, KOPPEL, D, STEWART AM. Psychological consequences of maxillofacial trauma: a preliminary study. *Br J Oral Maxillofac Surg* 2003;**41**:317–22.

23. REISINE ST, LOCKER D. Social, psychological and economic impacts of oral conditions and treatments. In: Cohen LK, Gift HC. eds. *Disease prevention and oral health promotion. Socio-dental sciences in action.* Copenhagen: Munksgaard, 1995:33–71.

24. SHEIHAM A, CROOG SH. The psychosocial impact of dental diseases on individuals and communities. *J Behav Med* 1981;**4**:257–72.

25. LOCKER D. Measuring oral health: a conceptual framework. *Community Dent Health* 1988;**5**:3–18.

26. CORTES MI. *Epidemiology of traumatic injuries to the permanent teeth and the impact of the injuries on the daily living of Brazilian schoolchildren.* Thesis. London, 2000.

27. HELM S, KREIBORG S, SOLOW B. Psychosocial implications of malocclusion: a 15-year follow-up study in 30-year-old Danes. *Am J Orthod* 1985;**87**:110–18.

28. NIKIAS M. Oral disease and quality of life. *Am J Public Health* 1985;**75**:11–12.

29. CHEN MS, HUNTER P. Oral health and quality of life in New Zealand: a social perspective. *Soc Sci Med* 1996:1213–22.

30. LANSDOWN R, LLOYD J, HUNTER J. Facial deformity in childhood: severity and psychological adjustment. *Child Care Health Dev* 1991;**17**:165–71.

31. LE BT, DIERKS EJ, UEECK BA, HOMER LD, POTTER BF. Maxillofacial injuries associated with domestic violence. *J Oral Maxillofac Surg* 2001;**59**:1277–83.

32. DYREGROV A. Katastrofpsykiatri. Studentlitteratur, 1992.

33. RUTTER M, TAYLOR E, HERSOV E. *Child and adolescent psychiatry.* Oxford: Blackwell, 2002.

34. BRESLAU N, DAVIS GC, ANDRESKI P. Traumatic events and posttraumatic stress disorder in an urban population of young adults. *Arch Gen Psychiatry* 1991;**48**:216–22.

35. BLANCHARD EB, HICKLING EJ, MITNICK N, TAYLOR AE, LOOS WR, BUCKLEY TC. The impact of severity of physical injury and perception of life threat in the development of post-traumatic stress disorder in motor vehicle accident victims. *Behav Res Ther* 1995;**33**:529–34.

36. SHALEV AY, FREEDMAN S, PERI T, BRANDES, D, SAHAR T. Predicting PTSD in trauma survivors: prospective evaluation of self-report and clinician-administered instruments. *Br J Psychiatry* 1997;**170**:558–64.

37. TYANO S, IANCU I, SOLOMON Z, SEVER J, GOLDSTEIN I, TOUVIANA Y, BLEICH A. Seven-year follow-up of child survivors of a bus-train collision. *J Am Acad Child Adolesc Psychiatry* 1996;**35**:365–73.

38. YULE W, BOLTON D, UDWIN O, BOYLE S, O'RYAN D, NURRISH J. The long-term psychological effects of a disaster experienced in adolescence: I: The incidence and course of PTSD. *J Child Psychol Psychiatry Allied Disciplines* 2000;**41**:503–11.

39. SHALEV AY. Acute stress reactions in adults. *Biol Psychiatry* 2002;**51**:532–43.

40. MARCENES W, AL BEIRUTI N, TAYFOUR D, ISSA D. Epidemiology of traumatic injuries to the permanent incisors of 9–12-year-old schoolchildren in Damascus, Syria. *Endod Dent Traumatol* 1999;**15**:117–23.

41. MARCENES W, ZABOT NE, TRAEBERT J. Socio-economic correlates of traumatic injuries to the permanent incisors in schoolchildren aged 12 years in Blumenau, Brazil. *Dent Traumatol* 2001;**17**:222–6.

42. MARCENES W, MURRAY S. Social deprivation and traumatic dental injuries among 14-year-old schoolchildren in Newham, London. *Dent Traumatol* 2001;**17**:17–21.

43. HAMILTON FA, HILL FJ, HOLLOWAY PJ. An investigation of dento-alveolar trauma and its treatment in an adolescent population. Part 2: Dentists' knowledge of management methods and their perceptions of barriers to providing care. *Br Dent J* 1997;**182**:129–33.

44. FRAIBERG S. *The magic years.* New York: Charles Scriber's Sons, 1959.

45. Koch G, Poulsen S. *Pediatric dentistry: a clinical approach*. Copenhagen: Munksgaard, 2001.

46. Schechter DN, Berde C, Yaster M. *Pain in infants, children and adolescents*. Baltimore MD: Lippincott Williams & Wilkins, 2002.

47. Bush AJ, Harkins S. *Children in pain: clinical and research issues from developmental perspective*. New York: Springer Verlag, 1991.

48. Piaget J. *The language and thought of the child*. London: Routledge & Kegan Paul, 1959.

49. Lagerheim B. 'Why me?' A depressive crisis at the age of nine in handicapped children. In: Gyllensvärd Å, Lauren K, eds. *Psychosomatic diseases in childhood*. Stockholm: Sven Jerring Foundation, 1983.

50. Brännström M. Dentin and pulp in restorative dentistry. *Dental therapeutics*. Stockholm: Wolfe Medical Publications, 1981;127.

51. Robertson A, Noren JG. Subjective aspects of patients with traumatized teeth. A 15-year follow-up study. *Acta Odontol Scand* 1997;**55**:142–7.

52. Oosterhaven SP, Westert GP, Schaub RM, van der Bilt A. Social and psychologic implications of missing teeth for chewing ability. *Community Dent Oral Epidemiol* 1988;**16**:79–82.

53. Schuurs AH, Duivenvoorden HJ, Thoden van Velzen SK, Verhage F, Makkes PC. Value of the teeth. *Community Dent Oral Epidemiol* 1990;**18**:22–6.

54. Kayser AF. How much reduction of the dental arch is functionally acceptable for the ageing patient? *Int Dent J* 1990;**40**:183–8.

55. Albino JE, Cunat JJ, Fox RN, Lewis EA, Slakter MJ, Tedesco LA. Variables discriminating individuals who seek orthodontic treatment. *J Dent Res* 1981;**60**:1661–7.

56. Soderfeldt B, Palmqvist S, Arnbjerg D. Factors affecting attitudes toward dental appearance and dental function in a Swedish population aged 45–69 years. *Community Dent Health* 1993;**10**:123–30.

57. Tuominen ML, Tuominen RJ. Factors associated with subjective need for orthodontic treatment among Finnish university applicants. *Acta Odontol Scand* 1994;**52**:106–10.

58. Burden DJ, Pine CM. Self-perception of malocclusion among adolescents. *Community Dent Health* 1995;**12**:89–92.

59. Pietila T, Pietila I. Dental appearance and orthodontic services assessed by 15–16-year-old adolescents in eastern Finland. *Community Dent Health* 1996;**13**:139–44.

60. Shaw WC, O'Brien KD, Richmond S. Quality control in orthodontics: factors influencing the receipt of orthodontic treatment. *Br Dent J* 1991;**170**:66–8.

61. Shaw WC, Jones BM. The expectations of orthodontic patients in South Wales and St Louis, Missouri. *Br J Orthod* 1979;**6**:203–5.

62. Dunin-Wilczynska I. Reactions of school children to the appearance of teeth. *Czasopismo Stomatologiczne* 1990;**43**:629–32.

63. Locker D. *An introduction to behavioral science and dentistry*. London: Routledge, 1989.

64. Gift HC. Quality of life – an outcome of oral health care? *J Public Health Dent* 1996;**56**:67–8.

65. Slade GD. *Measuring oral health and quality of life*. Chapel Hill, University of North Carolina, Dental Ecology, 1997.

66. Cohen LK, Jago JD. Toward the formulation of sociodental indicators. *Int J Health Serv* 1976;**6**:681–98.

67. Gift HC, Atchison KA. Oral health, health, and health-related quality of life. *Med Care* 1995;**33**:NS57–77.

68. WHO. *International classification of impairments, disabilities and handicaps*. Geneva: World Health Organization, 1980.

69. Locker D. *Measuring oral health and quality of life*. London: Routledge, 1989.

70. Gift HC, Atchison KA, Dayton CM. Conceptualizing oral health and oral health-related quality of life. *Soc Sci Med* 1997;**44**:601–8.

71. Mahler M. The meaning of health for all by the year 2000. *World Health Forum* 1981;**2**:5–22.

72. Slade GD, Strauss RP, Atchison KA, Kressin NR, Locker D, Resisine ST. Conference summary: assessing oral health outcomes – measuring health status and quality of life. *Community Dent Health* 1998;**15**:3–7.

73. Gherunpong S, Tsakos G, Sheiham A. Developing and evaluating an oral health related quality of life index for children. The CHILD OIDP. *Community Oral Health* 2004;**21**:161–9.

74. Jokovic A, Locker D, Stephens M, Kenny D, Tompson B. Validity and reliability of a questionnaire to measure child oral health related quality of life. *J Dent Res* 2002;**81**:159–63.

75. Jokovic A, Locker D, Stephens M, Kenny D, Tompson B, Guyatt G. Measuring parental perceptions of child oral health-related quality of life. *J Public Health Dent* 2003;**63**:67–72.

76. Socialstyrelsen. *Barn och Smärta (State of the art) 2003*, 2003.

77. Hwang P. Spadbarnets psykologi. *Natur & Kultur*, 1993.

78. Mahler M, Pine F, Bergman, A. *The psychological birth of the human infant*. New York: Basic, 1975.

79. Feiglin B, Andreasen JO, Rydå V. The psychological implications of traumatic dental injuries. 2006. In preparation.

80. Cortes MI, Marcenes W, Sheiham A. Psychologic impact of crown fractures upon patient satisfaction and teasing experience. 2006. In preparation.

# 7
# Child Physical Abuse

R. R. Welbury

## Child physical abuse – a definition

A child is considered to be abused if he or she is treated in a way that is unacceptable in a given culture at a given time. The last two clauses are important, because not only are children treated differently in different countries, but also within a country and even within a city there are subcultures of behavior and variations of opinion as to what constitutes abuse.

## Child physical abuse – historical aspects

Violence towards children has been noted between cultures and at different times within the same culture since early civilization. Infanticide has been documented in almost every culture so that it can almost be considered a universal phenomenon (1). Ritualistic killing, maiming and severe punishing of children in an attempt to educate them, exploit them or rid them of evil spirits has been reported since early biblical times and ritualistic surgery or mutilation of children has been recorded as part of religious and ethnic traditions (2).

With the advent of urbanization and technological advancement in the 18th century, more economic value was placed upon the child by society and they were often used as a cheap source of labor. Harsh punishments for relatively minor misdemeanors were accepted and indeed expected in the courts, the school and the home (3).

In the 19th century, Western societies became more protective towards children, and their lot gradually improved. However, the mortality rate remained high, and the isolated death of a child probably did not arouse suspicion. Lord Shaftesbury, who campaigned to create better conditions in Britain for children at work, recognized the problem of child abuse at home, but was powerless to intervene: 'The evils are enormous and indisputable, but they are so private, internal and domestic a character as to be beyond the reach of legislation and the subject would not, I think, be entertained in either House of Parliament.' (Lord Shaftesbury 1880).

As more effective health care became available in the developed countries, more children survived poor living and working conditions. But in the middle of the 20th century reports appeared in the USA of unexplained skeletal injury to children (4, 5). These reports described unexpected skeletal trauma, sometimes associated with subdural hematoma. The possibility that these injuries could have been inflicted by a parent was recognized by some authors; but there appears to have been a general reluctance to accept that parents could wilfully abuse their offspring (6). However, when Kempe et al. published their paper 'The battered-child syndrome' in 1962 (7), the full impact of the physical maltreatment of children was brought to the attention of the medical community and subsequently the general public. The battered-child syndrome, or non-accidental injury (NAI) is now usually referred to as child physical abuse. Its recognition had such a profound effect upon the professions and the public that within a few years the majority of states in the USA had introduced laws which made it mandatory for physicians, dentists and other health related professionals to report suspected cases. The primary aim of all professionals involved in the child protection process is to ensure the safety of the child. The secondary aim is to provide help and counselling for the parents or caregivers so that the abuse stops.

## Prevalence

Child physical abuse is part of the spectrum of child abuse that also involves emotional abuse, sexual abuse and neglect. Physical abuse is now recognized as an international issue and has been reported in many countries (8–18). However, despite this global recognition, prevalence rates in most countries are still not available. In the USA in 2000 there were 12.2 victims of maltreatment per 1000 children (19); and this is a major threat to children's mental health (20). It was reported in 1989 that in Britain most departments of social services and child welfare were notified of more than 20 times as many cases of suspected child abuse as they were 10 years previously (21). Although some of these reports would prove to be unfounded, the common experience was that proven cases of child abuse were four or five times as common as they were a decade previously (21).

In Britain, at least 1 child per 1000 under 4 years of age per year suffers severe physical abuse – for example fractures, brain hemorrhage, severe internal injuries or mutilation (22); and in the USA more than 95% of serious intracranial injuries during the first year of life are the result of abuse (23). Studies analyzing the attendance of children in accident and emergency departments of hospitals have shown that in the USA 10% of children younger than 5 (24) and in Denmark 1.3 children per 1000 per year (25) will have injuries that were wilfully inflicted. Each year as many as 1200 children in the USA (19) and 200 children in Britain (26) will die as a result of abuse or neglect. In Scandinavia, the estimated number of deaths from physical abuse is much lower, at about 10 annually, giving an estimated frequency of 0.5 child deaths per million inhabitants per year (27). A common finding in all countries is that the workers concerned with child abuse believe that many cases remain undetected and the real mortality figures are considerably higher.

Children of all ages are subject to physical abuse; but the majority of cases occur in younger children (22) (Fig. 7.1). This is partly because they are more vulnerable and partly because they cannot seek help elsewhere. Children under 2 years of age are most at risk from severe physical abuse. Death from abuse is rare after the age of 1 year. The number of boys subjected to violence slightly exceeds that of girls; and first-born children are more often affected. Within a family, it is common for just one of the children to be abused and the others to be free from such abuse.

## Etiology

The etiology of physical abuse is based on the interaction between the personality traits of the parents or the abusing adult, the child's characteristics and the environmental conditions (28). Due to the wide variation in behavioral characteristics, personality traits and psychiatric symptoms among abusive adults, a specific abusive personality does not exist. However, certain commonly recurring traits can be recognized (8, 22, 29–31).

Physical abuse encompasses all social classes; but more cases have been identified in the poorer socio-economic groups. Many cases of physical abuse are by the child's parents or by persons known to the child (25). Often the mother of the affected child may be divorced or single. It is also common for a cohabitant who is living in the home, but who is not related to the child, to be the perpetrator. Young parents, often of low intelligence, are more likely to be abusers. This is especially true if they have been exposed to

such behavior during their own childhood (32). Indeed, abuse is thought to be 20 times more likely if one of the parents was abused as a child (21). A significant proportion of the perpetrators have a criminal record of some kind; and although they usually do not have an identified mental illness, they may exhibit personality traits predisposing to violent behavior. Contributing factors to abuse on behalf of the adults involved include alcohol and other drug misuse, poverty, unemployment and marital problems. Children already at risk may add to the stress by continually crying, throwing tantrums, or soiling their clothes. In addition, the child may be handicapped, be the result of an unwanted pregnancy or may fail to attain the expectations of the parents. These factors can provoke frustration in the most stable parent. But in association with other stresses, they may lead to physical neglect or injury.

## Diagnosis

The most important step in recognizing the possibility that an injury in a child has been caused on purpose is to believe that it can happen in the first place. The diagnosis is a difficult intellectual and emotional exercise; and is one of the most consuming tasks for a pediatrician, requiring time, experience and emotional energy. Failure to spot the signs and make the diagnosis can vitally influence a child's future life. At worst, it is a matter of life or death for the child. Short of death, there may still be possible brain damage or handicap.

Physical abuse is not a full diagnosis; it is merely a symptom of disordered parenting. The aim of intervention is to diagnose and cure (if possible) the disordered parenting and abnormal family dynamics. It is not the intention to take children away from their natural parents unless there is serious risk of physical injury. In practice only about 1–4% of all children who are the subject of referrals are taken out of the home to a place of safety. In the 1970s it was estimated that in the USA 5% of abused children who were returned to the home environment without some form of intervention died following further trauma (33) and 35–50% sustained serious re-injury (33, 34). However, by 1986 it was recognized that probably as many as 50% of severely abused children returned to the abuser would die of recurrent abuse if proper therapeutic measures were not introduced (35). In some cases, the occurrence of physical abuse may provide an opportunity for intervention. If this opportunity is missed, there may be no further opportunity for many years.

There are no hard-and-fast rules to make the diagnosis of physical abuse easier (36). The following list constitutes seven classic indicators to the diagnosis. None of them is pathognomonic on its own; neither does the absence of any of them preclude the diagnosis of physical abuse (37).

(1) There is a delay in seeking medical help (or medical help is not sought at all).

(2) The story of the 'accident' is vague, is lacking in detail, and may vary with each telling and from person to person.

(3) The account of the accident is not compatible with the injury observed.

(4) The parents' mood is abnormal. Normal parents are full of creative anxiety for the child; while abusing parents tend to be more pre-occupied with their own problems – for example, how they can return home as soon as possible.

(5) The parents' behavior gives cause for concern – for example they may become hostile and rebut accusations that have not been made.

(6) The child's appearance and the interaction with their parents are abnormal. The child may look sad, withdrawn, or frightened.

(7) The child may say something concerning the injury that is different to the parents' story.

## Types of orofacial injuries in child physical abuse

At least 50% of cases diagnosed as child physical abuse have orofacial trauma, which may or may not be associated with injury elsewhere (8, 38–43). Although the face often seems to be the focus of impulsive violence, facial fractures are not frequent. The most detailed studies were those reported by Becker et al. (1978) (40), da Fonseca et al. (1992) (41), Jessee (1995) (42) and Cairns et al. (2005) (43). In Becker's study the medical records of 260 cases of child abuse admitted to The Children's Hospital in Boston between 1970 and 1975 were reviewed. One-hundred-and-twenty-eight (49%) of the patients had facial and/or intra-oral trauma. An additional 16% of the children had injuries to the head, such as skull fractures, subdural hematomas, contusions and lacerations of the scalp. Of the 236 injuries sustained by the orofacial structures, 61% involved the face (66% contusions and ecchymoses, 28% abrasions and lacerations, 4% burns and bites, 2% fractures) and 6% the intraoral structures (43% contusions and ecchymoses, 28% abrasions and lacerations, 28% dental trauma). In da Fonseca's study the number of cases was higher (1248) but the spectrum of injuries was similar. The incidence of orofacial signs in physical abuse was 78%, sexual abuse 13%, and neglect 24%. In all types of abuse the average incidence of orofacial signs was 34%. Jessee's study undertaken in Texas found that out of 266 patients with physical abuse some 65% had orofacial injuries, and Cairns et al. in Scotland found a figure of 59% with orofacial injuries in a similar population of 390 children. In all the studies it was found that soft tissue injuries, most frequently bruises, were the most common injury sustained to the orofacial structures in physical abuse.

It is extremely important to state that there are no injuries which are pathognomonic of child abuse. Any text that suggests so is incorrect.

**Table 7.1** Typical sites for inflicted bruises.

| |
| --- |
| Buttocks and lower back (paddling) |
| Genitals and inner thigh |
| Cheek (slap marks) |
| Earlobe (pinch marks) |
| Upper lip and frenum (forced feeding) |
| Neck (choke marks) |

## Bruising

Accidental falls rarely cause bruises to the soft tissues of the cheek; but instead involve the skin overlying bony prominences such as the forehead or cheekbone. Inflicted bruises occur at typical sites and/or fit recognizable patterns (Table 7.1) (25). The clinical dating of bruises according to color is inaccurate (44, 45). However bruises of different vintage indicate more than one episode of abuse and, together with extensive bruising and a history of minimal trauma, bruises of different vintages are very suggestive of physical abuse (Fig. 7.1).

Bruises on the ear are commonly due to the child being pinched or pulled by the ear (Fig. 7.1); and there will usually be a matching bruise on the posterior surface of the ear.

Bruises or cuts on the neck are almost always due to being choked or strangled by a human hand, cord or some sort of collar. Accidents to this site are extremely rare and should be looked upon with suspicion. 'Resuscitation' attempts do not leave bruises on the face or neck. Bruising and laceration of the upper labial frenum of a young child can be produced by forcible bottle feeding and is another injury of physical abuse, but one which may remain hidden unless the lip is carefully everted (Fig. 7.2). The same injury can also be caused by gagging or gripping and violent rubbing of the face; and may be accompanied by facial bruising/abrasions. A frenum tear is not uncommon in the young child who accidentally falls while learning to walk (generally between 8–18 months). However, a frenum tear in a very young non-ambulatory patient (less than 1 year) should arouse one's suspicion as to the possibility of this injury being non-accidental (46).

## Human hand marks

The human hand can leave various types of pressure bruises: grab marks or fingertip bruises, linear marks or finger-edge bruises, handprints, slap marks and pinch marks (25). The most common types are grab marks or squeeze marks which leave oval-shaped bruises that resemble fingerprints. Grab mark bruises can occur on the cheeks if an adult squeezes a child's face in an attempt to get food or medicine into his mouth. This action leaves a thumb mark bruise on one cheek and 2–4 finger mark bruises on the other cheek. Linear marks are caused by pressure from the entire finger.

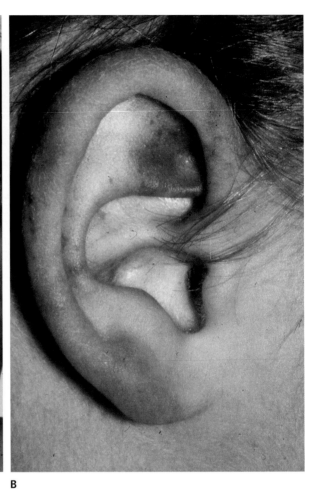

A                                                                    B

**Fig. 7.1** Three-year-old boy suffering from physical abuse. Note bruising of different vintages involving the skin overlying the bony prominences of the cheekbones and the soft tissue areas of the cheek and circumoral region. This history was inconsistent with the amount, degree and vintage of the bruising. The 'pinch' type bruises on the superior surface of the right ear was a result of the ear being held between the fingers and thumb of the abuser and then pulled.

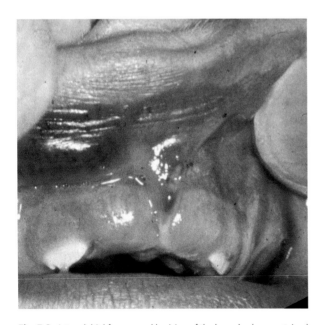

**Fig. 7.2** A torn labial frenum and bruising of the buccal sulcus, sustained during forceful feeding.

In slap marks to the cheek, parallel linear bruises at finger-width spacing will be seen to run through a more diffuse bruise (Fig. 7.3). These linear bruises are due to the capillaries rupturing at the edge of the injury (between the striking fingers), as a result of being stretched and receiving a sudden influx of blood.

## Bizarre bruises

Bizarre-shaped bruises with sharp borders are nearly always deliberately inflicted. If there is a pattern on the inflicting implement, this may be duplicated in the bruise – so-called tattoo bruising (Fig. 7.4).

## Abrasions and lacerations

Penetrating injuries to the palate, vestibule and floor of the mouth can occur during forceful feeding of young infants; these are usually caused by the feeding utensil.

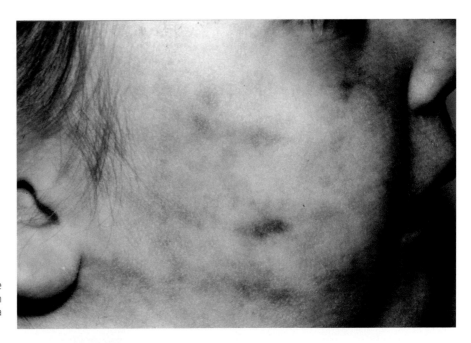

**Fig. 7.3** A slap mark bruise. Three parallel linear bruises at finger-width spacing can be seen to run through a more diffuse bruise.

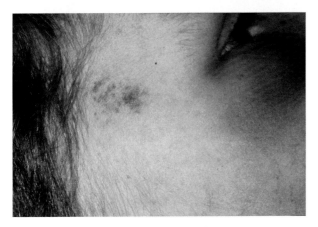

**Fig. 7.4** Tattoo bruising in the right forehead region of the child in Fig. 7.1. The exact object causing this injury was not known.

Abrasions and lacerations on the face may be caused by a variety of objects, but are most commonly due to rings or fingernails on the inflicting hand and injuries are rarely confined to the orofacial structures (Figs 7.1 and 7.5).

## Burns

Approximately 10% of physical abuse cases involve burns (47). Burns of the oral mucosa can be the result of forced ingestion of hot or caustic fluids in young children. Burns from hot solid objects applied to the face are usually without blister formation and the shape of the burn often resembles its agent. Cigarette burns give circular, punched out lesions of uniform size (Figs 7.5 and 7.9). Lesions produced by cigarette burns may resemble bullous impetigo, hence it is critical to reiterate the point made earlier that no single type of lesion is pathognomonic of child abuse.

## Bite marks

Human bite marks are identified by their shape and size (Fig. 7.6). When necessary, serological techniques are available and may assist in identification (48). The nature and location of the bite is likely to change with increasing age of the child. In infants, bite marks tend to be punitive and are often a response to soiling or crying. As a result, bite marks may appear anywhere; but they tend to be concentrated on the cheek, arm, shoulders, buttocks or genitalia. In childhood, bite marks tend to be less punitive and more a function of assault or defense. Sexually orientated bite marks occur more frequently in adolescents and adults (49). However, a bite mark at any age should raise the suspicion of child sexual abuse.

The duration of a bite mark is dependent on the force applied and the extent of tissue damage. Teeth marks that do not break the skin are visible up to 24 hours. In those cases where the skin is broken, the borders or edges will be apparent for several days depending on the thickness of the tissue. Thinner tissues retain the marks longer (50).

## Dental trauma

Trauma either to the primary or permanent dentition in physical abuse can be due to blunt trauma (Fig. 7.7). A similar range of injuries to those found in accidental trauma is seen.

## Eye injuries

Most periorbital bruises caused by child physical abuse involve both sides of the face. Ocular damage in child

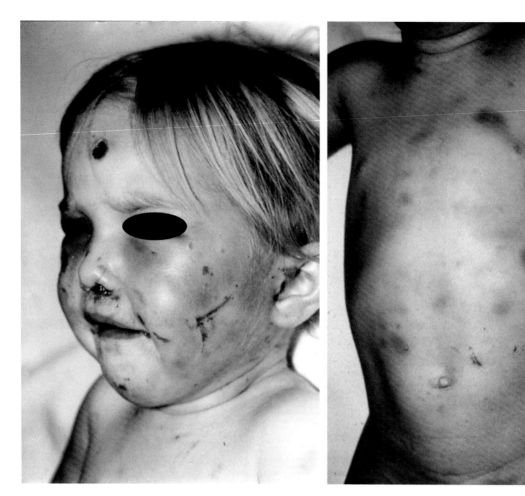

**Fig. 7.5** Multiple superficial lacerations, extensive facial bruising of different vintages, a cigarette burn of the forehead and a 'pinch' injury of the left ear in a child subjected to repeated physical abuse. There are numerous pinch mark bruises over the chest and abdomen, extensive bruising over the suprapubic region and a number of small abrasions and lacerations.

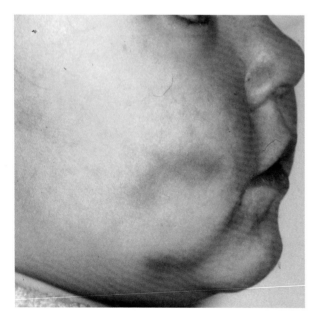

**Fig. 7.6** A human bite-mark injury on the right cheek.

physical abuse includes acute hyphema, dislocated lens, traumatic cataract and detached retina (51). More than half of these injuries result in permanent impairment of vision affecting one or both eyes.

## Bone fractures

Fractures are among the most serious injuries sustained in physical abuse. They may occur in almost any bone and may be single or multiple, clinically obvious, or occult and detectable only by radiography. Most fractures in physically abused children occur under the age of 3 (52). In contrast, accidental fractures occur more commonly in children of school age.

Facial fractures are relatively uncommon in children. They can, however, occur during physical assault with nasal fractures occurring most frequently (45%), followed by mandibular fractures (32%), and zygomatic maxillary complex and orbit fractures (20%) (53).

The presence of a fracture of the facial skeleton in a case of child physical abuse is an indication for a full skeletal

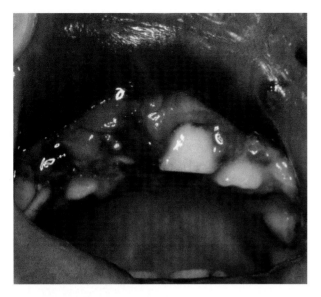

**Fig. 7.7** Luxation of four incisors and extensive bruising in the upper buccal sulcus sustained as a result of a blow to the mouth.

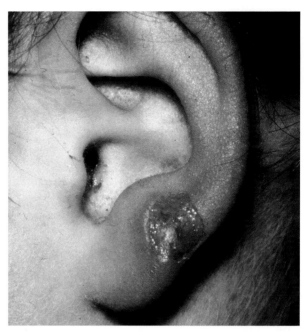

**Fig. 7.9** A discrete well demarcated lesion, typical of the appearance of a cigarette burn.

## Differential diagnosis

Although dental practitioners should be suspicious of all injuries to children, they should never consider the diagnosis of child physical abuse on the basis of one sign, as various diseases can be mistaken for child physical abuse. Impetiginous lesions may look similar to cigarette burns (Figs 7.9 and 7.10); birthmarks can be mistaken for bruising; and conjunctivitis can be mistaken for trauma. All children who are said to bruise easily and extensively should have a full blood count, platelet estimation and blood coagulation studies to eliminate a blood dyscrasia (e.g. leukemia), a platelet deficiency (e.g. thrombocytopenia) or other hemorrhagic disorders (e.g. hemophilia, von Willebrand's disease).

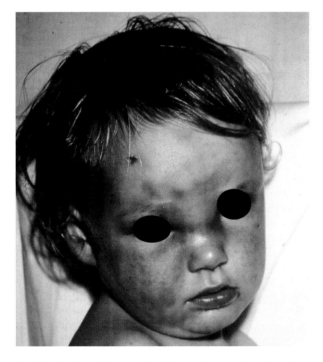

**Fig. 7.8** A fracture of the nasoethmoidal complex caused by a heavy blow to the midface.

## The dentist's role in the management of child physical abuse

radiographic survey (Fig. 7.8). Generally the force required to produce a facial fracture in a child is greater than that required to produce metaphyseal, epiphyseal, spiral, oblique and transverse fractures in long bones. A skeletal survey of a child who has suffered child physical abuse may show evidence of multiple fractures at different stages of healing.

In some instances, a number of the varied features mentioned above may be present at any one time and the diagnosis of child physical abuse will be clear. However, there are occasions when clinical evidence is inconclusive and the diagnosis merely suspected.

The dental practitioner may be the first professional to suspect physical abuse as a result of injuries involving the orofacial structures (54–63). The primary aim of all professionals involved is to ensure the safety of the child. The secondary aim is to provide help and counseling for the parents or care givers so that the abuse stops. The method of liaison and referral between dental practitioners and the other health care professionals involved in child abuse cases will vary, not only from country to country, but also between cities and different regions within one country. It is now law in a number of countries that regional child welfare

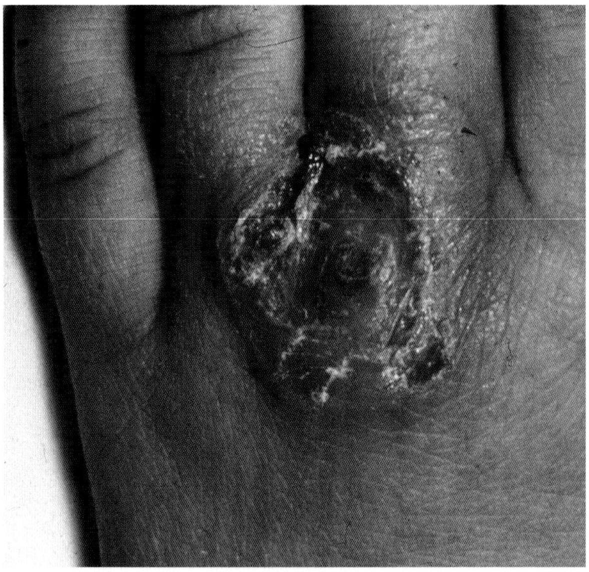

**Fig. 7.10** An impetiginous lesion which can resemble the appearance of a cigarette burn.

departments issue procedural guidelines for dental practitioners in suspected child abuse cases. A small number of studies have investigated general dental practitioners' views on their role within child protection or on possible barriers specifically related to child protection which militate against their undertaking such a role (64–71). They felt some reluctance to become involved because of their lack of knowledge both of the signs of child abuse and the workings of the other agencies involved in child protection. They also reported significant concerns about how notifying possible incidents might affect the child, family unit and practice. This suggests a lack of knowledge about the aim of the child protection agencies that are not only to protect children from further abuse but also to strengthen the family unit. It seems highly likely that unless this training issue is addressed, children will present to dentists with indicators of potential abuse and will receive an inadequate and/or inconsistent response to their need for protection. This is particularly disturbing as the consequences of such inadequate responses from health and social care professionals have recently been widely publicized in landmark cases (72).

A child with a severe injury should be referred immediately to a hospital-based consultant pediatrician. Where suspicions are aroused in other cases, the dentist should speak to the designated person in the local guidelines who will advise on the appropriate course of action.

Dental practitioners should ensure that their clinical records are completed immediately with illustrations of the size, position and type of injuries. Photographic documentation would be beneficial in this respect. These records may be referred to in any subsequent case conference or legal proceedings.

In law the needs of a child are paramount. Dental practitioners should not feel any guilt about referring a child in need to the child protection services as they are not accus-

ing either parent; they are simply asking for help and a second opinion on an important and difficult diagnosis. It is neither in the interest of the child nor the parents for child abuse to be covered up. To do so leaves the parents at greater risk of inflicting more severe injuries next time, being imprisoned for causing more severe injuries, and long-term loss of custody of their children. Early intervention may help to prevent these events. Failure to follow up suspicions is a form of professional negligence. Dental practitioners should be aware that in the United States a doctor who fails to report suspected child abuse is guilty of a federal offence that is punishable by imprisonment.

This said, it must be stressed that the diagnosis of child physical abuse is a difficult one to make with certainty. Because of the high frequency of intraoral and facial injuries, dental professionals comprise a very important part of the team necessary for identifying and reporting child abuse and neglect (41, 73). However, the team approach is absolutely necessary, whereby members of multiple specialties collaborate to confirm the diagnosis of child physical abuse. Successful child protection involves the sharing of albeit small pieces of information between the caring agencies to obtain a whole picture of that child and their environment. Without adequate training, dental staff will not feel empowered to take responsibility for referring a child to the protection services. This mismatch between dental practitioners' attitudes to and knowledge of the child protection process and the reality of child abuse poses of itself a significant risk to children.

In conclusion, the dental practitioner's contribution to the management of child physical abuse. should be to (31):

(1) recognize the possibility of physical abuse
(2) provide essential emergency dental treatment and arrange further treatment if required
(3) inform the appropriate authorities of his or her suspicions.

## Essentials

### Terminology

- Non-accidental injury (NAI) or child physical abuse.

### Frequency

- Prevalences in children range from 0.1% to 10% in various countries.

### Clinical findings

- Delay in seeking treatment
- Explanation for injury does not fit the clinical findings
- Explanation for injury may differ with each telling and from person to person
- Abnormal parental reaction and behavior
- Type of relationship between parents and child

- The child's reaction to other people
- The child's story may differ from parents'
- 50% of child physical abuse cases have orofacial findings
- Usually more than one sign present
- Hematomas of different vintage suggest repeated trauma.

## Treatment

- Recognize the possibility of physical abuse
- Provide emergency dental treatment
- Refer the patient for a medical examination.

## References

1. BAKAN D. *Slaughter of the innocents. A study of the battered child phenomenon.* Boston: Beacon Press, 1972.
2. RADBILL SX. A history of child abuse and infanticide. In: Herfer RE, Kempe CH. eds. *The battered child.* Chicago: University of Chicago Press, 1968.
3. SOLOMON T. History and demography of child abuse. *Paediatrics* 1973;**51**:773–6.
4. CAFFEY J. Multiple fractures in the long bones of infants suffering from chronic subdural haematoma. *Am J Roentgenol Radium Ther Nucl Med* 1946;**56**:162–73.
5. SILVERMAN FN. The roentgen manifestations of unrecognised skeletal trauma in infants. *Am J Roentgenol Radium Ther Nucl Med* 1953;**69**:413–27.
6. WOOLLEY PV, EVANS WA. Significance of skeletal lesions in infants resembling those of traumatic origin. *J Am Med Assoc* 1955;**158**:539–43.
7. KEMPE CH, SILVERMAN FN, STEELE BF, DROEGEMUELLER W, SILVER HK. The battered-child syndrome. *J Am Med Assoc* 1962;**181**:105–12.
8. BAETZ K, SLEDZIEWSKI W, MARGETTS D. Recognition and management of the battered child syndrome. *J Dent Assoc S. Afr* 1977;**32**:13–18.
9. AGATHONOS H, STATHACOPOULOU N, ADAM H, NAKOU S. Child abuse and neglect in Greece: sociomedical aspects. *Child Abuse Neglect* 1982;**6**:307–11.
10. CREIGHTON S. An epidemiological study of abused children and their families in the United Kingdom between 1977 and 1982. *Child Abuse Neglect* 1985;**9**:441–8.
11. FERRIER P, SCHALLER M, GIRARDET I. Abused children admitted to a paediatric in-patient service in Switzerland: a ten year experience and follow up evaluation. *Child Abuse Neglect* 1985;**9**:373–81.
12. MARZOUKI M, HADHFREDI A, CHELLI M. L'enfant battu et les attitudes culturelles: L'exemple de la Tunisie. *Child Abuse Neglect* 1987;**11**:137–41.
13. SYMONS AL, ROWE PV, ROMANIAK K. Dental aspects of child abuse: review and case reports. *Aust Dent J* 1987;**32**:427.
14. FINKELHOR D, KORBIN J. Child abuse as an international issue. *Child Abuse Neglect* 1988;**12**:3–23.
15. MERRICK J, MICHELSEN N. Children at-risk: child abuse in Denmark. *Int J Rehabil Res* 1985;**8**:181–8.
16. LARSSON G, EKENSTEIN G, RASCH E. Are the social workers prepared to assist a changing population of dysfunctional parents in Sweden? *Child Abuse Neglect* 1984;**8**:9–14.
17. PELTONIEMI T. Child abuse and physical punishment of children in Finland. *Child Abuse Neglect* 1983;**7**:33–6.
18. OLESEN T, EGEBLAD M, DIGE-PETERSEN H, AHLGREN P, NIELSEN AM, VESTERDAL J. Somatic manifestations in children suspected of having been maltreated. *Acta Paediatr Scand* 1988;**77**:154–60.
19. WALDMAN BH, PERLMAN SP. The rate of child abuse and neglect cases per population totals decreased since the mid 1990s. *ASDC J Dent Child* 2002;**69**:314–18.
20. HART SN, BRASSARD MR. A major threat to children's mental health: psychological maltreatment. *Amer Psychol* 1987;**42**:160–5.
21. MEADOW R. Epidemiology. The ABC of child abuse. *Br Med J*, 1989;**298**:727–30.
22. CREIGHTON SJ. The incidence of child abuse and neglect. In: Browne K, Davies C, Stratton P. eds. *Early prediction and prevention of child abuse.* Chichester, England: Wiley, 1988.
23. BILLMIRE ME, MYERS PA. Serious head injury in infants: accident or abuse? *Pediatrics* 1985;**75**:340–2.
24. HOLTER JC, FRIEDMAN SB. Child abuse, early case finding in the emergency department. *Pediatrics* 1968;**42**:128–38.
25. BREITING VB, HELWEG-LARSEN K, STAUGAARD H, et al. Injuries due to deliberate violence in areas of Denmark. *Forensic Sci Int* 1989;**41**:285–94.
26. CREIGHTON SJ, GALLAGHER B. *Child abuse deaths.* Information Briefing No.5 (revised). London: The National Society for the Prevention of Cruelty to Children, 1988.
27. GREGERSEN M, VESTERBY A. Child abuse and neglect in Denmark: medicolegal aspects. *Child Abuse Neglect* 1984;**8**:83–91.
28. GREEN AH, GAINES RW, SANDRUND A. Child abuse: pathological syndrome of family interaction. *Am J Psych* 1974;**131**:882–8.
29. LASKIN DM. The battered child syndrome. *J Oral Surg* 1973;**31**:903.
30. SOPHER IM. The dentist and the battered child syndrome. *Dent Clin North Am* 1977;**21**:113–22.
31. MacINTYRE DR, JONES GM, PINCKNEY RCN. The role of the dental practitioner in the management of non-accidental injury to children. *Br Dent J* 1986;**161**: 108–10.
32. POLLOCK VE, BRIERE J, SCHNEIDER L, KNOP J, MEDNICK SA, GOODWIN DW. Childhood antecedents of antisocial behaviour: parental alcoholism and physical abusiveness. *Am J Psych* 1990;**147**:1290–3.
33. SCHMITT BD, KEMPE CH. Neglect and abuse of children. In: Vaughan VC, Mckay RJ. eds. *Nelson textbook of paediatrics.* 10th edn. Philadelphia: WB Saunders, 1975:107–11.
34. LASKIN DM. The recognition of child abuse. *J Oral Surg* 1978;**36**:349.
35. KITTLE PE, RICHARDSON DS, PARKER JW. Examining for child abuse and neglect. *Pediatric Dentistry* 1986;**8**:80–2.
36. SILVER LB, DUBLIN CC, LAURIE RS. Child abuse syndrome. The 'grey areas' in establishing a diagnosis. *Paediatrics* 1969;**44**:594–600.
37. SPEIGHT N. Non-accidental injury. The ABC of child abuse. *Br Med J* 1989;**298**:879–81.

38. CAMERON JM, JOHNSON HR, CAMPS FE. The battered child syndrome. *Med Sci Law* 1966;**6**:1–36.

39. SKINNER AE, CASTLE RL. *78 battered children: a retrospective study*. London: National Society for the Prevention of Cruelty to Children 1969:1–21.

40. BECKER DB, NEEDLEMAN HL, KOTELCHUCK M. Child abuse and dentistry; orofacial trauma and its recognition by dentists. *J Am Dent Assoc* 1978;**97**:24–8 .

41. DA FONSECA MA, FEIGAL RJ, TEN BENSEL RW. Dental aspects of 1248 cases of child maltreatment on file at a major county hospital. *Paed Dent* 1992;**14**:152–7.

42. JESSEE SA. Physical manifestations of child abuse to the head, face and mouth: a hospital survey. *ASDC J Dent Child* 1995;**62**:245–9.

43. CAIRNS AM, MOK JYQ, WELBURY RR. Injuries to the head, face, mouth and neck in physically abused children in a community setting. *Int J Paed Dent* 2005;**5**:310–318.

44. STEPHENSON T, BIALAS Y. Estimation of the age of bruising. *Arch Dis Child* 1996;**74**:53–5.

45. MUNANG LA, LEONARD PA, MOQ JYQ. Lack of agreement on colour description between clinicians examining childhood bruising. *J Clini Foren Med* 2002;**9**:171–9.

46. WELBURY RR, MURPHY JM. The dental practitioner's role in protecting children from abuse: 2. The orofacial signs of physical abuse. *Br Dent J* 1998;**184**:61–5.

47. LENOSKI EF, HUNTER KA. Specific patterns of inflicted burn injuries. *J Trauma* 1977;**17**:842–6.

48. SWEET D, PRETTY IA. A look at forensic dentistry. Part 2: Teeth as weapons of violence – identification of bite mark perpetrators. *Br Dent J* 2001;**8**:415–18.

49. WAGNER GN. Bitemark identification in child abuse cases. *Paed Dent* 1986;**8**:96–100.

50. DINKEL EH. The use of bitemark evidence as an investigative aid. *J For Sci* 1974;**19**:535–47.

51. GAMMON JA. Ophthalmic manifestations of child abuse, In: Ellerstein NS. ed. *Child abuse and neglect: a medical reference*. New York: John Wiley and Sons, 1981:121–39.

52. WARLOCK P, STOWER M, BARBOR P. Patterns of fractures in accidental and non-accidental injury in children: a comparative study. *Br Med J* 1986;**293**:100–2.

53. KABAN LB, MULLIKEN JB, MURRAY JE. Facial fractures in children. *Plast Reconstr Surg* 1977;**59**:15–20.

54. HAZELWOOD AI. Child abuse. The dentist's role. *N Y State Dent J* 1970;**36**:289–91.

55. TATE RJ. Facial injuries associated with the battered child syndrome. *Br J Oral Surg* 1971;**9**:41–5.

56. DAVIS GR, DOMOTO PK, LEVY RM. The dentist's role in child abuse and neglect, issues, identification, and management. *ASDC J Dent Child* **46**:185–92.

57. BLUMBERG ML, KUNKEN FR. The dentist's involvement with child abuse. *N Y State Dent J* 1981;**47**:65–9.

58. CROLL TP, MENNA VJ, EVANS CA. Primary identification of an abused child in the dental office: a case report. *Paed Dent* 1981;**3**:339–41.

59. KITTLE PE, RICHARDSON DS, PARKER JW. Two child abuse/child neglect examinations for the dentist. *ASDC J Dent Child* 1981;**48**:175–80.

60. WRIGHT JT, THORNTON JB. Osteogenesis imperfecta with dentinogenesis imperfecta: a mistaken case of child abuse. *Paed Dent* 1983;**5**:207–9.

61. SOBEL RS. Child abuse: a case report. *Paed Dent* 1986;**8**:93–5.

62. TSANG A, SWEET D. Detecting child abuse and neglect – are dentists doing enough? *J Can Dent Assoc* 1999;**65**:387–91.

63. SENN DR, MCDOWELL JD, ALDER ME. Dentistry's role in the recognition and reporting of domestic violence, abuse, and neglect. *Dent Clin North Am* 2001;**45**:343–63.

64. NEEDLEMAN HL, MACGREGOR SS, LYNCH LM. Effectiveness of a statewide child abuse and neglect educational program for dental professionals. *Paed Dent* 1995;**17**:41–5.

65. ADAIR SM, WRAY IA, HANES CM, SAMS DR, YASREBI S, RUSSELL CM. Perceptions associated with dentists' decisions to report hypothetical cases of child maltreatment. *Paed Dent* 1997;**19**:461–5.

66. ADAIR SM, WRAY IA, HANES CM, SAMS DR, YASREBI S, RUSSELL CM. Demographic. educational, and experiential factors associated with dentists' decisions to report hypothetical cases of child maltreatment. *Paed Dent* 1997;**19**:466–9.

67. RAMOS-GOMEZ, F, ROTHMAN, D, BLAIN, S. Knowledge and attitudes among California dental care providers regarding child abuse and neglect. *J Am Dent Assoc* 1998;**129**(3):340–8.

68. KILPATRICK NM, SCOTT J, ROBINSON S. Child protection: a survey of experience and knowledge within the dental profession of New South Wales, Australia. *Paed Dent* 1999;**9**:153–9.

69. JOHN V, MESSER LB, ARORA R, FUNG S, HARZIS E, NGUYEN T, SAN A, THOMAS K. Child abuse and dentistry: a study of knowledge and attitudes among dentists in Victoria, Australia. *Aust Dent J* 1999;**44**:259–67.

70. WELBURY RR, MACASKILL SG, MURPHY JM, EVANS DJ, WEIGHTMAN KE, JACKSON MC, CRAWFOD MA. General dental practitioners' perception of their role within child protection: a qualitative study. *Eur J Paed Dent* 2003;**4**:89–95.

71. CAIRNS AM, MOK JYQ, WELBURY RR. The dental practitioner and child protection in Scotland. *Br Dent J* 2005;**199**:517–520.

72. Department of Health. *The Victoria Climbié Inquiry*. Report of an inquiry by Lord Laming. London: Her Majesty's Stationary Office, 2003.

73. RASMUSSEN P. *Tannlegens forhold til sykdom hos barn, barnemishandling og omsorgssvikt. Odontologi 1992*. Copenhagen: Munksgaard, 1992:81–92.

# 8

# Classification, Epidemiology and Etiology

U. Glendor, W. Marcenes & J. O. Andreasen

## Classification

A fundamental prerequisite for the study of a disease or condition is an accurate definition of the disease or condition under investigation. Traumatic dental injuries (TDI) have been classified according to a variety of factors, such as etiology, anatomy, pathology, therapeutic considerations (1–14, 62, 131, 132, 200–205), and degree of severity (151, 172, 188, 206–208).

### Classification in the clinic

The present classification is based on a system adopted by the World Health Organization (WHO) in its *Application of international classification of diseases to dentistry and stomatology* (133). However, for the sake of completeness, it was felt necessary to define and classify certain trauma entities not included in the WHO system. The following classification includes injuries to the teeth, supporting structures, gingival, and oral mucosa and is based on anatomical, therapeutic, and prognostic considerations and can be applied to both the primary and the permanent dentitions (Table 8.1, Figs 8.1 to 8.4). The code number is according to the International Classification of Diseases (1992) (133). This classification is appropriate to use in a dental surgery with diagnostic aids such as pulp sensibility tests, transillumination, and radiographic examination. In this text the WHO classification will be used to describe the various trauma types.

### Field screening

Epidemiological studies may also be performed as field screenings, but they lack some of the methods used in clinics, for example radiographic examination. A solution to this is to use a classification that is a compilation based on the most common classifications currently used in epidemiological surveys. It is very similar to the one proposed by Ellis and Davey in 1970 (6).

The second epidemiological classification (Table 8.2) presented here is not a new classification, but a compilation based on common classifications currently used in epidemiological surveys. It is similar to the one proposed by Ellis and Davey in 1970 (6). In addition, the current classification reorganized the categories into a logical system reflecting the level of severity of the injury and the complexity of the treatment required. The epidemiological classification includes 6 categories: no TDI, treated TDI, enamel fracture only, enamel and dentin fracture, pulp injury, and missing tooth due to TDI (Table 8.2). The prevalence of TDI obtained using this classification can be directly compared to those recorded in most studies carried out in several countries, for example, the UK (212) and USA (210) (Table 8.3). It is important to note that many signs and symptoms assessed in a dental surgery at the time of the injury (Table 8.2) cannot be identified in a survey. For example, injuries to the supporting structures are not included in any classification because they do not leave a visible permanent marker, such as tooth fractures. Similarly, other signs are excluded because surveys do not use diagnostic aids. Hospital or surgery based studies present a similar challenge as these do not record injuries in those who did not visit a dentist due to the injury. In the UK, two out of each three children presented with untreated TDI (212). Thus, the prevalence of TDI tends to be grossly underestimated unless one carries out a prospective study including a random sample from a population.

To assess the prevalence of TDI one needs to record both the presence of treated and untreated TDIs. Also, it may be of interest to know the type of treatment provided and needed.

**Table 8.1** Clinical classification of traumatic dental injuries (TDI) including codes of the WHO International Classification of Diseases to Dentistry and Stomatology.

### (a) Injuries to the hard dental tissues and the pulp (Fig. 8.1).

| Code | Injury | Criteria |
|---|---|---|
| N 502.50 | Enamel infraction | An incomplete fracture (crack) of the enamel without loss of tooth substance (Fig. 8.1, A). |
| N 502.50 | Enamel fracture (uncomplicated crown fracture) | A fracture with loss of tooth substance confined to the enamel (N 502.50) (Fig. 8.1, A). |
| N 502.51 | Enamel-dentin fracture (uncomplicated crown fracture) | A fracture with loss of tooth substance confined to enamel and dentin, but not involving the pulp (Fig. 8.1, B). |
| N 502.52 | Complicated crown fracture | A fracture involving enamel and dentin, and exposing the pulp (Fig. 8.1, C). |
| N 502.54 | Uncomplicated crown-root fracture | A fracture involving enamel, dentin and cementum, but not exposing the pulp (Fig. 8.1, D). |
| N 502.54 | Complicated crown-root fracture | A fracture involving enamel, dentin and cementum, and exposing the pulp (Fig. 8.1, E). |
| N 502.53 | Root fracture | A fracture involving dentin, cementum, and the pulp (Fig. 8.1, F). Root fractures can be further classified according to displacement of the coronal fragment, see under Luxation injuries. |

### (b) Injuries to the periodontal tissues (Fig. 8.2).

| Code | Injury | Criteria |
|---|---|---|
| N 503.20 | Concussion | An injury to the tooth-supporting structures without abnormal loosening or displacement of the tooth, but with marked reaction to percussion (Fig. 8.2, A). |
| N 503.20 | Subluxation (loosening) | An injury to the tooth-supporting structures with abnormal loosening, but without displacement of the tooth (Fig. 8.2, B). |
| N 503.20 | Extrusive luxation (peripheral dislocation, partial avulsion) | Partial displacement of the tooth out of its socket (Fig. 8.2, C). |
| N 503.20 | Lateral luxation | Displacement of the tooth in a direction other than axially. This is accompanied by comminution or fracture of the alveolar socket (Fig. 8.2, D). |
| N 503.21 | Intrusive luxation (central dislocation) | Displacement of the tooth into the alveolar bone. This injury is accompanied by comminution or fracture of the alveolar socket (Fig. 8.2, E). |
| N 503.22 | Avulsion (exarticulation) | Complete displacement of the tooth out of its socket (Fig. 8.2, F). |

### (c) Injuries to the supporting bone (Fig. 8.3).

| Code | Injury | Criteria |
|---|---|---|
| N 502.40 | Comminution of the maxillary alveolar socket | Crushing and compression of the alveolar socket. This condition is found concomitantly with intrusive and lateral luxations (Fig. 8.3, A). |
| N 502.60 | Comminution of the mandibular alveolar socket | |
| N 502.40 | Fracture of the maxillary alveolar socket wall | A fracture confined to the facial or oral socket wall (Fig. 8.3, B). |
| N 502.60 | Fracture of the mandibular alveolar socket wall | |
| N 502.40 | Fracture of the maxillary alveolar process | A fracture of the alveolar process which may or may not involve the alveolar socket (Figs 8.3, C and D). |
| N 502.60 | Fracture of the mandibular alveolar process | |
| N 502.42 | Fracture of the maxilla | A fracture involving the base of the maxilla or mandible and often the alveolar process (jaw fracture). The fracture may or may not involve the alveolar socket (Figs 8.3, E and F). |
| N 502.61 | Fracture of the mandible | |

### (d) Injuries to gingiva or oral mucosa (Fig. 8.4).

| Code | Injury | Criteria |
|---|---|---|
| S 01.50 | Laceration of gingiva or oral mucosa | A shallow or deep wound in the mucosa resulting from a tear, and usually produced by a sharp object (Fig. 8.4, A). |
| S 00.50 | Contusion of gingiva or oral mucosa | A bruise usually produced by impact with a blunt object and not accompanied by a break in the mucosa, usually causing submucosal hemorrhage (Fig. 8.4, B). |
| S 00.50 | Abrasion of gingiva or oral mucosal | A superficial wound produced by rubbing or scraping of the mucosa leaving a raw, bleeding surface (Fig. 8.4, C). |

**Table 8.2** Epidemiological classification of traumatic dental injuries (TDI) including codes of the WHO International Classification of Diseases to Dentistry and Stomatology.

| Code | Injury | Criteria |
|------|--------|----------|
| Code 0 | No injury | No evidence of treated or untreated dental injury. |
| Code 1 | Treated dental injury | Composite restoration, bonding of the tooth fragment, crown, denture or bridge pontics replacing missing teeth due to TDI, restoration located in the palatal/lingual surface of the crown suggesting endodontic treatment and no evidence of decay, or any other treatment provided due to TDI.<br>Note: Composite restorations may be difficult to recognize. It is crucial to use the CPI probe to detect any loss in continuity in the labial and/or lingual/palatal surfaces. |
| Code 2<br>(N 502.50) | Enamel fracture only<br>(Fig. 8.1, A) | Loss of a small portion of the crown, including only the enamel. |
| Code 3<br>(N 502.51) | Enamel/dentin fracture<br>(Fig. 8.1, B) | Loss of a portion of the crown, including enamel and dentin without pulp exposure. |
| Code 4<br>(N 502.52)<br>(N 502.53)<br>(N 502.54)<br>(N 503.20)<br>(N 503.21) | Pulp injury<br>(Fig. 8.1, C)<br>(Fig. 8.1, F)<br>(Fig. 8.1, E)<br>(Figs 8.2, C, D)<br>(Fig. 8.2, E) | Signs or symptoms of pulp involvement due to dental injury. It includes fractures with pulp exposure, dislocation of the tooth, presence of sinus tract and/or swelling in the labial or lingual vestibule without evidence of caries and discoloration of the crown. The examiner must check if pulp involvement was due to caries (presence of treated or untreated caries lesion, and ask the subject whether they have a history of a harmful incident involving the front teeth/mouth. |
| Code 5<br>(N 503.22) | Missing tooth due to trauma<br>(Fig. 8.2, F) | Absence of the tooth due to a complete avulsion. Code 5 should be used only for teeth judged to be missing due to trauma. A positive history of trauma is needed to record missing due to trauma and the examiner must ask the subject if the avulsion was due to a harmful incident involving the front teeth/mouth or have been extracted due to caries. |
| Code 9 | Excluded tooth | Signs of traumatic injury cannot be assessed, i.e. presence of appliances or all permanent incisors missing due to caries. |

**Table 8.3** Reported prevalence of traumatic dental injuries (TDI) in population based surveys.

| Examiner | Year | Country | Age groups | Sample size | No. with TDI | % |
|----------|------|---------|-----------|-------------|--------------|---|
| Holland et al. (236) | 1994 | Ireland | 16–24 | 400 | 54 | 13.5 |
|  |  |  | 25–34 | 346 | 52 | 15.0 |
| Josefsson & Lilja Karlander (373) | 1994 | Sweden[1] | 7–17 | 750 | 88 | 11.7 |
| Hargreaves et al. (245) | 1995 | USA | 11 | 1,035 | 160 | 15.4 |
| Kaste et al. (210) | 1996 | USA | 6–50 | 154 million | 39 million | 24.9 |
|  |  |  | 6–20 | 50 million | 9 million | 18.4 |
|  |  |  | 21–50 | 104 million | 29 million | 28.1 |
| Otuyemi et al. (246) | 1996 | Nigeria | 1–5 | 1,401 | 432 | 30.8 |
| Petti & Tarsitani (374) | 1996 | Italy | 6–11 | 824 |  | 20.3 |
| Borssén & Holm (225) | 1997 | Sweden | 16 | 3,007 | 1,040 | 35 |
| Hamilton et al. (201) | 1997 | England | 11–14 | 2,022 | 696 | 34.4 |
| Rodd & Chesham (274) | 1997 | UK | 14–15 |  | 557 | 44.2 |
| Carvalho et al. (262) | 1998 | Belgium | 3–5 | 750 |  | 18.0 |
| Chen et al. (220) | 1999 | Central Taiwan | 8 | 1,200 | 193 | 16.5 |
| Hargreaves et al. (255) | 1999 | South Africa | 1–5 | 1,466 | 220 | 15.0 |
| Marcenes et al. (215) | 1999 | Syria | 9 | 248 | 13 | 5.2 |
|  |  |  | 10 | 343 | 23 | 6.7 |
|  |  |  | 11 | 334 | 32 | 9.6 |
|  |  |  | 12 | 162 | 19 | 11.7 |
| Sgan-Cohen et al. (375) | 2000 | Israel | 10–11 | 1,195 |  | 32 |
| Al-Majed et al. (258) | 2001 | Saudi Arabia[3] | 5–6 | 354 | 116 | 32.8 |
|  |  |  | 12–14 | 862 | 296 | 34.3 |
| Cortes et al. (248) | 2001 | Brazil | 9 | 578 | 46 | 8.0 |
|  |  |  | 10 | 573 | 52 | 9.1 |
|  |  |  | 11 | 608 | 64 | 10.5 |
|  |  |  | 12 | 649 | 88 | 13.6 |
|  |  |  | 13 | 722 | 106 | 14.7 |
|  |  |  | 14 | 572 | 92 | 16.1 |
| Marcenes et al. (240) | 2001 | Brazil | 12 | 652 | 382 | 58.6 |
| Marcenes & Murray (242) | 2001 | England | 14 | 2,242 | 531 | 23.7 |
| Nicolau et al. (269) | 2001 | Brazil | 13 | 652 | 133 | 20.4 |
| Nik-Hussein (250) | 2001 | Malaysia | 16 | 4,085 | 169 | 4.1 |
| Perheentupa et al. (270) | 2001 | Finland | 31 | 5,737 |  | 43.3 |
| Marcenes & Murray (266) | 2002 | England | 14 | 411 |  | 43.8 |
| Kramer et al. (252) | 2003 | Brazil | 0–6 | 1,545 | 548 | 35.5 |
| Shulman & Peterson (237) | 2004 | USA | 8–50 | 15,364 |  | 23.5 |
|  |  |  | 6–20 | 6,558 |  | 16.0 |
|  |  |  | 21–50 | 8,806 |  | 27.1 |

[1] Rural population; [2] national survey; [3] urban males.

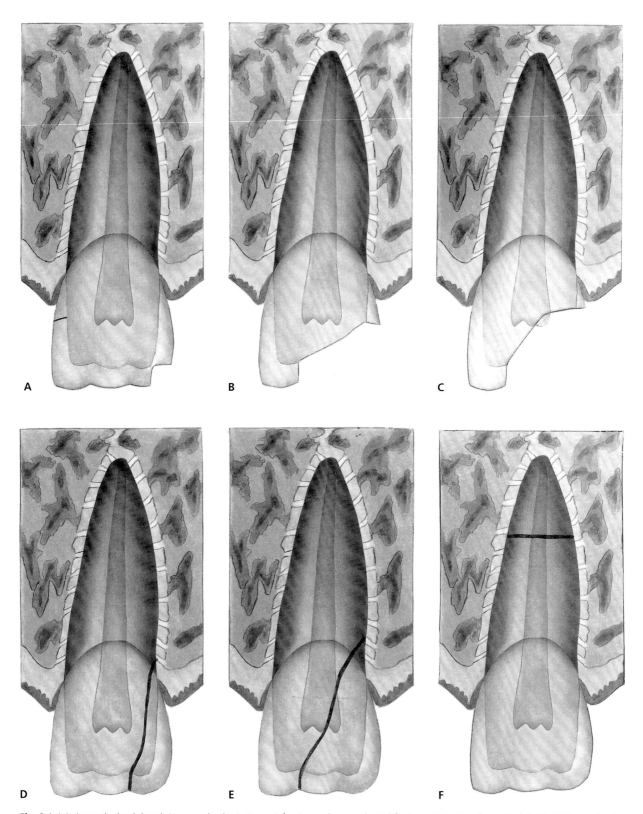

**Fig. 8.1** Injuries to the hard dental tissues and pulp. A. Crown infraction and uncomplicated fracture without involvement of dentin. B. Uncomplicated crown fracture with involvement of dentin. C. Complicated crown fracture. D. Uncomplicated crown-root fracture. E. Complicated crown-root fracture. F. Root fracture.

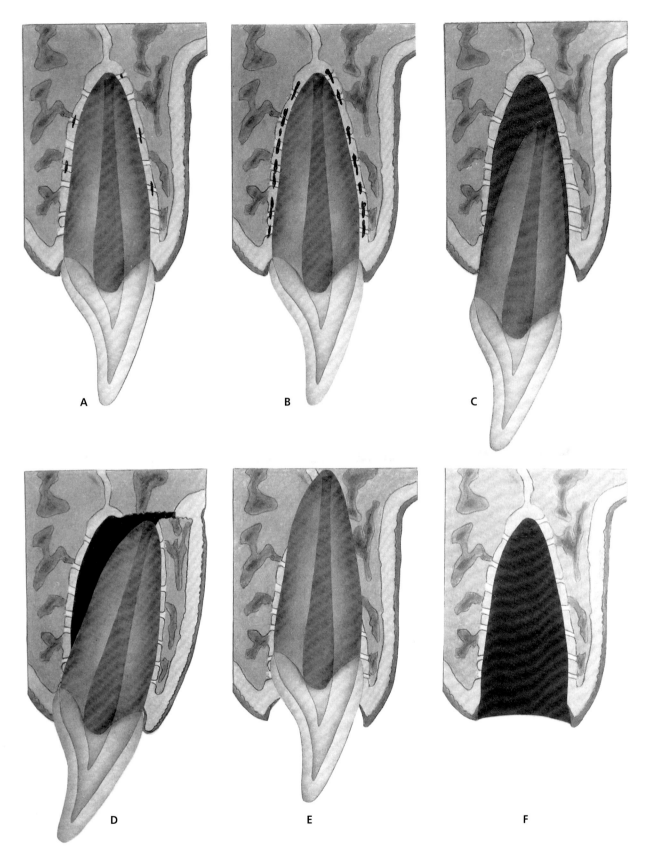

**Fig. 8.2** Injuries to the periodontal tissues. A. Concussion. B. Subluxation. C. Extrusive luxation. D. Lateral luxation. E. Intrusive luxation. F. Exarticulation.

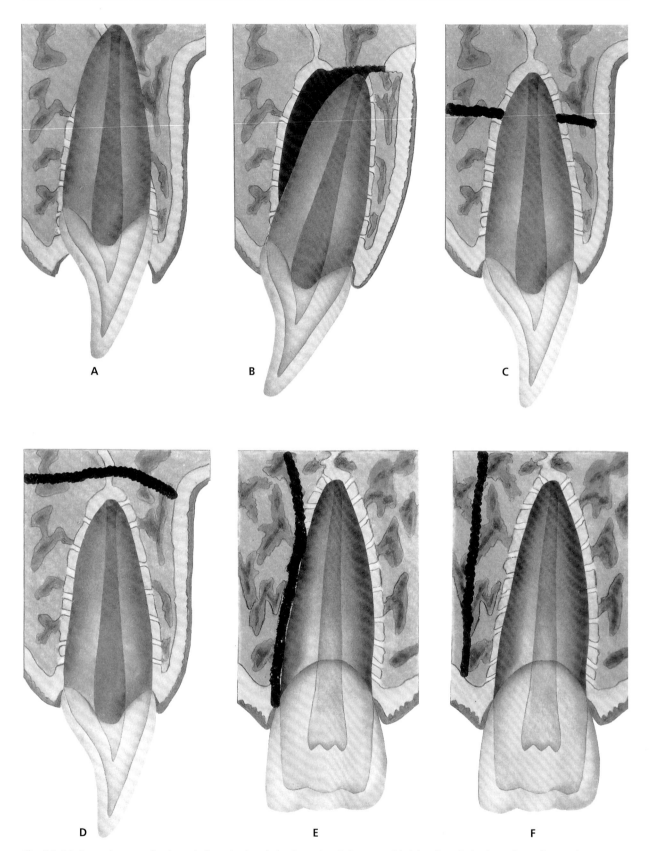

**Fig. 8.3** Injuries to the supporting bone. A. Comminution of alveolar socket. B. Fractures of facial or lingual alveolar socket wall. C. and D. Fractures of alveolar process with and without involvement of the tooth socket. E. and F. Fractures of mandible or maxilla with and without involvement of the tooth socket.

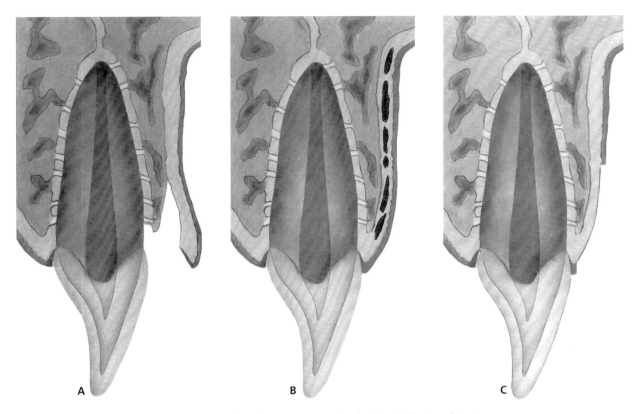

**Fig. 8.4** Injuries to gingiva or oral mucosa. A. Laceration of gingiva. B. Contusion of gingiva. C. Abrasion of gingiva.

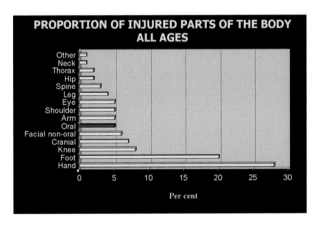

**Fig. 8.5** Proportion of injured parts of the body (all ages). From EILERT-PETERSSON et al. (216) 1997.

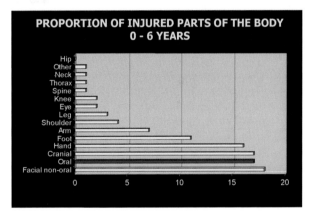

**Fig. 8.6** Proportion of injured parts of the body (ages 0–6 years). From EILERT-PETERSSON et al. (216) 1997.

## Epidemiology

TDI is a neglected oral condition despite its relatively high prevalence, significant impact on individuals and society, and sound body of knowledge about its causative factors and treatment. In addition, the remarkable decline of the prevalence and severity of dental caries amongst children in many countries (1–5) may have made TDI the most serious dental public health challenging among youth in those countries (215). This is because TDI affects mainly the front teeth, thus esthetic and facial attraction, while dental caries in children with low levels of the disease present only small occlusal caries in molars. Furthermore, most treatments needed for TDI are more complex and expensive than treatment of occlusal caries.

Although the oral region comprises as small an area as 1% of the total body area, a population based Swedish survey has shown that it accounts for 5% of all injuries in all ages (Fig. 8.5) (216). In pre-school children in Sweden, traumatic oral injuries may make up as much as 17% of all bodily injuries, with injuries to the head being the most common (Fig. 8.6) (216).

**Table 8.4** Prevalence of traumatic dental injuries to primary teeth in 5-year-olds (percent).

| Examiner | Year | Country | Male | Female |
|---|---|---|---|---|
| Andreasen & Ravn (64) | 1972 | Denmark | 31.3 | 24.6 |
| García-Godoy et al. (168) | 1983 | Dominican Republic | 33.6 | 28.9 |
| Forsberg & Tedestam (178) | 1990 | Sweden | 28.0 | 16.0 |
| Sanchez & García-Godoy (179) | 1990 | Mexico | 40.0 | – |
| Stecksén-Blicks & Holm (376)* | 1992 | Sweden | 27.0 (M + F) | |

\* 4-year-olds.

Worldwide the proportion of maxillofacial trauma in relation to all types of trauma reported from hospital accident and emergency departments varies from 9% (217) to 33% (218).

## Prevalence and incidence

References of prevalence and incidence of TDI up to the year 1993 are presented in the third edition of *Textbook and color atlas of traumatic injuries to the teeth* (213). As shown in Table 8.3, the prevalence of TDI still varies considerably. This variation reflects not only socio-economic, behavioral and cultural diversity, but also the lack of standardization of methods and classifications observed in the literature. The use of standardized epidemiological protocols would facilitate comparison between countries. For example, differences in age and sex distribution between population based studies examined have significantly contributed to the large variation observed in the literature.

The prevalence of TDI is high worldwide (Table 8.3). A large national survey in the USA in 6–50-year-olds showed that approximately 1 in 4 adults had evidence of TDI (210). In the UK, 1 in 5 children have experienced TDI to their permanent anterior teeth before leaving school (212). One way to eliminate the influence of age is to study the prevalence of TDI at given stages of development, such as for the primary dentition at the age of 5 (i.e. prior to the mixed dentition period) and at the age of 12 (i.e. after the mixed dentition period and the period of high trauma incidence) (see Tables 8.4 and 8.5).

The prevalence of TDI is likely to be much higher than the figures presented in Table 8.3. Apart from a few longitudinal studies, most reports are cross-sectional, which means that registration of previous injuries is to a certain extent dependent upon information from either the child or parents, which can entail a significant error. A clinical study demonstrated that parents in about half the cases of previously recorded injuries to primary teeth in a pre-school dental clinic denied in a questionnaire that such injuries had occurred (64). Furthermore, the lack of diagnostic aids in cross-sectional surveys implies missing several relevant signs of TDI, such as luxation injuries (concussion, subluxation, intrusion, extrusion), pulp injuries, root fractures and

**Table 8.5** Prevalence of traumatic dental injuries to permanent teeth in 12-year-olds (percent).

| Examiner | Year | Country | Male | Female |
|---|---|---|---|---|
| Andreasen & Ravn (64) | 1972 | Denmark | 25.7 | 16.3 |
| Clarkson et al. (114) | 1973 | England | 11.6 | 9.6 |
| Todd (182) | 1973 | England | 22.0 | 12.0 |
| Todd (183) | 1983 | England | 29.0 | 16.0 |
| Järvinen (108) | 1979 | Finland | 33.0 | 19.3 |
| Baghdady et al. (166) | 1981 | Iraq | 19.5 | 16.1 |
| Baghdady et al. (166) | 1981 | Sudan | 16.5 | 3.6 |
| García-Godoy et al. (170) | 1985 | Dominican Republic | 18.0 | 12.0 |
| García-Godoy et al. (171) | 1986 | Dominican Republic | 31.7 | 15.0 |
| Holland et al. (172) | 1988 | Ireland | 21.2 | 12.1 |
| Hunter et al. (177) | 1990 | England | 19.4 | 11.0 |
| Forsberg & Tedestam (178) | 1990 | Sweden | 27.0 | 12.0 |
| Marcenes et al. (244) | 2000 | Brazil | 20.7 | 9.3 |
| Cortes et al. (248) | 2001 | Brazil | 7.1 | 6.5 |
| Traebert et al. (233) | 2003 | Brazil | 22.4 | 15.1 |
| Hamdan & Rajab (341) | 2003 | Jordan | 17.1 | 10.5 |
| Soriano et al. (243) | 2004 | Brazil | 30.0 | 16.1 |

**Table 8.6** Reported incidence of traumatic dental injuries in longitudinal surveys during one year.

| Examiner | Year | Country | Age | Per 100 |
|---|---|---|---|---|
| Ravn & Rossen (20) | 1969 | Denmark | 7–16 | 3 |
| Andreasen & Ravn (64) | 1972 | Denmark | 0–14 | 4 |
| Hedegård & Stålhane (78) | 1973 | Sweden | 7–15 | 1.5 |
| Ravn (77) | 1974 | Denmark | 7–16 | 3 |
| Hansen & Lothe (185) | 1982 | Norway | 7–18 | 2.5 |
| Stockwell (159) | 1988 | Australia | 6–12 | 1.7 |
| Glendor et al. (206) | 1996 | Sweden | 0–19 | 1.3 |
| | | | 0–6 | 1.5 |
| | | | 7–19 | 1.3 |
| Borssén & Holm (225)* | 1997 | Sweden | 1–16 | 2.8 |
| Eilert-Petersson et al. (216)** | 1997 | Sweden | All ages | 0.4 |
| | | | 0–12 | 1.8 |
| Skaare & Jacobsen (219) | 2003 | Norway | 7–18 | 1.8 |

\* The yearly incidence of 16-year-olds born in 1975 and followed retrospectively until 1991.
\*\* Oral injuries including dental injuries, injuries to the mandible or maxilla and injuries of oral soft tissue.

resorptions, periapical lesions, replanted teeth and injuries to the supporting bone, gingiva and oral mucosa.

Very few studies assessed the incidence of TDI (Table 8.6). The findings of a prospective study, where all dental injuries occurring from birth to the age of 14 years were carefully registered, demonstrated that 30% of the children had sustained injuries to the primary dentition and 22% to the permanent dentition (Figs 8.7 and 8.8). Altogether, every second child had sustained a TDI by the age of 14 years (64). In another prospective study, carried out in Australia, an

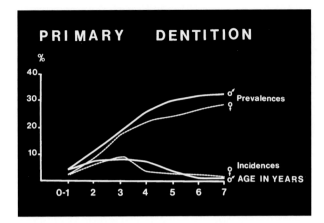

**Fig. 8.7** Prevalence and incidence of traumatic dental injuries to primary teeth among children in Copenhagen. Prevalence indicates frequency (in percentage) of children who have sustained dental injuries at the various ages examined. Incidence indicates the number of new dental injuries (in percentage) arising per year at the various ages examined. From ANDREASEN & RAVN (64) 1972.

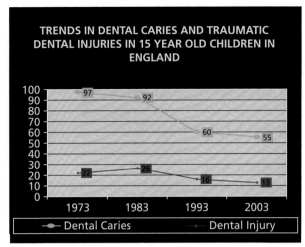

**Fig. 8.9** Trends (%) in dental caries and traumatic dental injuries in 15 year old children in England. From TODD (182) 1975, TODD & DODD (183) 1985, O'BRIEN (212) 1994 and PITTS (379) 2003.

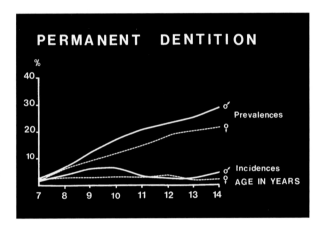

**Fig. 8.8** Prevalence and incidence of traumatic dental injuries to permanent teeth among children in Copenhagen. Prevalence indicates frequency (in percentage) of children who have sustained dental injuries at the various ages examined. Incidence indicates the number of new dental injuries (in percentage) arising per year at the various ages examined. From ANDREASEN & RAVN (64) 1972.

incidence of 20 cases of TDI per thousand per year in children aged 6–12 years was reported (181). In a Swedish prospective study, the mean incidence for boys was 1.6 and for girls 1.0 per 100 individuals per year in the age interval 0–19 years (206).

## Trends

The trend in TDI is not as clear and well documented as the trend in dental caries. Very few comparable studies allow identifying a trend in TDI. Data from the last 20–30 years suggest that there has not been a significant change in TDI in children and adolescents in Scandinavian countries (219). Similarly, data from the USA suggested small changes, 18.4% and 16% in 1996 and 2004 among 6–20-year-old individu-

als (Table 8.3). Data from the UK showed a small reduction, but not a clear trend (Fig. 8.9). Variations may be explained by variation in measuring TDI. Also, data from 1973 to 1993 refers to England and Wales, while in 2003 only England. It is of interest to compare trends in dental caries and TDI. It seems that the prevalence of dental caries is falling more rapidly than TDI. If this trend continues TDI may became more prevalent than dental caries.

## Repeated trauma episodes

Dental trauma affects children and adolescents unequally. Some individuals are not affected at all or just once, while others suffer from repeated trauma episodes (201, 210, 220, 222, 223, 378) (Fig. 8.10), with *no gender differences* (224–227), and with *repeated trauma episodes to the same teeth* (78, 181, 226, 228). Frequencies of repeated trauma episodes have been reported to range from 4 to 49% (16, 40, 54, 65, 77–79, 159, 201–220, 225–226, 229), while repeated trauma episodes *to the same teeth* have been reported to range from 8 to 45% (78, 181, 226, 229). The risk of sustaining a second TDI episode has been found to be eightfold for patients with their first trauma episode at 9 years of age, compared with 12 years of age (226). Due to the increased risk for some individuals of sustaining multiple trauma episodes during life, prevention and/or orthodontic treatment must be performed at an early stage in life (226, 228). Prevention should be based on behavioral and environmental changes. Orthodontic treatment should be provided if proved cost-effective.

## Distribution by sex, age, race and socio-economic status

The literature shows clearly that boys sustain more TDI than girls; and that the prevalence of TDI increases with age. The latter is due to a cumulative effect. The relationship between

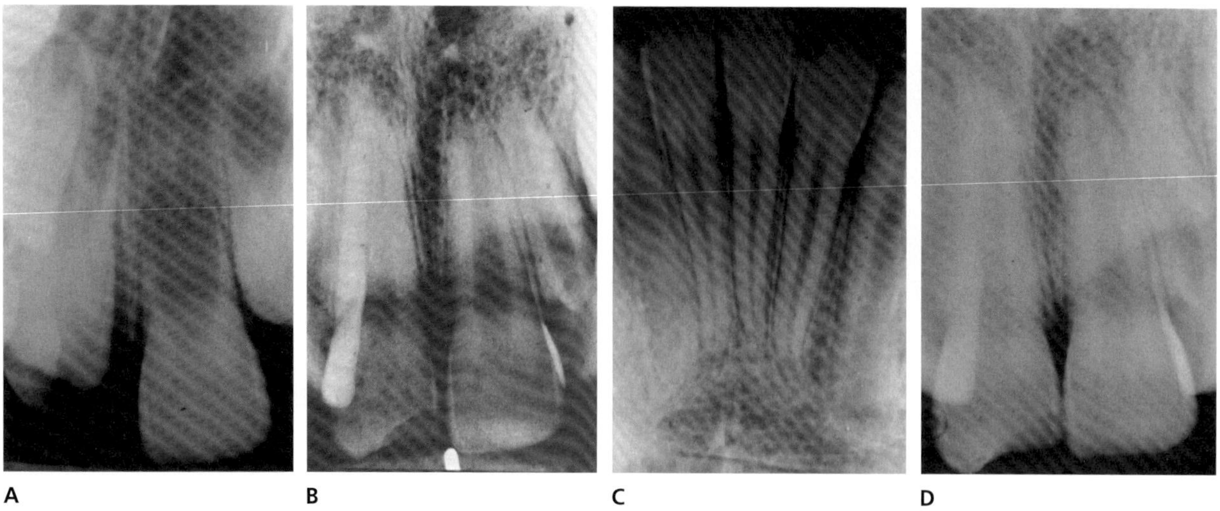

A          B          C          D

**Fig. 8.10** Individual with repeated trauma episodes. A. Avulsion of primary right maxillary central incisor at the age of 7. B. Crown fracture at the age of 9. C. Luxation of the right mandibular central incisor at the age of 10. D. New trauma to the right central incisor at the age of 12.

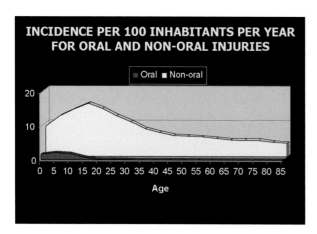

**Fig. 8.11** Incidence per 100 inhabitants per year for oral and non-oral injuries. From EILERT-PETERSSON et al. (216) 1997.

TDI and race and ethnicity is not clear. Ethnic minorities tend to experience more financial adversities and live in more deprived areas. Therefore, it is difficult to disentangle the effects of these factors. Furthermore, few studies recorded race or ethnicity of participants. Data from the USA showed a similar prevalence of TDI in different race-ethnicity categories (210).

In most countries, the boy to girl ratio of TDI differs significantly. The general finding that boys have almost twice TDI than girls in the permanent dentition seems to be related to their more active participation in contact games and sports (16, 56, 82, 112, 187, 219); but recent studies show a reduction in this difference, which may reflect a change in girls' behavior in playing sports traditionally regarded as boys' games such as ice hockey and soccer (222, 232, 233).

In a Swedish study oral injuries were most frequent during the first 10 years of life, decreasing gradually with age and were very rare after the age of 30, whereas non-oral injuries were seen most frequently in adolescents and were present throughout life (216) (Fig. 8.11).

Data from several studies demonstrated that the majority of TDI occurs at childhood and adolescence. It is estimated that 71–92% of all TDI sustained in a lifetime occur before the age of 19 years (194, 206, 234, 235). Holland et al. (236) reported a decrease of traumatic tooth injuries after the age of 24, and Shulman and Peterson (237) after the age of 30. Gassner et al. (238) also reported that 81.2% of all TDI occur before 30 years of age; of that, almost 50% before 10 years of age. The *prevalence* and *incidence* of TDI according to age and sex in a group of children from Copenhagen followed continuously from the age of 2 to 14 years is shown in Figs 8.7 and 8.8 (64). It can be seen that the first peak appears at 2 to 4 years of age. By the age of 7 years, 28% of the girls and 32% of the boys have suffered a TDI to the primary dentition. In the permanent dentition, a marked increase in the incidence of TDI is seen in boys aged 8 to 10 years; while the incidence is rather stable for girls (64, 77, 185). This peak incidence in boys is probably related to the more vigorous play characteristic of this age group compared to girls (20, 21, 23, 54, 56, 77). An increase in the rate and absolute number of oral and maxillofacial injuries was reported among persons aged 65 or more in New Zealand (239). This may be because an increasing proportion of older people are keeping their own natural teeth for life, and the risk of falling is high in old adults, which may lead to an increase in TDI. The scale of this problem is currently unknown, as research reports on prevalence of TDI in older people are scarce.

Very few reports on TDI have included socio-economic indicators and the results were conflicting. Intriguingly, some studies reported a higher prevalence of TDI among adolescents from higher compared to those from lower socio-economic groups. The higher risk of dental injuries among children from higher socio-economic backgrounds

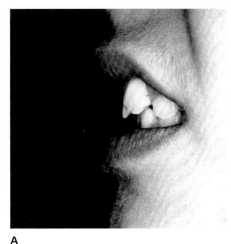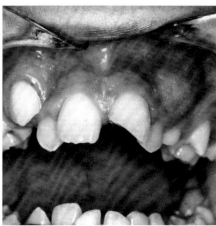

**Fig. 8.12** A. Protruding central incisors with incomplete lip coverage. B. Crown fracture of a left central incisor.  **A**  **B**

may be related to greater ownership of bicycles, access to skiing, skateboard, roller-skating, horse-riding and swimming pools than those from low socio-economic groups (240). Further research is needed to elucidate this relationship.

## Predisposing factors

Increased overjet with protrusion of upper incisors and insufficient lip closure are significant predisposing factors to TDI (79, 103, 186, 191, 228, 237, 241–243). Studies have shown that TDIs are approximately twice as frequent among children with protruding incisors as in children with normal occlusion (41, 46), and that the greatest number of injured teeth in the individual patient is associated with protrusive occlusion (43) (Fig. 8.12).

Inadequate lip coverage has been shown to result in a threefold risk for TDIs to the maxillary incisors, compared to adequate lip coverage (215, 232), while other studies show no significant relation between inadequate lip coverage and TDIs (244, 380). The study showing a significant association (215) did not account for other risk factors. The other study carried out by Marcenes et al. (244) accounted for the environment, and showed a significant association between lip coverage and TDI before accounting for other factors in the data analysis, but not after adjusting results for levels of deprivation experienced. Therefore, the conflicting findings may be due to the interaction between predisposing factors (size of the overjet and lip coverage) and environmental (playground design) and/or behavioral factors (risk taking). Unfortunately, very few studies accounted for all these factors together. Concerning orthodontic evaluation of these patients, the reader is referred to Chapter 24.

## Teeth involved

Irrespective of type of study, the majority of dental injuries involve the anterior teeth, especially the maxillary central incisors; while the mandibular central incisors and maxillary lateral incisors are less frequently involved (6, 16, 18, 21, 56, 63, 77–79, 219, 237, 249). This preference for location also applies to the primary dentition (61, 251, 254).

Dental injuries usually also affect only a single tooth (18, 20, 49, 63, 77, 210, 219, 249); however, certain trauma events, such as sports and automobile accidents, favor multiple tooth injuries (16, 78, 256), especially among teenagers (224, 256).

Concomitant injuries to teeth and oral tissues are also common in patients presenting with oral trauma due to violence and traffic accidents.

## Types of traumatic dental injuries

The most common type of traumatic injuries to permanent teeth is enamel fracture followed by enamel and dentin fracture (40, 49, 54, 56, 64, 77, 78, 210, 237, 253, 257). Other types of TDI are less common. However, soft tissue lesions were not assessed in the cross-sectional studies. In a prospective Swedish study, dental injuries were recorded in 92% of the patients, whereas soft tissue injuries were seen in 28%, and fractures involving the jawbone in only 6% of all patients presenting with oral injuries (216). Findings from hospital or surgery based studies presented a different picture (259). This is because many people who sustain a small fracture do not seek treatment; and soft tissue injuries and the most serious injuries end in hospital or dental surgeries for treatment. Hospital data tend to show facial bone fractures (37%), dentoalveolar injuries (50%) and soft tissue injuries (62%) (231). The number of injuries often exceeds the number of teeth due to multiple injuries for some teeth.

It appears that injuries to the primary dentition are usually confined to the supporting structures, i.e. luxation and exarticulation (16, 64, 191, 192, 257, 260, 261). In some studies, however, the primary dentition was dominated by enamel fractures instead of injuries to the supporting structures (227, 251–253, 255, 258, 262). This is probably due to the periodic visits of these patients to the emergency clinic, a fact that favors the recording of enamel fractures, which might normally go undetected (227).

## Place of injury

The great majority of population based studies reviewed showed that most TDIs occur at home, followed by at school and in the street or other public places (216, 220, 233, 264). It is disturbing that in most studies a high proportion reported that they could not remember where the injury event had occurred.

The place of injury varies in different countries according to local customs. In studies examining dental trauma in Iraq, India, Australia, Norway and England, it was found that the majority of injuries occurred outside school grounds (185, 193, 194, 264). Furthermore, a greater number of severe injuries occurred after school hours (195).

## Seasonal variations

A relationship seems to exist between the time of year and occurrence of TDI. This seasonal variation in TDI is dependent upon local customs. While several studies have shown that the frequency of TDI increases during the winter months (43, 54, 77, 116, 216, 231), other reports indicate an increase in the summer months (148, 154, 196, 197, 251, 253, 256, 265).

## Etiology

Clearly, TDIs are caused by a collision that can generate enough mechanical energy to produce the injury. Any object, animate or inanimate, in motion has energy that depends on its mass and speed. Increase in mass and/or speed increases energy. Thus, it is relevant to understand the vehicles and circumstances that generate mechanical energy, which in turn cause a TDI. Violence, sports, traffic incidents and falls are commonly cited in the literature as causes of TDI. In addition, it is important to learn about the 'causes of the causes' of TDIs. What makes people fall or having a collision? What makes people have an injury when driving, cycling or walking on the street? What makes people have an injury when playing sports? What makes people fight? The answer for these questions leads to the environmental and behavioural causes of TDIs (Fig. 8.13).

A major *environmental determinant* of TDI is materiel deprivation. Data from the UK showed a higher prevalence of TDI in deprived areas, such as 43.8% in Newham (266) and 34.4% in Bury and Salford (201) compared with the overall prevalence of 17% and 15% recorded in England (212). In addition, even within a deprived area, more deprived children have more TDI than their less deprived counterparts. Overcrowding was the major environment factor related to TDI (242, 266). This seems

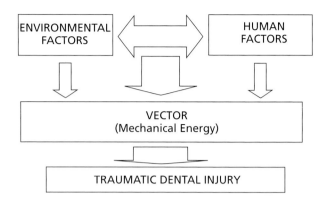

**Fig. 8.13** Environmental and behavioral causes of traumatic dental injuries.

logical, as deprived areas have more unsafe playgrounds, sport facilities, streets, schools and houses. This unsafe environment facilitates falls and collisions, which in turn leads to TDIs.

*Human behavior* also plays an important role in the occurrence of TDI. As expected, risk-taking children tend to have more TDI than their less risk-taking counterparts. Other problem behaviors have also been related to TDI. Odoi et al. (267) showed that children with peer relationship problems (e.g. being picked on or bullied by other children) have significantly more TDI than other children. Interestingly, the same study reported a tendency for children who show pro-social behaviour to have less dental injuries than their counterparts. Lalloo (268) reported that hyperactive children have significantly more TDI than non-hyperactive children. Conversely, Odoi et al. (267) failed to demonstrate a significant relationship between TDI and hyperactivity. This conflicting result is easy to understand and suggests that environment plays a stronger role in determining TDI than human behavior. A hyperactive child can express this without risk if the environment is safe.

Emotionally stressful states measured using biological markers or questionnaires have also been reported to be associated with TDI (221, 269, 270). Nicolau et al. (271) applied the life course approach to further elucidate the causes of TDI and concluded that adolescents who experienced adverse psychosocial environments along the life course had more traumatic dental injuries than their counterparts who experienced more favorable environments. This included living in a non-nuclear family and experiencing high levels of paternal punishment (271).

Worldwide, physical leisure activities, violent incidents and traffic accidents accounted for most TDIs among adolescents. Rough playing with others, biting hard items and inappropriate use of teeth also contribute to having a TDI, but to a lesser extent. Falls and collisions tend to be the most prevalent events associated with TDI reported in the literature (Table 8.7). These very broad categories may mask the actual causes of TDI, because it does not assess intention. For example, a fall from tripping (unintentional) differs from falls from pushing (intentional). The latter should be

**Table 8.7** Frequency of causes (in percent) of traumatic dental injuries. The variables presented follow WHO nomenclature.

| Study | Year | Country | Age | Physical leisure activity | Collision | Fall | Sport | Traffic accident | Violence | Inappropriate use of teeth or biting hard item | Other | Unknown |
|---|---|---|---|---|---|---|---|---|---|---|---|---|
| Baghdady et al. (166) | 1981 | Iraq | 6–12 | – | – | 54.0 | 3.0 | 2.4 | 35.8 | – | – | 4.9 |
| Baghdady et al. (166) | 1981 | Sudan | 6–12 | – | – | 18.3 | 3.3 | 2.8 | 70.6 | – | – | 5.0 |
| García Godoy et al. (383) | 1981 | Dominican Republic | 7–14 | – | 1.7 | 50.0 | – | 5.1 | – | – | 10.2 | 32.4 |
| García Godoy et al. (384)* | 1984 | Dominican Republic | 5–14 | 36.6 | – | – | 49.4 | 14.0 | – | – | – | – |
| Uji & Teramoto (385)* | 1988 | Japan | 6–18 | – | – | 37.7 | 29.2 | 1.6 | 7.9 | – | 23.6 | – |
| Chen et al. (220) | 1999 | Central Taiwan | Mean 8.2 | – | 65.3 | 26.9 | 3.6 | – | 2.6 | – | 1.6 | – |
| Marcenes et al. (215) | 1999 | Syria | 9–12 | – | 16.0 | 9.1 | – | 24.1 | 42.5 | – | 3.4 | 4.6 |
| Blinkhorn (264)* | 2000 | UK | 11–14 | 18.5 | – | 33.9 | 17.2 | 14.6 | 4.3 | – | – | 11.5 |
| Marcenes et al. (244) | 2000 | Brazil | 12 | – | 6.8 | 26.0 | 19.2 | 20.6 | 16.4 | – | 9.6 | 1.4 |
| Nicolau et al. (269)* | 2001 | Brazil | 13 | – | 15.0 | 24.1 | 2.3 | 10.5 | 1.5 | 6.0 | – | 40.6 |
| Traebert et al. (233) | 2003 | Brazil | 12 | – | 37.5 | 47.9 | – | 2.1 | – | 2.1 | – | 10.4 |

\* Population.

considered as a minor form of violence. Similarly, it is common to record collision when a child is pushed against another child or object, in particular, the school water fountain. If human intent was assessed in previous studies, these events would have been recorded as bullying, or a minor violence, rather than collision. Thus, it is possible that the role of violence in the occurrence of TDI has been terribly underestimated (233). Of further concern is the high proportion of children who tend to report 'unknown cause' in most studies. Victims tend to report unknown cause when an injury is due to violence. The overrepresentation of accidents at home, compared to violence (Table 8.7), may depend on a difficulty in finding the actual rate for injuries associated with child, spouse and elderly abuse.

TDI may be classified based on its etiology, taking into account the TDI event or the intent as proposed by WHO in the document *Dictionary for minimum data sets on injuries* (230). TDI event is defined as the activity related to the occurrence of the TDI. It includes falls, collisions, physical leisure activities, traffic accidents, rough playing with others, violence, inappropriate use of teeth, and biting hard items. Less common events are recorded as 'other events' (Table 8.7). The last two TDI events were added for the sake of completeness. They are relatively common TDI events; but not applicable to general injuries. Intent represents the human involvement in the occurrence of the TDI event. It includes unintentional TDI, intentional TDI (self-harm events and violent events) and iatrogenic (doctor's mistreatment) TDI.

## Unintentional traumatic dental injuries

### Falls and collisions

Falls are common among children and old adults. To primary teeth TDIs increase substantially with the child's

first efforts to move about. Due to lack of experience and coordination, frequency increases as the child begins to walk and tries to run. A prospective survey of injuries to pre-school children in a home setting showed that oral and head injuries were sustained following falls on or from stairs or pieces of furniture (272). They were incurred on stairs, in garages, or on/from verandas, and pre-school children aged 1 year were more often involved than expected by chance. The incidence of TDIs reaches its peak just before school age and consists mainly of injuries due to falls and collisions (16, 18, 63–65, 216) (Table 8.7). Home is the most common place of injury in pre-school (216, 224) and school age. Falls or being struck by an object tend to be reported as the most common causes of injury (216, 223, 233, 264, 273). This is not surprising. One cannot imagine any other way to sustain a dental injury. However, the event that caused the fall or collision is the actual cause of TDI; and should have been recorded. A refined assessment of the causes of TDI would identify a smaller proportion of TDI due to falls. The result may be a higher proportion of TDI due to violence. Victims of abuse tend to give a vague history when asked about the cause of the injury. Fall is a perfect vague history. Furthermore, falls among young children are mainly related to neglecting the child and can often be prevented by better supervision from parents and safe house design.

### Physical leisure activities

Injuries during the teenage years are often due to sports (21, 65, 78–84, 149–155, 216, 274). Federation Dentaire International (FDI) has organized sport in two categories due to risk for TDI: *High risk sports* that include American football, hockey, ice hockey, lacrosse, martial sports, rugby and skating; and *medium risk sports* including basketball, diving, squash, gymnastics, parachuting and waterpolo (275). Studies confirmed that contact sports, such as ice hockey, soccer, baseball, American football, basketball, rugby,

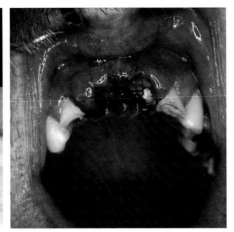

**Fig. 8.14** The unprotected ice hockey player runs a high risk of injuries due to collision with other players or being hit by a puck or a hockey stick.

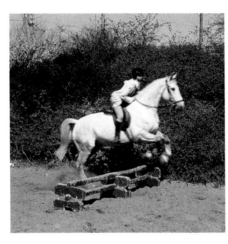

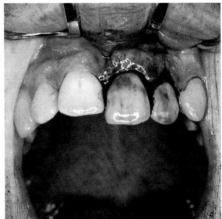

**Fig. 8.15** Horseback riding related injuries. In the jump, the rider's face can collide with the horse's neck, usually resulting in luxation injuries.

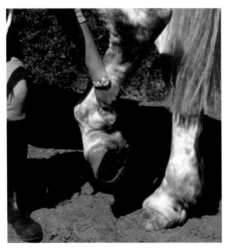

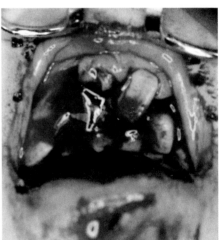

**Fig. 8.16** A kick by a horse normally results in serious injuries, e.g. exarticulation, intrusion and sometimes jaw fractures.

wrestling and handball (17, 23–27, 83, 85, 156–159, 276, 277) are the major TDI events (Fig. 8.14). The severity of this problem has been elucidated in a number of studies, which report that each year 1.5% to 3.5% of children participating in contact sports sustain dental injuries (26–29, 86); and as many as one-third of all dental injuries and up to 19% of injuries to the head and face are sports related

(278–283). Horseback riding, a popular sport in many countries, is a significant source of injury. In a single season, 23% of all riders sustained injuries of various types, including dental and maxillofacial injuries (87, 88). Figs 8.15 and 8.16 illustrate the typical trauma situations related to horseback riding. There is little doubt that special precautions, such as the use of sturdy helmets, can reduce the number and sever-

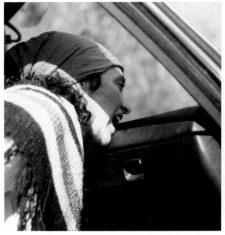

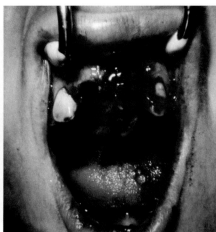

**Fig. 8.17** Automobile accidents in which the front seat passenger hits the dashboard result in soft tissue injuries and damage to the supporting bone.

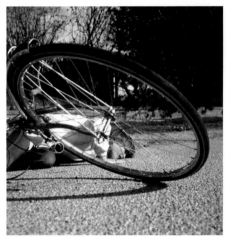

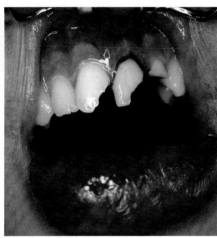

**Fig. 8.18** Bicycle accident usually results in multiple crown fractures and soft tissue injuries.

ity of these accidents (88). Similarly, the provision of a well-fitting mouth guard may possibly reduce the occurrence of TDI. However, there is still insufficient evidence that planned intervention is effective in reducing the prevalence or incidence of sports related injuries to the mouth and face (284); and much remains to be elucidated regarding attitude and effective use of protective equipment (283). The injury profiles of various types of sports, as well as measures for their prevention, are described in Chapter 30. Physical leisure activities at playgrounds also account for a significant proportion of TDI (20, 76, 77, 148, 224, 264). Most of the resultant injuries are characterized by a high frequency of crown fractures (16, 78). This type of TDI can be dramatically reduced through environmental changes. This includes better playground design and construction.

## Traffic accidents

Traffic accidents include pedestrian, bicycle and car related injuries. Facial and dental injuries resulting from automobile accidents are seen more frequently in the late teens (30, 31) (Fig. 8.17). The front seat passenger is particularly prone to facial injuries. This trauma group is dominated by mul-

tiple dental injuries, injuries to the supporting bone, and soft tissue injuries to the lower lip and chin (16, 89, 161). This pattern of injury is seen when the front seat passenger or the driver hits the steering wheel or dashboard (32, 90, 285). A study in road traffic accidents from Nigeria has shown that occupants of commercial vehicles were the ones most likely to receive maxillofacial injuries, especially the rear seat occupants (286). Children seated on, or standing on, the front seat are in a very dangerous position, as dental injuries often occur as a result of being thrown against the dashboard during sudden stops (33). Children with dental injuries and involved in traffic accidents have a 2.4-fold risk for bone fractures compared to accidents during play, sport and assaults (265). Enforcement of speed limits for cars, use of seat belts, air bags and special car seats for smaller children in motor vehicles have reduced severe injuries; but new types of facial trauma have been reported and are attributable to airbag deployment in cars (287, 288).

Bicycle related injuries have been widely reported. These injuries usually result in severe trauma to both the hard and soft tissues due to the high velocity at the time of impact (16, 151, 160, 289) (Fig. 8.18). Bicycle-related oral injuries

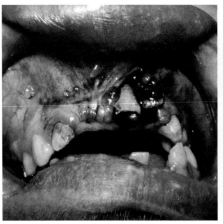 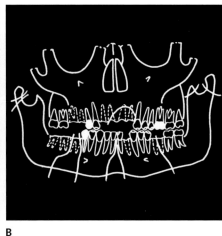

**Fig. 8.19** A 32-year-old male who has sustained 5 trauma episodes within 7 years due to epilepsy. These episodes involved multiple fractures of teeth and the mandible, as well as an alveolar fracture of the maxilla. A. Intruded maxillary incisors. B. Diagram with indication of fracture lines as well as missing teeth due to trauma. From BESSERMANN (93) 1978.

**A**                    **B**

seem to be more common up to the age of 14 years, compared to non-oral injuries (290). The use of bicycle helmets may reduce risk of serious facial injury to upper and middle face regions by approximately 65% compared to non-users, but no protection is provided for the lower face and jaw (291). Patients sustaining this type of trauma frequently experience severe facial and dentoalveolar trauma in addition to injuries to the upper lip and chin (16, 289, 292) (Fig. 8.18). To reduce dentoalveolar trauma there is a need to extend the area of helmet coverage (289, 292).

### Inappropriate use of teeth

Few studies have included this category. However, those that have included this category found that many individuals sustain a TDI when using the teeth as a tool. Nicolau et al. (269) reported that 6% of TDI were due to inappropriate use of teeth and Tapias (293) reported 8.5% while Traebert et al. (233) found smaller proportions, 3.3% (Table 8.7). The most common inappropriate uses of teeth reported in the literature are biting a pen, opening hair clips, opening packets of savoury snacks, trying to fix electronic equipment or changing batteries, cutting or holding objects and opening screw top bottles.

### Biting hard items

Another event related to the occurrence of TDI is biting hard items. Traumatic dental injuries have been shown among patients wearing piercing jewels. Patients and health care professionals should be informed of procedures and risks associated with tongue and oral piercing (294–296). Limited information has shown that piercing can result in chipping and fracturing of teeth and restorations, pulpal damage, cracked tooth syndrome and tooth abrasion (294, 297, 298). Information around dental/oral and systemic complications from tongue piercing has to date primarily been presented as case reports. Only one prevalence study has been published. Campbell et al. (296) showed a chipped teeth preva-

lence of 19.2% among individuals wearing tongue piercing, especially to molars and premolars, and to individuals wearing short stem barbells. They also showed an increased risk with years of wear.

### Presence of illness, physical limitations or learning difficulties

Attack of illness is an uncommon cause of TDI in the general population, but common in individuals suffering from epilepsy, cerebral palsy, anemia and dizziness. Epileptic patients present special risks and problems with regard to dental injuries (34, 93, 299–301). A study of 437 such patients in an institution showed that 52 % had suffered traumatic dental injuries, many of which were of a repetitive nature. In one-third of the cases, the injuries could be directly related to falls during epileptic seizures (93) (Fig. 8.19). Another study showed that of patients with epilepsy, who during the past year had suffered from seizures resulting in injury, 10% had suffered a TDI (299). Epileptic seizures have been shown to be the third most common medical incident in dental surgeries (302, 303). There is also a risk for the dental personnel to be infected from human bites of a patient suffering an epileptic seizure (304–306).

A very high frequency of dental injuries has been found among patients with learning difficulties (65, 123), a phenomenon probably related to various factors, such as lack of motor coordination, crowded conditions in institutions or concomitant epilepsy. O'Donnell (307) indicated that totally blind children and young adults in Hong Kong were at greater risk of sustaining anterior tooth injury than were sighted and partially sighted populations. Hearing impaired children, compared to visually impaired children, have been found to have significantly more TDI compared to children as a whole (308). This difference is probably due to greater opportunities to play and move around for the hearing impaired children, compared to the visually impaired children.

**Fig. 8.20** Spontaneous root fractures in a 15-year-old patient with osteogenesis and dentinogenesis imperfecta. A. Clinical view of incisors at the age of 14 years. The color of the teeth is bluish-brown. Note the marked attrition. The incisal edges of the incisors were later restored with cast inlays. B. Root fractures affecting three incisors and the left canine at the age of 15 years. There was no evidence of trauma in the history. The right central incisor was later extracted. From OVERVAD (38) 1969.

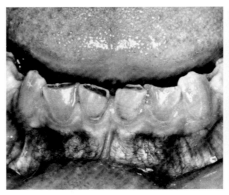

**A**

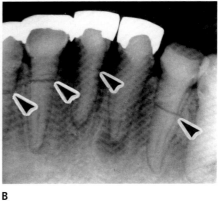

**B**

An unusual type of injury is root fracture without apparent reason affecting individuals with *dentinogenesis imperfecta* (36). The explanation for this phenomenon could be the decreased microhardness of dentin (37) and abnormal tapering of the roots (Fig. 8.20).

It has also been reported that many drug addicts suffer from crown fractures of molars and premolars, apparently resulting from violent tooth clenching 3 to 4 hours after drug intake. Up to 5 or 6 fractured teeth have been found in the same individual (35, 94).

## Intentional traumatic dental injuries

### Physical abuse

A tragic cause of oral injuries in small children is manifested in the battered child syndrome (or non-accidental injuries (NAI)), a clinical condition in infants who have suffered serious *physical abuse* (19, 66–68, 74, 75, 137–147, 309). It has been reported that child abuse occurs in approximately 0.6% of children (19, 142), and 10% of all injuries to children involve the teeth (142). In 1972, in New York City alone, 5200 cases were reported. Twenty years later, in the USA, an estimated 2 694 000 children were reported to child protection agencies as victims of abuse by parents and/or guardians (310). It has been estimated that in the entire USA, 4000–6000 children yearly die as a result of maltreatment (69, 140). Approximately 75% of all children being exposed to physical abuse and who visit a major county hospital suffer injuries to the head, face, mouth, or neck (311). The outcome is often fatal due to intracranial hemorrhage (19, 72–74) (Fig. 8.21). Facial trauma is often the principal reason for admission to a hospital (71, 74, 75). Multiple healed fractures in the teeth or jaws, especially with different stages of healing, are signs of abuse (312).

The official data regarding the number of children abused more often reflect reported cases rather than true incidence (313). Out of 16–29% of dentists claimed to have

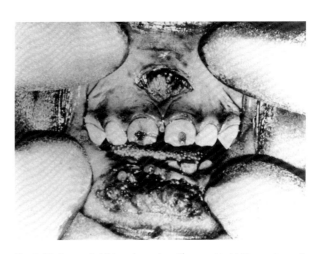

**Fig. 8.21** Battered child syndrome in a 2½-year-old girl. The mother suffered from depression and shook the child violently against a fireplace. The child died and was found to have contusion of the brain with intracranial hemorrhage. The child also had partly healed fractures at the lower end of each radius, which had been treated by an orthopedic consultant one month previously; but battering was not suspected at that time. The oral injuries consisted of laceration of the mucosa of the lower lip and tearing of the frenum. From TATE (19) 1971.

seen or suspected a case of child abuse; only 6–14% claimed to have reported such a case (314, 315). Physical abuse mainly happens at home (311), and dentists and dental personnel have an obligation to report occurrences of child abuse and neglect (316, 317). The etiologic and diagnostic aspects of child abuse are further described in Chapter 7.

*Assaults*, together with road accidents, comprised 71% of maxillofacial injuries in a study in the UK, as reported by Dimitroulis and Eyre (318). Injuries to the face represented 62% of all injuries due to assault (319). Injuries from fights are prominent in older age groups and are closely related to alcohol abuse (89, 91, 92, 124, 162, 270). This type of trauma usually results in a particular injury pattern characterized by luxation and exarticulation of teeth as well as fractures of roots and/or supporting bone (16) (Fig. 8.22).

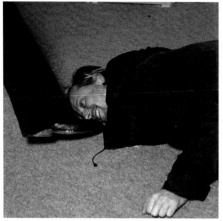
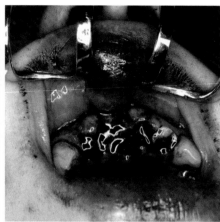

**Fig. 8.22** Kicks to the face during assaults result in severe damage to teeth and supporting structures.

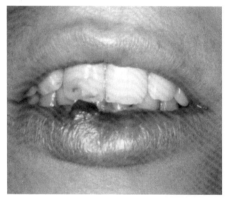
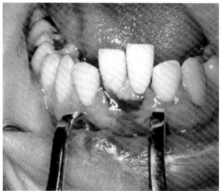

**Fig. 8.23** A 19-year-old woman battered by her husband. The patient was beaten around the face and suffered lacerations of the lower lip and an alveolar fracture confined to the mandibular incisor region.

In this context, it should be mentioned that recent evidence has shown that domestic violence is a universal problem (124–130, 163, 164). These assaults often result in trauma to the facial region (Fig. 8.23). Establishing the victim as a battered person is complicated by the fact that these victims will seldom volunteer that information. Social agencies for the care and counselling of these victims exist in many countries and should be used (128).

A disgraceful and apparently increasing type of injury is represented by trauma to the oral and facial regions of *tortured* prisoners. Investigations have shown that the majority of these victims, apart from other atrocities inflicted upon their persons, have suffered from torture involving the oral region (95–97) (Fig. 8.24). A study has described the findings from examinations of 34 former prisoners from 6 countries who had all been subjected to torture involving the facial region (95). The most common type of torture was beating, which resulted in loosening, avulsion or fracture of teeth and soft tissue laceration. Deliberate tooth fractures with forceps were also seen. Furthermore, electrical torture was described in which electrodes were attached to teeth, lips, tongue and the soft tissue over the temporomandibular joint. (Fig. 8.24) In the latter instance, very forceful occlusion resulted due to muscle spasm. The result was loosening and fracture of teeth as well as severe pain in the muscles and the temporomandibular joint.

Under the auspices of Amnesty International, working groups of dentists and physicians have been formed in several countries with the aim of gathering evidence to document the torture of prisoners.

## Iatrogenic procedures

*Prolonged intubation* is a procedure which is used in the care of prematurely born infants. The prolonged pressure of tubes against the maxillary alveolar process is an iatrogenic procedure that may lead to a high frequency of developmental enamel defects in the primary dentition (134–136, 320, 321) (see Chapter 20, p. 544) as well as injuries to the tooth germs of the first and second dentition and deformation of the maxillary skeleton (322).

The incidence of *perianesthetic dental injury* varies from 0.04% to 12% (323), and is considered to be the most frequent anesthesia-related cause for claims in the UK, representing approximately one-third of all confirmed claims (324). A restrospective study in France showed a mean incidence of 9.5 accidents/100 anesthetists/year (325), while other studies have shown a yearly incidence ranging from 1:150 to 1:1000 cases (326, 327). The maxillary incisors are the most commonly affected (326, 329–331), especially on the left side (326, 330, 331). Tooth injuries range from microfractures of natural tooth substance to actual avulsion

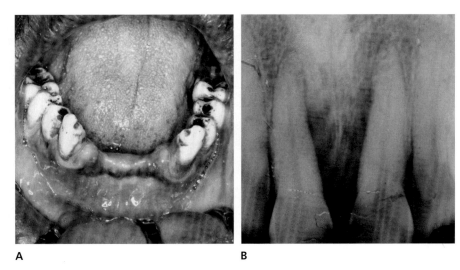

A                                                                              B

**Fig. 8.24** A 35-year-old political refugee who was tortured by having live electrodes attached to the oral mucosa. Furthermore, lower incisors were avulsed during 'interrogation'. The patient still suffers profound pain in the masticatory muscles, 9 years after being tortured. B. A 35-year-old male political refugee who had been tortured during his imprisonment. The man was beaten by security police. During torture, he fell and fractured and luxated two central incisors. No treatment was given. The radiograph is indicative of his condition one year after torture. It was taken at an examination by the medical board of Amnesty International. Courtesy Drs. P. MARSTRAND, B. JERLANG & P. JERLANG, Amnesty International, Copenhagen.

(326, 329, 331, 332); and include pulpal necrosis (331) and damage to crowns or bridges (326, 329, 331). Skeie and Schwartz (333) have shown a spectrum of fractured teeth in 47%, dislocated or mobile teeth in 41%, and avulsed teeth in 10% of patients with perianesthetic dental injuries. Givol et al. (334) showed that 72% of the patients were 50–70 years of age; and the most common injury was to upper (87%) and lower incisors (12.5%). Avulsion of teeth was the most common type of injury (48%), followed by crown fracture (22%); and 65% of the teeth could not be restored. The major risk factor for dental injury seems to be pre-existing poor dentition (334). The risk of injuries to the teeth can be reduced by a pre-surgical inspection of the oral cavity and evaluation of the individual anatomical conditions in the head and neck region, which might interfere with endotracheal intubation (322, 335). Using a toothguard has been shown to be a simple way of preventing dental trauma during general anesthesia and has a low effect on the difficulty of intubation (336); but such recommendations would have to be subject to controlled cost–benefit analysis prior to their widespread application (323), especially since Skeie and Schwartz (333) have found that 0.062% of patients in general anesthesia suffered dental injury despite the use of a toothguard, compared to 0.063% not wearing a toothguard. At present, the use of a toothguard for each intubation does not seem reasonable; but tooth fragility must be researched (337). The cost of restoring a perianesthetic dental injury has been estimated to be approximately $2000 per patient in Israel (334).

## Mechanisms of traumatic dental injuries

The exact mechanisms that produce the mechanical energy leading to dental injuries are, for the most part, unknown

and without experimental evidence. A few experimental attempts have been made to make *in vitro* models for fracture resistance of extracted human teeth (381, 382). Injuries can be the result of either direct or indirect trauma (2). *Direct trauma* occurs when the tooth itself is struck, e.g. against playground equipment, a table or chair (Fig. 8.25). *Indirect trauma* is seen when the lower dental arch is forcefully closed against the upper, as by a blow to the chin in a fight or a fall. While direct trauma usually implies injuries to the anterior region, indirect trauma favors crown or crown-root fractures in the premolar and molar regions (Fig. 8.26), as well as the possibility of jaw fractures in the condylar regions and symphysis. Another effect of a blow to the chin can be the forceful whiplash effect to the head and neck, occasionally leading to cerebral involvement. This condition can be revealed during the clinical examination (see later).

The following factors characterize the impact and determine the extent of injury (42):

(1) *Energy of impact.* This factor includes both mass and velocity. Examples of these combinations are a force of high velocity and low mass (gunshot) (Fig. 8.27) or of high mass and minimal velocity (striking the tooth against the ground). Experience has shown that low velocity blows cause the greatest damage to the supporting structures, whereas tooth fractures are less pronounced. In contrast, in high velocity impacts the resulting crown fractures are usually not associated with damage to the supporting structures. In these cases, the energy of the impact is apparently expended in creating the fracture and is seldom transmitted to any great extent to the root or supporting structures of the tooth (16).

(2) *Resilience of the impacting object.* If a tooth is struck with a resilient or cushioned object, such as an elbow during

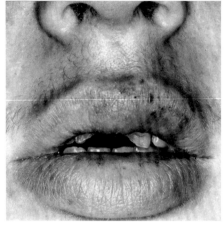
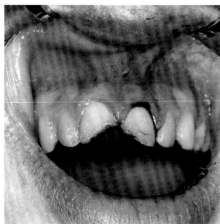

**Fig. 8.25** Direct tooth trauma without soft tissue injury. The impact was absorbed by the protruding central incisors leading to fractures. From ANDREASEN (16) 1970.

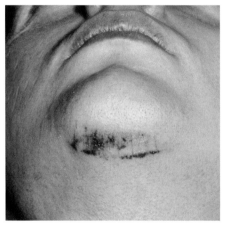
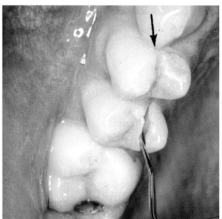

**Fig. 8.26** Induced tooth trauma. The impact was transferred via the chin to the dental arches and inflicted crown-root fractures in both right premolars by the forceful occlusion. From ANDREASEN (16) 1970.

play, or if the lip absorbs and distributes the impact, the chance of crown fracture is reduced while the risk of luxation and alveolar fracture is increased (16) (Figs 8.28 and 8.29).

(3) *Shape of the impacting object.* Impact with a sharp object favors clean crown fractures with a minimum of displacement of the tooth, as the energy is spread rapidly over a limited area. On the other hand, with a blunt object, impact increases the area of resistance to the force in the crown region and allows the energy to be transmitted to the apical region, causing luxation or root fracture.

(4) *Direction of the impacting force.* The impact can meet the tooth at different angles, most often hitting the tooth facially and perpendicular to the long axis of the root. In this situation, typical cleavage lines will be encountered, as demonstrated in Fig. 8.30. With other angles of impact, other fracture lines will arise.

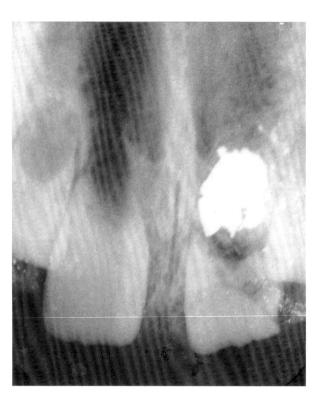

**Fig. 8.27** Multiple dental fractures caused by a gunshot.

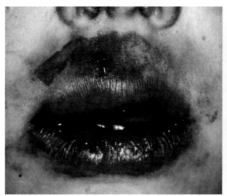

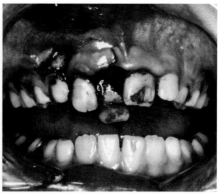

**Fig. 8.28** Direct trauma to the upper lip. The impact was transmitted through the lip, resulting in extrusive luxation of right incisors and laceration of gingiva. The upper surface of the lip shows minor lacerations in the area which was in contact with the tooth surfaces during transmission of the trauma. From ANDREASEN (16) 1970.

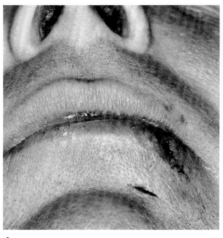

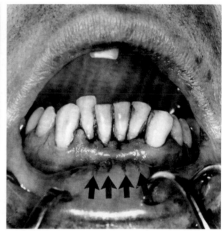

A                                        B

**Fig. 8.29** Direct trauma to the lower lip. A. Force of a frontal blow to the lower lip was transmitted through the lip to the lower incisor region, resulting in a fracture of the alveolar process. B. The oral mucosa is lacerated in areas where the incisal edges contacted the labial mucosa during impact (arrows). From ANDREASEN (16) 1970.

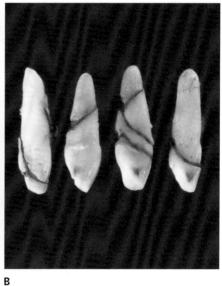

A                                        B

**Fig. 8.30** Fracture lines in four extracted maxillary incisors inflicted by a frontal impact from an ice-hockey puck. A. Labial aspect. B. Lateral aspect; note that the courses of the crown-root fractures and the root fractures are approximately perpendicular to each other.

When considering the direction and position of fracture lines caused by frontal impacts, the fractures fall easily into four categories (Fig. 8.31):

(1) Horizontal crown fractures
(2) Horizontal fractures at the neck of the tooth
(3) Oblique crown-root fractures
(4) Oblique root fractures.

Engineering principles can provide a description of the forces involved in injuries caused by frontal impacts.

Frontal impacts to anterior teeth generate forces which tend to displace the coronal portion orally. Under certain conditions, such as blunt impacts and high resilience of tooth supporting structures in young individuals, a tooth is more likely to be displaced orally without fracturing, as the energy of the impact is absorbed by the supporting structures during displacement (Fig. 8.32).

A different situation arises if the bone and periodontal ligament resist displacement (Fig. 8.33A). The root surface is forced against bone marginally and apically (a and b), creating high compressive forces. As the tensile and shearing strength of the brittle dental tissues are much lower than the compressive strength, shearing strains develop between the two zones of the opposing forces, and the root is fractured along the plane joining the two compression areas (a and b) (Fig. 8.33B) (105).

Fig. 8.34 illustrates a condition presumably leading to horizontal fractures at the level of the gingival margin. The tooth is firmly locked in its socket so that stresses in the shearing zone will not be as high as that shown in Fig. 8.33. The impact will, therefore, induce a pure bending fracture at the site of maximum bending stress, i.e. where the tooth emerges from its supporting structures (Fig. 8.34B). Tensile strains on the facial surface of the crown usually result in horizontal infraction lines in the cervical enamel (Fig. 8.35). Horizontal fractures at the cervical area usually affect the maxillary lateral incisors, probably due to their firm, deep anchorage in alveolar bone.

In Fig. 8.36, the stresses presumably causing oblique crown-root fractures are illustrated. The oblique fracture line follows a course along the inclined tensile stress lines developed between the compressive areas a and c. This line of fracture is supported by experiments using brittle materials, such as concrete (Fig. 8.37).

In Fig. 8.38, the same compressive forces and tensile strains as in Fig. 8.36 are presumably present, but are not great enough to cause an oblique fracture, so that the cleavage line follows the shortest possible route, resulting in a horizontal fracture of the crown. The area of contact between the impacting object and the enamel may show a shallow notch surrounded by radiating infraction lines (see Chapter 10, p. 281). The orientation of the enamel prisms determines the course of the fracture line in enamel, while the direction of the fracture in dentin is primarily perpendicular to the dentinal tubules (Fig. 8.39). The theoretical

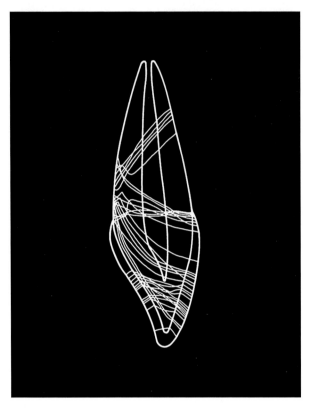

**Fig. 8.31** Facio-lingual orientation of 33 fracture lines.

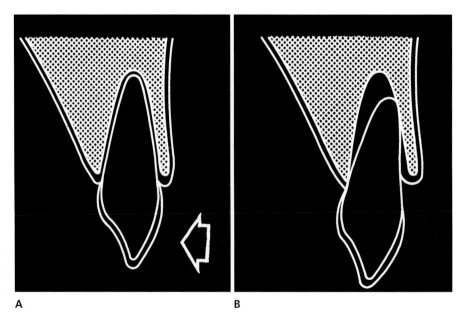

**Fig. 8.32** Pathogenesis of extrusive luxation. A. Frontal impact to the facial surface of an anterior tooth tends to displace the tooth lingually. B. If the energy is absorbed by the tooth-supporting structures, the tooth is displaced.

A                                        B

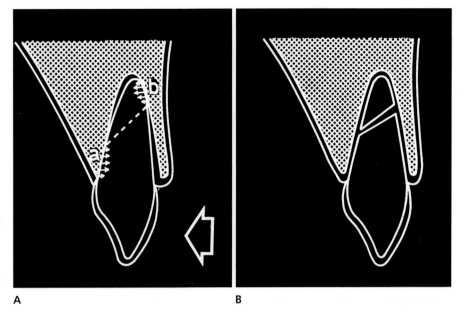

**Fig. 8.33** Pathogenesis of a midroot fracture. A. Bone and periodontal ligament resist displacement from a frontal impact. Compressive forces are exerted upon the root surface at a and b and tensile strains develop across the line connecting a and b. B. A root fracture occurs in the shearing zone, at the area of tensile strain.

**A**                                  **B**

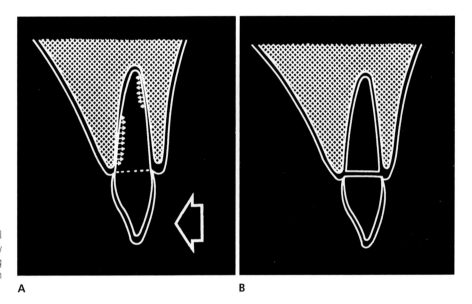

**Fig. 8.34** Pathogenesis of a cervical root fracture. A. The tooth is firmly locked in its socket. B. A pure bending fracture occurs at the site of maximum bending stress.

**A**                                  **B**

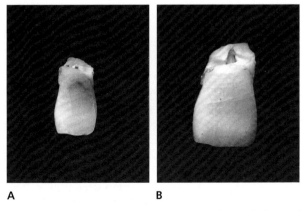

**A**              **B**

**Fig. 8.35** A. Horizontal infraction lines in the cervical area of a fractured maxillary incisor. B. High magnification of the cervical area.

explanation for this has been sought in experimental procedures testing the fracture properties of enamel and dentin (106, 107). It has been found that enamel is weakest parallel to the enamel rods and that dentin is most easily fractured perpendicularly to the dentinal tubules (107).

Penetrating lip lesions occur when the direction of impact is parallel to the axis of the mandibular or maxillary incisors (Figs 8.40 and 8.41). In these cases, foreign bodies such as gravel and tooth fragments are frequently found in the lip lesion. The management of this type of wound is described in Chapter 21.

## Treatment need

Epidemiological studies have demonstrated that the treatment needs of TDI are not properly met. This applies

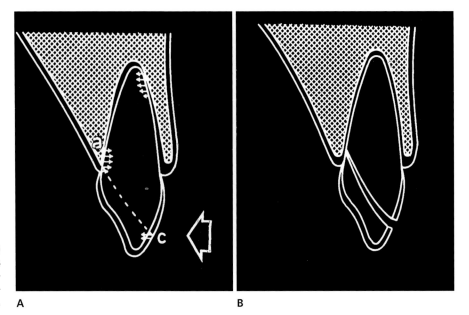

**Fig. 8.36** Pathogenesis of a crown root fracture. A. Tensile strain develops across the line between the compressive areas a and c. B. An oblique fracture occurs in the area of tensile strain.

**A**                                        **B**

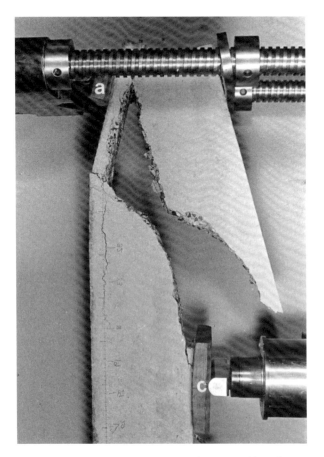

**Fig. 8.37** Experimental model in concrete showing an oblique fracture connecting the area of compression c and supporting area a. Courtesy of Dr. H. H. KRENCHEL, Structural Research Laboratory, Technical University, Copenhagen.

to both poor developing countries and rich developed countries.

In Britain only 10–15% (183, 199) and in Finland only 25% of children who sustained TDI had received treatment (198). Onetto et al. (224) reported a tendency for neglecting treatment of serious TDI in very young patients. In a study from Tanzania, 21% of the children had at least one type of untreated TDI, where the highest percentage (26%) was observed among children with high socio-economic status (338). However, almost all (94%) of the teeth showing untreated TDI were enamel- or enamel-dentin fractures. The low rates of treatment provided observed worldwide may be because TDI is not perceived as a disease. Another aspect that could enhance treatment neglect is the dentists' lack of knowledge regarding the treatment of TDI (340). In addition, dental school curricula and health authorities tend to focus resources on other oral health conditions but not on treatment of TDIs.

One may argue that these studies did not assess normative treatment need and that most injuries may be too small, therefore they need no treatment. Alternatively, it may be argued that epidemiological studies too often include only visual assessment and therefore tend to underestimate the need for treatment. Marcenes and Murray (242, 266) evaluated the need for treatment in addition to assessing only untreated damage, and showed that not all untreated dental injuries needed treatment because some injuries were minor. Conversely, the study also showed that not all treated injuries were satisfactory and some needed retreatment. A more accurate estimation of treatment need used in these studies confirmed that the treatment of TDIs was neglected, as 56% of incisors that sustained damage were assessed as needing treatment. Another study, using radiographs to assess the treatment provided, found that only 47% of

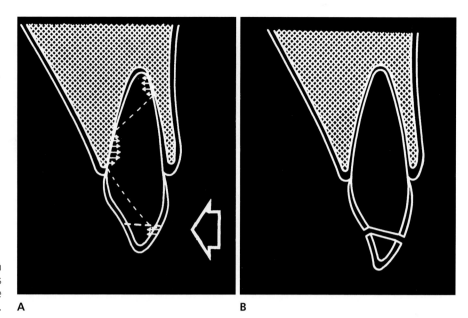

**Fig. 8.38** Pathogenesis of a crown fracture. A and B. Cleavage line takes the shortest route, resulting in a pure horizontal shear fracture of the crown.

**A**

**B**

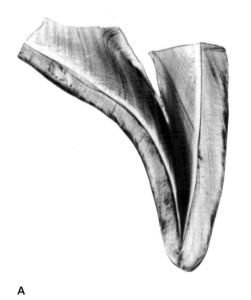

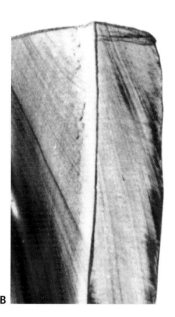

**Fig. 8.39** Fracture line orientation in enamel and dentine. A. The orientation of the enamel prisms and, to a certain degree, the dentinal tubules determine the course of the fracture line. B. Ground section of a fractured maxillary central incisor.

**A**

**B**

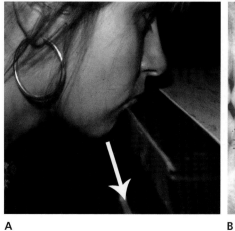

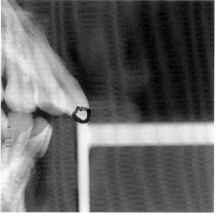

**Fig. 8.40** Etiology of a penetrating lip lesion. A. Impact direction parallel to the axis of the maxillary incisors. B. The lower lip has been interposed between the incisal edges and the staircase.

**A**

**B**

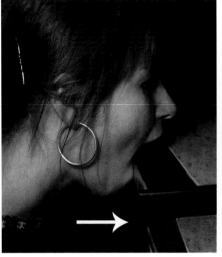
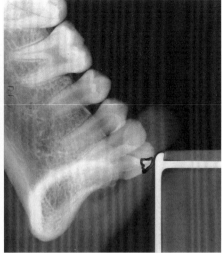

**Fig. 8.41** Etiology of a penetrating lip lesion. A. Impact direction is parallel to the axis of the mandibular incisors. B. The lower lip has been interposed between incisal edges and the staircase.

**A**                                    **B**

damaged teeth had received treatment, of which 59% was inadequate (340). A study carried out in a developing country (Jordan) has shown that only 3% of the injured teeth were treated, while 64% of the teeth needed treatment (341).

Several studies confirmed that treatment of TDI often is neglected. Marcenes et al. (215, 240) have shown in studies in Brazil and Syria that a majority of the traumatized teeth were not treated. In another study it was reported that nearly half of the sample who had experienced injuries to the permanent anterior teeth were not taken to the dentist for evaluation or treatment (244). A study from Central Taiwan also showed that a minor number of the subjects had sought dental or medical help (220).

## Lay knowledge in society

The prognosis of some injuries, especially avulsed teeth, depends on the correct measures taken immediately after injury. Research findings have defined correct first aid measures. Thus, it is of importance that not only professionals have access to this knowledge, but also lay people who are likely to provide the first aid to the injured person, e.g. parents, teachers, school nurses, health care professionals and physical trainers. They should know first aid procedures related to an avulsed permanent tooth. However, studies on lay knowledge on the management of TDI generally report a low level of knowledge (342–348). Physicians, medical students or physical education teachers have also been found lacking in knowledge of how to manage TDI (349, 350).

The prognosis for some of the dental injuries, e.g. avulsion injuries, depends on early treatment (351). However, many studies have shown that there is a significant delay before patients seek treatment (247, 352, 353), especially among low socio-economic populations (222, 354). It should be noted that it is essential that professional advice is sought from a dentist following all dental injuries; and not just for injuries which cause pain or result in poor esthetics (264). Campaigns with brochures or posters are, therefore, important tools for informing the general population about what to do in dental trauma situations and have been conducted in many countries including Argentina, Australia, Brazil, Denmark, Sweden, the UK and the USA. Such campaigns must also be repeated. In the scientific literature to date only a few studies have measured the effects of such campaigns (355–357). Better public awareness of emergency care may significantly improve long-term prognosis of treatment of many TDIs.

## Organization of emergency care

TDIs account for a large proportion of oral related emergency treatment. Analysis of after-hours emergency dental service data during one calendar year at the Royal Belfast Hospital for Sick Children reveal that traumatic injuries to teeth, supporting structures, gingiva, and oral mucosa represent the second most frequent complaint. While 39% visited the service due to dental injuries, 49% visited it due to all types of toothache including abscess (358). Similar proportions are reported in other studies. Oral injuries tend to occur in leisure time (359), in the middle of the week and in the afternoon (0–15 years) and during week-end and late evening (16–30 years) (216). Emergency room reports also indicated a greater frequency of TDIs in the summer months, whereas reports from Scandinavian public dental health services indicated a drop in the same period (20, 153, 176, 206, 216). This discrepancy could be related to the fact that most people tend to leave the bigger cities for summer vacations and if a TDI occurs, they visit a local dental surgery.

For this reason it is important that a dental emergency service is organized in each geographic region. Ideally, such a service should be provided on a 24-hour basis. During office hours, dental clinics can provide emergency service. However, because the majority of dental injuries occur outside office hours, other solutions must also be provided. An emergency service should be provided via a central dental emergency clinic or hospital.

Studies have shown that treatment of dental trauma in emergency care services is often inadequate (201, 215, 340, 360–362), and that patients are not always satisfied with the care provided (201, 363). For this reason it is important that emergency dental staff have experience in dental trauma treatment and preferably be regularly exposed to such situations (359). Manuals and guidelines for emergency treatment are valuable tools and will facilitate the treatment of dental trauma for dentists serving in the emergency service. (364–368).

Prevention of TDIs is also largely neglected. This may be because injuries have traditionally been regarded as random events, unavoidable 'accidents'. This assumption is incorrect, as a body of knowledge now exists on the etiology of TDI. For example, it is well established that human factors, such as increased incisal overjet, and environmental factors, such as playgrounds, coupled with a vector, such as tough sports are significant factors predisposing to TDI. Therefore, TDI has causal factors and can often be prevented. Nevertheless, few health professionals provide appropriate information to the public on how to prevent and manage a TDI event. A public survey conducted in Australia reported that, while most parents would seek emergency dental care if necessary, only 10% were informed on the correct emergency procedures if a permanent tooth was avulsed (199).

## Future research

While learning how to care for a patient is a continuously ongoing process, a goal for the future would be to increase lay knowledge in managing a TDI, and to increase the accessibility and the quality of emergency care. A model to follow would be the *WHO Healthy Cities Programme*, where a healthy city is defined as one that continually creates and improves the physical and social environment and expands community resources for enabling the mutual support among population groups for living (369). The WHO *Health Promoting Schools Programme* offers a broad solution for dental trauma as a public health problem, where a Health Promoting School constantly strengthens its capacity as a healthy setting for living, learning and working (370). A wide range of actions and policies are possible, including personal and social education aimed at developing life skills, school policy against bullying and violence, physical environment, school health policy, alcohol policy, provision of mouth guards, and links with health services (371). Moysés et al. (372) showed that 10% fewer children in Brazil had TDI in Health Promoting Schools that demonstrated a commitment towards health and society.

## Essentials

### Injuries to the hard dental tissues and the pulp (Fig. 8.1)

- Enamel infraction
- Enamel fracture
- Enamel-dentin fracture
- Complicated crown fracture (i.e. with pulp exposure)
- Uncomplicated crown-root fracture
- Complicated crown-root fracture (i.e. with pulp exposure)
- Root fracture

### Injuries to the periodontal tissues (Fig. 8.2)

- Concussion
- Subluxation (loosening)
- Extrusive luxation (peripheral dislocation, partial avulsion)
- Lateral luxation
- Intrusive luxation (central dislocation)
- Avulsion (exarticulation)

### Injuries to the supporting bone (Fig. 8.3)

- Comminution of alveolar socket
- Fracture of alveolar socket wall
- Fracture of alveolar process
- Fracture of mandible or maxilla (jaw fracture)

### Injuries to the gingiva or oral mucosa (Fig. 8.4)

- Laceration of gingiva or oral mucosa
- Contusion of gingiva or oral mucosa
- Abrasion of gingiva or oral mucosa

### Prevalence and incidence (Table 8.3)

- 1 in 5 children and 1 in 4 adults have evidence of dental injuries to permanent anterior teeth

### Trends

- Dental trauma may become more prevalent than dental caries in some countries

### Repeated episodes

- If a trauma episode occurs at an early age (9 years) there is an eight-fold increase in risk for new trauma
- Increased risk for trauma to the same teeth

### Sex and age

- Boys affected almost twice as often as girls
- Peak incidence of dental injuries at 2–4 and 8–10 years of age

- Incidence per year (1–18 years of age): 1.3–4 (Table 8.6)

### Prevalence in primary dentition (at 5 years of age) (Table 8.4)

- Boys (31–40%)
- Girls (16–30%)

### Prevalence in permanent dentition (at 12 years of age) (Table 8.5)

- Boys (12–33%)
- Girls (4–19%)

Prevalence of dental injuries decreases significantly at around 30 years of age (Fig. 8.11).

## Predisposing factors

- Increased overjet
- Protrusion of upper incisors
- Insufficient lip closure

## Types of dental injuries

- Primary dentition: most often luxations
- Maxillary central incisors most commonly involved
- Permanent dentition: most often uncomplicated crown fractures

## Place of injury

- At home
- In the street or in public places

## Seasonal variations

- Dependent on local customs

### Etiology

- Human behavior
  a. Risk-taking
  b. Peer relationship problems
  c. Hyperactivity
  d. Stress behavior
- Environmental factors
  a. Deprivation
  b. Overcrowding
- Unintentional injuries
  a. Falls and collisions
  b. Physical leisure activities (sports)
  c. Traffic accidents
  d. Inappropriate use of teeth
  e. Biting hard itims
  f. Presence of illness, physical limitations or learning difficulties

- Intentional injuries
  a. Physical abuse
  b. Iatrogenic procedures

## Mechanism of dental injuries

### Trauma type

- Direct trauma
- Indirect trauma

## Factors characterizing an impact to the teeth

- Energy of impact
- Resilience of the impacting object
- Shape of the impacting object
- Angle of direction of the impacting force

## Treatment need

- Treatment needs are insufficiently met in most countries

## Lay knowledge in society

- Professionals and lay people usually have a low level of knowledge of how to take care of a traumatic dental injury

## Organization of emergency care

- Dental emergency service should be provided on a 24-hour basis by emergency dental staff regularly exposed to such situations

## Future research

- Increase professional and lay knowledge in managing dental trauma by including the WHO Health Promoting Schools Programme and WHO Healthy Cities Programme

## Public health

- Need to standardize the assessment and the classification of dental trauma and its etiology

## References and further reading

1. ADAMS FR. Traumatized and fractured young teeth. *J Am Dent Assoc* 1944;**31**:241–8.
2. BENNETT DT. Traumatised anterior teeth. I – Assessing the injury and principles of treatment. *Br Dent J* 1963;**115**:309–11.
3. BRAUER JC. Treatment and restoration of fractured permanent anterior teeth. *J Am Dent Assoc* 1936;**23**:2323–36.
4. CAWSON RA. *Essentials of dental surgery and pathology.* 2nd edn. London: J & A Churchill, 1968:90–9.
5. COOKE C, ROWBOTHAM TC. Treatment of injuries to anterior teeth. *Br Dent J* 1951;**91**:146–52.

6. Ellis RG, Davey KW. *The classification and treatment of injuries to the teeth of children*. 5th edn. Chicago: Year Book Publishers Inc., 1970.

7. Eschler J, Schilli W, Witt E. *Die traumatischen Verletzungen der Frontzähne bei Jungendlichen*. 3rd edn. Heidelberg: Alfred Hilthig Verlag, 1972.

8. Hogeboom FE. *Practical pedodontia or juvenile operative dentistry and public health dentistry*. 5th edn. St. Louis: CV Mosby Company, 1946:288–314.

9. McBride WC. *Juvenile dentistry*. 5th edn. London: Henry Kimpton, 1952:247–62.

10. Ingle JI, Frank AL, Natkin E, Nutting EE. Diagnosis and treatment of traumatic injuries and their sequelae. In: Ingle JI, Beveridge EE. eds. *Endodontics*. 2nd edn. Philadelphia: Lea & Febiger, 1976:685–741.

11. Soleil J. Essai de classification des lésions traumatiques des dents. *Rev Stomatol* 1960;**61**:633–6.

12. Sweet CA. A classification and treatment for traumatized anterior teeth. *ASDC, J Dent Child* 1955;**22**:144–9.

13. Toverud G. Traumatiske beskadigelser av incisiver i barnealderen og deres behandling. *Odontologisk Tidskrift* 1947;**55**:7182.

14. Thoma KH, Goldman HM. *Oral pathology*. 5th edn. St. Louis: CV Mosby Company, 1960:231–41.

15. World Health Organization. *Application of the international classification of diseases to dentistry and stomatology, ICD-DA*. 2nd edn. Geneva: WHO, 1978:88–9.

16. Andreasen JO. Etiology and pathogenesis of traumatic dental injuries. A clinical study of 1298 cases. *Scand J Dent Res* 1970;**78**:339–42.

17. Nord C-E. Tandskador hos skolbarn och ishockeyspelare. *Odontologisk Förenings Tidskrift* 1966;**30**:15–25.

18. Schützmannsky G. Unfallverletzungen an jugendlichen Zähnen. *Dtsch Stomatol* 1963;**13**:919–27.

19. Tate RJ. Facial injuries associated with the battered child syndrome. *Br J Oral Surg* 1971;**9**:41–5.

20. Ravn JJ, Rossen I. Hyppighed og fordeling of traumatiske beskadigelser of tænderne hos københavnske skolebørn 1967/68. *Tandlægebladet* 1969;**73**:1–9.

21. Magnusson B, Holm A-K. Traumatised permanent teeth in children – a follow-up. I. Pulpal complications and root resorption. In: Nygaard J, Ostby B, Osvald O. eds. *Nordisk Klinisk Odontologi*. Copenhagen: A/S Forlaget for Faglitteratur 1964: Chapter 11, 1–40.

22. Ravn JJ. Dental injuries in Copenhagen school children, school years 1967–1972. *Community Dent Oral Epidemiol* 1974;**2**:231–45.

23. Edward S, Nord C-E. Dental injuries of school-children. *Sver Tandläkarförb Tidn* 1968;**61**:511–6.

24. Grimm G. Kiefer- und Zahnverletzungen beim Sport. *Zahnärztl* 1967;**76**:115–35.

25. Hawke JE. Dental injuries in rugby football. *N Z Dent J* 1969;**65**:173–5.

26. Kramer LR. Accidents occurring in high school athletics with special reference to dental injuries. *J Am Dent Assoc* 1941;**28**:1351–2.

27. Roberts JE. *Wisconsin Interscholastic Athletic Association 1970. Benefit plan summary*. Supplement to the 47th Official Handbook of the Wisconsin Interscholastic Athletic Association 1970:1–77.

28. Roberts JE. *Dental guard questionaire summary*. Wisconsin Interscholastic Athletic Association report to the National Alliance Football Rules Committee, 1962.

29. Cohen A, Borish AL. Mouth protector project for football players in Philadelphia high schools. *J Am Dent Assoc* 1958;**56**:863–4.

30. Kulowski J. Facial injuries; a common denominator of automobile casualties. *J Am Dent Assoc* 1956;**53**:32–7.

31. Kulowski J. *Crash injuries*. Springfield, Illinois: CT Thomas, 1960:306–22.

32. Schultz RC. Facial injuries from automobile accidents: a study of 400 consecutive cases. *Plast Reconstr Surg* 1967;**40**:415–25.

33. Straith CL. Guest passenger injuries. *J Am Dent Assoc* 1948;**137**:348–51.

34. Russell BG. Personal communication, 1969.

35. Wikström L. Narkotika och tänder. *Sver Tandläkarforb Tidn* 1970;**62**:1152–5.

36. Wilson GW, Steinbrecher M. Heriditary hypoplasia of the dentin. *J Am Dent Assoc* 1929;**16**:866–86.

37. Hodge HC. Correlated clinical and structural study of hereditary opalescent dentin. *J Dent Res* 1936;**15**:316–7.

38. Overvad H. Et tilfaelde of osteogenesis imperfecta med dentinogenesis imperfecta. *Tandlægebladet* 1969;**73**:840–50.

39. Glucksman DD. Fractured permanent anterior teeth complicating orthodontic treatment. *J Am Dent Assoc* 1941;**28**:1941–3.

40. Hardwick JL, Newmann PA. Some observations on the incidence and emergency treatment of fractured permanent anterior teeth of children. *J Dent Res* 1954;**33**:730.

41. Lewis TE. Incidence of fractured anterior teeth as related to their protrusion. *Angle Orthod* 1959;**29**:128–31.

42. Hallet GEM. Problems of common interest to the paedodontist and orthodontist with special reference to traumatised incisor cases. *Eur Orthod Soc Trans* 1953;**29**:266–77.

43. Eichenbaum IW. A correlation of traumatized anterior teeth to occlusion. *ASDC J Dent Child* 1963;**30**:229–36.

44. Büttner M. Die Häufigkeit von Zahnunfällen im Schulalter. *Zahnärztl Prax* 1968;**19**:286.

45. Wallentin I. Zahnfrakturen bei Kindern and Jugendlichen. *Zahnärztl Mitt* 1967;**57**:875–7.

46. McEwen JD, McHugh WD, Hitchin AD. Fractured maxillary central incisors and incisal relationships. *J Dent Res* 1967;**46**:1290.

47. Kessler W. *Kinder-Zahnheilkunde und, Zugendzahnpflege*. 3rd edn. München: Carl Hanser Verlag, 1953:144.

48. Kessler W. Fratture dentarie nell'infanzia. *Riv Ital Stomatol* 1959;**14**:251–5.

49. Grundy JR. The incidence of fractured incisors. *Br Dent J* 1959;**106**:312–4.

50. Beck JJ. *Dental health status of the New Zealand population in late adolescence and young adulthood*. Department of Health. Special report series 29. Wellington: RE Owen Government Printer, 1968: 65–9.

51. AKPATA ES. Traumatised anterior teeth in Lagos school children. *J Nigeria Med Assoc* 1969;**6**:1–6.

52. GAARE A, HAGEN AR, KANSTAD S. Tannfrakturer hos barn. Diagnostiske og prognostiske problemer og behandling. *Norske Tannlegeforenings Tidende* 1958;**68**:364–78.

53. PARKIN SF. A recent analysis of traumatic injuries to children's teeth. *ASDC J Dent Child* 1967;**34**:323–5.

54. GELBIER S. Injured anterior teeth in children. A preliminary discussion. *Br Dent J* 1967;**123**:331–5.

55. LIEBAN EA. Traumatic injuries to children's teeth. *N Y State Dent J* 1947;**13**:319–34.

56. ABRAHAM G. Über unfallbedingte Zahnschädigungen bei Jugendlichen. Thesis. Zürich, 1963.

57. SCHREIBER CK. The effect of trauma on the anterior deciduous teeth. *Br Dent J* 1959;**106**:340–3.

58. NORD C-E. Traumatiska skador i det primära bettet. *Odontologisk Förenings Tidende* 1968;**32**:157–63.

59. DOWN CH. The treatment of permanent incisor teeth of children following traumatic injury. *Aust Dent J* 1957;**2**:9–24.

60. KRETER F. Klinik und Therapie extraalveolärer Frontzahnfrakturen. *Zahnärztl Prax* 1967;**18**:257–60.

61. TAATZ H. Verletzungen der Milchzähne und ihre Behandlung. In: Reichenback E. ed. *Kinderzahnheilkunde im Vorschulalter. Zahnärztliche Fortbildung*. No. 16. Leipzig: Johann Ambrosius Barth Verlag, 1967:363–86.

62. STICH E. Dentoalveoläre Verletzungen. *Zahnärztl Welt* 1970;**79**:554–6.

63. SCHÜTZMANNSKY G. Statistisches über Häufigkeit und Schweregrad von Unfalltraumen an der Corona Dentis im Frontzahnbereich des kindlichen und jugendlichen Gebisses. *Z Gesamte Hyg* 1970;**16**:133–5.

64. ANDREASEN JO, RAVN JJ. Epidemiology of traumatic dental injuries to primary and permanent teeth in a Danish population sample. *Int J Oral Surg* 1972;**1**:235–9.

65. JOHNSON JE. Causes of accidental injuries to the teeth and jaws. *J Public Health Dent* 1975;**35**:123–31.

66. LASKIN DM. The battered-child syndrome. *J Oral Surg* 1973;**31**:903.

67. SCHWARTZ S, WOOLRIDGE E, STEGE D. Oral manifestations and legal aspects of child abuse. *J Am Dent Assoc* 1977;**95**:586–91.

68. LASKIN DM. The recognition of child abuse. *J Oral Surg* 1978;**36**:349.

69. BENSEL RW, KING KJ. Neglect and abuse of children; historical aspects, identification, and management. *ASDC J Dent Child* 1975;**42**:348–58.

70. O'NEILL JA Jr, MEACHAM WF, GRIFFIN PP, SAWYERS JL. Patterns of injury in the battered child syndrome. *J Trauma* 1973;**13**:332–9.

71. HOLTER JC, FRIEDMAN SB. Child abuse; early case finding in the emergency department. *Pediatrics* 1968;**42**:128–38.

72. CAMERON JM, JOHNSON HRM, CAMPS FE. The battered child syndrome. *Med Sci Law* 1966;**6**:2–21.

73. SKINNER AE, CASTLE RL. *A retrospective study*. London: National Society for the Prevention of Cruelty to Children, 1969.

74. BECKER DB, NEEDLEMAN HL, KOTELCHUCK M. Child abuse and dentistry; orofacial trauma and its recognition by dentist. *J Am Dent Assoc* 1978;**97**:24–8.

75. HAZLEWOOD AI. Child abuse. The dentist's role. *N Y Dent J* 1970;**36**:289–91.

76. CARTER AP, ZOLLER G, HARLIN VK, JOHNSON CJ. Dental injuries in Seattle's public school children – school year 1969–1970. *J Public Health Dent* 1972;**32**:251–4.

77. RAVN JJ. Dental injuries in Copenhagen schoolchildren, school years 1967–1972. *Community Dent Oral Epidemiol* 1974;**2**:231–45.

78. HEDEGÅRD B, STÅLHANE I. A study of traumatized permanent teeth in children aged 7–15 years. Part I. *Swed Dent J* 1973;**66**:431–50.

79. O'MULLANE DM. Some factors predisposing to injuries of permanent incisors in school children. *Br Dent J* 1973;**134**:328–32.

80. KNYCHALSKA-KARWAN Z. Trauma to the anterior teeth in sportsmen in the light of statistics. *Czas Stomatol* 1975;**28**:479–84.

81. HAAVIKKO K, RANTANEN L. A follow-up study of injuries to permanent and primary teeth in children. *Proc Finn Dent Soc* 1976;**72**:152–62.

82. O'MULLANE DM. Injured permanent incisor teeth; An epidemiological study. *J Irish Dent Assoc* 1972;**18**: 160–73.

83. LEES GH, GASKELL PH. Injuries to the mouth and teeth in an undergraduate population. *Br Dent J* 1976;**140**:107–8.

84. SZYMANSKA-JACHIMCZAK EI, Szpringernodzak M. Statistical analysis of traumatic damage to permanent teeth in children and adolescents treated at the outpatient clinic of the department of pediatric stomatology institute of the medical academy in Warsaw in the years 1960–1975. *Czas Stomatol* 1977;**30**:689–93.

85. GRIMM G. Kiefer und Zahnverletzungen beim Sport. *Zahnärtzl Rdsch* 1967;**76**:115–35.

86. DENNIS CG, PARKER DAS. Mouthguards in Australian sport. *Aust Dent J* 1972;**17**:228–35.

87. LIE HR, LUCHT U. Ridesportsulykker. I. Undersøgelse af en rytterpopulation med særligt henblik på ulykkesfrekvensen. *Ugeskr Læger* 1977;**139**:1687–9.

88. LUCHT U, LIE HR. Ridesportsulykker. II. Ulykkerne belyst gennem en prospektiv sygehusundersøgelse. *Ugeskr Læger* 1977;**139**:1689–92.

89. LINDAHL L, GRØNDAHL H-G. Traumatiserade tänder hos vuxna. *Tandläkartidningen* 1977;**69**:328–32.

90. HUELKE DF, SHERMAN HW. Automobile injuries – the forgotten area of public health dentistry. *J Am Dent Assoc* 1973;**86**:384–93.

91. LINDAHL L. Tand-och käskador i Göteborg. Epidemiologisk och behandlingsmässig kartläggning. *Svensk Tandläkares Tidning* 1974;**66**:1019–30.

92. LINDAHL L. Tand-och käskador i Göteborg. Några sociala faktorers inverkan. *Svensk Tandläkares Tidning* 1974;**66**:1011–4.

93. BESSERMANN K. Frequency of maxillo-facial injuries in a hospital population of patients with epilepsy. *Bull Nord Soc Dent Handicap* 1978;**5**:12–26.

94. VON GERLACH D, WOLTERS HD. Zahn- and Mundschleimhautbefunde bei Rauschmittelkonsumenten. *Dtsch Zahnärtztl Z* 1977;**32**:400–4.

95. BOLLING P. Tandtortur. *Tandlægebladet* 1978;**82**; 571–4.

96. DIEM CR, RICHLING M. Dental problems in Navy and Marine Corps repatriated prisoners of war before and after captivity. *Milit Med* 1978;**143**:532–7.

97. DIEM CR, RICHLING M. Improvisational dental first aid used by American prisoners of war in Southeast Asia. *J Am Dent Assoc* 1979;**98**:535–7.

98. BERZ H, BERZ A. Schneidezahnfrakturen und sagitale Schneidezahnstufe. *Dtsch Zahnärtztl Z* 1971;**26**:941–4.

99. WOJCIAK L, ZIOLKIEWICS T, ANHOLCER H, FRANKOWSKALENARTOWSKA M, HABER-MILEWSKA T, ZYNDA B. Trauma to the anterior teeth in school-children in the city of Poznân with reference to masticatory anomalies. *Czas Stomatol* 1974;**27**:1355–61.

100. ANTOLIC I, BELIC D. Traumatic damages of teeth in the intercanine sector with respect to the occurrence with school children. *Zoboz Vestn* 1973;**28**:113–20.

101. PATKOWSKA-INDYKA E, PLONKA K. The effect of occlusal anomalies on fractures of anterior teeth. *Stomatol* 1974;**24**:375–9.

102. DE MUNIZ BR, MUNIZ MA. Crown fractures in children. Relationship with anterior occlusion. *Rev Asoc Odont Argent* 1975;**63**:153–7.

103. JÄRVINEN S. Incisal overjet and traumatic injuries to upper permanent incisors. A retrospective study. *Acta Odontol Scand* 1978;**36**:359–62.

104. FERGUSON FS, RIPA LW. Incidence and type of traumatic injuries to the anterior teeth of preschool children. *J Dent Res* 1975;**58**: I.A.D.R. Abstracts no. 401, 1979.

105. LEHMAN ML. Bending strength of human dentin. *J Dent Res* 1971;**50**:691.

106. RENSON CE, BOYDE A, JONES SJ. Scanning electron microscopy of human dentin specimens fractured in bend and torsion tests. *Arch Oral Biol* 1974;**19**:447–54.

107. RASMUSSEN ST, PATCHIN RE, SCOTT DB, HEUER AH. Fracture properties of human enamel and dentin. *J Dent Res* 1976;**55**:154–64.

108. JÄRVINEN S. Fractured and avulsed permanent incisors in Finnish children. A retrospective study. *Acta Odontol Scand* 1979;**37**:47–50.

109. MARCUS M. Delinquency and coronal fractures of anterior teeth. *J Dent Res* 1951;**30**:513.

110. HARGREAVES JA, CRAIG JW. *The management of traumatised anterior teeth in children.* London: E. & S. Livingstone Publishers, 1970.

111. LIND V, WALLIN H, EGERMARK-ERIKSSON I, BERNHOLD M. Indirekta traumaskador. Kliniska skador på permanenta incisiver som följd av trauma mot temporära incisiver. *Sver Tandläkarforb Tidn* 1970;**62**:738–56.

112. GUTZ DP. Fractured permanent incisors in a clinic population. *ASDC J Dent Child* 1971;**38**:94–121.

113. BERGINK AH. Tandbeschadigungen. *Maandschr Kindergeneesk* 1972;**40**:278–93.

114. CLARKSON BH, LONGHURST P, SHEIHAM A. The prevalence of injured anterior teeth in English school children and adults. *J Int Assoc Dent Child* 1973;**4**:21–4.

115. HOLM AK, ARVIDSSON S. Oral health in preschool Swedish children. 1. Three-year-old children. *Odontologisk Revy* 1974;**25**:81–98.

116. WIESLANDER I, LIND V. Traumaskador på permanenta tänder. Något om förekomst och behandlingsproblem. *Tandläkartidningen* 1974;**66**:716–19.

117. ZADIK D. A survey of traumatized primary anterior teeth in Jerusalem preschool children. *Community Dent Oral Epidemiol* 1976;**4**:149–51.

118. YORK AH, HUNTER RM, MORTON JG, WELLS GM, NEWTON BJ. Dental injuries in 11–13-year-old children. *N Z Dent J* 1978;**74**:218–20.

119. IRMISCH B, HETZER G. Eine klinische Auswertung akuter Traumen im Milchgebiss und permanenten Gebiss. *Dtsch Stomatol* 1971;**21**:28–34.

120. HERFORTH A. Zur Frage der Pulpavitalität nach Frontzahntrauma bei Jugendlichen- eine Longitudinaluntersuchung. *Dtsch Zahnärztl Z* 1976;**31**;938–46.

121. WORLE M. Katamnestische Erhebung zur Prognose des Frontzahntraumas. *Dtsch Zahnärzl Z* 1976;**31**:635–7.

122. ZADIK D, CHOSACK A, EIDELMAN E. A survey of traumatized incisors in Jerusalem school children. *ASDC J Dent Child* 1972;**39**:185–8.

123. SNYDER JR, KNOOPS JJ, JORDAN WA. Dental problems of non-institutionalized mentally retarded children. *North-West Dent* 1960;**39**:123–33.

124. GAYFORD JJ. Wife battering: a preliminary survey of 100 cases. *Br Med J* 1975;**I(5951)**:194–7.

125. PARKER B, SCHUMACHER DN. The battered wife syndrome and violence in the nuclear family of origin. A controlled pilot study. *Am J Public Health* 1977;**67**:760–1.

126. SCOTT PD. Battered wives. *Br J Psychiatry* 1974;**125**:433–41.

127. ROUNSAVILLE B, WEISSMANN MM. Battered women; A medical problem requiring detection. *Int J Psychiatry* 1977–78;**8**:191–202.

128. ROUNSAVILLE BJ. Battered wives. Barriers to identification and treatment. *Am J Orthopsychiatry* 1978;**48**:487–94.

129. PETRO JA, QUANN PL, GRAHAM WP. Wife abuse. The diagnosis and its implications. *J Am Dent Assoc* 1978;**240**:240–1.

130. PETERSSON B, JACOBSEN AT. Mishandlede kvinder (battered wives). *Ugeskr Læger* 1980;**142**:469–71.

131. JOHNSON R. Descriptive classification of traumatic injuries to the teeth and supporting structures. *J Am Dent Assoc* 1981;**102**:195–7.

132. GARCÍA-GODOY F. A classification for traumatic injuries to primary and permanent teeth. *J Pedodont* 1981;**5**:295–7.

133. WORLD HEALTH ORGANIZATION. *Application of the international classification of diseases to dentistry and stomatology, ICD-DA.* 3rd edn. Geneva: WHO, 1992.

134. MOYLAN FMB, SELDEN EB, SHANNON DC, TODRES JD. Defective primary dentition in survivors of neonatal mechanical ventilation. *J Paediatr* 1980;**96**:106–8.

135. BOICE JB, KROUS HF, FOLEY JM. Gingival and dental complication of orotracheal intubation. *J Am Med Assoc* 1976;**236**:957–8.

136. SEOW WK, BROWN JP, TUDEHOPE DI, O'CALLAGHAN M. Developmental defects in the primary dentition of low birthweight infants: adverse effects of laryngoscopy and prolonged endotracheal intubation. *Pediatr Dent* 1984;**6**:28–31.

137. BECKER DB, NEEDLEMAN HL, KOTELCHUCK M. Child abuse and dentistry: orofacial trauma and its recognition by dentists. *J Am Dent Assoc* 1978;**27**:24–8.

138. Malecz RE. Child abuse, its relationship to pedodontics: a survey. *ASDC J Dent Child* 1979;**46**:193–4.

139. Davis GR, Domoto PK, Levy RL. The dentist's role in child abuse and neglect. *ASDC J Dent Child* 1979;**46**:185–92.

140. Kittle PE, Richardson DS, Parker JW. Two child abuse/child neglect examinations for the dentist. *ASDC J Dent Child* 1981;**48**:175–80.

141. Schmitt BD. Types of child abuse and neglect: an overview for dentists. *Pediatr Dent* 1986;**8**:67–71.

142. Needleman HL. Orofacial trauma in child abuse: types, prevalence, management, and the dental professions involvement. *Pediatr Dent* 1986;**8**:71–80.

143. Kittle PE, Richardson DS, Parker JW. Examining for child abuse and child neglect. *Pediatr Dent* 1986;**8**:80–2.

144. Schmitt BD. Physical abuse: specifics of clinical diagnosis. *Pediatr Dent* 1986;**8**:83–7.

145. Dubowitz H. Sequelae of reporting child abuse. *Pediatr Dent* 1986;**8**:88–92.

146. Wagner GN. Bitemark identification in child abuse cases. *Pediatric Dent* 1986;**8**:96–100.

147. Casamassimo PS. Child sexual abuse and the pediatric dentist. *Pediatr Dent* 1986;**8**:102–6.

148. Oneil DW, Clark MV, Lowe JW, Harrington MS. Oral trauma in children: a hospital survey. *Oral Surg Oral Med Oral Pathol* 1989;**68**:691–6.

149. Nysether S. Dental injuries among Norwegian soccer players. *Community Dent Oral Epidemiol* 1987;**15**:141–3.

150. Nysether S. Tannskader i norsk idrett. *Norske Tannlegeforenings Tidende* 1987;**97**:512–4.

151. Järvinen S. On the causes of traumatic dental injuries with special reference to sports accidents in a sample of Finnish children. A study of a clinical patient material. *Acto Odontol Scand* 1980;**38**:151–4.

152. Häyrinen-Immonen R, Sane J, Perkki K, Malmström M. A six-year follow-up study of sports-related dental injuries in children and adolescents. *Endod Dent Traumatol* 1990;**6**:208–12.

153. Brat M, Li S-H. Consumer product-related tooth injuries treated in hospital emergency rooms: United States, 1979–87. *Community Dent Oral Epidemiol* 1990;**18**:133–8.

154. Kenrad B. Tandlægetjeneste på en spejderlejr. *Tandlægebladet* 1991;**95**:583–5.

155. Sandham A, Dewar I, Craig J. Injuries to incisors during sporting activities at school. *Tandlægebladet* 1986;**90**:661–3.

156. Hill CM, Crocher RF, Mason DA. Dental and facial injuries following sports accidents: a study of 130 patients. *Br J Oral Maxillofac Surg* 1985;**23**:268–74.

157. Linn EW, Vrijhoef MMA, de Wijn JR, Coops RPHM, Cliteur BF, Meerloo R. Facial injuries sustained during sports and games. *J Maxillofac Surg* 1986;**14**:83–8.

158. Seguin P, Beziat JL, Breton P, Freidel M, Nicod C. Sports et traumatologie maxillo-faciale. Aspects étiologiqes et cliniqes à propos de 46 cas. Mesures de prévention. *Rev Stomatol Chir Maxillofac* 1986;**87**:372–5.

159. Stockwell AJ. Incidence of dental trauma in the Western Australian School Dental Service. *Community Dent Oral Epidemiol* 1988;**16**:294–8.

160. Wiens JP. Acquired maxillofacial defects from motor vehicle accidents: statistics and prosthodontic considerations. *J Prosthet Dent* 1990;**63**:172–81.

161. Lamberg MA, Tasanen A, Kotilainen R. Maxillofacial fractures caused by assault and battery. Victims and their injuries. *Proc Finn Dent Soc* 1975;**71**:162–75.

162. Korsgaard GM, Carlsen A. 'Hustruvold'. En prospektiv opgørelse of vold mod kvinder i parforhold. *Ugeskrift for Læger* 1983;**145**:443–6.

163. Laskin DM. Looking out for the battered woman. *J Oral Surg* 1981;**39**:405.

164. Young GH, Gerson S. New psychoanalytic perspectives on masochism and spouse abuse. *Psychotherapy* 1991;**28**:30–8.

165. Sanchez JR, Sanchez R, García-Godoy F. Traumatismos de los dientes anteriores en ninos pre-escolares. *Acta Odontol Pediatr* 1981;**2**:17–23.

166. Baghdady VS, Ghose LJ, Enke H. Traumatized anterior teeth in Iraqi and Sudanese children – a comparative study. *J Dent Res* 1981;**60**:677–80.

167. García-Godoy F, Sanchez R, Sanchez JR. Traumatic dental injuries in a sample of Dominican schoolchildren. *Community Dent Oral Epidemiol* 1981;**9**:193–7.

168. García-Godoy F, Morbán-Laucher F, Corominas LR, Franjul RA, Noyola M. Traumatic dental injuries in preschoolchildren from Santo Domingo. *Community Dent Oral Epidemiol* 1983;**11**:127–30.

169. García-Godoy FM. Prevalence and distribution of traumatic injuries to the permanent teeth of Dominican children from private schools. *Community Dent Oral Epidemiol* 1984;**12**:136–9.

170. García-Godoy F, Morbán-Laucher F, Corominas LR, Franjul RA, Noyola M. Traumatic dental injuries in schoolchildren from Santo Domingo. *Community Dent Oral Epidemiol* 1985;**13**:177–9.

171. García-Godoy F, Dipres FM, Lora IM, Vidal ED. Traumatic dental injuries in children from private and public schools. *Community Dent Oral Epidemiol* 1986;**14**:287–90.

172. Holland T, O'Mullane DO, Clarkson J, O'Hickey SO, Whelton H. Trauma to permanent teeth of children aged 8, 12 and 15 years, in Ireland. *Paediatr Dent* 1988;**4**:13–6.

173. Uji T, Teramoto T. Occurrence of traumatic injuries in the oromaxillary region of children in a Japanese prefecture. *Endod Dent Traumatol* 1988;**4**:63–9.

174. Yagot KH, Nazhat NY, Kuder SA. Traumatic dental injuries in nursery schoolchildren from Baghdad, Iraq. *Community Dent Oral Epidemiol* 1988;**16**:292–3.

175. Kaba AD, Maréchaux SC. A fourteen-year follow-up study of traumatic injuries to the permanent dentition. *ASDC J Dent Child* 1989;**56**:417–25.

176. Ravn JJ. Dental traume epidemiologi i Danmark: en oversigt med enkelte nye oplysninger. *Tandlægebladet* 1989;**93**:393–6.

177. Hunter ML, Hunter B, Kingdon A, Addy M, Dummer PMH, Shaw WC. Traumatic injury to maxillary incisor teeth in a group of South Wales schoolchildren. *Endod Dent Traumatol* 1990;**6**:260–4.

178. Forsberg C, Tedestam G. Traumatic injuries to teeth in Swedish children living in an urban area. *Swed Dent J* 1990;**14**:115–22.

179. SANCHEZ AV, GARCÍA-GODOY F. Traumatic dental injuries in 3–13-year-old boys in Monterrey, Mexico. *Endod Dent Traumatol* 1990;**6**:63–5.

180. BIJELLA MFTB, YARED FNFG, BIJELLA VT, LOPES ES. Occurrence of primary incisor traumatism in Brazilian children: a house-by house survey. *ASDC J Dent Child* 1990;**57**:424–7.

181. STOCKWELL AJ. Incidence of dental trauma in the Western Australian School Dental Service. *Community Dent Oral Epidemiol* 1988;**16**:294–8.

182. TODD JE. *Children's dental health in England and Wales 1973*. London: Social Survey Division and Her Majesty's Stationery Office, 1975.

183. TODD JE, DODD T. *Children's dental health in the United Kingdom 1983*. London: Social Survey Division and Her Majesty's Stationery Office, 1985.

184. RAVN JJ. Stiger antallet of akutte trandtraumer? *Odontologia Practica* 1991;**3**:103–5.

185. HANSEN M, LOTHE T. Tanntraumer hos skolebarn og ungdom i alderen 7–18 år i Oslo. *Norske Tannlægeforenings Tidende* 1982;**92**:269–73.

186. GHOSE LJ, BAGHDADY VS, ENKE H. Relation of traumatized permanent anterior teeth to occlusion and lip condition. *Community Dent Oral Epidemiol* 1980;**8**:381–4.

187. OLUWOLE TO, LEVERETT DH. Clinical and epidemiological survey of adolescents with crown fractures of permanent anterior teeth. *Pediatr Dent* 1986;**8**:221–3.

188. HOLLAND T, O'MULLANE D, CLARKSON J, HICKEY SO, WHELTON H. Trauma to permanent teeth of children aged 8, 12 and 15 years, in Ireland. *J Paediat Dent* 1988;**4**:13–6.

189. GALEA H. An investigation of dental injuries treated in an acute care general hospital. *J Am Dent Assoc* 1984;**109**:434–8.

190. ANDREASEN FM, ANDREASEN JO. Diagnosis of luxation injuries: The importance of standardized clinical, radiographic and photographic techniques in clinical investigations. *Endod Dent Traumatol* 1985;**1**:160–9.

191. TETSCH P. Statistische Auswertung von 1588 traumatisierten Zähnen. *Dtsch Zahndrztl Z* 1983;**38**:474–5.

192. MORGANTINI J, MARÉCHAUX SC, JOHO JP. Traumatismes dentaires chez l'enfant en âge préscolaire et répercussions sur les dents permanentes. *Rev Mens Suisse Odontostomatol* 1986;**96**:432–40.

193. BAGHDADY VS, GHOSE LJ, ALWASH R. Traumatized anterior teeth as related to their cause and place. *Community Dent Oral Epidemiol* 1981;**9**:91–3.

194. DAVIS GT, KNOTT SC. Dental trauma in Australia. *Aust Dent J* 1984;**29**:217–21.

195. LIEW VP, DALY CG. Anterior dental trauma treated after hours in Newcastle, Australia. *Community Dent Oral Epidemiol* 1986;**14**:362–6.

196. GARCÍA-GODOY F, GARCÍA-GODOY F, OLIVO M. Injuries to primary and permanent teeth treated in a private paedodontic practice. *J Canad Dent Assoc* 1979;**45**: 281–4.

197. GARCÍA-GODOY F, GARCÍA-GODOY F, GARCÍ-GODOY FM. Primary teeth traumatic injuries at a private pediatric dental center. *Endod Dent Traumatol* 1987;**3**:126–9.

198. JÄRVINEN S. Extent to which treatment is sought for children with traumatized permanent anterior teeth. An epidemiological study. *Proc Finn Dent Soc* 1979;**75**:103–5.

199. RAPHAEL LSJ, GREGORY PJ. Parental awareness of the emergency management of avulsed teeth in children. *Australian Dent J* 1990;**35**:130–5.

200. DUMSHA TC. Luxation injuries. *Dent Clin North Am* 1995;**39**:79–91.

201. HAMILTON FA, HILL FJ, HOLLOWAY PJ. An investigation of dento-alveolar trauma and its treatment in an adolescent population. Part 1: The prevalence and incidence of injuries and the extent and adequacy of treatment received. *Br Dent J* 1997;**182**:91–5.

202. DEWHURST SN, MASON C, ROBERTS GJ. Emergency treatment of orodental injuries: a review. *Br J Oral Maxillofac Surg* 1998;**6**:165–75.

203. DiANGELIS AJ, BAKLAND LK. Traumatic dental injuries: current treatment concepts. *J Am Dent Assoc* 1998; **129**:1401–14.

204. BASTONE EB, FREER TJ, McNAMARA JR. Epidemiology of dental trauma: a review of the literature. *Aust Dent J* 2000;**45**:2–9.

205. ELLIS SGS. Incomplete tooth fracture – proposal for a new definition. *Br Dent J* 2001;**190**:424–8.

206. GLENDOR U, HALLING A, ANDERSSON L, EILERT-PETERSSON E. Incidence of traumatic tooth injuries in children and adolescents in the county of Västmanland, Sweden. *Swed Dent J* 1996;**20**:15–28.

207. ENGELHARDTSEN S, JACOBSEN I, MOLVEN O, MYRHAUG I, NYSETHER S, OKSTAD A, RÖYNESDAL K, STÖEN GKB, STÖRMER K, THORGERSEN A. *Tannskader hos barn och ungdom. En undersökelse i Nord-Trøndelag og Oslo i 1992/93. Utredning (IK-2600)*. Oslo: Statens helsetilsyn (in Norwegian), 1998.

208. GLENDOR U. On dental trauma in children and adolescents. Incidence, risk, treatment, time and costs. *Swed Dent J* Suppl. 2000;**140**:1–52. http://www.ep.liu.se/diss/med/06/24/index.html

209. BHAT M, NELSON KB, SWANGO PA. Lack of stability in enamel defects in primary teeth of children with cerebral palsy or mental retardation. *Pediatr Dent* 1989;**11**: 118–20.

210. KASTE LM, GIFT HC, BHAT M, SWANGO PA. Prevalence of incisor trauma in persons 6 to 50 years of age: United States, 1988–1991. *J Dent Res* 1996;**75**:696–705.

211. NAQVI A, OGIDAN O. Classification for traumatic injuries to teeth for epidemiological purposes. *Odontostomatol Trop* 1990;**13**:115–6.

212. O'BRIEN M. *Children's dental health in the United Kingdom 1993*. London: Her Majesty's Stationery Office, 1994.

213. ANDREASEN JO, ANDREASEN FM. *Textbook and color atlas of traumatic injuries to the teeth*. 3rd edn. Copenhagen: Munksgaard, 1994.

214. CORTES MIS. Epidemiology of traumatic injuries to the permanent teeth and the impact of the injuries on the daily living of Brazilian schoolchildren. PhD thesis, University of London, 2000, 2001.

215. MARCENES W, AL BEIRUTI N, TAYFOUR D, ISSA S. Epidemiology of traumatic injuries to the permanent

incisors of 9–12-year-old schoolchildren in Damascus, Syria. *Endod Dent Traumatol* 1999;**15**:17–123.

216. EILERT-PETERSSON E, ANDERSSON L, SÖRENSEN S. Traumatic oral vs non-oral injuries. An epidemiological study during one year in a Swedish county. *Swed Dent J* 1997;**21**:55–68.

217. NAIR KB, PAUL G. Incidence and etiology of fractures of the facio-maxillary skeleton in Trivandrum: a retrospective study. *Br J Oral Maxillofac Surg* 1986;**24**:40–3.

218. HAYTER JP, WARD AJ, SMITH EJ. Maxillofacial trauma in severely injured patients. *Br J Oral Maxillofac Surg* 1991;**29**:370–3.

219. SKAARE AB, JACOBSEN I. Dental injuries in Norwegians aged 7–18 years. *Dent Traumatol* 2003;**19**:67–71.

220. CHEN YL, TSAI TP, SEE LC. Survey of incisor trauma in second grade students of Central Taiwan. *Chan Gung Med J* 1999;**22**:212–9.

221. VANDERAS AP, PAPAGIANNOULIS AP. Urinary catecholamine levels and incidence of dento-facial injuries in children: 2-year prospective study. *Endod Dent Traumatol* 2000;**16**:222–8.

222. ROCHA MJC, CARDOSO M. Traumatized permanent teeth in Brazilian children assisted at the Federal University of Santa Catarina, Brazil. *Dent Traumatol* 2001;**17**:245–9.

223. CARDOSO M, DE CARVALHO ROCHA MJ. Traumatized primary teeth in children assisted at the Federal University of Santa Catarina, Brazil. *Dent Traumatol* 2002;**18**:129–133.

224. ONETTO JE, FLORES MT, GARBARINO ML. Dental trauma in children and adolescents in Valparaiso, Chile. *Endod Dent Traumatol* 1994;**10**:223–227.

225. BORSSÉN E, HOLM AK. Traumatic dental injuries in a cohort of 16-year-olds in northern Sweden. *Endod Dent Traumatol* 1997;**13**:276–280.

226. GLENDOR U, KOUCHEKI B, HALLING A. Risk evaluation and type of treatment of multiple dental trauma episodes to permanent teeth. *Endod Dent Traumatol* 2000;**16**:205–210.

227. CUNHA RF, PUGLIESI DMC, VIEIRA AED. Oral trauma in Brazilian patients aged 0–3 years. *Dent Traumatol* 2001;**17**:210–12.

228. BAUSS O, ROHLING J, SCHWESTKA-POLLY R. Prevalence of traumatic injuries to the permanent incisors in candidates for orthodontic treatment. *Dent Traumatol* 2004;**20**:61–6.

229. AL-JUNDI, SH. Type of treatment, prognosis, and estimation of time spent to manage dental trauma in late presentation cases at a dental teaching hospital: a longitudinal and retrospective study. *Dent Traumatol* 2004;**20**:1–5.

230. WORLD HEALTH ORGANIZATION. *Dictionary for minimum data sets on injuries*. WHO, 2001.

231. GASSNER R, TARKAN T, HÄCHL O, RUDISH A, ULMER H. Cranio-maxillofacial trauma: a 10 year review of 9543 cases with 21 067 injuries. *J Craniomaxillofac Surg* 2003;**31**:51–61.

232. BURDEN DJ. An investigation of the association between overjet size, lip coverage, and traumatic injury to maxillary incisors. *Eur J Orthod* 1995;**17**:513–7.

233. TRAEBERT J, PERES MA, BLANK V, BOELL RD, PIETRUZA JA. Prevalence of traumatic dental injury and associated factors among 12-year-old school children in Florianópolis, Brazil. *Dent Traumatol* 2003;**19**:15–18.

234. IANETTI G, MAGGIORE C, RIPARI M, GRASSI P. Studio statistico sulle lesioni traumatiche dei denti. *Minerva Stomatol* 1984;**33**:933–43.

235. REDFORS Å, OLSSON B. Tandskador i norra Älvsborg 940201–95013: en delstudie i 'Skaderegistreringen i Norra Älvsborg'. Vänersborg: Landstinget i Älvsborg, 1996.

236. HOLLAND TJ, O'MULLANE DM, WHELTON HP. Accidental damage to incisors amongst Irish adults. *Endod Dent Traumatol* 1994;**10**:191–4.

237. SHULMAN JD, PETERSON J. The association between incisor trauma and occlusal characteristics in individuals 8–50 years of age. *Dent Traumatol* 2004;**20**:67–74.

238. GASSNER R, BOSCH R, TULI T, EMSHOFF R. Prevalence of dental trauma in 6000 patients with facial injuries: implications for prevention. *Oral Surg Oral Med Oral Pathol Oral Radiol Endod* 1999;**87**:27–33.

239. THOMSON WM, STEPHENSON S, KIESER JA, LANGLEY JD. Dental and maxillofacial injuries among older New Zealanders during the 1990s. *Int J Oral Maxillofac Surg* 2003;**32**:201–5.

240. MARCENES W, ZABOT NE, TRAEBERT J. Socio-economic correlates of traumatic injuries to the permanent incisors in schoolchildren aged 12 years in Blumenau, Brazil. *Dent Traumatol* 2001;**17**:222–6.

241. FORSBERG CM, TEDESTAM G. Etiological and predisposing factors related to traumatic injuries to permanent teeth. *Swed Dent J* 1993;**17**:183–90.

242. MARCENES W, MURRAY S. Social deprivation and traumatic dental injuries among 14-year-old schoolchildren in Newham, London. *Dent Traumatol* 2001;**17**:17–21.

243. SORIANO EP, CALDAS AF Jr, GÓES PSA. Risk factors related to traumatic dental injuries in Brazilian schoolchildren. *Dent Traumatol* 2004;**20**:246–50.

244. MARCENES W, ALESSI ON, TRAEBERT J. Causes and prevalence of traumatic injuries to the permanent incisors of school children aged 12 years in Jaragua do Sul, Brazil. *Int Dent J* 2000;**50**:87–92.

245. HARGREAVES JA, MATEJKA JM, CLEATON-JONES PE, WILLIAMS S. Anterior tooth trauma in 11-year-old South-African children. *J Dent Child* 1995;**62**:353–5.

246. OTUYEMI OD, SEGUN-OJO IO, ADEGBOYE AA. Traumatic anterior dental injuries in Nigerian preschool children. *East Afr Med J* 1996;**73**:604–6.

247. ALTAY N, GÜNGÖR HC. A retrospective study of dento-alveolar injuries of children in Ankara, Turkey. *Dent Traumatol* 2001;**17**:201–4.

248. CORTES MI, MARCENES W, SHEIHAM A. Prevalence and correlates of traumatic injuries to the permanent teeth of schoolchildren aged 9–14 years in Belo Horizonte, Brazil. *Dent Traumatol* 2001;**17**:22–6.

249. CALDAS AD, BURGOS MEA. A retrospective study of traumatic dental injuries in a Brazilian dental trauma clinic. *Dent Traumatol* 2001;**17**:250–3.

250. NIK-HUSSEIN NN. Traumatic injuries to anterior teeth among schoolchildren in Malaysia. *Dent Traumatol* 2001;**17**:149–52.

251. Wood EB, Freer TJ. A survey of dental and oral trauma in south-east Queensland during 1998. *Aust Dent J* 2002;**47**:142–6.

252. Kramer PF, Zembruski C, Ferreira SH, Feldens CA. Traumatic dental injuries in Brazilian preschool children. *Dent Traumatol* 2003;**19**:299–303.

253. Kargul B, Caglar E, Tanboga I. Dental trauma in Turkish children, Istanbul. *Dent Traumatol* 2003;**19**:72–5.

254. Glendor U, Halling A, Andersson L, Andreasen JO, Klitz I. Type of treatment and estimation of time spent on dental trauma. A longitudinal and retrospective study. *Swed Dent J* 1998;**22**:47–60.

255. Hargreaves JA, Cleaton-Jones PE, Roberts GJ, Williams S, Matejka JM. Trauma to primary teeth of South African pre-school children. *Endod Dent Traumatol* 1999;**15**:73–6.

256. Schatz JP, Joho JP. A retrospective study of dento-alveolar injuries. *Endod Dent Traumatol* 1994;**10**:11–14.

257. Borssén E, Holm AK. Treatment of traumatic dental injuries in a cohort of 16-year-olds in northern Sweden. *Endod Dent Traumatol* 2000;**16**:276–81.

258. Al-Majed I, Murray JJ, Maguire A. Prevalence of dental trauma in 5–6-and 12–14-year-old boys in Riyadh, Saudi Arabia. *Dent Traumatol* 2001;**17**:153–8.

259. Wong FSL, Kolokotsa K. The cost of treating children and adolescents with injuries to their permanent incisors at a dental hospital in the United Kingdom. *Dent Traumatol* 2004;**20**:327–33.

260. Borum MK, Andreasen JO. Sequelae of trauma to primary maxillary incisors. 1. Complications in the primary dentition. *Endod Dent Traumatol* 1998;**14**:31–44.

261. Flores MT. Traumatic injuries in the primary dentition. *Dent Traumatol* 2002;**18**:287–98.

262. Carvalho JC, Vinker F, Declerck D. Malocclusion, dental injuries and dental anomalies in the primary dentition of Belgian children. *Int J Paediatr Dent* 1998;**8**:137–41.

263. LaBella CR, Smith BW, Sigurdsson A. Effect of mouthguards on dental injuries and concussions in college basketball. *Med Sci Sport Exerc* 2002;**34**:41–4.

264. Blinkhorn FA. The etiology of dento-alveolar injuries and factors influencing attendance for emergency care of adolescents in the north west of England. *Endod Dent Traumatol* 2000;**16**:162–5.

265. Gassner R, Tuli T, Hachl O, Moreira R, Ulmer H. Craniomaxillofacial trauma in children: a review of 3,385 cases with 6,060 injuries in 10 years. *J Oral Maxillofac Surg* 2004;**62**:399–407.

266. Marcenes W, Murray S. Changes in prevalence and treatment need for traumatic dental injuries among 14-year-old children in Newham, London: a deprived area. *Community Dent Health* 2002;**19**:104–8.

267. Odoi R, Croucher R, Wong F, Marcenes W. The relationship between problem behaviour and traumatic dental injury amongst children aged 7–15 years old. *Community Dent Oral Epidemiol* 2002;**30**:392–6.

268. Lalloo R. Risk factors for major injuries to the face and teeth. *Dent Traumatol* 2003;**19**:12–14.

269. Nicolau B, Marcenes W, Sheiham A. Prevalence, causes and correlates of traumatic dental injuries among 13-year-olds in Brazil. *Dent Traumatol* 2001;**17**:213–17.

270. Perheentupa U, Laukkanen P, Veijola J, Joukamaa M, Jarvelin MR, Laitinen J, Oikarinen K. Increased lifetime prevalence of dental trauma is associated with previous non-dental injuries, mental distress and high alcohol consumption. *Dent Traumatol* 2001;**17**:10–16.

271. Nicolau B, Marcenes W, Sheiham A. The relationship between traumatic dental injuries and adolescents' development along the life course. *Community Dent Oral Epidemiol* 2003;**31**:306–13.

272. Laflamme L, Eilert-Petersson E. Injuries to pre-school children in a home setting: patterns and related products. *Acta Paediatr* 1988;**87**:206–11.

273. Celenk S, Sezgin B, Ayna B, Atakul F. Causes of dental fractures in the early permanent dentition: A retrospective study. *J Endo* 2002;**28**:208–10.

274. Rodd HD, Chesham DJ. Sports-related oral injury and mouthguard use among Sheffield school children. *Community Dent Health* 1997;**14**:25–30.

275. Federation Dentaire International (FDI), Commission on Dental Products, Working Party No. 7:1990.

276. Chapman PJ, Nasser BP. Prevalence of orofacial injuries and use of mouthguards in high school Rugby Union. *Aust Dent J* 1996;**41**:252–5.

277. Lang B, Pohl Y, Filippi A. Knowledge and prevention of dental trauma in team handball in Switzerland and Germany. *Dent Traumatol* 2002;**18**:329–34.

278. Meadow D, Lindner G, Needleman H. Oral trauma in children. *Pediatr Dent* 1984;**6**:248–51.

279. Lephart SM, Fu FH. Emergency of athletic injuries. *Dent Clin North Am* 1991;**35**:707–17.

280. US Department of Health and Human Services. *Understanding and improving health and objectives for improving health.* 2nd edn. Washington, DC: Healthy People, 2010, 2000.

281. US Department of Health and Human Services. *Oral health in America: a report of the surgeon general.* Rockville, MD: US National Institutes of Health, National Institute of Dental and Craniofacial Research, 2000.

282. Burt CW, Overpeck MD. Emergency visits for sports-related injuries. *Ann Emerg Med* 2001;**37**:301–8.

283. Billings RJ, Berkowitz RJ, Watson G. Teeth. *Pediatrics* 2004;**113**:*(Suppl 4)*:1120–7.

284. Nowjack-Raymer RE, Gift HC. Use of mouthguards and headgear in organized sports by school-aged children. *Public Health Rep* 1996;**111**:82–6.

285. Worrall SF. Mechanisms, pattern and treatment costs of maxillofacial injuries. *Injury* 1991;**22**:25–8.

286. Fasola AO, Lawoyin JO, Obiechina AE, Arotiba FT. Inner city maxillofacial fractures due to road traffic accidents. *Dent Traumatol* 2003;**19**:2–5.

287. Roccia F, Servadio F, Gerbino G. Maxillofacial fractures following airbag deployment. *J Cranio Maxillofac Surg* 1999;**27**:335–8.

288. Mouzakes J, Koltai PJ, Kuhar S, Bernstein DS, Wing P, Salsberg E. The impact of airbags and seat belts on the incidence and severity of maxillofacial injuries in automobile accidents in New York State. *Arch Otolaryngol Head Neck Surg* 2001;**127**:1189–93.

289. Gassner RJ, Hackl W, Tuli T, Fink C, Waldhart E. Differential profile of facial injuries among

mountainbikers compared with bicyclists. *J Trauma* 1999;**47**:50–4.

290. EILERT-PETERSSON E, SCHELP L. An epidemiological study of bicycle-related injuries. *Accid Anal Prev* 1997;**29**:363–72.

291. THOMPSON DC, RIVARA FP, THOMPSON R. Helmets for preventing head and facial injuries in bicyclists (Cochrane Review). In: *The Cochrane Library*, Issue 1, 2003. Oxford: Update Software.

292. ACTON CH, NIXON JW, CLARK RC. Bicycle riding and oral/maxillofacial trauma in young children. *Med J Aust* 1996;**165**:249–51.

293. TAPIAS MA. Prevalence of traumatic crown fractures to permanent incisors in a childhood population: Mostoles, Spain. *Dent Traumatol* 2003;**19**:119–22.

294. BOTCHWAY C, KUC I. Tongue piercing and associated tooth fracture. *J Can Dent Assoc* 1998;**64**:803–5.

295. FEHRENBACH MJ. Tongue piercing and potential oral complications. *J Dent Hyg* 1998;**72**:23–5.

296. CAMPBELL A, MOORE A, WILLIAMS E, STEPHENS J, TATAKIS DN. Tongue piercing: impact of time and barbell stem length on lingual gingival recession and tooth chipping. *J Periodontol* 2002;**73**:289–97.

297. REICHL RB, DAILEY JC. Intraoral body piercing: a case report. *Gent Dent* 1996;**44**:346–7.

298. DE MOORE RJG, DE WITTE AMJC, DE BRUYNE MAA. Tongue piercing and associated oral and dental complications. *Endod Dent Traumatol* 2000;**16**:232–7.

299. BUCK D, BAKER GA, JACOBY A, SMITH DF, CHADWICK DW. Patients' experiences of injury as a result of epilepsy. *Epilepsia* 1997;**38**:439–44.

300. OGUNBODEDE EO, ADAMOLEKUN B, AKINTOMIDE AO. Oral health and dental treatment needs in Nigerian patients with epilepsy. *Epilepsia* 1998;**39**:590–4.

301. PICK L, BAUER J. Zahnmedicin und Epilepsi. *Nervenarzt* 2001;**72**:946–9.

302. CHAPMAN PJ. Medical emergencies in dental practice and choice of emergency drugs and equipment: a survey of Australien dentists. *Aust Dental J* 1997;**42**:103–8.

303. GIRDLER NM, SMITH DG. Prevalence of emergency events in British dental practice and emergency management skills of British dentists. *Resuscitation* 1999;**41**:159–67.

304. MANN RJ, JOFFELD TA, FARMER CB. Human bites of the hand: twenty years of experience. *J Hand Surg* 1977;**2**:97–104.

305. TSOUKAS CM, HADJIS T, SHUSTER J. Lack of transmission of HIV through human bites and scratches. *J Acquired Imm Def Syn* 1988;**1**:505–7.

306. STORNELLO C. Hepatitis B virus transmitted via bite. *Lancet* 1991;**338**:1024–5.

307. O'DONNELL D. The prevalence of nonrepaired fractured incisors in visually impaired Chinese children and young adults in Hong Kong. *Quintessence Int* 1992;**23**:363–5.

308. ALSARHEED M, BEDI R, HUNT NP. Traumatised permanent teeth in 11–16-year-old Saudi Arabian children with a sensory impairment attending special schools. *Dent Traumatol* 2003;**19**:123–5.

309. HAUG RH, Foss J. Maxillofacial injuries in the pediatric patient. *Oral Surg Oral Med Oral Pathol Oral Radiol Endod* 2000;**90**:126–34.

310. MOUDEN LD, BROSS JD. Legal issues affecting dentistry's role in preventing child abuse and neglect. *J Am Dent Assoc* 1995;**126**:1173–80.

311. DA FONSECA MA, FEIGAL RJ, TEN BENSEL RW. Dental aspects of 1248 cases of child maltreatment on file at a major county hospital. *Pediatr Dent* 1992;**14**:152–7.

312. COUNCIL ON DENTAL PRACTICE. *The dentist's responsibility in identifying and reporting child abuse.* Chicago: American Dental Association, 1987.

313. MILLER CA, FINE A, ADAMS-TAYLOR S. *Monitoring children's health: key indicators.* 2nd edn. Washington DC: American Public Health Association, 1989:144–52.

314. MCDOWELL JD, KASSEBAUM DK, FRYER GE Jr. Recognizing and reporting dental violence: a survey of dental practitioners. *Spec Care Dentist* 1994;**14**:49–53.

315. RAMOS GOMEZ F, ROTHMAN D, BLAIN S. Knowledge and attitudes among California dental care providers regarding child abuse and neglect. *J Am Dent Assoc* 1998;**129**:340–8.

316. RUPP RP. Conditions to be considered in the differential diagnosis of child abuse and neglect. *Gen Dent* 1998;**46**:96–100.

317. WELBURY RR, MURPHY JM. The dental practitioner's role in protecting children from abuse. 2. The orofacial signs of abuse. *Br Dent J* 1998;**184**:61–5.

318. DIMITROULIS G, EYRE J. A 7-year review of maxillofacial trauma in a central London hospital. *Br Dent J* 1991;**170**:300–2.

319. SHEPHERD JP, SHAPLAND M, PEARCE N, SCULLY C. Pattern, severity and etiology of injuries in victims of assault. *J R Soc Med* 1990;**83**:75–8.

320. MACDONALD E, AVERY DR. *Dentistry for the child and adolescent.* 6th edn. St. Louis: Mosby, 1994.

321. SEOW WK, AMARATUNGE A, BENNET R. Dental health of aboriginal pre-school children in Brisbane, Australia. *Community Dent Oral Epidem* 1996;**24**:187–90.

322. FOLWACZNY M, HICKEL R. Oro-dental injuries during intubation anesthesia. *Anaesthesist* 1998;**47**:707–31.

323. CHADWICK RG, LINDSAY SM. Dental injuries during general anaesthesia. *Br Dent J* 1996;**180**:255–8.

324. CHADWICK RG, LINDSAY SM. Dental injuries during general anaesthesia: can the dentist help the anaesthetist? *Dent Update* 1998;**25**:76–8.

325. GERSON C, SICOT C. Dental accidents in relation to general anesthesia. Experience of mutual medical insurance group. *Ann Fr Anesth Reanim* 1997;**16**: 918–21.

326. LOCKHART PB, FELDBAU EV, GABEL RA, CONNOLY SF, SILVERSIN JB. Dental complications during and after tracheal intubation. *J Am Dent Assoc* 1986;**112**:480–3.

327. HYODO M, KURIMOTO KM. Statistical observation about the injury to the teeth caused by endotracheal intubation. *Masui* 1991;**20**:1064–7.

328. WRIGHT RB, MANFIELD FFV. Damage to teeth during the administration of general anaesthetic. *Anesth Analg* 1974;**53**:405–8.

329. BURTON JF, BAKER AB. Dental damage during anaesthesia and surgery. *Anaesth Intens Care* 1987;**15**:262–8.

330. CHEN J-J, SUSETIO L, CHAO C-C. Oral complications associated with endotracheal general anaesthesia. *Anaesth Sinica* 1990;**28**:163–9.

331. Bory E-N, Goudard V, Magnin C. Les traumatismes dentaires lors des anesthesies generales, des endoscopies orales et des sismotherapies. *Actualites Odonto-Stomatologiques* 1991;**45**:107–20.

332. Singleton RJ, Ludbrook GL, Webb RK, Fox MAL. Physical injuries and environmental safety in anaesthesia: an analysis of 2000 incident reports. *Anaesth Intens Care* 1993;**21**:659–63.

333. Skeie A, Schwartz O. Traumatic injuries of the teeth in connection with general anaesthesia and the effect of use of mouthguards. *Endod Dent Traumatol* 1999;**15**:33–6.

334. Givol N, Gershtansky Y, Halamish-Shani T, Taicher S, Perel A, Segal E. Perianesthetic dental injuries: Analysis of incident reports. *J Clin Anesth* 2004;**16**:173–6.

335. Mebius C, Soras A, Raf L. Tooth injuries in connection with intubation anesthesia: severity of the disease and dental status. *Läkartidningen* 1998;**95**:2848–9.

336. Brosnan C. Radford P. The effect of a toothguard on the difficulty of intubation. *Anaesthesia* 1997;**52**: 1011–4.

337. Lacau Saint Guily J, Boisson-Bertrand D, Monnier P. Lesions to lips, oral and nasal cavities, pharynx, larynx, trachea and esophagus due to endotracheal intubation and its alternatives. *Ann Fr Anesth Reanim* 2003;**22**:81–96.

338. Kahabuka FK, Plasschaert A, Van't Hof M. Prevalence of teeth with untreated dental trauma among nursery and primary school pupils in Dar es Salaam, Tanzania. *Dent Traumatol* 2001;**17**:109–13.

339. Hamilton FA, Hill FJ, Holloway PJ. An investigation of dento-alveolar trauma and its treatment in an adolescent population. Part 1: The prevalence and incidence of injuries and the extent and adequacy of treatment received. *Br J Dent* 1997;**182**:91–5.

340. Hamilton FA, Hill FJ, Holloway PJ. An investigation of dento-alveolar trauma and its treatment in an adolescent population. Part 2: Dentists' knowledge of management methods and their perceptions of barriers to providing care. *Br Dent J* 1997;**182**:129–33.

341. Hamdan MAM, Rajab LD. Traumatic injuries to permanent anterior teeth among 12-year-old schoolchildren in Jordan. *Community Dent Health* 2003;**20**:89–93.

342. Osuji OO. Traumatised primary teeth in Nigerian children attending University Hospital: the consequences of delays in seeking treatment. *Int Dent J* 1996;**46**:165–70.

343. Hamilton FA, Hill FJ, Mackie IC. Investigation of lay knowledge of the management of avulsed permanent incisors. *Endod Dent Traumatol* 1997;**13**:19–23.

344. Sae-Lim V, Chulaluk K, Lim LP. Patient and parental awareness of the importance of immediate management of traumatised teeth. *Endod Dent Traumatol* 1999;**15**:37–41.

345. Adekoya-Sofowora CA. Traumatized anterior teeth in children: a review of the literature. *Niger J Med* 2001;**10**:151–7.

346. Blakytny C, Surbuts A, Thomas A, Hunter L. Avulsed permanent incisors: knowledge and attitudes of primary school teachers with regard to emergency management. *Int J Paediatr Dent* 2001;**11**:327–32.

347. Sae-Lim V, Lim LP. Dental trauma management awareness of Singapore pre-school teachers. *Dent Traumatol* 2001;**17**:71–6.

348. Pacheco LF, García PF, Letra A, Menezes R, Villoria GEM, Ferreira SM. Evaluation of the knowledge of the treatment of avulsions in elementary school teachers in Rio de Janeiro, Brazil. *Dent Traumatol* 2003;**19**:76–8.

349. Chan AWK, Wong TKS, Cheung GSP. Lay knowledge of physical education teachers about the emergency management of dental trauma in Hong Kong. *Dent Traumatol* 2001;**17**:77–85.

350. Holan G, Shmueli Y. Knowledge of physicians in hospital emergency rooms in Israel on their role in cases of avulsion of permanent incisors. *Int J Paediatr Dent* 2003;**13**:13–9.

351. Andreasen JO, Andreasen FM, Skeie A, Hjørting-Hansen E, Schwartz O. Effect of treatment delay upon pulp and periodontal healing of traumatic dental injuries – a review article. *Dent Traumatol* 2002;**18**:116–128.

352. Oulis CJ, Berdouses ED. Dental injuries of permanent teeth treated in private practice in Athens. *Endod Dent Traumatol* 1996;**12**:60–5.

353. Saroglu I, Sönmez H. The prevalence of traumatic injuries treated in the pedodontic clinic of Ankara University, Turkey, during 18 months. *Dent Traumatol* 2002;**18**:299–303.

354. Rajab LD. Traumatic dental injuries in children presenting for treatment at the Department of Pediatric Dentistry, Faculty of Dentistry, University of Jordan, 1997–2000. *Dent Traumatol* 2003;**19**:6–11.

355. Jolly KA, Messer LB, Manton D. Promotion of mouthguards among amateur football players in Victoria. *Aust N Z J Public Health* 1996;**20**:630–9.

356. Kahabuka FK, Willemsen W, Van't Hof M, Burgersdijk R. The effect of a single educational input given to school teachers on patient's correct handling after dental trauma. *S Afr Dent J* 2001;**6**: 284–7.

357. Kahabuka FK, Ntabaye MK, Van't Hof MA, Plasschaert A. Effect of a consensus statement on initial treatment for traumatic dental injuries. *Dent Traumatol* 2001;**17**:159–62.

358. Fleming P, Gregg TA, Saunders ID. Analysis of an emergency dental service provided at a children's hospital. *Int J Paediatr Dent* 1991;**1**:25–30.

359. Wood GD, Herion S. Oral and maxillofacial surgery: should a district service be retained? *Arch Emerg Med* 1991;**8**:257–62.

360. Kahabuka FK, Willemsen W, Van't Hof M, Ntabaye MK, Burgersdijk R, Frankenmolen F. Initial treatment of traumatic dental injuries by dental practitioners. *Endod Dent Traumatol* 1998;**14**: 206–9.

361. Kahabuka FK, Willemsen W, Van't Hof M, Ntabaye MK, Plasschaert A, Frankenmolen F, Burgersdijk R. Oro-dental injuries and their management among children and adolescents in Tanzania. *East Afr Med J* 1999;**76**:160–2.

362. Maguire A, Murray JJ, Al-Majed I. A retrospective study of treatment provided in the primary and

secondary care services for children attending a dental hospital following complicated crown fracture in the permanent dentition. *Int J Paediatr Dent* 2000;**10**:182–90.

363. ROBERTSON A, NORÉN JG. Subjective aspects of patients with traumatized teeth. A 15-year follow-up study. *Acta Odontol Scand* 1997;**55**:142–7.

364. FLORES MT, ANDREASEN JO, BAKLAND LK, FEIGLIN B, GUTMANN JL, OIKARINEN K, PITT FORD TR, SIGURDSSON A, TROPE M, VANN WF Jr. Guidelines for the evaluation and management of traumatic dental injuries. *Dent Traumatol* 2001;**17**:1–4.

365. FLORES MT, ANDREASEN JO, BAKLAND LK, FEIGLIN B, GUTMANN JL, OIKARINEN K, PITT FORD TR, SIGURDSSON A, TROPE M, VANN WF Jr. Guidelines for the evaluation and management of traumatic dental injuries. *Dent Traumatol* 2001; **17**:49–52.

366. FLORES MT, ANDREASEN JO, BAKLAND LK, FEIGLIN B, GUTMANN JL, OIKARINEN K, PITT FORD TR, SIGURDSSON A, TROPE M, VANN WF Jr, ANDREASEN FM. Guidelines for the evaluation and management of traumatic dental injuries. *Dent Traumatol* 2001;**17**:97–102.

367. FLORES MT, ANDREASEN JO, BAKLAND LK, FEIGLIN B, GUTMANN JL, OIKARINEN K, PITT FORD TR, SIGURDSSON A, TROPE M, VANN WF Jr, ANDREASEN FM. Guidelines for the evaluation and management of traumatic dental injuries. *Dent Traumatol* 2001;**17**:193–196.

368. ANDERSSON L, AMIR F, AL-ASFOUR A. *Oral trauma guide for dentists in Kuwait.* Kuwait: Kuwait University Press, 2003.

369. GOLDSTEIN G, KICKBUSCH I. WHO Healthy Cities Programme. *Urban Health Newsl* 1996;**28**:7–13.

370. WORLD HEALTH ORGANIZATION. *Health promoting schools: a healthy setting for living, learning and working.* Geneva: WHO, 1998.

371. SHEIHAM A, WATT RG. The common risk factor approach: a rational basis for promoting oral health. *Community Dent Oral Epidemiol* 2000;**28**:399–406.

372. MOYSÉS ST, MOYSÉS SJ, WATT RG, SHEIHAM A. Associations between health promoting schools' policies and indicators of oral health in Brazil. *Health Promot Int* 2003;**18**:209–18.

373. JOSEFSSON E, LILJA KARLANDER E. Traumatic injuries to permanent teeth among Swedish School children living in a rural area. *Swed Dent J* 1994;**18**:87–94.

374. PETTI S, TARSITANI G. Traumatic injuries to anterior teeth in Italian schoolchildren: Prevalence and risk factors. *Endod Dent Traumatol* 1996;**12**:294–2.

375. SGAN-COHEN HD, JAKOBY Y, MEGNAGI G. The prevalence of dental trauma and associated variables among 10–11 yr-old Jerusalem children. *J Dent Res 796 (IADR Abstracts)*, 2000.

376. STECKSÉN-BLICKS C, HOLM AK. Dental caries, tooth trauma, malocclusion, fluoride usage, toothbrushing and dietary habits in 4-year-old Swedish children: changes between 1967 and 1992. *Int J Paediatr Dent* 1995;**5**:143–8.

377. HANSEN M, LOTHE T. Tanntraumer hos skolebarn og ungdom i alderen 7–18 år i Oslo. *Nor Tannlegeforen Tid* 1982;**92**:269–73.

378. VANDERAS AP, PAPAGIANNOULIS L. Incidence of dentofacial injuries in children: a 2-year longitudinal study. *Endod Dent Traumatol* 1999;**15**:235–8.

379. PITTS N. *Children's dental health in the United Kingdom 2003.* London: Her Majesty's Stationery Office.

380. STOKES AN, LOH T, TEO CS, BAGRAMIAN RA. Relation between incisal overjet and traumatic injury: a case control study. *Endod Dent Traumatol* 1995;**11**:2–5.

381. FABRA-CAMPOS H, DALMASES F, BUENDIA M, CIBIRIÀN R. Dynamic resistance of teeth: technical considerations and applications of an experimental device. *Endod Dent Traumatol* 1991;**7**:10–14.

382. SCHATZ D, ALFTER G, GÖZ G. Fracture resistance of human incisors and premolars: morphological and patho-anatomical factors. *Dent Traumatol* 2001;**17**:167–73.

383. GARCÍA-GODOY F, SANCHEZ R, SANCHEZ JR. Traumatic dental injuries in a sample of Dominican school children. *Community Dent Oral Epidemiol* 1981;**9**:193–7.

384. GARCÍA-GODOY F. Prevalence and distribution of traumatic injuries to the permanent teeth of Dominican children from private schools. *Community Dent Oral Epidemiol* 1984;**12**:136–9.

385. UJI T, TERAMOTO T. Occurrence of traumatic injuries in the oromaxillary region of children in a Japanese prefecture. *Endod Dent Traumatol* 1988;**4**:63–9.

# 9

# Examination and Diagnosis of Dental Injuries

F. M. Andreasen, J. O. Andreasen & M. Tsukiboshi

A dental injury should be considered an emergency and should ideally be treated immediately to relieve pain, facilitate reduction of displaced teeth and for some injuries also improve prognosis. However, minor injuries can very well be treated with some delay. This issue is further discussed in Chapter 35.

Rational therapy depends upon a correct diagnosis, which can be achieved with the help of various examination techniques. While a dental injury can often present a complex picture, most injuries can be broken down into several smaller components. Information gained from the various examination procedures will assist the clinician in defining these trauma components and determining treatment priorities (1–18, 57–65, 97–107). It must be understood that an incomplete examination can lead to inaccurate diagnosis and less successful treatment (102). Surveys of examination procedures in children have been published by Hall (108) (1986), Newton (148) (1992) and Bakland and Andreasen (147) (2004).

An adequate history is essential to the examination and should include answers to the questions listed below. In order to save time, standardized charts are recommended for acute examination and follow-ups (149) (See Appendices 1–3, pp. 876–881 and Fig. 9.1). The recorded information is of value in insurance claims and for other medico-legal considerations.

Despite the importance of a systemic approach, which begins with an adequate medical and dental history, acute bleeding or respiratory problems and replantation of avulsed teeth will change this sequence.

The *pattern of injury* observed depends primarily upon factors such as (a) the energy of impact, (b) the direction and location of impact, and (c) the resilience of the periodontal structures (see Chapter 8).

Resilience of the periodontal structures appears to be the most significant factor in determining the *extent of injury*. Thus, impact in the very resilient skeleton supporting the primary dentition usually results in tooth displacement rather than fracture of hard tissues.

The opposite is true of injuries in the permanent dentition. Thus, with impact against the ground in an adult,

either a *crown, crown-root* or *root fracture* may result, as the energy of impact will tend to produce a combination of zones of compression and tensile stress.

In the event that the lips intercept the initial blow, the energy delivered may be distributed over several teeth, resulting in *concussions, subluxations, lateral luxations* or *intrusions*.

If the course of impact is steeper and there is direct impact against the teeth, *crown fractures* can result. An indirect impact with the lips intervening may result in *extrusive luxation* with or without a *penetrating lip wound*.

In case of an axially directed impact against the chin, energy may be absorbed by the mandibular condyles or symphysis, and the premolars or molars of both dental arches. Such an impact can result in *fracture* or luxation of the mandible or *temporomandibular joint*, as well as *crown-* or *crown-root fractures* of the involved teeth. In the event of this type of impact, it should also be borne in mind that the axis of rotation of the head can be at the base of the skull. In these cases, *cerebral involvement* should also be considered. (See also under History, p. 256).

The extent of the above-mentioned injuries will naturally be altered by the relative binding strength of the teeth to their supporting structures.

In conclusion, when examining a dental trauma, consider the following features with respect to determining the pattern of injury and the subsequent extent of injury:

(1) The direction of impact (its relationship to the occlusal plane)
(2) Possible lip involvement
(3) Resilience of the periodontal structures. In this regard, the patient's history will be valuable.

## History

(1) Patient's name, age, sex, address, and telephone number
(2) When did injury occur?
(3) Where did injury occur?
(4) How did injury occur?

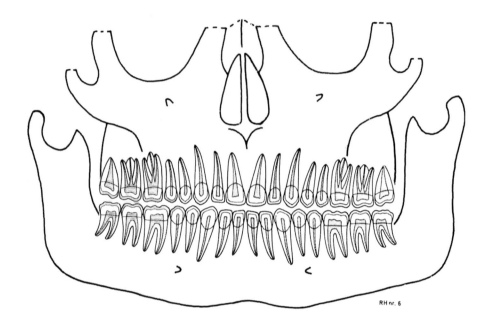

UNIVERSITY HOSPITAL
(RIGSHOSPITALET)
Copenhagen

Diagram for dental and
maxillo-facial injuries

Name:

Date:

RH nr. 6

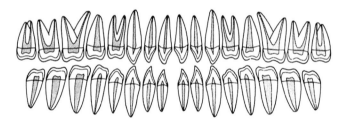

**Fig. 9.1** Diagram used for recording dental and maxillo-facial injuries.

(5) Treatment elsewhere
(6) History of previous dental injuries
(7) General health

The implications of the answers to these questions are discussed separately:

**Item 1.** Apart from the obvious necessity of such information, the ability of the patient to provide the desired information might also provide clues to possible cerebral involvement or general mental status (e.g. inebriation) (see also Item 8).

**Item 2.** The time interval between the injury and treatment significantly influences the result of replantation of avulsed teeth (see Chapter 17). Furthermore, the result of treatment of luxated teeth (20), crown fractures with and without pulp exposures (21–23), as well as bone fractures, may be influenced by delay in treatment (24, 25). This issue is, however, uncertain as a recent study has shown conflicting data (178). It is further discussed on p. 273.

**Item 3.** The place of accident may indicate a need for tetanus prophylaxis.

**Item 4.** As already indicated, the nature of the accident can yield valuable information on the type of injury to be expected, e.g. a blow to the chin will often cause fracture at the mandibular symphysis or condylar region as well as crown-root fractures in the premolar and molar regions (Fig. 9.2). Accidents in which a child has fallen with an object in its mouth, e.g. a pacifier or toy, tend to cause dislocation of teeth in a labial direction.

In young children and women presenting multiple soft tissue injuries at different stages of healing, and where there is a marked discrepancy between the clinical findings and the past history, the battered child or battered wife syndromes should be considered (see Chapter 7). In such cases the patient should be referred for a medical examination.

**Item 5.** Previous treatment, such as immobilization, reduction or replantation of teeth, should be considered before further treatment is instituted. It is also important to ascertain how the avulsed tooth was stored, e.g. tap water, sterilizing solutions, or dry.

**Item 6.** A number of patients may have sustained repeated injuries to their teeth. This can influence pulpal sensibility

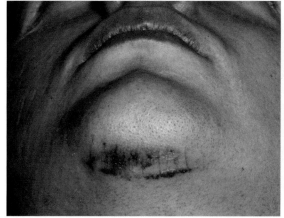 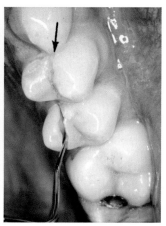

**Fig. 9.2** Induced trauma. A soft tissue bruise under the chin can imply a complicated injury pattern, often involving fractures of premolars and molars, the temporomandibular joint and symphysis, as well as risk of cerebral involvement. In this case, a blow to the chin has resulted in multiple crown-root fractures of premolars.

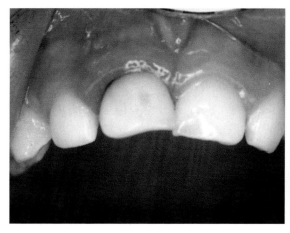 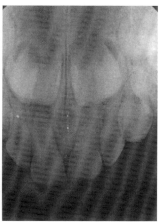

**Fig. 9.3** Previous injury, primary dentition. This 4-year-old girl has suffered subluxation of her right central incisor. At the age of 1 year there was an injury affecting both central incisors resulting in pulp necrosis of the right central incisor and pulp canal obliteration of the left incisor.

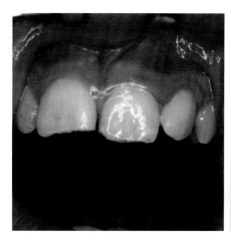 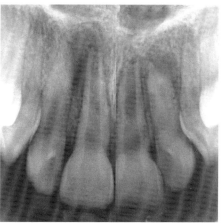

**Fig. 9.4** Previous injury, permanent dentition. The patient has just suffered enamel fractures of the incisors. However, a dental injury 4 years earlier has resulted in pulp necrosis of both central incisors and pulp canal obliteration, arrested root formation and secondary pulp necrosis of the left lateral incisor.

tests and the recuperative capacity of the pulp and/or periodontium (Figs 9.3 and 9.4).

**Item 7.** A short medical history is essential for providing information about a number of disorders such as allergic reactions, epilepsy, or bleeding disorders, such as hemophilia (66–68). These conditions can influence emergency as well as later treatment (Fig. 9.5).

The subjective complaints can provide the examiner with a clue to the injury. The following questions should be addressed:

(1) Did the trauma cause amnesia, unconsciousness, drowsiness, vomiting, or headache?
(2) Is there spontaneous pain from the teeth?
(3) Do the teeth react to thermal changes, sweet or sour foods?
(4) Are the teeth tender to touch, or during eating?
(5) Is there any disturbance in the bite?

**Item 8.** Episodes of amnesia, unconsciousness, drowsiness, vomiting or headache indicate cerebral involvement.

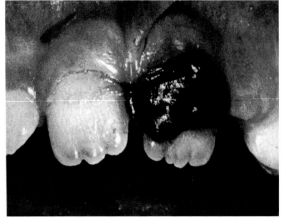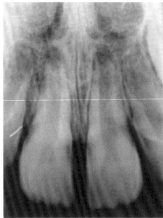

**Fig. 9.5** An 8-year-old boy with known hemophilia experiencing prolonged bleeding from the periodontal ligament around the left central incisor. The patient had suffered a subluxation injury 22 hours earlier. From BESSERMAN-NIELSEN (67) 1974.

Amnesia can be disclosed by the patient's response to questions (e.g. Item 1), repetition of questions (e.g. 'Where am I?', 'What's happened?') and inability to recall events immediately before or after the accident. In such cases, the patient should immediately be referred for medical examination to establish priorities for further treatment (109). It should be noted, however, that most acute dental treatment (e.g. radiographic examination, repositioning of displaced teeth, application of fixation) can be performed at the patient's bedside. And, as previously mentioned, early treatment will help to improve the long-term prognosis of dental injury.

Another type of trauma may occur in patients under general anesthesia who are slowly regaining consciousness. At a certain stage of recovery, strong masticatory muscle activity can take place with resultant clenching and biting which can lead to injury of the tongue, lips and teeth (108, 111).

**Item 9.** Spontaneous pain can indicate damage to the tooth-supporting structures, e.g. hyperemia or extravasation of blood into the periodontal ligament. Damage to the pulp due to crown or crown-root fractures can also give rise to spontaneous pain.

**Item 10.** Reaction to thermal or other stimuli can indicate exposed dentin or pulp. This symptom is to some degree proportional to the area of exposure.

**Items 11 and 12.** If the tooth is painful during mastication or if the occlusion is disturbed, injuries such as extrusive or lateral luxation, alveolar or jaw fractures, or crown-root fractures should be suspected.

## Clinical examination

An adequate clinical examination depends upon a thorough examination of the entire injured area and the use of special examination techniques. The use of standardized examination charts can aid data registration (see Appendices 1–3, pp. 876–881). These diagnostic procedures can be summarized as follows:

(1) Recording of extraoral wounds and palpation of the facial skeleton
(2) Recording of injuries to oral mucosa or gingiva.
(3) Examination of crowns of teeth for the presence and extent of fractures, pulp exposures, or changes in color
(4) Recording of displacement of teeth (i.e. intrusion, extrusion, lateral displacement, or avulsion)
(5) Disturbances in occlusion
(6) Abnormal mobility of teeth or alveolar fragments
(7) Palpation of the alveolar process
(8) Tenderness of teeth to percussion and change in percussion (ankylosis) tone
(9) Reaction of teeth to pulpal sensibility testing.

**Item 13.** Extraoral wounds are usually present in cases resulting from traffic accidents. The location of these wounds can indicate where and when dental injuries are to be suspected, e.g. a wound located under the chin suggests dental injuries in the premolar and molar regions and/or concomitant fracture of the mandibular condyle and/or symphysis. Palpation of the facial skeleton can disclose jaw fractures. Subcutaneous hematomas can also be an indication of fracture of the facial skeleton.

**Item 14.** Injuries of the oral mucosa or gingiva should be noted. Wounds penetrating the entire thickness of the lip can frequently be observed, often demarcated by two parallel wounds on the inner and/or outer labial surfaces (Fig. 9.6). If present, the possibility of tooth fragments buried between the lacerations should be considered (26, 27, 69–72). Such embedded fragments can cause acute or chronic infection and disfiguring fibrosis. The probable mechanism for these injuries is that the tooth, having penetrated the full thickness of the lip, is fractured as it emerges from the skin and strikes a hard object. The tooth fragment is retained within the soft tissue, which then envelops it at the moment of impact (26). These fragments can seldom be palpated, irrespective of size. Careful radiographic examination of the involved soft tissues is therefore necessary to disclose these fragments (Fig. 9.6). Along with tooth fragments, other foreign bodies can often be found within the soft tissue.

**Fig. 9.6** Penetrating lip lesion. Two parallel lesions, either in the mucosa and skin or mucosa only, are an indication that teeth have penetrated tissue and that tooth fragments and other foreign bodies can be expected deep within the wound. A radiographic film is placed between the lips and the dental arch. The exposure time is 25% of the normal for a dental exposure.

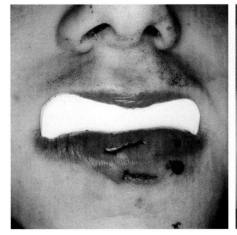
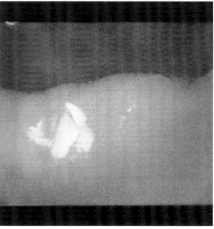

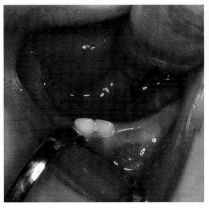
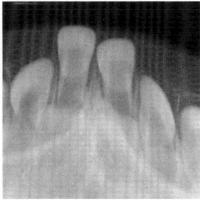
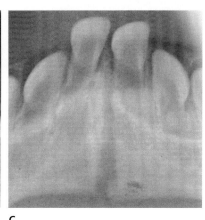

A                              B                              C

**Fig. 9.7** A 10-month-old child referred for a luxated left primary central incisor. The clinical examination revealed slight loosening of the incisor and a sublingual hematoma (arrow). B. Radiographic examination of the involved incisors revealed no sign of jaw fracture. C. Because of the finding of a sublingual hematoma, a new radiograph including the border of the mandible was taken. This radiograph clearly demonstrated fracture of the symphysis.

Gingival lacerations are often associated with displaced teeth. Bleeding from non-lacerated marginal gingiva indicates damage to the periodontal ligament.

Submucosal hematomas sublingually, in the vestibular region or in the palate can be indicative of a jaw fracture. Thorough radiographic examination, including examination of the border of the mandible and mobility of jaw segments *en bloc*, must accompany this finding, as a jaw fracture could otherwise be overlooked (Fig. 9.7).

Finally, it is essential that blood covering the alveolar process be removed, as this can sometimes reveal displacement of the mucoperiosteum into the buccal sulcus. Typically these patients demonstrate severe edema of the upper lip and sharp pain upon palpation of the exposed periosteal surface (108).

**Item 15.** Before examining traumatized teeth, the crowns should be cleaned of blood and debris.

Infraction lines in the enamel can be visualized by directing a light beam parallel to the long axis of the tooth or by shadowing the light beam with a finger or mouth mirror (see Chapter 10, p. 280). When examining crown fractures, it is important to note whether the fracture is confined to enamel or includes dentin. The fracture surface should be

carefully examined for pulp exposures; if present, the size and location should be recorded. In some cases, the dentin layer may be so thin that the outline of the pulp can be seen as a pinkish tinge beneath dentin. One should take care not to perforate the thin dentinal layer during the examination.

Crown-root fractures in the molar and premolar regions should be expected in the case of indirect trauma (see Chapter 11, p. 314). It is important to remember that crown-root fractures in one quadrant are very often accompanied by similar fractures on the same side of the opposing jaw. It is therefore necessary to examine occlusal fissures of all molars and premolars to confirm the presence or absence of possible fractures.

Depending on the stage of eruption, fractures below the gingival margin can involve the crown alone or the cervical third of the root.

Color of the traumatized tooth should be noted, as changes can occur in the post-injury period. These color changes are most often prominent on the oral aspect of the crown at the cingulum. Moreover, examination with transillumination can reveal changes in translucency (see Chapter 13, p. 380).

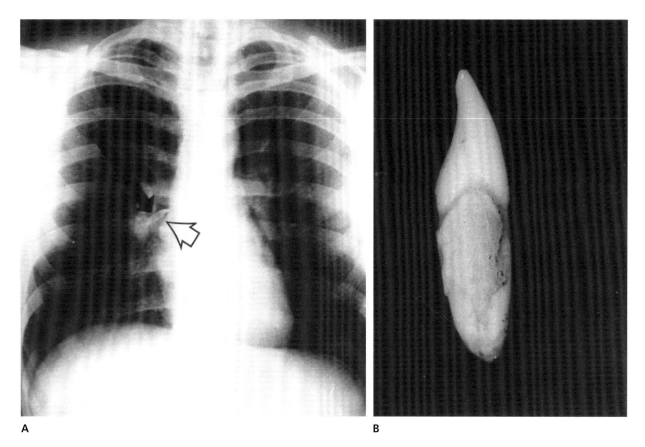

**Fig. 9.8** A. Posteroanterior radiograph of chest showing foreign body in right middle lobe intermediate bronchus after maxillofacial injury. B. Tooth recovered from right lung via bronchoscopy. From GILLILAND et al. (76) 1972.

**Item 16.** Displacement of teeth is usually evident by visual examination; however, minor abnormalities can often be difficult to detect. In such cases, it is helpful to examine the occlusion as well as radiographs taken at various angulations (see p. 267).

The possibility of inhaling or swallowing teeth at the time of injury should always be considered when teeth or prosthetic appliances are missing and their presence elsewhere cannot be established (73–76).

Although inhalation of foreign bodies in connection with traumatic injuries is normally associated with a loss of protective reflexes in an unconscious patient, it may also occur in a conscious patient without producing symptoms (76). Consequently, if there is reason to suspect inhalation or swallowing of a tooth or dental appliance, it is important that radiographs of the chest and the abdomen be taken as soon as possible (Fig. 9.8).

In case of tooth luxation, the direction of the dislocation as well as extent (in mm) should be recorded. In the primary dentition, it is of utmost importance to diagnose oral dislocation of the apex of a displaced primary tooth, as it can impinge upon the permanent successor.

It is important to remember that, apart from displacement and interference with occlusion, laterally luxated and intruded teeth present very few clinical symptoms. Moreover, these teeth are normally firmly locked in their displaced position and do not usually demonstrate tenderness to percussion. While radiographs can be of assistance, diagnosis is confirmed by the percussion tone (see Chapter 13, p. 372).

**Item 17.** Abnormalities in occlusion can indicate fractures of the jaw or alveolar process. In the former case, abnormal mobility of the jaw fragments can be demonstrated.

**Item 18.** All teeth should be tested for abnormal mobility, both horizontally and axially. Disruption of the vascular supply to the pulp should be expected in case of axial mobility.

It should be remembered that erupting teeth and primary teeth undergoing physiologic root resorption always exhibit some mobility.

The typical sign of alveolar fracture is movement of adjacent teeth when the mobility of a single tooth is tested.

In case of root fracture, location of the fracture determines the degree of tooth mobility. However, without radiographic examination, it is usually not possible to discriminate between luxation injuries and root fractures.

**Item 19.** Uneven contours of the alveolar process usually indicate a bony fracture. Moreover, the direction of the dislocation can sometimes be determined by palpation.

**Item 20.** Reaction to percussion is indicative of damage to the periodontal ligament (77). The test may be performed by tapping the tooth lightly with the handle of a mouth mirror, in a vertical as well as horizontal direction. Injuries to the periodontal ligament will usually result in pain. As with all examination techniques used at the time of injury, the percussion test should be begun on a non-injured tooth to assure a reliable patient response. In smaller children, the use of a fingertip can be a gentler diagnostic tool. In infants, this is neither possible nor reliable.

The sound elicited by percussion is also of diagnostic value. Thus, a hard, metallic ring elicited by percussion in a horizontal direction indicates that the tooth is locked into bone; while a dull sound indicates subluxation or extrusive luxation. However, it should be noted that teeth with apical and marginal periodontal lesions can also give a dull percussion sound (77). Dental trauma has also been found to be associated with increased touch thresholds in permanent teeth with recovery towards healthy control values after 3–12 months (150).

A calibrated percussion instrument has been introduced, Periotest®, which is an electronic device that measures the dampening (shock absorbing) characteristics of the periodontium (112, 113, 151, 152, 177). However, the force imparted by such an instrument might contribute a new trauma, possibly leading to damage to the neurovascular supply of the pulp. In the follow-up period, however, this instrument could be of value in the diagnosis of post-traumatic sequelae, such as ankylosis (153).

## Sensitivity and specificity

A dental trauma implies a number of examination procedures, whose purpose is to determine the extent of injury and the status of healing processes or healing complications in the follow-up period. Each of these procedures has a certain *sensitivity* (i.e. the capacity to diagnose healing complications (e.g. pulp necrosis). Thus, a sensitivity value of 1.0 implies 100% effectiveness that all cases with pathologic change (e.g. pulp necrosis) were identified. *Specificity* is the capacity to diagnose correctly a healthy status (e.g. healthy pulp). A specificity value of 1.0 implies 100% effectiveness in that regard. An ideal testing method should, therefore, have 100% sensitivity (i.e. no false pathologic changes) and 100% specificity (i.e. no false healthy cases), a utopian situation which presently does not exist (154). This concept will be applied in the description of the various examination procedures.

In selecting examination procedures, it is important to consider the consequences of the value of specificity. If a method is chosen which favors high *sensitivity*, this will imply that a certain number of teeth with vital or healing pulps will be subjected to endodontic treatment if *precision* is not reasonably high at the same time.

If all attention is paid to the *precision* (i.e. avoiding endodontic treatment of vital or healing teeth), a certain number of teeth with pulp necrosis will not be detected or treated. In case of pulp-related root resorption, this is an unfortunate situation; so in this situation, a high *specificity* of a test procedure should be used (see later).

**Item 21.** Pulp testing following traumatic injuries is a controversial issue. These procedures require cooperation and a relaxed patient, in order to avoid false reactions. However, this is often not possible during initial treatment of injured patients, especially children.

Pulpal sensibility testing at the time of injury is important for establishing a point of reference for evaluating pulpal status at later follow-up examinations. A number of tests have been proposed. However, the value of these has recently been questioned (28–30, 114, 116). The principle of these tests involves transmitting stimuli to the sensory receptors of the dental pulp and registering the reaction; while others register the vascular component in the pulp canal.

## Pulp testing principles

In the evaluation of various pulp testing procedures, it should be considered that most procedures (e.g. thermal tests, electronic pulp testing (EPT)) assess the nerve supply to the pulp (which is naturally dependent upon an intact vascular supply); whereas laser Doppler flowmetry (LDF) assesses the presence of a functioning vascular supply.

A disturbing fact then comes to mind, that neural regeneration in a traumatized pulp is slower than vascular regeneration and sometimes is even lacking (159–162). Thus, a priori vascular detecting systems (e.g. LDF) are more sensitive than EPT and thermal testing devices, which are specifically related to nerve regeneration.

In a recent, very detailed study on the sensitivity and specificity of various pulp testing methods, LDF was compared to other pulp testing methods in vital teeth and teeth with known pulp necrosis. LDF was found to be far better than EPT and ethyl chloride (i.e. higher sensitivity and specificity) (154) (Fig. 9.9).

## Mechanical stimulation

In crown fractures with exposed dentin, pulpal sensibility can be tested by scraping with a dental probe. Some authors have proposed drilling a test cavity in the tooth in order to register the pain reaction when the bur advances into the dentin. However, in a study on sensibility reactions of replanted teeth, it was found that a pain reaction was not noted until the dentin-pulp border was reached (31).

In the case of crown fractures with exposed pulp tissue, the reaction of the pulp to mechanical stimuli can be tested by applying a cotton pellet soaked in saline. Exploration with a dental probe must not be attempted as it may provoke severe pain and inflict additional injury to the pulp.

## Thermal tests

Thermal stimulation of teeth has been used for many years and various methods have been advocated. Among these, the most frequently used are heated gutta-percha, ethyl chloride, ice, carbon dioxide snow, and dichlor-difluormethane.

Thermal pulp testing results are not reproducible in terms of graded intensity, and normal pulp tissue may yield a negative response (29, 79). A positive reaction usually indicates a vital pulp, but it may also occur in a non-vital pulp, especially in cases of gangrene when heat produces thermal expansion of fluids in the pulp space, which in turn presumably exerts pressure on inflamed periodontal tissues (38).

**HOW FREQUENTLY WILL HISTORY, CLINICAL OR RADIOGRAPHIC FINDINGS OR A DIAGNOSTIC TEST REVEAL TRUE PULP NECROSIS (SENSITIVITY)**

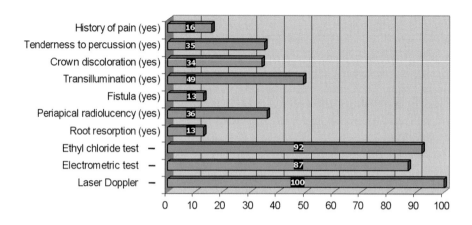

**HOW FREQUENTLY WILL HISTORY, CLINICAL OR RADIOGRAPHIC FINDINGS OR A DIAGNOSTIC TEST REVEAL TRUE PULP VITALITY (SPECIFICITY)**

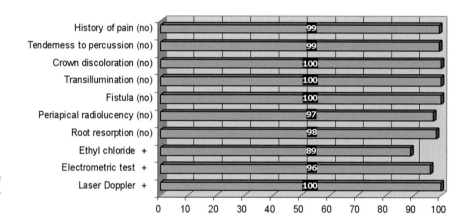

**Fig. 9.9** Sensitivity and specificity of various pulp testing procedures. After EVANS et al. (154) 1999.

## Heated gutta-percha

The following standardization has been advocated by Mumford (29). A stick of gutta-percha is heated by holding about 5 mm of its length in a flame for 2 seconds, whereupon it is applied to the tooth on the middle third of the facial surface (Fig. 9.10). The value of this test has been questioned, as the intensity of sensation reported by the patient is not reproducible, and even non-injured teeth may fail to respond (29, 79). The sensitivity of this test has been found to be 0.86 and specificity to be 0.41 (155).

## Ice

This method involves the application of a cone of ice to the facial surface of the tooth (Fig. 9.11). Reaction depends on the duration of application; a period of 5 to 8 seconds increases the sensitivity of this test (33). The reliability of this procedure has also been questioned as non-injured teeth may not respond (32, 33, 78).

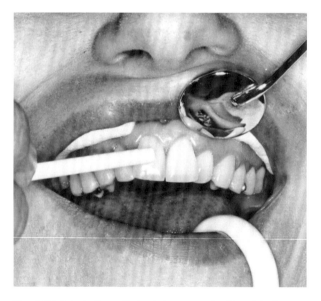

**Fig. 9.10** Pulp testing with heated gutta-percha. The stick of gutta-percha is applied to the middle third of the facial surface.

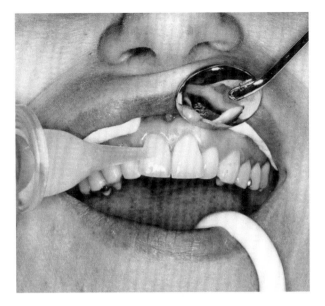

**Fig. 9.11** Pulp testing with ice. A cone of ice is applied to the middle third of the facial surface of the tooth: 5 to 8 seconds may be required to elicit a reaction.

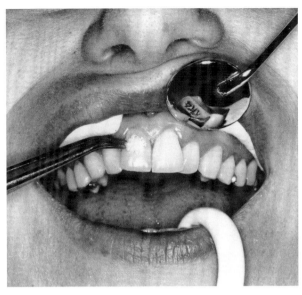

**Fig. 9.12** Pulp testing with ethyl chloride. A pledget of cotton is saturated with ethyl chloride and applied to the middle third of the facial surface.

**Fig. 9.13** Pulp testing with carbon dioxide snow. A. Pulp testing with carbon dioxide snow of a fractured incisor covered with a stainless steel crown. B. Disassembled model of a carbon dioxide snow pulp tester (Odontotest®, Fricar A. G., Zürich 1, Switzerland).

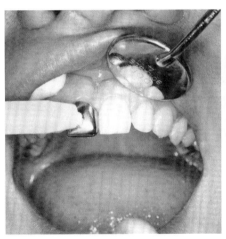

**A**

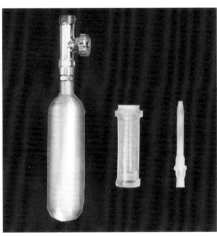

**B**

### Ethyl chloride

Ethyl chloride can be applied by soaking a cotton pledget and then placing it on the facial surface of the tooth to be tested (Fig. 9.12) (CAUTION! flammable). The limitations described for heated gutta-percha also apply to this method, although ethyl chloride gives more consistent results (29, 80, 81). The sensitivity for this test has been found to be 0.83 and specificity 0.93 (116).

### Carbon dioxide snow

Because of its low temperature (−78°C, −108°F), carbon dioxide snow gives very consistent and reliable results, even in immature teeth (34–37, 78, 79, 82, 83) (Fig. 9.13). This method also allows pulp testing in cases where an injured tooth is completely covered with a temporary crown or splint (32, 82) (Fig. 9.11). However, a serious drawback to

this procedure is that the very low temperature of the carbon dioxide snow can result in new infraction lines in the enamel (84, 85) (Fig. 9.14), although this finding has not been substantiated in later studies (116, 118). Furthermore, no changes could be found in the pulp in animal experiments (119). Only prolonged exposure to very low temperatures (i.e. −80°C for 1 to 3 minutes) has been shown to elicit transient pulpal changes (secondary dentin formation) (120).

### Dichlor-difluormethane

This is another cold test (e.g., Frigen®, Provotest®) in which an aerosol is released at a temperature of −28°C (−18°F) onto the enamel surface (85–87, 109). Like carbon dioxide snow, it elicits a very reliable and consistent response from both mature and immature teeth (88). However, the same drawback has been recorded with this test as with carbon

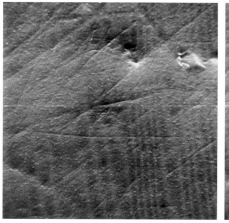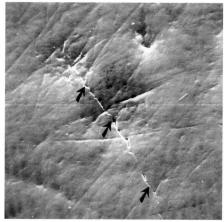

**Fig. 9.14** Scanning electron microscope view of the enamel surface before (A) and after (B) pulp testing with carbon dioxide snow. It is apparent that an infraction line has developed after testing (arrows). ×1200. From BACHMANN & LUTZ (85) 1976.

**A**                                    **B**

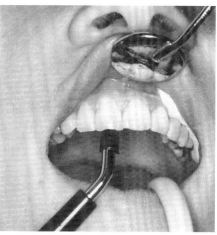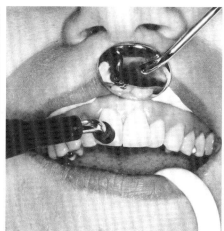

**Fig. 9.15** Electrometric pulp testing. The tooth is air-dried and isolated with cotton rolls. The electrode is placed on the incisal edge or on the incisal third of the facial surface of the crown.

dioxide snow, although to a lesser degree; namely, infraction lines in the enamel caused by the thermal shock (85).

## Electric pulp testing (EPT)

### Electric pulp testers

Electric pulp testing should employ a current measurement instrument that allows control of the mode, duration, frequency, and direction of the stimulus (38, 121). Voltage measurement is not satisfactory because a given voltage produces varying currents as a result of differences in the electrical resistance of the tissues, especially enamel. Such variations can result from fissures, caries, and restorations (39). Experimental studies have shown that the current is presumably carried ionically through the electrolytes of the tooth (40, 41). Moreover, immediate changes in the vascular flow after a luxation injury are reflected in loss of EPT response, which with time can return to normal (163).

The stimulus should be clearly defined, as it significantly affects nerve excitation (42). Furthermore, the electrode area should be as large as the tooth shape will permit, allowing maximum stimulation (39, 43, 122). Stimulus duration of 10 milliseconds or more has been advocated (43). Recently, a digital pulp tester has been introduced which appears to produce very reliable readings (123).

Electrical sensibility testing is usually carried out in the following way (Fig. 9.15).

(1)  The patient is informed as to the purpose and nature of the test and is instructed to indicate when a sensation is first experienced.

(2)  The tooth surface is isolated with cotton rolls and air-dried. Saliva on the tooth surface can divert the current to the gingiva and periodontal tissue, giving false readings. However, the tooth should not be desiccated for long periods, as enamel can lose moisture with a resultant increase in electrical resistance (44, 45). Several media such as saline and toothpaste can be used as conductor between electrode and tooth surface (146).

(3)  The electrode is placed as far from the gingiva as possible, preferably on a fracture area or the incisal edge, where the strongest response can be obtained (124, 125). The neutral electrode can be held by the patient. A modification of this system involves the examiner completing the circuit by touching the patient's mouth with a finger or a mouth mirror. A metal dental instrument (e.g. dental explorer) can also serve as an electric conductor to the tooth (126). The use of rubber gloves presents a clinical problem, as the correct use of the pulp tester requires that the dentist completes the electrical circuit by direct physical contact with the patient. One

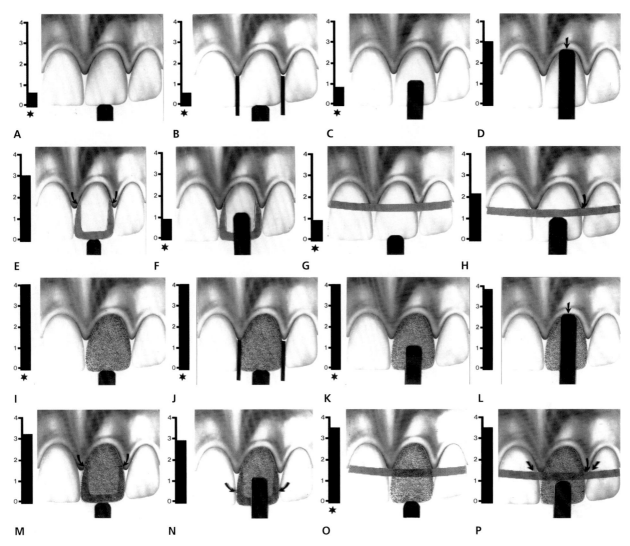

**Fig. 9.16** Influence of splints and temporary crowns upon electric pulp testing procedures. The schematic drawings illustrate the reactions recorded with a Siemens pulp tester (Sirotest II®) which has a scale from 0 to 4. The columns next to the drawing of the teeth indicate the average reaction to the specific testing circumstances. A to H illustrate testing of a vital tooth and I to P illustrate testing of a tooth with pulp necrosis. A. Electrode placed upon the incisal edge. B. Tooth isolated with an acetate strip. C. Electrode placed upon the middle third of the labial surface. D. Electrode contacting gingiva. E. Electrode contacting an open faced steel crown. F. Electrode placed upon enamel on a tooth with an open faced steel crown. G. Electrode placed upon the incisal edge of a tooth splinted with a metal arch bar. H. Electrode placed upon the metal arch bar. I. Electrode placed upon the incisal edge of a tooth with pulp necrosis. J. Tooth isolated with acetate strips. K. Electrode placed upon the middle third of the labial surface. L. Electrode contacting gingiva. M. Electrode contacting an open faced steel crown. The current is passed on to the gingiva, giving a weak response. N. Electrode placed upon enamel on a tooth with an open-faced steel crown. The current is passed on to the adjacent teeth. O. Electrode placed upon the incisal edge of a tooth splinted with a metal arch bar. Current is passed on to neighboring vital teeth. P. Electrode placed upon the metal arch bar. The current is passed on to neighboring vital teeth. NOTE: all testing situations revealing a reliable response are indicated with an asterisk. From FULLING & ANDREASEN (79) 1976.

study has indicated that this problem can be overcome if the patient grasps the end of the pulp tester after it is positioned on the tooth (128); however, other studies suggest that such a procedure can produce unreliable results (129, 130). Recently, a clip to the lip has been developed which permits the dentist to conduct a test wearing rubber gloves (131).

(4) The rheostat of the tester is advanced continuously until the patient reacts. If the current is then maintained at the existing level, adaptation occurs and the patient feels that the pain has disappeared, so that a further increase of current gives a higher threshold value. This phenomenon implies that the pain threshold cannot be regarded as constant (43). The threshold value should therefore be determined by a quick rather than a slow increase in current. However, the current should not be increased so quickly that it is painful. The value of the pain threshold of the tooth should be recorded for later comparison.

(5) Splints and temporary crowns used in the treatment of traumatic dental injuries can alter the response to both thermal and electrometrical tests (79). Thus, contact between the gingiva and a stainless steel crown, a metal cap splint or arch bar significantly increases the pain threshold, as the current bypasses the tooth and is conducted to the gingiva or adjacent teeth (79). In order to obtain a reliable sensibility response to electrometric pulp testing, the electrode must be placed upon enamel and the tooth isolated from adjacent vital teeth

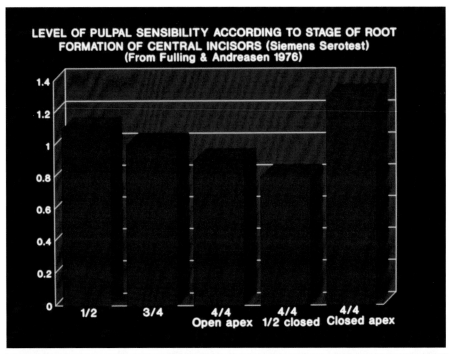

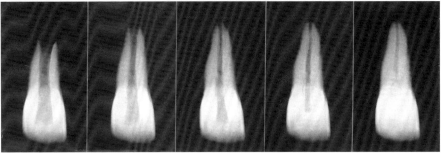

**Fig. 9.17** Variation in sensibility level according to stage of root development of permanent incisors. The diagram illustrates the reactions recorded with a Siemens pulp tester (Sirotest 77® which has a scale from 0 to 4). It appears that early and late stages of root development are related to higher sensibility levels. From FULLING & ANDREASEN (78) 1976.

(Fig. 9.16). A distance of at least 1 millimeter between the electrode and metal is recommended. If the temporary crown or splint cannot be altered in the above-mentioned manner, thermal pulp testing with carbon dioxide snow is a reliable alternative (79) (Fig. 9.16).

The value and reliability of electrometric pulp testing have been evaluated by comparison of the pain threshold with the histologic condition of the pulp (30, 46, 89–92). Apparently, there is not always a direct relationship; thus teeth which fail to respond to stimulation with maximum current can show a histologically normal pulp, while inflamed or even necrotic pulps can respond electrometrically within the normal range. A common belief has been that low readings indicate hyperemia or acute pulpitis while high readings indicate chronic pulpitis or degenerative changes. However, recent investigations do not support this view (30, 47).

The interpretation of pulpal sensibility tests performed immediately after traumatic injuries is complicated by the fact that sensitivity responses can be temporarily or permanently decreased, especially after luxation injuries (132–135). However, repeated testing has shown that normal reactions can return after a few weeks or months (1, 32, 48–51, 81, 93, 133–135). Moreover, teeth which have

been loosened can elicit pain responses merely from pressure of the pulp testing instrument. It is therefore important to reposition and immobilize, e.g. root-fractured or extruded incisors prior to pulp testing. If local anesthetics are to be administered for various treatment procedures, pulp testing should be performed prior to doing this.

Another factor to consider is the stage of eruption. Teeth react differently at various stages, sometimes showing no reaction at all when root formation is not complete (52–54, 78, 94, 95). However, the excitation threshold is gradually lowered to the normal range as maturation proceeds, although it increases again in adulthood when the pulp canal becomes partly obliterated (78, 136, 137) (Fig. 9.17). One explanation could be incomplete communication between odontoblastic processes and nerve fibers in immature teeth (55). However, this has been questioned in a recent study where numerous myelinated nerve fibers were found in the coronal odontoblast layer irrespective of stage of development (138). Moreover, it is often difficult to isolate partially erupted teeth and the current may circumvent the tooth, passing directly to the gingiva (56).

Finally, teeth undergoing orthodontic movement display higher excitation thresholds (96).

The sensitivity of EPT has been found in the range of 0.72 and specificity 0.93 (154–158).

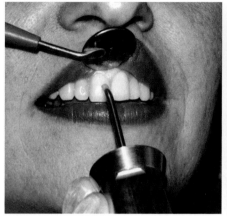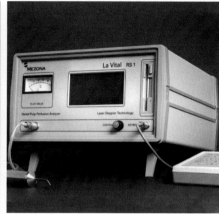

**Fig. 9.18** Pulp testing using a laser Doppler flowmeter. The probe is placed on the labial surface of the tooth.

## Laser Doppler flowmetry (LDF)

A method has been developed whereby a laser beam can be directed at the coronal aspect of the pulp. The reflected light scattered by moving blood cells undergoes a Doppler frequency shift. The fraction of light scattered back from the pulp is detected and processed to yield a signal (Fig. 9.18). The value of this method has been demonstrated in several clinical studies where it was possible to diagnose the state of pulp revascularization approximately 3–4 months before EPT (Figs 9.19 and 9.20). (139, 140, 154, 164–171) The design of the probes (169, 170), wave length, band width and laser power have been found to influence the sensitivity and specificity of LDF (172–174). Furthermore, it has been found that the optimal position of the probe should be 2–3 mm from the facial gingiva (173).

### Improved diagnosis of pulp necrosis by the use of LDF compared to other methods

An experimental study has demonstrated the superiority of this procedure in evaluation of the revascularization process in replanted dog incisors (166). In a clinical study it was found that in traumatized incisors which showed no electrometric sensibility reactions and where laser Doppler flowmetry (LDF) indicated no pulp vitality the *sensitivity* of LDF was 97%. Conversely in electrometric non-sensible teeth, where LDF showed the presence of blood perfusion, the *specificity* of LDF in regard to pulp vitality was 100% (164, 165).

In several clinical studies, it has been found that LDF was able to advance detection of the revascularization process of a damaged pulp due to a luxation injury compared to other examination procedures (e.g. $CO_2$ and EPT), i.e. from 6 months to 3 months after injury (139, 140, 164–166, 168). In a recent and very comprehensive study, the sensitivity and specificity of LDF was tested in 80 patients with luxated maxillary incisors. In this study, the control teeth demonstrated pulpal blood flow values (PBF) of 9.9 at the time of injury. The final status 6 months after trauma showed that the cases which at that time could be classified as having obvious signs of pulp necrosis (Type 4, loss of sensitivity and periapical radiolucency; and Type 5, loss of sensitivity,

periapical radiolucency and grey discoloration) had the maximum predictive values (high sensitivity (70%) and specificity (93%)) if a PBU value of 2.9 at the time of splint removal was chosen to separate pulps which would become revascularized and those which would become necrotic (175, 176).

However, several problems must be solved before this method can be of general use. First it has been found that blood pigment within a discolored tooth crown can interfere with laser light transmission (145). Second, the equipment necessary for this procedure needs further refinement before it can be of general clinical value. Thus, the time required to test a single tooth must be reduced significantly (presently, 10–15 min). Third, the price of the equipment must be considerable lower than it is at present.

## Radiographic examination

All injured teeth should be examined radiographically. This examination serves two purposes: it reveals the stage of root formation and it discloses injuries affecting the root portion of the tooth and the periodontal structures. Most root fractures are disclosed by radiographic examination, as the fracture line usually runs parallel to the central beam (102, 141) (see Chapter 12, p. 339).

The clinical diagnosis of tooth displacement is corroborated radiographically. There is a widening of the periodontal space in lateral and extrusive luxations, whereas intruded teeth often demonstrate a blurred periodontal space. However, determination of dislocation on the basis of radiographs is highly dependent on the angle of the central beam (20, 102). Radiographic demonstration of dislocation of permanent teeth normally requires the use of more than one exposure at differing angulations. The ideal method is the use of 3 different angulations for each traumatized tooth, using a standardized projection technique (102). Thus, a traumatized anterior region is covered by one occlusal film and 3 periapical exposures, where the central beam is directed between the lateral and central incisors and the two central incisors. This procedure ensures diagnosis of even minor dislocations or root fractures (Fig. 9.21). In this

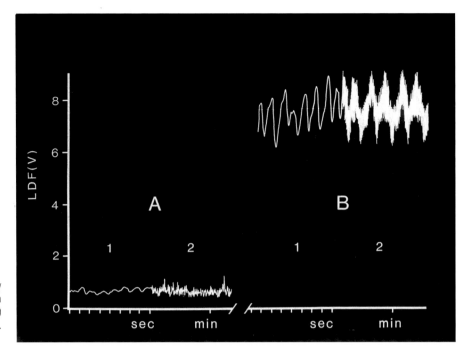

**Fig. 9.19** Laser Doppler flowmetry (LDF) recording from a non-vital tooth (A) and adjacent normal (control) tooth (B). Chart speed 600 mm/min. From GAZELIUS et al. (139) 1986.

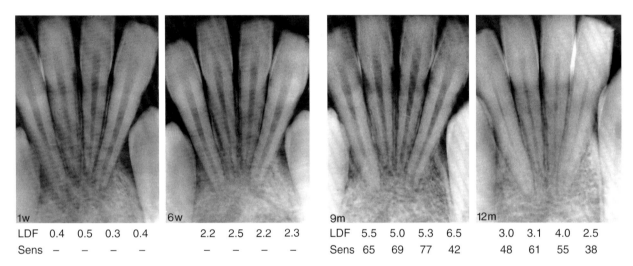

| | | | | | | | | | | | | |
|---|---|---|---|---|---|---|---|---|---|---|---|---|
| **1w** | | | | **6w** | | | | **9m** | | | | **12m** |
| LDF | 0.4 | 0.5 | 0.3 | 0.4 | 2.2 | 2.5 | 2.2 | 2.3 | LDF | 5.5 | 5.0 | 5.3 | 6.5 | 3.0 | 3.1 | 4.0 | 2.5 |
| Sens | – | – | – | – | – | – | – | – | Sens | 65 | 69 | 77 | 42 | 48 | 61 | 55 | 38 |

**Fig. 9.20** Comparison of LDF and EPT. Follow-up of 4 luxated incisors at 1 and 6 weeks, 9 and 12 months. LDF represents laser Doppler flow values and electrometric settings (EPT) (Analytic Technology® pulp tester) at which sensory responses were obtained in each tooth. Indicates absence of sensory response at highest stimulus level. From GAZELIUS et al. (139) 1986.

context, it is important to bear in mind that a steep occlusal exposure is of special value in the diagnosis of root fractures and lateral luxations with oral displacement of the crown (102, 141) (see Chapter 12, p. 338 and Chapter 14).

Children under 2 years of age are often difficult to examine radiographically because of fear or lack of cooperation. With the parents' help and the use of film holders, it is usually possible to obtain a radiograph of the traumatized area. (Fig. 9.22) It should also be noted that exposure time can be reduced by 30% for each 10 KVP increase (Fig. 9.23). In this way, radiographs of diagnostic quality can be taken even with uncooperative patients.

Extraoral radiographs are of value in determining the direction of dislocation of intruded primary incisors (Fig. 9.24 and Chapter 19, p. 523). Bone fractures are usually dis-

cernible on intraoral radiographs unless the fracture is confined to the facial or lingual bone plate.

Dislocated tooth fragments within a lip laceration can be demonstrated radiographically by the use of an ordinary film placed between the dental arches and the lips. A short exposure time (i.e. one-quarter to one-half normal exposure time) or the use of low kilovoltage is advocated for these exposures. At follow-up it is essential that radiogrphic controls are taken at times when the chance of detecting pathology is optimal (see Appendix 3, p. 881).

### Panoramic technique

This procedure is always indicated in cases where a jaw fracture is suspected or a TM-J problem is found. Sensitivity and

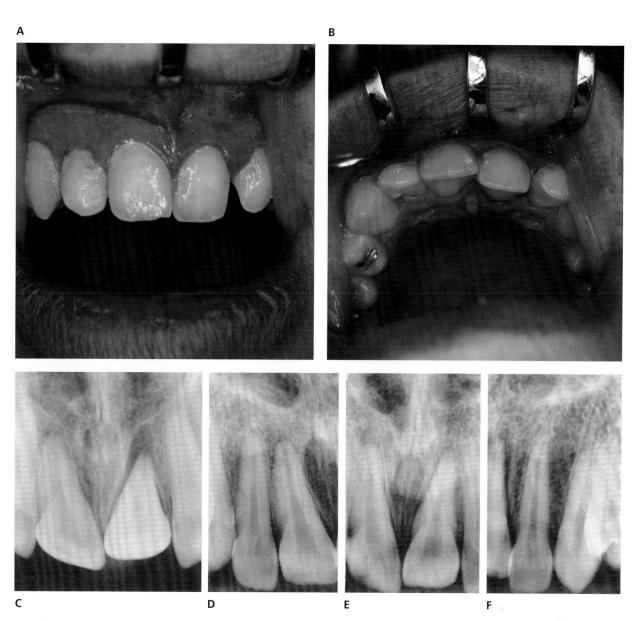

**Fig. 9.21** Radiographic intraoral exposures in suspected luxation injuries in the anterior region. A and B. Clinical examination reveals displacement of a left central incisor. C. to F. The radiographic examination of the anterior region consists of one occlusal film (C) and three periapical exposures, where the central beam is directed between the lateral and central incisors (D) and (F) and between the central incisors (E). Note that the displacement of the left central incisor is clearly shown on the occlusal exposure (C), whereas an apical exposure (E) shows hardly any displacement.

**Fig. 9.22** Radiographic examination of infants. A special film holder is used in combination with a standard dental film (3.8 × 5.1 cm) (Twix film holder®, AIB Svenska Dental Instrument, Stockholm, Sweden). The film holder is held between two fingers and the film placed between the dental arches. The mother holds the infant in position with her left arm while steadying the child's head with her right hand. The projection angle should be more vertical than normal in order not to have the index finger projected onto the film. Note that both mother and child are protected by lead aprons.

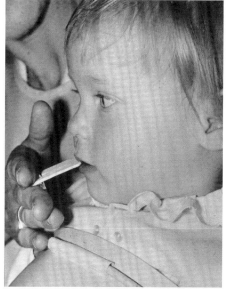
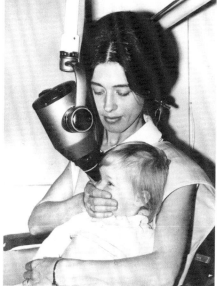

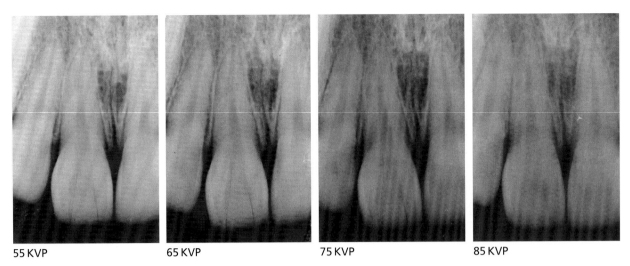

| 55 KVP | 65 KVP | 75 KVP | 85 KVP |

**Fig. 9.23** An increase in KVP slightly reduces the contrast. The right central incisor in a skull was radiographed using ranges from 55–85 KVP. The infraction line in the crown which is clearly shown at 55 KVP is not so prominent at 85 KVP.

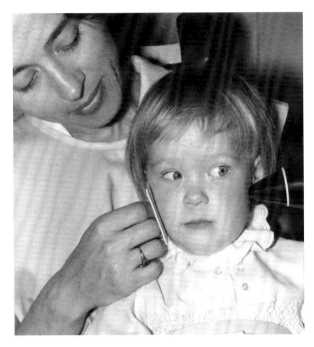

**Fig. 9.24** Extraoral lateral projection used to determine the position of displaced anterior teeth. The central beam is directed against the apical area and is parallel to the occlusal plane. A 6 × 7.5 cm film is held against the cheek perpendicular to the central beam.

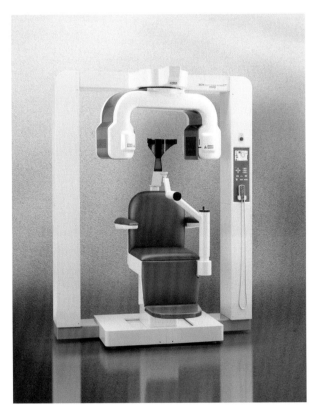

**Fig. 9.25** Micro CT scanning equipment (J. Morita Mfg. Corp.).

specificity values of this technique have not been studied in relation to dental trauma.

### Conventional computed tomograph (CT) scanning

This is a very useful method in the diagnosis of maxillofacial injuries, especially in cases of LeFort 1, 2 and 3 fractures. However, the resolution is not optimal and radiation exposure too high to make it useful for dental trauma diagnosis. Recently, a micro CT scanning technique has been introduced.

### Micro CT scanning

Conventional dental and panorama images have limited diagnostic ability due to their two-dimensional character. Recently, a micro CT scanner has been developed and the clinical efficacy has been evaluated in a variety of clinical situations (180–185) (Fig. 9.25).

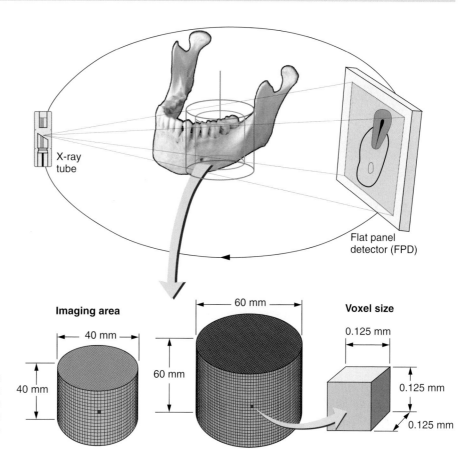

**Fig. 9.26** Exposure principle for the 3DX Multi Image Micro CT (J. Morita Mfg. Corp.). The smaller voxel size makes it possible to create an 8 times clearer 3-dimensional image than conventional medical CT.

Micro CT (3DX: J. Morita Mfg. Corp.) is small in size, which means that it can also be used in smaller offices. The cone-shaped X-ray beam is received by a high sensitivity and high resolution light intensifying tube (Fig. 9.25). As the beam passes through only a very limited region of the body, the result is a three-dimensional image with extremely high resolution, but requiring only a very small radiation dose (180–183) (Fig. 9.26). The tube is usually set at 12–30 μSv, which is the equivalent of approximately 4 dental film exposures or a single panorama exposure; and represents only 1/50 of the dosage for a conventional CT – and the resolution is much higher, 2 line pair/mm, minimum; which is 8 times greater than a conventional CT (Figs 9.26 and 9.27).

The image processing software is able to reconstruct a three-dimensional image in only 1 or 2 minutes. The X, Y and Z axes of the three-dimensional image can be observed at 0.25 to 1 mm slice intervals. (Fig. 9.27)

While the 3DX has a wide range of applications, the examples presented here have been limited to trauma cases. In Fig. 9.28, fracture of the labial bone plate is very evident in the micro CT scan. Fig. 9.29 shows root fractures of two central incisors. A fracture line was observed only on the left incisor at the first visit using conventional radiographic techniques. Four months later, a second fracture line became obvious in the right central incisor. The micro CT revealed very clear images of the fracture lines of both teeth. Oblique fracture lines seem difficult to be detected with conventional methods; but micro CT appears useful in their detection.

### Magnetic resonance scanning

Recently, magnetic resonance scanning with administration of a contrast medium was found to be able to demonstrate signs of revascularization of transplanted teeth earlier than a $CO_2$ test (186). However, the complexity of this procedure appears prohibitive as a suitable method for monitoring the healing status of traumatized teeth.

All radiographs should be stored carefully as they provide a record for comparison at future controls.

## Effect of treatment delay

Rather few studies have been found to have examined possible relationships between treatment delay and pulpal and periodontal ligament healing complications. It has been commonly accepted that all injuries should be treated

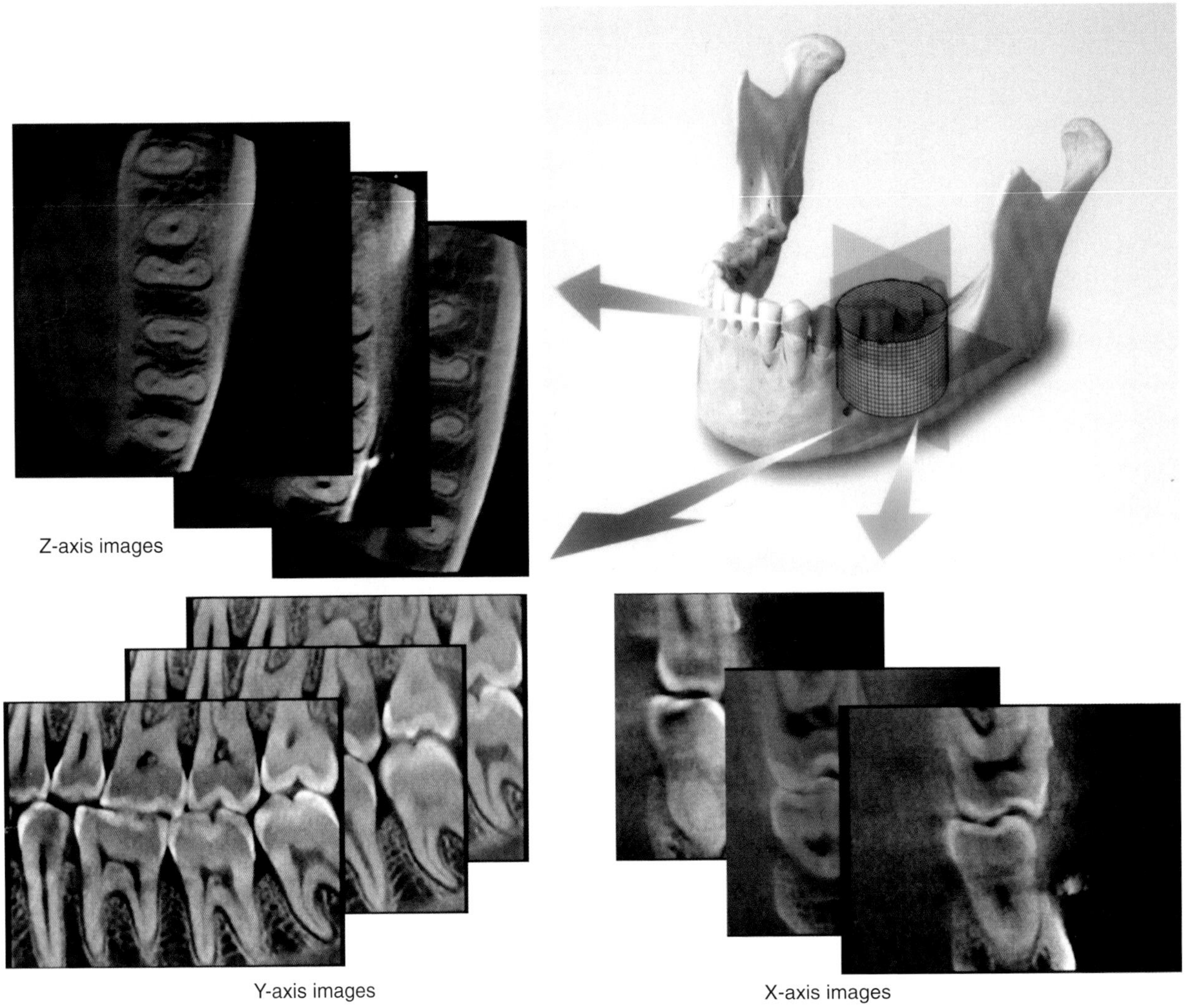

**Fig. 9.27** Principles of a Micro CT scan. Cross-section images of the cylindrical imaging area. Images of a tooth model demonstrate the 3DX's 3-dimensional feature. The imaging area is a cylinder 40 mm in diameter and 30 mm high. Within this area, slices at 1-mm intervals can be viewed for all three dimensions: the X axis (right-left or buccal lingual), the Y axis (back-front or mesial-distal) and the Z axis (vertical).

on an emergency basis, for the comfort of the patient and also to reduce wound healing complications. For practical and especially economical reasons, various approaches can be selected to fulfill such a demand, such as *acute treatment* (i.e. within a few hours), *subacute treatment* (i.e. within the first 24 hours) and *delayed treatment* (i.e. after the first 24 hours). In a recent study, the consequences of treatment delay on pulpal and periodontal healing have been analyzed for the various dental trauma groups (179). Applying such a treatment approach to the various types of injuries, the following guidelines can be recommended, based on our present, rather limited knowledge of the effect of treatment delay upon wound healing.

*Crown and crown-root fractures*: Subacute or delayed approach.

*Root fractures*: Acute or subacute approach.

*Alveolar fractures*: Acute approach (evidence however questionable).

*Concussion and subluxation*: Subacute approach.

*Extrusion and lateral luxation*: Acute approach (evidence however questionable).

*Intrusion*: Subacute approach (evidence however questionable).

*Avulsion*: If the tooth is not replanted at the time of injury, acute approach; otherwise subacute.

*Primary tooth injury*: Subacute approach, unless the primary tooth is displaced into the follicle of the permanent tooth or occlusal problems are present; in the latter instances, an acute approach should be chosen.

These treatment guidelines are based on very limited evidence from the literature and should be revised as soon as more evidence about the effect of treatment delay becomes available.

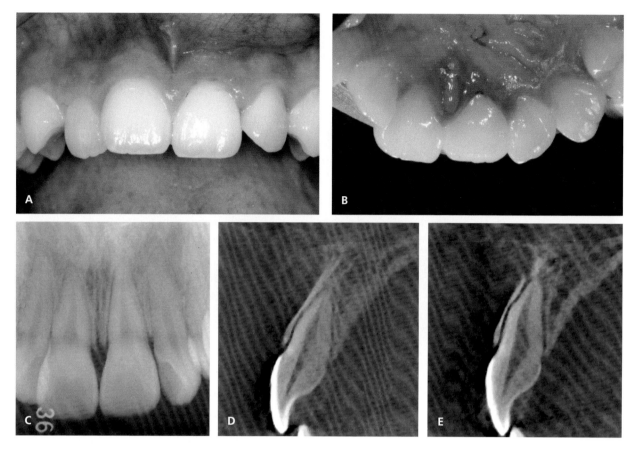

**Fig. 9.28** Lateral luxation. A. The buccal aspect at the first examination of a 13-year-old girl. The left central incisor has suffered a trauma. She visited the dental office after she repositioned the tooth herself. B. The palatal aspect at the first examination. C. A conventional radiograph at the first examination shows no apparent displacement. The left central incisor shows negative EPT. D. The cross-sectioned image of the left central incisor shows a labial bone fracture near the apex, indicating an initial diagnosis of lateral luxation.

## Essentials

### History

- Patient's name, age, sex, address, and telephone number
- When did the accident occur?
- Where did the accident occur?
- How did the accident occur?
- Treatment elsewhere
- History of previous dental injuries and general health
- Did the trauma cause amnesia, unconsciousness, drowsiness, vomiting, or headache?
- Is there spontaneous pain from the teeth?
- Do the teeth react to thermal changes, sweet or sour foods?
- Are the teeth painful to touch or during eating?
- Is there any disturbance in the bite?

### Clinical examination

- Recording of extraoral wounds and palpation of the facial skeleton

- Recording of injuries to oral mucosa or gingiva
- Examination of the tooth crowns for the presence and extent of fractures, pulp exposures, or changes in tooth color
- Recording of displacement of teeth (i.e. intrusion, extrusion, lateral displacement, or avulsion)
- Abnormalities in occlusion
- Abnormal mobility of teeth or alveolar fragments
- Palpation of the alveolar process
- Reaction and sound of teeth to percussion

### Reaction of teeth to sensibility tests

- Mechanical stimulation
- Heated gutta-percha (Fig. 9.10)
- Ice (Fig. 9.11)
- Ethyl chloride (Fig. 9.12)
- Carbon dioxide snow (Fig. 9.13)
- Dichlor-difluormethane
- Electric pulp testers (EPT) (Figs 9.15 and 9.16)
- Laser Doppler flowmetry (LDF) (Fig. 9.18)

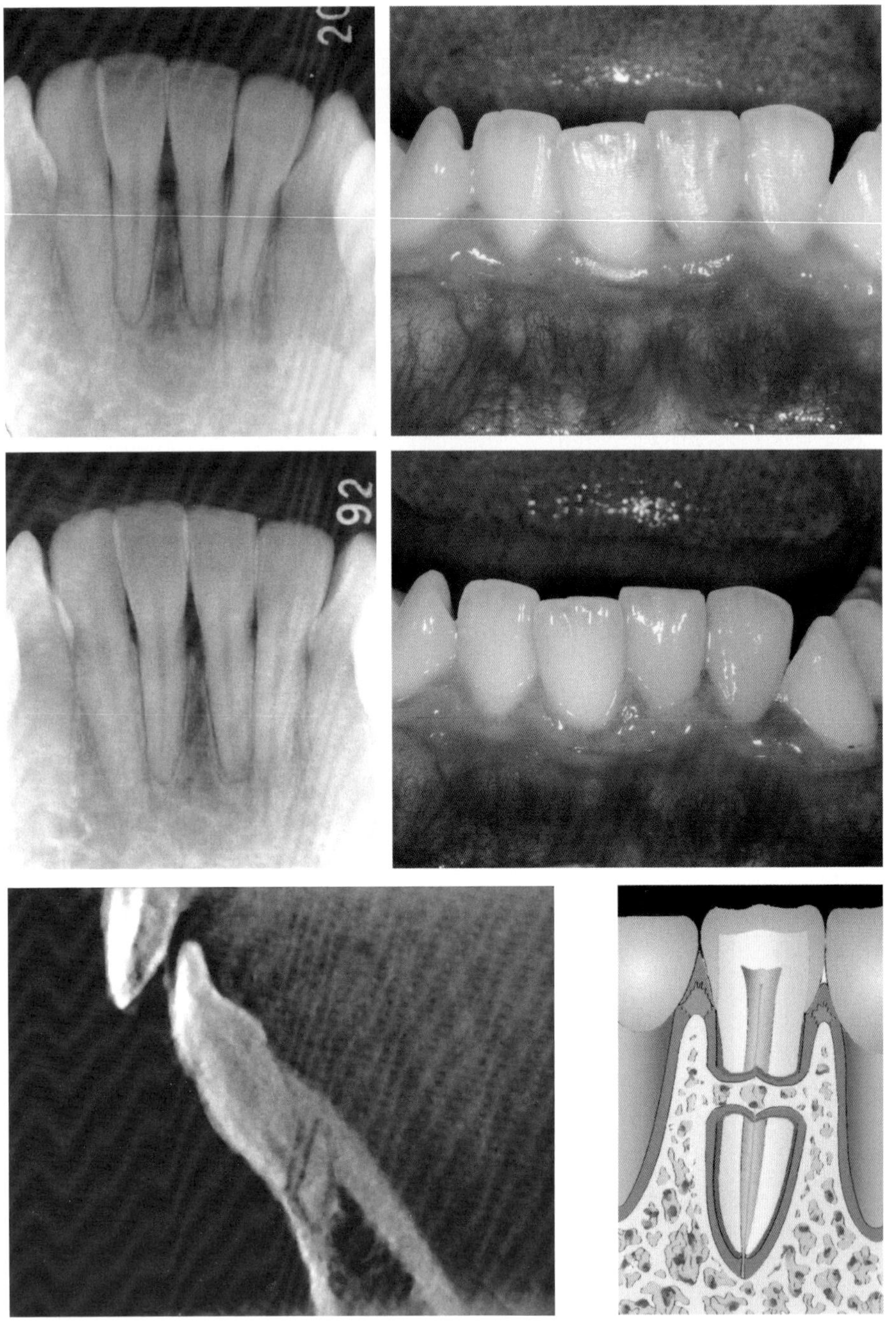

**Fig. 9.29** Micro CT scan of a root fracture. A and B. Conventional radiograph and clinical photograph taken at the initial examination of a 17-year-old male referred 2 months after injury. Although there were no symptoms, the patient's history disclosed that the right central incisor had suffered a subluxation injury. Examination revealed a root fracture at the apical third of the right lateral incisor. The crowns of the teeth were very slightly discolored. Both teeth showed negative EPT. C and D. Six months later, both teeth showed positive EPT. E. One year later, a Micro CT scan showed root fracture healing with interposition of PDL and bone. F. Schematic illustration of this healing type.

## Radiographic examination

- Intraoral radiographs (Figs 9.21 and 9.22)
- Extraoral radiographs (Fig. 9.24)
- CT scanning
- Micro CT scanning (Fig. 9.27)
- MR scanning

## References

1. GAARE A, HAGEN AR, KANSTAD S. Tannfrakturer hos barn. Diagnostiske og prognostiske problemer og behandling. *Norske Tannlægeforenings Tidende* 1958;**68**:364–78.
2. MALONE AJ, MASSLER M. Fractured anterior teeth. Diagnosis, treatment, and prognosis. *Dent Dig* 1952;**58**:442–7.
3. ELLIS RG. Treatment of fractured incisors. *Int Dent J* 1953;**4**:196–208.
4. COOKE C, ROWBOTHAM TC. Treatment of injuries to anterior teeth. *Br Dent J* 1951;**91**:146–52.
5. CURRY VL. Fractured incisors. *Dent Practit Dent Rec* 1951;**1**:341–6.
6. DOÜNIAU R. Traumatismes dentaires accidentels. *J Dent Belge* 1960;**5**:603–15.

7. RIPA LW, FINN SB. The care of injuries to the anterior teeth in children. In: Finn SB. ed. *Clinical pedodontics*. Philadelphia: W B Saunders Company, 1967:324–62.

8. SUNDVALL-HAGLAND 1. Olycksfallsskador på tænder och parodontium under barnaåren. In: Holst JJ, Nygaard Ostby B, Osvald O. eds. *Nordisk Klinisk Odontologi*. Copenhagen: A/S Forlaget for Faglitteratur, 1964:Chapter 11, III, 1–40.

9. RAVN JJ. Ulykkesskadede fortænder på børn. Klassifikation og behandling. *Odontologisk Forening*, Copenhagen 1966.

10. INGLE JI, FRANK AL, NATKIN E, NUTTING EE. Diagnosis and treatment of traumatic injuries and their sequelae. In: Ingle JI, Beveridge EE. eds. *Endodontics*. 2nd edn. Philadelphia: Lea & Febiger, 1976:685–711.

11. ANDREWS RG. Emergency treatment of injured permanent anterior teeth. *Dent Clin North Am* 1965;**11**:703–10.

12. DOWN CH. The treatment of permanent incisor teeth of children following traumatic injury. *Aust Dent J* 1957;**2**:9–24.

13. KISLING E. Om behandlingen af skader som følge af akutte mekaniske traumer på unge permanente incisiver. *Tandlægebladet* 1953;**57**:61–9, 109–29.

14. KISLING E. Beskadigelser af tænder og deres ophængningsapparat ved akutte mekaniske traumata. In: Toverud G. ed. *Nordisk Lærebog i Pedodonti*. Stockholm: Sveriges Tandläkarförbunds Förlagsförening, 1963:266–87.

15. WILBUR HM. Management of injured teeth. *J Am Dent Assoc* 1952;**44**:1–9.

16. BROWN WE. The management of injuries to young teeth. *J Dent Assoc South Afr* 1963;**18**:247–51.

17. OHLSSON Å. Behandling av olycksfallsskadade incisiver på barn. *Odontologisk Tidskrift* 1957;**65**:105–15.

18. ESCHLER J. *Die traumatischen Verletzungen der Frontzähne bei Jugendlichen*. Heidelberg: Alfred Hüthig Verlag, 1966.

19. ANDREASEN JO. Luxation of permanent teeth due to trauma. *Scand J Dent Res* 1970;**78**:273–86.

20. ANDREASEN JO. Luxation of permanent teeth due to trauma. A clinical and radiographic follow-up study of 189 injured teeth. *Scand J Dent Res* 1970;**78**:273–86.

21. FIALOVA S, JURECEK B. Orazy zubu u deti a nase zkusenosti s jejich lécenim. *Prakt Zubni Lék* 1968;**16**:171–6.

22. ROZKOVCOVA E, KOMINEK J. Zhodnoceni vitâlni amputace pri osetrovâni úrazu stálych zubu u deti. *Cs. Stomatol* 1959;**59**:30–5.

23. HALLET GEM, PORTEOUS JR. Fractured incisors treated by vital pulpotomy. A report on 100 consecutive cases. *Br Dent J* 1963;**115**:279–87.

24. ANDREASEN JO. Fractures of the alveolar process of the jaw. A clinical and radiographic follow-up study. *Scand J Dent Res* 1970;**78**:263–72.

25. ROED-PETERSEN B, ANDREASEN JO. Prognosis of permanent teeth involved in jaw fractures. A clinical and radiographic follow-up study. *Scand J Dent Res* 1970;**78**:343–52.

26. ALLEN FJ. Incisor fragments in the lips. *Dent Practit Dent Rec* 1960;61;**11**:390–1.

27. JACOWSKI & COLAS. Incarcération dentaire d'origine traumatique dans la langue et sous la muqueuse vestibulaire. *Rev Stomatol* 1952;**53**:909–12.

28. DEGERING CI. Physiologic evaluation of dental pulp testing methods. *J Dent Res* 1962;**41**:695–700.

29. MUMFORD JM. Evaluation of gutta-percha and ethyl chloride in pulp-testing. *Br Dent J* 1964;**116**:338–42.

30. MUMFORD JM. Pain perception threshold on stimulating human teeth and the histological condition of the pulp. *Br Dent J* 1967;**123**:427–33.

31. ÖHMAN A. Healing and sensitivity to pain in young replanted human teeth. An experimental, clinical, and histological study. *Odontologisk Tidskrift* 1965;**73**:165–228.

32. EHRMANN EH. Pulp testers and pulp testing with particular reference to the use of dry ice. *Aust Dent J* 1977;**22**:272–9.

33. DACHT SF, HALEY JV, SANDERS JE. Standardization of a test for dental sensitivity to cold. *Oral Surg Oral Med Oral Pathol* 1967;**24**:687–92.

34. OBWEGESER H, STEINHAUSER E. Ein neues Gerät für Vitalitätsprüfung der Zähne mit Kohlensäureschnee. *Schweiz Monatschr Zahnheilk* 1963;**73**:1001–12.

35. FUHR K, SCHERER W. Prüfmethodik und Ergebnisse vergleichender Untersuchungen zur Vitalitätsprüfung von Zähnen. *Dtsch Zahnärztl Z* 1968;**23**:1344–9.

36. SCHILLER F. Ist die Vitalitätsprüfung mit Kohlensäureschnee unschädlich. *Öst Z Stomatol* 1937;**35**:1056–63.

37. SAUERMANN G. Die Vitalitätsprüfung der Pulpa bei überkronten Zähnen. *Zahnärztl Rdsch* 1952;**61**:14–9.

38. MUMFORD JM. Thermal and electrical stimulation of teeth in the diagnosis of pulpal and periapical disease. *Proc Roy Soc Med* 1967;**60**:197–200.

39. MUMFORD JM. Pain threshold of normal human anterior teeth. *Arch Oral Biol* 1963;**8**:493–501.

40. MUMFORD JM. Path of direct current in electric pulp-testing using two coronal electrodes. *Br Dent J* 1959;**106**:243–5.

41. MUMFORD JM. Path of direct current in electric pulp-testing using one coronal electrode. *Br Dent J* 1959;**106**:23–6.

42. MUMFORD JM, BJORN H. Problems in electric pulp-testing and dental algesimetry. *Int Dent J* 1962;**12**:161–79.

43. MUMFORD JM. Pain perception threshold and adaptation of normal human teeth. *Arch Oral Biol* 1965;**10**:957–68.

44. NEWTON AV, MUMFORD JM. Transduction of square wave stimuli through human teeth. *Arch Oral Biol* 1968;**13**:831–2.

45. MUMFORD JM. Drying of enamel under rubber dam. *Br Dent J* 1966;**121**:178–9.

46. SELTZER S, BENDER IB, ZIONTZ M. The dynamics of pulp inflammation: Correlations between diagnostic data and actual histologic findings in the pulp. *Oral Surg Oral Med Oral Pathol* 1963;**16**:846–71, 969–77.

47. REYNOLDS RL. The determination of pulp vitality by means of thermal and electrical stimuli. *Oral Surg Oral Med Oral Pathol* 1966;**22**:231–40.

48. ANEHILL S, LINDAHL B, WALLIN H. Prognosis of traumatised permanent incisors in children. A clinical-

roentgenological after-examination. *Svensk Tandläkaras Tidning* 1969;**62**:367–75.

49. SKIELLER V. Om prognosen for unge tænder med løsning efter akut mekanisk læsion. *Tandlægebladet* 1957;**1**:657–73.

50. MAGNUSSON B, HOLM A-K. Traumatised permanent teeth in children – a follow-up. I. Pulpal complications and root resorption. *Svensk Tandläkaras Tidning* 1969;**62**:61–70.

51. KRÖNCHE A. Über die Vitalerhaltung der gefährdeten Pulpa nach Fraktur von Frontzahn-kronen. *Dtsch Zahnärztebl* 1957;**11**:333–6.

52. ELOMAA M. Oireettomien ehjien ja pinnalta karioituneiden hampaiden reaktio sähköstimulaattoriin. *Suomi Hammaslääk Toim* 1963;**59**:316–31.

53. ELOMAA M. Alaleuan pysyvien etuhampaiden reaktio sähköstimulaattoriin 6–15 vuoden idssä. *Suomi Hammaslääk Toim* 1968;**64**:13–17.

54. STENBERG S. Vitalitetsprövning med elektrisk ström av incisiver i olika genombrottsstadier. *Svensk Tandläkaras Tidning.* 1950;**43**:83–6.

55. FEARNHEAD RW. The histological demonstration of nerve fibres in human dentine. In: Anderson DJ. ed. *Sensory mechanisms in dentine.* London: Pergamon Press, 1963:15–26.

56. MUMFORD JM. Personal communication, 1969.

57. ESCHLER J, S CHILLI W, WITT E. *Die Verletzungen der Frontzähne bei Jugendlichen.* Heidelberg: Alfred Hülthig Verlag, 1972.

58. HARGIS HW. Trauma to permanent anterior teeth and alveolar processes. *Dent Clin North Am* 1973;**17**:505–21.

59. HERFORTH A. Notfall: Frontzahntrauma. Hinweise zur Therapie der esten Stunde. *Zahnärztl Mitt* 1973;**63**:317–320.

60. HARGREAVES JA. Emergency treatment for injuries to anterior teeth. *Int Dent J* 1974;**24**:18–29.

61. INGLE JJ, FRANK AL, NATKIN E, NUTTING EE. Diagnosis and treatment of traumatic injuries and their sequelae. In: Ingle JJ, Beveridge EE. eds. *Endodontics.* Philadelphia: Lea & Febiger, 1976.

62. SNAWDER KD. Traumatic injuries to teeth of children. *J Prev Dent* 1976;**3**:13–20.

63. BRAHAM RL, ROBERTS MW, MORRIS ME. Management of dental trauma in children and adolescents. *J Trauma* 1977;**17**:857–65.

64. GRANATH L-E. Traumatologi. In: Holst JJ, Nygaard-Östby B, Osvald O. eds. *Nordisk Klinisk Odontologi.* Copenhagen: A/S Forlaget for Faglitteratur, 1978: Chapter 11:79–100.

65. RAVN JJ. *Ulykkesskadede fortænder på børn. Klassifikation og behandling.* Copenhagen: Odontologisk Boghandels Forlag, 1970.

66. SHUSTERMAN S. Treatment of Class III fractures in the hemophiliac patient. A case report. *J Acad Gen Dent* 1973;**21**:25–8.

67. BESSERMANN-NIELSEN M. Orale blødninger hos hæmofilipatienter. *Tandlægebladet* 1974;**78**:756–61.

68. POWELL D. Management of a lacerated frenum and lip in a child with severe hemophilia and an inhibitor: report of case. *J Dent Child* 1976;**43**:272–5.

69. SNAWDER KD, BASTAWI AE, O'TOOLE TJ. Tooth fragments lodged in unexpected areas. *J Am Med Assoc* 1976;**236**:1378–9.

70. SNAWDER KD, O'TOOLE TJ, BASTAWI AE. Broken-tooth fragments embedded in soft tissue. *ASDC J Dent Child* 1979;**46**:145–8.

71. MAYER C. Restoration of a fractured anterior tooth. *J Am Dent Assoc* 1978;**96**:113–5.

72. GILBERT JM. Wrinkle corner traumatic displacement of teeth into the lip. *Injury* 1977;**9**:64–5.

73. BOOTH NA. Complications associated with treatment of traumatic injuries of the oral cavity – aspiration of teeth – report of case. *J Oral Surg* 1953;**11**:242–4.

74. BUSCHINDER K. Dens in pulmone. *Dtsch Zahnärztl Z* 1955;**10**:1302–4.

75. BOWERMAN JE. The inhalation of teeth following maxillo-facial injuries. *Br Dent J* 1969;**127**:132–4.

76. GILLILAND RF, TAYLOR CG, WADE WM Jr. Inhalation of a tooth during maxillofacial injury: report of a case. *J Oral Surg* 1972;**30**:839–40.

77. REICHBORN-KJENNERUD I. Development, etiology and diagnosis of increased tooth mobility and traumatic occlusion. *J Periodontol* 1973;**44**:326–38.

78. FULLING H-J, ANDREASEN JO. Influence of maturation status and tooth type of permanent teeth upon electrometric and thermal pulp testing. *Scand J Dent Res* 1976;**84**:286–90.

79. FULLING H-J, ANDREASEN JO. Influence of splints and temporary crowns upon electric and thermal pulp-testing procedures. *Scand J Dent Res* 1976;**84**:291–6.

80. TEITLER D, TZADIK D, EIDELMAN E, CHOSACK A. A clinical evaluation of vitality tests in anterior teeth following fracture of enamel and dentin. *Oral Surg Oral Med Oral Pathol* 1972;**34**:649–52.

81. ZADIK D, CHOSACK A, EIDELMAN E. The prognosis of traumatized permanent anterior teeth with fracture of the enamel and dentin. *Oral Surg Oral Med Oral Pathol* 1979;**47**:173–5.

82. MAYER R, HEPPE H. Vergleichende klinische Untersuchungen unterschiedlicher Mittel und Methoden zur Prüfung der Vitalität der Zähne. *Zahnärztl Welt* 1974;**83**:777–81.

83. HERFORTH A. Zur Frage der Pulpavitalität nach Frontzahntrauma bei Jugendlichen – eine Longitudinaluntersuchung. *Dtsch Zahnärztl Z* 1976;**31**:938–46.

84. LUTZ R, MÖRMANN W, LUTZ T. Schmelzsprünge durch die Vitalitätsprüfung mit Kohlensäureschnee. *Schweiz Monatsschr Zahnheilk* 1974;**84**:709–25.

85. BACHMANN A, LUTZ F. Schmelzsprünge durch die Sensibilitätsprüfung mit $CO_2$- Schnee und Dichlor – difluormethan – eine vergleichende In-vivo-Untersuchung. *Schweiz Monatsschr Zahnheilk* 1976;**86**:1042–59.

86. MAYER R. Neues über die Vitalitätsprüfung mit Kältemitteln. *Dtsch Zahnärztl Z* 1971;**26**:423–8.

87. FERGER P, MATTHIESSEN J. Untersuchungen über die Sensibilitätsprilfung mit Provotest. *Zahnärztl Welt* 1974;**83**:422–3.

88. EIFINGER FF. Sensibilitätstest am menschlichen Zahn mit Kälteaerosolen. *Dtsch Zahnärztebl* 1970;**70**:26–32.

89. JOHNSON RH, DACHI SF, HALEY JV. Pulpal hyperemia – a correlation of clinical and histological data of 706 teeth. *J Am Dent Assoc* 1970;**81**:108–17.

90. BHASKAR SN, RAPPAPORT HM. Dental vitality tests and pulp status. *J Am Dent Assoc* 1973;**86**:409–11.

91. MATTHEWS B, SEARLE BN, ADAMS D, LINDEN R. Thresholds of vital and non-vital teeth to stimulation with electric pulp testers. *Br Dent J* 1974;**137**:352–5.

92. CONSTANTIN I, SEVERINEAU V, TUDOSE N. Die Prüfung des elektrischen Widerstandes als objektiver Diagnosetest bei Pulpaerkrankungen. *Zahn Mund Kieferheilkd* 1976;**64**:550–60.

93. BARKIN PR. Time as a factor in predicting the vitality of traumatized teeth. *ASDC J Dent Child* 1973;**40**: 188–92.

94. BADZIAN-KOBOS K, WOCHNA SOBANSKA M, SZOSLAND E, CICHOCKA D. Application of certain tests for assessment of reactions of dental pulp in permanent anterior teeth of children aged from 7 to 11. *Czas Stomatol* 1975;**28**:1155–62.

95. KLEIN H. Pulp responses to an electric pulp stimulator in the developing permanent anterior dentition. *ASDC J Dent Child* 1978;**45**:199–202.

96. BURNSIDE RR, SORENSON FM, BUCK DL. Electric vitality testing in orthodontic patients. *Angle Orthod* 1974;**44**:213–7.

97. HAUN F. Unfallfolgen mit Spätkomplikationen bei Kindern und Jugendlichen. *ZWR* 1974;**83**:927–31.

98. VEIGEL W, GARCIA C. Möglichkeiten und Grenzen der Erhaltung traumatisch geschädigter Milchzähne. *Dtsch Zahnärztl Z* 1976;**31**:271–3.

99. KRETER F, KLAHN K-H. Das akute extraalveoläre Zahntrauma des Milch- und Wechselgebisses. *Zahnärztl Prax* 1975;**26**:228–32.

100. JOHO J-P, MARECHAUX SC. Trauma in the primary dentition: a clinical presentation. *ASDC J Dent Child* 1980;**47**:167–74.

101. JACOBSEN I. Clinical problems in the mixed dentition: traumatized teeth – evaluation, treatment and prognosis. *Int Dent J* 1981;**31**:99–104.

102. ANDREASEN FM, ANDREASEN JO. Diagnosis of luxation injuries: The importance of standardized clinical, radiographic and photographic techniques in clinical investigations. *Endod Dent Traumatol* 1985;**1**:160–9.

103. CAPRIOGLIO D, FALCONI A. I traumi dei denti anteriori in stomatologia infantile. *Dental Cadmos* 1985;**52**:21–47 and 1986;**53**:21–44.

104. MOSS SJ, MACCARO H. Examination, evaluation and behavior management following injury to primary incisors. *N Y State Dent J* 1985;**51**:87–92.

105. MACKIE IC, WARREN VN. Dental trauma: 1. General aspects of management, and trauma to the primary dentition. *Dent Update* 1988;**15**:155–9.

106. HOTZ PR. Accidents dentaires. Accidents aux dents permanentes en denture jeune. *Rev Mens Odontostomatol* 1990;**100**:859–63.

107. FRENKEL G, ADERHOLD L. Das Trauma im Frontzahnbereich des jugendlichen Gebisses aus chirurgischer Sicht. *Fortschr Kieferorthop* 1990;**51**:138–44.

108. HALL RK. Dental management of the traumatized child patient. *Ann Roy Aust Coll Dent Surg* 1986;**9**:80–99.

109. KOPEL HM, JOHNSON R. Examination and neurologic asssessment of children with oro-facial trauma. *Endod Dent Traumatol* 1985;**1**:155–9.

110. TURLEY PK, HENSON JL. Self-injurious lip-biting etiology and management. *J Pedodont* 1983;**7**:209–20.

111. NGAN PWH, NELSON LP. Neuropathologic chewing in comatose children. *Pediatr Dent* 1985;**7**:302–6.

112. GUDAT H, MARKL M, LUKAS D, SCHULTE W. Analyse von Perkussionssignalen an Zähnen. *Dtsch Zahnärztl Z* 1977;**32**:169–72.

113. WEISMAN MI. The use of a calibrated percussion instrument in pulpal and periapical diagnosis. *Oral Surg Oral Med Oral Pathol* 1984;**57**:320–2.

114. CHAMBERS IG. The role and methods of pulp testing in oral diagnosis: a review. *Int Endod J* 1982;**15**:1–5.

115. LADO EA, RICHMOND AF, MARKS RG. Reliability and validity of a digital pulp tester as a test standard for measuring sensory perception. *J Endod* 1988;**14**: 352–6.

116. ROWE AHR, PITT FORD TR. The assessment of pulpal vitality. *Int Endod J* 1990;**23**:77–83.

117. PETERS DD, LORTON L, MADER CL, AUGSBURGER RA, INGRAM TA. Evaluation of the effects of carbon dioxide used as a pulpal test. 1. *In vitro* effect on human enamel. *J Endod* 1983;**9**:219–27.

118. PETERS DD. MADER CI, DONNELLY JC. Evaluation of the effects of carbon dioxide used as a pulpal test. 3. *In vivo* effect on human enamel. *J Endod* 1986;**12**:13–20.

119. INGRAM TA, PETERS DD. Evaluation of the effects of carbon dioxide used as a pulpal test. Part 2. *In vivo* effect of canine enamel and pulpal tissues. *J Endod* 1983;**9**:296–303.

120. DOWDEN WE, EMMINGS F, LANGELAND K. The pulpal effect of freezing temperatures applied to monkey teeth. *Oral Surg Oral Med Oral Pathol* 1983;**55**:408–18.

121. MCGRATH PA, GRACELY RH, DUBNER R, HEFT MW. Non-pain and pain sensations evoked by tooth pulp stimulation. *Pain* 1983;**15**:377–88.

122. COOLEY RL, ROBINSON SF. Variables associated with electric pulp testing. *Oral Surg Oral Med Oral Pathol* 1980;**50**:66–73.

123. COOLEY RL, STILLEY J, LUBOW RM. Evaluation of a digital pulp tester. *Oral Surg Oral Med Oral Pathol* 1984;**58**:437–42.

124. JACOBSON JJ. Probe placement during electric pulp-testing procedures. *Oral Surg Oral Med Oral Pathol* 1984;**58**:242–7.

125. BENDER IB, LANDAU MA, FONSECCA S, TROWBRIDGE HO. The optimum placement-site of the electrode in electric pulp testing of the 12 anterior teeth. *J Am Dent Assoc* 1989;**118**:305–10.

126. PANTERA EA, ANDERSON RW, PANTERA CT. Use of dental instruments for bridging during electric pulp testing. *J Endod* 1992,**18**:37–41.

127. KOLBINSON DA, TEPLITSKY PE. Electric pulp testing with examination gloves. *Oral Surg Oral Med Oral Pathol* 1988;**65**:122–6.

128. ANDERSON RW, PANTERA EA. Influence of a barrier technique on electric pulp testing. *J Endod* 1988;**14**:179–80.

129. BOOTH DQ, KIDD EAM. Unipolar electric pulp testers and rubber gloves. *Br Dent J* 1988;**165**:254–5.

130. TREASURE P. Capacitance effect of rubber gloves on electric pulp testers. *Int Endod J* 1989;**22**:236–40.

131. STEIMAN HR. Endodontic diagnostic techniques. *Current Science* 1991;**1**:723–8.

132. BHASKAR SN, RAPPAPORT HM. Dental vitality tests and pulp status. *J Am Dent Assoc* 1973;**86**:409–11.

133. ANDREASEN FM, PEDERSEN BV. Prognosis of luxated permanent teeth – the development of pulp necrosis. *Endod Dent Traumatol* 1985;**1**:207–20.

134. ANDREASEN FM. Transient apical breakdown and its relation to color and sensibility changes after luxation injuries to teeth. *Endod Dent Traumatol* 1986;**2**:9–19.

135. ANDREASEN FM. Pulpal healing after luxation injuries and root fracture in the permanent dentition. *Endod Dent Traumatol* 1989;**5**:111–31.

136. BRANDT K, KORTEGAARD U, POULSEN S. Longitudinal study of electrometric sensitivity of young permanent incisors. *Scand J Dent Res* 1988;**96**:334–8.

137. ANDREASEN JO, PAULSEN HU, YU Z, AHLQUIST R, BAYER T, SCHWARTZ O. A long-term study of 370 autotransplanted premolars. Part 1. Surgical procedures and standardized techniques for monitoring healing. *Eur J Orthod* 1990;**12**:313.

138. PECKHAM K, TORABINEJAD M, PECKHAM N. The presence of nerve fibres in the coronal odontoblast layer of teeth at various stages of root development. *Int Endod J* 1991;**24**:3037.

139. GAZELIUS B, OLGART L, EDWALL B, EDWALL L. Non-invasive recordings of blood blow in human dental pulp. *Endod Dent Traumatol* 1986;**2**:219–21.

140. WILDER-SMITH PEEB. A new method for the non-invasive measurement of pulpal blood flow. *Int Endod J* 1988;**21**:307–12.

141. ANDREASEN FM, ANDREASEN JO. Resorption and mineralization processes following root fracture of permanent incisors. *Endod Dent Traumatol* 1988;**4**:202–14.

142. ANDREASEN JO, BORUM M, JACOBSEN HL, ANDREASEN FM. Replantation of 400 avulsed permanent incisors. II. Factors related to pulp healing. *Endod Dent Traumatol* 1995;**11**:59–68.

143. ANDREASEN JO, BORUM M, JACOBSEN HL, ANDREASEN FM. Replantation of 400 avulsed permanent incisors. IV. Factors related to periodontal ligament healing. *Endod Dent Traumatol* 1995;**11**:76–89.

144. BOOTH JM. 'It's a knock-out' – an avulsed tooth campaign. *J Endod* 1980;**6**:425–7.

145. HEITHERSAY GS, HIRSCH RS. Tooth discoloration and resolution following a luxation injury: Significance of blood pigment in dentin to laser Doppler flowmetry readings. *Quintess Int* 1993;**24**:669–76.

146. MARTIN H, FERRIS C, MAZZELLA W. An evaluation of media used in electric pulp testing. *Oral Surg Oral Med Oral Pathol* 1969;**27**:374–8.

147. BAKLAND LK, ANDREASEN JO. Dental traumatology: essential diagnosis and treatment planning. *Endod Topics* 2004;**7**:14–34.

148. NEWTON CW. Trauma involving the dentition and supporting tissues. *Prosthod and Endod* 1992; 108–14.

149. DAY PF, DUGGAL MS. A multicentre investigation into the role of structured histories for patients with tooth avulsion at their initial visit to a dental hospital. *Dental Traumatol* 2003;**19**:243–7.

150. GAUBERT SA, HECTOR MP. Periodontal mechano-sensory responses following trauma to permanent incisor teeth in children. *Dent Traumatol* 2003;**19**:145–53.

151. ANDRESEN MH, MACKIE IC, WORTHINGTON H. The periotest in traumatology. I. Does it have the properties necessary for use as a clinical device and can the measurements be interpreted? *Dent Traumatol* 2003;**19**:214–17.

152. ANDRESEN M, MACKIE I, WORTHINGTON H. The Periotest in traumatology. Part II. The Periotest as a special test for assessing the periodontal status of teeth in children that have suffered trauma. *Dent Traumatol* 2003;**19**:218–20.

153. PLODER O, PARTIK B, RAND T, FOCK N, VORACEK M, UNDT G, BAUMANN A. Reperfusion of autotransplanted teeth – comparison of clinical measurements by means of dental magnetic resonance imaging. *Oral Surg Oral Med Oral Pathol Oral Radiol Endod* 2001;**92**: 335–40.

154. EVANS D, REID J, STRANG R, STIRRUPS D. A comparison of laser Doppler flowmetry with other methods of assessing the vitality of traumatised anterior teeth. *Endod Dent Traumatol* 1999;**15**:284–90.

155. PETERSSON K, SÖDERSTRÖM C, KIANI-ANARAKI M, LÉVY G. Evaluation of the ability of thermal and electrical tests to register pulp vitality. *Endod Dent Traumatol* 1999;**15**:127–31.

156. HYMAN JJ, COHEN ME. The predictive value of endodontic diagnostic tests. *Oral Surg Oral Med Oral Pathol* 1984;**58**:343–6.

157. FUSS Z, TROWBRIDGE H, BENDER IB, RICKOFF B, SOLOMON S. Assessment of reliability of electrical and thermal pulp testing agents. *J Endod* 1986;**12**: 301–5.

158. PETERS DD, BAUMGARTNER JC, LORTON L. Adult pulpal diagnosis. I. Evaluation of the positive and negative responses to cold and electrical pulp tests. *J Endod* 1994;**20**:506–11.

159. KVINNSLAND I, HEYERAAS KJ, BYERS MR. Regeneration of calcitonin gene-related peptide immunoreactive nerves in replanted rat molars and their supporting tissues. *Arch Oral Biol* 1991;**36**: 815–26.

160. ÖHMAN A. Healing and sensitivity to pain in young replanted human teeth. An experimental, clinical and histological study. *Odontologisk Tidsskrift* 1965;**73**:165–228.

161. PAULSEN H-U, ANDREASEN JO. Autotransplantation of premolars in orthodontic treatment: Initial pulp and periodontal healing, root development and tooth eruption subsequent to transplantation. A long-term study. In Davidovitch Z. ed. *The biological mechanisms of tooth eruption, resorption and replacement by implants.* Boston, Mass: Harvard Society for the Advancement of Orthodontics, 1994:513–25.

162. SCHENDEL KU, SCHWARTZ O, ANDREASEN JO, HOFFMEISTER B. Reinnervation of autotransplanted teeth. A histological investigation in monkeys. *Int J Oral Maxillofac Surg* 1990;**19**:247–9.

163. PILEGGI R, DUMSHA TC, MYSLINKSI NR. The reliability of the electric pulp test after concussion injury. *Endod Dent Traumatol* 1996;**12**:16–19.

164. OLGART L, GAZELIUS B, LINDH-STRÖMBERG U. Laser Doppler flowmetry in assessing vitality in luxated permanent teeth. *Int Endod J* 1988;**21**: 300–6.

165. GAZELIUS B, OLGART L, EDWALL B. Restored vitality in luxated teeth assessed by laser Doppler flowmetry. *Endod Dent Traumatol* 1988;**4**:265–8.

166. YANPISAT K, VONGSAVAN N, SIGURDSSON A, TROPE M. The efficacy of laser Doppler flowmetry for the diagnosis of revascularization of reimplanted immature dog teeth. *Dent Traumatol* 2001;**17**:63–70.

167. MESAROS SV, TROPE M. Revascularization of traumatized teeth assessed by laser Doppler flowmetry: case report. *Endod Dent Traumatol* 1997;**13**:24–30.

168. LEE JY, YANPISET K, SIGURDSSON A, VANN JR WF. Laser Doppler flowmetry for monitoring traumatized teeth. *Dent Traumatol* 2001;**17**:231–5.

169. INGÓLFSON ÆR, TRONSTAD L, HERSH E, RIVA CE. Effect of probe design on the suitability of laser Doppler flowmetry in vitality testing of human teeth. *Endod Dent Traumatol* 1993;**9**:65–70.

170. INGÓLFSON ÆR, TRONSTAD L, HERSH E, RIVA CE. Efficacy of laser Doppler flowmetry in determining pulp vitality of human teeth. *Endod Dent Traumatol* 1994;**10**:83–7.

171. INGÓLFSSON ÆR, TRONSTAD L, RIVA CE. Reliability of laser Doppler flowmetry in testing vitality of human teeth. *Endod Dent Traumatol* 1994;**10**:185–7.

172. ODOR TM, PITT FORD TR, MCDONALD F. Effect of wavelength and bandwidth on the clinical reliability of laser Doppler recordings. *Endod Dent Traumatol* 1996;**12**:9–15.

173. ROEBUCK EM, EVANS DJP, STIRRUPS D, STRANG R. The effect of wavelength, bandwidth, and probe design and position on assessing the vitality of anterior teeth with laser Doppler flowmetry. *Int J Paediatric Dent* 2000;**10**:213–20.

174. SASANO T, ONODERA D, HASHIMOTO K, IIKUBO M, SATOH-KURIWADA S, SHOJI N, MIYAHARA T. Possible application of transmitted laser light for the assessment of human pulp vitality. Part 2. Increased laser power for enhanced detection of pulpal blood flow. *Dent Traumatol* 2005;**21**:37–41.

175. EMSHOFF R, EMSHOFF I, MOSCHEN I, STROBL H. Diagnostic characteristics of pulpal blood flow levels associated with adverse outcomes of luxated permanent maxillary incisors. *Dent Traumatol* 2004;**20**:270–5.

176. STROBL H, HAAS M, NORER B, GERHARD S, EMSHOFF R. Evaluation of pulpal blood flow after tooth splinting of luxated permanent maxillary incisors. *Dent Traumatol* 2004;**20**:36–41.

177. OIKARINEN K, KAUPPINEN P, HERRALA E. Mobility and percussion sound of healthy upper incisors and canines. *Endod Dent Traumatol* 1992;**8**:21–5.

178. ANDREASEN JO, ANDREASEN FM, SKEIE A, HJØRTING-HANSEN E, SCHWARTZ O. Effect of treatment delay upon pulp and periodontal healing of traumatic dental injuries – a review article. *Dent Traumatol* 2002;**18**:116–28.

179. ARAI Y, TAMMISALO E, IWAI K, HASHIMOTO K, SHINODA K. Development of ortho cubic super high resolution CT (Ortho-CT). *Car'98 CARS*, Elsevier, Amsterdam, 1998, 780–5.

180. ARAI Y, HASHIMOTO K, IWAI K, SHINODA K. Fundamental efficiency of limited cone-beam X-ray CT (3DX, multi image micro CT) for practical use. *Jpn Dent Radiol* 2000;**40**:145–54.

181. HONDA K, ARAI Y, SHINODA K. Fundamental efficiency of new-style limited cone-beam CT (3DX): comparison with spherical CT. *Jpn J Tomogr* 2001;**27**:193–8.

182. IWAI K, ARAI Y, HASHIMOTO K, NISHIZAWA K. Estimation of effective dose from limited cone beam X-ray CT examination. *Jpn Dent Radiol* 2001;**40**:251–9.

183. ARAI Y, HONDA K, SHINODA K. Practical model '3DX' of limited cone-beam X-ray CT for dental use. *Cars 2001*, Elsevier Science, 2001, 671–5.

184. SHINODA K, ARAI Y. *The application of the cone beam computed tomography in dentistry.* Ishiyaku Publishers, Inc. Tokyo, 2003.

185. TSUKIBOSHI M. *Treatment planning for traumatized teeth.* Chicago: Quintessence Publishing Co, Inc, 2000.

# 10
# Crown Fractures

F. M. Andreasen & J. O. Andreasen

## Terminology, frequency and etiology

The following classification of crown fractures is based upon anatomic, therapeutic and prognostic considerations (Fig. 10.1).

(1) *Enamel infraction*, an incomplete fracture (crack) of the enamel without loss of tooth substance
(2) *Enamel fracture*, a fracture with loss of tooth substance confined to enamel (uncomplicated crown fracture)

(3) *Enamel-dentin fracture*, a fracture with loss of tooth substance confined to enamel and dentin, but not involving the pulp (uncomplicated crown fracture)
(4) *Enamel-dentin fracture involving the pulp* (complicated crown fracture).

In the permanent dentition, crown fractures comprise 26 to 76% of dental injuries (1–4, 111–113, 339).

The most common etiologic factors of crown and crown-root fractures in the permanent dentition are injuries caused by falls, contact sports, automobile accidents or foreign bodies striking the teeth (1, 112).

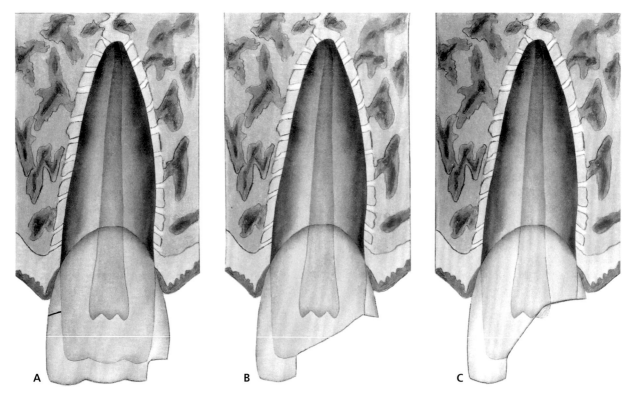

**A**  **B**  **C**

**Fig. 10.1** Schematic drawings illustrating different types of crown fractures. A. Crown infraction and uncomplicated crown fracture without involvement of dentin. B. Uncomplicated crown fracture with involvement of dentin. C. Complicated crown fracture.

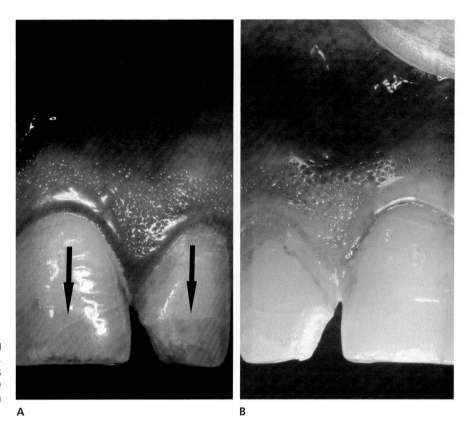

**Fig. 10.2** Infraction lines involving the right central and lateral incisors. The use of indirect illumination reveals the infraction lines (A) although they are barely visible by direct illumination (B).

A  B

Enamel fractures comprise a very common occupational hazard among glassblowers, presumably due to impact by the blowpipe (192).

## Clinical findings

*Enamel infractions* are very common but often overlooked. These fractures appear as crazing within the enamel substance which do not cross the dentinoenamel junction and may appear with or without loss of tooth substance (i.e. uncomplicated or complicated crown fractures) (5, 6, 114, 194). Infractions are caused by direct impact to the enamel, e.g. traffic accidents and falls, which explains their frequent occurrence on the labial surface of upper incisors (194). Various patterns of infraction lines can be seen depending on the direction and location of the trauma, i.e. horizontal, vertical or diverging. Infractions are often overlooked if direct illumination is used, but are easily visualized when the light beam is directed perpendicular to the long axis of the tooth from the incisal edge (Fig. 10.2). Fiber optic light sources are also very useful in detecting infractions. By modifying the intensity of the light beam, many infractions become readily visible (193). Infractions are often the only evidence of trauma, but can be associated with other types of injury. Thus the presence of infraction lines should draw attention to the possible presence of associated injuries, especially to the supporting structures.

*Enamel* and *enamel-dentin fractures* without pulpal involvement occur more often than complicated crown fractures in both the permanent and primary dentitions (3, 7–9, 111, 115, 116). They are often confined to a single tooth, usually the maxillary central incisors (7, 10, 115), especially the mesial or distal corners (7) (Fig. 10.3). Fractures can be horizontal, extending mesiodistally. Occasionally only the central lobe of the incisal edge is involved (Fig. 10.4). In rare cases, the fracture can involve the entire facial or oral enamel surface.

Although not frequently found in combination with luxation injuries (195, 196), crown fractures can be seen concomitant to subluxations, extrusions and especially intrusions (1, 197, 198). This combination of luxation injury and crown fracture is of prognostic importance (see later).

A very unusual finding is crown fractures of non-erupted permanent teeth due to trauma transmitted from impact to the primary dentition (118, 119, 336) (see p. 284).

Examination of fractured teeth should be preceded by thorough cleansing of the injured teeth with a water spray. This is followed by an assessment of the extent of exposed dentin as well as a careful search for minute pulp exposures.

Dentin exposed after crown fracture usually gives rise to symptoms such as sensitivity to thermal changes and mastication, which are to some degree proportional to the area of dentin exposed and the maturity of the tooth (199).

The layer of dentin covering the pulp may be so thin that the outline of the pulp is seen as a pinkish tinge. In such cases, it is important not to perforate the dentin with a

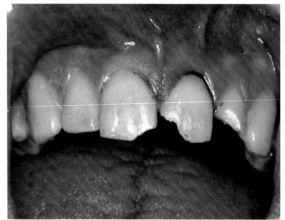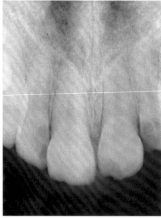

**Fig. 10.3** Central and lateral incisors with typical uncomplicated crown fractures involving the mesial corners.

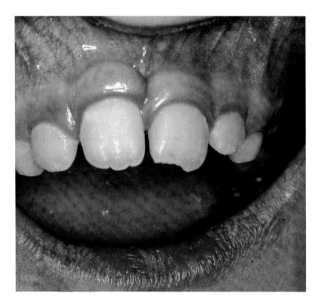

**Fig. 10.4** Uncomplicated crown fracture involving the central lobe of the incisal edge.

dental probe during the search for pulp exposures. Clinical examination should also include sensibility testing as a point of reference for later evaluation of pulpal status (120) (see Chapter 9, p. 255).

*Complicated crown fractures* usually present slight hemorrhage from the exposed part of the pulp (Fig. 10.5). Proliferation of pulp tissue (i.e. pulp polyp) can occur when treatment in young teeth is delayed for days or weeks (Fig. 10.6). Pulp exposure is usually followed by symptoms, such as sensitivity to thermal changes.

## Radiographic findings

The radiographic examination adds important information to the clinical evaluation which can influence future treatment, such as the size of the pulp and the stage of root development (200–202). Moreover, the radiograph serves as a record for comparison at later visits. This is especially true

in the verification of a hard tissue barrier over an exposed pulp when clinical verification is not possible. However, it should be borne in mind that a radiograph can only provide an estimate of pulpal dimensions; and that the pulp cavity is usually larger and the distance of pulp horns from the incisal edge is usually smaller than that shown radiographically (200). In rare cases, displacement of primary teeth may lead to a crown fracture of a permanent successor, a finding which can be shown radiographically (Fig. 10.7).

## Healing and pathology

*Enamel infractions* can be seen in ground sections, where they appear as dark lines running parallel to the enamel rods and terminate at the dentinoenamel junction (11) (Fig. 10.8).

*Enamel-dentin crown fractures* expose a large number of dentinal tubules. It has been estimated that the exposure of $1 mm^2$ of dentin exposes 20 000 to 45 000 dentinal tubules (12, 121). Dentinal tubules constitute a pathway for bacteria and thermal and chemical irritants which can provoke pulpal inflammation, for which reason dentin-covering procedures described later in this chapter and in Chapter 22 are necessary. The speed of bacterial penetration into prepared dentin left exposed to saliva and plaque formation *in vivo* was found by Lundy and Stanley (203) to be 0.03–0.36 mm 6–11 days after preparation and 0.52 mm after approximately 84 days. No studies have so far studied the progress of bacteria after fracture exposure of dentin (205). In one experimental study in monkeys, bacteria were formed in dentinal tubules after 3 months in both treated (composite and fragment bonding) and non-treated teeth. Presence of bacteria in tubules was related to significant hard tissue formation in the coronal part of the pulp (377).

These findings are supported by a recent study in monkeys, where induced fractures were either restored with Dycal® and resin composite or by reattachment of the crown fragment with GLUMA® dentin bonding system. After 3 months, the general appearance was hard tissue deposition in the coronal portion of the pulp and inflammatory

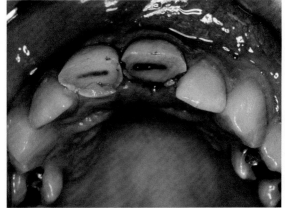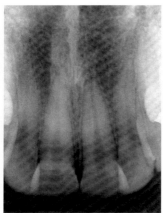

**Fig. 10.5** Complicated crown fractures showing difference in pulp circulation illustrated by differences in color of the exposed pulp.

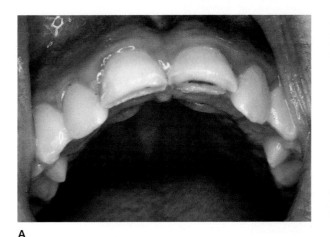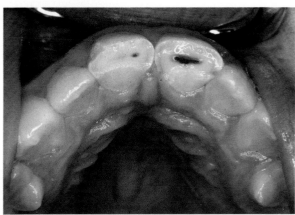

A

B

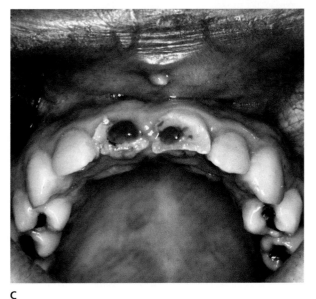

C

**Fig. 10.6** Complicated crown fractures of permanent incisors. A and B. Small pulp exposures of central incisors. C. Pulp proliferation in a case of complicated crown fractures left untreated for 21 days.

infiltrates were seen in only a few teeth and then as clusters of mononuclear leukocytes. More extensively hard tissue formation correlated with the presence of bacteria in dentinal tubules (337).

The ingrowth of bacteria is to a certain degree inhibited by an outward flow of dentinal fluid within the tubules due to a positive pulpal pressure (338, 367, 368). In contrast, bacterial penetration is more rapid where impeding hydrostatic pressure from an outward pulpal fluid flow is minimal or nonexistent, as after concomitant luxation injuries where there is a compromised pulpal blood supply (205–210). Experimental studies *in vivo* in cats have thus demonstrated an increased fluid flow from exposed dentinal tubules with an intact pulpal blood supply, presumably due to a chain of

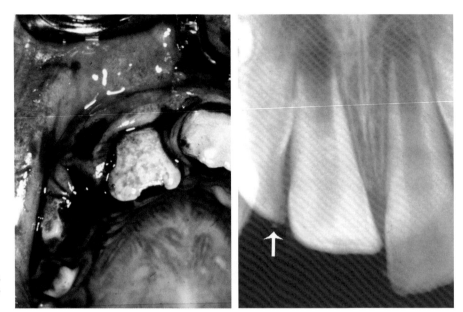

**Fig. 10.7** A primary tooth injury has resulted in an enamel fracture of the non-erupted, lateral incisor (arrow).

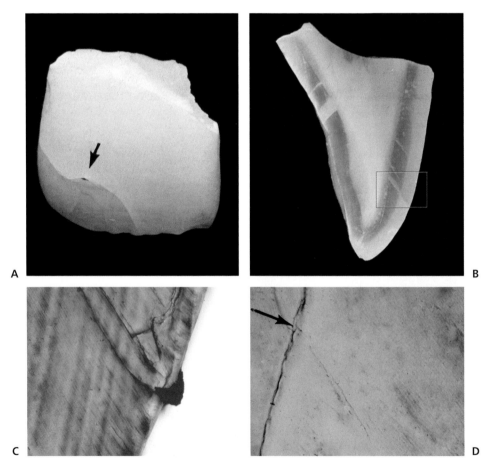

**Fig. 10.8** Histologic features of a permanent central incisor showing crown infractions. A. Gross specimen. Note the point of impact (arrow) with irradiating infraction lines. B. Low power view of ground section through the impact area. ×8. C. Facial aspect of the crown exhibiting an infraction line. ×30. D. Higher magnification of (C) reveals that the line follows the direction of the enamel prisms. ×195.

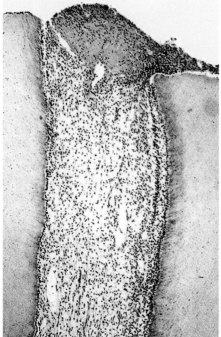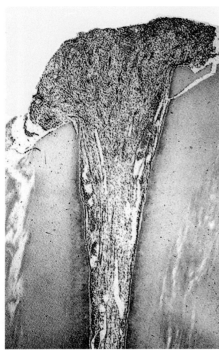

**Fig. 10.9** Immediate and histologic response to a crown fracture in a monkey. A. The inflammation is very superficial after 24 hours. B. After 1 week the pulp shows proliferation and still very limited inflammation.

**A**

**B**

events involved in neurogenic inflammation arising from dentinal irritation following exposure and subsequent stimulation of, e.g., the inferior alveolar nerve (206–210). This fluid flow might mechanically inhibit bacterial ingress through patent dentinal tubules, and also distribute antibodies (205).

This increase in fluid flow after dentin exposure might also have clinical implications with respect to moisture control in the use of dentin bonding agents. Thus, it might seem advisable to administer a local anesthetic prior to such procedures to reverse dentinal fluid flow due to neurogenic stimulation (211). However, further investigation is necessary to test this theory before it can be advocated universally.

Little information exists about pulpal changes after *enamel-dentin crown fractures*. Experimental studies have demonstrated inflammatory changes when artificially exposed dentin was left uncovered for one week (13, 14). However, recent research suggests that the inflammatory changes are of a transient nature, if the pulpal vascular supply remains intact and bacterial invasion is prevented (212) (see later).

Histologically, exposed pulp tissue in *complicated crown fractures* is quickly covered by a layer of fibrin. Eventually the superficial part of the pulp shows capillary budding, numerous leukocytes and proliferation of histiocytes. This inflammation spreads apically with increasing observation periods. However, experimental studies in permanent teeth of monkeys have shown that the inflammatory process does not usually penetrate more than approximately 2 mm in an apical direction (122, 213), a finding which is of clinical significance in treatment planning (see Chapter 22).

Complicated crown fractures which are left untreated for longer periods of time normally show extensive proliferation of granulation tissue at the exposure site (Fig. 10.9).

However, rare cases of spontaneous closure of the perforation with hard tissue have been reported (15, 123).

## Treatment

Many authors have discussed treatment principles for crown fractures in the *permanent dentition* (16–59). For reviews the reader is referred to excellent reports published by Rauchenberger and Hovland 1995 (339), Blatz 2001 (340) and Olsburgh et al. 2002 (341). Therapeutic considerations comprise *pulpal* response to injury and treatment as well as the *prosthetic* considerations arising at the time of injury and final, definitive treatment. The reader is referred to Chapter 22 regarding pulpal considerations following crown fracture; while emphasis in the present chapter will be placed upon emergency treatment procedures. Final restorative treatment using composite resin will be described in Chapter 25.

### Enamel infractions

While infractions in enamel, dentin and cementum in the *posterior* region are often implicated in 'the cracked tooth syndrome', enamel infractions in *anterior* teeth following acute trauma do not appear to imply the same risk to tissue integrity due to the fact that these infractions are usually limited to enamel and stop at the dentinoenamel junction (Fig. 10.8). However, due to frequently associated injuries to periodontal structures, sensibility tests should be carried out in order to disclose possible damage to the pulp.

As a rule, enamel infractions do not require treatment. However, in case of multiple infraction lines, the indication might be to seal the enamel surface with an unfilled resin and acid etch technique, as these lines might otherwise take up stain from tobacco, food, drinks, or other liquids (e.g. tea, red wine, cola drinks and chlorhexidine mouthwashes).

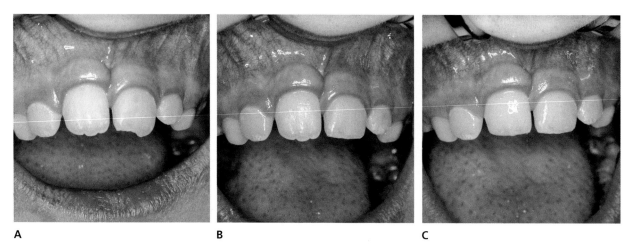

**A**                                   **B**                                   **C**

**Fig. 10.10** Grinding procedure used in the treatment of an uncomplicated crown fracture confined to enamel. A. Before treatment. B. After grinding of injured tooth. C. Grinding of the non-injured incisor in order to restore symmetry.

## Enamel and enamel-dentin crown fractures

Immediate treatment of crown fractures *confined to enamel* can be limited to smoothing of sharp enamel edges to prevent laceration of the tongue or lips. Selective reduction can be undertaken at the same time or at a later visit with good esthetic results, especially in imitating an accentuated rounding of a distal corner (47, 60) (Fig. 10.10). However, because of esthetic demands for midline symmetry, a fractured mesial corner can usually not be corrected in the same way. Selective reduction can in some cases be combined with orthodontic extrusion of the fractured tooth in order to restore incisal height. However, cervical symmetry must also be considered (61, 214) (see Chapter 29).

When the shape or extent of the fracture precludes recontouring, a restoration is necessary.

Whatever treatment is decided, it is essential that the crown's anatomy and occlusion be restored immediately in order to prevent labial protrusion of the fractured tooth, drifting or tilting of adjacent teeth into the fracture site (6, 34, 63, 124) or over eruption of opposing incisors (60, 64) (Fig. 10.11).

Immediate reattachment of the original fragment (see p. 290) or restoration with a composite resin (see Chapter 25) is normally to be preferred over a temporary crown for several reasons. These procedures are usually esthetically superior and are probably less traumatic to the injured tooth than adaptation of temporary crowns. The most significant disadvantage of temporary crowns is the potential risk of leakage which permits access of bacteria to the exposed dentin and thereby represents a significant threat to the recovery of the pulp.

An isolated fracture of enamel does not appear to represent any hazard to the pulp (see p. 302). However, in crown fractures with *exposed dentin*, therapeutic measures should be directed towards dentin coverage in order to avoid bacterial ingress and thereby permit the pulp to recover and elicit repair.

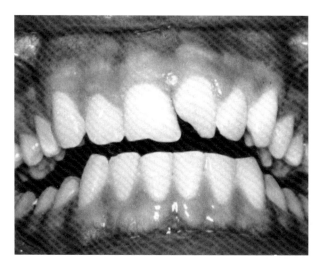

**Fig. 10.11** Untreated crown fracture. Note drifting and tilting of adjacent teeth into the fracture area. Courtesy of Dr. J. J. RAVN, Department of Pedodontics, Royal Dental College, Copenhagen, Denmark.

It was in the 1970s that the impact on pulpal healing of bacterial invasion and colonization in the gap between the tooth and the restorative material after exposure of dentin was first appreciated (204, 215–240, 342, 343).

Thus, when bacteria are excluded from the tooth/restoration interface experimentally by placement of a superficial layer of zinc oxide-eugenol cement over the restorations or liners, healing with formation of a hard tissue bridge can be achieved even after direct pulp capping with silicate cement, zinc-phosphate cement, amalgam and light-cured composite resin (236, 237, 241–244) (Fig. 10.11). It would therefore seem that the initial cytotoxic effect of these materials placed on or near the human pulp is not greater than that which is seen after capping with calcium hydroxide (199).

Experimentally it has been found that in teeth with vital pulp tissue, dentin can provide considerable resistance to bacterial invasion and that dentin which has been exposed to the oral environment for longer periods of time appears to be less permeable than fresh dentinal wounds (240). Furthermore, bacterial irritation via an area of exposed dentin causes limited pulpal inflammation and with little permanent damage (245).

As support for these findings, long-term clinical studies have shown very little pulpal response (e.g. pulp necrosis, or pulp canal obliteration) to either crown fracture with or without pulp exposure or subsequent restorative procedures as long as there was not a concomitant periodontal injury (233, 246–253) (see p. 302).

### Treatment strategy

Survey articles (339–341) have addressed this problem and should be consulted. In light of current knowledge concerning the role of bacterial influences associated with marginal leakage, one must conclude that the primary objective of restorative procedures following crown fractures which expose dentin is to prevent injury to the pulp that is initiated by bacteria and bacterial components in the event that the restoration will not provide an adequate marginal seal (250).

## The use of dentin bonding agents: should exposed dentin be lined?

Until recently, strategy for the treatment of enamel-dentin fractures without pulp exposure has been dentin coverage with a hard-setting calcium hydroxide containing liner. Clinical experience, however, indicates that hard setting calcium hydroxide cements disintegrate beneath dental restorations with time. This finding has been confirmed both experimentally *in vitro* (255, 256) and *in vivo* (230, 257). Moreover, cultivable and stainable bacteria have been found within the calcium hydroxide liners used in both exposed and pulp capped and non-exposed control teeth and these are thus unable to provide a permanent barrier against microleakage (230, 257). Finally, it has been found *in vitro* that calcium hydroxide liners can have the same softening effect on composite resins as zinc oxide-eugenol liners (258). The long-term benefit of their use is therefore questionable (259). While a light-cured calcium hydroxide liner might prove more stable clinically, no long-term data exists at present.

What appears to be critical to pulpal healing is how effectively the dentin is sealed from bacterial irritants. If deeply exposed dentin is adequately sealed, the non-exposed pulp will form reparative dentin even without calcium hydroxide.

Microleakage around composite resin restorations is one of the major causes of restoration failure (260). Microleakage can be counteracted in part by a strong micromechanical bond arising between a composite resin and acid-etched *enamel* (261–263). If *dentin* bonding is also employed, it has been shown experimentally that the bonding strength of

reattached crown fragments is approximately 3 times greater than if only acid-etched enamel is the only source of retention (264).

The goal of a dentin bonding agent is, therefore, to supplement enamel acid etching by mediating a bond between an adhesive resin and the dentin surface. This would imply a hermetic seal against the oral flora and optimize pulpal healing after fracture.

As the bond strength of any dentin bonding system is proportional to the surface area of available unlined dentin for bonding, it is important that any calcium hydroxide liner does not cover more dentin than is absolutely necessary.

Research into the impact of bacteria on pulpal healing (versus the impact of restorative material toxicity) has led to the concept of a single-step total etch technique (i.e. simultaneous enamel and dentin conditioning) (265).

Such an approach greatly simplifies the bonding procedures. Moreover, experimental results indicate little adverse pulpal response (266). However, long-term clinical pulpal response to such procedures has not yet been documented. An important key to the success of either the total etch or dual step approach appears to be the chemical and physicochemical aspects of the (dentin) bonding system employed.

Thus, it has been demonstrated that the chemical reactions needed for dentin bonding require compatibility between dentin or conditioned dentin and the adhesive resin with respect to polarity and solubility parameters (269). For example, to achieve minimum gap formation (270) and maximum bond strength with the original GLUMA® dentin bonding system (Bayer Corp., Leverkusen BRD), a neutral dentin surface is necessary (271, 272). Simultaneous acid etching the dentin and enamel thus lowers the pH of the dentin surface and weakens bond strength (273, 274).

The above findings might imply that a calcium hydroxide liner could be eliminated and a dentin bonding agent used to maximize bonding area and minimize gap formation between the tooth surface and the composite resin restoration to ensure pulpal healing. However, at present, the clinical durability of the bond achieved is unknown. Clinical failure might arise due to polymerization contraction, thermally induced dimensional changes or mechanical stress or fatigue of the material used. This may imply renewed contamination of the dentin surface and subsequent risk to pulpal integrity. Until further data exists, treatment strategy of deep dentin fractures would, therefore, imply application of *glass ionomer cement* to the deepest aspect of the fracture and then use of a dentin bonding agent to complete the hermetic seal against the oral environment. The advantages of glass ionomer liners are many. The material does not require etching, which simplifies application. It is hydrophilic, which implies that it can adhere to newly exposed dentin, with an outward flow of dentinal fluid (342). Moreover, little microleakage is found compared to other liners (344). Finally, there is good pulpal biocompatibility, which has been demonstrated in many studies (345–348). In summary, these findings indicate that glass ionomer cement may be an ideal material for temporary coverage (bandage), as a liner for deep fractures prior to restoration with resin composite or for restoration of crown-fractured teeth.

While the use of dentin bonding agents would immediately appear to be easier, modern restorative dentistry involves the use of uncompromisingly demanding dental materials. And such an approach implies great sensitivity of technique and places responsibility upon the clinician for meticulous tissue and moisture control and attention to detail that is required for treatment success.

## Enamel-dentin crown fractures with pulp exposure

The principles for the restoration of crown fractures with pulpal involvement differ from those of uncomplicated crown fractures only with respect to treatment of the exposed dental pulp. This implies pulp capping, partial pulpotomy or pulpal extirpation, which are described in Chapter 22.

## Provisional treatment of crown fractures

### Uncomplicated fractures

Several approaches exist, depending on the trauma setting (i.e. whether private practice or an emergency room) and the need for an immediate esthetic solution. All approaches rest on the premise of creating a hermetic seal against bacterial invasion into dentinal tubules.

### Glass ionomer cement 'bandage'

This is a very simple procedure, whereby light- or chemically activated glass ionomer cement is used to cover the exposed dentin and adjacent enamel (Fig. 10.12). The advantage of using glass ionomer instead of composite in this situation is that no etching is required and that the relatively low bond strength of glass ionomer to enamel and dentin facilitates its removal.

Before application, the tooth surfaces are rinsed with a water spray or saline. Increments of glass ionomer cement can be used to build up the 'bandage' esthetically. This procedure is especially useful in the case of multiple fractures and limited resources for definitive restorative procedures (e.g. emergency room settings).

All of these findings indicate that glass ionomer may be an ideal material for temporary coverage (bandage) or as a liner for deep fractures before restoration with composite restoration.

### Resin or celluloid crowns

When esthetic demands are foremost, a temporary acrylic crown should be considered. Various types of prefabricated temporary crowns are available. Resin or celluloid crown forms have too little strength for this purpose and should only be used as a mould for the crown. After placement of a calcium hydroxide liner or glass ionomer over the fracture surface, a suitable crown form is selected and contoured to fit the fractured tooth. A hole is made with a sharp explorer through the mesial or distal incisal corner to permit escape of excess crown material during placement. The fitted form is then filled with a composite resin or resin material, seated, and excess resin removed. When polymerized, the crown is removed, finished and cemented (60, 186). The crown is finished short of the gingival margin in order to permit optimal gingival health and prevent the restorative material from being forced into the injured periodontal ligament.

## Splints as coverage

In case of concomitant injuries to the periodontium, dentin and pulp protection must be incorporated into the splint. In these instances, it is a good idea for ease of splint removal and later restoration to cover the exposed enamel and dentin with a calcium hydroxide liner or glass ionomer before application of an acid-etch/resin splint. Enamel coverage with a liner is especially important in the case of later reattachment of the fractured crown fragment to ensure an intact enamel margin to which the fragment can be bonded (see later). In the case of profound crown fracture and simultaneous need for splinting, a fiber-reinforced splint can be the solution for satisfactory retention until splint removal and final restoration (276, 277).

## Definitive treatment of crown fractures

Because of the recent improvements in dental materials available, the boundary between provisional and definitive treatment has become less and less distinct.

Various cast semipermanent restorations (e.g. basket crowns, gold-acrylic open-faced crowns and pinledge inlays) have been designed in the past to meet the esthetic demands of a young traumatized permanent dentition until such time as definitive treatment was considered appropriate (60, 64, 70, 74–87, 99–110, 188). However, with the advent of composite resin materials and the acid etch technique (129–169, 180, 181, 261–263, 278, 279), the indications for these restorations has been eliminated. Moreover, in many situations, considering the life expectancy of these new materials, other definitive treatments of the past might not be necessary or might actually be over treatment.

Definitive restoration of crown fractures presently consists of composite restorations (375) (see Chapter 25, p. 716), reattachment of the original crown fragment (see later), full crown coverage (70, 76, 80, 94, 99–110), partial crown coverage or laminate veneers (280, 281) (see later).

**Fig. 10.12 Provisional coverage of an enamel dentin fracture with glass ionomer cement**
A glove-covered finger can be used to mould the palatal surface of the glass ionomer.

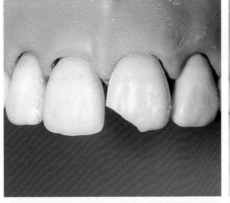
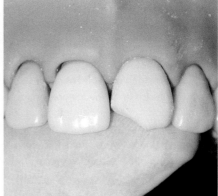

Application of glass ionomer.

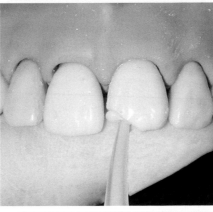
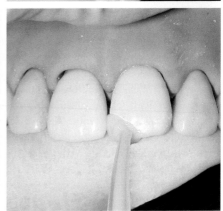

Moulding and curing the glass ionomer.

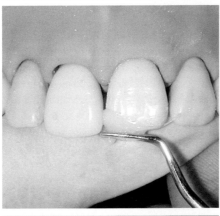
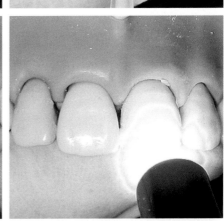

The finished glass ionomer bandage.

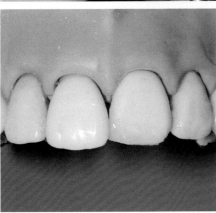
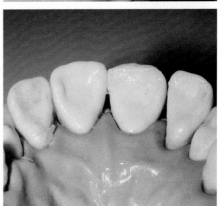

## Reattachment of the original crown fragment

Reattachment of the fragment provides several advantages over other forms of dental restoration following crown fracture. It results in exact restoration of crown and surface morphology in a material that abrades at the same rate as adjacent teeth. Chair time for the completion of the restoration is minimal, normally requiring less time than that needed for completion of a temporary restoration (Fig. 10.13).

Prior to the advent of dentin bonding agents, the only available method of fragment reattachment was by the use of enamel acid etching. Preparation of the tooth and avulsed fragment included either an internal bevel of enamel on both fracture surfaces (282) or simply hollowing out of the dentin of the fragment fracture surface to accommodate a thickness of hard-setting calcium hydroxide liner on the fracture surface of the tooth. This was then followed by enamel etching and adhesion of fragments using a creamy mixture of unfilled and filled composite resin on both fracture surfaces (282–295). Reports of these procedures have been anecdotal and with mixed long-term success. The concept of fragment reattachment was, therefore, re-evaluated with the development of the new dentin bonding agents in the mid-1980s (296–303, 350).

Reattachment of fractured enamel-dentin crown fragments using the original GLUMA® dentin bonding system was begun as a routine treatment of complicated and uncomplicated crown fractures by the authors and co-workers in 1984 (304, 305). As already mentioned, in vitro studies demonstrated a three-fold increase in fracture strength if a dentin bonding agent supplemented retention from acid-etched enamel (264). However, the bonding strengths achieved were only 50–60% that of intact teeth (264).

Recently it has been shown in in vitro testings that beveling along the fracture line may increase the fracture resistance (359, 360, 369).

In animal studies, the bonding system has been proved safe for pulpal tissues as long as a 0.2 mm thickness of dentin remained between the pulp and the bonding surface. However, the adverse pulpal response seen after 8 days when the remaining dentin thickness was less than 0.2 mm was not evident at 90 days (306).

At the time the GLUMA® dentin bonding system was introduced and crown fracture bonding initiated, it was one of the most promising of the dentin bonding agents available. Since then, significant advances have been made in the area of dentin bonding agents and bond strength to dentin (307–311, 351–358, 370, 371). Fracture strengths have been achieved, which are not significantly different from that of intact teeth (352). However, it should be considered that present laboratory tests cannot simulate a traumatic injury (353). But, at least in the case of reattachment of crown fragments, recent experiments have shown that successful frag-ment bonding can be achieved irrespective of the dentin bonding agent used as long as the manufacturer's directions are followed closely (264, 312).

## Indications

It goes without saying that successful fragment reattachment is dependent upon fragment retrieval at the time of injury. As in the correct treatment of tooth avulsions, fragment retrieval requires an informed public. In Scandinavia, public information campaigns in the form of television spots and posters have proved successful in informing patients of their role in treatment success.

An intact enamel-dentin fragment is the sole indication for reattachment. That is, the majority of the enamel margin should be present so that the fragment can rest firmly against the fracture surface when it is tried against the fractured tooth. Small defects, however, can be restored with composite resin at the time of or following the bonding procedure. Moreover, if the fragment is in 2 pieces, these fragments can be bonded together prior to bonding the final fragment (Fig. 10.13).

## Treatment strategy

In 1994, at the time of publication of the third edition, treatment strategy for fragment reattachment was defined according to eventual pulpal involvement and thickness of remaining dentin in the case of no pulpal involvement. However, since then, a clinical study has been published which indicates that enamel-dentin tooth fragments can be reattached without a hazard to pulpal vitality at the time of injury (362). Immediate fragment reattachment has several advantages: short treatment time (often compared to traditional temporary/emergency measures), an immediate hermetic seal of dentinal tubules, immediate restoration of function and esthetics. The bonding procedure is illustrated in Fig. 10.13.

However, there can be situations that are not conducive to this approach, e.g. an unruly patient, where the traumatic event should be put at a distance prior to successful definitive treatment or a concomitant luxation injury, which would imply difficulties in maintaining a dry operating field.

If provisional treatment is the chosen strategy and there is an uncomplicated crown fracture, the entire fracture surface (enamel and dentin) can be covered with glass ionomer cement and a provisional restoration placed for approximately one month to permit hard tissue deposition in the pulp horn. The use of a calcium hydroxide liner has been found to lower the strength of future fragment bonding and should, therefore, be avoided (355). Placement of provisional restorations can be incorporated in the necessary splints and bonding performed at the time of splint removal. In the interim period, the crown fragment is kept moist, e.g. in tap water or physiologic saline which is changed weekly. If the coronal fragment has been allowed to

**Fig. 10.13 Reattaching a crown fragment with a dentin bonding agent and reinforcement of the bonding site with composite resin**
This 10-year-old boy has fractured his central incisor after a fall from his skateboard. The fracture is very close to the mesial pulp horn.

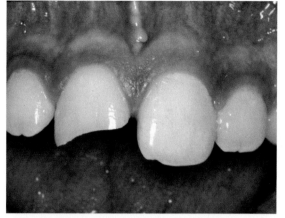
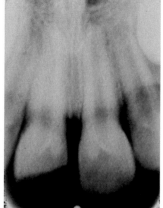

**Testing pulpal sensibility**
Pulpal response to sensibility testing is normal. The radiographic examination shows no displacement or root fracture.

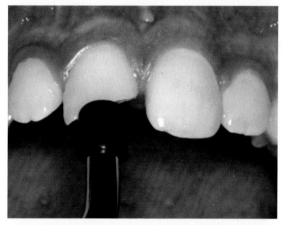
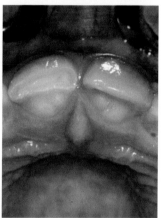

**Testing the fit of the fragment**
The fragment fits exactly. The enamel surface is intact, with no apparent defect at the enamel margins.

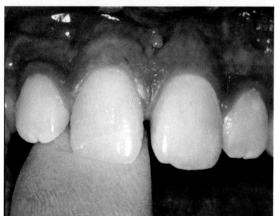
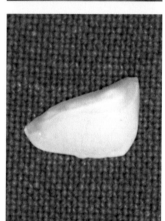

**Temporary dentin coverage with calcium hydroxide**
Due to the close proximity of the fracture surface to the pulp, a temporary glass ionomer lining is placed on the exposed dentin and enamel prior to placement of the temporary restoration.

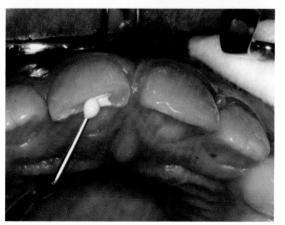
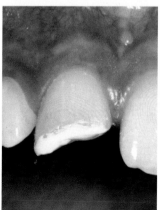

### Etching the enamel

A 2-mm wide zone of enamel around the fracture surface is etched.

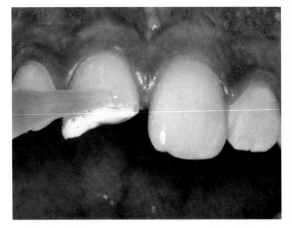 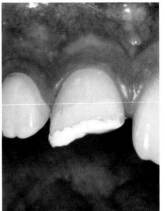

### Covering the fracture surface

The tooth is temporarily restored with a temporary crown and bridge material. To provide greater stability, the restoration may be extended to adjacent teeth.

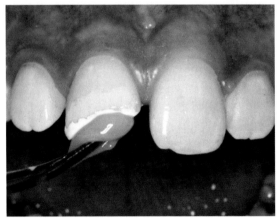 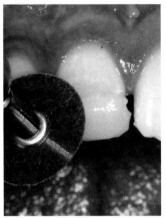

### Storage of the crown fragment

The tooth is stored in physiologic saline for 1 month. The patient is given the fragment and is instructed to change the solution once a week to reduce contamination.

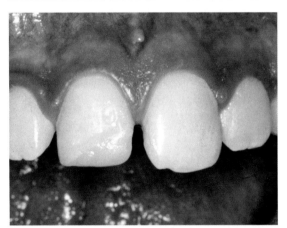 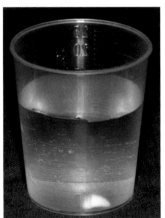

### Bonding of the fragment after 1 month

The temporary cover is removed and the fragment is fastened to a piece of sticky wax for ease of handling.

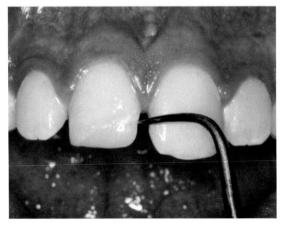 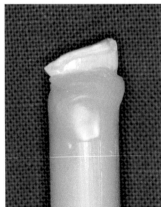

## Preparing for bonding

Pulpal sensibility is monitored and the fracture surfaces (of the tooth and crown fragment) are cleansed with a pumice-water slurry and a rubber cup.

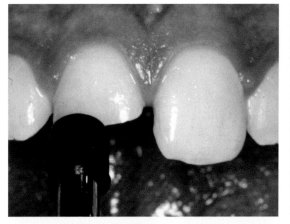 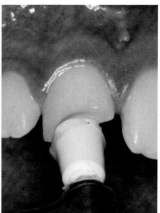

## Etching enamel

Enamel on both fracture surfaces as well as a 2-mm wide collar of enamel cervical and incisal to the fracture are etched for 30 seconds with 35% phosphoric acid being sure that the etchant does not come in contact with dentin.

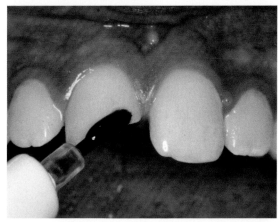 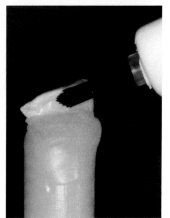

## Removal of the etchant

The fracture surfaces are rinsed thoroughly with a copious flow of water for 20 seconds.

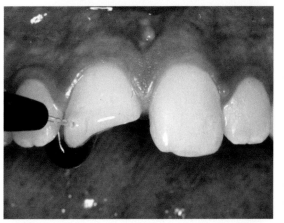 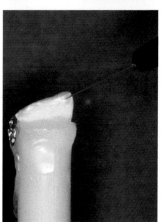

## Drying the fracture surfaces

The fracture surfaces are air-dried for 10 seconds. NOTE: To avoid entrapment of air in the dentinal tubules and a subsequent chalky mat discoloration of the fragment, the air stream must be directed parallel with the fracture surface and not perpendicular to it.

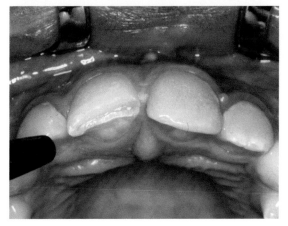 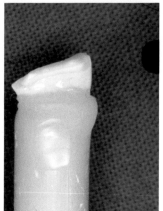

### Conditioning the dentin with EDTA and GLUMA®

The fracture surfaces are conditioned with EDTA for 20 seconds, followed by 10 seconds water rinse and 10 seconds air drying. Thereafter 20 seconds GLUMA® and 10 seconds air drying.

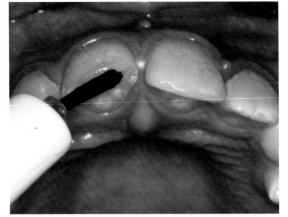 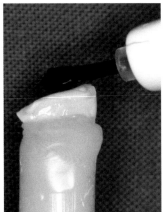

### Bonding the fragment

The fracture surfaces are covered with a creamy mixture of a filled composite and its unfilled resin. After repositioning of the fragment, the composite is light-polymerized.

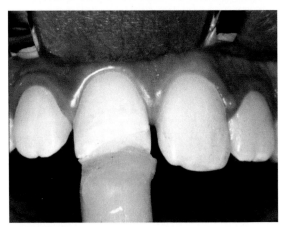 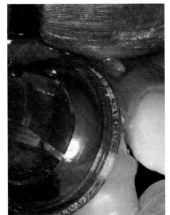

### Light polymerization

The composite is light polymerized 60 seconds facially and 60 seconds orally.

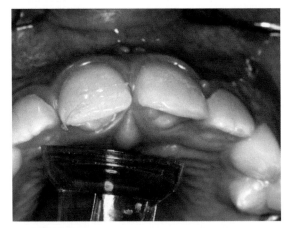 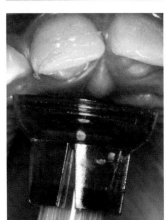

### Removal of surplus composite

With a straight scalpel blade or composite finishing knives surplus composite is removed from the fracture site. The interproximal contacts are finished with finishing strips.

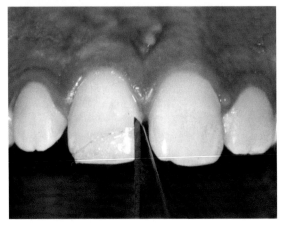 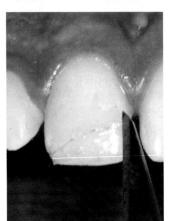

### Reinforcing the labial aspect of the fracture site

A round diamond bur is used to create a 'double chamfer' margin 1 mm coronally and apically to the fracture line. To achieve optimal esthetics, the chamfer follows an undulating path along the fracture line.

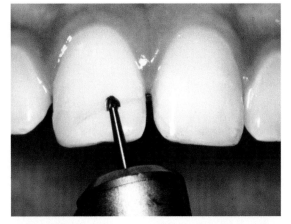
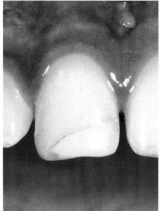

### Finishing the labial surface

After restoring the labial aspect with composite, the restoration is contoured using abrasive discs.

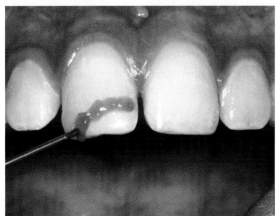
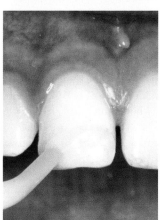

### Reinforcing the palatal aspect of the fracture

The palatal aspect of the fracture is reinforced using the same procedure. Due to its position, esthetic consideration is less. The preparation can, therefore, follow the fracture line exactly.

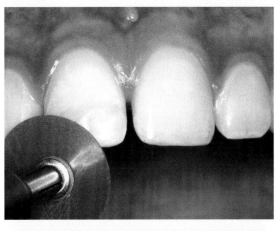
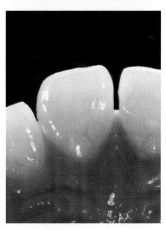

### Final restoration

The condition 1 month after reattachment of the crown fragment.

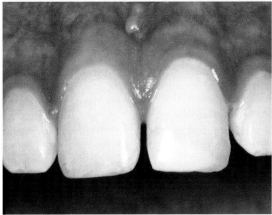
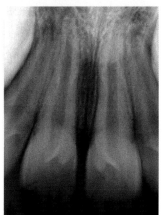

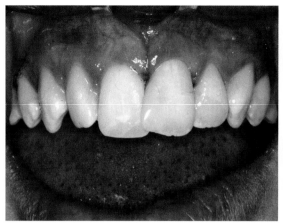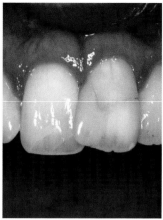

**Fig. 10.14** Esthetic problems following crown fragment reattachment due to discoloration of the composite bonding material at the fracture line. Left: appearance at the time of fragment bonding of the maxillary left central incisor. Right: appearance one year later. There is discoloration of the bonding material.

dry out prior to bonding, the fragment will whiten; and *in vitro* tests have shown a decreased bonding strength of such a fragment (354, 356). In these cases, wet storage of at least 24 hours can normalize the situation (354).

It should be considered that the use of eugenol-containing liners or cements is not recommended on teeth where dentin/resin bonding is anticipated, as bonding strength can be reduced (301) presumably due to the complexing action of eugenol with calcium in sound dentin (313). However, the deleterious effect of eugenol-containing provisional cements on *enamel bonding* is presumably eliminated if the bonding surface is cleaned with pumice and etched with phosphoric acid prior to restoration due to the mechanical nature of the bond (314). Thus, non-eugenol cement is recommended in situations where provisional therapy is indicated (e.g. crown fractures with concomitant luxation injuries and cases of multiple dental injuries).

Treatment strategy for crown fractures with pulpal involvement includes pulpotomy (see Chapter 22, p. 605), provisional restoration and a 3-month observation period to permit formation of a hard tissue barrier at the exposure site; or direct bonding of the fragment can be performed after pulpotomy.

Lately, a series of new bonding procedures have been developed and appear to yield increased bond strength (352). The early dentin bonding agents worked on a dry dentin surface. Drying of the etched surface apparently leads to collapse of the collagen meshwork, making it difficult for an adhesive primer to penetrate due to limited porosity (364) Thus, the newer dental adhesives which bond to a moist dentin surface have led to improved results (363–365). Another benefit of the newer dental adhesives and their action on moist dentin is the expanded area of application in the treatment of fractures close to the gingival crevice.

## Clinical results of fragment reattachment

With respect to the long-term success of fragment reattachment, factors such as pulpal response, esthetics and retention of the fragment should be considered.

## Pulpal response to fragment reattachment

The reattachment of enamel-dentin crown fragments has not been found to lead to pulpal complications in a larger long-term study (250). The few cases of pulp necrosis and pulp canal obliteration were all found in relation to concomitant luxation injuries. This low complication rate is more likely a response to the injury itself than to the treatment procedure.

## Esthetics following fragment reattachment

Approximately half of the teeth bonded demonstrate acceptable esthetics at long-term follow-up (250). Esthetic problems at the follow-up controls include discoloration or degradation of the composite bonding material at the fracture line (Fig. 10.14) or discoloration of the incisal fragment with time. The problem of discoloration of the fracture line is most pronounced in earlier cases of bonding, due to discoloration of the catalyst system of the chemically-cured resins used. This problem has been solved in part by the use of light-cured composite materials. Esthetics have also been enhanced by the use of a double chamfer preparation along the fracture line after fragment bonding and restoration with a composite resin (see Fig. 10.13).

The problem of fragment discoloration, usually to a mat white color, is presumably due to dehydration of the underlying dentin (250). This is more difficult to manage clinically, as direct composite facings tend not to mask the color disharmony between the tooth and bonded fragment.

## Fragment retention

Results from a Scandinavian study indicate that 60% of the bonded fragments were lost after 5 years due primarily to a new trauma or nonphysiological use of the restored teeth (252) (Fig. 10.15). Fragment debonding occurred irrespective of the use of enamel acid etch alone or supplemented with GLUMA dentin bonding agent; also irrespective of the use of composite resin along the fracture line for esthetic revision and reinforcement of the restoration. While fragment debonding represents a practical inconvenience, it has

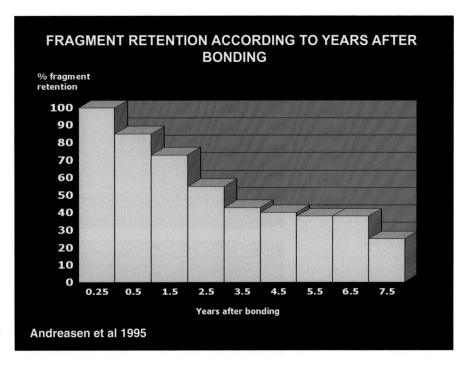

**FRAGMENT RETENTION ACCORDING TO YEARS AFTER BONDING**

Andreasen et al 1995

**Fig. 10.15** Survival of fragment bonding. From ANDREASEN et al. (252) 1995.

no impact on pulpal vitality since debonding occurs as a cohesive failure within the bonding resin and not in dentin. Thus, the fracture surfaces of teeth with debonded fragments are glossy from retained resin plugs within the treated dentin. For this reason, the dentin must be freed of bonded resin, e.g. with a slurry of pure pumice and water, prior to rebonding of fragments.

It would seem that at present reattachment of the original incisal fragment can only be considered as an acceptable semi-permanent anterior restoration whereby gross and surface anatomy are restored perfectly with a material that abrades at a rate identical to adjacent teeth and which does not threaten pulpal vitality (305, 315, 316). Development of new dentin bonding systems and/or resins might provide improved fragment retention.

Fragment reattachment or restoration with a composite build-up is a realistic treatment alternative in the young (preteen and teenage) patient groups. These treatments serve to postpone the time of definitive treatment until an age when the gingival marginal contours are relatively stable (i.e. 20 years of age).

Finally, it should be mentioned that laminate veneers under laboratory conditions can restore or even increase the strength of a fractured incisor treated by reattachment of the original fragment to attain the strength of an intact tooth (see later) (280, 281) (Figs 10.16 and 10.17).

## Laminate veneers in the treatment of crown fractures

### Indications

Clinical experience seems to indicate expanded areas of application for ceramic veneering (Fig. 10.16). Ceramic veneers can be used with advantage in the treatment of trau-

matic dental injuries in cases of acquired discoloration (pulp necrosis and pulp canal obliteration), crown fractures and crown defects due to developmental disturbances, as well as restoration of autotransplanted premolars to the anterior region due to anterior tooth loss (see Chapter 27). Furthermore, veneers can be used as an important supplement in the treatment of crown fractures following reattachment of the enamel-dentin fragment. Thus, recent experimental studies demonstrated that fracture strength of fractured incisors with bonded fragments can be increased from half, to equal to or sometimes exceeding the fracture strength of intact teeth if restored with porcelain or cast ceramic veneers respectively, as long as the preparation was limited to enamel (281) (see later). Moreover, the fracture strength of a fractured incisor restored *in vitro* with a cast ceramic veneer alone (i.e. no preliminary composite build-up or fragment reattachment) is on average more than 1.5 times greater than intact control teeth (281). These experimental studies indicate that a conservative treatment approach (i.e. versus full crown coverage) might be justified in restoring esthetics and function to the traumatized anterior dentition and at the same time preserve tooth substance, maintain occlusal relationships and maintain pulpal vitality.

Because of optical properties which are similar to enamel, ceramic veneers have the advantage over direct composite veneering of consistently good esthetic results. Moreover, there is good marginal adaptation, minimal plaque retention, long-term stability with respect to color and anatomy, inherent strength of veneering material and reasonably limited chair time to complete treatment in comparison to direct composite veneering (318–320). Fabrication of ceramic veneers, however, is a technically demanding procedure. There must be a high level of cooperation and communication between patient, dentist and laboratory technician if the patient's subjective and objective functional and esthetic needs are to be fulfilled (321).

### Fig. 10.16 Use of veneer to improve esthetics after fragment reattachment

Clinical appearance after fragment reattachment following a complicated crown fracture in a 9-year-old girl. Six years after treatment, there is discoloration of the composite bonding resin.

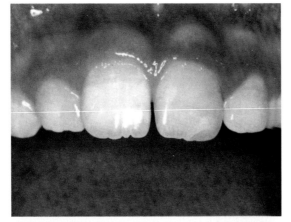
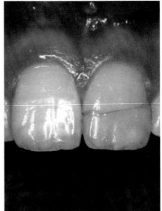

### Preparation of tooth

Gingival retraction cord is used to permit a slightly subgingival placement of margins to ensure optimal esthetics. Mounted diamonds used for enamel reduction.

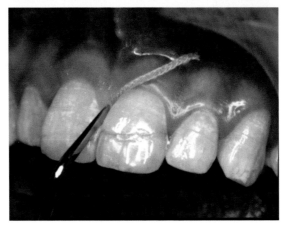
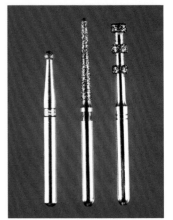

### Initial enamel reduction

The incisor is isolated with a dead soft metal matrix strip and the triple cutting diamond is used for initial depth cuts of 0.5 mm facially.

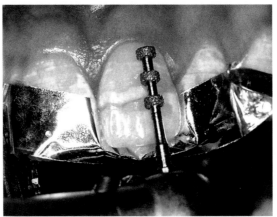
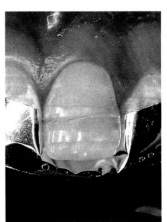

### Final enamel reduction

To ensure uniform enamel reduction, the tapered diamond is used to reduce only one-half of the facial surface at a time. Approximately 1 mm is removed incisally to permit optimal porcelain translucency in this region. Finishing lines are enhanced using a round diamond, which also permits additional veneer bulk at the margins.

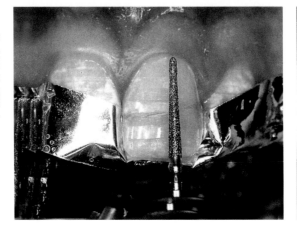
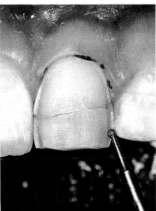

**Completed preparation**
Note uniform tissue reduction following the curve of the tooth. A second cord is placed to ensure adequate tissue retraction, which is removed immediately prior to impression taking, while the first cord is removed once a satisfactory impression has been obtained.

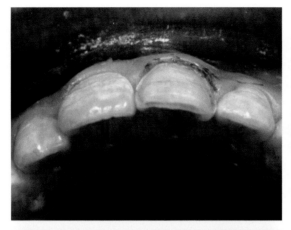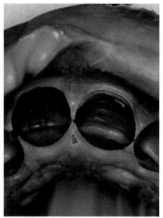

**Final restoration**
Dicor veneer cemented using a light-activated dual cement (Dicor LAC®) (Technique: Flügge's Dental Laboratory, Copenhagen). Radiographic condition 6 years after injury. Pulp vitality has been maintained.

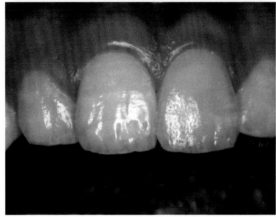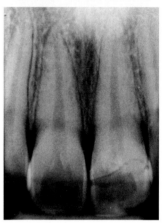

## Contraindications

In cases of malposed teeth, where a direct access line of insertion cannot be secured, veneering is not recommended (322, 323). Moreover, ceramic veneers are contraindicated in patients who are bruxers or with parafunctional activity or habits (e.g. nail biters, pipe smokers) (317, 324, 325). Ceramic veneers are fragile and the shearing stresses elicited by such habits may be too great for the veneer to withstand. Moreover, they are contraindicated in teeth that are composed predominantly of dentin and cementum (317, 322). This is due to compromised bonding to dentin with the presently available dentin bonding agents. Finally, teeth showing grey discoloration are very difficult to mask, and the success of ceramic veneers in these cases can be limited (325).

While some reports seem to indicate acceptable success as long as the bulk of the preparation and margins remain in enamel under experimental conditions (317, 322, 326), preparation into dentin has shown reduced strength (281). Furthermore greater microleakage was recorded at the cervical dentin/composite resin interface than at the cervical enamel/composite interface of bonded ceramic veneers (327).

There has been some debate concerning whether or not cervical enamel should be reduced prior to the taking of impressions (328–332). It would seem that at least gingival health is improved if enamel is reduced in order to diminish the risk of over contouring of the restoration as well as to provide a well-defined finishing line for the fabrication of the restoration. The resultant accuracy of fit, especially with castable ceramics (333), reduces the need for marginal finishing at the time of cementation and thereby produces a smooth surface which is less plaque-retentive.

## Patient selection: treatment problems to be solved

As many crown fractures occur in the younger age groups, the question arises as to when to provide ceramic veneering as a treatment option. The porcelain veneer has been considered a useful cosmetic procedure for correction of minor functional problems in the young dentition (e.g. rotated or lingually inclined incisors, spacing and defects in mineralization) (321).

If it is decided to build the incisor up in a composite resin prior to veneering (e.g. to achieve uniform ceramic thickness in the final restoration), at least 2 weeks should elapse prior to taking impressions for the veneer to allow for dimensional stability of the composite (334).

In the patient illustrated in Fig 10.17, the fractured crown fragments were bonded and the tooth thereafter veneered. However, experimental results might justify a more direct treatment approach in adult patients (281).

Some situations require earlier definitive treatment. This can be in the situation of congenital enamel malformations where due to their superior esthetic properties and very low plaque retention ceramic veneers can be a realistic treatment option.

### Fig. 10.17 Improved esthetics achieved by ceramic veneering after fragment reattachment

Clinical and radiographic condition one year after fragment following an uncomplicated enamel-dentin fracture in a 25-year-old man. Note color harmony between tooth and fragment. Because of porcelain's very low affinity for stain and plaque accumulation, it is necessary to determine shade prior to stain removal, otherwise there is a serious risk that the veneer will always be too light in relation to adjacent teeth.

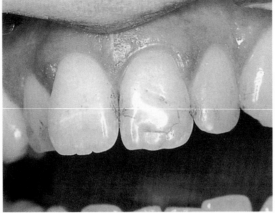 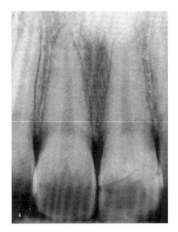

### Veneer preparation

There is uniform enamel reduction mesiodistally following the curve of the facial surface and the proximal contacts.

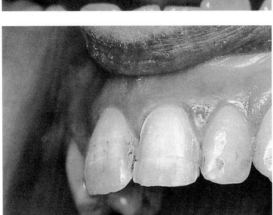 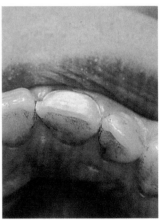

### Finished restoration

The veneer in place after cementation. Note the facial 'discoloration' incorporated into the surface to mimic tobacco stain, as well as the hypoplastic striae, similar to those seen on the surface of the right central incisor. Note gingival health and harmony of the restoration within the dental arch at the one-year follow-up. (Technique: Flügge's Dental Laboratory, Copenhagen).

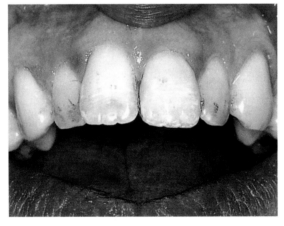 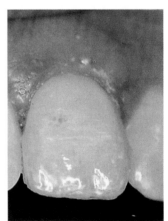

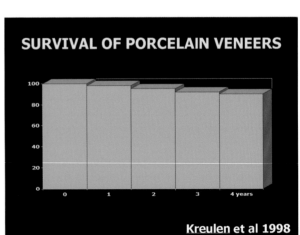

**Fig. 10.18** Survival of laminate veneers. From KREULEN et al. (366) 1998.

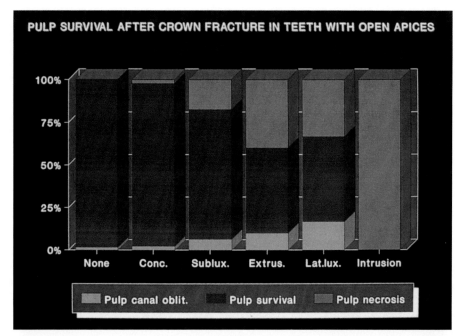

**Fig. 10.19** Pulp survival following crown fracture in the permanent dentition with immature root formation (open apices) in relation to concomitant luxation injuries. From ANDREASEN & ANDREASEN (376) 2006.

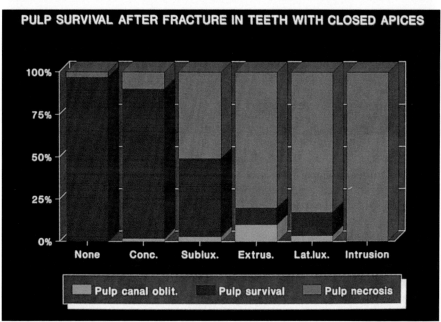

**Fig. 10.20** Pulp survival following crown fracture in the permanent dentition with mature root formation (closed apices) in relation to concomitant luxation injuries. From ANDREASEN & ANDREASEN (376) 2006.

In the case of severe trauma leading to anterior tooth loss, autotransplantation can be a treatment solution. Such teeth can also be restored with veneers (see Chapter 27).

Clinical evaluation of porcelain veneers has shown very promising results with respect to longevity of restorations, fractures, and secondary caries (322, 325, 329, 331, 332, 335). Thus a meta-analysis of 1552 porcelain veneer restorations derived from 9 studies showed a 92% survival after 3 years (366) (Fig. 10.18).

## Prognosis of crown fractures

### Pulp survival

Pulpal sensibility reactions in crown fractured teeth are often lowered immediately after injury (7, 72, 187, 195).

Usually 1 to 8 weeks can elapse before a normal pulpal response can be elicited. However, longer observation periods can be required. Pulp testing can usually be carried out during this observation period without removing the temporary restoration (see Chapter 9, p. 265). In the following the risk of pulp necrosis is presented for the various types of fracture. It appears that the most important factor is an associated luxation injury (Figs 10.19, 10.20).

### Enamel infractions

The prognosis of isolated infractions with respect to risk of pulp necrosis appears to be very good (Table 10.1). Thus, three studies have shown risks between 0 and 3.5%, which is about the same as for 'non-injured control teeth' (193, 195–197); which implies that the few cases with pulp necro-

**Table 10.1** Prevalence of pulp necrosis after crown infraction.

| Examiner | No. of teeth | Pulp necrosis |
|---|---|---|
| Stålhane & Hedegård (116) 1975 | 656 | 23 (3.5%) |
| Ravn (194) 1981 | 174 | 0 (0%) |
| Robertson (372) 1998 | 16 | 0 (0%) |

**Table 10.2** Prevalence of pulp necrosis after enamel fracture.

| Examiner | No. of teeth | Pulp necrosis |
|---|---|---|
| Fialova & Jurecek (62) 1968 | 31 | 0 (0%) |
| Stålhane & Hedegård (116) 1975 | 876 | 2 (0.2%) |
| Ravn (195) 1981 | 2862 | 29 (1%) |
| Robertson (372) 1998 | 46 | 0 (0%) |

**Table 10.3** Prevalence of pulp necrosis after crown fracture with exposed dentin.

| Examiner | No. of teeth | Pulp necrosis |
|---|---|---|
| Stålhane & Hedegård (116) 1975 | 413 | 3 (1%) |
| Zadik et al. (120) 1979 | 123 | 7 (6%) |
| Ravn (196) 1981 | 3144 | 250 (6%) |
| Robertson (372) 1998 | 60 | 2 (2%) |
| Robertson et al. (373) 2000 | 106 | 0 (0%) |

**Table 10.4** Relation between associated luxation injuries to enamel-dentin fractures upon frequency pulp necrosis. After RAVN (196) 1981.

| | No. of teeth | Pulp necrosis |
|---|---|---|
| Enamel-dentin fracture | 3144 | 100 (3%) |
| Enamel-dentin fracture + concussion | 327 | 19 (6%) |
| Enamel-dentin fracture + subluxation | 423 | 106 (25%) |

**Table 10.5** Relation between extent of enamel-dentin fracture upon pulp necrosis. After RAVN (196) 1981.

| | No. of teeth | No. with pulp necrosis |
|---|---|---|
| Small mesial fracture | 1034 | 26 (0.2%) |
| Comprehensive mesial fracture | 435 | 30 (7%) |
| Fracture involving the entire incisal edge | 1019 | 38 (0.4%) |

**Table 10.6** Relation between treatment upon frequency of pulp necrosis in teeth with extensive mesial or distal enamel-dentin fractures. After RAVN (196) 1981.

| | No. of teeth | No. with pulp necrosis |
|---|---|---|
| No treatment | 24 | 13 (54%) |
| Dentin coverage | 620 | 30 (8%) |

sis possibly reflect overlooked concussion or subluxation injuries.

## Enamel fractures

In two sets of studies, the risk of pulp necrosis was found to range from 0.2 to 1.0% (Table 10.2, Figs 10.19, 10.20). Using the above-mentioned rationale, these figures would imply virtually no risk to the pulp.

## Enamel-dentin fractures without pulpal involvement

The overall risk of pulp necrosis irrespective of the extent of fracture and type of treatment ranges from 1 to 6% (Table 10.3, Figs 10.19, 10.20). In this regard, it should be noted that factors, such as associated luxation injuries, stage of root development, type of treatment and extent of fracture exert significant influence upon the risk of pulp necrosis. A detailed study on the combined effects of these factors has been reported by Ravn (196).

With respect to the effect of *stage of root development* on the risk of pulp necrosis after uncomplicated crown fracture

with or without concomitant luxation injury, it has been found that teeth with constricted apices have a significantly greater risk of pulp necrosis than do teeth with open apices (316, 373, 376). Furthermore that the extent of periodontal ligament injury as revealed by the *luxation diagnosis* is significantly related to pulp survival after injury (373) (Table 10.4 and Figs 10.19 and 10.20).

Another factor to be considered is the *extent* and *location* of the fracture. Thus, horizontal and proximal superficial (corner) fractures demonstrate a very low frequency of pulp necrosis; whereas deep proximal fractures show increased risk (Table 10.5).

Only a single study has examined the *effect of treatment* (i.e. untreated versus treated crown fractures). A treatment effect was only in operation for deep proximal fractures (Table 10.6). In this connection, *no treatment* was found to be associated with 54% pulp necrosis; whereas *dentin coverage* resulted in a decrease to 8% (196).

The effect of time interval between injury and dentin coverage and subsequent risk of pulp necrosis has yet to be examined (374). A certain relationship has been claimed in one study but associated luxation injuries were not monitored (196).

In Fig. 10.21 the predictors for pulp necrosis are shown.

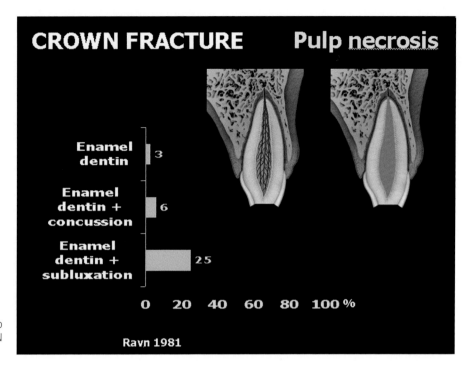

**Fig. 10.21** Predictors for pulp necrosis after crown fracture. RAVN (194–196) 1981.

**Table 10.7** Prevalence of pulp canal obliteration and root resorption after crown fracture. After STÅLHANE & HEDEGÅRD (116) 1975.

|  | No. of teeth | No. with pulp canal obliteration | No. with external root resorption |
|---|---|---|---|
| Enamel infraction | 174 | 0 (0%) | 0 (0%) |
| Enamel fracture | 876 | 4 (0.5%) | 2 (0.2%) |
| Enamel and dentin fracture | 413 | 2 0.5% | 1 (0.2%) |

## Pulp canal obliteration

In one study, pulp canal obliteration (PCO) was analyzed subsequent to crown fractures without associated luxation injury (116) (Table 10.7). The paucity of PCO cases possibly implies non-diagnosed luxation injuries. It seems safe to assume that a crown fracture *per se* does not elicit PCO.

## Root resorption

In one study, where only crown fractures without associated luxation injuries were examined, root resorption was a rare finding (116) (Table 10.7). Thus, like pulp canal obliteration, root resorption is probably not related to crown fractures *per se*.

## Reattachment of the crown fragment

With respect to pulp survival, fragment retention and esthetics, preliminary findings from a long-term clinical study indicate the following (251, 252).

## Pulp survival

Pulp survival without radiographic change was the predominant finding, whereby only 1 out of 198 bonded incisors (0.5%) developed pulp necrosis and 4 developed pulp canal obliteration (2%). All 5 teeth had suffered concomitant luxation injuries (251, 252).

## Essentials

### Terminology (Fig. 10.1)

- Enamel infraction
- Enamel fracture
- Enamel-dentin fracture
- Enamel-dentin fracture with pulp exposure

### Frequency

Permanent dentition: 26–76% of dental injuries

### Etiology

- Usually falls with direct impact on the crown

### History

- Symptoms

### Clinical examination

- Extent of fracture
- Pulp exposure

- Dislocation of tooth
- Reaction to sensibility tests

## Radiographic examination

- Size of pulp cavity
- Stage of root development
- Concomitant root fracture or luxation

## Pathology

- If the pulp is exposed, pulp inflammation normally confined close to the exposure site

## Enamel infraction

### Treatment

- Pulpal sensibility control after 6 to 8 weeks
- Eventual sealing of infraction lines with resin

### Prognosis

- Pulp necrosis (0 to 3.5%)

## Enamel fracture (no dentin exposed)

### Treatment

- Removal of sharp enamel edges
- Corrective grinding (Fig. 10.10) or restoration with a composite resin
- Radiographic and sensibility controls

### Prognosis

- Pulp necrosis (0 to 1.0%)

## Enamel-dentin fracture, no pulp exposure

### Immediate (provisional) treatment (Fig. 10.12)

- Place glass ionomer cement over the exposed dentin and enamel to permit optimal bonding of the restorative material at the time of definitive therapy (Fig. 10.12).
- Alternatively adapt a temporary crown (e.g. acrylic crown). Crown cemented with a non-eugenol containing luting agent.
- Check the occlusion.
- Control the tooth radiographically and with sensibility tests after 6 to 8 weeks.

## Permanent treatment

- Reattachment of the crown fragment (Fig. 10.13)
- Restoration with laminate veneer (Fig. 10.17)
- Restoration with composite resin (see Chapter 25)
- Restoration with full crown coverage

### Prognosis

- Pulp necrosis (0–6%)

## Enamel-dentin fracture with pulp exposure

### Immediate treatment

- Exposed pulp tissue is treated by pulp capping, pulpotomy or pulpectomy (see Chapters 22 and 23).

## References

1. ANDREASEN JO. Etiology and pathogenesis of traumatic dental injuries. A clinical study of 1,298 cases. *Scand J Dent Res* 1970;**78**:329–42.
2. SUNDVALL-HAGLAND I. Olycksfallsskador på tænder och parodontium under barnaåren. In: Holst JJ, Nygaard-Östby B, Osvald O. eds. *Nordisk Klinisk Odontologi*. Copenhagen: A/S Forlaget for Faglitteratur, 1964: Chapter 11, III:1–40.
3. RAVN JJ, ROSSEN I. Hyppighed og fordeling af traumatiske beskadigelser af tænderne hos københavnske skolebørn 1967/68. *Tandlægebladet* 1969;**78**:1–9.
4. MAGNUSSON B, HOLM A-K. Traumatised permanent teeth in children – a follow-up. I. Pulpal complications and root resorption. *Svensk Tandläkaras Tidning* 1969;**62**:61–70.
5. SUTTON PRN. Transverse crack lines in permanent incisors of Polynesians. *Aust Dent J* 1961;**6**:144–50.
6. SUTTON PRN. Fissured fractures; 2501 transverse crack lines in permanent incisors. *Aust Dent J* 1969;**14**:18–21.
7. KRÖNCKE A. Über die Vitalerhaltung der gefährdeten Pulpa nach Fraktur von Frontzahn-Kronen. *Dtsch Zahnärztebl* 1957;**11**:333–6.
8. HARDWICK JL, NEWMAN PA. Some observations on the incidence and emergency treatment of fractured permanent anterior teeth of children. *J Dent Res* 1954;**33**:730.
9. GELBIER S. Injured anterior teeth in children. A preliminary discussion. *Br Dent J* 1967;**123**:331–5.
10. SOBKOWIAK E-M. Unser Standpunkt zur Versorgung frakturierter jugendlicher Zähne. *Zahnärztl Welt* 1965;**66**:502–9.
11. BODECKER CF. Enamel lamellae. A consultant article. *Oral Surg Oral Med Oral Pathol* 1951;**4**:787–98.
12. ORBAN B. *Oral histology and embryology*. 3rd edn. St. Louis: CV Mosby Company, 1953:124.
13. BRÄNNSTRÖM M. Observations on exposed dentine and the corresponding pulp tissue. A preliminary study with replica and routine histology. *Odontologisk Revy* 1962;**13**:235–45.
14. BRÄNNSTRÖM M, ÅSTROM A. A study on the mechanism of pain elicited from the dentin. *J Dent Res* 1964;**43**:619–25.
15. WILLIGER. Zähne und Trauma: *Deutsche Zahnheilkunde in Vortragen*, No. 16. Leipzig: Verlag von Georg Thieme, 1911.
16. DOW PR, THOMPSON ML. Pulp management for the immature fractured anterior tooth. *J Canad Dent Assoc* 1960;**26**:59.

17. KOMINEK J. Urazy frontdlnich zubu u deti. *Cs. Stomatol* 1954;239–60.

18. MALONE AJ, MASSLER M. Fractured anterior teeth. Diagnosis, treatment, and prognosis. Dent Dig 1952;**58**:442–7.

19. HARRIS SD. Fractured incisors. Primary and permanent. *ASDC J Dent Child* 1954;**21**:205–7.

20. BERK H. Maintaining vitality of injured permanent anterior teeth. *J Am Dent Assoc* 1954;**49**:391–401.

21. FRENTZEN H. Die prothetische Behandlung von Frontzahnfrakturen bei Kindern und Jugendlichen. *Dtsch Stornatol* 1964;**14**:904–11.

22. DUNN NA, EICHENBAUM IW. Diagnosis and treatment of fractured anterior teeth. *J Am Dent Assoc* 1952;**44**:166–72.

23. KISLING E. Om behandlingen of skader som følge of akutte mekaniske traumer på unge permanente incisiver. *Tandlægebladet* 1953;**57**:61–9, 109–29.

24. ROTTKE R. Zeitgerechte Behandlung der Schneidezahnfraktur im Wechselgebiss. *Zahnärztl Prax* 1954;**5**:1–4.

25. ANDREWS RG. Emergency treatment of injured permanent anterior teeth. *Dent Clin North Am* 1965;703–10.

26. NOLDEN R. Die konservierende Behandlung der Traumafolgen im Wachstumsalter. *Zahnärztl Welt* 1967;**68**:19–24.

27. RABINOWITCH BZ. The fractured incisor. *Pediatr Clin North Am* 1956;**3**:979–94.

28. NOTERMAN F. Restauration des traumatismes dentaires chez les jeunes. *Rev Belge Stomatol* 1951;**48**:367–81.

29. NOTERMAN F. Les fractures d'incisives en pratique courante. *Rev Belg Sci Dent* 1961;**16**:499–513.

30. CURRY VL. Fractured incisors. *Dent Practit Dent Rec* 1951;**1**:341–6.

31. BROGLIA ML, RE G. Le lesioni traumatiche dei denti permanenti nell'età infantile. *Minerva Stomatatol* 1959;**8**:161–80.

32. SWEET CA. A classification and treatment for traumatized anterior teeth. *ASDC J Dent Child* 1955;**22**:144–9.

33. BRAUER JC. The treatment of children's fractured permanent anterior teeth. *J Am Dent Assoc* 1950;**41**:399–407.

34. BENNETT DT. Traumatised anterior teeth. *Br Dent J* 1963;**115**:346–8, 392–4, 432–5, 487–9.

35. BENNETT DT. Traumatised anterior teeth. *Br Dent J* 1964;**116**:96–8.

36. LENCHNER NH. A diagnosis and treatment plan for traumatized anterior teeth. *ASDC J Dent Child* 1957;**24**:197–205.

37. PALMER JD. Simple emergency treatment of fractured incisors. *Dent Practit Dent Rec* 1969;**20**:102–4.

38. PARKET J, VINCENT R. Fracture de l'incisive centrale permanente entre 7 et 12 ans. *Odont Stomatol Maxillofacial* 1950;**6**:74–7.

39. BROWN WE. The management of injuries to young teeth. *Aust Dent J* 1967;**12**:99–104.

40. TOVERUD G. Traumatiske beskadigelser av incisiver i barnealderen og deres behandling. *Odontologisk Tidskrift* 1947;**55**:7182

41. ELLIS RG. Treatment of fractured incisors. *Int Dent J* 1953;**4**:196–208.

42. OHLSSON A. Behandling av olycksfallsskadade incisiver pa barn. *Odontologisk Tidskrift* 1957;**65**:105–15.

43. MCBRIDE WC. *Juvenile dentistry*. 5th edn. London: Henry Kimpton, 1952:247–62.

44. ADAMS FR. Traumatized and fractured young teeth. *J Am Dent Assoc* 1944;**31**:241–8.

45. COOKE C, ROWBOTHAM TC. Treatment of injuries to anterior teeth. *Br Dent J* 1951;**91**:146–52.

46. BRUCE RH. Inlays for fractured teeth. *Dent J Aust* 1947;**19**:309–14.

47. PANTKE H. Kronenfrakturen permanenter Frontzähne bei Jugendlichen. *Zahnärztl Prax* 1963;**14**:253–6.

48. RIPA LW, FINN SB. The care of injuries to the anterior teeth in children. In: Finn SB. ed. *Clinical Pedodontics*. 3rd edn. Philadelphia: W B Saunders Company, 1967:324–62.

49. HARTSOOK JT. Management of young anterior teeth which have been involved in accidents. *J Am Dent Assoc* 1948;**37**:554–64.

50. RAVN JJ. Ulykkesskadede fortænder på børn. *Klassifikation og behandling*. Copenhagen: Odontologisk Forening, 1966.

51. HORSNELL AM. Everyday procedure. Trauma to the incisor teeth. *Br Dent J* 1952, **93**:105–10.

52. RITZE H. Die Traumen im Frontzahngebiet. *Zahnärztl Prax* 1964;**15**:1–4.

53. STRASSBURG M. Zahnerhaltung nach Trauma im kindlichen Gebiss. *Dtsch Zahnärztl Z* 1968;**23**: 1235–43.

54. NEGRO GC. Contributo alla conoscenza dell'eziologia e del trattamento conservativo delle fratture traumatiche dentarie nella eta infantile. *Minerva Stomatol* 1967;**16**:165–9.

55. MUGNIERA. Traumatologie dentaire en stomatologie infantile. *Actual Odontostamtol* 1967;**77**:87–119.

56. OVERDIEK HF. Die Versorgung tiefer Kronenfrakturen an bleibenden Frontzähnen bei jugendlichen Patienten. *Zahnärztl Welt* 1956;**11**:56–7.

57. GIUSTI C. Contributo alla conoscenza delle affezioni traumatiche dei denti. *Minerva Stomatol* 1957;**6**:10–25.

58. RAPP R. Restoration of fractured primary incisor teeth. *Bull Acad Gen Dent* 1968;**2**:6–31.

59. HAWES RR. Traumatized primary teeth. *Dent Clin North Am* 1966;391–404.

60. ELLIS RG, DAVEY RG. *The classification and treatment of injuries to the teeth of children*. 5th edn. Chicago: Year Book Publishers Inc., 1970.

61. KISLING E. Beskadigelser of tænder og deres ophængningsapparat ved akutte mekaniske traumata. In: Toverud G. ed. *Nordisk Lærebog i Pedodonti*. Stockholm: Sveriges Tandläkarförbunds Förlagsförening, 1963:266–87.

62. FIALOVA S, JURECEK B. Llrazy zubu udeti a nase zkusenosti s jejich lécenim. *Prakt Zubni Lék* 1968;**16**:171–6.

63. BERGER H. Do fractured incisors migrate? *ASDC J Dent Child* 1964;**27**:178–9.

64. PROPHET AS, ROWBOTHAM TC, JAMES PMC. Symposium: Traumatic injuries of the teeth. *Br Dent J* 1964;**116**:377–85.

65. Winter GB. Temporary restoration of fractured incisor teeth. *Br Dent J* 1966;**120**:249–50.

66. Starkey P. The use of self-curing resin in the restoration of young fractured permanent anterior teeth. *ASDC J Dent Child* 1967;**34**:25–9.

67. Stewart DJ. Protective caps for fractured incisors. *Br Dent J* 1957;**102**:404–6.

68. Dana F, Pejrone CA. Uso delle corone fenestrate per la ricostruzione degli incisivi fratturati nei giovani pazienti. *Minerva Stomatol* 1967;**16**:775–80.

69. Glucksmand D. Fractured permanent anterior teeth complicating orthodontic treatment. *J Am Dent Assoc* 1941;**28**:1941–3.

70. Down CH. The treatment of permanent incisor teeth of children following traumatic injury. *Aust Dent J* 1957;**2**:9–24.

71. Dannenberg JL. Emergency covering for a fractured anterior tooth in children. *J Am Dent Assoc* 1965;**71**:853–5.

72. Gaare A, Hagen A, Kanstad S. Tannfrakturer hos barn. Diagnostiske og prognostiske problemer og behandling. *Norske Tannlegeforenings Tidende* 1958;**68**:364–78.

73. Lieban EA. Traumatic injuries to children's teeth. *N Y State Dent J* 1947;**13**:319–34.

74. Lawrence KE. Restoration of fractured anterior teeth for the young patient. *North West Dent* 1965;**44**: 269–73.

75. Kelsten LB. Modern methods of managing injuries of children's anterior teeth. *Dent Dig* 1952;**58**:310–5.

76. Kelsten LB. A simple and rapid technic for restoring the fractured young incisor. *J Am Dent Assoc* 1950;**40**:455–6.

77. Magnusson B, Holm A-K, Berg H. Traumatised permanent teeth in children – a follow-up. II. The crown fractures. *Svensk Tandläkaras Tidning* 1969;**62**:71–7.

78. Gausch K, Waldhart E. Zur vitalerhaltenden Therapie der Kronenfrakturen bei Frontzähnen Jugendlicher. *Zahnärztl Welt* 1969;**78**:718–21.

79. Goldstein-Jourdan VB. Contribution a la dentisterie opératioire infantile – Traitement des fractures dentaires chez l'enfant. *Rev Fr Odontostomatol* 1954;**1**:62–70.

80. Noonan MA. A shoulder preparation and veneered gold jacket for fractured young vital permanent incisors. *ASDC J Dent Child* 1955;**22**:167–9.

81. Warnick ME. The use of porcelain-fused-to-gold in the restoration of fractured young permanent anterior teeth. *ASDC J Dent Child* 1962;**29**:3–8.

82. Mumford JM, Goose DH. Anterior crowns for young people. *Dent Practit Dent Rec* 1967;**18**:45–8.

83. Holloway PJ. The basket crown. *Dent Practit Dent Rec* 1953;**4**:308–11.

84. Slotosch H, Eschrich D, Stanka E. Die Versorgung frakturierter Frontzahnkronen mit vitaler Pulpa bei jugendlichen Patienten. *Zahnärztl Welt* 1968;**69**:473–7.

85. Anehill S, Lindahl B, Wallin H. Prognosis of traumatised permanent incisors in children. A clinical-roentgenological after-examination. *Svensk Tandlakaras Tidning* 1969;**62**:367–75.

86. Gelbier S. Stainless-steel preformed crowns in children's dentistry. *Dent Practit Dent Rec* 1965;**15**:448–50.

87. Humphrey WP, Fleece F. Restoration of fractured anterior teeth with steel crowns. *ASDC J Dent Child* 1953;**20**:178–9.

88. Dogon L. A technic for long term temporary repair of fractured anterior teeth. *ASDC J Dent Child* 1968;**35**:322–7.

89. Goldstein PM. Retention pins are friction locked without use of cement. *J Am Dent Assoc* 1966;**73**:1103–6.

90. McCormich EM. Use of stainless steel pins in the esthetic repair of fractured anterior teeth. *Dent Dig* 1968;**74**:218–20.

91. Sutter W. Frakturierte Frontzahn-Ecke bei Kindern. *Schweiz Monatsschr Zahnheilk* 1957;**67**:823.

92. Dietz WH. Means of saving mutilated teeth. *J Prosthet Dent* 1961;**11**:967–72.

93. Johnson DF. Anterior tooth fracture repair using Addent 12. *Dent Dig* 1968;**74**:340–2.

94. Kanter JC, Kanter EL. A restoration for fractured anterior teeth. *Dent Dig* 1964;**70**:159–63.

95. Liatukas EL. Branched pin restoration of anterior teeth with one penetration into tooth structure. *J Am Dent Assoc* 1969;**78**:1010–2.

96. Watson RJ. Pin retention in pedodontics. *ASDC J Dent Child* 1968;**35**:476–82.

97. Starkey P. Personal communication, 1971.

98. Laswell HR, Welk DA, Regenos JW. Attachment of resin restorations to acid pretreated enamel. *J Am Dent Assoc* 1971;**82**:558–63.

99. Kreter F. Klinik and Therapie extraalveolärer Frontzahnfrakturen. *Zahnärztl Prax* 1967;**18**: 257–60.

100. Hogeboom FE. *Practical pedodontia or juvenile operative dentistry and public health dentistry*. 5th edn. St. Louis: CV Mosby Company, 1946:288–314.

101. Engelhardt JP. Die prothetische Versorgung des traumatisch geschädigten Jugendgebisses aus klinischer Sicht. *Zahnärztl Welt* 1968;**69**:264–70.

102. Marxkors R. Die prothetische Versorgung traumatisch geschädigter Frontzähne Jugendlicher. *Dtsch Zahnärztebl* 1965;**19**:74–6.

103. Brown WE. The management of injuries to young teeth. *J Dent Assoc South Afr* 1963;**18**:247–51.

104. Crabb HSM. Direct acrylic restorations in fractured incisors. Their use and limitations. *Int Dent J* 1952;**3**:10–2.

105. Wilbur HM. Management of injured teeth. *J Am Dent Assoc* 1952;**44**:1–9.

106. Vest G. Über die Behandlung von Unfallschäden des Gebisses mit Kronen- and Brüchenprothesen bei Jugendlichen. *Schweiz Monatsschr Zahnheilk* 1941;**51**:369–79.

107. Hampson EL. Fractured anterior teeth. *Dent Practit Dent Rec* 1950;**1**:34–41.

108. Voss R. Die Möglichkeiten der prothetischen Versorgung von Traumafolgen im Wachstumsalter. *Zahnärztl Welt* 1967;**68**:11–5.

109. Olsen NH. The family dentist and injured teeth in children. *Practical dental monographs*. Chicago: Year Book Medical Publishers, Inc, 1964:1–29.

110. Law DB. Prevention and treatment of traumatized permanent anterior teeth. *Dent Clin N Am* 1973;**66**:431–50.

111. ANDREASEN JO, RAVN JJ. Epodemiology of tramatic dental injuries to primary and permanent teeth in a Danish population sample. *Int J Oral Surg* 1972;**1**:235–39.

112. HEDEGÅRD B, STÅLHANE I. A study of traumatized permanent teeth in children aged 7–15 years. Part I. *Swed Dent J* 1973;**66**:431–50.

113. RAVN JJ. Dental injuries in Copenhagen school children, school years 1967–1972. *Community Dent Oral Epidemiol* 1974;**2**:231–45.

114. DOMINKOVICÉ T. Total reflection in tooth substance and diagnosis of cracks in teeth: A clinical study. *Swed Dent J* 1977;**1**:163–72.

115. GUTZ DP. Fractured permanent incisors in a clinic population. *ASDC J Dent Child* 1971;**38**:94–121.

116. STÅLHANE I, HEDEGÅRD B. Traumatized permanent teeth in children aged 7–15 years. Part II. *Swed Dent J* 1975;**68**:157–69.

117. MACKO DJ, GRASSO JE, POWELL EA, DOHERTY NJ. A study of fractured anterior teeth in a school population. *ASDC J Dent Child* 1979;**46**:130–3.

118. ANDREASEN JO, SUNDSTRÖM B, RAVN JJ. The effect of traumatic injuries to primary teeth on their permanent successors. I. A clinical and histologic study of 117 injured permanent teeth. *Scand J Dent Res* 1971;**79**:219–83.

119. CLAUSEN BR, CRONE AS. To tilfælde af kronefraktur på permanente tænder som følge af traume på tilsvarende primære tænder. *Tandlægebladet* 1973;**77**:611–5.

120. ZADIK D, CHOSACK A, EIDELMAN E. The prognosis of traumatized permanent anterior teeth with fracture of the enamel and dentin. *Oral Surg Oral Med Oral Pathol* 1979;**47**:173–5.

121. GARBEROGLIO R, BRÄNNSTRÖM M. Scanning electron microscopic investigation of human dentinal tubules. *Arch Oral Biol* 1976;**21**:355–62.

122. CVEK M, CLEATON-JONES PE, AUSTIN JC, ANDREASEN JO. Pulp reactions to exposure after experimental crown fractures in adult monkeys. *J Endod* 1982;**8**:391–7.

123. MICRON FJ, CARR RF. Repair of a coronal fracture that involved the pulp of a deciduous incisor: report of case. *J Am Dent Assoc* 1978;**87**:1416–7.

124. BARRETT BE, O MULLANE D. Movement of permanent incisors following fracture. *J Irish Dent Assoc* 1973;**19**:145–8.

125. MJØR IA. Histologic demonstration of bacteria subjacent to dental restorations. *Scand J Dent Res* 1977;**85**:169–74.

126. MJØR IA. Bacteria in experimentally infected cavity preparations. *Scand J Dent Res* 1977;**85**:599–605.

127. QVIST J, QVIST V, LAMBJERG-HANSEN H. Bacteria in cavities beneath intermediary base materials. *Scand J Dent Res* 1977;**85**:313–9.

128. ERIKSEN HM, LEIDAHL TI. Monkey pulpal response to composite resin restorations in cavities treated with various cleansing agents. *Scand J Dent Res* 1979;**87**:309–17.

129. BUONOCORE MG. *The use of adhesives in dentistry.* Illinois: CC Thomas, 1975.

130. LASWELL HR, WELK DA, REGENOS JW. Attachment of resin restorations to acid pretreated enamel. *J Am Dent Assoc* 1972;**82**:558–63.

131. GOURION GRE. Une nouvelle méthode de restauration des fractures d'angles incisifs. Etude comparative des forces d'adhesion developpees entre une resine auto-polymerisante et l'email dentaire traite a l'acide orthophosphorique. *Rev Odontostomatol* 1972;**19**:19–25.

132. ROBERTS MW, MOFFA JP. Restoration of fractured incisal angles with an ultraviolet-light-activated sealant and a composite resin – a case report. *ASDC J Dent Child* 1972;**39**:36–45.

133. STAFFANOU RS. Restoration of fractured incisal angles. *J Am Dent Assoc* 1972;**84**:146–50.

134. WARD GT, BUONOCORE MG, WOOLRIDGE ED. Preliminary report of a technique using Nuva-seal in the treatment and repair of anterior fractures without pins. *N Y State Dent J* 1972;**38**:264–74.

135. BUONOCORE MG, DAVILA J. Restoration of fractured anterior teeth with ultraviolet-light-polymerized bonding materials: a new technique. *J Am Dent Assoc* 1973;**86**:1349–54.

136. DOYLE WA. Acid etching in pedodontics. *Dent Clin North Am* 1973;**17**:93–104.

137. HELLE A, SIRKKANEN R, EVÄLAHTI M. Repair of fractured incisal edges with UV-light polymerized and self-polymerized fissure sealants and composite resins. Two-year report of 93 cases. *Proc Finn Dent Soc* 1975;**71**:87–90.

138. HINDING JH. The acid-etch restoration: a treatment for fractured anterior teeth. *ASDC J Dent Child* 1973;**40**:21–4.

139. LEE HL Jr, ORLOWSKI JA, KOBASHIGAWA A. *In vitro* and *in vivo* studies on a composite resin for the repair of incisal fractures. *J Calif Dent Assoc* 1973;**1**:42–7.

140. ULVESTAD H, KEREKES K, DANMO C. Kompositkronen. En ny type semipermanent krone. *Norske Tannlægeforenings Tidende* 1973;**83**:281–4.

141. GOLAND U, KOCH G, PAULANDER J, RASMUSSEN C-G. Principper for 'självretinerende' plastmaterial jämte nogra användingsområden. *Tandläkartidningen* 1974;**66**:109–14.

142. MEURMAN JH, HELMINEN K J. Repair of fractured incisal edges with ultraviolet-light activated fissure sealant and composite resin. *Proc Finn Dent Soc* 1974;**70**:186–90.

143. OPPENHEIM MN, WARD GT. The restoration of fractured incisors using a pit and fissure sealant resin and composite material. *J Am Dent Assoc* 1974;**89**:365–8.

144. RAVN JJ, NIELSEN LA, JENSEN IL. Plastmaterialer til restaurering af traumebeskadigede incisiver. En foreløbig redegørelse. *Tandlægebladet* 1974;**78**:233–40.

145. RAVN JJ, NIELSEN LA, JENSEN IL. Plastmateriale til restaurering af traumebeskadigede incisiver. Fortsatte observationer. *Tandlægebladet* 1976;**80**:185–6.

146. THYLSTRUP A. Ætsteknik og plastmaterialer anvendt som semipermanent erstatning på traumatiserede fortænder. *Tandlægebladet* 1974;**78**:225–32.

147. McLUNDIE AC, MESSER JG. Acid-etch incisal restorative materials. A comparison. *Br Dent J* 1975;**138**:137–40.

148. MANNERBER GF. Etsningsteknik ved klas IV restaurationer. Några synpunkter. *Tandläkartidningen* 1975;**67**:735–40.

149. RULE DC, ELLIOTT B. Semi-permanent restoration of fractured incisors in young patients. A clinical evaluation of one 'acid-etch' technique. *Br Dent J* 1975;**139**:272–5.

150. SCHEER B. The restoration of injured anterior teeth in children by etch-retained resin. A longitudinal study. *Br Dent J* 1975;**139**:465–8.

151. BROWN JP, KEYS JC. The clinical assessment of two adhesive composite resins. *J Dent* 1976;**4**:179–282.

152. KOCH G, PAULANDER J. Klinisk uppföljning av compositrestaureringar utförda med emaljetsningsmetodik. *Swed Dent J* 1976;**69**:191–6.

153. SHEYKHOLESLAM Z, OPPENHEIM M, HOUPT MI. Clinical comparison of sealant and bonding systems in the restoration of fractured anterior teeth. *J Am Dent Assoc* 1977;**95**:1140–4.

154. HILL. FJ, SOETO PO. A simplified acid-etch technique for the restoration of fractured incisors. *J Dent* 1977;**5**:207–12.

155. JORDAN RE, SUZUKI M, GWINNETT AJ, HUNTER JK. Restoration of fractured and hypoplastic incisors by the acid etch resin technique: a three-year report. *J Am Dent Assoc* 1977;**95**:795–803.

156. LUTZ F, OCHSENBEIN H, LÜSCHER B. Nachkontrolle von 11/4 jährigen Adhäsivfüllungen. *Schweiz Monatsschr Zahnheilk* 1977;**87**:125–36.

157. RAU G. Klinische Erfahrungen mit der adhäsiven Restauration nach dem Nuva-System. *Zahnärztl Welt* 1977;**86**:296–304.

158. SMALES RJ. Incisal angle adhesive resins: a two-year clinical survey of three materials. *Aust Dent J* 1977;**22**:267–71.

159. STOKES AN, BROWN RH. Clinical evaluation of the restoration of fractured incisor teeth by an acid-etch retained composite resin. *N Z Dent J* 1977;**73**:31–3.

160. WATKINS JJ, ANDLAW RJ. Restoration of fractured incisors with an ultra-violet light-polymerised composite resin: a clinical study. *Br Dent J* 1977;**142**:249–52.

161. FUKS AB, SHAPIRA J. Acid-etch/composite resin restoration of fractured anterior teeth. *J Prosthet Dent* 1977;**37**:639–42.

162. FUKS AB, SHAPIRA J. Acid-etch/composite resin restoration of fractured anterior teeth: Part II. *J Prosthet Dent* 1978;**39**:637–9.

163. WEGELIN H. Die Behandlung traumatisch geschädigter Frontzähne. *Schweiz Monatsschr Zahnheilk* 1978;**88**:623–9.

164. GWINNET AJ. Structural changes in enamel and dentin of fractured anterior teeth after acid conditioning *in vivo*. *J Am Dent Assoc* 1973;**86**:117–22.

165. JÖRGENSEN KD, SHIMOKOBE H. Adaptation of resinous restorative materials to acid etched enamel surfaces. *Scand J Dent Res* 1975;**83**:31–6.

166. JÖRGENSEN KD. Contralateral symmetry of acid etched enamel surfaces. *Scand J Dent Res* 1975;**83**:26–30.

167. ASMUSSEN E. Penetration of restorative resins into acid etched enamel. I. Viscosity, surface tension and contact angle of restorative resin monomers. *Acta Odontol Scand* 1977;**35**:175–82.

168. ROBERTS MW, MOFFA JP. Repair of fractured incisal angles with an ultraviolet-light-activated fissure sealant and a composite resin: two-year report of 60 cases. *J Am Dent Assoc* 1973;**87**:888–91.

169. CRIM GA. Management of the fractured incisor. *J Am Dent Assoc* 1978;**96**:99–100.

170. BROSE J, COOLEY R, MOSER JB, MARSHAL GW, GREENER EH. *In vitro* strength of repaired fractured incisors. *Dent J* 1976;**45**:273–7.

171. BRÄNNSTRG MM, NYBORG H. Pulpal reaction to composite resin restorations. *J Prosthet Dent* 1972;**27**:181–9.

172. ERIKSEN HM. Protective effect of different lining materials placed under composite resin restorations in monkeys. *Scand J Dent Res* 1974;**82**:373–80.

173. STANLEY HR, GOING RE, CHAUNCEY HH. Human pulp response to acid pretreatment of dentin and to composite restoration. *J Am Dent Assoc* 1975;**91**:817–25.

174. VOJNVOVLC O, NYBORG H, BRÄNNSTRÖM M. Acid treatment of cavities under resin fillings: bacterial growth in dentinal tubules and pulpal reactions. *J Dent Res* 1973;**52**:1189–93.

175. RETIEF DH, AUSTIN JC, FATTI LP. Pulpal response to phosphoric acid. *J Oral Pathol* 1974;**3**:114–22.

176. KARJALAINEN S, FORSTEN L. Sealing properties of intermediary bases and effect on rat molar pulp. *Scand J Dent Res* 1975;**83**:293–301.

177. HEYS DR, HEYS RJ, COX CF, AVERY JK. Pulpal response to acid etching agents. *J Michigan Dent Assoc* 1976;**58**:221–32.

178. MACKO DJ, RUTBERG M, LANGELAND K. Pulpal response to the application of phosphoric acid to dentin. *Oral Surg Oral Med Oral Pathol* 1978;**45**:930–46.

179. SUZUKI M, GOTO B, JORDAN RE. Pulpal response to pin placement. *J Am Dent Assoc* 1973;**87**:636–40.

180. ULVESTAD H. A 5-year evaluation of semipermanent composite resin crowns. *Scand J Dent Res* 1978;**86**:163–8.

181. BROWN JP, KEYS JC. The clinical assessment of two adhesive composite resins. *J Dent* 1976;**4**:279–82.

182. STANLEY HR, SWERDLOW H, BUONOCORE MG. Pulp reactions to anterior restorative materials. *J Am Dent Assoc* 1967;**75**:132–41.

183. PLANT CG. The effect of polycarboxylate cement on the dental pulp. *Br Dent J* 1970;**129**:424–6.

184. TRUELOVE EL, MITCHELL DF, PHILLIPS RW. Biologic evaluation of a carboxylate cement. *J Dent Res* 1971;**50**:166.

185. JENDRESEN MP, TROWBRIDGE HO. Biologic and physical properties of a zinc polycarboxylate cement. *J Prosthet Dent* 1972;**28**:264–71.

186. KOPEL HM, BATTERMAN SC. The retentive ability of various cementing agents for polycarbonate crown. *ASDC J Dent Child* 1976;**43**:333–9.

187. BARKIN PR. Time as a factor in predicting the vitality of traumatized teeth. *ASDC J Dent Child* 1973;**40**:188–92.

188. PALMER JD. The care of fractured incisors and their restoration in children. *Dent Pract* 1971;**21**:395–400.

189. ASMUSSEN E. Factors affecting the color stability of restorative resins. *J Dent Res* 1981;**60** *(Spec Issue A)* (Abstract):1088.

190. WILLIAMS HA, GARMAN TA, FAIRHURST CW, ZWEMER JD, RINGLE RD. Surface characteristics of resin-coated composite restorations. *J Am Dent Assoc* 1978;**97**:463–7.

191. SIMONSEN RJ. *Clinical applications of the acid etch technique*. Chicago: Quintessence Publishing Co. Inc., 1978.

192. Schiødt M, Larsen V, Bessermann M. Oral findings in glassblowers. *Community Dent Oral Epidemiol* 1980;**8**:195–200.

193. Bedi R. The use of porcelain veneers as coronal splints for traumatised anterior teeth in children. *Restorative Dentistry* 1989;August:55–8.

194. Ravn JJ. Follow-up study of permanent incisors with enamel cracks as a result of an acute trauma. *Scand J Dent Res* 1981;**89**:117–23.

195. Ravn JJ. Follow-up study of permanent incisors with enamel fractures as a result of acute trauma. *Scand J Dent Res* 1981;**89**:213–7.

196. Ravn JJ. Follow-up study of permanent incisors with enamel-dentin fractures after acute trauma. *Scand J Dent Res* 1981;**89**:355–65.

197. Andreasen FM, Vestergaard Pedersen B. Prognosis of luxated permanent teeth – the development of pulp necrosis. *Endod Dent Traumatol* 1985;**1**:207–20.

198. Andreasen FM, Noren JG, Andreasen JO, Engelhardtsten S, Lindh-Strömberg U. Long-term survival of crown fragment bonding in the treatment of crown fractures. A multi-center clinical study of fragment retention. *Quintess Int* 1995;**26**:669–81.

199. Brännström M. *Dentin and pulp in restorative dentistry.* Nacka, Sweden: Dental Therapeutics AB, 1981:127.

200. Jung OJ. The value of radiographs in the preparation of teeth for crowns. *Proceedings of 3rd International Congress of Maxillofacial Radiology,* Kyoto, Japan, 1974.

201. Andreasen FM, Andreasen JO. Diagnosis of luxation injuries. The importance of standardized clinical, radiographic and photographic techniques in clinical investigations. *Endod Dent Traumatol* 1985;**1**:160–9.

202. Andreasen FM, Yu Z, Thomsen BL. The relationship between pulpal dimensions and the development of pulp necrosis after luxation injuries in the permanent dentition. *Endod Dent Traumatol* 1986;**2**:90–8.

203. Lundy T, Stanley HR. Correlation of pulpal histopathology and clinical symptoms in human teeth subjected to experimental irritation. *Oral Surg Oral Med Oral Pathol* 1969; **27**:187–201.

204. Vojinovic Q, Nyborg H, Brännström M. Acid treatment of cavities under resin fillings: bacterial growth in dentinal tubules and pulp reactions. *J Dent Res* 1973;**52**:1189–93.

205. Olgart L, Brännström M, Johnson G. Invasion of bacteria into dentinal tubules. Experiments *in vivo* and *in vitro. Acta Odontol Scand* 1974;**32**:61–70.

206. Vongsavan N, Matthews B. The permeability of cat dentine *in vivo* and *in vitro. Archs Oral Biol* 1991;**36**:641–6.

207. Vongsavan N, Matthews B. Fluid flow through cat dentine *in vivo. Arch Oral Biol* 1992;**37**:175–85.

208. Vongsavan N, Matthews B. Changes in pulpal blood flow and in fluid flow through dentine produced by autonomic and sensory nerve stimulation in the cat. *Proc Finn Dent Soc* 1992;**8**:(Suppl 1):491–7.

209. Vongsavan N, Matthews RW, Matthews B. The permeability of human dentine in vitro and in vivo. *Arch Oral Biol* 2000;**45**:931–5.

210. Matthews B. Sensory physiology: a reaction. *Proc Finn Dent Soc* 1992;**8**:(Suppl 1):529–32.

211. Matthews B. Personal communication 1992.

212. Cox CF. Effects of adhesive materials on the pulp. Presented at the International Symposium on Adhesives in Dentistry, Creighton University, Omaha, Nebraska, 11–13 July 1992. *Operative Dentistry* 1992;(Suppl 5):156–76.

213. Heide S, Mjör IA. Pulp reactions to experimental exposures in young permanent monkey teeth. *Int Endod J* 1983;**16**:11–9.

214. Ingber JS. Forced eruption: Part II. A method of treating nonrestorable teeth – periodontal and restorative considerations. *J Periodont* 1976;**47**:203–16.

215. Waerhaug J, Zander HA. Reaction of gingival tissues to self-curing acrylic restorations. *J Am Dent Assoc* 1957;**54**:760–8.

216. Zander HA. Pulp response to restorative materials. *J Am Dent Assoc* 1959;**59**:911–5.

217. Brännström M, Nyborg H. The presence of bacteria in cavities filled with silicate cement and composite resin materials. *Swed Dent J* 1971;**64**:149–55.

218. Brännström M, Nyborg H. Cavity treatment with a microbicidal fluoride solution: growth of bacteria and effect on the pulp. *J Prosthet Dent* 1973;**30**:303–10.

219. Brännström M, Nyborg H. Pulp reaction to a temporary zinc oxide/eugenol cement. *J Prosthet Dent* 1976;**35**:185–91.

220. Frank RM. Reactions of dentin and pulp to drugs and restorative materials. *J Dent Res* 1975;**54**:(Spec Issue B):176–87.

221. Heys RJ, Heys DR, Cox CF, Avery JK. The histological effects of composite resin materials on the pulps of monkey teeth. *J Oral Pathol* 1977;**6**:63–81.

222. Heys RJ, Heys DR, Cox CF, Avery JK. Histopathologic evaluation of three ultraviolet-activated composite resins on monkey pulps. *J Oral Pathol* 1977;**6**:317–30.

223. Qvist J, Qvist V, Lambjerg-Hansen H. Bacteria in cavities beneath intermediary base materials. *Scand J Dent Res* 1977;**85**:313–9.

224. Mejàre B, Mejàre I, Edwardsson S. Bacteria beneath composite restorations – a culturing and histobacteriological study. *Acta Odontol Scand* 1979;**37**:267–75.

225. Bergenholtz G, Cox CF, Loesche WJ, Syed SA. Bacterial leakage around dental restorations: its effect on the dental pulp. *J Oral Pathol* 1982;**11**:439–50.

226. Cox CF, Bergenholtz G, Fitzgerald M, et al. Capping of the dental pulp mechanically exposed to the oral microflora – a 5 week observation of wound healing in the monkey. *J Oral Pathol* 1982;**11**:327–39.

227. Heys RJ, Heys DR, Cox CF, Avery JK. Experimental observations on the Biocompatibility of composite resins. In: Smith DC, Williams DF. eds. *Biocompatibility of dental materials* Vol. III. Boca Raton, FL: CRC Press, 1982:131–50.

228. Torstenson B, Nordenvall KJ, Brännström M. Pulpal reaction and microorganisms under Clearfil Composite Resin in deep cavities with acid etched dentin. *Swed Dent* 1982;**6**:167–76.

229. Browne RM, Tobias RS, Crombie IK, Plant CG. Bacterial microleakage and pulpal inflammation in experimental cavities. *Int Endod J* 1983;**16**:147–55.

230. Cox CF, Bergenholtz G, Heys DR, Syed SA, Fitzgerald M, Heys RJ. Pulp capping of dental pulp

mechanically exposed to oral microflora: a 1–2 year observation of wound healing in the monkey. *J Oral Pathol* 1985;**14**:156–68.

231. LEIDAHL TI, ERIKSEN HM. Human pulpal response to composite resin restorations. *Endod Dent Traumatol* 1985;**1**:66–8.

232. BROWNE RM, TOBIAS RS. Microbial microleakage and pulpal inflammation: a review. *Endod Dent Traumatol* 1986;**2**:177–83.

233. GERKE DC. Pulpal integrity of anterior teeth treated with composite resins. A long-term clinical evaluation. *Aust Dent Assoc* 1988;**33**:133–5.

234. HÖRSTED PB, SIMONSEN A-M, LARSEN MJ. Monkey pulp reactions to restorative materials. *Scand J Dent Res* 1986;**94**:154–63.

235. COX CF. Biocompatibility of dental materials in the absence of bacterial infection. *Oper Dent* 1987;**12**:146–52.

236. COX CF, KEALL CL, KEALL HJ, OSTRO E, BERGENHOLTZ G. Biocompatability of surface-sealed dental materials against exposed pulps. *J Prosthet Dent* 1987;**57**:1–8.

237. CVEK M, GRANATH L, CLEATON-JONES P, AUSTIN J. Hard tissue barrier formation in pulpotomized monkey teeth capped with cyanoacrylate or calcium hydroxide for 10 and 60 minutes. *J Dent Res* 1987;**66**:1166–74.

238. FUSAYAMA T. Factors and prevention of pulp irritation by adhesive composite resin restorations. *Quintessence Int* 1987;**18**:633–41.

239. COX CF, WHITE KC, RAMUS DL, FARMER JB, SNUGGS HM. Reparative dentin: factors affecting its deposition. *Quintessence Int* 1992;**23**:257–70.

240. BERGENHOLTZ G. Bacterial leakage around dental restorations – impact on the pulp. In: Anusavice KJ. ed. *Quality evaluation of dental restoration. Criteria for placement and replacement of dental restorations.* Chicago: Quintessence Publishing Co. Inc., 1989:243–54.

241. BRÄNNSTRÖM M, NYBORG H. Pulpal reaction to polycarboxylate and zinc phosphate cements used with inlays in deep cavity preparations. *J Am Dent Assoc* 1977;**94**:308–10.

242. BRÄNNSTRÖM M, VOJINOVIC O, NORDENVALL K-J. Bacteria and pulpal reactions under silicate cement restorations. *Prosthet Dent* 1979;**41**:290–4.

243. WATTS A. Bacterial contamination and the toxicity of silicate and zinc phosphate cements. *Br Dent J* 1979;**146**:7–13.

244. COX CF, WHITE KC. Biocompatability of amalgam on exposed pulps employing a biological seal. *J Dent Res* 1992;**71** *(AADR Abstracts)*: Abstract no. 656.

245. WARFVINGE J, BERGENHOLTZ G. Healing capacity of human and monkey dental pulps following experimentally-induced pulpitis. *Endod Dent Traumatol* 1986;**2**:256–62.

246. KISLING E. Om behandlingen of skader som følge af akute mekaniske traumer på unge permanente incisiver. *Tandlægebladet* 1953;**57**:61–9, 109–29.

247. GAARE A, HAGEN A, KANSTAD S. Tannfrakturer hos barn, Diagnostiske og prognostiske problemer og behandling. *Norske Tannl Tid* 1958;**68**:364–78.

248. STÅLHANE I, HEDEGÅRD B. Traumatized permanent teeth in children aged 7–15. Part II. *Svenske Tandläk-T* 1975;**68**:157–69.

249. ZADIK D, CHOSAK A, EIDELMAN E. The prognosis of traumatized permanent incisor teeth with fracture of the enamel and dentin. *Oral Surg Oral Med Oral Path* 1979;**47**:173–5.

250. ROBERTSON A, ANDREASEN FM, ANDREASEN JO, NOREN JG. Long-term prognosis of crown fractures: the effect of stage of root development and associated luxation injury. *Int J Paediatric Dent* 2000;**10**:191–9.

251. ANDREASEN FM, RINDUM JL, MUNKSGAARD EC, ANDREASEN JO. Bonding of enamel-dentin crown fractures with Gluma® and resin. Short communication. *Endo Dent Traumatol* 1986;**2**:277–80.

252. ANDREASEN FM, NOREN JG, ANDREASEN JO, ENGELHARDTSEN S, LINDH-STRÖMBERG U. Long-term survival of crown fragment bonding in the treatment of crown fractures. A multi-center clinical study of fragment retention. *Quintessence Int* 1995;**26**: 669–81.

253. LINDH-STRÖMBERG U, CVEK M, MEJÀRE I. Long-term prognosis of crown fractures treated by reattachment of the original fragment using enamel acid-etch retention. Report from Scandinavian Trauma Study Group, 1992.

254. BERGENHOLTZ G. Iatrogenic injury to the pulp in dental procedures: Aspects of pathogenesis, management and preventive measures. *Int Dent J* 1991;**41**:99–110.

255. McCOMB D. Comparison of physical properties of commercial calcium hydroxide lining cements. *J Am Dent Assoc* 1983;**107**:610–13.

256. HWAS M, SANDRICK JL. Acid and water solubility and strength of calcium hydroxide bases. *J Am Dent Assoc* 1984;**108**:46–8.

257. COX CF, SUBAY RK, OSTRO E, SUZUKI S, SUZUKI SH. Tunnel defects in dentin bridges: their formation following direct pulp capping. *Oper Dent* 1996;**21**: 4–11.

258. REINHARDT JW, CHALKEY Y. Softening effects of bases on composite resins. *Clinical Preventive Dentistry* 1983;**5**:9–12.

259. HÖRSTED PB, SIMONSEN A-M, LARSEN MJ. Monkey pulp reactions to restorative materials. *Scand J Dent Res* 1986;**94**:154–63.

260. RETIEF DH. Dentin bonding agents: a deterrent to microleakage? In: Anusavice KJ. ed. *Quality evaluation of dental restorations. Criteria for placement and replacement.* Chicago: Quintessence Publishing Co. Inc., 1989:185–98.

261. BUONOCORE MG. A simple method of increasing the adhesion of acrylic filling materials to enamel surfaces. *J Dent Res* 1955;**34**:849.

262. BUONOCORE MG. Adhesives in the prevention of caries. *J Am Dent Assoc* 1973;**87**:1000–5.

263. BUONOCORE MG, SHEYKHOLESI AM Z, GLENA R. Evaluation of an enamel adhesive to prevent marginal leakage: an *in vitro* study. *J Dent Child* 1973;**40**:19–24.

264. MUNKSGAARD EC, HÖJTVED L, JÖRGENSEN EHW, ANDREASEN FM, ANDREASEN JO. Enamel-dentin crown fractures bonded with various bonding agents. *Endod Dent Traumatol* 1991;**7**:73–7.

265. FUSAYAMA T. *New concepts in operative dentistry.* Chicago: Quintessence Publishing Co. Inc., 1980.

266. INOKOSHI S, IWAKU M, FUSAYAMA T. Pulpal response to a new adhesive restorative resin. *J Dent Res* 1982;**61**:1014–9.

267. KANKA J. A method for bonding to tooth structure using phosphoric acid as a dentin-enamel conditioner. *Quintessence Int* 1991;**22**:285–90.

268. WHITE KC, COX CF, KANCA III J, FARMER JB, RAMUS DL, SNUGGS HM. Histologic pulpal response of acid etching vital dentin. *J Dent Res* 1992;**71**:*(AADR Abstracts)*:188, Abstr. no. 658.

269. ASMUSSEN E, UNO S. Adhesion of restorative resins to dentin: chemical and physico-chemical aspects. Proceedings of the International Symposium on Adhesives in Dentistry, Creighton University, Omaha, Nebraska, 11–13 July 1991. *Operative Dentistry* 1992; *(Suppl)* 5:68–74.

270. HANSEN EK. Effect of Gluma in acid-etched dentin cavities. *Scand J Dent Res* 1987;**95**:181–4.

271. ASMUSSEN E, BOWEN RL. Effect of acid pretreatment on adhesion to dentin mediated by Gluma. *J Dent Res* 1987;**66**:1386–8.

272. ASMUSSEN E, BOWEN RL. Adhesion to dentin mediated by Gluma: Effect of pretreatment with various amino acids. *Scand J Dent Res* 1987;**95**:521–5.

273. NATHANSON D, AMIN F, ASHAYERI N. Dentin etching vs. priming: effect on bond strength *in vitro*. *J Dent Res* 1992;**71**:*(AADR Abstracts)*: Abstract no. 1192.

274. NATHANSON D, L HERAULT R, FRANKL S. Dentin etching vs priming: surface element analysis. *J Dent Res* 1992;**71**:*(AADR Abstracts)*: Abstract no. 1193.

275. ANDREASEN FM, YU Z, THOMSEN BL, ANDERSEN PK. The occurrence of pulp canal obliteration after luxation injuries in the permanent dentition. *Endod Dent Traumatol* 1987;**3**:103–15.

276. HENRY PJ, BISHOP BM, PURT RM. Fiber-reinforced plastics for interim restorations. *Quintessence Dental Technology (QDT)* 1990/1991:110–23.

277. OIKARINEN K, ANDREASEN JO, ANDREASEN FM. Rigidity of various fixation methods used as dental splints after tooth dislocation. *Endod Dent Traumatol* 1992;**8**: 113–9.

278. BEECH DR. Adhesion to teeth: Principles and mechanism. In: Smith DC, Williams DF. eds. *Biocompatibility of dental materials* Vol. II. Boca Raton, FL: CRC Press, 1982:87.

279. SILVERSTONE CM. The structure and characteristics of human dental enamel. In: Smith DC, Williams DF. eds. *Biocompatibility of dental materials* Vol. I. Boca Raton, FFL: CRC Press, 1982:39.

280. ANDREASEN FM, DAUGAARD-JENSEN J, MUNKSGAARD EC. Reinforcement of bonded crown fractures with porcelain laminate veneers. *Endod Dent Traumatol* 1991;**7**:78–83.

281. ANDREASEN FM, FLÜGGE E, DAUGAARD-JENSEN J, MUNKSGAARD EC. Treatment of crown fractured incisors with laminate veneer restorations. *Endod Dent Traumatol* 1992;**8**:30–35.

282. SIMONSEN RJ. Restoration of a fractured central incisor using original tooth fragment. *J Am Dent Assoc* 1982;**105**:646–8.

283. MADER C. Restoration of a fractured anterior tooth. *J Am Dent Assoc* 1978;**96**:113–5.

284. TENNERY TN. The fractured tooth reunified using the acid etch bonding technique. *Texas Dent J* 1978;**96**:16–17.

285. SIMONSEN RJ. Traumatic fracture restoration: an alternative use of the acid-etch technique. *Quintess Int* 1979;**10**:15–22.

286. STARKEY PE. Reattachment of a fractured fragment to a tooth. *J Indiana Dent Assoc* 1979;**58**:37–8.

287. MCDONALD RE, AVERY DR. *Dentistry for the child and adolescent.* 4th edn. St. Louis: CV Mosby Co., 1983:436–8.

288. AMIR E, BAR-GIL B, SARNAT H. Restoration of fractured immature maxillary central incisors using the crown fragments. *Pediatr Dent* 1986;**8**:285–8.

289. DEAN JA, AVERY DR, SWARTZ ML. Attachment of anterior tooth fragments. *Pediatr Dent* 1986;**8**:139–43.

290. RICCITIELLO F, CARLOMAGNO F, INGENITO A, DE FAZIO P. Nuova metodica di reincollamento di un frammento di corona su dente tirattato endodonticamente. *Min Stom* 1986;**35**:1057–63.

291. DIANGELIS AJ, JUNGBLUTH MA. Restoration of an amputated crown by the acid-etch technique. *Quintessence Int* 1987;**18**:829–33.

292. LIEW VP. Re-attachment of original tooth fragment to a fractured crown. Case report. *Aust Dent J* 1988;**33**:47–50.

293. EHRMANN EH. Restoration of a fractured incisor with exposed pulp using original tooth fragment: report of case. *J Am Dent Assoc* 1989;**118**:183–5.

294. KOTSANOS N. Restoring fractured incisors with the original fragments. Abstract, 12th Congress of the International Association of Dentistry for Children, Athens, Greece, June 1989. p. 83.

295. BARATIERI LN, MONTEIRO S JR, CALDEIRA DE ANDRADA MA. The 'sandwich' technique as a base for reattachment of dental fragments. Quintessence International 1991;**22**:81–5.

296. ASMUSSEN E, MUNKSGAARD EC. Formaldehyde as bonding agent between dentin and restorative resins. *Scand J Dent Res* 1984;**92**:480–3.

297. MUNKSGAARD EC, ASMUSSEN E. Bond strength between dentin and restorative resins mediated by mixtures of HEMA and glutaraldehyde. *J Dent Res* 1984;**63**:1087–90.

298. MUNKSGAARD EC, HANSEN EK, ASMUSSEN E. Effect of five adhesives on adaptation of resin in dentin cavities. *Scand J Dent Res* 1984;**92**:187–91.

299. MUNKSGAARD EC, IRIS M, ASMUSSEN E. Dentin-polymer bond promoted by Gluma and various resins. *J Dent Res* 1985;**64**:1409–11.

300. FINGER WJ, OHSAWA M. Effect of bonding agents on gap formation in dentin cavities. *Operative Dentistry* 1987;**12**:100–4.

301. HANSEN EK, ASMUSSEN E. Comparative study of dentin adhesives. *Scand J Dent Res* 1985;**93**:280–7.

302. MUNKSGAARD EC, IRIS M. Dentin-polymer bond established by Gluma and tested by thermal stress. *Scand J Dent Res* 1987;**95**:185–90.

303. ALBERS HF. ed. Dentin-resin bonding. *ADEPT Report* 1990;**1**:33–41.

304. RINDUM JL, MUNKSGAARD EC, ASMUSSEN E, HÖRSTED P, ANDREASEN JO. Pålimning af tandfragmenter efter fraktur: en foreløbig redegørelse. *Tandlægebladet* 1986;**90**:397–403.

305. ANDREASEN FM, RINDUM JL, MUNKSGAARD EC, ANDREASEN JO. Bonding of enamel-dentin crown fractures with Gluma® and resin. Short communication. *Endod Dent Traumatol* 1986;**2**:277–80.

306. HÖRSTED-BINDSLEV P. Monkey pulp reactions to cavities treated with Gluma Dentin Bond and restored with a microfilled composite. *Scand J Dent Res* 1987;**95**:347–55.

307. SETCOS JC. Dentin bonding in perspective. *Am J Dent* 1988;**1**:*(Spec Issue)*:173–5.

308. ROULET J-F, BLUNCK U. Effectiveness of dentin bonding agents. *Scanning Microscopy* 1989;**3**:1013–22.

309. EICK JD. Materials interaction with smear layer. *Proc Finn Dent Soc* 1992;**88**:*(Suppl 1)*:225–42.

310. EICK JD, COBB CM, CHAPPELL RP, SPENCER P, ROBINSON SJ. The dentin surface – its influence on dentin adhesion. Part I. *Quintessence Int* 1991; **22**:967–77.

311. GWINNETT AJ, KANCA III J. The micromorphology of the bonded dentin interface and its relationship to bond strength. *Am J Dent* 1992;**5**:73–7.

312. ANDREASEN FM, STEINHARDT U, BILLE M, MUNKSGAARD EC. Bonding of enamel-dentin crown fragments after crown fracture. An experimental study using bonding adhesives. *Endod Dent Traumatol* 1993;**3**:111–4.

313. ROTBERG SJ, DESHAZER DO. The complexing action of eugenol on sound dentin. *J Dent Res* 1966;**45**:307–10.

314. SCHWARTZ R, DAVIS R, MAYHEW R. The effect of a ZOE temporary cement on the bond strength of a resin luting cement. *Am J Dent* 1990;**3**:28–30.

315. ANDREASEN FM, ANDREASEN JO, RINDUM JL, MUNKSGAARD EC. Preliminary clinical and histological results of bonding dentin-enamel crown fragments with GLUMA technique. Presented at the Nordic Association of Pedodontology, Annual Congress, Bergen, Norway, June 1988.

316. ANDREASEN JO, ANDREASEN FM. *Essentials of traumatic injuries to the teeth*. Copenhagen: Munksgaard, 1990:168.

317. GARBER DA, GOLDSTEIN RE, FEINMAN RA. *Porcelain laminate veneers*. Chicago: Quintessence Publishing Co. Inc., 1988:136.

318. SMITH DC, PULVER F. Aesthetic dental veneering materials. *Int Dent J* 1982;**32**:223–9.

319. WALLS AWG, MURRAY JJ, MCCABE JF. Composite laminate veneers: a clinical study. *J Oral Rehab* 1988;**15**:439–54.

320. MEUNINGHOFF LA, O NEAL SJ, RAMUS DL. Six months evaluation of clinical esthetic veneers. *J Dent Res* 1990;**69**:Abstr. no. 1542.

321. MCLEAN JW. Ceramics in clinical dentistry. *Br Dent J* 1988;**164**:187–94.

322. CLYDE JS, GILMOUR A. Porcelain veneers: a preliminary review. *Br Dent J* 1988;**164**:9–14.

323. NASEDKIN JN. Current perspectives on esthetic restorative dentistry. Part I. Porcelain laminates. *J Canad Dent Assoc* 1988;**54**:248–55.

324. QUINN F, MCCONNELL RJ, BYRNE D. Porcelain laminates: a review. *Br Dent J* 1986;**161**:61–5.

325. ANDREASEN FM, FLÜGGE E, DAUGAARD JENSEN J, MUNKSGAARD EC. Reinforcement of crown fractured incisors with laminate veneer restorations. Presented at the Nordic Pedodontic Association, Turku, Finland, August 15, 1992.

326. DOERING JV, JENSEN ME, SHETH J, TOLLIVER D, CHAN DCN. Fracture resistance of resin-bonded etched porcelain full veneer crowns. *J Dent Res* 1987;**66**:207 (Abstr. no. 803).

327. TJAN AHL, DUNN JR, SANDERSON IR. Microleakage patterns of porcelain and castable ceramic laminate veneers. *J Prosthet Dent* 1989;**61**:276–82.

328. PLANT CG, THOMAS GD. Do we need to prep porcelain veneers? *Br Dent J* 1987;**163**:231–4.

329. CALAMIA JR, CALAMIA S, LEMLER J, HAMBURG M, SCHERER W. Clinical evaluation of etched porcelain laminate veneers: Results at (6 months–3 years). J Dent Res 1987;**66**:*(Spec issue)*:245 (Abstr. no. 1110).

330. NORDBO H. Individuelle porselenslaminater – et alternativ til komposittfasader og kroner? *Norske Tannlægeforenings Tid* 1987;**97**:194–200.

331. REID JS, MURRAY MC, POWER SM. Porcelain veneers – a four-year follow-up. *Restorative Dentistry* 1988;August:60–6.

332. STRASSLER HE, NATHANSON D. Clinical evaluation of etched porcelain veneers over a period of 18 to 42 months. *Esthetic Dent* 1989;**1**:21–8.

333. TAY WM, LYNCH E, AUGER D. Effects of some finishing techniques on cervical margins of porcelain laminates. *Quintessence Int* 1987;**18**:599–602.

334. OLIVA RA, LOWE JA. Dimensional stability of composite used as a core material. *J Prosthet Dent* 1986;**56**:554–61.

335. JORDAN RE, SUZUKI M, SENDA A. Four year recall evaluation of labial porcelain veneer restorations. *J Dent Res* 1989;**68**:*(Spec issue)*:240 (Abstr. no. 544).

336. WILSON CM. Fracture of a developing permanent central incisor prior to eruption. *Br Dent J* 1981;**151**:426.

337. ROBERTSON A, ANDREASEN FM, BERGENHOLTZ G, ANDREASEN JO, MUNKSGAARD C. Pulp reactions to restoration of experimentally induced crown fractures. *J Dent* 1998;**26**:409–16.

338. CIUCCHI B, BOUILLAGUET S, HOLZ J, PASHLEY D. Dentinal fluid dynamics in human teeth, *in vivo*. *J Endod* 1995;**21**:191–4.

339. RAUSCHENBERGER CR, HOVLAND EJ. Clinical management of crown fractures. *Dent Clin N Amer* 1995;**39**:25–51.

340. BLATZ MB. Comprehensive treatment of traumatic fracture and luxation injuries in the anterior permanent dentition. *Pract Proced Aesthet Dent* 2001;**13**:273–9.

341. OLSBURGH S, JACOBY T, KREJCI I. Crown fractures in the permanent dentition: pulpal and restorative considerations. *Dent Traumatol* 2002;**18**:103–15.

342. COX CF. Microleakage related to restorative procedures. *Proc Finn Dent Soc* 1992;**88**:*(Suppl 1)*:83–93.

343. COX CR, SUZUKI S, SUZUKI SH. Biocompatibility of dental adhesives. *CDA Journal* 1995;August:35–41.

344. MITCHEM JC, TERKLA LG, GRONAS DG. Bonding of resin dentin adhesives under simulated physiological conditions. *Dent Mater* 1988;**4**:351–3.

345. BULLARD RH, LEINFELDER KF, RUSSELL CM. Effect of coefficient of thermal expansion on microleakage. *J Am Dent Assoc* 1988;**116**:871–4.

346. FELTON DA, COX CF, ODOM M, KANOY BE. Pulpal response to chemically cured and experimental

light-cured glass ionomer cavity liners. *J Prosthet Dent* 1991;**65**:704–12.

347. Heys RJ, Fitzgerald M, Heys DR, Charbeneau GT. An evaluation of a glass ionomer luting agent: pulpal histologic response. *J Am Dent Assoc* 1987;**114**:607–11.

348. Mjör IA, Nordahl I, Tronstad L. Glass ionomer cements and the dental pulp. *Endod Dent Traumatol* 1991;**7**:59–64.

349. Tobias RS, Browne RM, Plant CG, et al. Pulpal response to a glass ionomer cement. *Br Dent J* 1978;**144**:345–50.

350. Murchison DF, Burke FJT, Worthington RB. Incisal edge reattachment: indications for use and clinical technique. *Brit Dent J* 1999;**186**:614–19.

351. Badame AA, Dunne SM, Scheer B. An *in vitro* investigation into the shear bond strengths of two dentine-bonding agents used in the reattachment of incisal edge fragments. *Endod Dent Traumatol* 1995;**11**:129–35.

352. Farik B, Munksgaard EC, Kreiborg S, Andreasen JO. Adhesive bonding of fragmented anterior teeth. *Endod Dent Traumatol* 1998;**14**:119–23.

353. Farik B, Munksgaard EC. Fracture strength of intact and fragment-bonded teeth at various velocities of the applied force. *Eur J Oral Sci* 1999;**107**:70–3.

354. Farik B, Munksgaard EC, Andreasen JO, Kreiborg S. Drying and rewetting anterior crown fragments prior to bonding. *Endod Dent Traumatol* 1999;**15**:113–16.

355. Farik B, Munksgaard EC, Andreasen JO. Fracture strength of fragment-bonded teeth. Effect of calcium hydroxide lining before bonding. *Am J Dent* 2000;**13**:98–100.

356. Farik B, Munksgaard EC, Byoung IS, Andreasen JO, Kreiborg S. Adhesive bonding of fractured anterior teeth: effect of wet technique and rewetting agent. *Am J Dent* 1998;**11**:251–3.

357. Aldridge D, Wilder JR, Swift EJ Jr, Waddel SL. Bond strengths of conventional and simplified bonding systems. *Am J Dent* 1998;**11**:114–17.

358. Al-Salehi SK, Burke FJ. Methods used in dentin bonding tests: an analysis of 50 investigations on bond strength. *Quintessence Int* 1997;**28**:717–23.

359. Demarco FF, Fay R-M, Pinzon LM, Powers JM. Fracture resistance on re-attached coronal fragments – influence of different adhesive materials and bevel preparation. *Dent Traumatol* 2004;**20**:157–63.

360. Reis A, Francci C, Loguercio AD, Carrilho MRO, Rodrigues Filho LE. Re-attachment of anterior fractured teeth: Fracture strength using different techniques. *Oper Dent* 2001;**26**:287–94.

361. Andreasen FM, Steinhardt U, Bille M, Munksgaard EC. Bonding of enamel-dentin crown fragments after crown fracture. An experimental study using bonding agents. *Endod Dent Traumatol* 1993:111–14.

362. Andreasen FM, Norén JG, Andreasen JO, Engelhardtsen S, Lindh-Strömberg. Long-term survival of fragment bonding in the treatment of fractured crowns: A multicenter clinical study. *Quintessence Int* 1995;**26**:669–81.

363. Kanca J III. Improving bond strength through acid etching of dentin and bonding to wet dentin surfaces. *J Am Dent Assoc* 1992;**123**:35–42.

364. de Goes MR, Ferrari Pachane GC, Garcia-Godoy F. Resin bond strength with different methods to remove excess water from the dentin. *Am J Dent* 1997;**10**:298–301.

365. Tay F, Gwinnett AJ, Pang KM, et al. Resin permeation into acid-conditioned, moist and dry dentin: A paradigm using water-free adhesive primers. *J Dent Res* 1996;**75**:1034–44.

366. Kreulen CM, Creugers NHJ, Meijering AC. Meta-analysis of anterior veneer restorations in clinical studies. *J Dent* 1998;**26**:345–3.

367. Nagaoka S, Miyazaki Y, Liu HJ, Iwamoto Y, Kitano M, Kawagoe M. Bacterial invasion into dentinal tubules of human vital and nonvital teeth. *J Endod* 1995;**21**:70–3.

368. Olgart L, Brännström M, Johnson G. Invasion of bacteria into dentinal tubules: experiments *in vivo* and *in vitro*. *Acta Odontol Scand* 1974;**32**:61–70.

369. Worthington RB, Murchison DF, Vandewalle KS. Incisal edge reattachment: the effect of preparation utilization and design. *Quintessence Int* 1999;**30**:637–43.

370. Liebenberg WH. Reattachment of coronal fragments: Operative considerations for the repair of anterior teeth. *Pract Periodontics Aesthet* 1997;**9**:761–72.

371. DiAngelis AJ, Jungbluth M. Reattaching fractured tooth segments: an esthetic alternative. *J Am Dent Assoc* 1992;**123**:58–62.

372. Robertson A. A retrospective evaluation of patients with uncomplicated crown fractures and luxation injuries. *Endod Dent Traumatol* 1998;**14**:245–56.

373. Robertson A, Andreasen FM, Andreasen JO, Norén JG. Long-term prognosis of crown-fractured permanent incisors. The effect of stage of root development and associated luxation injury. *Int J Paed Dent* 2000;**10**:191–9.

374. Andreasen JO, Andreasen FM, Skeie A, Hjørting-Hansen E, Schwartz O. Effect of treatment delay upon pulp and periodontal healing of traumatic dental injuries – a review article. *Dent Traumatol* 2002;**18**:116–28.

375. Spinas E. Longevity of composite restorations of traumatically injured teeth. *Am J Dent* 2004;**17**:407–11.

376. Andreasen FM, Andreasen JO. Long-term prognosis of crown fractues: pulp survival after injury. 2006. Manuscript in preparation.

377. Robertson A, Andreasen FM, Bergenholtz G, Andreasen JO, Munksgaard C. Pulp reactions to restoration of experimentally induced crown fractures. *J Dent* 1998;**26**:409–16.

# 11

# Crown-Root Fractures

## J. O. Andreasen, F. M. Andreasen & M. Tsukiboshi

## Terminology, frequency and etiology

A crown-root fracture is defined as a fracture involving enamel, dentin, and cementum. The fractures may be grouped according to pulpal involvement into *uncomplicated* and *complicated*.

In some studies this type of injury is not recognized as a special entity and is, therefore, classified as either a crown or a root fracture. In the authors' material, however, crown-root fractures comprised 5% of injuries affecting the permanent dentition and 2% in the primary dentition (1).

The most common etiologic factors are injuries caused by falls, bicycle and auto mobile accidents and foreign bodies striking the teeth (1).

Crown-root fractures in the anterior region are usually caused by *direct trauma* (see Chapter 8, p. 236). The direction of the impacting force determines the type of fracture. A frontal blow results in the typical fracture line shown in Fig. 11.1. In the posterior regions, fractures of the buccal or oral cusps of premolars and molars may occur (2, 21). These fractures extend below the gingival attachment, often without

pulp exposure (uncomplicated) (Fig. 11.2). The causes of such injuries are often *indirect trauma* (see Chapter 8, p. 240).

Although not caused by accident trauma, for the sake of completeness, it should be mentioned that crown-root fractures can also have an iatrogenic etiology, such as longitudinal crown-root fractures, especially in the premolar and molar regions, caused by lateral pressure during root filling procedures, cementation of posts, corrosion of posts or improperly designed restorations (22–33). The clinical and radiographic signs of these fractures have been previously described (54).

## Clinical findings

Most commonly, the fracture line begins a few millimeters incisal to the marginal gingiva facially and follows an oblique course below the gingival crevice orally. The fragments are usually only slightly displaced, the coronal fragment being kept in position by fibers of the periodontal ligament orally and/or the dental pulp (Fig. 11.3).

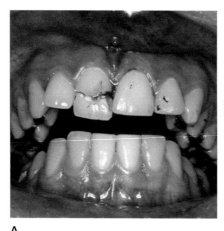
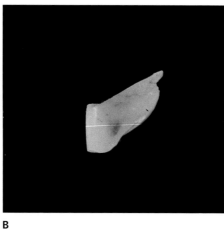

**Fig. 11.1** Complicated crown-root fracture of a right central incisor due to direct trauma. A. Clinical condition. B. Lateral view of crown portion after removal. Note extension below gingival crevice palatally.

**A**

**B**

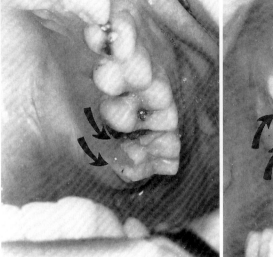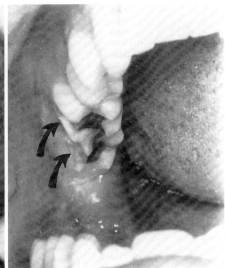

**Fig. 11.2** Uncomplicated crown-root fractures involving palatal cusps in the maxilla and buccal cusps in the mandible (arrows) due to forceful occlusion from a blow to the chin. Note that the fractures of the lingual cusps in the maxilla correspond to the fractures of the buccal cusps in the mandible.

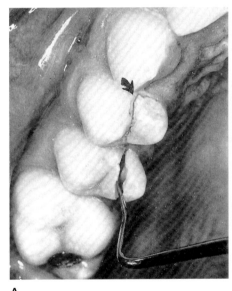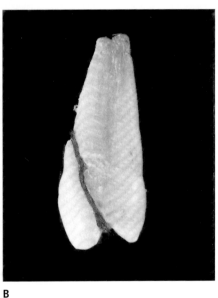

**Fig. 11.3** Complicated crown-root fractures of right first and second premolars (arrow) following indirect trauma (blow to the chin). A. Minimal displacement of fragments in the first premolar. B. Lateral view of the extracted tooth.

A                                                    B

Displacement of the coronal fragment is often minimal, which explains why these fractures are frequently overlooked, particularly in the posterior regions (Fig. 11.3).

In rare cases, a crown-root fracture may occur prior to eruption of the permanent tooth due to a trauma transmitted by displacement of a primary incisor (55).

The fracture line is usually *single*, but *multiple* fractures can occasionally be seen (Fig. 11.4A). A rare type of injury is a vertical fracture running along the long axis of the tooth (34) (Fig. 11.4B), or deviating in a mesial or distal direction.

Crown-root fractures of anterior teeth often expose the pulp in fully erupted teeth, while fractures of teeth in earlier stages of eruption can be uncomplicated.

Even with pulp exposure, symptoms are normally few, and are usually limited to slight pain due to mobility of the crown fragment during function.

## Radiographic findings

Radiographic examination of crown-root fractures following the usual course seldom contributes to the clinical diagnosis, as the oblique fracture line is almost perpendicular to the central beam (Fig. 11.5). Radiographic determination of the oral limit of the fracture is frequently unsuccessful due to the close proximity of fragments at this level. On the other hand, the facial limit is always visible (Fig. 11.6).

Vertical fractures are easily demonstrated if oriented in a facio-oral direction. This also applies to superficial vertical fractures deviating in a mesial or distal direction (chisel fractures) (Fig. 11.7). However, vertical root fractures running in a mesio-distal direction can seldom be seen radiographically (see Fig. 11.10).

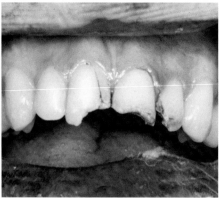

**Fig. 11.4** A. Multiple complicated crown-root fractures of left central incisor. B. Complicated crown-root fracture of a right central incisor running along the long axis of the tooth.

A                                    B

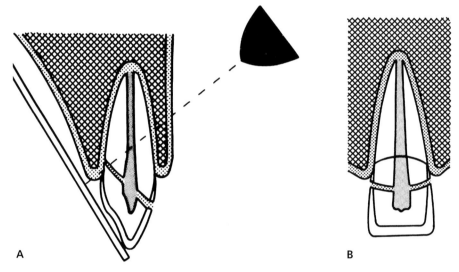

**Fig. 11.5** Schematic drawings of radiographic orientation in a complicated crown-root fracture. A. The normal projection angle is almost perpendicular to the fracture surface. B. Radiographic determination of the lingual part of the fracture is obscured due to the perpendicular relationship between fracture line and central X-ray beam.

A                                    B

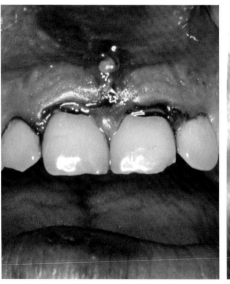
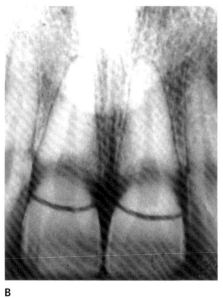

**Fig. 11.6** A. Crown-root fractures involving both central incisors. B. In contrast to the lingual aspect of the fractures, the facial aspect is clearly visible.

A                                    B

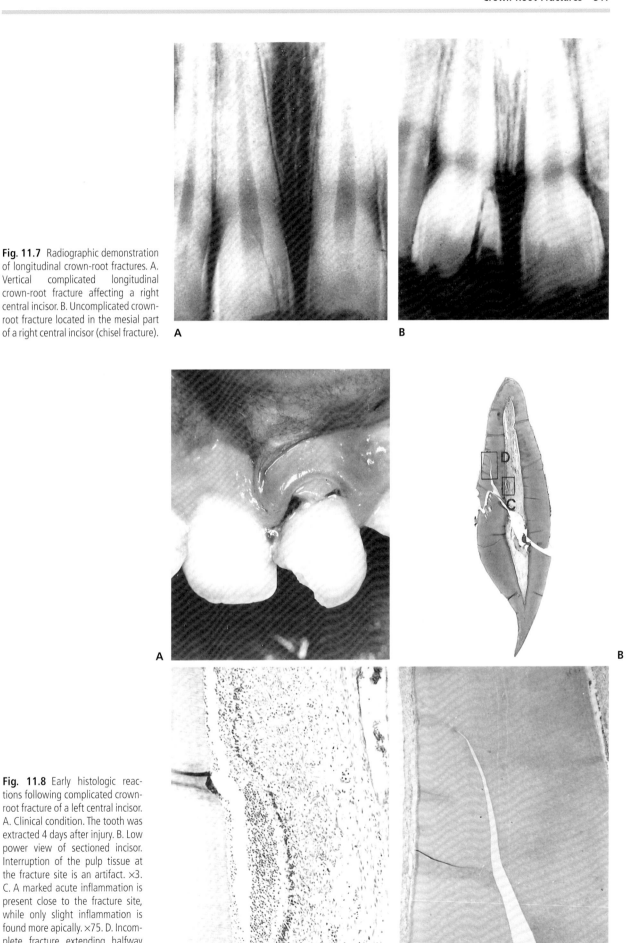

**Fig. 11.7** Radiographic demonstration of longitudinal crown-root fractures. A. Vertical complicated longitudinal crown-root fracture affecting a right central incisor. B. Uncomplicated crown-root fracture located in the mesial part of a right central incisor (chisel fracture).

**Fig. 11.8** Early histologic reactions following complicated crown-root fracture of a left central incisor. A. Clinical condition. The tooth was extracted 4 days after injury. B. Low power view of sectioned incisor. Interruption of the pulp tissue at the fracture site is an artifact. ×3. C. A marked acute inflammation is present close to the fracture site, while only slight inflammation is found more apically. ×75. D. Incomplete fracture extending halfway through the dentin. ×20.

## Healing and pathology

Communication with the oral cavity to the pulp and periodontal ligament in these fractures permits bacterial invasion and subsequent inflammation (3–5). For this reason fracture healing cannot be expected in crown-root fractures, in contrast to root fractures where the fracture is located entirely within the alvelous.

Early histological changes consist of acute pulpal inflammation located close to the fracture caused by invasion of bacteria (56) (Fig. 11.8). Later, proliferation of marginal gingival epithelium into the pulpal chamber can be seen (Figs 11.9 and 11.10). Repair of the fracture by deposition of osteodentin along the fracture line is exceptionally rare (5–7) (Fig. 11.11) and should not govern a treatment decision. Instead the coronal fragment is usually removed and the treatment should be focused on the possibility of using the remaining fragment.

## Treatment

In the *emergency treatment* of crown-root fractures in the *anterior region* it is possible to stabilize of the coronal fragment with an acid etch/resin splint to adjacent teeth (Fig. 11.12) as a temporary measure. Despite contamination from saliva along the fracture line to the pulp, the tooth will generally remain without symptoms. However, it is essential that definitive treatment is initiated within a few days after injury. In case of multiple uncomplicated crown-root fractures in the *premolar and molar region*, immediate provisional treatment can include removal of loose fragments and coverage of exposed supragingival dentin with a glass ionomer cement.

*Vertical crown-root fractures* must generally be extracted. However, it should be mentioned that cases have been reported where bonding of the coronal fragment has led to consolidation of the intraalveolar part of the fracture (58, 59). The tissue involved in this type of healing has not yet been established.

Finally, it should be mentioned that in the case of vertical fractures of *immature permanent incisors*, the fractures are usually incomplete, stopping at or slightly apical to the level of the alveolar crest. These fractures are amenable to orthodontic extrusion, whereby the level of the fracture is brought to a level where pulp capping and restoration are possible (see Chapter 24, p. 684).

Definitive conservative therapy in the *permanent dentition* comprises one of four treatment alternatives. The choice is primarily determined by exact information on the site and type of fracture, but cost and complexity of treatment can also be deciding factors (Table 11.1). In the following, conservative treatment of various types of crown-root fractures will be described.

## Removal of coronal fragment and supragingival restoration

### Treatment principle

This is to allow gingival healing (presumably with formation of a long junctional epithelium), whereafter the coronal portion can be restored (Fig. 11.13). With respect to restoration, the following procedures can be used: bonding the original tooth fragment, where the subgingival portion of the fragment has been removed, composite build-up using dentin and enamel bonding agents; or full crown coverage.

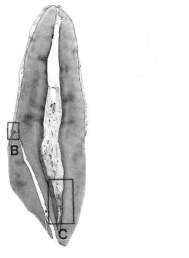
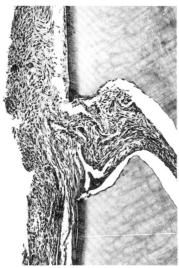
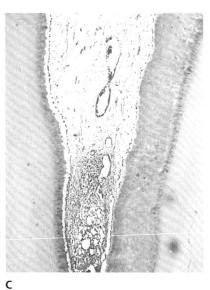

A　　　　　　　　　　　　　　B　　　　　　　　　　　　　　C

**Fig. 11.9** Late histologic reactions following uncomplicated crown-root fracture of a right central incisor. The tooth was left untreated and extracted 3 weeks after injury. A. Low power view of sectioned incisor. ×3. B. Proliferation of connective tissue into the fracture line. ×75. C. Marked inflammation in the coronal part of the pulp. ×30.

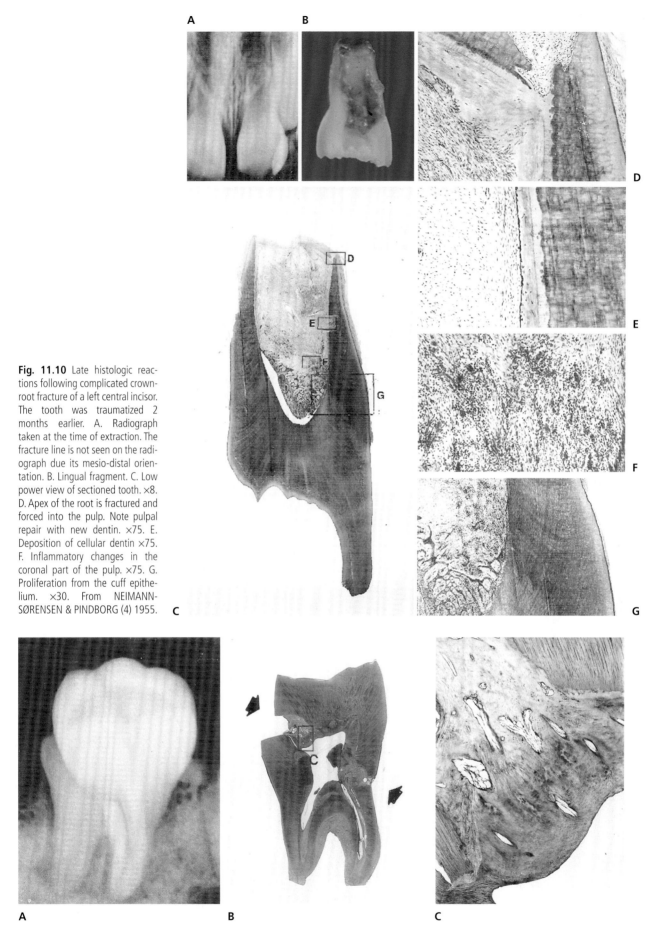

**Fig. 11.10** Late histologic reactions following complicated crown-root fracture of a left central incisor. The tooth was traumatized 2 months earlier. A. Radiograph taken at the time of extraction. The fracture line is not seen on the radiograph due its mesio-distal orientation. B. Lingual fragment. C. Low power view of sectioned tooth. ×8. D. Apex of the root is fractured and forced into the pulp. Note pulpal repair with new dentin. ×75. E. Deposition of cellular dentin ×75. F. Inflammatory changes in the coronal part of the pulp. ×75. G. Proliferation from the cuff epithelium. ×30. From NEIMANN-SØRENSEN & PINDBORG (4) 1955.

**Fig. 11.11** Healing of a crown-root fracture with calcified tissue. A. Radiograph of a right second molar taken 10 months after crown-root fracture. The tooth was immobilized after the injury. Fourteen months after injury, the tooth was extracted for prosthetic reasons. B and C. Note that the fracture communicating with the oral cavity is united by new dentin with vascular inclusions. C ×30. From LOSEE (7) 1948.

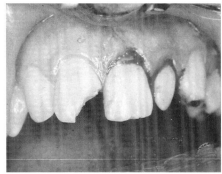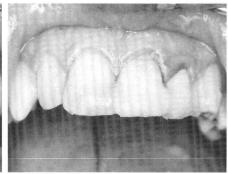

**Fig. 11.12** Emergency treatment of a crown-root fracture of a right central incisor. The coronal fragment was stabilized using an acid-etch/resin splint.

**Table 11.1** Comparison between various treatment modalities of crown-root fractures.

| Procedure | Indications | Advantages | Disadvantages |
|---|---|---|---|
| Fragment removal only | Superficial fractures (chisel fractures). | Easy to perform. Definitive restoration can be completed soon after injury. | Long-term prognosis has not been established. |
| Fractures where denudation of the fracture site does not compromise esthetics (i.e. fractures with palatal extension) | Fragment removal and gingivectomy (sometimes ostectomy). | Relatively easy procedure. Restoration can be completed soon after injury. | The restored tooth may migrate labially due to accumulation of granulation tissue in the deep palatal pocket (45). |
| Orthodontic extrusion of apical fragment | All types of fractures, assuming that reasonable root length can be achieved. | Stable position of the restored tooth. Optimal gingival health. Can be performed in complicated crown-root fractures. | Technically time consuming procedure, with late completion of final treatment.* |
| Surgical extrusion of apical fragment | All types of fractures (except uncomplicated crown-root fractures where vitality should be preserved) assuming that reasonable root length can be achieved. | Rapid procedure. Stable position of the tooth. The method allows inspection of the root for additional fractures. | Limited risk of the root resorption and marginal breakdown of periodontium. Cannot be performed in uncomplicated crown-root fractures where vitality should be preserved. |

\* Note: Cervical gingival fibers must be incised once tooth is at desired position to prevent return of tooth to original position.

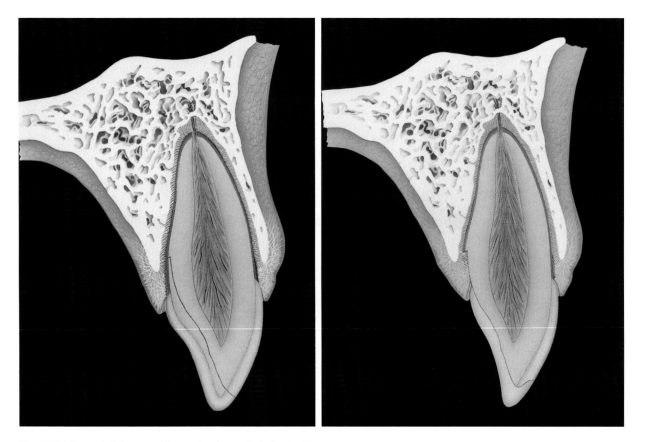

**Fig. 11.13** Removal of the coronal fragment and supragingival restoration.

**Fig. 11.14 Removal of the coronal fragment and supragingival restoration**
This 16-year-old girl has suffered a crown-root fracture which has exposed the palatal root surface. The clinical condition is shown after fragment removal.

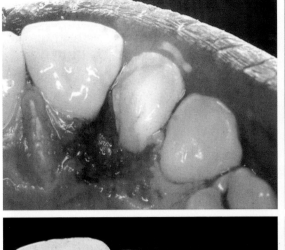

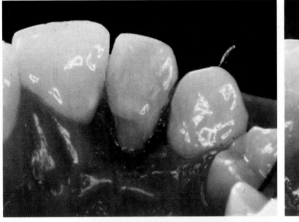
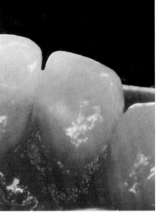

**Condition 1 week later**
(Left) The palatal fragment has been removed and the exposed root dentin smoothed with a chisel; the exposed dentin covered with calcium hydroxide and a temporary crown. Two weeks later (right) creeping reattachment is seen and the palatal of the crown restored with a dentin-bonded composite resin restoration.

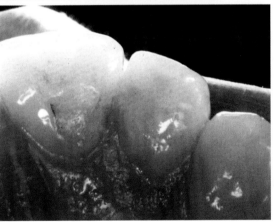
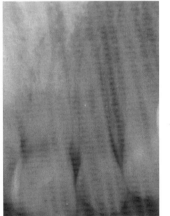

**Follow-up**
Clinical and radiographic condition 4 years after treatment. (Courtesy of Dr. B. MALMGREN Eastman Institute, Stockholm, Sweden).

Pulpal considerations are identical to those that apply to treatment of crown fractures (see Chapter 10).

### Indication

This procedure should be limited to superficial fractures that do not involve the pulp (i.e. chisel fractures).

### Treatment procedure

The loose fragment is removed as soon as possible after injury. Rough edges along the fracture surface below the gingiva may be smoothed with a chisel. The remaining crown is temporarily restored supragingivally (Fig. 11.14). Optimal oral hygiene should be maintained during the healing period (e.g. daily chlorhexidine rinsing). Once gingival healing is seen (after 2–3 weeks), the crown can be restored with a dentin and enamel-bonded composite.

Reattachment of an incisal fragment of a crown-root fractured tooth basically follows the same principles as reattachment of the incisal fragment of a crown-fractured incisor (see Chapter 10). However, due to the subgingival placement of the fracture margin palatally, certain preliminary steps must be followed (Fig. 11.15). The subgingival aspect of the incisal fragment should be reduced to a sharp, smooth margin ending at the free gingival margin and then bonded to the remaining tooth (Fig. 11.15).

**Fig. 11.15 Fragment bonding**
The subgingival part of the fragment is reduced with diamonds and aluminum oxide discs. As the facio-oral dimension of the fracture surface exceeded 5 mm, thereby exceeding the maximum depth of light penetration by a curing lamp (2.5 mm from each direction), a self-curing composite resin is chosen.

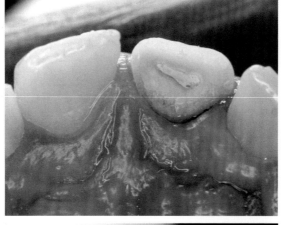
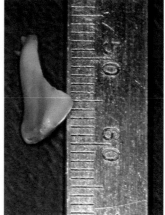

**Condition after fragment bonding**
Treatment resulted in complete restoration of coronal dental anatomy.

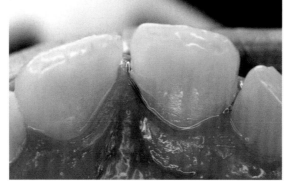
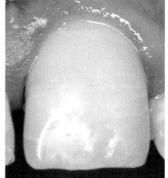

## Cost–benefit

While the pulp has been shown to respond well to this form of conservative treatment, the immediate shortcoming is frequent re-fracture of the reattached fragment or loss of the composite resin build-up due to the steep, non-retentive inclination of the fracture surface. Thus, these treatments probably can best be described as temporary until definitive treatment can be provided.

## Surgical exposure of fracture surface

### Treatment principle

This is to convert the subgingival fracture to a supragingival fracture with the help of gingivectomy and osteotomy (8–11, 37–42, 57) (Fig. 11.16).

### Indication

This should only be used where the surgical technique does not compromise the esthetic result, i.e. only the palatal aspect of the fracture must be exposed by this procedure.

### Treatment procedure

After administration of a local anesthetic, the coronal fragment is removed and the fracture surface carefully exam-ined. It is important to remember that most crown-root fractures contain a lingual step (Fig. 11.16). In some cases, this step is a part of an incomplete or complete fracture extending more apically (Fig. 11.8). It is therefore essential to determine whether the lingual step in the root is part of a secondary fracture. This can be done during the gingivectomy by placing a sharp explorer or similar instrument at the base of the step and, with a gentle palatal movement, check whether abnormal mobility can be detected. Axial fracture lines running from the pulp chamber to the root surface should also be carefully explored. If these fractures are overlooked, an inflammatory reaction in the periodontium will develop after completion of the restoration (43, 45). The use of a conventional cast core and separate crown instead of a single unit restoration has the advantage that future changes in the position of the gingiva and subsequent loss of esthetics can easily be corrected.

## Cost–benefit

Treatment time is short. The long-term prognosis of these restorations has been evaluated and the following results obtained (45). After gingivectomy, and despite good marginal adaptation, re-growth of the gingiva often takes place, leading to development of a pathologic pocket palatally and inflammation of the surrounding gingiva. After some years, this can result in labial migration of the restored teeth. Migration has been found to be approximately 0.8 mm over a 5-year period (45) (Fig. 11.17).

### Fig. 11.16 Removal of the coronal fragment and surgical exposure of the fracture

Clinical and radiographic appearance of a complicated crown-root fracture.

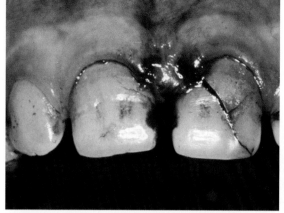
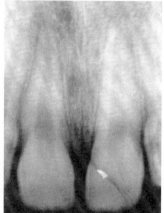

### Exposing the fracture site

The coronal fragment is removed. A combined gingivectomy and osteotomy expose the fracture surface.

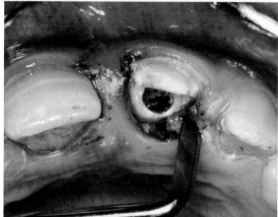
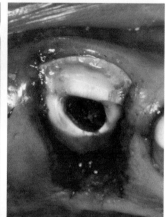

### Constructing a post-retained crown

After taking an impression, a post-retained full crown is fabricated.

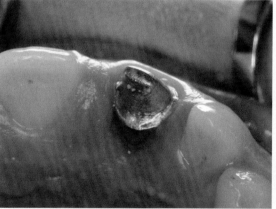
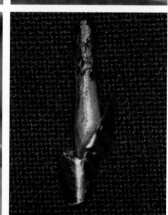

### The finished restoration

The clinical and radiographic condition 2 months after insertion of the crown.

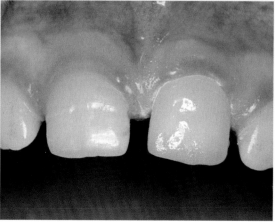
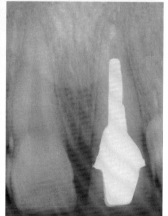

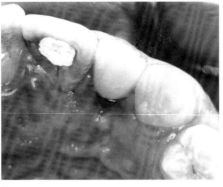 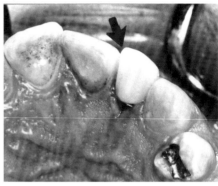

**Fig. 11.17** Labial movement of a crown-root fractured tooth, restored after surgical exposure of the fracture surface. A. Condition immediately after restoration of the right lateral incisor. B. Condition after 6 years. From BESSERMANN (45) 1980.

A                    B

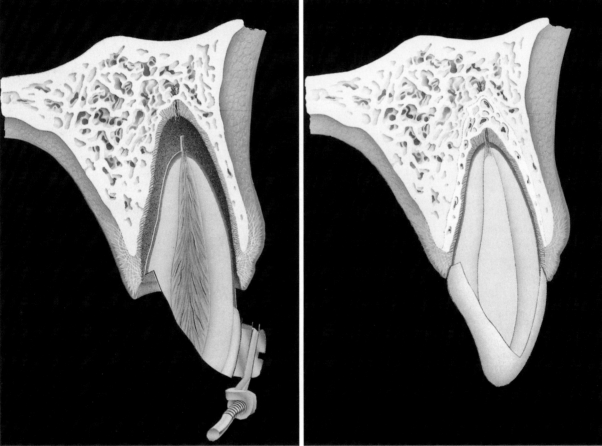

**Fig. 11.18** Removal of the coronal fragment and orthodontic extrusion of the root.

## Orthodontic extrusion of apical fragment

### Treatment principle

This is to move the fracture to a supragingival position orthodontically (Fig. 11.18).

This treatment procedure was introduced in 1973 by Heithersay (44). Since then several clinical studies have supported its value (42, 46–50, 60–67).

### Indication

This is the only method for uncomplicated crown-root fractures if pulp vitality is to be preserved. Can also be used for complicated crown-root fractures but is more time-consuming than surgical extrusion. In cases where it is desirable to reconstruct osseous and/or gingival defects, slow orthodontic extrusion can be used to guide downgrowth of these tissues. The cervical diameter after extrusion is essential and should be analyzed before extrusion (Fig. 11.19).

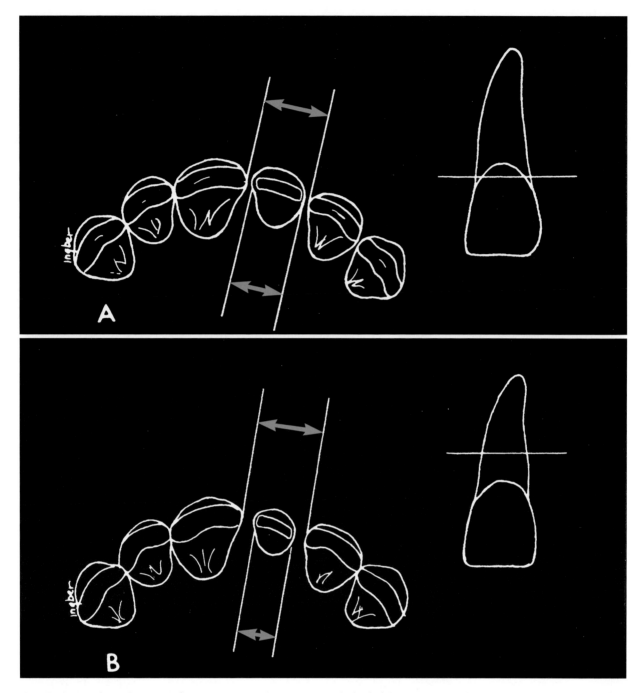

**Fig. 11.19** Cervical root dimensions after extrusion. A. Tooth preparation at the level of the cemento-enamel junction is directly related to the fixed amount of space between the teeth. B. Tooth preparation after eruption of the apical root fragment; the diameter of the preparation is small relative to the fixed amount of space between the teeth. Restoration will thus require greater attention. From INGBER (47) 1976.

### Treatment procedure

In teeth with *completed root formation* and a crown-root fracture, endodontic therapy can be performed prior to removal of the coronal fragment (i.e. while the coronal fragment is splinted to the adjacent teeth). Fragment retention can facilitate the endodontic procedure, whereby placement of a rubber dam and tissue control of the operative field is improved (in contrast to fragment removal). Thereafter orthodontic extrusion is performed (83) (Fig. 11.20). Recent

esthetic improvements have been achieved whereby the extrusion devices have been masked by using either the hollowed out crown portion of the tooth or a pontic fastened to adjacent teeth with wire (78). The orthodontic procedure is described in Chapter 24, p. 684.

In teeth with *incomplete root formation*, pulp capping or pulpotomy may be performed. Thereafter, orthodontic traction is initiated; this technique is further described in Chapter 24, p. 684. Recently, a new method of orthodontic extrusion with magnets has been described. One or two

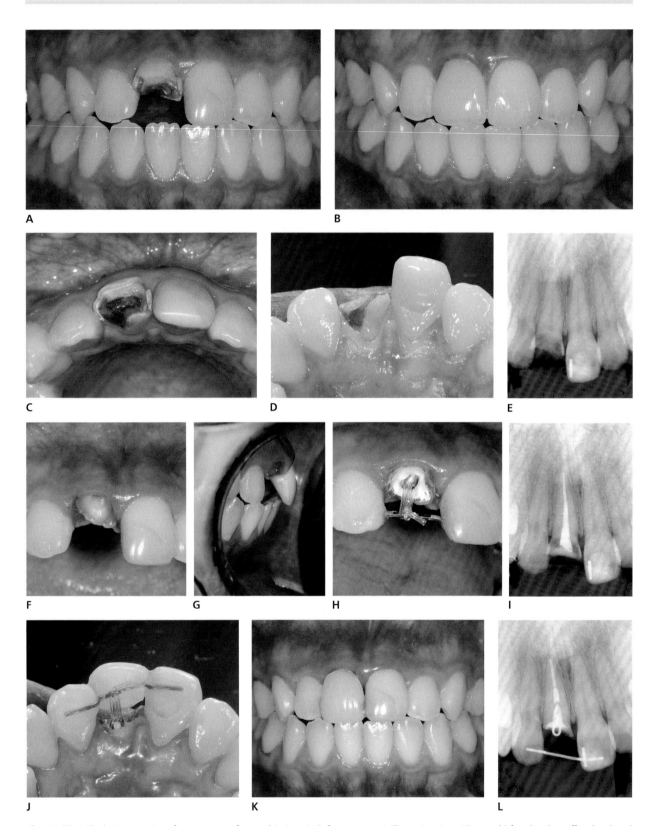

**Fig. 11.20** Orthodontic extrusion of a crown-root fractured incisor. A. Before treatment. The patient is a 16-year-old female who suffered a dental trauma 7 years ago. The two central incisors were fractured and were restored with composite. However, the restoration of the right central incisor failed due to secondary caries. B. After treatment. The right extruded central incisor was restored with a porcelain jacket crown after orthodontic extrusion and the left incisor was restored with new composite. C and D. Incisal and palatal aspect at the first examination. E. Radiograph at the first examination. Caries has invaded to the crest of the alveolar bone. Buccal aspect after endodontic treatment and before orthodontic extrusion. There seems no sound tooth structure preserved above the alveolar crest. F. Condition after endodontic treatment G. The occlusal relation; enough space is found to accommodate an orthodontic appliance. H. After placing an orthodontic appliance, a hook is placed in the canal. Elastic is placed between the wire and the hook. The distance between the hook and the wire is 4 mm. I. Radiograph before extrusion. J and K. Palatal and buccal aspect at the start of extrusion. A laminate is bonded to neighboring teeth. Note there is enough space between the gingival margin and the cervical margin of the temporary crown. L. Radiograph taken at the start of extrusion. (*continued*)

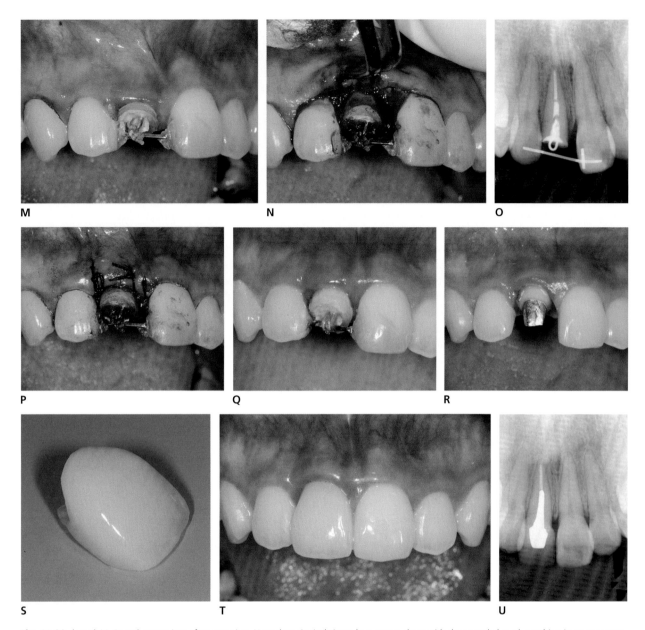

**Fig. 11.20** (*cont.*) M. Buccal aspect just after extrusion. Note that gingival tissue has grown along with the extruded tooth resulting in an unacceptable gingival topography. N. Apically repositioned flap. A gingival flap was raised and positioned apically after osseous resection of excessive bone around the extruded tooth. O. Radiograph taken 6 weeks later at the end of the extrusion. A slight amount of bone seems to have regenerated along with extrusion. P. Immediately after surgery. Q. Three months after extrusion. R. Four months after extrusion. S. A porcelain jacket crown to be seated. T. Buccal view after setting of the crown. U. Radiograph after the restoration.

neodymium-iron-boron magnets were attached to the remaining root and a second, larger magnet was incorporated in a removal appliance. The roots were extruded over a treatment period of 9–11 weeks; 2 patients were successfully treated using this method (79).

In cases of *incomplete vertical fracture* of *immature incisors* (see later), it can be difficult to gain access to the pulp and to control moisture and hemorrhage in order to perform a pulpotomy. It could then be an advantage to seal the fracture lines facially and orally with an acid-etch technique and an unfilled resin while the tooth is being extruded. Once the fracture is at a level where access is pos-

sible, the fragment can be removed, and pulp capping or pulpotomy performed (see Chapter 24, p. 684) and the crown restored.

An important question is: how much can a tooth be extruded and still maintain reasonable periodontal support? This can best be answered by considering the crown-root ratio. If the goal of extrusion is a crown-root ratio of approximately 1:1, a central incisor can be extruded 2–4 mm, while a lateral incisor can be extruded 4–6 mm. However, it should be noted that, as yet, no study has confirmed that a crown-root ratio of 1:1 cannot be exceeded while maintaining stable periodontal support. Clinical experience with long-term observations of root fractures showing healing with interposition of connective tissue (i.e. a shortened root, see Chapter 8) indicates that a relatively large deviation from a crown-root ratio of 1:1 can be accepted without resulting in excessive mobility or breakdown of the periodontium.

After extrusion and stabilization, restorative procedures can be carried out as described under the surgical approach. However, special restorative problems arise when dealing with a root which has been moved coronally. Thus, it should be realized that the extruded root will normally present a smaller cervical diameter for restoration than a root in its normal position (47, 65) (Fig. 11.19). If conventional restorative techniques are employed, the final restoration will have greater divergence from the gingival margin incisally. However, experience gained by the restoration of single tooth implants has shown that conventional porcelain techniques can be used to restore anterior symmetry.

Concerning the prognosis of teeth treated by forced eruption, nothing definite can be said at the present time. However, experience to date has shown that this procedure can result in stable periodontal conditions (45).

### Cost–benefit

The procedure is slow and cumbersome (Table 11.1). However, it can provide excellent esthetic results and the gingival health appears to be optimal. Moreover, pulpal vitality can in some cases be maintained where indicated.

## Surgical extrusion of apical fragment

### Treatment principle

This is to surgically move the fracture to a supragingival position (Fig. 11.20).

This treatment procedure was introduced by Tegsjö et al. (53, 69) in 1978, and the method further developed by Bühler (70, 71) and Kahnberg (72–76).

### Indication

This should only be used where there is completed root development and the apical fragment is long enough to accommodate a post-retained crown. Surgical extrusion results in loss of pulp vitality if performed in uncomplicated crown-root fractures. In such cases orthodontic extrusion may be a better alternative if there is a desire to keep the pulp vital.

### Treatment

Clinical experience has shown that the time factor for removal of the coronal fragment is not critical for success of treatment. Thus, fragment removal can be instituted days or weeks after injury. The pulp can be extirpated and the tooth root filled at this time. However, clinical studies have shown that postponement of endodontic therapy for 3–4 weeks gives better results (76). If the latter approach is chosen, the pulp canal is sealed with zinc oxide-eugenol cement. Moreover, experience has shown that postponement of the surgical procedure for 2–3 weeks facilitates atraumatic extraction due to inflammatory processes arising in the periodontal ligament.

The apical fragment is luxated with a thin periosteal elevator (Fig. 11.21). The extracted root is then inspected for incomplete fractures which will contraindicate repositioning of the root. The root is moved into a more coronal position and stabilized in the new position with interproximal sutures and/or a splint. In case of palatally inclined fractures, 180° rotation can often imply that /only slight extrusion is necessary to accommodate crown preparation due to the difference in position of the cemento-enamel junction labially and palatally. The exposed pulp is covered with a zinc oxide-eugenol cement. After 3–4 weeks, the tooth can be treated endodontically. After another 1–2 months, the tooth can be restored with a post-retained crown.

### Prognosis

In the reported series of patients treated, with up to 5-year observation periods, either no or slight root resorption (surface resorption) was seen (Table 11.2 and Figs 11.22–11.25) (69, 74). In a recent 10-year follow-up study of 19 surgically extruded teeth, Kahnberg showed that all teeth survived; and only one showed cervical resorption (81).

### Cost–benefit

Several clinical studies have indicated that this is a safe and rapid method for the treatment of crown-root fractures. However, pulp vitality must be sacrificed (Table 11.1).

## Vital root submergence

In cases not considered restorable in young individuals, it might be indicated to keep the root portion in place in order to maintain the alveolar width and height (84, 85). This procedure is described in Chapter 24.

## Extraction

This alternative is relevant when none of the above mentioned treatment procedures is indicated. With respect to subsequent tooth replacement, it should be remembered that the supporting bone is very rapidly resorbed (see Chapter 28). For this reason the apical root fragment may be preserved submerged to keep the volume of the alveolar process. Provided the patient has finished growth, implant treatment may be a good alternative (Chapter 28). In still growing patients orthodontic space closure (Chapter 24) or autotransplantation (Chapter 27) are better alternatives.

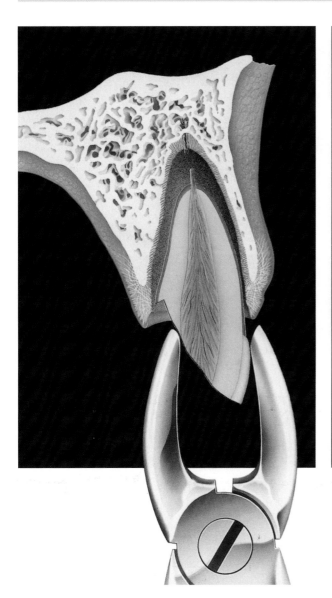
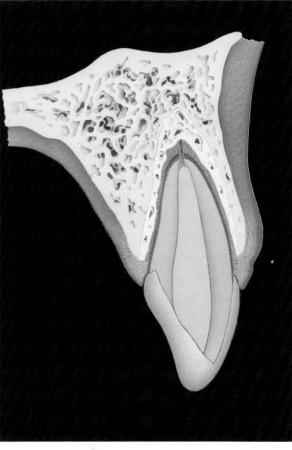

**Fig. 11.21** Removal of the coronal fragment and surgical extrusion of the root.

**Table 11.2** Long-term results of surgical extrusion of crown-root fractured anterior teeth.

| | Observation period yr. (mean) | Age of patient yr. (mean) | No. of teeth | Tooth survival (%) | PDL healing[3] (%) | Apical healing (%) | Gingival healing (%) |
|---|---|---|---|---|---|---|---|
| Tegsjö et al. (69) 1987 | 4 (4.0) | 9–33 (15.0) | 56 | 91 | 88 | 98 | |
| Kahnberg (74) 1988 | 5.5 (2.4) | 13–75 (31.0) | 17[1] | 100 | 65 | 94 | 100 |
| | | 13–75 (31.0) | 41[2] | 100 | 74 | 95 | 100 |
| Caliskan et al. (80) 1999 | 1.2 | 10–45 (21.5) | 20 | 100 | 90 | 100 | 95 |

[1] Transplant performed via apical exposure; [2] Transplant performed via coronal approach; [3] Non-healing represents cases with surface resorption that results in a slight shortening of the root.

**Fig. 11.22 Removal of the coronal fragment and surgical extrusion of the root**

A complicated crown-root fracture in a 13-year-old boy. The loose fragment is stabilized immediately after injury with a temporary crown and bridge material using the acid-etch technique.

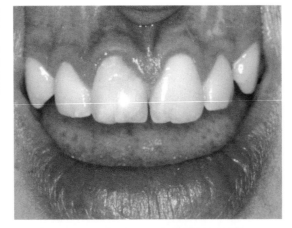 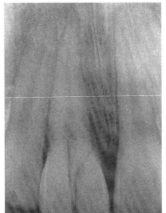

**Incision of the PDL**

After a local anesthesia the PDL is incised using a specially contoured surgical blade. The PDL is incised as far apically as possible.

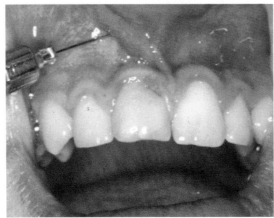 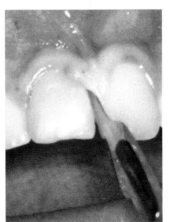

**Luxation of the root**

The root is then luxated with a narrow elevator which is placed at the mesiopalatal and distopalatal corners respectively.

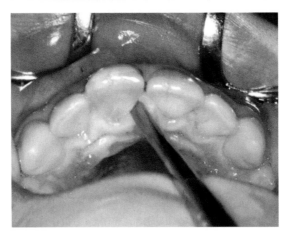 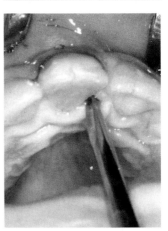

**Extracting the root**

The root is extracted and inspected for additional fractures.

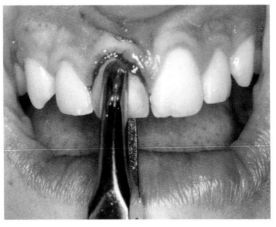 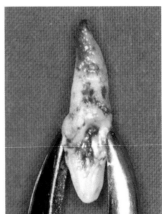

**Replanting the apical fragment**
The root is tried in different positions in order to establish where the fracture is optimally exposed, yet with minimal extrusion. In this instance, optimal repositioning was achieved by rotating the root 45°.

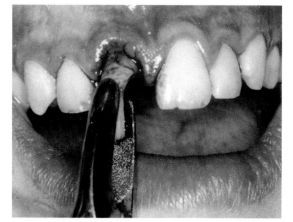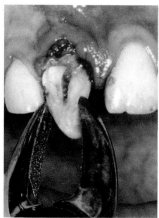

**Stabilization of the apical fragment during healing**
The root is splinted to adjacent teeth. The pulp is extirpated and the access cavity to the root canal closed.

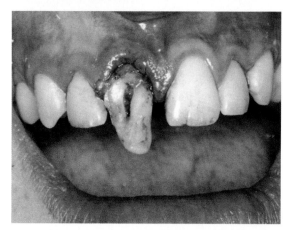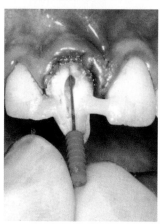

**Root filling**
Two weeks after initial treatment, endodontic therapy can be continued, in the form of an interim dressing with calcium hydroxide. The root canal is obturated with gutta-percha and sealer as far apically as possible 1 month after surgical extrusion.

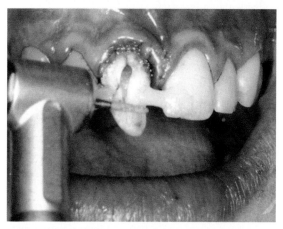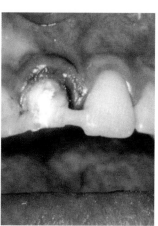

**Completion of the restoration**
Two months after surgical extrusion, healing has occurred and it is possible to complete the restoration.

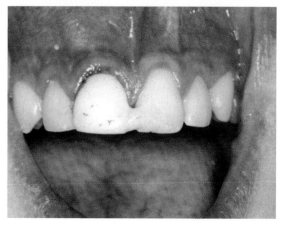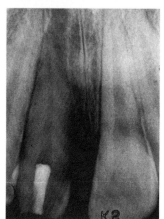

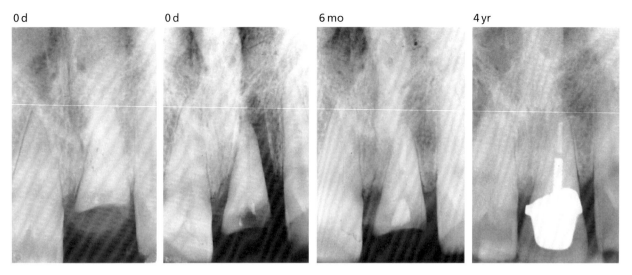

| 0 d | 0 d | 6 mo | 4 yr |

**Fig. 11.23** Intra-alveolar transplantation of a crown-root fractured central incisor. No sign of root resorption is seen 4 years after transplantation. From KAHNBERG (73) 1985.

## Essentials

### Treatment of permanent teeth

#### *Emergency procedures*

Fragments of crown-root fractured teeth can be temporarily splinted to alleviate pain from mastication (Fig. 11.12). Definitive treatment should be provided within a few days.

#### *Definitive treatment*

The level of the fracture determines the type of therapy (i.e. extraction of the root, surgical exposure of the fracture surface or orthodontic or surgical extrusion of the root).

### Extraction of the tooth

Indicated in teeth where the coronal fragment comprises more than 1/3 of the clinical root and in case of fractures following the long axis of the tooth.

### Removal of coronal fragment and supragingival restoration

Indicated in superficial fractures that do not involve the pulp (Figs 11.13 and 11.14).

(1) Administer local anesthesia.
(2) Remove loose fragments.
(3) Smooth rough subgingival fracture surface with a chisel.
(4) Cover supragingival exposed dentin.
(5) When gingival healing has occurred a supragingival restoration is made using bonded composite or the original fragment where the subgingival portion has been removed.

### Surgical exposure of fracture surface

Indicated in teeth where the coronal fragment comprises 1/3 or less of the clinical root (Fig. 11.16).

(1) Administer local anesthesia.
(2) Remove loose fragments.
(3) Perform a pulpectomy and obturate the root canal with gutta percha and a sealer.
(4) Expose the fracture surface with a gingivectomy and ostectomy.
(5) Restore the tooth with a post-retained porcelain jacket crown.

### Orthodontic extrusion of apical fragment

Indicated in teeth where the coronal fragment comprises 1/3 or less of the clinical root (Figs 11.18 and 11.20).

(1) Administer local anesthesia.
(2) Remove loose fragments.
(3) In teeth with *mature root formation*, perform pulpectomy and obturate the root canal with gutta-percha and a sealer. In teeth with *immature root formation*, perform a cervical pulpotomy (see Chapter 22, p. 646).
(4) Expose the fracture surface via orthodontic extrusion of the root (see also Chapter 24, p. 684).
(5) When the root is extruded, perform a gingivectomy and ostectomy, if needed, to restore symmetry of gingival contour.
(6) Restore the tooth temporarily and splint to adjacent teeth for a retention period of 6 months.
(7) After the retention period, restore definitively.

### Surgical extrusion of apical fragment

Indicated in teeth where the coronal fragment comprises less than half root length (Figs 11.20 and 11.22).

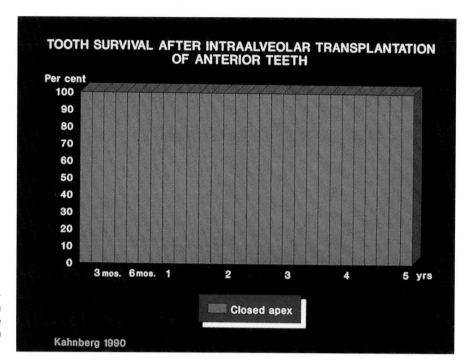

**Fig. 11.24** Tooth survival of 68 intra-alveolar transplanted anterior teeth with completed root formation at time of surgery. From KAHNBERG (75) 1990.

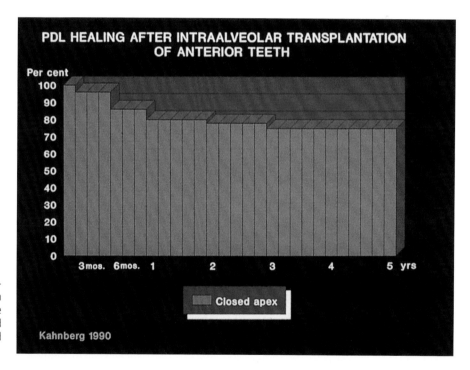

**Fig. 11.25** PDL healing of 68 intra-alveolar transplanted anterior teeth with completed root formation at time of surgery. Complications involved surface resorption of the repositioned tooth. From KAHNBERG (75) 1990.

(1) Administer antibiotics and local anesthesia.

(2) The pulp can be extirpated and the root canal filled with gutta percha and a sealer prior to intra-alveolar transplantation; or endodontics can be postponed and the root canal entrance sealed with a zinc oxide-eugenol cement.

(3) The PDL is incised, the tooth luxated with an elevator and the tooth extracted with forceps.

(4) The root surface is inspected for incomplete root fractures, which would contraindicate transplantation.

(5) The root is repositioned at a level 1 mm coronal to the alveolar crest. If desirable, the root can be rotated to achieve a maximum periodontal surface area within the socket.

(6) The tooth is stabilized using interproximal sutures.

(7) Take a postoperative radiograph.

(8) After 2 to 3 weeks, the transplant is usually firm. If the root canal has not been filled, calcium hydroxide can be used as an interim dressing which will ensure apical hard tissue closure. A temporary restoration can now be fabricated.

(9) After 6 months, a permanent root filling as well as a definitive crown restoration can be completed.

(10) If a gutta-percha root filling has been made prior to transplantation, the tooth can be restored after 2 months.

## Vital root submergence

Indicated in young individuals where the abovementioned treatment alternatives cannot be carried out in order to maintain the dimensions of the alveolar process.

(1) Administer a local anesthetic.

(2) A flap is raised.

(3) The supra-alveolar fragments of the tooth are removed.

(4) The flap is closed over the exposed root including the pulp.

(5) Insert a space maintainer.

## Extraction

Indicated in cases where none of the above mentioned treatments can be performed.

## References

1. ANDREASEN JO. Etiology and pathogenesis of traumatic dental injuries. A clinical study of 1,298 cases. *Scand J Dent Res* 1970;**78**:329–42.

2. SUTHER T, FIXOTT HC. Multiple accidental fractures of posterior primary teeth. *A case report. ASDC J Dent Child* 1952;**19**:115–7.

3. BEVELANDER G. Tissue reactions in experimental tooth fracture. *J Dent Res* 1942;**21**:481–7.

4. NEIMANN-SÖRENSEN E, PINDBORG JJ. Traumatisk betingede forandringer i ikke fäirdigdannede tinder. *Tandlaegebladet* 1955;**59**:230–43.

5. LINDEMANN H. Histologische Untersuchung einer geheilten Zahnfraktur. *Dtsch Zahn Mund Kieferheilk* 1938;**5**:915–25.

6. RITCHIE GM. Repair of coronal fractures in upper incisor teeth. *Br Dent J* 1962;**112**:459–60.

7. LOSEE FL. Untreated tooth fractures. Report of three cases. *Oral Surg Oral Med Oral Pathol* 1948;**1**: 464–73.

8. CLYDE JS. Transverse-oblique fractures of the crown with extension below the epithelial attachment. *Br Dent J* 1965;**119**:402–6.

9. LANGDON JD. Treatment of oblique fractures of incisors involving the epithelial attachment. A case report. *Br Dent J* 1968;**125**:72–4.

10. FELDMAN G, SOLOMON C, NOTARO PJ. Endodontic management of traumatized teeth. *Oral Surg Oral Med Oral Pathol* 1966;**21**:100–12.

11. NATKIN E. Diagnosis and treatment of traumatic injuries and their sequelae. In: Ingle JI. ed. *Endodontics*. Philadelphia: Lea & Febiger, 1965;566–611.

12. ELLIS RG. Fractured anterior teeth. Natural crown restoration. *J Canad Dent Assoc* 1940;**6**:339–44.

13. GRAZIDE, COULOMB, BOISSET & DASQUE. L'embrochage et le collage dans le traitement des fractures dentaires. *Rev Stomatol (Paris)* 1956;**57**:428–44.

14. KISLING E. Om behandlingen of skader som fölge of akutte mekaniske traumer på unge permanente incisiver. *Tandlægebladet* 1953;**57**:61–9, 109–29.

15. LEE EC. Total fracture of the crown. *Br Dent J* 1966;**120**:139–40.

16. CURRY VL. Fractured incisors. *Dent Practit Dent Rec* 1951;**1**:341–6.

17. PROPHET AS, ROWBOTHAM TC, JAMES PMC. Traumatic injuries of the teeth. *Br Dent J* 1964;**116**:377–85.

18. RAVN JJ. Ulykkesskadede fortänder på börn. Klassifikation og behandling. Copenhagen: Odontologisk Forening, 1966.

19. CHOSACH A, EIDELMAN E. Rehabilitation of a fractured incisor using the patient's natural crown. Case report. *ASDC J Dent Child* 1964;**31**:3119–21.

20. TAMUCHI H, NOBUHARAA, NOHMI A. Repair of the total fracture of anterior tooth crown and its fluorination. Three case reports. *Epn J Conserv Dent* 1967;**10**:37–41.

21. NEEDLEMAN HL, WOLFMAN MS. Traumatic posterior dental fractures Report of a case. *ASDC J Dent Child* 1976;**43**:262–4.

22. RUD J, OMNELL K-AA. Root fractures due to corrosion. Diagnostic aspect. *Scand J Dent Res* 1970;**78**:397–403.

23. PIETROKOVSKI J, LANTZMANE. Complicated crown fractures in adults. *J Prosthet Dent* 1973;**30**:801–7.

24. SNYDER DE. The cracked tooth syndrome and fractured posterior cusp. *Oral Surg Oral Med Oral Pathol* 1976;**41**:698–704.

25. CAMERON CE. The cracked tooth syndrome: additional findings. *J AmDent Assoc* 1976;**93**:971–5.

26. SILVESTRI AR Jr. The undiagnosed split-root syndrome. *J Am Dent Assoc* 1976;**92**:930–5.

27. BOUCHON F, HERVÉ M, MARMASSE A. Propos empiriques fractures dentaires spontanées. *Actual Odontostomatatol* 1977;**118**:221–39.

28. HIATT WH. Incomplete crown-root fracture in pulpal-periodontal disease. *J Periodontol* 1973;**44**:369–79.

29. MAXWELL EH, BRALY BV. Incomplete tooth fracture. Prediction and prevention. *J Calif Dent Assoc* 1977;**5**:51–5.

30. POLSON AM. Periodontal destruction associated with vertical root fracture. Report of four cases. *J Periodontol* 1977;**48**:27–32.

31. LOMMEL TJ, MEISTER F Jr, GERSTEIN H, DAVIES EE, TILK MA. Alveolar bone loss associated with vertical root fractures. Report of six cases. *Oral Surg Oral Med Oral Pathol* 1978;**45**:909–19.

32. WECHSLERS M, VOGEL RI, FISHELBERG G, SHOWLING FE. Iatrogenic root fractures: a case report. *J Endod* 1978;**4**:251–3.

33. WEISMAN MI. The twenty-five cent crack detector. *J Endod* 1978;**4**:222.

34. MICHANOWICZ AE, PERCHERSKY JL, McKIBBEN DH. A vertical fracture of the crown and root. *ASDC J Dent Child* 1978;**45**:54–6.

35. TODD HW. Avulsed natural crown as a temporary crown: report of case. *J Am Dent Assoc* 1971;**82**:1398–400.

36. STERN N. Provisional restoration of a broken anterior tooth, with its own natural crown. *J Dent* 1975;**2**: 217–8.

37. FELDMAN G, SOLOMON C, NOTARO P, MOSKOWITZ E. Endodontic management of the subgingival fracture. *Dent Radio Photogr* 1972;**45**:3–9.

38. GOLDSTEIN RE, LEVITAS TC. Preservation of fractured maxillary central incisors in an adolescent: report of case. *J Am Dent Assoc* 1972;**84**:371–4.

39. TALIM ST, GOHIL KS. Management of coronal fractures of permanent posterior teeth. *J Prosthet Dent* 1974;**31**:172–8.

40. GOERIG AC. Restoration of teeth with subgingival and subosseous fractures. *J Prosthet Dent* 1975;**34**:634–9.

41. FEDERICK DR. Klinische Wiederherstellung der Kronenlänge durch parodontal-prothetische Verfahren. *Quintessence* 1976;**3**:47–53.

42. BESSERMANN M. Ny behandlingsmetode af krone-rodfrakturer. *Tandlaegebladet* 1978;**82**:441–4.

43. LIMABURG RG, MARSHALL FJ. The diagnosis and treatment of vertical root fractures. Report of case. *J Am Dent Assoc* 1973;**86**:679–83.

44. HEITHERSAY GS. Combined endodontic-orthodontic treatment of transverse root fractures in the region of the alveolar crest. *Oral Surg Oral Med Oral Pathol* 1973;**36**:404–15.

45. BESSERMANN-NIELSEN M. Personal communication, 1980.

46. WOLFSON EM, SEIDEN L. Combined endodontic-orthodontic treatment of subgingivally fractured teeth. *J Canad Dent Assoc* 1975;**11**:621–4.

47. INGBER JS. Forced eruption Part II. A method of treating nonrestorable teeth – periodontal and restorative considerations. *J Perodontol* 1976;**47**:203–16.

48. PERSSON M, SERNEKE D. Ortodontisk framdragning av tand med cervikal rotfraktur för att möjliggöra kronersättning. *Tandläkartidningen* 1977;**69**: 1263–9.

49. DELIVANIS P, DELIVANIS H, KUFTINEC MM. Endodontic-orthodontic management of fractured anterior teeth. *J Am Dent Assoc* 1978;**97**:483–5.

50. SIMON JHS, KELLY WH, GORDON DG, ERICKSEN GW. Extrusion of endodontically treated teeth. *J Am Dent Assoc* 1978;**97**:17–23.

51. STENVIK A. The effect of extrusive orthodontic forces on human pulp and dentin. *Scand J Dent Res* 1971;**79**: 430–5.

52. REITAN K. Initial tissue behavior during apical root resorption. *Angle Orthod* 1974;**44**:68–82.

53. TEGSJÖ U, VALERIUS-OLSSON H, OLGART K. Intra-alveolar transplantation of teeth with cervical root fractures. *Swed Dent J* 1978;**2**:73–82.

54. PITTS DL, NATKIN E. Diagnosis and treatment of vertical root fractures. *J Endod* 1983;**9**:338–46.

55. BODNER L, LUSTMANN J. Intra-alveolar fracture of a developing permanent incisor. *Pediatr Dent* 1988;**10**: 1379.

56. WALTON RE, MICHELICH RJ, SMITH GM. The histopatogenesis of vertical root fractures. *J Endod* 1984;**10**:48–56.

57. MCDONALD FL, DAVIS SS, WHITBECK P. Periodontal surgery as an aid to restoring fractured teeth. *J Prosthet Dent* 1982;**47**:366–72.

58. MICHANOWICZ AE, PERCHERSKY JL, MCKIBBEN DH. A vertical fracture of the crown and root. *ASDC J Dent Child* 1978;**45**:310–12.

59. SPETALEN E. Behandling av komplisert vertikal krone-rot fraktur. Kasusrapport. *Norske Tannlegeforenings Tidende* 1985;**95**:301–3.

60. BIELAK S, BIMSTEIN E, EIDELMAN E. Forced eruption: the treatment of choice for subgingivally fractured permanent incisors. *ASDC J Dent Child* 1982;**49**:186–90.

61. LEMON RR. Simplified esthetic root extrusion techniques. *Oral Surg Oral Med Oral Pathol* 1982;**54**:93–9.

62. COOKE MS, SCHEER B. Extrusion of fractured teeth. The evolution of practical clinical techniques. *Brit Dent J* 1980;**149**:50–7.

63. MANDEL RC, BINZER WC, WITHERS JA. Forced eruption in restoring severely fractured teeth using removable orthodontic appliances. *J Prosthet Dent* 1982;**47**:269–74.

64. GARRETT GB. Forced eruption in the treatment of transverse root fractures. *J Am Dent Assoc* 1985;**111**:270–2.

65. FEIGLIN B. Problems with the endodontic-orthodontic management of fractured teeth. *Int Endod J* 1986;**19**:57–63.

66. WILLIAMS S, DIETZ B. Kieferorthopädische Zahnverlängerung im Rahmen der Restaurierung eines frakturierten Frontzahns. *J Stomatol* 1986;**83**:555–9.

67. INGBER JS. Forced eruption: alteration of soft tissue cosmetic deformities. *Int J Periodont Rest Dent* 1989;**9**:417–25.

68. MALMGREN O, MALMGREN B, FRYKHOLM A. Rapid orthodontic extrusion of crown-root and cervical root fractured teeth. *Endod Dent Traumatol* 1991;**7**:49–54.

69. TEGSJÖ U, VALERIUS-OLSSON H, FRYKHOLM H, OLGART K. Clinical evaluation of intra-alveolar transplantation of teeth with cervical root fractures. *Swed Dent J* 1987;**11**:235–50.

70. BÜHLER H. Nachuntersuchung wurzelseparierter Zähne. (Eine röntgenologische Langzeitstudie). *Quintessence Int* 1984;**35**:1825–37.

71. BÜHLER H. Intraalveolaere Transplantation von Einzelwurzeln. *Quintessence Int* 1987;**38**:1963–70.

72. KAHNBERG K-E, WARFVINGE J, BIRGERSSON B. Intraalveolar transplantation (I). The use of autologous bone transplants in the periapical region. *Int J Oral Surg* 1982;**11**:372–9.

73. KAHNBERG K-E. Intraalveolar transplantation of teeth with crown-root fractures. *J Oral Surg* 1985;**43**:38–42.

74. KAHNBERG K-E. Surgical extrusion of root-fractured teeth – a follow-up study of two surgical methods. *Endod Dent Traumatol* 1988;**4**:85–9.

75. KAHNBERG 1990. Personal communication.

76. WARFVINGE J, KAHNBERG K-E. Intraalveolar transplantation of teeth. IV. Endodontic considerations. *Swed Dent J* 1989;**13**:229–33.

77. BORUM MK, ANDREASEN JO. Therapeutic and economic implications of traumatic dental injuries in Denmark: an estimate based on 7549 patients treated at a major trauma center. *Int J Paediatr Dent* 2001;**11**:249–58.

78. TSUKIBOSHI M. *Minimal tooth movement* (In Japanese). Illinois: Quintessence International, 2002.

79. BONDEMARK L, KUROL J, HALLONSTEN A-L, ANDREASEN JO. Attractive magnets for orthodontic extrusion of crown-root fractured teeth. *Am J Orthod Dentofac Orthop* 1997;**112**:187–93.

80. CALISKAN MK, TÜRKÜN M, GOMEL M. Surgical extrusion of crown-root-fractured teeth: a clinical review. *Int Endod J* 1999;**32**:146–51.

81. KAHNBERG K-E. Intra-alveolar transplantation. I. A 10-year follow-up of a method for surgical extrusion of root fractured teeth. *Swed Dent J* 1996;**20**:165–72.

82. BÜHLER H. Extraoral apical elongation of deeply damaged roots with titanium posts. A comparison of 2 methods. *J Clin Periodontol* 1996;**23**:1117–26.

83. OLSBURGH S, JACOBY T, KREJCI I. Crown fractures in the permanent dentition: pulpal and restorative considerations. *Dent Traumatol* 2002;**18**:103–15.

84. MACKIE JC, QUAYLE AA. Alternative management of a crown-root fractured tooth in a child. *Br Dent J* 1992;**173**:60–2.

85. RODD HD, DAVIDSON LE, LIVESEY S, COOKE ME. Survival of intentionally retained permanent incisor roots following crown-root fractures in children. *Dent Traumatol* 2002;**18**:92–97.

# 12
# Root Fractures

F. M. Andreasen, J. O. Andreasen & M. Cvek

## Terminology, frequency and etiology

Root fractures, defined as fractures involving dentin, cementum and pulp, are relatively uncommon among dental traumas, comprising 0.5 to 7% of the injuries affecting the permanent dentition (1–8, 88, 89, 132, 163, 164) and 2–4% in the primary dentition (1, 4, 162, 163). Frequent causes of root fractures in the permanent dentition are fights and foreign bodies striking the teeth (1).

The mechanism of root fractures is usually a frontal impact which creates compression zones labially and lingually. The resulting shearing stress zone then dictates the plane of fracture (see Chapter 8, p. 236). The result on a histologic level is a periodontal ligament injury (rupture and/or compression) confined to the coronal fragment and stretching or lacerating the pulp at the level of fracture (Figs 12.1 and 12.2).

## Clinical findings

Root fractures involving the *permanent dentition* predominantly affect the maxillary central incisor region in the age group of 11 to 20 years (1, 9–12, 136). In younger individuals, with the permanent incisors in various stages of eruption and with incomplete root development, root fractures are unusual (13, 136, 170), a finding possibly related to the elasticity of the alveolar socket which renders such teeth more susceptible to luxation injuries than to fractures (90). However, careful scrutiny of radiographs following luxation injuries in this age group can sometimes reveal incomplete (partial) root fractures (see later). In the *primary dentition*, root fractures are also uncommon before completion of root development and are most frequent at the age of 3–4 years where physiologic root resorption has begun, thereby weakening the root (91).

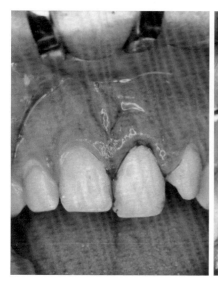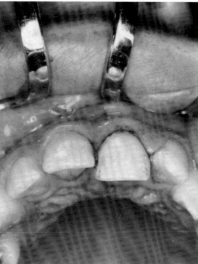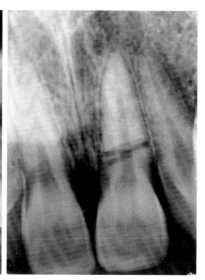

**Fig. 12.1** Palatal and incisal displacement of left central incisor due to root fracture.

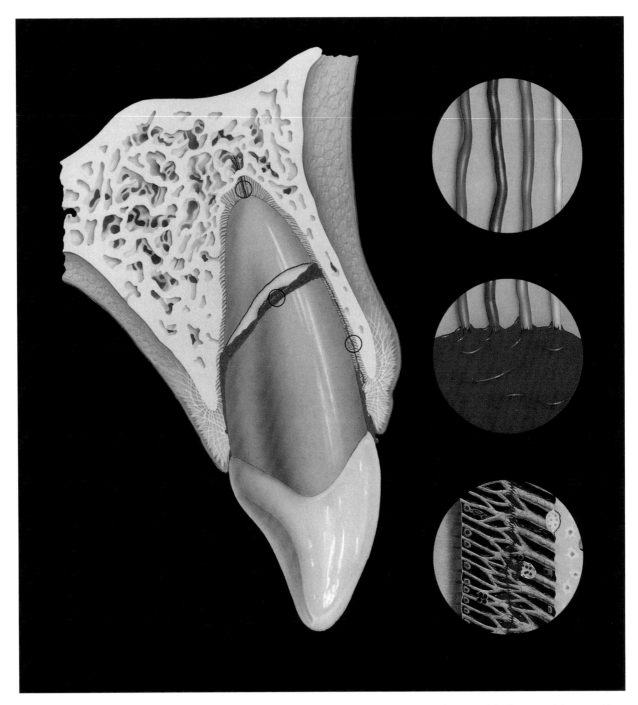

**Fig. 12.2** Pathogenesis of a root fracture. A frontal impact displaces the tooth orally and results in a root fracture and displacement of the coronal fragment. This results in both pulpal and PDL damage coronally. The pulp in the apical part of the root usually remains vital.

Root fractures can often be associated with other types of injuries; among these, concomitant fracture of the alveolar process, especially in the mandibular incisor region, is a common finding (1).

Clinical examination of teeth with root fractures usually reveals a slightly extruded tooth, frequently displaced in an oral direction (Fig. 12.1). While the site of the fracture determines the degree of tooth mobility, it is usually not possible to distinguish clinically between displacement due to a root fracture and a luxation injury. Diagnosis is entirely dependent upon radiographic examination (see later).

## Radiographic findings

Radiographic demonstration of root fractures is facilitated by the fact that the fracture line is most often oblique and at an optimal angle for radiographic disclosure (13) (Figs 12.3 and 12.4). In this context, it should be remembered that a root fracture will normally be visible only if the central beam is directed within a maximum range of 15–20° of the fracture plane (133, 134). Thus, if an ellipsoid radiolucent line is seen on a radiograph, two additional periapical

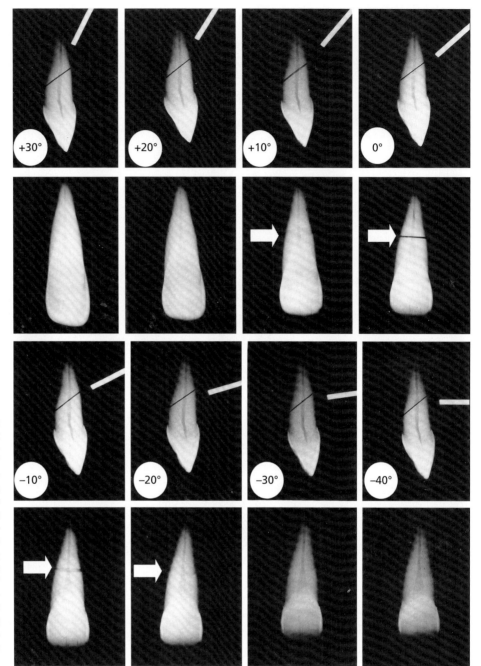

**Fig. 12.3** Radiographs taken of a human tooth with an artificial root fracture. The top row of radiographs indicates the direction of the central beam. The 0° beam corresponds to the direction of the central beam used in ordinary occlusal exposures. It appears from the bottom row that the fracture line was only disclosed with an angulation of the central beam from +10° to –20° in relation to the occlusal angulation of 0° (arrows). It also appears that deviations of the central beam from the fracture plane tend to depict the fracture as an ellipsoid structure mimicking an intermediary fragment.

radiographs should be taken – one with an increased angulation of 15° to the original and the second at a negative angulation of 15° to the original (92) (Fig. 12.3). However, the direction of the fracture can vary considerably. Thus, the typical apical or mid-root fracture follows a steep course facio-orally in an incisal direction, while fractures of the cervical third tend to be more horizontal. This change in direction dictates a radiographic technique which involves multiple exposures, including a steep occlusal exposure, which is optimal for detecting fractures of the apical third of the root (134); there is no significant difference in the sensitivity of digital radiography and conventional radiography in their capacity (165).

Root fractures occasionally escape detection immediately after injury, while later radiographs clearly reveal the fracture (4, 16–18, 93, 94) (Fig. 12.5). This can be due to the development of either hemorrhage or granulation tissue between the fragments, which displaces the coronal fragment incisally or due to resorption at the fracture line which is a part of the healing process (see later) (134).

In previous clinical studies, root fractures were seen to occur most often in the apical or middle third of the root, and only rarely in the coronal one-third (11–13, 93, 94). However, in more recent clinical studies, fractures of the middle third of the root were the most frequent, while fractures of the apical and cervical thirds occurred with equal

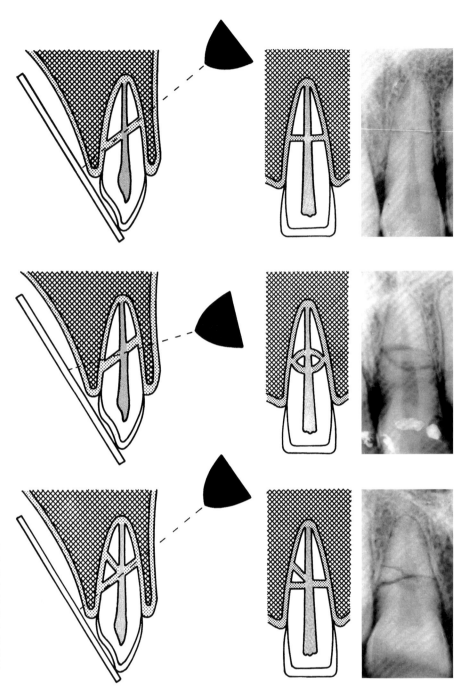

**Fig. 12.4** Radiographic demonstration of root fractures. The normal projection angle is parallel to the fracture surface, resulting in a single transverse line on the radiograph. Decrease or increase of the projection angle results in an ellipsoid fracture line on the radiograph. The fracture line in multiple root fractures shows an irregular shape on the radiograph. After ANDREASEN & HJÖRTING-HANSEN (13) 1967.

frequency (135, 136). A single transverse fracture is the usual finding; however, oblique or multiple fractures can occur (Fig. 12.6).

Root fractures of teeth with incomplete root formation can demonstrate a partial root fracture, a possible analogue to 'green stick' fractures of long bones (4, 19). They are usually seen as a unilateral break in the continuity of the thin root canal wall/root surface of the immature root (Fig. 12.7). In a recent clinical study, these fractures were subsequently seen to heal with hard tissue formation (136).

## Healing and pathology

### Root fracture healing

Healing events following root fracture are initiated at the site of pulpal and periodontal ligament involvement and lead to two types of wound healing response (22–24, 96, 134–139) (Fig. 12.8). These processes apparently occur independently of each other and are sometimes even

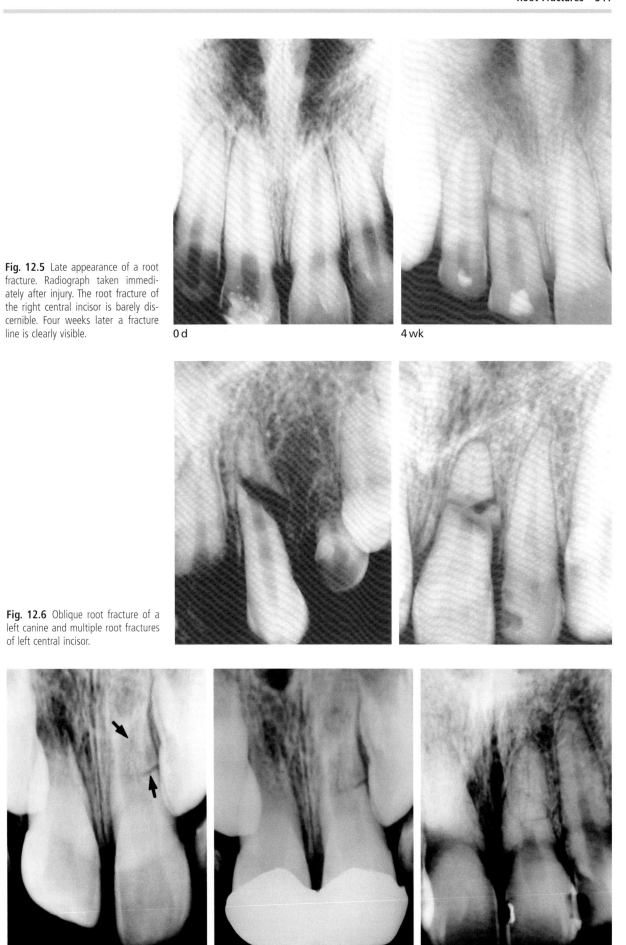

**Fig. 12.5** Late appearance of a root fracture. Radiograph taken immediately after injury. The root fracture of the right central incisor is barely discernible. Four weeks later a fracture line is clearly visible.

0 d

4 wk

**Fig. 12.6** Oblique root fracture of a left canine and multiple root fractures of left central incisor.

0 d

0 d

12 yr

**Fig. 12.7** Incomplete root fracture of a left central incisor. Twelve years later the fracture line is hardly visible.

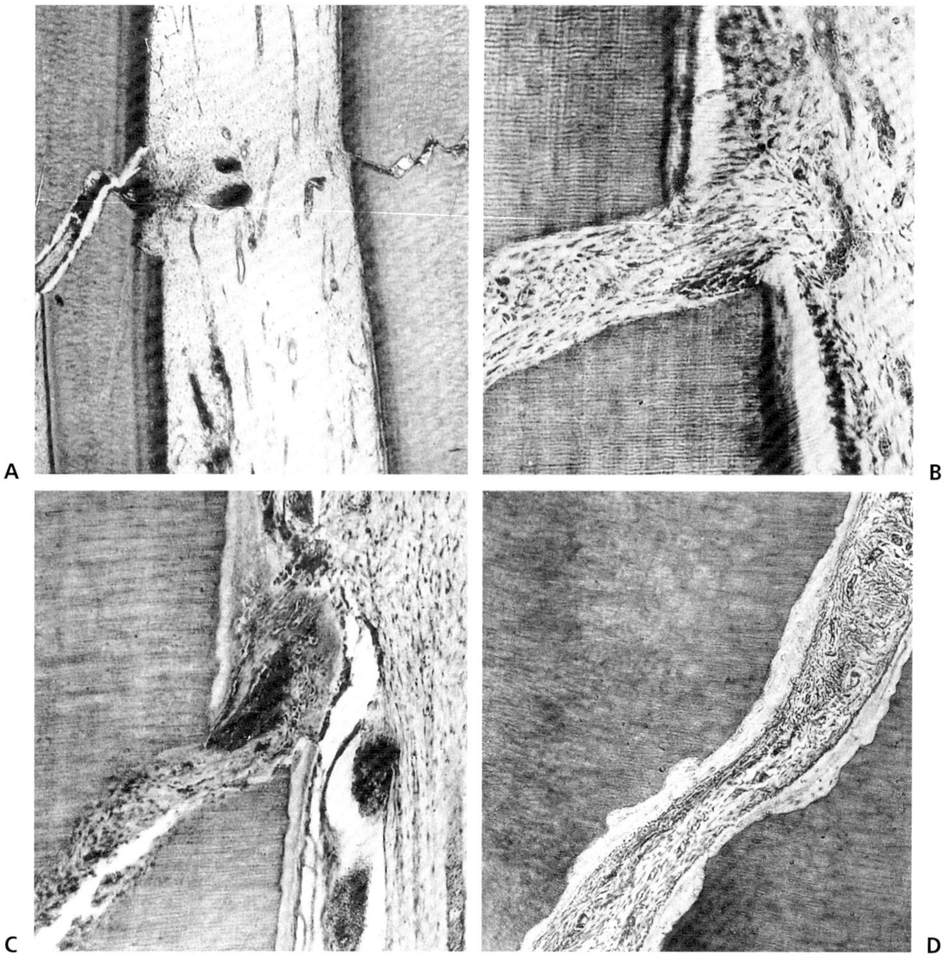

A

B

**Fig. 12.8** Healing sequence after experimental root fractures in dogs. A. Eight days postoperatively, proliferation of odontoblasts and pulpal cells. B. and C. After 2 weeks a dentinal callus is formed, uniting the fragments. D. Nine months after experimental fracture, connective tissue separates the fragments in the peripheral part of the fracture. From HAMMER (23) 1939.

C

D

competitive in their endeavor to close the injury site with either pulpal or periodontally derived tissue.

On the pulpal side of the fracture, two healing events might occur, depending upon the integrity of the pulp at the level of fracture. Thus, if the pulp is intact at the fracture site, it will react in a manner analogous to a coronal pulp exposure under optimal conditions (i.e. with an intact vascular supply and absence of infection). Odontoblast progenitor cells will be recruited and create a small hard tissue dentin bridge which will unite the apical and coronal fragments after 2 weeks in dogs (23) (Figs 12.8 and 12.10). This bridge forms the initial callus and will possibly stabilize the fracture (Figs 12.8 and 12.9). Callus formation is followed by deposition of cementum derived by ingrowth of tissue from the periodontal ligament (23) at the fracture line, first centrally and gradually obliterating the fracture site (23). Hard tissue union of the fractured root fragments cannot be diagnosed radiographically earlier than 3 months after injury and may take several years to be completed (134–136) (see p. 347).

In the event that the pulp is severed or severely stretched at the level of the fracture, a revascularization process in the coronal aspect of the pulp is initiated (167). In the absence of bacteria, this process will result in obliteration of the coronal pulp canal. While this revascularization process is under way, periodontally derived cells can dominate root fracture healing, resulting in 'union' of the coronal and apical root fragments by interposition of connective tissue (167) (Fig. 12.10).

Finally, if bacteria gain access – usually to the coronal pulp – an infected pulp necrosis results, with accumulation of inflamed, granulation tissue between the two root fragments (Fig. 12.11). The source of these bacteria is still subject to debate. Presently three points of entry are discussed: (1) through a tear in the coronal aspect of the periodontal ligament; (2) through exposed dentinal tubules (e.g. an associated crown fracture, or denuded neck of the tooth); or (3) via the invading neovasculature (anachoresis).

During the initial stages of wound healing, traumatized pulpal and hard dental tissues can stimulate an inflammatory response and thereby trigger the release of a series of osteoclast-activating factors (138) (see Chapter 4, p. 148).

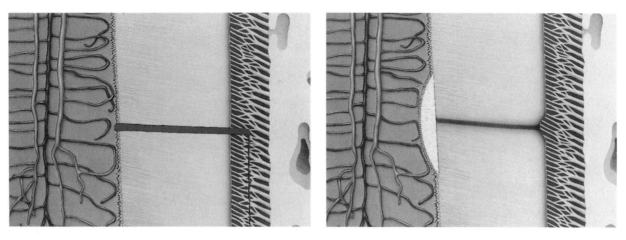

**Fig. 12.9** Hard tissue healing after root fracture. Due to minimal displacement of the coronal fragment, the pulp is probably only slightly stretched at the level of the fracture. Fracture healing with ingrowth of cells originating from the apical half of the pulp ensures hard tissue union of the fracture.

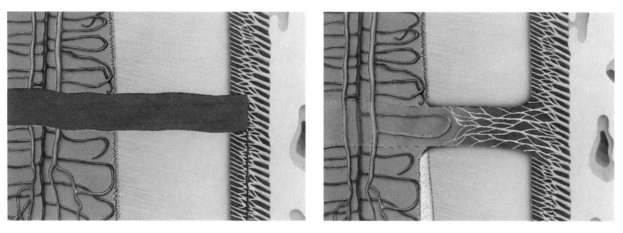

**Fig. 12.10** Connective tissue healing after root fracture. The pulp is ruptured or severely stretched at the level of the fracture following displacement of the coronal fragment. Healing is dominated by ingrowth of cells originating from the periodontal ligament and results in interposition of connective tissue between the two fragments.

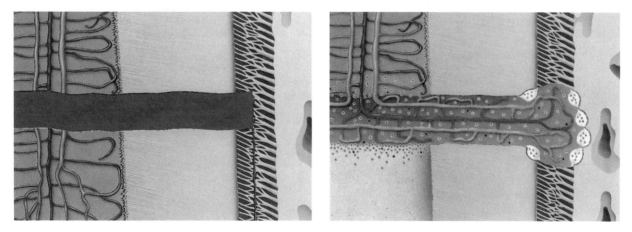

**Fig. 12.11** Non-healing due to infection in the line of fracture. Infection occurs in the avascular coronal aspect of the pulp. Granulation tissue is soon formed which originates from the apical pulp and periodontal ligament. Accumulation of granulation tissue between the two fragments causes separation of the fragments and loosening of the coronal fragment.

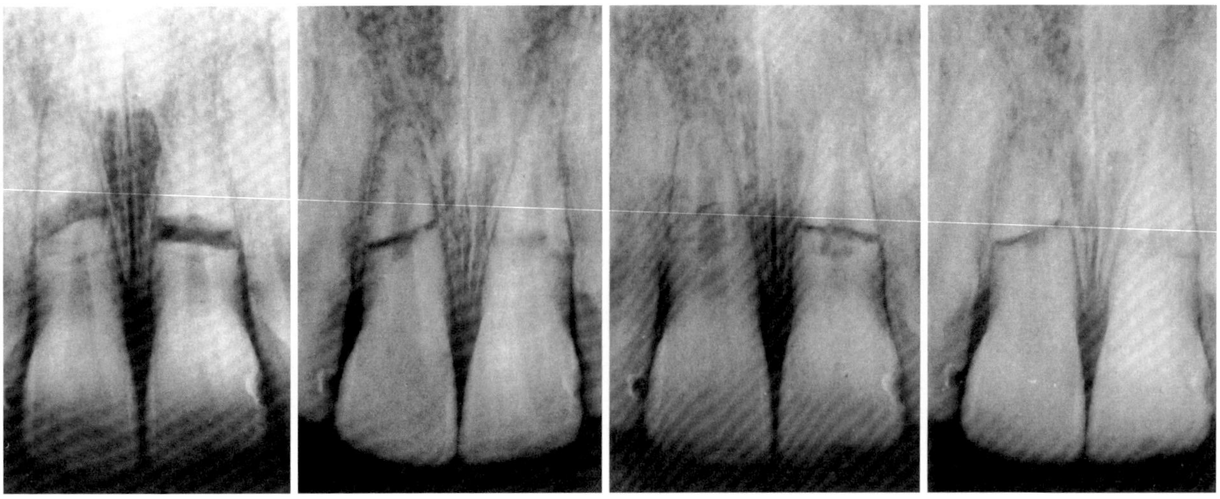

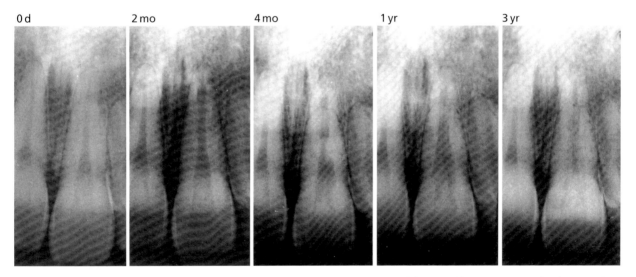

0 d                3 mo                6 mo                3 yr

**Fig. 12.12** Root fracture of the right and left maxillary central incisors of a 22-year-old woman, with extrusion of the fragments after 3 and 6 months. There is evidence of internal surface resorption (ISR) at the junction of the pulp canal and fracture line of both teeth and external surface resorption (ESR) of the right central incisor. After 3 years, there is resolution of ISR and pulp canal obliteration of the coronal canal can be seen. Healing is by interposition of connective tissue. From ANDREASEN & ANDREASEN (134) 1988.

0 d          2 mo          4 mo          1 yr          3 yr

**Fig. 12.13** Root fracture of the left maxillary central incisor in a 19-year-old man with extrusion of the coronal fragment. Two months after injury, there is evidence of resorption of the pulp canal walls (internal surface resorption (ISR)). Six months after injury, simultaneous resorption and deposition of hard tissue can be seen. Internal tunneling resorption (ITR) can be clearly seen after 1 year. After 2 years, arrest of the resorption process and obliteration of the apical and coronal pulp canals can be seen. Healing is by interposition of connective tissue. From ANDREASEN & ANDREASEN (134) 1988.

Thus, root resorption processes beginning either at the periphery of the fracture line adjacent to the periodontal ligament or centrally at the border of the root canal were observed in 60% of a clinical material of root-fractured permanent incisors (134).

These processes could usually be detected within the 1st year after injury and preceded fracture healing and obliteration of the apical and/or coronal portions of the root canals. The changes observed represented three resorption entities:

(1) *External surface resorption (ESR)* (i.e. rounding of proximal fracture edges at the periodontal side of the fracture) (Fig. 12.12)
(2) *Internal surface resorption (ISR)* (i.e. rounding of fracture edges centrally, at the pulpal side of the fracture) (Figs 12.12 and 12.13)
(3) *Internal tunnelling resorption (ITR)* (i.e. resorption which burrows behind the predentin layer and along the root canal walls of the coronal fragment) (Figs 12.13 and 12.14).

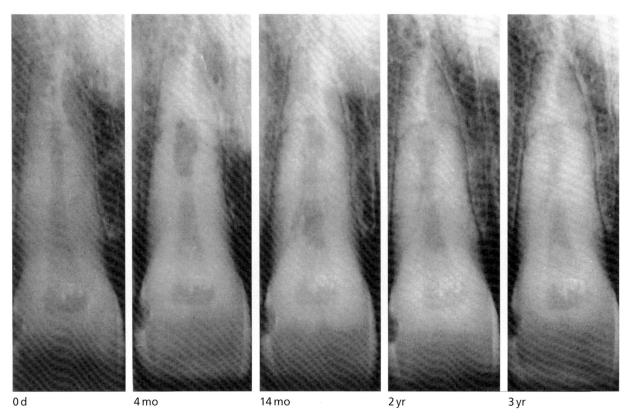

0 d          4 mo          14 mo          2 yr          3 yr

**Fig. 12.14** Root fracture of the right maxillary central incisor in a 32-year-old man with extrusion of the coronal fragment. Four months after injury, there is evidence of ISR. One year after injury, ITR can be seen. After 2 years, arrest of the resorption process and obliteration of the apical and coronal pulp canals can be seen. Healing is by interposition of connective tissue. From ANDREASEN & ANDREASEN (134) 1988.

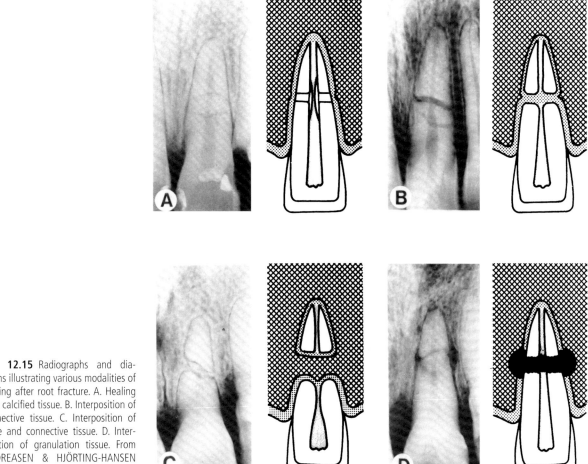

**Fig. 12.15** Radiographs and diagrams illustrating various modalities of healing after root fracture. A. Healing with calcified tissue. B. Interposition of connective tissue. C. Interposition of bone and connective tissue. D. Interposition of granulation tissue. From ANDREASEN & HJÖRTING-HANSEN (13) 1967.

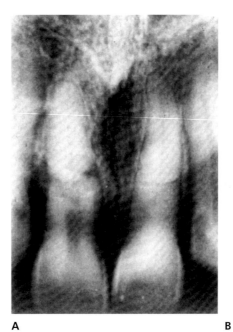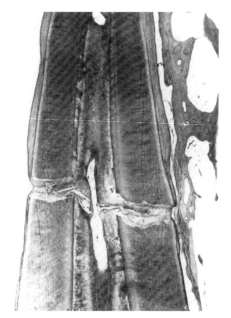

**Fig. 12.16** Complete healing with calcified tissue after root fracture. A. Radiographic condition 8 years after root fracture of both central incisors. Fracture lines are still visible. B. Histologic examination of left central incisor reveals a complete hard tissue callus. From SCHULZE (36) 1957.

**A**                                    **B**

It has been speculated that the various root resorption entities represent osteoclastic activity connected with ingrowth of new highly vascularized connective tissue into the fracture site or coronal aspect of the root canal, as revascularization processes are known to elicit transient osteoclast activity (134) (see Chapter 4, p. 148).

The resorption processes were all self-limiting, usually resolving within the first 1–2 years after injury, and therefore requiring no interceptive treatment. The pattern of resorption and pulp canal obliteration appeared to be decisive for fracture healing. Thus, all resorption entities collectively were significantly related to healing by interposition of connective tissue between fragments. However, when seen alone, internal surface resorption was significantly related to hard tissue union. Pulp canal obliteration in both aspects of the root canal indicated interposition of connective tissue; when seen only in the apical aspect, healing was by hard tissue union (134).

It should be emphasized that the pathogenesis of root fracture healing, while suggested by retrospective clinical studies (13, 93, 134), is only weakly supported by experimental research. Revision of this hypothesis could therefore be expected when future studies examine the specific roles of the pulp and periodontium in root fracture healing.

So far, radiographic and histological observations in *human subjects* have revealed that the final outcome after root fracture can be divided into the events listed below (13, 26) (Fig. 12.15).

## Healing with calcified tissue

A uniting callus of hard tissue has been demonstrated histologically in a number of cases (9, 13, 19, 27–36, 97–100) (Figs 12.16 and 12.17). Varying opinions exist on the nature of the hard tissue found uniting the fragments. Dentin (36),

osteodentin (27), or cementum (28, 29, 33, 34) have all been found at the repair site. In most cases, the innermost layer of repair seems to be dentin (Fig. 12.17F), while the more peripheral part of the fracture is incompletely repaired with cementum (9, 13, 30–32, 36) (Fig. 12.17E, F). The first layer of dentin is often cellular and atubular, later followed by normal tubular dentin (31, 36). Cementum deposition in the fracture line is often preceded by resorptive processes both centrally and peripherally (Fig. 12.17E). Most often, cementum will not completely bridge the gap between the fracture surfaces, but is interspersed with connective tissue originating from the periodontal ligament (Fig. 12.17G). This, combined with the greater radiodensity of cementum as compared with dentin, could explain why a fracture line is often discernible radiographically although the fragments are in close apposition and the fracture is completely consolidated (Fig. 12.18).

Occasionally, a slight widening of the root canal close to the fracture site is seen (i.e. *internal surface resorption* (134)), followed by hard tissue formation (101, 102) (Fig. 12.18). Moreover, it is characteristic that there is limited peripheral rounding of the fracture edges (*external surface resorption* (134)) (Fig. 12.18).

*Partial pulp canal obliteration*, confined to the apical fragment, is a frequent finding. Clinical examination of teeth within this healing group reveals normal mobility, as compared with non-injured adjacent teeth; moreover, there is normal reaction to percussion and normal or slightly decreased response to pulpal sensibility testing (13, 103, 134).

This type of healing is dependent upon an intact pulp and is seen primarily in cases with little or no dislocation (i.e. concussion or subluxation) of the coronal fragment and most often in teeth with immature root formation (13, 90, 103, 134) (Fig. 12.19).

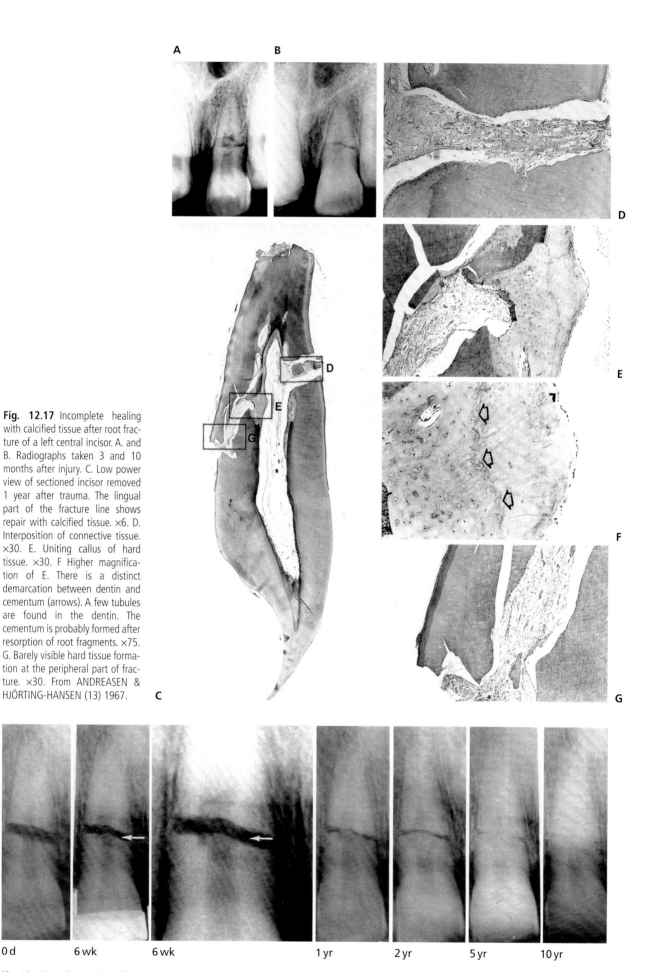

**Fig. 12.17** Incomplete healing with calcified tissue after root fracture of a left central incisor. A. and B. Radiographs taken 3 and 10 months after injury. C. Low power view of sectioned incisor removed 1 year after trauma. The lingual part of the fracture line shows repair with calcified tissue. ×6. D. Interposition of connective tissue. ×30. E. Uniting callus of hard tissue. ×30. F Higher magnification of E. There is a distinct demarcation between dentin and cementum (arrows). A few tubules are found in the dentin. The cementum is probably formed after resorption of root fragments. ×75. G. Barely visible hard tissue formation at the peripheral part of fracture. ×30. From ANDREASEN & HJÖRTING-HANSEN (13) 1967.

| 0 d | 6 wk | 6 wk | 1 yr | 2 yr | 5 yr | 10 yr |

**Fig. 12.18** Healing with calcified tissue of a fracture located at the gingival third of the root of a left lateral incisor. At the 6-week control, evidence of widening of the root canal close to the fracture site (arrow) is apparent. At controls 1 and 2 years later, the resorption cavity in the pulp canal as well as the fracture site show repair with calcified tissue. After 5 and 10 years, the fracture site is almost occluded with hard tissue.

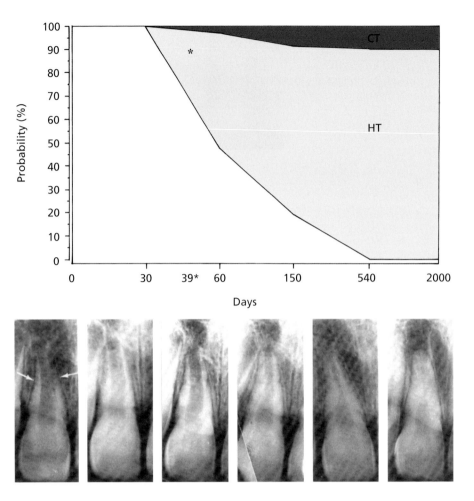

**Fig. 12.19** Upper. Probability of the various healing modalities after root fracture of the maxillary right central incisor (arrows) in an 8-year-old boy based on the following information from the time of injury: the coronal fragment was *subluxated*, with *first-degree loosening*; the diameter of the apical foramen was *2.8 mm*; *antibiotics* were administered due to avulsion and replantation of the maxillary left central incisor. Fixation was with an *acid-etch splint*. The times on the horizontal axis of the probability curves are the intervals defined in the statistical analysis. The times given on the radiographs are the exact observation periods, which correspond to the defined intervals. Lower. The radiographic appearance at the various observation periods. At 39 days, the diagnosis of hard tissue union (HT) was made (asterisk). From ANDREASEN et al. (136) 1989.

## Interposition of connective tissue

This type of healing is apparently related to a moderate pulpal injury (i.e. extrusion or lateral luxation of the coronal fragment), whereby pulpal revascularization and/or reinnervation must be completed prior to pulpal participation in fracture healing. In the interim, periodontal ligament cells are able to dominate the healing process (13, 136). Histologically, this is characterized by the presence of connective tissue between the fragments (13, 37, 48) (Fig. 12.20). The fracture surfaces are covered by cementum, often deposited after initial resorption (38, 39, 43, 99, 168), with connective tissue fibers running parallel to the fracture surface or from one fragment to the other. By means of secondary dentin formation, a new 'apical foramen' is created at the level of fracture (32, 45, 134, 135, 169). A common finding is peripheral rounding of the fracture edges (*external surface resorption* (134)), sometimes with slight ingrowth of bone into the fracture area from the lateral side (13, 27) (Fig. 12.18). The width of the periodontal space around the fragments reflects the functional activity of the two fragments. The periodontal space surrounding the apical fragment is narrow, with fibers oriented parallel to the root surface, while the space around the coronal fragment is wide, with normal fiber arrangement (37, 41).

The radiographic features in this type of healing consist of peripheral rounding of the fracture edges and a radiolucent line separating the fragments (Fig. 12.15B). Initially, *external* and *internal surface resorption* are often seen (134), as well as *pulp canal obliteration* of both apical and coronal aspects of the root canal (136).

Clinically, the teeth are normally firm or slightly mobile and with a weak pain response to percussion. The response to sensibility testing is usually within the normal range (13, 93, 134–135). Although no interceptive therapy is required at the appearance of the above-mentioned resorption processes, it should be mentioned that a few cases have been observed whereby the post-resorptive mineralization process resulted in *ankylosis*. Thus, longer observation periods as well as more frequent follow-up examinations during the 1st year after injury might be advisable when these resorption processes are diagnosed. (See Appendix 3, p. 881).

## Interposition of bone and connective tissue

Histologically teeth in this healing group demonstrate interposition of a bony bridge and connective tissue between the

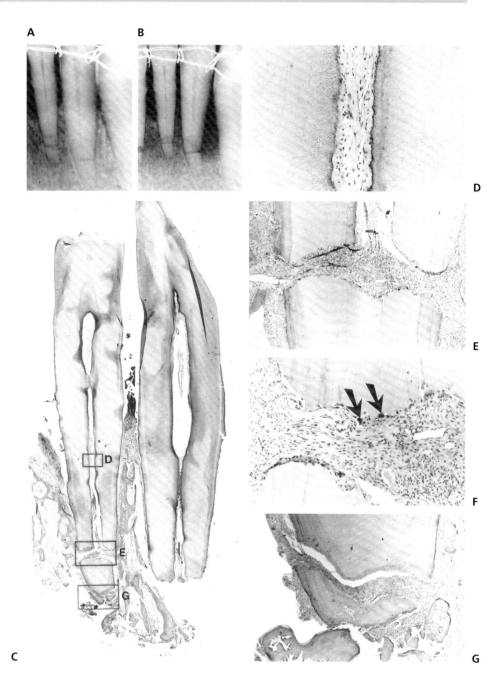

**Fig. 12.20** Interposition of connective tissue after root fracture of left central and lateral incisors. A. One week after injury. B. Radiograph at time of removal 6 weeks after injury. C. Low power view of sectioned central incisor shows interposition of connective tissue. ×30. D. Vital pulp tissue in crown portion. ×75. E. Connective tissue in fracture line. ×30. F. Higher magnification of E. Note active resorption on surface of fragments (arrows) ×75. G. Comminuted fracture in apical region. Note formation of cementum on fragments. ×30. From ANDREASEN & HJÖRTING-HANSEN (13) 1967.

apical and coronal fragments, with a normal periodontal ligament surrounding both fragments (27, 49–53). In some instances, bone can be seen extending into the root canals (49–51) (Fig. 12.21).

This mode of healing is apparently a result of trauma prior to completed growth of the alveolar process, thus the coronal fragment continues to erupt, while the apical fragment remains stationary in the jaw (13) (Figs 12.22 and 12.23).

Radiographically, a bony bridge is seen separating the fragments, with a periodontal space around both fragments. Total *pulp canal obliteration* of the root canals in both fragments is a common finding (Fig. 12.15C).

Clinically, the teeth are firm and react normally to pulp tests.

## Interposition of granulation tissue

Histologic examination of teeth in this group reveals inflamed granulation tissue between the fragments (13, 37, 53–57, 140) (Figs 12.24 and 12.25). The coronal portion of the pulp is necrotic and infected, while the apical fragment usually contains vital pulp tissue (13) (Fig. 12.24D and G). The necrotic and infected pulp tissue is responsible for the inflammatory changes along the fracture line (13). In some cases, however, communication between the fracture line and the gingival crevice is the source of inflammation (13, 47, 57) (Fig. 12.25).

Radiographically, widening of the fracture line, loss of lamina dura and rarefaction of the alveolar bone corresponding to the fracture line are typical findings (141) (Fig. 12.15D). If the tooth is not splinted, the coronal fragment is loose, slightly extruded and sensitive to percussion. If splinted, the apical fragment becomes displaced in apical direction. Fistulae at a level on the buccal mucosa corresponding to the fracture line are an occasional finding (13).

It has been found that negative pulpal sensibility at the time of injury was significantly related to later pulp necrosis, presumably a reflection of severe pulpal injury. However, a positive pulpal response was not able to predict healing by hard tissue union or interposition of connective tissue (136). Moreover, fixation by the forceful application of orthodon-

tic bands (a splinting technique employed prior to the advent of the passively applied acid-etch splints) (136) or cap splints (170) played an important role in the development of coronal pulp necrosis following root fracture. This

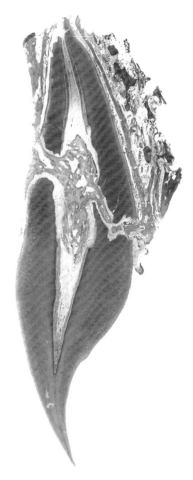

**Fig. 12.22** Interposition of bone and connective tissue between fragments of a permanent incisor removed 6 months after root fracture. Note extension of bone into the pulp canal. ×7. From BLACKWOOD (49) 1959.

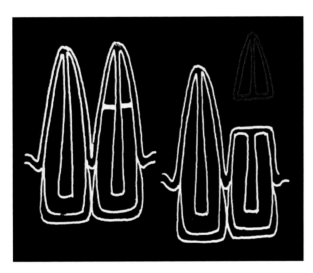

**Fig. 12.21** The growth of the alveolar process leaves the apical fragment behind in its original position.

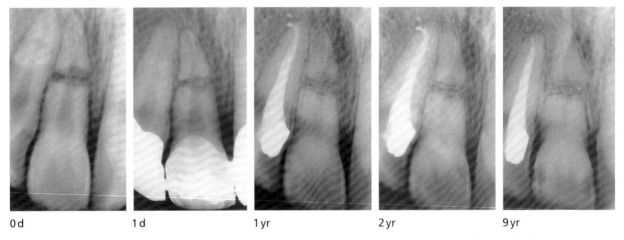

0 d          1 d          1 yr          2 yr          9 yr

**Fig. 12.23** Healing of fracture with interposition of bone and PDL. On the day of injury; there is a fracture with diastasis of about 1.8 mm and not optimal splinting. At controls after 1, 2, and 9 years, respectively, there is ingrowth of bone between the two fragments, further eruption of the coronal fragment and pulp canal obliteration in both fragments. From CVEK et al. (177) 2002.

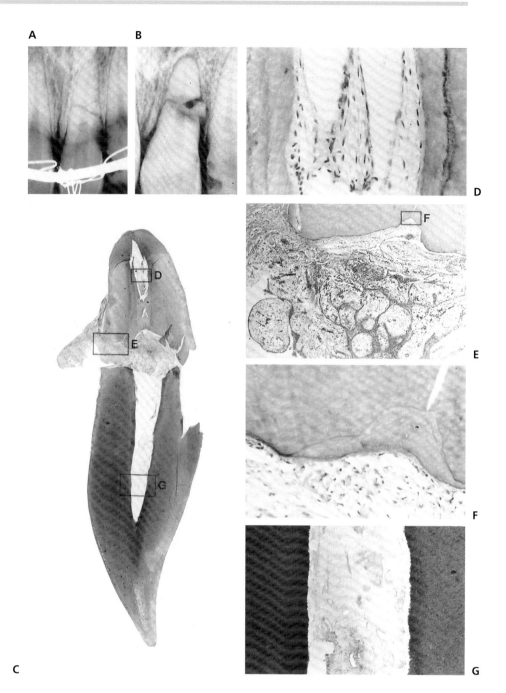

**Fig. 12.24** Non-healing with interposition of granulation tissue between fragments of a left central incisor. A. Immediately after injury. B. Radiographs at the time of removal 6 months after injury. C. Low power view of sectioned incisor. ×6. D. Vital pulp tissue in apical fragment. ×75. E. Granulation tissue with epithelial proliferation and chronic inflammation. ×30. F. Higher magnification of E. Area with newly formed cementum. ×195. G. Necrotic pulp tissue in coronal fragment. ×30. From ANDREASEN & HJÖRTING-HANSEN (13) 1967.

adverse effect was presumably due to an additional trauma, including possible dislocation of the coronal fragment, during splint application (170).

## Treatment

The principles of treating *permanent teeth* are reduction of displaced coronal fragments and immobilization (Fig. 12.26). Surveys of treatment principles have recently been published (171, 172). If treatment is instituted immediately after injury, repositioning of the fragment by digital manipulation is easily achieved (Fig. 12.27). If resistance is felt upon repositioning, it is most likely due to fracture of the labial socket wall. In this case, repositioning of the fractured bone is necessary before further attempts are made to reduce the root fracture (Fig. 12.28). After reduction, the position should be checked radiographically.

Immobilization of teeth with root fractures is achieved with semi-rigid fixation, e.g. an acid etch/resin splint (170) (see Chapter 32). As previously mentioned, forceful

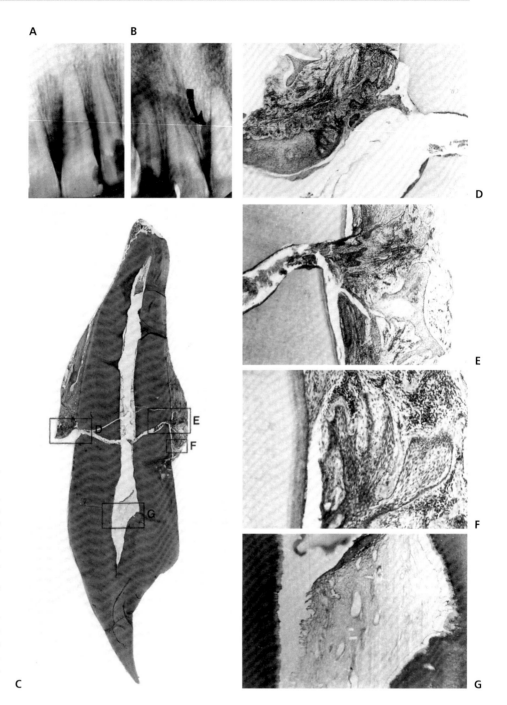

**Fig. 12.25** Non-healing with interposition of granulation tissue between fragments of a left central incisor. A. and B. Radiographs taken 2 months after trauma. Note the periradicular radiolucency adjacent to the fracture line (arrow). C. Low power view of sectioned incisor. The tooth was removed 2 months after injury. ×6. D. Downward proliferation of epithelium from gingival crevice. ×75. E and F. Palatal fracture with epithelial proliferation. ×30 and ×75. G. Necrotic pulp tissue in coronal fragment. ×30. From ANDREASEN & HJØRTING-HANSEN (13) 1967.

application of, e.g., orthodontic bands for the purpose of immobilizing the coronal fragment is contraindicated, due to its traumatic influence on the already traumatized pulp that could result in pulp necrosis. A passively applied splint (e.g. using the acid-etch technique) is advised. The fixation period should be about 1 month to ensure sufficient hard tissue consolidation; longer splinting periods have not been found to be of value (170).

It should be noted that immature teeth with incomplete root fractures require no fixation and will heal by hard tissue union (136). However, these teeth may be included in a splint if multiple tooth injuries so require. During this period, it is important that the tooth be observed radiographically and with sensibility tests in order to detect pulp necrosis. See Appendix 4, p. 882 for a suggested schedule for recall examinations.

If the fracture is located at the cervical third of the root and below the alveolar crest, various studies have shown that healing is possible and a conservative approach justified (13, 26, 58, 177) (Figs 12.29 and 12.30). In cases where oral hygiene is optimal, treatment can be permanent fixation of the coronal fragment to adjacent non-injured teeth at the contact areas proximally with a filled composite resin (Fig. 12.30). However, very close proximity of the root

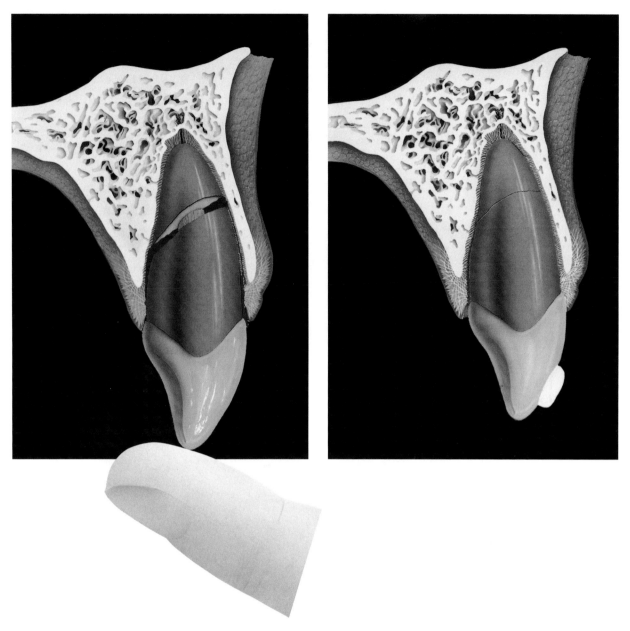

**Fig. 12.26** Principles for treatment of root fractures. Treatment of root fractures consists of complete repositioning and firm, immobile splinting, preferably with a passively applied splint until a hard tissue callus is formed, usually after 3 months.

fracture to the gingival crevice may dictate alternative treatment, as the chance of healing with calcified tissue is poorest when a cervical fracture line is close to or communicating with the gingival crevice. A treatment option which could then be considered is the removal of the coronal fragment and subsequent orthodontic (106) or surgical extrusion of the remaining apical fragment. These techniques are described in more detail in relation to treatment of complicated crown-root fractures (see Chapters 11 and 24).

In cases where it is not possible to treat the fractured tooth conservatively and the tooth must be extracted, it should be remembered that careless extraction procedures will result in extensive damage to the alveolar process and subsequent severe atrophy, especially in the labio-lingual direction, ultimately resulting in a compromised esthetic restorative treatment. This problem can be prevented to a certain degree by careful removal of the apical fragment with no or minimal sacrifice of labial bone. Thus, if removal of the apical fragment is not possible via the socket, surgical removal should be undertaken by raising a flap and making an osteotomy over the apical area, thereby pushing the apex out of its socket. Under no circumstance should the marginal socket wall be removed, as this can lead to labio-lingual collapse of the alveolar process (Fig. 12.31).

### Fig. 12.27 Treatment of a laterally luxated root fracture

This 13-year-old boy received a horizontal blow to the left maxillary central incisor.

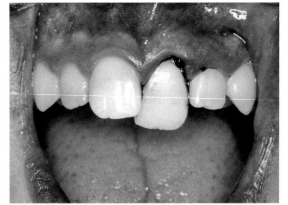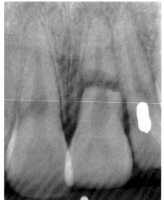

### Examining the tooth

The tooth reacts to SENSITIVITY TESTING, indicating an intact vascular supply. There is a high metallic sound elicited by the PERCUSSION TEST, indicating lateral luxation of the coronal fragment. The tooth is locked firmly in its displaced position, confirming the lateral luxation diagnosis.

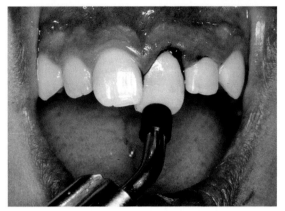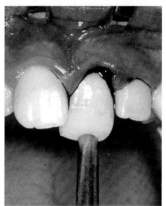

### Repositioning

Because of the force necessary to reposition a laterally luxated tooth, local anesthesia is administered prior to repositioning. Firm pressure is applied to the facial bone plate at the fracture level in order to displace the coronal fragment out of its alveolar 'lock.' This is followed by horizontal (forward) pressure at the palatal aspect of the incisal edge, which repositions the coronal fragment into its original position.

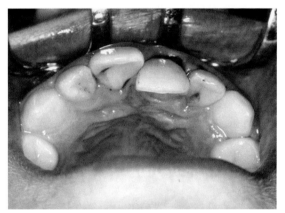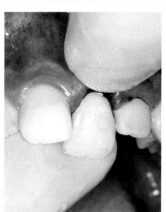

### Verifying repositioning

The correct position of the coronal fragment is confirmed radiographically.

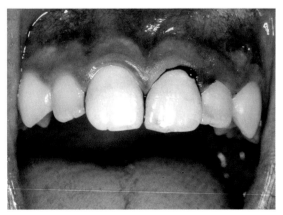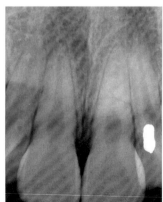

## Splinting procedure

The acid-etch technique and a temporary crown and bridge material are used. Phosphoric acid gel is applied for 30 seconds to the facial surfaces of the injured and adjacent non-injured teeth. The tooth surfaces are then rinsed thoroughly with a stream of water for 20–30 seconds and blown dry. A mat white enamel surface indicates adequate etching.

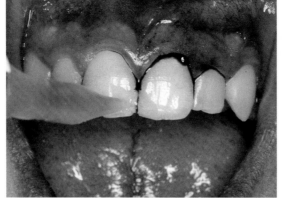 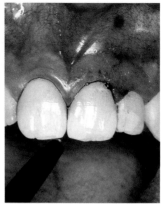

## Applying the splinting material

Temporary crown and bridge material is applied to the etched enamel surfaces (Luxatemp®). The bulk of the material should be placed on the mesial and distal corners of the traumatized and adjacent, non-injured incisors. After setting, any irregularity in the surface is removed with abrasive discs or a scalpel blade.

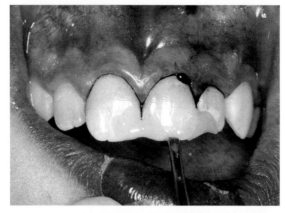 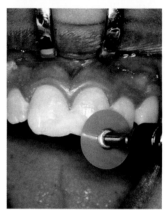

## Removing the splint

The healing events are monitored radiographically. If the tooth reacts to sensibility testing and there is no sign of infection in the bone at the level of the fracture, the splint may be removed.

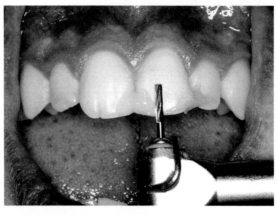 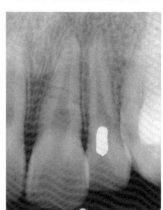

## One year after injury

The tooth responds normally to sensibility testing and the radiograph shows increasing radiopacity of the fracture line.

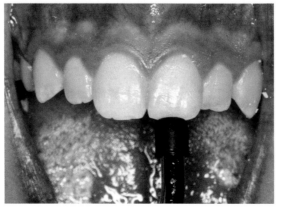 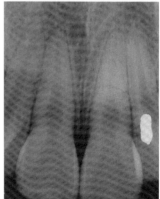

### Fig. 12.28 Treatment of a severely extruded root fracture

This 20-year-old woman has suffered a frontal blow to the left central incisor, resulting in extreme displacement of the coronal fragment.

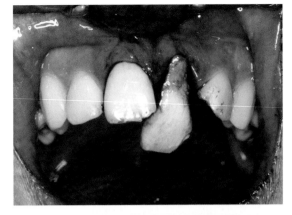 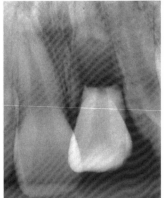

### Examining the displaced coronal fragment

After cleansing the exposed root surface with saline, it can be seen that the coronal fragment has been forced past the cervical margin of the labial bone plate. The stretched and displaced pulp is seen within the socket area.

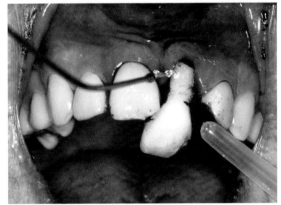 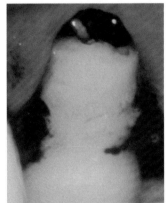

### Repositioning

After local anesthetic infiltration, the coronal fragment is repositioned. To guide the root fragment into place, an amalgam carver is inserted beneath the cervical bone margin and used like a shoe horn.

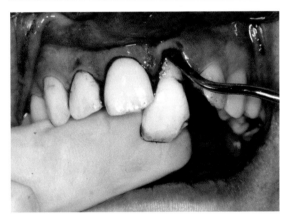 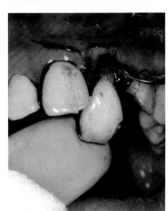

### Splinting

The acid-etch technique is employed once optimal repositioning has been verified radiographically. The labial surfaces are etched and a flexible splinting material is applied. The patient is given penicillin for 4 days to safeguard healing.

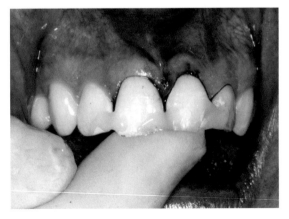 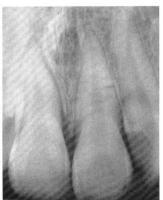

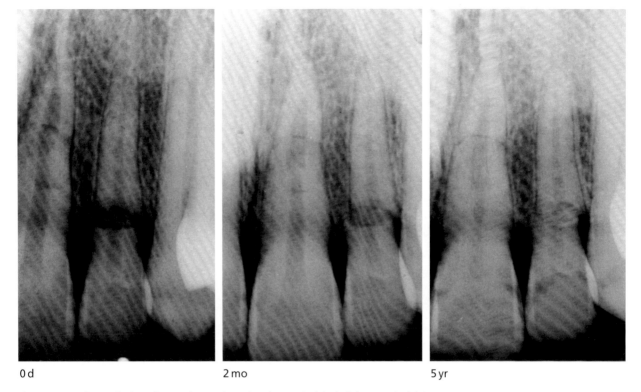

0 d       2 mo       5 yr

**Fig. 12.29** Hard tissue healing of a root fracture located at the marginal third of the root of a left incisor.

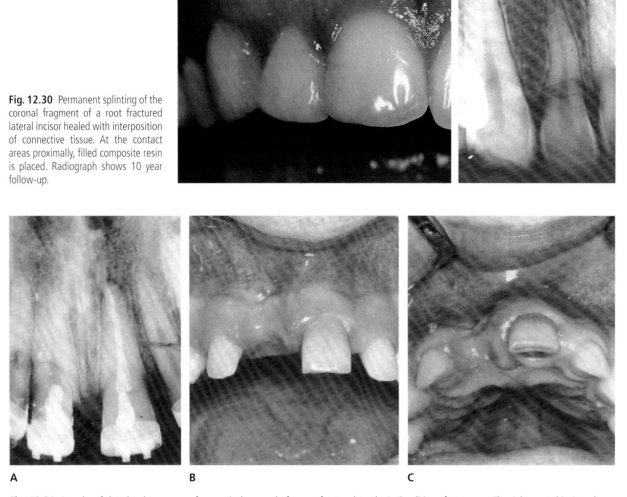

**Fig. 12.30** Permanent splinting of the coronal fragment of a root fractured lateral incisor healed with interposition of connective tissue. At the contact areas proximally, filled composite resin is placed. Radiograph shows 10 year follow-up.

A       B       C

**Fig. 12.31** Atrophy of the alveolar process after surgical removal of a root fractured tooth. A. Condition after trauma. The right central incisor shows a root fracture close to the gingival crevice. The tooth was surgically removed. During this procedure the labial bone plate was also removed. B and C. Marked atrophy of the alveolar process is evident 1 year later.

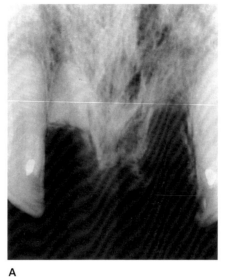
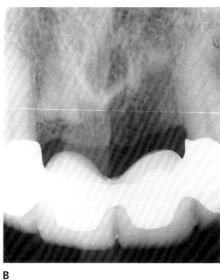

**Fig. 12.32** Apical fragment left *in situ* after root fracture. The two central incisors were avulsed. A. Condition at the time of injury. B. At a follow-up 5 years after injury, the pulp canal in the apical fragment shows complete obliteration and bone covers the fractured surface of the root.

**A**

**B**

A preferred alternative to the above situation is the preservation of the apical fragment, which normally contains vital pulp tissue. Experimental evidence seems to indicate that intentionally submerged root fragments with vital pulps prevent or retard resorption of the alveolar process. These roots are usually covered along the fractured surface with a new layer of cementum as well as a thin layer of new bone. Moreover, the pulp retains its vitality (107–109). Preliminary clinical experience seems to indicate that the intentionally buried apical fragment resulting from root fracture acts similarly (Fig. 12.32). This is presumably analogous to the submergence of the apical fragment which is seen after healing by interposition of bone and connective tissue. Whether this treatment procedure is reliable must await the results of long-term clinical studies.

## Prognosis

Several clinical reports have demonstrated successful treatment of root fractures (13, 26, 37, 59–71, 90–92, 100, 103, 110, 111, 133, 136, 142–144, 166, 170). However, follow-up examinations can disclose deviations in pulpal and periodontal healing. In this context, radiographic findings, such as *pulp canal obliteration, external and internal surface resorption* have been found to be related to specific healing modalities (134).

## Follow-up

A standard follow-up strategy using clinical information based on sensibility testing is used, see Chapter 9, p. 261. In that regard, a recent laser Doppler study has shown that this approach could be advantageous in demonstrating early revascularization of the coronal pulp (174). Furthermore,

radiographic examination should be included using standardized exposures (see Chapter 9, p. 267).

## Pulpal healing

Clinical experience has shown that the pulp is more likely to survive after root fracture than after luxation with no fracture of the root (41, 61, 65, 72–74, 135) (Fig. 12.33). An explanation could be that the fate of the injured pulp depends in part upon revascularization from the periodontal ligament. Such revascularization in luxation injuries is limited to the periapical tissues through the apical foramen, whereas a fractured root offers broader communication from the pulp canal to the periodontal tissues, facilitating re-establishment of the blood supply. Moreover, if one assumes that only the coronal aspect of the pulp has been damaged, the extent of tissue requiring revascularization is considerably reduced following root fracture than after luxation injuries. Another important factor could be the development of pulpal edema, which can escape through the fracture, minimizing pressure upon the delicate pulpal vessels. Furthermore, the root fracture itself could prevent transmission of the impact to the apical area, thus reducing damage to the vulnerable area at the constricted apical foramen (65).

Close clinical and radiographic follow-ups are necessary to disclose pulp necrosis (141). Extrusion of the coronal fragment, tenderness to percussion and, most significantly, radiographic signs of pulp necrosis, such as development of radiolucencies within bone adjacent to the fracture line (Figs 12.34 and 12.35), can usually be detected within the first 2 months after injury.

A negative sensibility response immediately after injury does not necessarily indicate pulp necrosis, as a slow return to normal vitality is often observed (103). However, it has been found that teeth which did not respond to pulp testing immediately following root fracture demonstrated a significantly greater risk of later pulp necrosis than those which

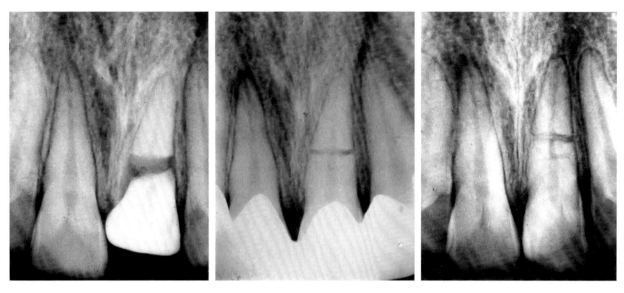

**Fig. 12.33** Pulp necrosis and periapical involvement after subluxation and pulp survival after root fracture. Left central incisor showed root fracture and dislocation while the right central incisor was subluxated. The subluxated tooth has developed pulp necrosis but the tooth with the root fracture has remained vital.

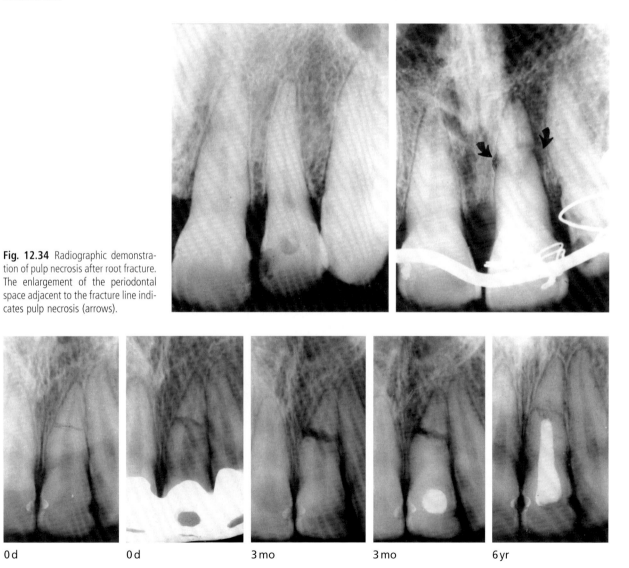

**Fig. 12.34** Radiographic demonstration of pulp necrosis after root fracture. The enlargement of the periodontal space adjacent to the fracture line indicates pulp necrosis (arrows).

0 d  0 d  3 mo  3 mo  6 yr

**Fig. 12.35** No healing after root fracture. The root fracture was splinted on the day of injury. At control 3 months after injury a perioradicular radiolucency is seen adjacent to the fracture, and there is no reaction to sensibility testing and there is discoloration of the crown. Treatment of the coronal fragment is instituted with calcium hydroxide. Control after 6 years shows periodontal healing after treatment and filling of the root canal in the coronal fragment with gutta-percha. From CVEK et al. (177) 2002.

responded positively at the time of injury (136, 166, 170). The diagnosis of pulp necrosis should therefore always be based upon a combined clinical and radiographic evaluation.

Table 12.1 lists various reports on the prevalence of pulp necrosis after root fracture. Factors related to healing events (hard tissue, connective tissue and non-healing) can be divided into *pre-injury* and *injury factors* and *treatment dependent factors* (166, 170).

### Pre-injury and injury factors

The pre-injury or injury factors which had the greatest influence upon healing (i.e. whether hard tissue fusion of pulp necrosis) were *age* (166), *stage of root development* (i.e. the size of the pulpal lumen at the fracture site) (90, 93, 136, 166, 170, 177), *mobility of the coronal fragment* (166), *dislocation of the coronal fragment* (13, 93, 136, 166) and *diastasis between fragments* (i.e. rupture or stretching of the pulp at the fracture site (166) (Fig. 12.36).

It has previously been supposed that root fractures located at the marginal one-third of the root had a very poor long-term prognosis, thus indicating extraction therapy. However, this assumption has not been supported by recent studies where no relationship could be demonstrated between the frequency of pulp necrosis and the position of the fracture line (13, 90, 93, 94, 103, 177, 178).

In this regard, it should be considered that these teeth are at risk of a new trauma which easily could lead to loss of the coronal fragment; or excessive mobility being an indication for extraction (176, 177) (Fig. 12.37). In such situations it is important to consider whether the fracture is strictly horizontal or oblique and thus involving both the cervical or middle thirds of the root (Fig. 12.38). In a recent long-term study of 94 cervical root fractures, 44% were lost. In comparison, only 8% horizontal and oblique fractures were lost when located mid-root (177).

Other factors which have been found to be predictive of the type of fracture healing have included the presence of *restorations* at the time of injury as well as the presence of *marginal periodontitis* (136). Thus, if either of these factors were present, there was a significantly greater risk of healing by interposition of connective tissue than healing by hard tissue union. It was impossible to determine whether this finding reflected an age phenomenon or reduced pulpal defence due to disease or operative procedures (136).

**Table 12.1** Frequency of pulp necrosis after root fracture of permanent teeth.

| Examiner | No. of teeth | Pulp necrosis |
|---|---|---|
| Austin (12) 1930 | 40 | 8 (20%) |
| Doniau & Werelds (10) 1955 | 24 | 5 (21%) |
| Lindahl (11) 1958 | 25 | 6 (24%) |
| Andreasen & Hjörting-Hansen (13) 1967 | 48 | 21 (44%) |
| Stålhane & Hedegård (111) 1975 | 18 | 4 (18%) |
| Zachrisson & Jacobsen (93) 1975 | 64 | 13 (20%) |
| Ravn (94) 1976 | 50 | 11 (22%) |
| Krenkel et al. (173) 1985 | 26 | 1 (4%) |
| Andreasen et al. (136) 1989 | 95 | 25 (26%) |
| Yates (164) 1992 | 22 | 5 (23%) |
| Caliskan & Pehlivan (175) 1996 | 56 | 21 (37%) |
| Majorana et al. (162) 2002 | 31 | 13 (40%) |
| Welbury et al. (176) 2002 | 84 | 46 (55%) |
| Feely et al. (73) 2003 | 34 | 7 (21%) |
| Andreasen et al. (166, 170) 2004 | 400 | 88 (22%) |

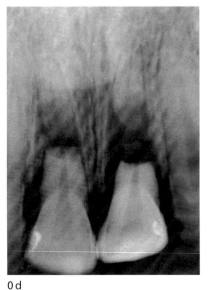 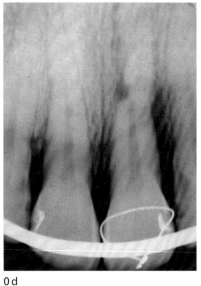 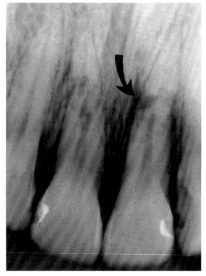

0 d                    0 d                    3 mo

**Fig. 12.36** Dislocation of a root fracture leading to pulp necrosis. Note that the left maxillary incisor is dislocated more than the right incisor. Three months later, the right central incisor was found to be vital whereas pulp necrosis and periapical rarefaction was diagnosed in the left central incisor (arrow).

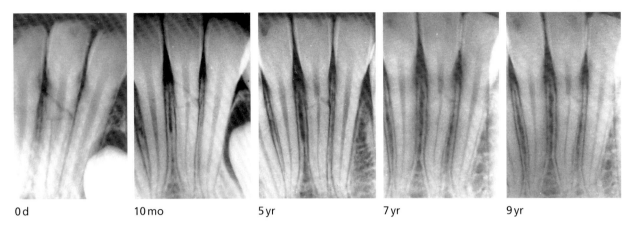

0 d          10 mo          5 yr          7 yr          9 yr

**Fig. 12.37** Healing of a cervical fracture with hard tissue. A transverse oblique and complicated fracture of a mandibular incisor involving the cervical part of the root healed by the formation of hard tissue between the fragments. The tooth was splinted with a cap-splint for 49 days. Control radiographs show slowly progressing healing with the formation of hard tissue; note formation of hard tissue at the fracture site in the pulpal lumen. From CVEK et al. (177) 2002.

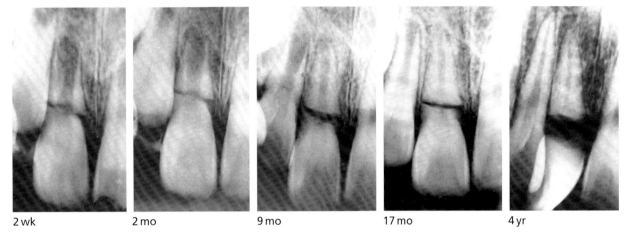

2 wk          2 mo          9 mo          17 mo          4 yr

**Fig. 12.38** Healing of a cervical fracture with connective tissue. Immature incisor with a transverse root fracture in the cervical one-third, healed with interposition of soft tissue between the fragments, followed by a secondary injury and tooth extraction. Treatment was delayed by the patient's fear of treatment. The tooth was immobilized with a cap-splint for 2 months. Control radiographs taken 2, 9 and 17 months after injury show healing with interposition of soft tissue and continued root development. After 4 years, the tooth suffered a new luxation injury and had to be extracted. From CVEK et al. (177) 2002.

## Treatment factors

Concerning treatment factors, the following had a negative influence upon healing: *forceful application of splints* (136) and the type of splint, rigid splints giving the poorest results (170). The length of splinting period appeared to be of no significance; and 4 weeks appeared to be acceptable (170). Furthermore, *treatment delay* of a few days did not have a negative effect on healing (170). Finally, *antibiotics* did not improve healing. In fact an unexplained inverse relation to healing has been found (136, 170).

Many types of treatment have been proposed for the management of pulp necrosis in root-fractured teeth (26, 179) (Fig. 12.39). The most important feature to consider is that the apical fragment normally contains vital pulp tissue (13). This is the basis for treatment where only the coronal fragment is root-filled, a treatment form which has been shown to result in a high rate of healing (26, 83, 112, 141,

179). This form of therapy is described in detail in Chapter 22, p. 612.

If the fracture line is situated in the cervical third of the root and the pulp is necrotic, the coronal fragment will become quite mobile. Intraradicular splinting, with a metal pin uniting the fragments and serving as a root canal filling has been tried (111, 115–118, 145–147). So far, only limited clinical data have been reported concerning long-term prognosis of these forms of therapy. However, the failure rate appears to be as high as half of all treated cases (146, 147).

Another suggested method of stabilizing the coronal fragment involves using metal endodontic implants which replace the apical fragment (74, 85–87, 104, 119–126, 148–156). Prefabricated implants are normally used in association with standardized endodontic intracanal instruments (85) (Fig. 12.40). The purpose of the implant is to shift the fulcrum of transverse movements to a more apical position. Clinically, this shift is evident in the stability of the

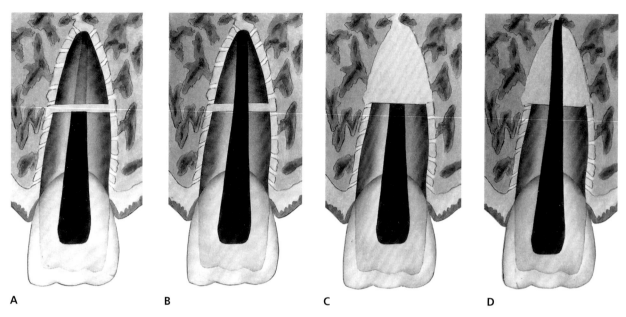

**A**                    **B**                    **C**                    **D**

**Fig. 12.39** Schematic drawings illustrating various types of treatments of pulp necrosis after root fracture. A. Root canal filling of coronal fragment. B. Intraradicular splinting with a metal pin used as root canal filling. C. Surgical removal of apical fragment together with root canal filling of coronal fragment. D. Metal implant replacing the apical fragment and acting as root canal filling. From ANDREASEN (87) 1968.

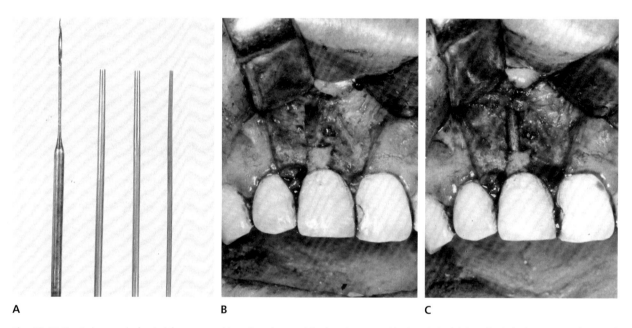

**A**                              **B**                              **C**

**Fig. 12.40** Surgical removal of apical fragment and insertion of a metal implant in a central incisor. A. Prefabricated cobalt-chromium implants and standardized endodontic instruments (Endodontic implant Starter Kit-B3, Star Dental Mfg. Co. Inc., Philadelphia, Pa., 19139, USA). B. A mucoperiosteal flap has been raised and the apical fragment removed. The entire root canal of the coronal fragment is enlarged to the level of the fracture. C. A cobalt-chromium implant of proper size is inserted into the root canal and the course taken by the implant noted. Subsequently, a cavity is created in the alveolar bone, ensuring that the length of the implant exceeds the original length of the root by 2–4 mm. The length of the implant is adjusted to the bone cavity and, in addition, to the level of the lingual surface of the crown. Finally, the implant is cemented into the root canal with a root canal sealer and special care is taken to remove excess cement.

fractured tooth immediately after implantation. However, successful long-term prognosis for these implants is dubious. Thus, in the authors' experience, 12 implants which originally were considered to have a good prognosis failed at later follow-ups (87) (Fig. 12.41). Moreover, increasing numbers of experimental studies have demonstrated evidence of corrosion of the pins as well as severe inflammation in the soft tissues adjacent to these implants (127–130,

157). Only a single experimental study found implants in teeth with no initial periapical inflammation to be accepted with no evidence of inflammation after 6 months (157).

Another treatment procedure has been advocated whereby the coronal fragment is extracted and the apical fragment removed. The root canal in the coronal fragment is enlarged and a combined root filling/root elongation is

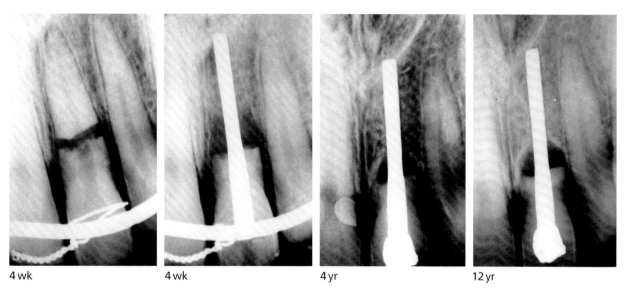

4 wk          4 wk          4 yr          12 yr

**Fig. 12.41** Treatment of root fracture by removal of apical fragment and insertion of a metal implant. At a follow-up 12 years later, inflammation around the implant is evident and a fistula is present.

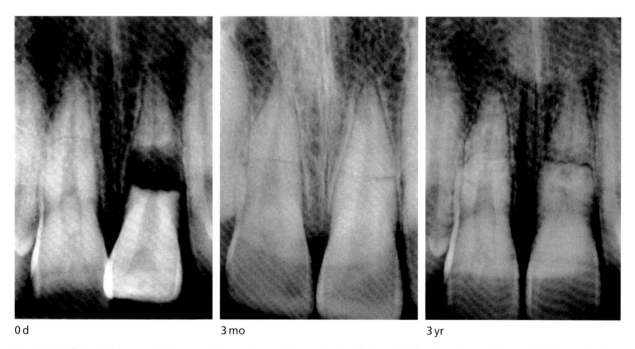

0 d                  3 mo                  3 yr

**Fig. 12.42** Effect of displacement of the coronal fragment on root fracture healing. Pulp canal obliteration after root fracture of both central incisors. The teeth were repositioned and splinted for 3 months. At the control appointment 3 years later, the right central incisor showed healing, with calcified tissue and partial pulp canal obliteration confined to the apical fragment and at the fracture site whereas the left central incisor demonstrated healing with interposition of connective tissue and complete pulp canal obliteration.

performed using an aluminum oxide or titanium implant which extends outside the apical foramen (see Chapter 17, p. 464). However, to date (15, 159) the long-term results of this procedure do not suggest that this procedure will be better than endodontic treatment of the coronal fragment only (112, 179). In this connection it should be borne in mind that root fractured incisors which heal after endodontic treatment of the coronal fragment tend to show decreasing mobility because of the physiologic decrease in tooth mobility with age (131, 160).

## Pulp canal obliteration

Partial or complete obliteration of the pulp canal is a common finding after root fracture (Fig. 12.42) (132, 134, 135, 166, 175). Thus, in clinical studies of root-fractured permanent incisors, pulp canal obliteration was found in 69–73% of the teeth (93, 103, 136). *Partial pulp canal obliteration* is seen most often in the fracture region and the apical fragment. In addition, partial obliteration extends 1–2 mm into the coronal fragment. *Complete pulp canal*

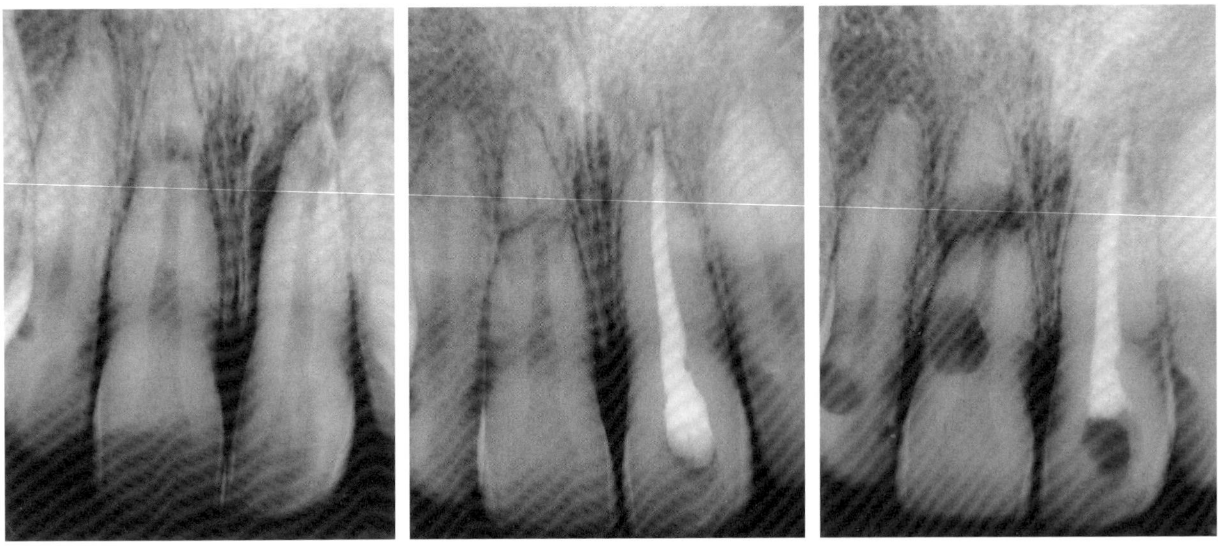

0 d                                    9 mo                                  2 yr

**Fig. 12.43** External inflammatory resorption following root fracture of a right central incisor. External resorption is evident at re-examination 2 years after injury (arrow). Mesial and distal radiographic projections revealed the external nature of this resorption process. Pulp necrosis was diagnosed at the clinical examination.

*obliteration* is seen as an even decrease in the size of the entire pulp cavity, leading to total obliteration. Both obliteration types progress at the same rate and are normally well advanced after 9–12 months and approach full density 1–2 years later (103). Obliteration of the apical root canal alone is commonly seen in cases of healing with hard tissue, while obliteration of the apical and coronal aspects of the root canal is often seen in cases with interposition of connective tissue, as well as in teeth with interposition of connective tissue and bone (103, 134). In this context, however, one should be aware that in cases of pulp necrosis, while the coronal root canal is usually the only part of the root canal affected, the apical root canal can be completely obliterated. Thus, one must use other criteria (i.e. resorption of bone and loss of lamina dura at the level of the fracture, loss of sensibility, loosening of the coronal fragment) for the determination of pulp status. Clinically, a slight yellowish discoloration of the crown is sometimes seen in the case of coronal pulp canal obliteration. Pulpal sensibility testing is in most cases normal, but a negative response can be registered. In contrast to pulp canal obliteration after luxation injuries, secondary pulp necrosis is a rare finding (103).

### Root resorption

Root resorption has been found to occur in approximately 60% of root-fractured permanent incisors and can usually be detected within 1 year after injury. These processes often precede fracture healing and obliteration of the coronal and/or apical aspects of the root canal and should be distinguished from resorption of bone at the level of root fracture which is indicative of coronal pulp necrosis. Root resorption appears in the following types:

(1) *External surface resorption* (ESR), characterized by the rounding of the fracture edges medially and/or distally (Fig. 12.12)

(2) *External inflammatory resorption* (Fig. 12.43)
(3) *External replacement resorption* (Fig. 12.44)
(4) *Internal surface resorption* (ISR), manifested as rounding of the fracture edges centrally, in the apical and coronal root canals, at the intersection between the root canal and fracture line (Figs 12.12 to 12.14)
(5) *Internal tunnelling resorption* (ITR), going behind the pre-dentin layer and burrowing along the root canal walls of the coronal fragment (Figs 12.13 and 12.14).

Only external inflammatory resorption needs treatment (pulp extirpation and root filling). External replacement resorption (ankylosis) cannot be treated. The other types of resorption just require observation.

## Orthodontic treatment of root fractured teeth

This problem is discussed in detail in Chapter 24.

## Predictors of healing

In this respect, the following three events will be present: development of *pulp necrosis* and *healing by hard or connective tissue.*

Basic information about these topics has been disclosed by two larger clinical studies (166, 170). As it appears from Fig. 12.45, the healing events are generally controlled by the *extent of injury* (± rupture / stretching of the pulp at the level of fracture) and the *anatomy of the pulp* (size and vascularity). Concerning treatment effects, *optimal repositioning* and the use of *flexible* (versus rigid) *splinting* has been found to favor healing.

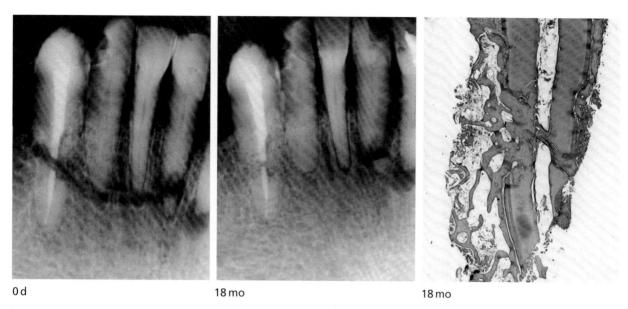

0 d                    18 mo                    18 mo

**Fig. 12.44** External replacement resorption following root fracture of right canine as well as fracture of the alveolar process. At re-examination 18 months later, external replacement resorption is evident. Histologic examination of extracted canine demonstrates marked replacement resorption. ×6.

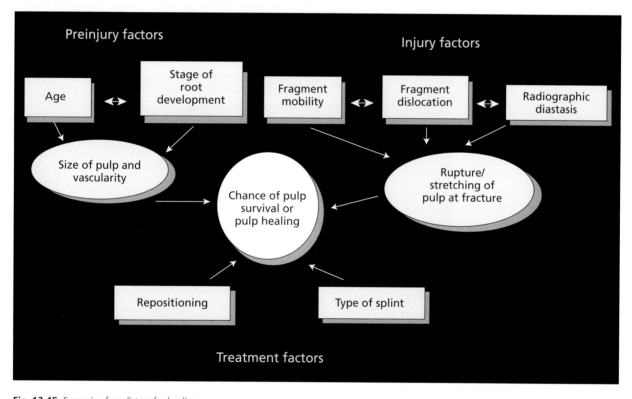

**Fig. 12.45** Synopsis of predictors for healing.

In the following, diagrams, the relative influence of the various factors is presented, based on a recent study of 400 root fractured incisors (166, 170) (Fig. 12.46). By entering the diagram with information from the time of injury, the likelihood of the following healing events can be ascertained.

## Type of healing

The following *pre-injury and injury factors* had a positive influence upon healing (i.e. hard tissue versus non-healing/pulp necrosis): immature root formation, lower age,

less displacement of the coronal fragment. The *treatment factors* which had a positive influence upon healing were: optimal repositioning and a flexible splinting.

## Tooth survival

Only a single study has examined this factor; and it was found that there was good long-term survival (Fig. 12.47). However, more studies are needed concerning this parameter, especially concerning fractures located at the cervical third (176).

A single study has shown an 83% 10-year survival (178).

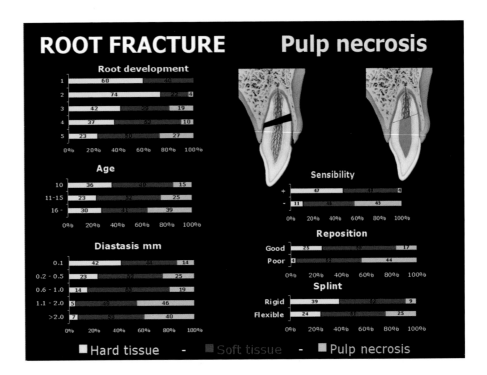

**Fig. 12.46** Predictors for healing.

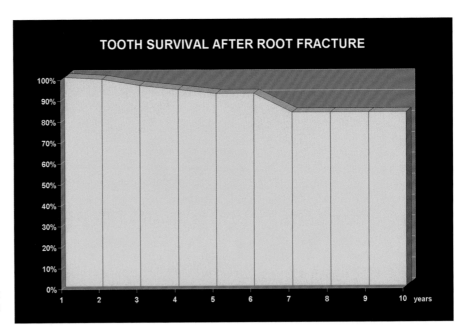

**Fig. 12.47** Long-term survival of root fractures. From ANDREASEN & ANDREASEN (180) 2006.

## Essentials

### Terminology

- Root fracture

### Frequency

- Primary dentition: 2 to 4% of dental injuries
- Permanent dentition: 0.5 to 7% of dental injuries

### Etiology

- Fight injuries
- Foreign bodies striking the teeth

### History

- Symptoms
- Tenderness from occlusion

## Clinical examination

- Mobility
- Dislocation
- Reaction to sensibility tests
- Radiographic examination
- Stage of root development
- Fracture site
- Dislocation
- Single, comminuted fracture

## Healing and pathology

- Healing with calcified tissue
- Interposition of PDL
- Interposition of bone and PDL
- Non-healing with interposition of granulation tissue

## Treatment

(1) Reposition the coronal fragment, if displaced (Figs 12.27 and 12.28).
(2) Check position of the coronal fragment radiographically.
(3) Immobilize the tooth with a semi-rigid splint (e.g. acid-etch/resin splint).
(4) Control the tooth radiographically and with sensibility tests.
(5) Maintain the splint for 4 weeks.
(6) Follow-up period minimum 1 year.
(7) If the fracture is located very close to the gingiva, extraction of the coronal fragment may be indicated, followed by orthodontic or surgical extrusion of the apical fragment (see Chapter 24). However, in the case of optimal oral hygiene, a conservative approach comprising permanent proximal fixation may be attempted.

## Prognosis

- Pulp necrosis: 20–40% (age dependent)
  — Treatment of pulp necrosis
  — Root canal treatment of coronal fragment (see Chapter 22, p. 612)
- Pulp canal obliteration: 69–73%
- Root resorption: 60%
  — Surface resorption (internal and/or external) is considered to be a link in fracture healing and requires no treatment
  — External inflammatory resorption and ankylosis (replacement resorption): very rare

## References

1. ANDREASEN JO. Etiology and pathogenesis of traumatic dental injuries. A clinical study of 1,298 cases. *Scand J Dent Res* 1979;**78**:329–42.
2. HARDWICK JL, NEWMAN PA. Some observations on the incidence and emergency treatment of fractured permanent anterior teeth of children. *J Dent Res* 1954;**33**:730.
3. DOWN CH. The treatment of permanent incisor teeth of children following traumatic injury. *Aust Dent J* 1957;**2**:9–24.
4. SUNDVALL-HAGLAND I. Olycksfallsskador på tänder och parodontium under barnaåren. In: Holst JJ, Nygaard Ostby B, Osvald O. *Nordisk Klinisk Odontologi.* Copenhagen: A/S Forlaget for Faglitteratur, 1964, Chapter 11, 111:1–40.
5. GELBIER S. Injured anterior teeth in children. A preliminary discussion. *Br Dent J* 1967;**123**:331–5.
6. RAVN JJ, ROSSEN I. Hyppighed og fordeling af traumatiske beskadigelser of tænderne hos københavnske skolebørn 1967/68. *Tandlægebladet* 1969;**73**:1–9.
7. FIALOVÁ S, JURECEK B. Urazy zubu udeti a nase zkusenosti s jejich lécenim. *Prakt Zubni Lék* 1968;**16**:171–6.
8. MAGNUSSON B, HOLM A-K. Traumatised permanent teeth in children – a follow-up. I. Pulpal complications and root resorption. *Svensk Tandläkars Tidning* 1969;**62**:61–70.
9. ENGELHARDT H-G, HAMMER H. Pathologie und Therapie der Zahnwurzelfrakturen. *Dtsch Zahnärztl Z* 1959;**14**:1278–89.
10. DONIAU R, WERELDS RJ. La consolidation des fractures radiculaires. Observations cliniques, radiographiques et histologiques. *Rev Belge Stomat* 1955;**52**:621–43.
11. LINDAHL B. Transverse intra-alveolar root fractures: Roentgen diagnosis and prognosis. *Odontologisk Revy* 1958;**9**:10–24.
12. AUSTIN LT. A review of forty cases of retained fractured roots of anterior teeth. *J Am Dent Assoc* 1930;**17**:1930–2.
13. ANDREASEN JO, HJÖRTING-HANSEN E. Intraalveolar root fractures: radiographic and histologic study of 50 cases. *J Oral Surg* 1967;**25**:414–26.
14. FREZIERES H, PONS J, LARTIGAU G. Traumatismes accidentels des incisives superieures chez l'adulte jeune. *Rev Fr Odonto-Stomatol* 1965;**12**:1017–27.
15. DUCLOS J, BRUGIRARD J. Diagnostic radiologique des fractures radiculaires (Loi des épasseurs du Professeur Duclos). *Ann Odontostomatol* 1955;**12**:59–71.
16. MARSHALL FJ. Root fracture. Report of a case. *Oral Surg Oral Med Oral Pathol* 1960;**13**:1485–7.
17. BOUCHER A. Fractures dentaires et radiographie. *Rev Fr Odontostomatol* 1956;**3**:1015–7.
18. GOOSE DH. Invisible root fracture. *Dent Practit Dent Rec* 1964;**14**:271–2.
19. BLACKWOOD HJJ. Metaplasia or repair of the dental pulp as a response to injury. *Br Dent J* 1957;**102**:87–92.
20. SARNAT BG, SCHOUR I. Effect of experimental fracture on bone, dentin, and enamel. Study of the mandible and the incisor in the rat. *Arch Surg* 1944;**49**:23–38.
21. DREYER CJ, GLUM L. Effect of root fracture on the epithelial attachment. *J Dent Assoc South Afr* 1967;**22**:103–5.
22. BEVELANDER G. Tissue reactions in experimental tooth fracture. *J Dent Res* 1942;**21**:481–7.
23. HAMMER H. Die Heilungsvorgänge bei Wurzelbrücken. *Dtsch Zahn Mund Kieferheilk* 1939;**6**:297–317.
24. ROTTKE B, HATIFOTIADIS D. Spätergebnisse experimentell gesetzter Zahnfrakturen im Tierversuch. *Fortschr Kiefer Gesichtschir* 1967;**12**:271–4.

25. BROSCH F. Über die Anwendbarkeit der Gesetze der traumatischen Entzündung auf die Vorgänge nach dem Zahnwurzelbruch. *Dtsch Zahn Mund Kieferheilk* 1961;**36**:169–86.

26. ANDREASEN JO. Treatment of fractured and avulsed teeth. *ASDC J Dent Child* 1971;**38**:29–48.

27. ARWILL T. Histopathologic studies of traumatized teeth. *Odontologisk Tidsskrift* 1962;**70**:91–117.

28. BOUYSSOU M, CHANCHUS P, BADER J, VIVES J. Observations histologiques sur deux fractures radiculo-dentaires spontanément consolidées. *Rev Stomatol* (Paris) 1956;**57**:417–27.

29. BRAUER JC. Treatment and restoration of fractured permanent anterior teeth. *J Am Dent Assoc* 1936;**23**:2323–36.

30. OMNELL KA. Study of a root fracture. *Br Dent J* 1953;**95**:181–5.

31. OTTOLENGUI R. Further consideration of the possible results of the fracture of the root of a tooth which contains a living pulp. *Dent Items Interest* 1927;**49**:79–90.

32. PRITCHARD GB. The reparative action of the dental tissues following severe injury. *Br Dent J* 1933;**54**:517–25.

33. REITAN K. Om vevsreaksjonen ved tilheling av rotfrakturer. *Norske Tannlægeforenings Tidende* 1947;**57**:367–73.

34. ZILKENS K. Beiträge zur traumatischen Zahnschädigung. In: Wannenmacher E. ed. *Ein Querschnitt der deutschen wissenschaftlichen Zahnheilkunde*. No. 33. Leipzig: Hermann Meusser Verlag, 1938:43–70.

35. SCHULZE C. Klinisch-röntgenologischer Beitrag zur Frage der Heilungsvorgänge bei Wurzelbrüchen vitaler Zähne. *Dtsch Zahnärztl Z* 1951;**6**:595–601.

36. SCHULZE C. Über die Heilungsvorgänge nach intraalveolären Frakturen vitaler Zähne. *Dtsch Zahnärztl Z* 1957;**12**:666–73.

37. PINDBORG JJ. Clinical, radiographic and histological aspects of intraalveolar fractures of upper central incisors. *Acta Odontol Scand* 1955;**13**:41–71.

38. BENNETT DT. Repair following root fracture. *Br Dent J* 1959;**107**:217–20.

39. BOULGER EP. Histologic studies of a specimen of fractured roots. *J Am Dent Assoc* 1928;**15**:1778–89.

40. EVERETT CC, ORBAN B. Fractured vital teeth. *Oral Surg Oral Med Oral Pathol* 1953;**6**:605–13.

41. KRONFELD R. A case of tooth fracture, with special emphasis on tissue repair and adaptation following traumatic injury. *J Dent Res* 1936;**15**:429–46.

42. KÖNIG A. Über Heilungsvorgänge bei Zahnfrakturen. *Dtsch Zahn Mund Kieferheilk* 1939;**6**:273–87.

43. LEHNERT S. Ein Beitrag zur Pathologie der Zahnwurzelfrakturen. *Dtsch Zahnärztebl* 1964;**18**:451–8.

44. MALLESON HC. Fractured upper lateral incisor extracted after being splinted for three months. *Dent Cosmos* 1923;**65**:492–4.

45. MANLEY EB, MARSLAND EA. Tissue response following tooth fracture. *Br Dent J* 1952;**93**:199–203.

46. GOLDMAN HM, BLOOM J. A collective review and atlas of dental anomalies and diseases. *Oral Surg Oral Med Oral Pathol* 1949;**2**:874–905.

47. DAWKINS J. Two transverse root fractures. *Aust Dent J* 1959;**4**:27–30.

48. BOUYSSOU M, WERELDS RJ. Histomorphologic assessment of the three possible patterns of hard callus in the healing of dental root fractures. *J Dent Res* 1969;**48**:1143–4.

49. BLACKWOOD HJJ. Tissue repair in intra-alveolar root fractures. *Oral Surg Oral Med Oral Pathol* 1959;**12**:360–70.

50. AISENBERG MS. Repair of a fractured tooth. *Dent Cosmos* 1932;**74**:382–5.

51. GOTTLIEB B. Histologische Untersuchung einer geheilten Zahnfraktur. Ein weiterer Beitrag zur Biologie der Zähne. *Z Stomatol* 1922;**20**:286–300.

52. LEFKOWITZ W. The formation of cementum. *Am J Orthod* 1944;**30**:224–40.

53. TULLIN B. Three cases of root fractures. *Odontol Rev* 1968;**19**:31–43.

54. KOVÁCS G, REHAK R. Das Verhalten wurzelfrakturierter Zähne. *Österr Z Stomatol* 1955;**52**:570–6.

55. OVERDIEKH F. Zur Auswirkung von Traumen auf Wurzeln bleibender Zähne unter besonderer Berücksichtigung der histologischen Befunde. *Dtsch Zahnärztl Z* 1957;**12**:1057–61.

56. STEINHARDT G. Pathologisch-anatomische Befunde nach Wurzelspitzenresektionen und Wurzelfrakturen beim Menschen. *Dtsch Zahnärztl Wochenschr* 1933;**36**:541–5.

57. MILES AEW. Resolution of the pulp following severe injury. *Br Dent J* 1947;**82**:187–9.

58. VERGARA-EDWARDS I. Fractures radiculaires au tiers cervical. *Rev Stomatol (Paris)* 1960;**61**:794–8.

59. ROY M. Les fractures radiculaires intra-alvéolaires. *Odontologie* 1938;**6**:601–13.

60. SCHUG-KOSTERS M. Frakturen und Subluxationen der Zähne mit lebender Pulpa und ihre Behandlung. *Dtsch Zahn Mund Kieferheilk* 1954;**21**:187–96.

61. SIBLEY LC. Management of root fracture. *Oral Surg Oral Med Oral Pathol* 1960;**13**:1475–84.

62. FLIEGE H, MÖLLENHOFF P. Ueber die Ausheilung interalveohirer Zahnfrakturen bei lebender Pulpa. *Dtsch Zahnärztl Wochenschr* 1933;**36**:479–81.

63. SCHINDLER J. Kasuistischer Beitrag zum Problem der Heilung von Zahnwurzelfrakturen mit Erhaltung der Vitalität der Pulpa. *Schweiz Monatschr Zahnheilkd* 1941;**51**:474–86.

64. HERVÉ M. Les fractures dentaires classification et traitement. *Actual Odontostomatol* 1951;**4**:157–91.

65. ANDERSON BG. Injuries to the teeth: Contusions and fractures resulting from concussion. *J Am Dent Assoc* 1944;**31**:195–200.

66. BRUSZT P. Intraalveoläre Frakturen der bleibenden Zähne und deren Behandlung. *Schweiz Monatschr Zahnheilkd* 1955;**65**:1103–10.

67. DRIAK F. Kasuistischer Beitrag zur Heilung von Zahnwurzelfrakturen. *Österr Z Stomatol* 1958;**55**:2–7.

68. JUNG F. Therapie bei Luxationen und Wurzelfrakturen. *Zahnärztl Prax* 1953;**4**:1–4.

69. OVERDIEK HF. Ein Beitrag zur Frage der Wurzelfrakturen insbesondere an Frontzähnen jugendlicher Patienten. *Dtsch Zahnärztl Z* 1957;**12**:1172–8.

70. FISCHER R. Zur Behandlung von Zahnwurzelfrakturen bei Jugendlichen. *Österr Z Stomatol* 1968;**65**:104–10.

71. Cwiora F, Rzeszutko R. Przyczynek do leczenia zlaman korzeni zebow przednich. *Czas Stomatol* 1968;**21**:199–203.

72. Ellis RG, Davey KW. *The classification and treatment of injuries to the teeth of children.* 5th edn. Chicago: Year Book Publishers Inc, 1970.

73. Feely I, Mackie IC, MacFarlane T. An investigation of root-fractured permanent incisor teeth in children. *Dent Traumatol* 2003;**19**:52–4.

74. Brugirard MJ. Réflexions sur 100 cas de traumatismes des régions incisives et canine. *Ann Odontostomatol* 1960;**17**:5572.

75. Grazid E, Coulomb, Boisset & Dasque. L'embrochage et le collage dans le traitement des fractures dentaires. *Rev Stomatol (Paris)* 1956;**57**:428–44.

76. Stacy GC. Intra-alveolar root re-fracture treated by internal splinting. *Br Dent J* 1965;**118**:210–2.

77. Naujoks R. Zahnfrakturen und ihre Therapie. *Dtsch Zahnärztebl* 1957;**11**:408–11.

78. Nolden R. Die konservierende Behandlung der Traumafolgen im Wachstumsalter. *Zahnärztl Welt* 1967;**68**:19–24.

79. Eschler J, Schilli W, Witt E. *Die traumatischen Verletzungen der Frontzähne bei Jugendlichen.* 3rd edn. Heidelberg: Alfred Hüthig Verlag, 1972.

80. Ingle JI, Frank AL, Natkin E, Nutting EE. Diagnosis and treatment of traumatic injuries and their sequelae. In: Ingle JI, Beveridge EE. eds. *Endodontics.* 2nd edn. Philadelphia: Lea & Febiger, 1976:685–741.

81. Weiskopf J, Gehre G, Graichen K-H. Ein Beitrag zur Behandlung von Luxationen und Wurzelfrakturen im Frontzahngebiet. *Stoma (Heidelberg)* 1961;**14**:100–13.

82. Cohen S. A permanent internal splint for a fractured incisor root. *Dent Dig* 1968;**74**:162–5.

83. Michanowicz AE. Root fractures. A report of radiographic healing after endodontic treatment. *Oral Surg Oral Med Oral Pathol* 1963;**16**:1242–8.

84. Feldman G, Solomon C, Notaro PJ. Endodontic management of traumatized teeth. *Oral Surg Oral Med Oral Pathol* 1966;**21**:100–12.

85. Frank AL. Improvement of the crown-root ratio by endodontic endosseous implants. *J Am Dent Assoc* 1967;**74**:451–62.

86. Frank AL, Abrams AM. Histologic evaluation of endodontic implants. *J Am Dent Assoc* 1969;**78**:520–24.

87. Andreasen JO. Treatment of intra-alveolar root fractures by cobalt-chromium implants. *Br J Oral Surg* 1968;**6**:141–6.

88. Hedegard B, Stalhane I. A study of traumatized permanent teeth in children aged 7–15 years. Part 1. *Swed Dent J* 1973;**66**:431–50.

89. Ravn JJ. Dental injuries in Copenhagen schoolchildren, school years 1967–1972. *Community Dent Oral Epidemiol* 1974;**2**:231–45.

90. Jacobsen I. Root fractures in permanent anterior teeth with incomplete root formation. *Scand J Dent Res* 1976;**84**:210–17.

91. Dynesen H, Ravn JJ. Rodfrakturer i det primære tandsæt. *Tandlægebladet* 1973;**77**:865–8.

92. Degering CI. Radiography of dental fractures. An experimental evaluation. *Oral Surg Oral Med Oral Pathol* 1970;**30**:213–19.

93. Zachrisson BU, Jacobsen I. Long-term prognosis of 66 permanent anterior teeth with root fracture. *Scand J Dent Res* 1975;**83**:345–54.

94. Ravn JJ. En klinisk og radiologisk undersøgelse af 55 rodfrakturer i unge permanente incisiver. *Tandlægebladet* 1976;**80**:391–6.

95. Hargreaves JA, Craig JW. *The management of traumatised anterior teeth in children.* London: E. & S. Livingstone, 1970.

96. Waldhart E. Röntgenologische und histologische tierexperimentelle Untersuchungen nach Zahnwurzelverletzungen. *ZWR* 1973;**82**:624–8.

97. Bouyssou M. Les calc de fractures dentaires compares aux calc de fracture osseuses. *Rev Fr Odontostomatol* 1970;**17**:1293–316.

98. Bouyssou M, Werelds RJ, Lepp FH, Soleilhavoup JP, Peyre J. Histologie comparative de la formation d'un cal dans les fractures dentaires et dans les fractures osseuses. *Bull Group Int Rech Soc Stomatol* 1970;**13**:317–68.

99. Fischer C-H. Beobachtungen bei intra- und extraalveolärer Verletzung der Pulpa nach einem Frontzahntrauma. *Dtsch Zahnärztl Z* 1970;**25**:1135–40.

100. Michanowicz AE, Michanowicz JP, Abou-Bass M. Cementogenic repair of root fractures. *J Am Dent Assoc* 1971;**82**:569–79.

101. Hansen P. Et tilfælde of rodfraktur med usædvanligt helingsforlöb. *Tandlægebladet* 1971;**75**:28–31.

102. Hartness JD. Fractured root with internal resorption, repair and formation of callus. *J Endod* 1975;**1**:73–5.

103. Jacobsen I, Zachrisson BU. Repair characteristics of root fractures in permanent anterior teeth. *Scand J Dent Res* 1975;**83**:355–64.

104. Tetsch P, Esser E. Die transdentale Fixation traumatisch geschädigter Frontzähne. *Österr Z Stomatol* 1974;**71**:59–65.

105. Fischer R, Kellner G. Klinische und histologische Befunde bei Zahnwurzelfrakturen. *Zahnärztl Welt* 1971;**80**:501–11.

106. Heithersay GS. Combined endodontic-orthodontic treatment of transverse root fractures in the region of the alveolar crest. *Oral Surg Oral Med Oral Pathol* 1973;**36**:404–15.

107. Johnson DL, Kelly JF, Flinton RJ, Cornell MT. Histologic evaluation of vital root retention. *J Oral Surg* 1974;**32**:829–33.

108. Whitaker DD, Shankle RJ. A study of the histologic reaction of submerged root segments. *Oral Surg Oral Med Oral Pathol* 1974;**37**:919–35.

109. Cook RT, Hutchens LH, Burkes EJ Jr. Periodontal osseous defects associated with vitally submerged roots. *J Periodontol* 1977;**48**:249–60.

110. Lustmann J, Azaz B. Roentgenographic study of mid root fractures. *Israel J Dent Med* 1976;**24**:23–8.

111. Stålhane I, Hedegard B. Traumatized permanent teeth in children aged 7–15 years. Part II. *Swed Dent J* 1975;**68**:157–69.

112. Cvek M. Treatment of non-vital permanent incisors with calcium hydroxide. IV. Periodontal healing and closure of the root canal in the coronal fragment of teeth with intra-alveolar fracture and vital apical fragment. A follow-up. *Odontologisk Revy* 1974;**25**:239–46.

113. Kröncke A. Zur Problematik der endodontalen Schienung frakturierter Zahnwurzeln. *Dtsch Zahnärztl Z* 1969;**24**:49–53.

114. Kozlowska I, Gratkowska H. Transverse fractures of roots of permanent teeth. *Czas Stomatol* 1975;**28**:681–6.

115. Lütterberg B, Götze G. Die Behandlung intraalveolärer Frakturen sowie parodontalgeschädigter Frontzähne mit der Stiftverbolzung. *Zahn Mund Kieferheilkd* 1978;**66**:669–73.

116. Luhr H-G. Endodontale Kompressionsverschraubung bei Zahnwurzelfrakturen. *Dtsch Zahnärztl Z* 1972;**27**:927–8.

117. Galitzien M-A. Die perkanaläre Kompressionschraube zur Versorgung von Zahnwurzelfrakturen im mittleren Drittel. *Dtsch Zahnärztl Z* 1978;**33**:665–7.

118. Luhr H-G, Bull H-G, Mohaupt K. Histologische Untersuchungen nach endodontaler Kompressionsverschraubung bei Zahnwurzelfrakturen. *Dtsch Zahnärztl Z* 1973;**28**:365–9.

119. Frank AL. Resorption, perforations and fractures. *Dent Clin North Am* 1974;**18**:465–87.

120. Dietz G. Apex und periapikales Parodont endodontisch enossal stiftfixierter Zähne. *Dtsch Zahnärztl Z* 1975;**30**:481–2.

121. Dietz G. Endodontischer enossaler Fixations – und Stumpfaufbaustift. *Dtsch Zahnärztl Z* 1975;**30**:483–5.

122. Cranin AN, Rabkin M. Endosteal oral implants. A retrospective radiographic study. *Dent Radio Photography* 1976;**49**:3–12.

123. Cranin AN, Rabkin MF, Garfinkel L. A statistical evaluation of 952 endosteal implants in humans. *J Am Dent Assoc* 1977;**94**:315–20.

124. Dietz G. Perkanaläre Schienung im Knochen von Frontzähnen mit horizontaler Wurzelfraktur im mittleren Drittel. *Dtsch Zahnärztl Z* 1977;**32**:450–2.

125. Gödde HJ. Ein kasuistischer Beitrag zur transdentalen Fixation. *ZWR* 1978;**87**:841–3.

126. Silverband H, Rabkin M, Cranin AN. The uses of endodontic implant stabilizers in posttraumatic and periodontal disease. *Oral Surg Oral Med Oral Pathol* 1978;**45**:920–9.

127. Seltzer S, Green DB, de la Guardia R, Maggio J, Barnett A. Vitallium endodontic implants: a scanning electron microscope, electron microscope, histologic study. *Oral Surg Oral Med Oral Pathol* 1973;**35**:828–60.

128. Langeland K, Spangberg L. Methodology and criteria in evaluation of dental endosseous implants. *J Dent Res* 1975;**54**:*(Spec Issue B)*:158–65.

129. Neuman G, Spangberg L, Langeland K. Methodology and criteria in the evaluation of dental implants. *J Endod* 1975;**1**:193–202.

130. Seltzer S, Maggio J, Woilard R, Green D. Titanium endodontic implants: a scanning electron microscope, electron microprobe and histologic investigation. *J Endod* 1976;**2**:267–76.

131. Scopp IW, Dictrow RL, Lichtenstein B, Blechman H. Cellular response to endodontic endosseous implants. *J Periodontol* 1971;**42**:717–20.

132. Birch R, Rock WP. The incidence of complications following root fracture in permanent anterior teeth. *Br Dent J* 1986;**160**:119–22.

133. Bender IB, Freedland JB. Clinical considerations in the diagnosis and treatment of intra-alveolar root fractures. *J Am Dent Assoc* 1983;**107**:595–600.

134. Andreasen FM, Andreasen JO. Resorption and mineralization processes following root fracture of permanent incisors. *Endod Dent Traumatol* 1988;**4**:202–14.

135. Andreasen FM. Pulpal healing after luxation injuries and root fracture in the permanent dentition. *Endod Dent Traumatol* 1989;**5**:111–31.

136. Andreasen FM, Andreasen JO, Bayer T. Prognosis of root-fractured permanent incisors – prediction of healing modalities. *Endod Dent Traumatol* 1989;**5**:11–22.

137. Michanowicz AE. Histologic evaluation of experimentally produced intra-alveolar root fractures. In: Gutmann JL, Harrison JW. eds. *Proceedings of the International Conference on Oral Trauma*. American Association of Endodontists Endowment & Memorial Foundation, Chicago, Illinois 1986:101–28.

138. Andreasen JO. Review of root resorption systems and models. Etiology of root resorption and the homeostatic mechanisms of the periodontal ligament. In: Davidovitch Z. ed. *The biological mechanisms of tooth eruption and root resorption*. 1988:9–21.

139. Herweijer JA, Torabinejad M, Bakland LK. Healing of horizontal root fractures. *J Endod* 1992;**18**:118–22.

140. Schmitz R, Donath K. Morphologische Veränderungen an traumatisierten Zähnen. Eine klinische und patho-histologische Studie. *Dtsch Zahnärztl Z* 1983;**38**:462–5.

141. Jacobsen I, Kerekes K. Diagnosis and treatment of pulp necrosis in permanent anterior teeth with root fracture. *Scand J Dent Res* 1980;**80**:370–6.

142. Engelhardtsen S. Rotfraktur i midtre tredjedel på rotåpen tann med luksasjon av koronale fragment. *Norske Tannlegeforenings Tidende* 1990;**100**:102–3.

143. Hagen SO. Rotfraktur i cervikale tredjedel på rotåpen tann – med tilheling. *Norske Tannlegeforenings Tidende* 1990;**100**:104–5.

144. Sundnes SK. Rotfraktur i midtre tredjdel med luksasjon og utvikling av pulpanekrose. *Norske Tannlegeforenings Tidende* 1990;**100**:106–7.

145. Bull H, Neugebauer W. Transdentale Kompressionsverschraubung zur Stabiliserung wurzelfrakturierter Zähne. *Zahnärztl Prax* 1983;**34**:258–60.

146. Reuter E, Weber W. Sekundäre Schienung von Zahnwurzelfrakturen durch endodontale Zugschraube. Langzeitergebnisse. *Dtsch Zahnärztl Z* 1987;**42**:308–10.

147. Bechtold H, Bull H-G, Schubert F. Ergebnisse der transdentalen Stabilisierung gelockerter und wurzelfrakturierter Zähne. *Dtsch Zahnärztl Z* 1987;**42**:295–8.

148. Berger F. Transdental Fixation bei noch weitem Apikalforamen. *Zahnärztl Prax* 1980;**31**:456–7.

149. Zinner R, Glien W. Die transdentale Fixation mit Aluminiumoxidkeramik. *Stomatol DDR* 1986;**36**:385–8.

150. Herforth A. Zur Stabilisierung gelockerter Zähne durch transdentale Fixation. *Dtsch Zahnärztl Z* 1983;**38**:129–30.

151. Schramm-Scherer B, Tetsch P, Tripplers, Broderle U. Stabilisierung einwurzeliger Zähne durch Transfixationsstifte. *Dtsch Zahnärztl Z* 1987;**42**:302–4.

152. HAUSSLER F, MAIER KH. Indikationen und Erfahrungen der chirurgischen Zahnerhaltung durch transdentale Fixation. *Dtsch Zahnärztl Z* 1987;**42**:290–1.

153. VOSS A. Kronen- und Wurzelfrakturen im bleibenden Gebiss. *Zahnärztl Mitt* 1989;**79**:2600–5.

154. FRENKEL G, ADERHOLD L. Das Trauma im Frontzahnbereich des jugendlichen Gebisses aus chirurgischer Sicht. *Fortschr Kieferorthop* 1990;**51**:138–44.

155. HERFORTH A. Wurzelfrakturen und Luxationen von Zähnen – I. Teil. *ZWR* 1990;**99**:440–4.

156. HERFORTH A. Wurzelfrakturen und Luxationen von Zähnen – II. Teil. *ZWR* 1990;**99**:604–8.

157. STRUNZ V, KIRSCH A. TransfizATION von Zähnen mit Titanplasma-beschichteten Stiften im Tierexperiment. *Dtsch Zahnärztl Z* 1987;**42**:292–4.

158. BRINKMANN E. Indikation und Anwendung der chirurgischen Zahnerhaltung. *Zahnärztl Mitt* 1982;**72**:1–12.

159. HERFORTH A. Zur Stabilisierung gelockerter Zähne durch transdental Fixation. *Dtsch Zahnärztl Z* 1983;**38**:129–30.

160. ANDREASEN JO, ANDREASEN FM. Long term tooth mobility testings of non-healed root fractures. A study of 50 cases. In preparation.

161. DIETZ G. Experimentel horizontal wurzelfrakturierte Affenfrontzähne und deren perkanaläre enossale Stiftfixation. *Dtsch Zahnärztl Z* 1976;**31**:89–91.

162. MAJORANA A, PASINI S, BARDELLINI E, KELLER E. Clinical and epidemiological study of traumatic root fractures. *Dent Traumatol* 2002;**18**:77–80.

163. BORUM MK, ANDREASEN JO. Therapeutic and economic implications of traumatic dental injuries in Denmark; an estimate based on 7549 patients treated at a major trauma centre. *Int J Paediatr Dent* 2001;**11**:116–28.

164. YATES JA. Root fractures in permanent teeth: a clinical review. *Int Endodont J* 1992;**25**:150–7.

165. KOCITBOWORNCHAI S, NUANSAKUL R, SIKRAM S, SINAHAWATTANA S, SAENGMONTRI S. Root fracture detection: a comparison of direct digital radiography with conventional radiography. *Dentomaxillofac Radiol* 2001;**30**:106–9.

166. ANDREASEN JO, ANDREASEN FM, MEJARE I, CVEK M. Healing of 400 intra-alveolar fractures. 1. Effect of pre-injury and injury factors such as sex, age, stage of root development, fracture type, location of fracture and severity of dislocation. *Dent Traumatol* 2004;**20**:192–202.

167. JIN H, THOMAS HF, CHEN J. Wound healing and revascularization. *Oral Surg Oral Med Oral Pathol Oral Radiol Endod* 1996;**81**:26–30.

168. POI WR, MANFRIN TM, HOLLAND R, SONODA CK. Repair characteristics of horizontal root fracture: a case report. *Dent Traumatol* 2002;**18**:98–102.

169. TZIAFAS D, MARGELES I. Repair of entreated root fracture: a case report. *Endod Dent Traumatol* 1993;**9**:40–3.

170. ANDREASEN JO, ANDREASEN FM, MEJARE I, CVEK M. Healing of 400 intra-alveolar fractures. 2. Effect of treatment factors, such as treatment delay, repositioning, splinting type and period and antibiotics. *Dent Traumatol* 2004;**20**:203–11.

171. HOVLAND EJ. Horizontal root fractures. Treatment and repair. *Dent Clin North Am* 1992;**36**:509–25.

172. FEIGLIN B. Clinical management of transverse root fractures. *Dent Clin North Am* 1995;**39**:53–78.

173. KRENKEL C, GRUNERT I, MESSAWARATI S. Nachuntersuchung von wurzelfrakturierten Zähnen versorgt mit Silcadraht-Klebeschienen. *Z Stomatol* 1985;**82**:325–36.

174. EPILIARA A, TOKITA Y, IZAWA T, SUDA H. Pulpal blood flow assessed by laser Doppler flowmetry in a tooth with a horizontal root fracture. *Oral Surg Oral Med Oral Pathol Oral Radiol Endod* 1996;**81**:229–33.

175. CALISKAN MK, PEHLIVAN Y. Prognosis of root-fractured permanent incisors. *Endod Dent Traumatol* 1996;**12**:129–36.

176. WELBURY RR, KINIRONS MJ, DAY P, HUMPHREYS K, GREGG TA. Outcomes for root-fractured permanent incisors: a retrospective study. *Pediatric Dentistry* 2002;**24**:98–102.

177. CVEK M, MEJARE I, ANDREASEN JO. Healing and prognosis of teeth with intra-alveolar fractures involving the cervical part of the root. *Dent Traumatol* 2002;**18**:57–65.

178. CVEK M, ANDREASEN JO, BORUM MK. Healing of 208 intraalveolar root fractures in patients aged 7–17 years. *Dent Traumatol* 2001;**17**:53–62.

179. CVEK M, MEJARE I, ANDREASEN JO. Conservative endodontic treatment of teeth fractured in the middle or apical part of the root. *Dent Traumatol* 2004;**20**:261–9.

180. ANDREASEN JO, ANDREASEN FM. Prognosis of 95 root fractured permanent teeth, 2006. Study in progress.

# 13

# Luxation Injuries of Permanent Teeth: General Findings

F. M. Andreasen & J. O. Andreasen

## Terminology, frequency and etiology

Depending on the direction of impact, a variety of luxation injuries may occur. From a therapeutic, anatomic and prognostic point of view, five different types of luxation injuries can be recognized (Fig. 13.1).

(1) *Concussion*: An injury to the tooth-supporting structures without abnormal loosening or displacement but with marked reaction to percussion (Fig. 13.1A).
(2) *Subluxation (loosening)*: An injury to the tooth-supporting structures with abnormal loosening but without clinically or radiographically demonstrable displacement of the tooth (Fig. 13.1B).
(3) *Extrusive luxation (peripheral displacement, partial avulsion)*: Partial displacement of the tooth following the axis of the tooth out of its socket but without leaving the socket (Fig. 13.1C). Radiographic examination always reveals increased width of the periodontal ligament space.
(4) *Lateral luxation*: Eccentric displacement (other than axial) of the tooth. This is accompanied by comminution or fracture of the alveolar socket (Fig. 13.1D, E). Depending on the angulation of the central beam, radiographic examination may or may not demonstrate increased width of the periodontal ligament space (148).
(5) *Intrusive luxation (central dislocation)*: Displacement of the tooth deeper into the alveolar bone. This injury is accompanied by comminution or fracture of the alveolar socket (Fig. 13.1F). The direction of dislocation follows the axis of the tooth. Radiographic examination reveals dislocation of the tooth and sometimes a missing or diminished periodontal space. In the adult dentition, an apical shift of the cemento-enamel junction of the involved tooth can be seen.

The most important clinical difference between intrusive and extrusive luxation is that in the latter the apex is displaced out of its socket and not through the alveolar bone socket as in intrusive luxation. Moreover, extrusive luxation can imply complete rupture or stretching/tearing of the neurovascular supply to the pulp at the apical foramen and the periodontal ligament fibers are to a great extent severed; whereas the supporting bone is not affected.

The factors which determine the type of luxation injury appear to be the force and direction of impact (Fig. 13.2).

Luxation injuries comprise 15–61% of dental traumas to permanent teeth (1–5).

## Clinical findings

In both the primary and permanent dentitions, tooth luxations primarily involve the maxillary central incisor region and are seldom seen in the mandible (1–5).

With increasing age, the frequency and pattern of injury change. In the primary dentition, intrusions and extrusions comprise the majority of all injuries, a finding which is possibly related to the high resilience of the alveolar bone at this age. In contrast, in the permanent dentition the number of intrusive luxation injuries is considerably reduced and usually seen in younger individuals (5).

Most frequently, two or more teeth are luxated simultaneously and a number of luxations show concomitant crown or root fractures (1, 2).

Clinical and radiographic findings for different luxation injuries are summarized in Table 13.1. While the diagnosis of luxation injuries is based on the combination of radiographic and clinical findings including sensibility testing (Table 13.1), diagnostic accuracy increases with multiple radiographic exposures, where angulation of the central beam is altered (148).

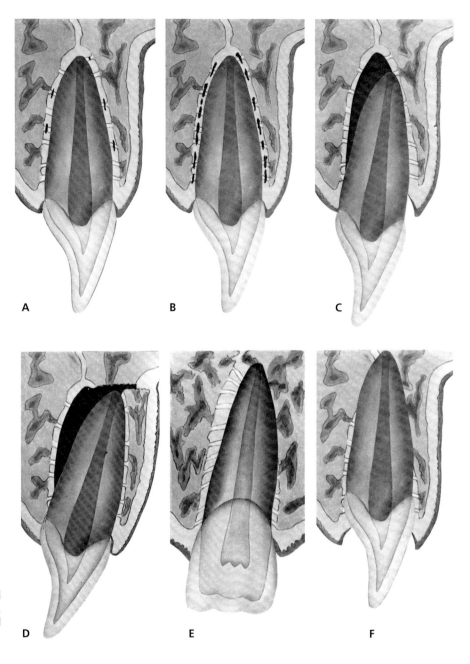

**Fig. 13.1** Injuries to the periodontal tissues. A. Concussion. B. Subluxation. C. Extrusive luxation. D and E. Lateral luxation. F. Intrusive luxation.

A　　　B　　　C

D　　　E　　　F

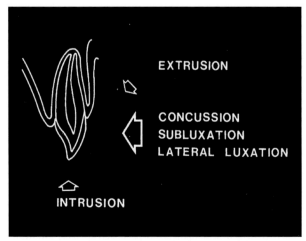

**Fig. 13.2** The energy and direction of the impact determine the type of luxation injury.

## Radiographic findings

Radiographic examination is an important adjunct to the clinical examination, as it can disclose minor dislocations. It has been shown experimentally that error in the radiographic recording of the distance of dislocation is minimal if the bisecting angle technique is used (254). Moreover, in order to obtain reproducible radiographs, film holders should be employed to standardize exposure technique. Thus, an average of 6.9% error in measurement of tooth length was encountered if film holders were not used compared to a 2.0% average error if they were (254). And the probability of diagnosing displacement (irrespective of direction) is increased if multiple radiographic exposures

**Table 13.1** Typical clinical and radiographic findings with different types of luxation injuries.

| | Type of luxation injury | | | | |
| --- | --- | --- | --- | --- | --- |
| | Concussion | Subluxation | Extrusion | Intrusion | Lateral luxation |
| Abnormal mobility | – | + | + | –(+)[1] | –(+) |
| Tenderness to percussion | + | +(–) | +(–) | – | – |
| Percussion sound | normal[2] | dull | dull | metallic | metallic |
| Positive response to sensibility testing | +/– | +/– | – | – | – |
| Radiographic dislocation | – | –(+) | + | + | + |

[1] A sign in parentheses indicates a finding of rare occurrence.
[2] Teeth with incomplete root formation and teeth with marginal or periapical inflammatory lesions will elicit a dull percussion sound.

with varying vertical and horizontal angulations of the central beam are taken of the injured region (254).

## Healing and pathology

Most luxations represent a combined injury to the pulp and periodontium. However, the pathology of luxation injuries has received little attention. At present, only a few specific changes can be ascribed to the periodontal ligament after luxation injury (153–158, 236, 237); whereas pulpal changes have been studied to a certain extent (6, 91, 99–102, 157–160, 236–238).

## Periodontal ligament (PDL)

The histologic response in the periodontal ligament has only been sparsely studied experimentally. *Concussion* and *subluxation* have been induced in rat molars (153, 157, 158) and in dog incisors (155). Furthermore, *extrusive luxations* have been studied in monkeys (156) and rats (157, 158, 238), whereas *intrusions* have been analyzed in dogs (154, 236, 237). These studies have revealed the following PDL changes after trauma (see also Chapter 2, p. 79).

### Concussion/subluxation

The general feature is edema, bleeding and sometimes laceration of PDL fibers. The neurovascular supply to the pulp may or may not be intact. The PDL changes 1 hour after trauma were characterized by hemorrhage, stretched, torn or compressed PDL fibers, cell destruction and edema (158). After 1 day, cell-free zones could be seen in the PDL, bordered by a zone of inflammation. In the bony socket 1 day after trauma, osteoclastic activity had begun. After 1 week, this had reached the root surface. After 10 days, the resorption activity was arrested, leaving healed surface resorption cavities along the root surface (158).

## Extrusive luxation

Immediate changes are characterized by a complete rupture of the PDL fibers and the neurovascular supply to the pulp. After 3 days, in monkeys, the split in the PDL, which is usually seen midway between bone and root surface, is filled in with a tissue dominated by endothelial cells and young fibroblasts. In some areas, cell-free zones indicate infarcted tissue. After 2 weeks, newly formed collagen fibers are seen. After 3 weeks, the PDL appears normal (156).

## Lateral luxation

This comprises a complex injury involving rupture or compression of PDL fibers, severance of the neurovascular supply to the pulp and fracture of the alveolar socket wall.

## Intrusive luxation

The immediate response to intrusion in monkeys appears to be an extensive crushing injury to the PDL and alveolar socket and rupture of the neurovascular supply to the pulp (162). After an observation period of 3 months, some intruded teeth in dogs showed extensive ankylosis; whereas others showed areas with surface resorption and otherwise normal PDL (154, 236, 237).

## Pulp

Changes seen in the pulp soon after injury are edema and disorganization of the odontoblast layer as well as nuclear pyknosis of pulp cells (6, 238). Perivascular hemorrhage can be demonstrated within a few hours in human subjects (Fig. 13.3). Such bleeding could be the result of a partially severed vascular supply. However, in most cases a complete arrest of pulpal circulation occurs, which leads to ischemia, breakdown of vessel walls, escape of erythrocytes and the eventual conversion of hemoglobin to red granular debris which permeates the pulp tissue and gives it a scarlet red color

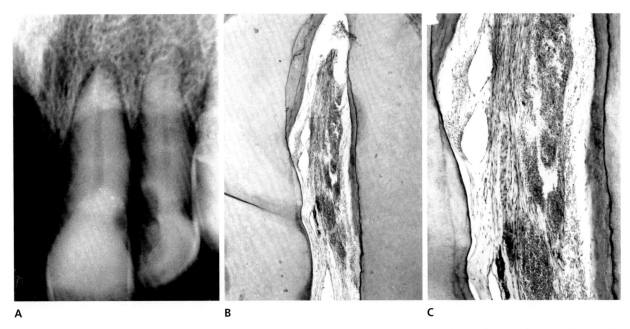

A                                    B                                    C

**Fig. 13.3** Early histologic changes following subluxation of a permanent central incisor. A. Radiograph of left central incisor following subluxation. The tooth was extracted 6 hours after injury. B. Perivascular bleeding is evident in the apical part of the pulp. ×30. C. Higher magnification of B. ×75.

(102). Ultrastructurally as well, blood vessels with disrupted or absent endothelium and erythrocyte remnants can be seen (159).

Histologic evidence of pulp necrosis, including nuclear pyknosis, disappearance of odontoblasts and stromal elements can be seen 6 days after injury (Fig. 13.3). This response is related to either partial or total rupture of the pulpal neurovascular supply. The later events of pulpal healing after luxation injury are presently unknown. However, based on experimental findings after extraction and replantation of teeth, it might be expected that a gradual revascularization and reinnervation of the pulp occurs if the size of the apical foramen is adequate to permit vascular ingrowth and that intervening infection of the ischemic pulp does not occur. This process is further described in Chapter 2, p. 84.

If the pulp survives or becomes revascularized, a number of regressive pulp changes can occur, such as hyalinization and deposition of amorphous, diffuse calcifications (6, 9, 10). Furthermore, the injury usually interferes with normal dentin formation. This interference is apparently related to a number of clinical factors, among which the stage of root formation and the type of luxation injury seem to be decisive (104, 105, 163, 164).

In teeth with incomplete root development, a distinct incremental line usually indicates arrest of normal tubular dentin formation at the time of injury. Most of the dentinal tubules stop at this line, while the original predentin layer is often preserved.

After a certain period, apposition of new hard tissue is resumed, but without the normal tubular structure. This tissue often contains cell inclusions which maintain their tubular connections with dentin formed before the injury (11, 15), as well as vascular inclusions. The junction between old and new dentin is rather weak, explaining the separation

which may occur in this area during extraction (12–14). This hard tissue formation often continues to the point of total obliteration of the root canal (15, 17–25, 106).

Although the calcified cellular tissue which is formed in response to the injury may resemble bone and cementum, it lacks the cellular organization characteristic of these tissues. Due to its tendency to convert to tubular dentin, the repair tissue has been termed cellular dentin (16). This tendency to return to tubular dentin could be related to differentiation of new odontoblasts from the primitive mesenchymal cells of the pulp. This response is especially marked in the apical portion of the root canal, possibly due to the rapid re-establishment of blood supply in this area after injury (16).

The rate of hard tissue formation is accelerated after injury, resulting in large amounts of newly formed hard tissue, especially in the coronal portion.

In the case of luxation of young permanent teeth, bone can be deposited within the pulp after trauma and is usually connected to the root canal walls by a collagenous fiber arrangement imitating a periodontal ligament (239). (See Chapter 2, p. 90.) This form of healing has been found to be related to damage or destruction of Hertwig's epithelial root sheath (HERS). Such damage can arise from either incomplete repositioning, whereby HERS suffers injury due to ischemia, or by forceful repositioning, whereby all or parts of HERS are crushed (165).

In mature teeth, the disturbance of the odontoblast layer can be more severe, with resorption sometimes preceding deposition of new hard tissue (16–18). Presumably, the time required for re-establishing vascularization after injury is longer in a tooth with complete root formation, thus increasing the damage to the pulp. The cellular hard tissue formed after the injury rarely assumes a tubular appearance; this applies especially to the coronal portion.

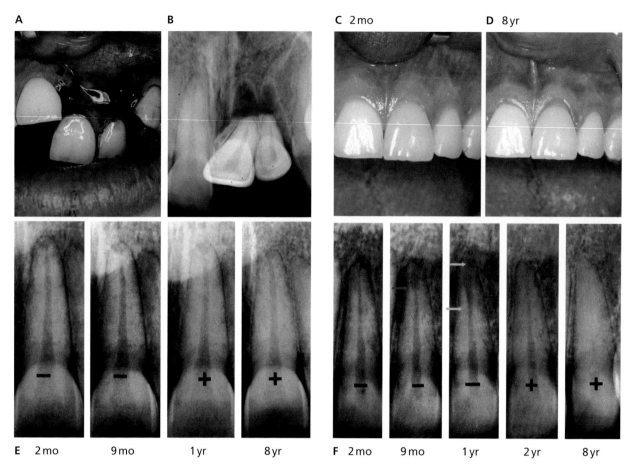

**Fig. 13.4** Root canal surface resorption of the apical foramen after fracture of the alveolar process and extrusion of the left maxillary central and lateral incisors in a 21-year-old woman. A and B. Clinical and radiographic appearance at the time of injury. C. Clinical appearance 2 months after injury. The crown of the left central incisor has become gray. E and F. Orthoradial exposures of the central and lateral incisors respectively at 2 months, 9 months, 1 year, 2 years and 8 years after injury. Plus and minus signs on the radiographs indicate positive or negative responses to pulp testing. Red arrows indicate the start of root canal surface resorption and green arrows an arrest of resorption. At the 8-year control, the color of the left central incisor is almost normal. From ANDREASEN (193) 1989.

In a clinical luxation material, temporary resorption of bone surrounding the root apex and of dentin within the apical foramen of extruded and laterally luxated mature incisors has been described (transient apical breakdown). Mineralization of these resorption processes could be associated with normalization of coronal discoloration and/or restoration of pulpal sensibility and was significantly related to later pulp canal obliteration (166) (Figs 13.4, 13.5) (see Chapter 2, p. 84).

Teeth with incomplete root formation at the time of injury sometimes show pulp necrosis confined to the coronal part of the pulp, while the apical portion apparently survives for some time, ensuring occlusion of the wide apex with calcified tissue (8, 103) (see Chapter 2, p. 84).

## Treatment

Therapeutic measures vary greatly from the primary to the permanent dentitions and according to the type of injury to the tooth-supporting structures. In this context, it should be borne in mind that repositioning and sometimes even splinting procedures can elicit further trauma. Before repositioning of a displaced tooth, it is therefore worth considering whether the repositioning procedure achieves any of the following goals:

(1) Facilitates pulpal healing?
(2) Facilitates periodontal ligament healing?
(3) Eliminates occlusal interferences?
(4) Improves esthetics?

At least one or more of these objectives should be achieved by the repositioning procedure, especially if this procedure, as in the case of lateral luxation, results in further damage to the site of injury. The use of and effect of treatment procedures are described in the following chapters on the various types luxation injury.

## Prognosis

The follow-up period can disclose a number of complications, such as pulp canal obliteration, pulp necrosis, root

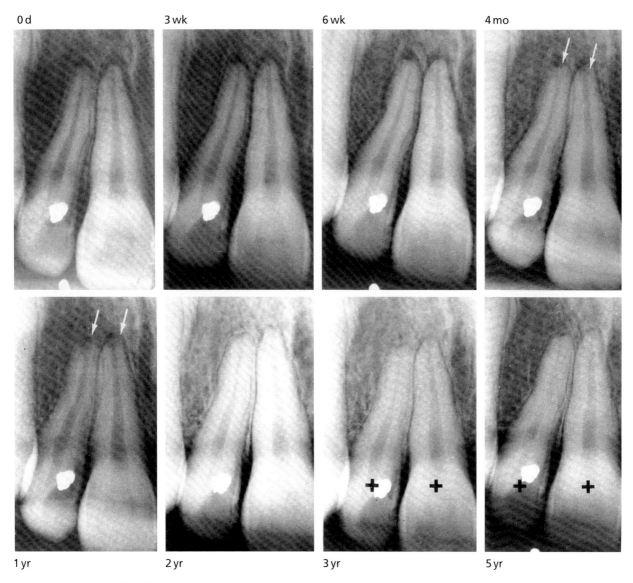

0 d       3 wk       6 wk       4 mo

1 yr       2 yr       3 yr       5 yr

**Fig. 13.5** Transient apical breakdown after extrusive luxation of the maxillary right central and lateral incisors in a 19-year-old man. There is coronal discoloration of both teeth at the 1- and 2-year controls. Note internal surface resorption of both teeth at the apical foramina (arrows) 4 months and 1 year after injury, which is later followed by apical blunting (external surface resorption) and pulp canal obliteration of the lateral incisor. Plus signs on radiographs indicate when the incisors regained normal pulpal sensibility. From ANDREASEN (193) 1989.

resorption and loss of marginal bone support. A good survey of these complications has been published by Dumsha (242). A follow-up schedule whereby healing complications can be diagnosed and interceptively treated is presented in Appendix 3, p. 881. However, in order to utilize the suggested recall schedule to full advantage, certain information must be gathered at the time of injury in order to identify those cases in which healing complications can be anticipated. The information needed for such clinical decisions will be discussed in the following.

'Tooth luxation' as a clinical diagnosis covers a broad spectrum of injury from a therapeutic, anatomic and prognostic point of view. A multivariate analysis of clinical and radiographic data registered at the time of injury confirmed the relevance of the current classification system, in that each type of injury could be described by a unique survival curve with respect to the development of pulp necrosis

following injury (163) (see later). The same classification system was found useful in describing the luxation injury to the coronal fragment of a root fracture (193, 194) (see Chapter 12).

## Pulp necrosis

The frequency of pulp necrosis after luxation injuries in the permanent dentition has been found to range from 15 to 59% (Table 13.2).

Two factors have been found to be significantly related to the development of pulp necrosis: the *type of luxation injury* and *stage of root development* (3, 163, 196, 197, 242) (Tables 13.3 and 13.4). In these investigations, it was not possible to demonstrate any effect of treatment upon the development

**Table 13.2** Prevalence of pulp necrosis after luxation of permanent teeth irrespective type of luxation injury.

| Examiner | No. of teeth | Pulp necrosis |
|---|---|---|
| Skieller (7) 1960 | 107 | 44 (41%) |
| Weiskopf et al. (74) 1961 | 121 | 72 (59%) |
| Anehill et al. (75) 1969 | 76 | 18 (24%) |
| Andreasen (3) 1970 | 189 | 98 (52%) |
| Stålhane & Hedegård (104) 1975 | 1116 | 172 (15%) |
| Rock et al. (97) 1974 | 200 | 75 (38%) |
| Rock & Grundy (178) 1981 | 517 | 192 (37%) |
| Wepner & Bukel (228) 1981 | 142 | 30 (21%) |
| Andreasen & Vestergaard Pedersen (163) 1985 | 637 | 156 (24%) |
| Oikarinen et al. (196) 1987 | 147 | 74 (50%) |
| Herforth (197) 1990 | 319 | 81 (25%) |
| Crona-Larsson et al. (240) 1991 | 104 | 24 (23%) |
| Robertson (241) 1997 | 196 | 34 (17%) |

**Table 13.3** Prevalence of pulp necrosis according to type of luxation of permanent teeth. From ANDREASEN & VESTERGAARD PEDERSEN (163) 1985.

| Type of luxation | No. of teeth | Pulp necrosis |
|---|---|---|
| Concussion | 178 | 5 (3%) |
| Subluxation | 223 | 14 (6%) |
| Extrusive luxation | 53 | 14 (26%) |
| Lateral luxation | 122 | 71 (58%) |
| Intrusive luxation | 61 | 52 (85%) |

**Table 13.4** Prevalence of pulp necrosis after luxation of permanent teeth according to stage of root development. From ANDREASEN & VESTERGAARD PEDERSEN (163) 1985.

| Stage of root development | No. of teeth | Pulp necrosis |
|---|---|---|
| Incomplete | 279 | 21 (8%) |
| Complete | 358 | 135 (38%) |

of pulp necrosis (e.g. repositioning, fixation, antibiotic therapy).

## Type of luxation injury

The greatest frequency of pulp necrosis is encountered among intrusions followed by lateral luxation and extrusion (Fig. 13.6) while the least frequent occurrence of pulp necrosis was after concussion and subluxation (3, 7, 104, 136, 163, 197) (Table 13.3).

## Stage of root development

Pulp necrosis occurs more frequently in teeth with fully developed roots (3, 7, 104, 136, 163) (Table 13.4 and Fig. 13.6). In teeth with immature root development, slight movements of the apex can presumably occur without disruption of the blood vessels passing through the apical foramen. Moreover, the process of revascularization is more easily achieved in teeth with a wide apical foramen, thus favoring the chance of pulp survival.

Fig. 13.6 shows survival curves following luxation injury according to type of injury and stage of root development (defined by quarters of anticipated root growth and patency of the apical foramen). It can be seen that teeth with a constricted apical foramen which have been displaced run a greater risk of pulp necrosis than do teeth with patent root apices, where there is a greater possibility of pulpal revascularization. If the stage of root development is expressed as the mesiodistal diameter of the apical foramen at the time of injury it is also possible to demonstrate an improved revascularization potential following extrusion and lateral luxation with an increase in apical diameter, presumably reflecting the area of the pulpo-periodontal interface from which new vessels could proliferate (198).

Regarding the diagnosis of pulp necrosis following luxations, different chronological patterns are followed for the various luxation types. Thus, pulp necrosis can be diagnosed within the first 6 months after concussion and subluxation; and up to 2 years after injury following extrusion, lateral luxation and intrusion (163), presumably due to difficulties in radiographic diagnosis related to the extent of damage to the periodontal structures.

## Diagnosis of pulp necrosis

In the permanent dentition, the development of pulp necrosis can be associated with symptoms such as spontaneous pain or tenderness to percussion or occlusion. In clinical material, where it was possible to compare pulpal histology with clinical and radiographic parameters, it was found that *tenderness to percussion* was the only sign which was significantly related to infected pulp necrosis following tooth luxation (193). However, pulp necrosis following luxation injuries and root fractures is normally asymptomatic and the diagnosis must therefore be based on clinical and radiographic parameters alone. Transillumination might reveal *decreased translucency* (Fig. 13.7C). *Grey color change* in the crown can be seen, which is especially prominent on the oral surface (Fig. 13.7B). This may be accompanied by a *periapical radiolucency* which can be observed as early as 2–3 weeks after injury; but many cases show no sign of periodontal involvement radiographically. In these cases, a sterile necrosis might be suspected. Teeth with periapical rarefaction almost always represent pulpal infection, which is dominated by anaerobic microorganisms (133–135). The diagnosis of pulp necrosis should be further confirmed by pulpal *sensibility tests*. However, these findings can be difficult to interpret or can even be misleading. But if a pulpal response changes from positive to negative, pulp necrosis should be strongly suspected.

From previous studies, there appears to be general agreement that lack of pulpal sensibility alone (7, 199–202) or coronal discoloration alone (199, 201) are not enough to justify a diagnosis of pulp necrosis. The development of periapical radiolucency (199, 201, 202) has so far been considered the only 'safe' sign of pulp necrosis. However, more recent investigations have cast doubt on the validity of the presently accepted diagnostic criteria (193). Even the concomitant presence of all three classical signs of pulp necrosis (coronal discoloration, loss of pulpal sensibility and

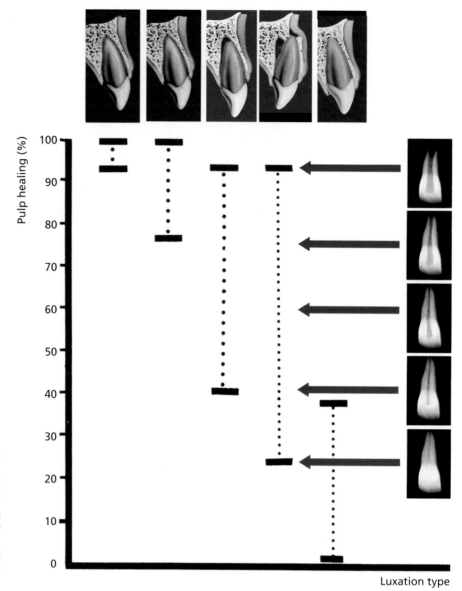

**Fig. 13.6** Relationship between luxation diagnosis, stage of root development and pulpal healing after trauma. The sequence of luxations is concussion, subluxation, extrusion, lateral luxation and intrusion. The upper lines indicate chance of pulpal healing for teeth with immature root formation, and the lower lines the chance for teeth with complete root formation. From ANDREASEN (193) 1989.

periapical radiolucency) could still, in rare cases, be followed by pulpal repair (193) (Figs 13.4 and 13.5). For practical reasons, guidelines for endodontic interventions after luxation injuries are necessary. In the following, the validity of various examination procedures will be described.

## Electrometric pulp testing

Pulpal sensibility tests have many limitations in diagnosing pulp necrosis after traumatic dental injuries. Immediately following trauma approximately half of the teeth with luxation injuries do not respond to sensibility tests (7, 130, 163, 164) (Fig. 13.8). In a recent clinical study, it was found that a negative response to pulp testing at the time of injury was closely related to the type of pulpal healing achieved. Thus, there were significantly more teeth that did not react to electrical stimulation at the time of injury whose root canals ultimately became obliterated than teeth that survived injury with no radiographic change (164, 193).

An explanation for the temporary loss of normal excitability could be pressure or tension on the nerve fibers

in the apical area. If complete rupture of nerve fibers has occurred, a period of at least 36 days is required before a positive response can be expected in immature permanent teeth (67, 130). In mature incisors, the observation period can be much longer (i.e. 1 year or more) prior to a return of a positive sensibility response (7, 66, 97, 131, 166, 193) (Fig. 13.8).

At later follow-up examinations, a previously negative reaction can return to positive, usually within the first 2 months after injury (130); but a period of at least 1 year can elapse before pulp excitability returns (7, 66, 166, 193). While this change in reaction is much more common in teeth with incomplete root formation than those with completely formed roots, longer observation periods can demonstrate restoration of pulpal sensibility in many mature permanent incisors (7, 97, 131, 193) (Fig. 13.8).

In rare cases, a previously positive response can become negative, a phenomenon usually evident within 2 months. However, cases have been reported in which a year or more elapsed before an avital response was recorded (7, 130).

**Fig. 13.7 Color changes following luxation injuries in the permanent dentition**
Gray discoloration 3 months after lateral luxation of a right central incisor.

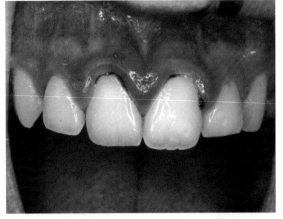 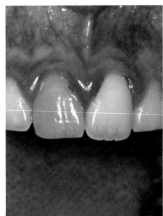

**Influence of the perpendicular direction of the light beam on the appearance of coronal discoloration**
The color of the left central incisor is almost normal when the beam of light is perpendicular to the long axis of the tooth. Only the palatal surface is discolored, whereas the labial surface of the tooth appears normal.

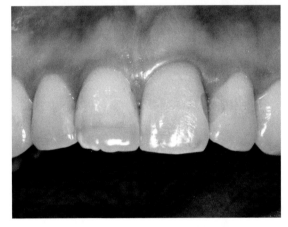 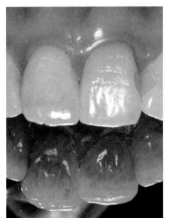

**Influence of the axial direction of the light beam**
A shift in color to gray appears when the light beam is parallel to the long axis of the same tooth as shown above. Furthermore, a change in translucency is evident.

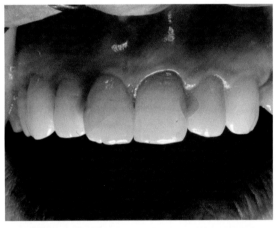 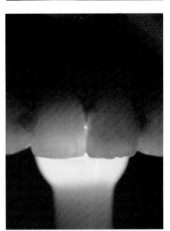

**Reversibility of gray discoloration**
This laterally luxated left central incisor shows marked grey discoloration which becomes normal at a later follow-up examination.

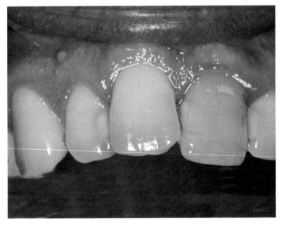 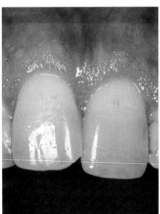

**Reversibility of red discoloration**
The clinical condition is shown 11 days after injury and at the 5-year follow-up.

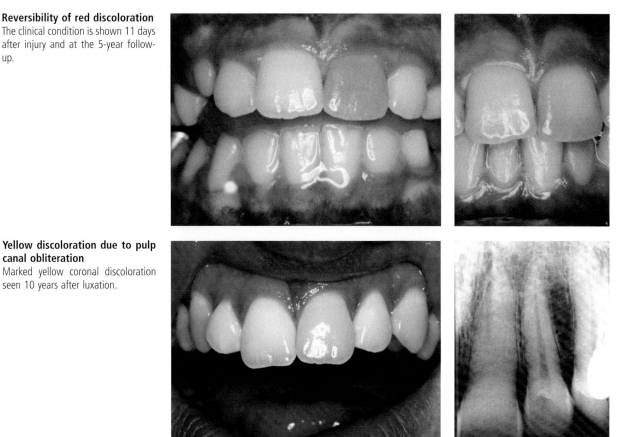

**Yellow discoloration due to pulp canal obliteration**
Marked yellow coronal discoloration seen 10 years after luxation.

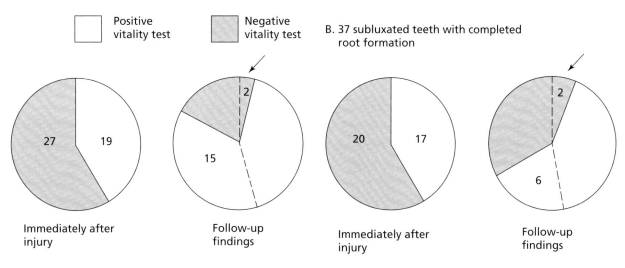

A. 46 subluxated teeth with incomplete root formation

☐ Positive vitality test

▨ Negative vitality test

B. 37 subluxated teeth with completed root formation

27  19

15  2

Immediately after injury

Follow-up findings

20  17

6  2

Immediately after injury

Follow-up findings

**Fig. 13.8** Diagrams illustrating electrometric sensibility reactions following subluxation of permanent teeth. After SKIELLER (7) 1960.

## Pulp testing using laser Doppler flowmetry

Lately, a new method has been developed whereby a laser beam can be directed against the coronal aspect of the pulp. The reflected light scattered by moving erythrocytes undergoes a Doppler frequency shift. The fraction of light scattered back from the pulp is detected and processed to yield a signal. The value of this method in determining pulp vitality has been demonstrated clinically (203–207) (see Chapter 9, p. 267). However, the equipment necessary for this procedure is quite costly and needs further refinement before it can be of general clinical value. Moreover, it has demonstrated false negative responses in the case of discolored vital teeth (see Chapter 9, p. 267).

Clearly, the diagnosis of pulp necrosis cannot be based upon sensibility tests alone, but should include additional findings, such as progressive grey discoloration of the crown, reaction to percussion, periapical radiolucency or cessation of root development.

## Color changes in the crown

Post-traumatic color change is a well-known phenomenon (9, 68–70). These changes can range from a lack of translucency to pink, bluish or grey discoloration (Fig. 13.7). Fish (71) offered an explanation for the pathogenesis of some of these changes, suggesting that an injury that was not strong enough to rupture the arteries passing through the apical foramen could occlude or sever the thin-walled veins. Hence, blood continues to be pumped into the canal, causing hemorrhage in the pulp and later diffusion into the hard dental tissues. Another explanation has been that occlusion or rupture of the apical vessels due to trauma leads to ischemia with breakdown of capillaries and subsequent escape of erythrocytes into the pulpal tissue (102).

When the injury displaces the tooth (e.g. intrusive or extrusive luxation), apical vessels are instantly severed with no extravasation of blood into the pulpal tissue and, thus, no immediate discoloration (73). In the case of moderate injury, where disruption of the vascular supply is less than total, ischemia can lead to increased vascular permeability. However, the same phenomenon could occur in the case of healing, as the immature vessels invading the avascular, traumatized pulp lack a basement membrane and are thereby incompetent until vessels mature (208–214). In this case, the ingrowing vessels can still carry blood to pulpal tissues, but blood and blood products could spill out into the stroma (193). In a recent clinical study, temporary grey coronal discoloration following luxation of mature permanent incisors was described (166, 193). These changes and their normalization could, in same cases, be associated with concomitant loss and restoration of pulpal sensibility, appearance and disappearance of apical radiolucencies and ultimately with pulp canal obliteration. It was suggested that, in the absence of infection, these transient changes could be links in a chain of events leading to pulpal healing. However, if bacteria gained access to the injured avascular pulp, permanent coronal discoloration might then be attributed to autolysis of the necrotic pulp and extravasation of these products into dentin.

Experimental findings indicate that hemoglobin breakdown products enter dentinal tubules (72). This penetration initially alters the crown color to a pinkish hue (Fig. 13.7E). As the hemocomponents disintegrate, the color turns bluish which, when seen through the grey enamel, gives a greyish-blue tinge (Fig. 13.7A, B). This shift from pink to greyish-blue takes approximately 2 weeks in the permanent dentition (9). A certain fading of the grey-blue tint can occur, or an opaque grey hue can persist (9). If the pulp survives, the stain can disappear (70) (Fig. 13.7D, E).

Late color changes can occur if the pulp canal becomes obliterated. In these cases, the color of the crown shifts to a yellow hue (3) (Fig. 13.7D–F).

## Radiographic changes

### Apical radiolucency

The typical change reflecting a necrotic and infected pulp is a widened periodontal ligament space or an apical radiolucency. These changes may develop as early as 2 to 3 weeks after injury and are caused by infection-induced release of a number of osteoclast activating factors (217) (see Chapter 4, p. 151).

### Transient apical breakdown (TAB)

In recent years, temporary apical radiographic changes in the region of the apical foramen following acute dental trauma and in connection with healing have been described and termed transient apical breakdown (TAB) (166, 193, 217, 243, 245) (Figs 13.4 and 13.5).

It would seem that as a result of displacement of the root after luxation (or of the coronal fragment of a root fracture), the vascular supply at the apical foramen (or 'fracture foramen' in a root fracture) could be partially or totally severed, leading to ischemic changes in the pulp. This would in turn lead to wound healing response and release of osteoclast-activating factors (see Chapter 4, p. 148). Subsequent resorption of hard tissue (dentin, cementum and alveolar bone), presumably at the interface between the vital and necrotic tissue, could then result either in an increase in the periodontal ligament space immediately adjacent to the injured apical foramen or an increase in the diameter of the apical foramen in the case of extrusion or lateral luxation of teeth with completed root formation. This event might be seen as a way to gain space to accommodate vascular ingrowth into the root canal. Presumably once repair has reached the remodelling phase, the resorption processes resolve. This can be seen as a normalization of the radiographic condition within the root canal (i.e. hard tissue deposition in the previous resorption process and occasionally pulp canal obliteration) and restoration of a normal apical periodontal ligament space (217, 243, 245) (Figs 13.4 and 13.5).

It might be speculated whether delay in treatment after the appearance of an apical radiolucent zone would worsen the prognosis of future endodontic therapy. However, it has been found that the success rate of endodontic therapy of teeth demonstrating periapical radiolucencies can be equal to the success rate of teeth treated before the development of manifest radiographic change, at least when the former are initially treated with calcium hydroxide prior to final gutta percha root filling (versus immediate gutta percha root filling) (218). Thus, it appears that there would be limited risk of healing complications in the event of late endodontic therapy (i.e. up to 1 year after injury), delayed in anticipation of pulpal repair in selected patient categories (i.e. extrusive and lateral luxation of mature incisors). However, a possible risk is the development of progressive root resorption in the obseeration period. The magnitude of this risk is not yet known.

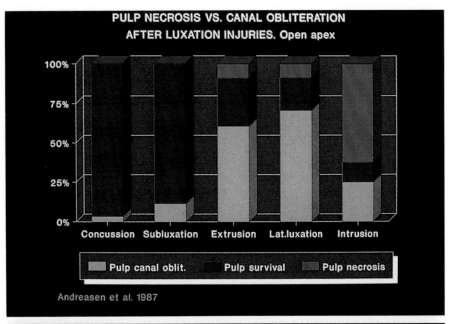

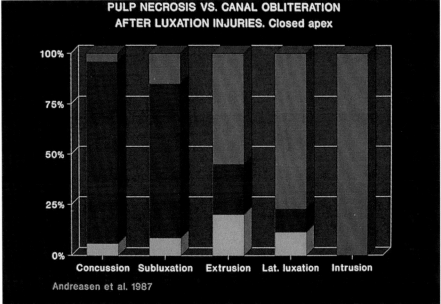

**Fig. 13.9** Relationship between pulp canal obliteration, pulp survival with no radiographic change and pulp necrosis in teeth with incomplete and completed root formation (open or closed apex). From ANDREASEN et al. (164) 1987.

## Guidelines for the diagnosis of irreversible pulp necrosis

The diagnosis of pulp necrosis should be based on primarily two or more of the following signs: crown discoloration, negative sensibility testing (electrometric and/or laser Doppler) and periapical radiolucency. In this regard, the importance of transient negative sensibility testing should be considered (i.e. a minimum of 2–3 months' observation). If these criteria are used, a certain percentage of mistakes will be made where pulps under revascularization are extirpated. The risk of this phenomenon is possibly about 1 in 10 cases (160). Finally, prophylactic active pulp extirpation may be indicated to prevent crown discoloration and/or progressive root resorption; this applies especially to teeth with completed root formation suffering from lateral luxation and intrusion (Fig. 13.9).

## Guidelines for observation without endodontic intervention

In selected cases, a conservative approach might be indicated, whereby active treatment can be avoided (193).

As long as the following conditions are met, a tooth with one or more signs of pulp necrosis could be observed for pulpal repair over a longer period of time (up to approximately 1 year):

(1) The patient is at low risk of inflammatory resorption (i.e. over 10 years of age, has completed root formation and has not suffered intrusive luxation) (193, 219).
(2) The injury type and stage of root development (extrusion and lateral luxation of teeth with completed root development) imply that transient apical changes might be anticipated (166).

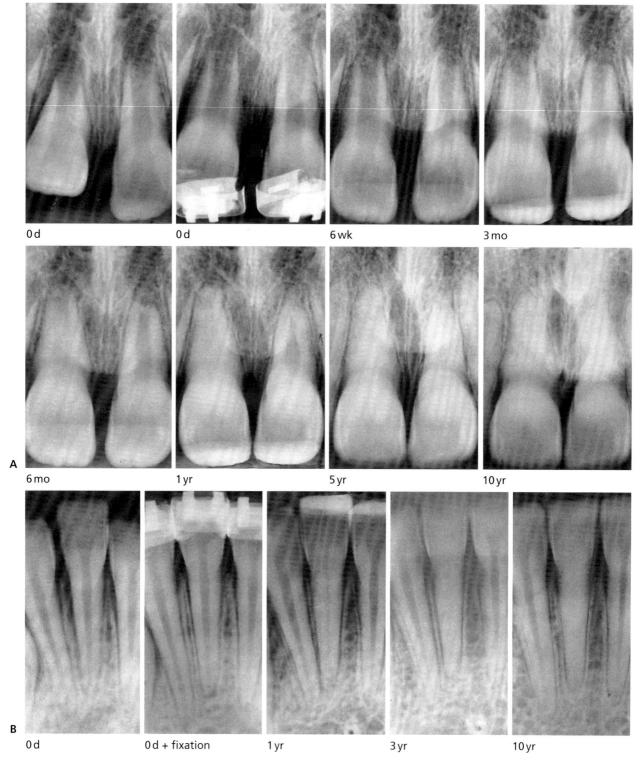

**Fig. 13.10** A. Radiographic illustration of the various stages in pulp canal obliteration (PCO). Extrusive luxation of the maxillary right central incisor and avulsion of the maxillary left central incisor in a 6-year-old boy. Onset of PCO is seen 6 months after injury. Total PCO of right incisor, partial PCO of left incisor is found 1 year after injury. B. Radiographic demonstration of the various stages in PCO. Lateral luxation of a mandibular right central incisor in a 10-year-old boy. Partial PCO is seen 1 year after injury and total PCO after 5 years. From ANDREASEN et al. (164) 1987.

(3) Neither prosthetic treatment nor orthodontic therapy is planned to immediately involve the injured tooth. As the clinical and radiographic signs previously described are assumed to reflect healing processes within the pulp, presumably because of a temporary disruption of the neurovascular supply, the additional trauma of crown preparation or orthodontic tooth movement might be anticipated to shift the balance of pulpal survival unfavorably.

(4) As it is not presently possible to adequately evaluate pulpal status following dental luxations, the possibility of *asymptomatic* sterile pulp necrosis must not be ignored.

It is therefore of utmost importance that the patient be thoroughly informed regarding the diagnostic problems involved and the consequent need for extra follow-up examinations – and is willing and able to cooperate. If there is any doubt as to the possibility of recalling the patient, endodontic therapy rather than 'observation therapy' should be the treatment of choice (193).

## Treatment of pulp necrosis

This subject is discussed in detail in Chapter 22, p. 598.

## Pulp canal obliteration

Pulp canal obliteration is related to the process of pulpal revascularization after tooth luxation. In that respect, the speed of obliteration appears to be associated with the degree of dislocation at the time of injury (Fig. 13.10).

Pulp canal obliteration can be regarded as a response to a severe injury to the neurovascular supply to the pulp which, after healing, leads to an accelerated dentin deposition and is frequently encountered after luxation injuries of permanent teeth (3, 20, 34, 35, 76, 77, 104–106, 141–143, 164, 178, 196, 225–227) (Table 13.5). Pulp canal obliteration is strongly related to the severity of the luxation injury, being especially common in severely mobile or dislocated teeth (104, 164, 178). It would appear to be a phenomenon which is closely related to the loss and reestablishment of pulpal neural supply (193), as it is rarely seen when there is no tooth displacement and thus little damage to the pulpal neurovascular supply (i.e. concussion and subluxation). Moreover, this complication mainly involves teeth injured before completion of root formation (3, 164) (Fig. 13.9).

A clinical manifestation of pulp canal obliteration is a yellow discoloration of the crown (Fig. 13.7F). Response to thermal sensibility tests has been reported to be lowered or absent (78, 130); and response to electrical stimulation is also reported decreased and often absent (78, 105, 141). However, a recent clinical investigation could find no difference in sensibility threshold between paired incisors with and without pulp canal obliteration up to 5 years after injury (164). Nevertheless, with longer observation periods there is a tendency to higher thresholds or absence of reaction in pulp canal obliterated teeth.

The first radiographic sign of obliteration is reduction in the size of the coronal pulp chamber, followed by gradual narrowing of the entire root canal, occasionally leading to partial or complete obliteration (Fig. 13.10). However, histologic examination of these teeth always shows a persisting narrow root canal. Normalization of temporary apical radiolucencies, as described earlier, has been found to be significantly related to pulp canal obliteration in mature permanent incisors. This apparently reflects the wound healing processes involved in revascularization and reinnervation of the injured pulp (166) (Fig. 13.4).

Pulp canal obliteration usually appears between 3 to 12 months after injury (Fig. 13.10). It has been shown that two types of pulp canal obliteration exist. In *partial canal obliteration*, the coronal part of the pulp chamber is not discernible, while the apical part is markedly narrowed but still discernible (Figs 13.10, 13.11). In *total canal obliteration*, the pulp chamber and root canal are hardly (or not at all) discernible (105) (Fig. 13.11).

As with pulp necrosis, pulp canal obliteration is determined by the *type of luxation injury* and stage *of root development* at the time of injury (164, 246) (Fig.13.9). Pulp canal obliteration appears to be more frequent after luxation injuries with displacement and in teeth with incomplete root formation (164, 246) (Fig.13.9).

In contrast to pulp necrosis, where no treatment effect at the time of injury could be established, pulp canal obliteration was found to be significantly related to the type of fixation used (164). Prior to the use of acid-etched splinting techniques, orthodontic bands were cemented onto the traumatized and adjacent teeth and united with cold-curing acrylic (Fig. 13.12). There was a significant relationship between the use of this type of splint and this healing complication, presumably reflecting additional injury to the already traumatized periodontium due to forceful placement of the bands. In some cases, displacement of initially non-displaced traumatized incisors could be demonstrated after orthodontic band/acrylic fixation (Fig. 13.12).

A late complication following pulp canal obliteration is the development of pulp necrosis and the occurrence of periapical changes and this has been found to occur in 7–16% of cases (3, 78, 79, 105, 141, 246) (Figs 13.13A,B and 13.14, Table 13.6). The pathogenesis of this complication is still obscure (246). Minor injuries are probably able to sever the vulnerable vascular supply at the constricted apical foramen, or the pulp vessels are progressively occluded due to hard tissue formation. Caries and restorative treatment have been suspected to lead to pulp necrosis; but no certain link could be demonstrated in a recent study (246) (Table 13.6). Several clinical investigations have recorded secondary pulp necrosis following pulp canal obliteration in 7–16% of cases. However, no distinction was made between new trauma, secondary caries and/or crown preparation. A recent clinical investigation with an average observation period of up to 10

**Table 13.5** Frequency of pulp canal obliteration after luxation injuries irrespective type of luxation.

| Examiner | No. of teeth | No. with pulp canal obliteration |
|---|---|---|
| Andreasen (3) 1970 | 189 | 42 (22%) |
| Gröndahl et al. (140) 1974 | 320 | 77 (24%) |
| Herforth (130) 1976 | 161 | 57 (35%) |
| Stålhane & Hedegård (104) 1975 | 1116 | 67 (6%) |
| Rock & Grundy (178) 1981 | 517 | 83 (16%) |
| Wepner & Bukel (228) 1981 | 142 | 12 (8%) |
| Lawnik & Tetsch (225) 1983 | 246 | 20 (8%) |
| Posukidist & Lehmann (226) 1983 | 162 | 25 (15%) |
| Andreasen et al. (164) 1987 | 637 | 96 (15%) |
| Oikarinen et al. (196) 1987 | 147 | 40 (27%) |
| Herforth (197) 1990 | 319 | 106 (33%) |
| Crona-Larsson et al. (240) 1991 | 103 | 3 (3%) |
| Robertson (241) 1997 | 196 | 36 (18%) |

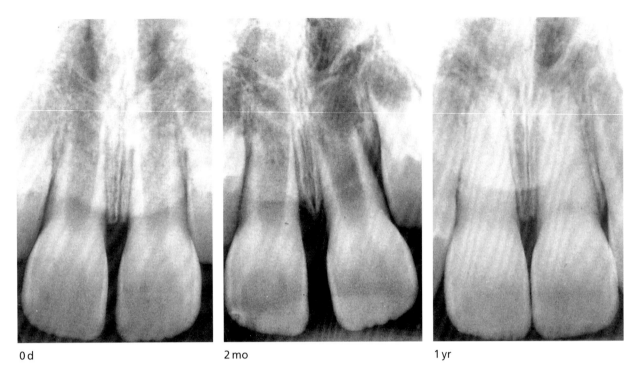

0 d                          2 mo                              1 yr

**Fig. 13.11** Partial pulp canal obliteration after extrusion of 2 central incisors. Partial canal obliteration is evident after one year.

years reported a frequency of 9%. No clear relationship could be made to factors, such as dental caries, crown preparation, orthodontics or new trauma (246). However, the general annual trauma incidence of approximately 1% could possibly explain that new traumas might present a hazard for a compromised dental pulp. It has also been reported that secondary pulp necrosis was only found in teeth with total canal obliteration and especially in those teeth which showed rapid obliteration after injury (i.e. total canal obliteration within 2 years after injury). Moreover, complicating pulp necrosis was common in teeth with completed root formation and with severe periodontal injury at the time of trauma (105).

While early prophylactic pulp extirpation and endodontic intervention can prevent periapical lesions, the rather low frequency of this complication does not support such early intervention measures (164, 229–232). The endodontic considerations of pulp canal obliteration are further discussed in Chapter 22, p. 639.

## Internal bone formation (pulp bone)

In cases with severe injury to both the pulp and the Hertwig's epithelial root sheath, invasion of bone and periodontal ligament into the pulpal cavity may be seen (239) (see Chapter 2).

## Treatment delay

Delay in treatment seems to play a questionable role in the frequency of healing complications. In cases of alveolar fractures, treatment delay appears to be related to pulp necrosis and root resorption (6). Concerning jaw fractures, four studies showed no significant difference between immediate and delayed treatment (126, 154–156). One study showed a

**Table 13.6** Frequency of necrosis secondary to pulp canal obliteration in permanent teeth irrespective of type of luxation injury.

| Examiner | Observation period yr. (mean) | No. of teeth | Pulp necrosis |
|---|---|---|---|
| Holcomb & Gregory (78) 1967 | 4 | 41 | 3 (7%) |
| Andreasen (3) 1970 | 1–12 (3.4) | 42 | 3 (7%) |
| Stålhane (141) 1971 | 13–21 | 76 | 12 (16%) |
| Jacobsen & Kerekes (105) 1977 | 10–23 (16.0) | 122 | 16 (13%) |
| Robertson et al. (246) 1996 | 7–22 (16) | 82 | 7 (9%) |

preference for healing for cases treated within 3 days (153), whereas another study indicated that treatment times between 3 and 5 days were optimal, with the lowest rate of complications (97). In conclusion, there is presently no strong evidence for either acute or delayed treatment of mandibular fractures in order to minimize healing complications; new studies including a number of cases treated on an acute basis are needed (157).

## Root resorption

A late complication following luxation injuries in the permanent dentition is root resorption (29, 70, 80, 163, 217, 233) (Table 13.7). The diagnosis of root resorption is entirely dependent upon a radiographic examination. *In vitro* studies have shown that radiographic demonstration of defects on the root surface is dependent upon the size and position of the defect, with 0.5 mm being the critical size

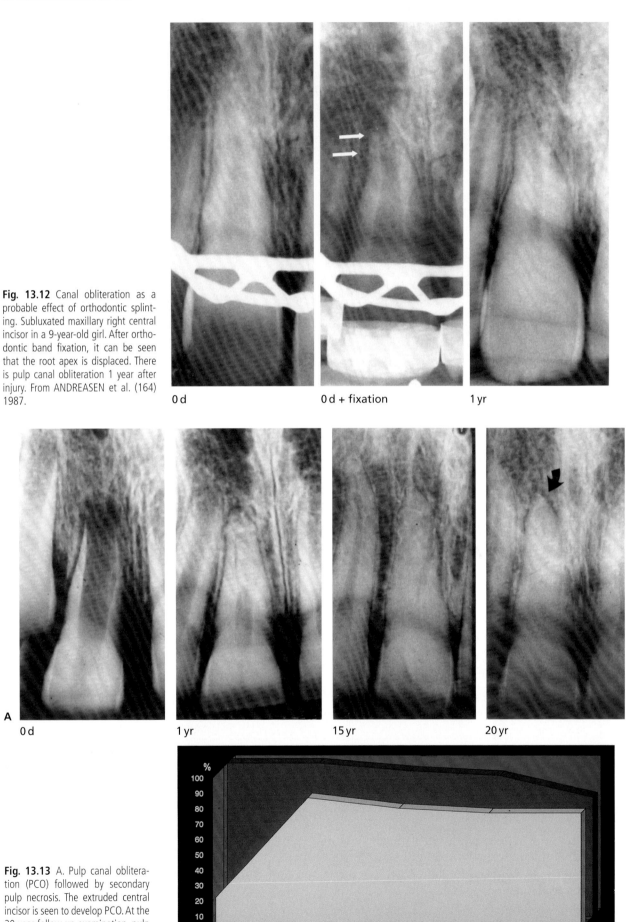

**Fig. 13.12** Canal obliteration as a probable effect of orthodontic splinting. Subluxated maxillary right central incisor in a 9-year-old girl. After orthodontic band fixation, it can be seen that the root apex is displaced. There is pulp canal obliteration 1 year after injury. From ANDREASEN et al. (164) 1987.

0 d                    0 d + fixation              1 yr

A

0 d            1 yr            15 yr            20 yr

**Fig. 13.13** A. Pulp canal obliteration (PCO) followed by secondary pulp necrosis. The extruded central incisor is seen to develop PCO. At the 20 year follow-up examination, pulp necrosis and a periapical rarefaction have developed. B. Pulp survival in relation to canal obliteration. From ROBERTSON et al. (246) 1996.

B

NEGATIVE SENSIBILITY   PULP SURVIVAL

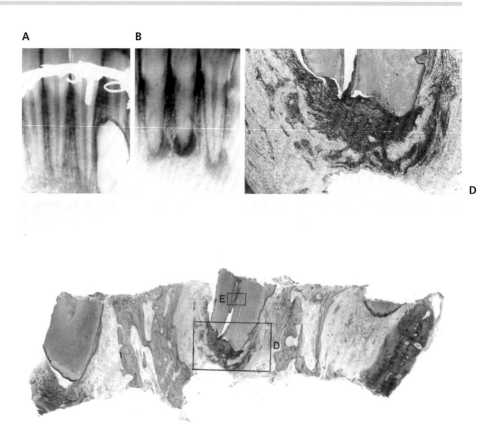

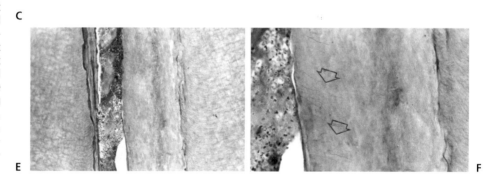

**Fig. 13.14** Extrusive luxation of permanent incisors leading to pulp obliteration and complicating pulp necrosis. A. Condition immediately after reduction and fixation. B. At follow-up 12 years later pulp canal obliteration and periapical inflammation are evident. C. Histologic specimen including apex of left central incisor. ×10. D. Periapical inflammation. ×30. E. Extensive hard tissue formation following injury. The pulp tissue is necrotic. ×75. F. Higher magnification of E. A few dentinal tubules in the post-traumatic hard tissue can be recognized (arrows). ×195.

**Table 13.7** Frequency of progressive root resorption after luxation of permanent teeth irrespective type of luxation.

| Examiner | No. of teeth | Progressive root resorption (ankylosis and inflammatory resorption) |
|---|---|---|
| Skieller (7) 1960 | 107 | 6 (6%) |
| Andreasen (3) 1970 | 189 | 21 (11%) |
| Stålhane & Hedegård (104) 1975 | 1116 | 16 (1%) |
| Rock & Grundy (178) 1981 | 517 | 37 (8%) |
| Andreasen & Vestergaard Pedersen (163) 1985 | 637 | 47 (7%) |
| Oikarinen et al. (196) 1987 | 147 | 27 (18%) |
| Crona-Larsson et al. (240) 1991 | 104 | 15 (14%) |

(254). Subtraction radiography does not seem to provide additional information (247, 248).

Root resorption can be classified into various types such as root surface resorption and root canal resorption (Figs 13.15 and 13.16).

## Root surface resorption (external root resorption)

The damage inflicted to the periodontal structures and the pulp by luxation injuries can result in various types of *root*

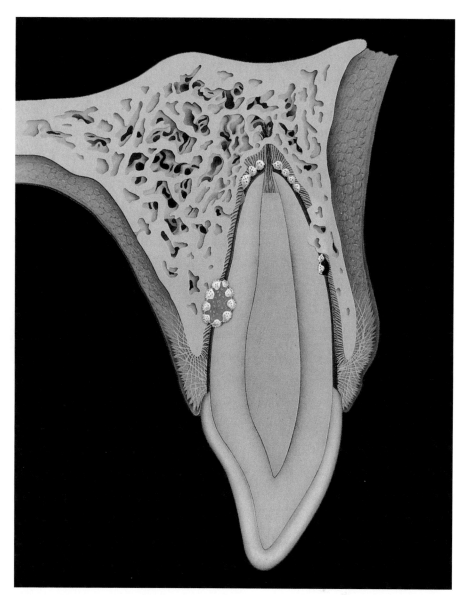

**Fig. 13.15** External root surface resorption. Three types of root surface (external) resorption may develop subsequent to trauma: surface resorption, inflammatory resorption and ankylosis. After ANDREASEN & ANDREASEN (217) 1991.

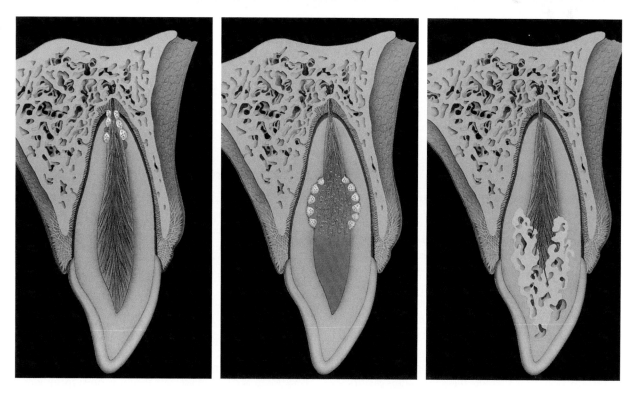

**Fig. 13.16** Root canal resorption. Three types of root canal (internal) resorption may develop subsequent to trauma: internal surface resorption, internal inflammatory resorption, and internal ankylosis. After ANDREASEN & ANDREASEN (217) 1991.

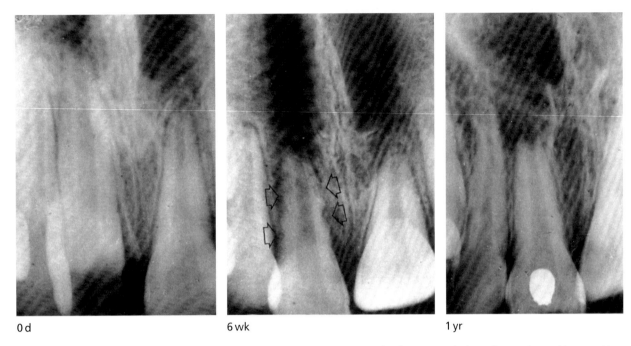

0 d                                        6 wk                                        1 yr

**Fig. 13.17** Surface resorption following intrusive luxation of right central incisor. Six weeks after injury multiple small resorption cavities are evident along the root surface (arrows). One year after injury repair is evident with re-establishment of the periodontal space adjacent to the resorption areas. From ANDREASEN (3) 1970.

**Table 13.8** Prevalence of external root resorption related to luxation diagnosis. From ANDREASEN & VESTERGAARD PEDERSEN (163) 1985.

|  | No. of teeth | Surface resorption | Inflammatory resorption | Ankylosis resorption |
|---|---|---|---|---|
| Concussion | 178 | 8 (4%) | 0 (0%) | 0 (0%) |
| Subluxation | 223 | 4 (2%) | 1 (0.5%) | 0 (0%) |
| Extrusive luxation | 53 | 3 (6%) | 3 (6%) | 0 (0%) |
| Lateral luxation | 122 | 32 (26%) | 4 (3%) | 1 (1%) |
| Intrusive luxation | 61 | 15 (24%) | 23 (38%) | 15 (24%) |

*surface resorption.* The etiology and pathogenesis of these complications seem to be identical to root resorption following replantation of avulsed teeth (see Chapter 17, p. 450). Three types of external root resorption can be recognized.

### Surface resorption (repair-related resorption)

The root surface shows superficial resorption lacunae repaired with new cementum. These lacunae have been termed surface resorption. It has been suggested that they occur as a response to a localized injury to the periodontal ligament or cementum (3, 81). In contrast to other types of resorption, surface resorption is not progressive, self-limiting and shows spontaneous repair. Surface resorptions are not usually seen on radiographs due to their small size; however, it is sometimes possible to recognize small excavations of the root surface delineated by a normal lamina dura (3) (Fig. 13.17). When visible, these resorption cavities are

usually confined to the lateral surfaces of the root, but may also be found apically, resulting in a slight shortening of the root.

### Ankylosis (replacement resorption)

Ankylosis is a rare finding with luxation injuries except for intrusive luxations (Table 13.8) A direct union between bone and root substance is seen, with the root substance gradually being replaced by bone (Figs 13.18 and 13.19). Disappearance of the periodontal space and progressive root resorption are typical radiographic findings (3) (Fig. 13.18).

### Inflammatory resorption

Histologically, bowl-shaped areas of resorption of both cementum and dentin are seen together with inflammation

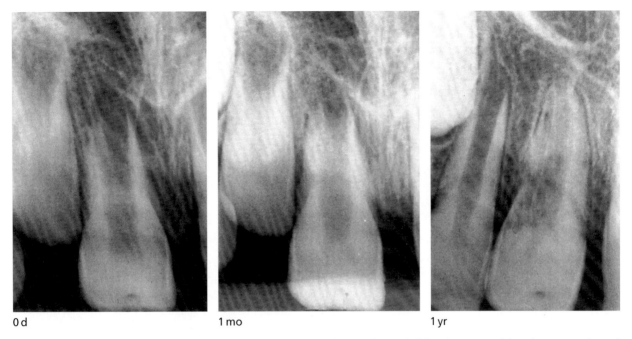

0 d    1 mo    1 yr

**Fig. 13.18** External replacement resorption as a sequel to lateral luxation. At the time of removal of the splint one month later there is no evidence of root resorption. At the 1 year follow-up, ankylosis is evident distally.

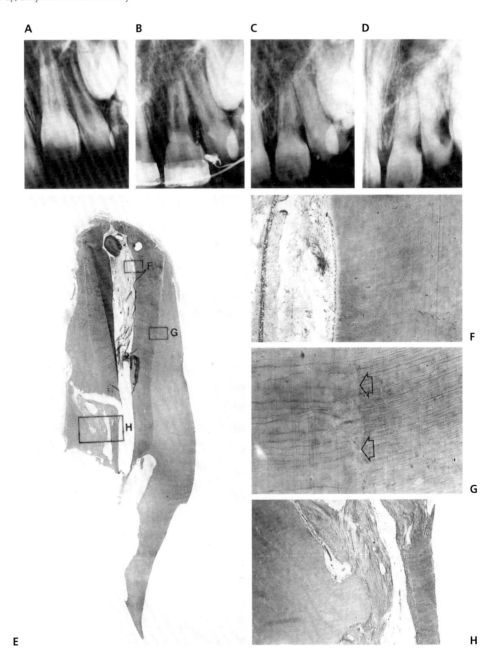

A    B    C    D

F

G

H

**Fig. 13.19** Replacement resorption following intrusive luxation of the left permanent incisors. Progression of replacement resorption is seen over 2$^1/_2$ year period. At this time both incisors were extracted. E. Low power view of sectioned lateral incisor. ×8. F. Vital pulp tissue. ×75. G. Marked posttraumatic dentin formation containing few dentinal tubules (arrows). ×75. H. Ankylosis area with apposition of bone. ×30.

E

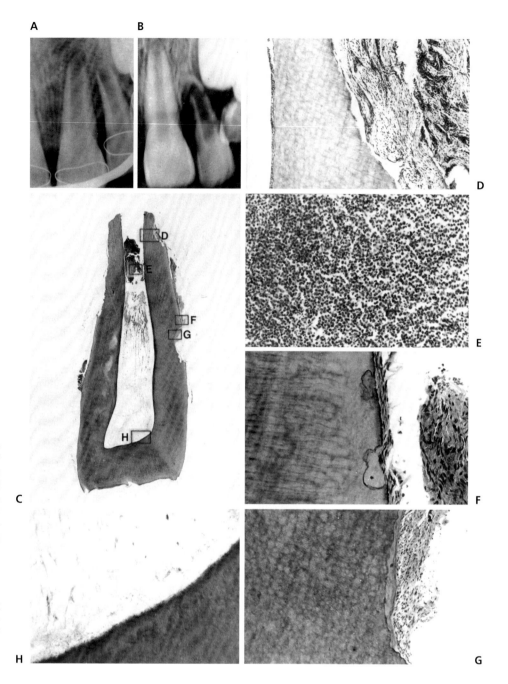

**Fig. 13.20** Inflammatory resorption following extrusive luxation of a left lateral incisor. A. Condition immediately after reduction and splinting. B. Six months later. Note periradicular radiolucency as well as root resorption. C. Low power view of sectioned incisor removed 6 months after injury. ×7. D. Resorption area with inflammation in the connective tissue and epithelial proliferation. ×75. E. Abscess bordering coronal necrotic pulp tissue. ×195. F and G. Surface resorption repaired with new cementum. ×195. H. Complete autolysis of pulp tissue. ×75.

of adjacent periodontal tissue. The inflammation and resorption activity are apparently related to the presence of infected, necrotic pulp tissue in the root canal (Fig. 13.20). Radiographically, root resorption with an adjacent radiolucency in bone is the typical finding (3) (Fig. 13.20).

In summary, *external root resorption* is most commonly seen after intrusive luxation. However, this can also be found following severe lateral luxations (163). Subluxation yields the lowest frequency of resorption, primarily in the form of surface resorption, and intrusion the highest frequency and with frequent occurrence of inflammatory and replacement resorption (3, 7, 93, 104, 163, 170) (Table 13.8). This reflects a correlation between the degree of injury to the periodontal structures and root resorption (see Chapter 2, p. 76).

For treatment of external root resorption, see Chapter 22, p. 632.

### *Cervical root surface resorption*

This resorption entity can have many etiologies, with trauma being one of the most frequent (249, 250). Bleaching has also been found to lead to this complication (249, 250). (See Chapters 22 and 33.)

## Root canal resorption (internal root resorption)

*Root canal resorption* is a rather unusual finding (35, 82, 83, 85, 217, 247) and has been recorded in only 2% of

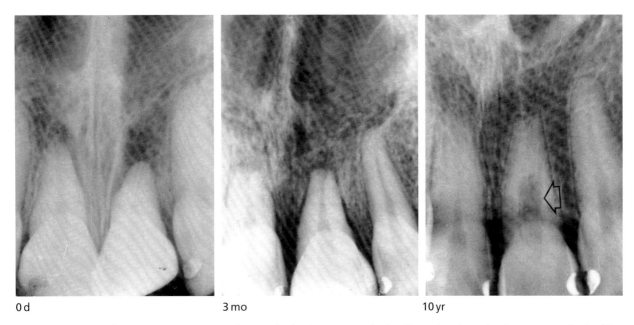

0 d                                  3 mo                               10 yr

**Fig. 13.21** Internal replacement resorption as a sequel to extrusive luxation. At re-examination 10 years later internal replacement resorption is evident (arrow). From ANDREASEN (3) 1970.

re-examined luxated permanent teeth (3). This resorption type is also seen in the primary dentition (144). In the radiographic diagnosis of internal root resorption, one must consider that root surface resorption located labially or lingually on the root can mimic internal resorption as it is superimposed over the root canal (145–147). It is therefore necessary to take supplementary mesial and distal eccentric radiographs of the root. If the resorption cavity does not change position, it is located centrally in the tooth indicating root canal resorption.

Root canal resorption can be classified as follows (Fig. 13.16).

### Root canal replacement resorption

This resorption type is characterized radiographically by an irregular enlargement of the pulp chamber (84, 85) (Fig. 13.21). A variant has been termed *internal tunnelling resorption*. This resorption is usually found in the coronal fragment of root fractures (234), but may also occur after luxation (Fig. 13.22). The typical feature of this resorption is a tunnelling resorption process next to the root canal. After some time the resorption process becomes arrested and complete pulp canal obliteration takes place.

Histologically, the teeth show metaplasia of the normal pulp tissue into cancellous bone. The continuous rebuilding of bone at the expense of dentin is responsible for the gradual enlargement of the pulp chamber (15, 86). This resorption type should just be observed as they tend not to progress (Fig. 13.22).

### Root canal inflammatory resorption

This resorption type is radiographically characterized by an oval-shaped enlargement within the pulp chamber (87–89,

91, 113, 129) (Fig. 13.23). This type of resorption is usually found in the cervical aspect of the pulp. If initial resorption is located in the apical aspect, it is often a sign of active revascularization (internal surface resorption) and not inflammatory resorption (166, 193, 234) (see p. 376).

Histologically, a transformation is seen of normal pulp tissue into granulation tissue with giant cells resorbing the dentinal walls of the root canal, advancing from the dentinal surface towards the periphery (Fig. 13.23). A zone of necrotic pulp tissue is usually found coronal to the resorbing tissue. This necrotic zone, or dentinal tubules containing bacteria, is apparently responsible for maintaining the resorptive process.

It should be emphasized that progression of root canal resorption depends upon the interaction between necrotic and vital pulp tissue at their interface. Consequently, root canal treatment should be instituted as soon as possible after root canal resorption has been diagnosed unless the resorption cavity is located in the vicinity of the apical foramen and suspected of being related to pulpal revascularization (see Chapter 22, p. 598).

## Loss of marginal bone support

The post-traumatic course following intrusive or lateral luxation is often complicated by temporary or permanent changes in the marginal periodontium. A frequency of 5–24% was found among luxated permanent teeth (163, 196) (Table 13.9). If broken down according to specific luxation categories, 5% of laterally luxated and 31% of intruded permanent incisors demonstrated this complication (163) (Table 13.10). It has been found that the repositioning procedure following intrusive luxation plays an important role

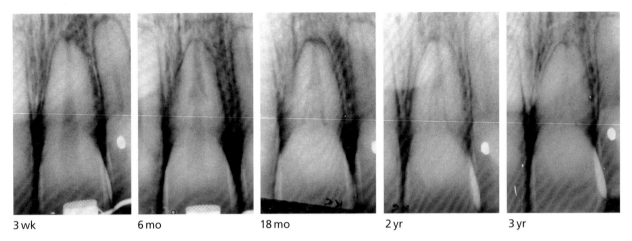

3 wk  6 mo  18 mo  2 yr  3 yr

**Fig. 13.22** Internal replacement resorption (tunnelling resorption variant) developed in an extruded and repositioned left central incisor. Tunnelling resorption is evident after 6 months, but gradually disappears. Courtesy of Dr. B. MALMGREN, Eastman Institute, Stockholm.

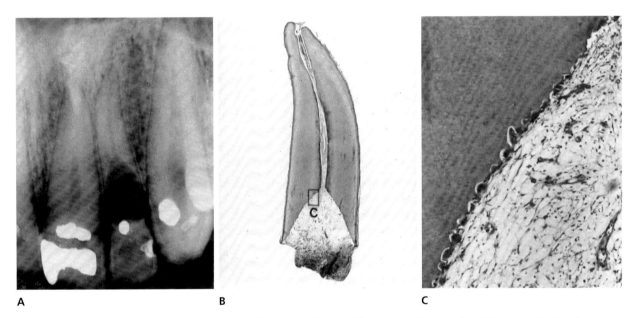

A  B  C

**Fig. 13.23** Internal inflammatory root resorption in a lateral incisor possibly caused by a luxation injury sustained 18 years previously. A. Radiograph showing marked internal inflammatory resorption. B. Histologic section of removed incisor. ×6. C. Active resorption of dentin by multinucleated cells. ×195.

in periodontal healing. Thus, immediate surgical repositioning (i.e. complete repositioning at the time of injury) of the intruded mature incisors results in slightly greater loss of marginal bone and a higher frequency of ankylosis compared to orthodontic extrusion. The best results have been found in relation to marginal bone healing (in case of spontaneous eruption) compared to surgical or orthodontic repositioning (251–253).

## Permanent or transient marginal breakdown

Loss of marginal support is a common healing complication following lateral luxation. It becomes clinically evident with the appearance of granulation tissue in the gingival crevice and sometimes secretion of pus from the pocket. Probing the pocket reveals a loss of attachment. Radiographically, rarefaction and loss of supporting bone is seen. This clinical situation might represent the first phase of the healing process in a traumatized periodontium, namely the resorption of traumatized bone. After 6–8 weeks, repair of the periodontium takes place with reattachment of new periodontal fibers (Fig. 13.24). This condition has been termed *transient marginal breakdown* (TMB) (251–253). If signs of marginal bone loss are evident, the fixation period following lateral luxation should be extended until the situation has resolved (Fig. 13.25).

If there has been injury to the marginal bone, it is essential that optimal oral hygiene be maintained throughout the healing period. If there is secretion of pus, the pocket should

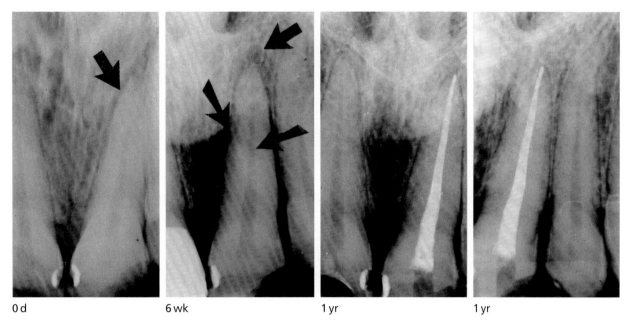

| | | | |
|---|---|---|---|
| 0 d | 6 wk | 1 yr | 1 yr |

**Fig. 13.24** Transient destruction of marginal bone around a left central incisor after lateral luxation. At time of injury there is displacement of the tooth in its socket (arrow). Six weeks later, extensive marginal and apical bone destruction is evident (arrows). Clinically, a pathologic deepening of the gingival crevice of 10 mm is found lingually. At follow-up one year later, marginal bone formation can be seen accompanied by normal pocket depth.

**Table 13.9** Frequency of loss of marginal bone support after luxation of permanent teeth irrespective type of luxation injury.

| Examiner | No. of teeth | Loss of marginal bone support |
|---|---|---|
| Andreasen & Vestergaard Pedersen (163) 1985 | 637 | 34 (5%) |
| Oikarinen et al. (196) 1987 | 147 | 35 (24%) |

**Table 13.10** Frequency of loss of marginal bone support related to type of luxation injury (Andreasen & Vestergaard Pedersen (163) 1985.

| | No. of teeth | Loss of marginal bone support |
|---|---|---|
| Concussion | 178 | 0 (0%) |
| Subluxation | 223 | 3 (1%) |
| Extrusive luxation | 53 | 3 (6%) |
| Lateral luxation | 122 | 9 (7%) |
| Intrusive luxation | 61 | 19 (31%) |

be rinsed with saline. Moreover, oral rinsing with chlorhexidine should be instituted.

Where sequestration of bone occurs during the healing period, permanent loss of marginal bone can be expected.

Delayed reduction of luxated teeth seems to increase the risk of damage to the supporting structures (3) (Fig. 13.26). Further, it has been found that loss of marginal bone support increases with increasing age of the patient, duration of the splinting period and the extent of displacement (140, 196, 252).

## Essentials

### Terminology (Fig. 13.1)

- Concussion
- Subluxation (loosening)
- Intrusive luxation (central dislocation)
- Extrusive luxation (peripheral dislocation, partial avulsion)
- Lateral luxation

### Frequency

- Permanent dentition: 15–40% of dental injuries
- Etiology
- Fall injuries
- Fight injuries
- History
- Symptoms
- Pain with occlusion

### Clinical examination (Table 13.1)

- Direction of dislocation
- Mobility testing
- Response to percussion
- Response to sensibility tests

### Radiographic examination

- Several projections necessary

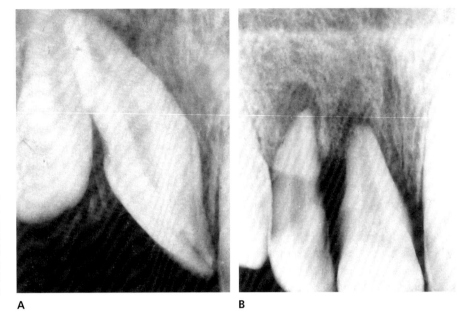

**Fig. 13.25** Loss of marginal supporting bone as a result of intrusive luxation. Radiograph at the time of injury reveals intrusive luxation of both right incisors. The teeth were repositioned and splinted. Three months later a marked loss of supporting marginal bone has occurred. From ANDREASEN (3) 1970.    **A**                                              **B**

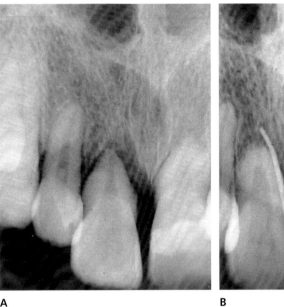
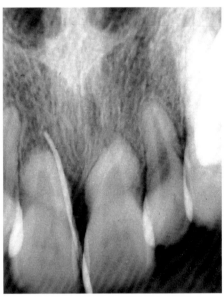

**Fig. 13.26** Loss of supporting bone as a result of delayed reduction of an extruded central incisor. A. Condition at time of admission. The tooth had been luxated 7 days previously. B. Two months later a periodontal pocket extends to the apex. A gutta-percha point is inserted in the periodontal pocket lingually.    **A**                                              **B**

## Pathology

- PDL changes varying from bleeding, PDL rupture to compression necrosis
- PDL changes, depending upon interference with the neurovascular supply (i.e. partial or total ischemia), leading to:
  — Pulpal healing
  — Pulpal revascularization
  — Partial pulp necrosis
  — Total pulp necrosis

## Root surface (external) resorption

- Surface resorption (repair-related resorption)
- Inflammatory resorption (infection-related resorption)
- Replacement resorption (ankylosis)

## Root canal (internal) resorption

- Internal replacement resorption
- Internal inflammatory resorption

## Prognosis

- Pulp necrosis: 15–52%
  — Risk groups: dislocated mature teeth
  — Treatment of pulp necrosis: see Chapters 22 and 23
- Pulp canal obliteration: 3–35%
  — Risk groups: extremely mobile or dislocated teeth with immature root formation
- Root surface resorption: 1–18%
  — Risk groups: intrusions
  — Treatment of external root resorption: see Chapter 22, p. 636
- Root canal resorption: 2%
  — Treatment of internal root resorption: see Chapter 22, p. 639
- Loss of supporting bone: 5%
  — Risk groups: intrusion and lateral luxation

## References

1. Andreasen JO. Etiology and pathogenesis of traumatic dental injuries. A clinical study of 1298 cases. *Scand J Dent Res* 1970;**78**:329–42.
2. Ravn JJ, Rossen I. Hyppighed og fordeling of traumatiserede beskadigelser af tænderne hos københavnske skolebörn 1967/68. *Tandlægebladet* 1969;**73**:1–9.
3. Andreasen JO. Luxation of permanent teeth due to trauma. A clinical and radiographic follow-up study of 189 injured teeth. *Scand J Dent Res* 1970;**78**:273–86.
4. Dobrzanska A, Szpringer M. Obserwacje zebow mlecznyck, dotknietych urazem mechanicznym. *Czas Stomatol* 1966;**19**:167–72.
5. Sundvall-Hagland I. Olycksfallsskador på tænder och parodontium under barnaåren. In: Holst JJ, Nygaard Ostby B, Osvald O. *Nordisk Klinisk Odontologi.* Copenhagen: A/S Forlaget for Faglitteratur, 1964: Chapter 11, 1–40.
6. Link K. Über Veränderungen der Pulpa bei luxierten Zähnen. *Frankfurt Z Pathol* 1957;**68**:596–612.
7. Skieller V. The prognosis for young teeth loosened after mechanical injuries. *Acta Odontol Scand* 1960;**18**:171–81.
8. Stewart DJ. Traumatised incisors. An unusual type of response. *Br Dent J* 1960;**108**:396–9.
9. Arwill T, Henschen B, Sundvall-Hagland 1. The pulpal reaction in traumatized permanent incisors in children aged 9–18. *Odontologisk Tidsskrift* 1967;**75**:130–47.
10. Chirnside IM. A bacteriological and histological study of traumatised teeth. *N Z Dent J* 1967;**53**:176–91.
11. Blackwood HJJ. Metaplasia or repair of the dental pulp as a response to injury. *Br Dent J* 1957;**102**:87–92.
12. Main DMG. Segmentation of teeth. *Br Dent J* 1968;**124**:275–7.
13. Payne JL. An unusual case of fracture of a tooth. *Proc Roy Soc Med* 1912;**5**:141–2.
14. Tammoscheit UG. The two-pieced tooth. *Quintessence Int* 1969;**1**:117–18.
15. Arwill T. Histopathologic studies of traumatized teeth. *Odontologisk Tidsskrift* 1962;**70**:91–117.
16. Blackwood HJJ. Tissue repair in intra-alveolar root fractures. *Oral Surg Oral Med Oral Pathol* 1959;**12**:360–70.
17. Rushton MA. Some late results of injury to teeth. *Br Dent J* 1956;**100**:299–305.
18. Morris ME. Pulpal changes in traumatized primary central incisors. *IADR Abstracts* 1966;**135**:135.
19. Herbert WE. Calcification of pulp following trauma. *Br Dent J* 1953;**94**:127–8.
20. Patterson SS, Mitchell DF. Calcific metamorphosis of the dental pulp. *Oral Surg Oral Med Oral Pathol* 1965;**20**:94–101.
21. Fischer C-H. Die Wurzelkanalbehandlung bei nichtinfiziertem Wurzelkanal. *Dtsch Zahnärztl Z* 1957;**12**:1729–42.
22. Harndt E. Die körpereigene Hartgewebsausfüllung des Wurzelkanals. *Dtsch Zahnärztl Z* 1960;**15**:392–9.
23. Harndt E. Milchzahnstudien. II. Zur Pathologie der Milchzahnpulpa. *Dtsch Zahn Mund Kieferheilk* 1948;**11**:97–121.
24. Lund G. Et tilfælde af tanddannelsesforstyrrelse på traumatisk basis. *Tandlægebladet* 1951;**55**:102–14.
25. Bubenik J. Der Heilungsprocess der verletzten Zahnpulpa nach einem Trauma der Milchzähne. *Dtsch Stomatol* 1966;**16**:159–66.
26. Eschler J, Schilli W, Witt E. *Die traumatischen Verletzungen der Frontzähne bei Jugendlichen.* 3rd edn. Heidelberg: Alfred Hüthig Verlag, 1972.
27. Kloeppel J. Diagnosis and treatment of traumatic injuries of the teeth among children. *Int Dent J* 1963;**13**:684–7.
28. Tränkmann J. Zur Prognose zentral luxierter Frontzähne im Wechselgebiss. *Dtsch Zahnärztl Z* 1966;**21**:999–1005.
29. Müller GH, Overdiek HF. Das parodontale Trauma beim Jugendlichen. *Dtsch Zahnärztl Z* 1965;**20**:94–105.
30. Bruszt P. Secondary eruption of teeth intruded into the maxilla by a blow. *Oral Surg Oral Med Oral Pathol* 1958;**11**:146–9.
31. Bruszt P. L'avenir des dents atteintes de luxation interne au niveau du maxillaire supérieur. Bilan dix ans après le traumatisme. *Actual Odontostomatol* 1967;**78**:139–46.
32. Andreasen JO, Ravn JJ. The effect of traumatic injuries to primary teeth on their permanent successors. II. A clinical and radiographic follow-up study of 213 injured teeth. *Scand J Dent Res* 1971;**79**:284–94.
33. Schreiber CK. The effect of trauma on the anterior deciduous teeth. *Br Dent J* 1959;**106**:340–3.
34. Ravn JJ. Sequelae of acute mechanical traumata in the primary dentition. *ASDC J Dent Child* 1968;**35**: 281–9.
35. Gaare A, Hagen A, Kanstad S. Tannfrakturer hos barn. Diagnostiske og prognostiske problemer og behandling. *Norske Tannlegeforenings Tidende* 1958;**68**:364–78.
36. Andreasen JO. Fiksation med ortodontisk bånd-akryl skinne. En ny fiksationsmetode til traumatisk løsnede permanente tænder. (Orthodontic band-acrylic splint: a new fixation method for luxated permanent teeth) *Tandlægebladet* 1971;**75**:404–7.

37. Shargus G. Experimentelle Untersuchungen über den Halt verschiedener Schienungssysteme. *Dtsch Zahn Mund Kieferheilk* 1969;**53**:378–88.

38. Humphrey WP. A simple technique for splinting displaced anterior teeth in children. *ASDC J Dent Child* 1967;**33**:359–62.

39. Burley MA, Crabs HSM. Replantation of teeth. *Br Dent J* 1960;**108**:190–3.

40. Smith DC. A new dental cement. *Br Dent J* 1968;**125**:381–4.

41. Hirschfeld L. The use of wire and silk ligatures. *J Am Dent Assoc* 1950;**41**:647–56.

42. Rud J. Provisoriske fiksationer med akryl. *Tandlægebladet* 1965;**69**:385–90.

43. Hamilton A. A method of arch wiring for displaced anterior teeth. In: Husted E, Hjörting-Hansen E. eds. *Oral Surgery Transactions, 2nd Congress of the International Association of Oral Surgeons.* Copenhagen: Munksgaard, 1967:333–5.

44. Behrman SJ. A new method of splinting loose, fractured and evulsed teeth. *N Y State Dent J* 1960;**26**:287–96.

45. Lehnert S. Zur chirurgischen Therapie traumatisch geschädigter Frontzähne. *Dtsch Zahnärztebl* 1964;**18**:352–8.

46. van de Vyver LM. Traumata van de fronttanden. *Acta Stomatol Belge* 1964;**61**:499–513.

47. Tillman HH. A method of stabilizing loosened and displaced anterior teeth. *J Am Dent Assoc* 1962;**65**:378–80.

48. Duclos J, Farouz R. Fixation des dents réimplantées apres luxations accidentelles. *Rev Stomatol (Paris)* 1947;**48**:434–6.

49. Wilbur HM. Management of injured teeth. *J Am Dent Assoc* 1959;**44**:1–9.

50. Schuchardt K. Ein Vorschlag zur Verbesserung der Drahtschienenverbände. *Dtsch Zahn Mund Kieferheilk* 1956;**24**:39–44.

51. Schuchardt K, Kapovits M, Spiessl B. Technik und Anwendung des Drahtbogenkunststoffverbandes. *Dtsch Zahnärztl Z* 1961;**16**:1241–9.

52. Rotzler J. Die Fixation von frakturierten oder luxierten Zähnen mit der Drahtkunstharzschiene. *Schweiz Monatschr Zahnheilk* 1962;**72**:162–5.

53. Rottke B, Shimizu M. Der Draht-Kunststoffschienenverband nach Schuchardt und seine Wirkung auf Gingiva und Periodontium. *Zahnärztl Rdsch* 1966;**75**:451–4.

54. Huget EF, Brauer GM, Kumpula JW, Cman S. A filled cold-curing acrylic resin as a splinting material. *J Am Dent Assoc* 1969;**79**:645–8.

55. Epstein LI. Traumatic injuries to anterior teeth in children. *Oral Surg Oral Med Oral Pathol* 1969;**15**:334–44.

56. Pfeifer G. Freihändige Kunststoffschienung bei Alveolarfortsatzfrakturen und Luxationen im Milchgebiss. *Fortschr Kiefer Gesichtschir* 1959;**5**:328–32.

57. Hering H-J, von Domarus H. Die Biegungsbelastbarkeit von Kieferbruchschienen aus Kunststoffen. *Stoma (Heidelberg)* 1968;**21**:231–6.

58. Hollmann K, Fischer R. Zur Schienung traumatisch gelockerter Zähne. *Österr Z Stomatol* 1965;**62**:452–5.

59. Ravn JJ. Fiksationsskinne i kunststof. En direkte fremstillingsmetode. *Tandlægebladet* 1968;**72**:264–6.

60. Freedman GL, Hooley JR. Immobilization of anterior alveolar injuries with cold curing acrylic resins. *J Am Dent Assoc* 1968;**76**:785–6.

61. Seela W. Eine freihändig anzufertigende, einfache Kappenschiene unter Verwendung selbsthärtender Kunststoffe. *Zahnärztl Rdsch* 1966;**75**:411–13.

62. Stewart DJ. Stabilising appliances for traumatised incisors. *Br Dent J* 1964;**115**:416–18.

63. Katterbach R. Eine einfache Methode zur Schienung traumatisch oder infektiös gelockerter Zähne sowie von Alveolarfortsatzfrakturen. *Dtsch Zahnärztebl* 1968;**22**:338–44.

64. Miller J. IX.-First aid for fractured permanent incisors. *Br Dent J* 1962;**112**:435–7.

65. Nordenram Å. Omnivac, en tandteknisk apparat med mangsidig användning. *Sveriges Tandläkaras Förbunds Tidning* 1966;**58**:961–3.

66. Tammoscheit U-G. Klassifikation und Behandlung unfallverletzter Milchfrontzähne. *Zahnärztl Rdsch* 1967;**76**:190–3.

67. Öhman A. Healing and sensitivity to pain in young replanted human teeth. An experimental, clinical and histological study. *Odontologisk Tidsskrift* 1965;**73**:165–228.

68. Auslander WP. Discoloration. A traumatic sequela. *N Y State Dent J* 1967;**33**:534–8.

69. Glucksman DD. Fractured permanent anterior teeth complicationg orthodontic treatment. *J Am Dent Assoc* 1941;**28**:1941–3.

70. Hotz R. Die Bedeutung, Beurteilung und Behandlung beim Trauma im Frontzahngebiet vom Standpunkt des Kieferorthopäden. *Dtsch Zahnärztl Z* 1958;**13**:42–51, 401–16.

71. Fish EW. *Surgical pathology of the mouth.* London: Isaac Pitman & Sons, 1948:123.

72. Forshufvud S. A study of the paracapillary nutrition canals and their possible sympathetic innervation. *Acta Odontol Scand* 1946;7;**7**:1–57.

73. Cooke C, Rowbotham TC. Treatment of injuries to anterior teeth. *Br Dent J* 1951;**91**:146–52.

74. Weiskopf J, Gehre G, Graichen K-H. Ein Beitrag zur Behandlung von Luxationen und Wurzelfrakturen im Frontzahngebiet. *Stoma (Heidelberg)* 1961;**14**:100–13.

75. Anehill S, Lindahl B, Wallin H. Prognosis of traumatised permanent incisors in children. A clinical-roentgenological after-examination. *Svensk Tandläkara Tidskrift* 1969;**62**:367–75.

76. Wenzel H. Ein Beitrag zur Patho-Biologie der Zahnpulpa nach Trauma. *Dtsch Zahn Mund Kieferheilk* 1934;**1**:278–83.

77. Smyth KC. Obliteration of the pulp of a permanent incisor at the age of 13–9/12 years. *Dent Rec* 1950;**70**:218–9.

78. Holcomb JB, Gregory WB. Calcific metamorphosis of the pulp: its incidence and treatment. *Oral Surg Oral Med Oral Pathol* 1967;**24**:825–30.

79. Luks S. Observed effects of traumatic injuries upon anterior teeth. *N Y State Dent J* 1962;**28**:65–70.

80. Langeland K. The histopathologic basis in endodontic treatment. *Dent Clin North Am* 1967;491–520.

81. Andreasen JO, Hjörting-Hansen E. Replantation of teeth. II. Histological study of 22 replanted anterior teeth in humans. *Acta Odontol Scand* 1966;**24**:287–306.

82. Cohen S. Internal tooth resorption. *ASDC J Dent Child* 1965;**32**:49–52.

83. Menzel G. Seltene Folgen eines Traumas an 2 Zähnen. *Dtsch Zahnärztl Wochenschr* 1942;**45**:249.

84. Zilkins K. Beiträge zur traumatischen Zahnschädigung. In: Wannenmacher E. *Ein Querschnitt der deutschen Wissenschaftlichen Zahnheilkunde.* No. 33. Leipzig: Verlag von Hermann Meusser, 1938:43–70.

85. Oehlers FAC. A case of internal resorption following injury. *Br Dent J* 1951;**90**:13–16.

86. Goldman HM. Spontaneous intermittent resorption of teeth. *J Am Dent Assoc* 1954;**49**:522–32.

87. Brauer JC, Lindahl RL. Fractured and displaced anterior teeth. In: Brauer JC, Higley LB, Lindahl RL, Massler M, Schour I. *Dentistry for children.* 5th edn. New York, Toronto, London: McGraw-Hill Book Company, 1964:530–53.

88. Hawes RR. Traumatized primary teeth. *Dent Clin North Am* 1966;391–404.

89. Bercher J, Parket J, Farouz R. Les effets des traumatismes sur les pulpes des dents en cours de croissance. *Rev Stomatol (Paris)* 1952;**53**:99–106.

90. Penick EC. The endodontic management of root resorption. *Oral Surg Oral Med Oral Pathol* 1963;**16**:344–52.

91. Lorber CG. Zur Behandlung bei Kiefergesichtsverletzungen traumatisch geschädigter Zähne unter besonderer Berücksichtigung ihres histologischen Befundes. *Stoma (Heidelberg)* 1968;**21**:25–34.

92. Andreasen JO, Ravn JJ. Epidemiology of traumatic dental injuries to primary and permanent teeth in a Danish population sample. *Int J Oral Surg* 1972;**1**: 235–9.

93. Hedegård B, Stålhane I. A study of traumatized permanent teeth in children aged 7–15 years. Part I. *Swed Dent J* 1973;**66**:431–50.

94. Ravn JJ. Dental injuries in Copenhagen schoolchildren, school years 1967–1972. *Community Dent Oral Epidemiol* 1974;**2**:231–45.

95. Haaviko K, Rantanen L. A follow-up study of injuries to permanent and primary teeth in children. *Proc Finn Dent Soc* 1976;**72**:152–62.

96. Guzner N, Lustmann J, Shteyer A. Trauma to primary teeth. *IADR Abstracts* 1978;**58**: abstract no. 469.

97. Rock WP, Gordon PH, Friend LA, Grundy MC. The relationship between trauma and pulp death in incisor teeth. *Br Dent J* 1974;**136**:236–9.

98. Reichborn-Kjennerud I. Development, etiology and diagnosis of increased tooth mobility and traumatic occlusion. *J Periodontol* 1973;**6**:326–38.

99. Lorber CG. Einige Untersuchungen zur Pathologie unfallgeschädigter Zähne. *Schweiz Monatschr Zahnheilk* 1973;**83**:990–1014.

100. Acetoze PA, Sabbag Y, Ramalho AC. Luxaçao dental. Estudo das Alteraçoes Teciduais em Dentes de Crescimento Continuo. *Rev Fac Farm Odont Araraquara* 1970;**4**:125–45.

101. Lorber CG. Röntgenologische und histologische Befunde an traumatisierten Zähnen. *Zahnärztl Welt* 1972;**81**:215–20.

102. Stanley HR, Weisman MI, Michanowicz AE, Bellizzi R. Ischemic infarction of the pulp: sequential degenerative changes of the pulp after traumatic injury. *J Endod* 1978;**4**:325–35.

103. Barker BCW, Mayne JR. Some unusual cases of apexification subsequent to trauma. *Oral Surg Oral Med Oral Pathol* 1975;**39**:144–50.

104. Stålhane I, Hedegård B. Traumatized permanent teeth in children aged 7–15 years. Part II. *Swed Dent J* 1975;**68**:157–69.

105. Jacobsen I, Kerekes K. Long-term prognosis of traumatized permanent anterior teeth showing calcifying processes in the pulp cavity. *Scand J Dent Res* 1977;**85**:588–98.

106. Künzel W. Die hartgewebige Metaplasie des Zahnmarkes nach akutem Trauma. *Dtsch Stomatol* 1970;**20**:617–24.

107. Ravn JJ. Intrusion of permanent incisors. *Tandlægebladet* 1975;**79**:643–6.

108. Andreasen JO. The influence of traumatic intrusion of primary teeth on their permanent successors. A radiographic and histologic study in monkeys. *Int J Oral Surg* 1976;**5**:207–19.

109. Thylstrup A, Andreasen JO. The influence of traumatic intrusion of primary teeth on their permanent successors in monkeys. A macroscopic, polarized light and scanning electron macroscopic study. *J Oral Pathol* 1977;**6**:296–306.

110. Selliseth N-E. The significance of traumatised primary incisors on the development and eruption of permanent teeth. *Trans Eur Orthod Soc* 1970;**46**:443–59.

111. Iranpour B. Application of enamel adhesives in oral surgery. *Int J Oral Surg* 1974;**3**:223–6.

112. McEvoy SA, Mink JR. Acid-etched resin splint for temporarily stabilizing anterior teeth. *ASDC J Dent Child* 1974;**41**:439–41.

113. Kelly JR, Webb EE, Newton JA. Use of acid-etch resins to splint traumatized anterior teeth. *Dent Surv* 1977; **53**:24–31.

114. Kin PJ. A simple technic for treatment of dental trauma. *Dent Surv* 1977;**53**:40–1.

115. Simonsen RJ. Splinting of traumatic injuries using the acid etch system. *Dent Surv* 1977;**53**:26–33.

116. Sayegh FS, Kim HW, Kazanoglu A. Pulp reactions to Scutan in monkeys' and dogs' teeth. *AADR Abstracts B* 1977:142.

117. Rothler G, Krenkel C, Richter M. Die Schienung luxierter Zähne mit Hilfe der Schmelzklebetechnik. *Zahnärztl Prax* 1977;**28**:507–8.

118. Wikkeling OE. Luxated teeth: a new way of splinting. *Int J Oral Surg* 1978;**7**:221–3.

119. Berman RG, Buch TM. Utilization of a splint combining bracket-type orthodontic bands and cold-curing resin for stabilization of replaced avulsed teeth: report of case. *ASDC J Dent Child* 1973;**40**: 475–8.

120. Hovland EJ, Gutmann JL. Atraumatic stabilization for traumatized teeth. *J Endod* 1976;**2**:390–2.

121. Macko DJ, Kazmierski MR. Stabilization of traumatized anterior teeth. *ASDC J Dent Child* 1977; **44**:46–8.

122. Fischer R. Nachuntersuchungen geschienter, traumatisch gelockerter Zähne. *Österr Z Stomatol* 1976;**67**:439–42.

123. Tasanen A. Eräs kappakiskomenatelmä hammasluksaatioiden ja dento-alveolaaristen murtumien hoidossa. *Suomi Hammaslääk Toim* 1971;**67**:199–201.

124. Megquier RJ. Splint technique for dental-alveolar trauma. *J Am Dent Assoc* 1972;**85**:634–6.

125. Biven GM, Ritchie GM, Gerstein H. Acrylic splint for intentional replantation. *Oral Surg Oral Med Oral Pathol* 1970;**30**:537–9.

126. Simpson TH, Harrington GW, Natkin E. A splinting method for replantation of teeth in a noncontiguous arch. *Oral Surg Oral Med Oral Pathol* 1974;**38**:104–8.

127. Kernohan DC, Beirne LR. Conservative treatment of severely displaced permanent incisors: a case report. *Br Dent J* 1971;**131**:111–12.

128. Saunders IDF. Removable appliances in the stabilisation of traumatised anterior teeth – a preliminary report. *Proc Br Paedod Soc* 1972;**2**:19–22.

129. Herforth A, Münzel H-J. Zur Frage der Atiologie intradentärer Resorptionen. *Dtsch Zahnärztl Z* 1974;**29**:971–80.

130. Herforth VA. Zur Frage der Pulpavitalität nach Frontzahntrauma bei Jugendlichen – eine Longitudinaluntersuchung. *Dtsch Zahnärztl Z* 1976;**31**:938–46.

131. Barkin PR. Time as a factor in predicting the vitality of traumatized teeth. *ASDC J Dent Child* 1973;**40**:188–92.

132. Schröder U, Wennberg E, Granath L-E, Möller H. Traumatized primary incisors – follow-up program based on frequency of periapical osteitis related to tooth color. *Swed Dent J* 1977;**70**:95–8.

133. Bergenholz G. Micro-organisms from necrotic pulp of traumatized teeth. *Odontol Revy* 1974;**25**:347–58.

134. Cvek M, Nord C-E, Hollender L. Antimicrobial effect of root canal debridement in teeth with immature root. A clinical and microbiologic study. *Odontol Revy* 1976;**27**:1–10.

135. Cvek M, Hollender L, Nord C-E. Treatment of non-vital permanent incisors with calcium hydroxide. VI. A clinical microbiological and radiological evaluation of treatment in one sitting of teeth with mature or immature root. *Odontol Revy* 1976;**27**:93–108.

136. Eklund G, Stålhane I, Hedegård B. A study of traumatized permanent teeth in children aged 7–15 years. Part III. A multivariate analysis of post-traumatic complications of subluxated and luxated teeth. *Swed Dent J* 1976;**69**:179–89.

137. Hetzer G, Irmisch B. Einige Beobachtungen nach Milschzahnintrusionen. *Dtsch Stomatol* 1971;**21**:35–9.

138. Veigel W, Garcia C. Möglichkeiten und Grenzen der Erhaltung traumatisch geschädigter Milchzähne. *Dtsch Zahnärztl Z* 1976;**31**:271–3.

139. Andreasen JO, Riis I. Influence of pulp necrosis and periapical inflammation of primary teeth on their permanent successors. Combined macroscopic and histologic study in monkeys. *Int J Oral Surg* 1978; **7**:178–87.

140. Gröndahl H-G, Kahnberg K-E, Olsson G. *Traumatiserade tænder. En klinisk och röntgenologisk efterundersökning.* Göteborg Tandläkare Sällskaps Årsbok, 1974:38–50.

141. Stålhane I. Permanente tænder med reducerat pulpalumen som följd av olycksfallsskada. *Svensk Tandläkare Tidskrift* 1971;**64**:311–6.

142. Fischer CH. Hard tissue formation of the pulp in relation to treatment of traumatic injuries. *Int Dent J* 1974;**24**:387–96.

143. Jacobsen I, Sangnes G. Traumatized primary anterior teeth. Prognosis related to calcific reactions in the pulp cavity. *Acta Odontol Scand* 1978;**36**:199–204.

144. Sharpe MS. Internal resorption in a deciduous incisor: an unusual case. *J Am Dent Assoc* 1970;**81**: 947–8.

145. Lepp FH. Progressive internal resorption. *Oral Surg Oral Med Oral Pathol* 1969;**27**:184–5.

146. Vincentelli R, Lepp FH, Bouyssou M. Les 'tàches rosées de la couronne' ('pink spots') – leurs localisations intra- et extra-camérales. *Schweiz Monatschr Zahnheilk* 1973;**83**:113–250.

147. Gartner AH, Mack T, Sommerlott RG, Walsh LC. Differential diagnosis of internal and external root resorption. *J Endod* 1976;**2**:329–34.

148. Andreasen FM, Andreasen JO. Diagnosis of luxation injuries: The importance of standardized clinical, radiographic and photographic techniques in clinical investigations. *Endod Dent Traumatol* 1985;**1**:160–9.

149. Haavikko K, Rantanen L. A follow-up study of injuries to permanent and primary teeth in children. *Proc Finn Dent Soc* 1976;**72**:152–62.

150. Crona-Larsson G, Norén JG. Luxation injuries to permanent teeth – a retrospective study of etiological factors. *Endod Dent Traumatol* 1989;**5**:176–9.

151. Kenwood M, Seow WK. Sequelae of trauma to the primary dentition. *J Pedodont* 1989;**13**:230–8.

152. von Arx T. Traumatologie im Milchgebiss (I). Kliniche and therapeutische Aspekte. *Schweiz Monatsschr Zahnmed* 1990;**100**:1195–204.

153. Birkedal-Hansen H. External root resorption caused by luxation of rat molars. *Scand J Dent Res* 1973; **81**:47–61.

154. Turley PK, Joiner MW, Hellström S. The effect of orthodontic extrusion on traumatically intruded teeth. *Am J Orthod* 1984;**85**:47–56.

155. Tziafas D. Pulpal reaction following experimental acute trauma of concussion type on immature dog teeth. *Endod Dent Traumatol* 1988;**4**:27–31.

156. Mandel U, Viidik A. Effect of splinting on the mechanical and histological properties of the healing periodontal ligament in the vervet monkey (cercopithecus aethiops). *Arch Oral Biol* 1989;**34**:209–17.

157. Miyashin M, Kato J, Takagi Y. Experimental luxation injuries in immature rat teeth. *Endod Dent Traumatol* 1990;**6**:121–8.

158. Miyashin M, Kato J, Takagi Y. Tissue reations after experimental luxation injuries in immature rat teeth. *Endod Dent Traumatol* 1991;**7**:26–35.

159. Cipriano TJ, Walton RE. The ischemic infarct pulp of traumatized teeth: a light and electron microscopic study. *Endod Dent Traumatol* 1986;**2**:196–204.

160. ANDREASEN FM. Histological and bacteriological study of pulps extirpated after luxation injuries. *Endod Dent Traumatol* 1988;**4**:170–81.

161. OIKARINEN K, ANDREASEN JO. Influence of conventional forceps extraction and extraction with an extrusion instrument on cementoblast damage and root resorption of replanted monkey incisors. *Periodont Res* 1996;**31**:337–44.

162. ANDREASEN JO, ANDREASEN FM. Immediate histologic periodontal ligament response to traumatic intrusion of incisors in monkeys. 2006. In preparation.

163. ANDREASEN FM, VESTERGAARD PEDERSEN B. Prognosis of luxated permanent teeth – the development of pulp necrosis. *Endod Dent Traumatol* 1985;**1**:207–20.

164. ANDREASEN FM, YU Z, THOMSEN BL, ANDERSEN PK. Occurrence of pulp canal obliteration after luxation injuries in the permanent dentition. *Endod Dent Traumatol* 1987;**3**:103–15.

165. ANDREASEN JO, KRISTERSON L, ANDREASEN FM. Damage to the Hertwigs epithelial root sheath: effect upon growth after autotransplantation of teeth in monkeys. *Endod Dent Traumatol* 1988;**4**:145–51.

166. ANDREASEN FM. Transient apical breakdown and its relation to color and sensibility changes after luxation injuries to teeth. *Endod Dent Traumatol* 1986;**2**: 9–19.

167. MORLEY KR, BELLIZZI R. Management of subluxative and intrusive injuries to the permanent dentition: a case report. *Ontario Dentist* 1981;**58**:28–31.

168. PEREZ B, BECKER A, CHOSACK A. The repositioning of a traumatically intruded mature rooted permanent incisor with a removable orthodontic appliance. *J Pedodontics* 1982;**6**:343–54.

169. HELING I. Intrusive luxation of an immature incisor. *J Endod* 1984;**10**:387–90.

170. JACOBSEN I. Long term evelution, prognosis and subsequent management of traumatic tooth injuries. In: Gutmann JL, Harrison JW. eds. *Proceedings of the International Conference on Oral Trauma*. Illinois: American Association of Endodontists Endowment & Memorial Foundation, 1986:129–38.

171. VINCKIER F, LAMBRECHTS W, DECLERCK D. Intrusion de l'incisive définitive. *Rev Belge Med Dent* 1989;**44**: 99–106.

172. KINIRONS MJ, SUTCLIFFE J. Traumatically intruded permanent incisors: a study of treatment and outcome. *Br Dent J* 1991;**170**:144–6.

173. SHAPIRA J, REGEY L, LIEBFELD H. Re-eruption of completely intruded immature permanent incisors. *Endod Dent Traumatol* 1986;**2**:113–6.

174. TRONSTAD L, TROPE M, BANK M, BARNETT F. Surgical access for endodontic treatment of intruded teeth. *Endod Dent Traumatol* 1986;**2**:75–8.

175. BELOSTOKY L, SCHWARTZ Z, SOSKOLNE WA. Undiagnosed intrusion of a maxillary primary incisor tooth: 15-year follow-up. *Pediatric Dent* 1986;**8**:294–6.

176. NIELSEN LA, RAVN JJ. Intrusion of primære tænder: et kasuistisk bidrag. *Tandlægebladet* 1989;**93**:441–4.

177. KRISTERSON L, ANDREASEN JO. The effect of splinting upon periodontal and pulpal healing after autotransplantation of mature and immature permanent incisors in monkeys. *Int J Oral Surg* 1983;**12**:239–49.

178. ROCK WP, GRUNDY MC. The effect of luxation and subluxation upon the prognosis of traumatized incisor teeth. *J Dent* 1981;**9**:224–30.

179. OIKARINEN K. Comparison of the flexibility of various splinting methods for tooth fixation. *J Oral Maxillofac Surg* 1988;**17**:125–7.

180. OIKARINEN K. Tooth splinting: a review of the literature and consideration of the versatility of a wire-composite splint. *Endod Dent Traumatol* 1990;**6**:237–50.

181. OIKARINEN K, ANDREASEN JO, ANDREASEN FM. Rigidity of various fixation methods used as dental splints. *Endod Dent Traumatol* 1992;**8**:113–19.

182. KRENKEL C, RICHTER M, ROTHLER G. Die Silcadraht-Klebeschiene – eine neue Methode zur Behandlung luxierter Zähne. *Dtsch Zahnärztl Z* 1979;**34**:280–2.

183. BELL O, STÖRMER K, ZACHRISSON B . Ny metode for fiksering av traumatiserte tenner. *Norske Tannlegeforenings Tidende* 1984;**94**:49–55.

184. LOWNIE JF, REA MA. Splinting a traumatically avulsed tooth. *J Dent* 1980;**8**:260–2.

185. WEISMAN MI. Tooth out! Tooth in! Simplified splinting. *CDS Review* **1984**:30–7.

186. HAGEN M, FRITZEMEIER CU. Unterschiedliche Schienungstechniken und deren Indikation zur chirurgischen Zahnerhaltung. *Dtsch Zahnärztl Z* 1987;**42**:194–7.

187. OIKARINEN K. Functional fixation for traumatically luxated teeth. *Endod Dent Traumatol* 1987;**3**:224–8.

188. ANTRIM DD, OSTROWSKI JS. A functional splint for traumatized teeth. *J Endod* 1982;**8**:328–32.

189. NORDENVALL K-J. Fixering av traumaskada. *Tandläkartidningen* 1991;**83**:770–1.

190. ANDERSSON L, FRISKOP J, BLOMLÖF L. Fiber-glass splinting of traumatized teeth. *ASDC J Dent Child* 1983;**50**:21–4.

191. FLEISCH L, CLEATON-JONES P, FORBES M, VAN WYK J, FAT C. Pulpal response to a bis-acryl-plastic (Protemp) temporary crown and bridge material. *J Oral Pathol* 1984;**13**:622–31.

192. POLSON AM, BILLEN JR. Temporary splinting of teeth using ultraviolet light-polymerized bonding materials. *J Am Dent Assoc* 1974;**89**:1137–9.

193. ANDREASEN FM. Pulpal healing after luxation injuries and root fracture in the permanent dentition. *Endod Dent Traumatol* 1989;**5**:111–31.

194. ANDREASEN FM, ANDREASEN JO, BAYER T. Prognosis of root-fractured permanent incisors – prediction of healing modalities. *Endod Dent Traumatol* 1989;**5**:11–22.

195. BUCHHORN I. *Følger efter behandling af palatinalt retinerede hjørnetænder. En efterundersøgelse.* Thesis: Royal Dental College, Copenhagen 1985.

196. OIKARINEN K, GUNDLACH KKH, PFEIFER G. Late complications of luxation injuries to teeth. *Endod Dent Traumatol* 1987;**3**:296–303.

197. HERFORTH A. Wurzelfrakturen und Luxationen von Zähnen – III. Teil. *ZWR* 1990;**99**:784–91.

198. ANDREASEN FM, YU Z, THOMSEN BL. Relationship between pulp dimensions and development of pulp necrosis after luxation injuries in the permanent dentition. *Endod Dent Traumatol* 1986;**2**:90–8.

199. MAGNUSSON B, HOLM A-K. Traumatised permanent teeth in children – a follow-up. I. Pulpal considerations

and root resorption. *Svensk Tandläk Tid* 1969;**62**: 61–70.

200. BHASKAR SN, RAPPAPORT HM. Dental vitality tests and pulp status. *J Am Dent Assoc* 1973;**86**:409–11.

201. JACOBSEN I. Criteria for diagnosis of pulp necrosis in traumatized permanent incisors. *Scand J Dent Res* 1980;**88**:306–12.

202. ZADIK D, CHOSAK A, EIDELMAN E. The prognosis of traumatized permanent anterior teeth with fracture of the enamel and dentin. *Oral Surg Oral Med Oral Pathol* 1979;**47**:173–5.

203. GAZELIUS B, OLGART L, EDWALL B, EDWALL L. Non-invasive recording of blood flow in human dental pulp. *Endod Dent Traumatol* 1986;**2**:219–22.

204. GAZELIUS B, OLGART L, EDWALL B. Restored vitality in luxated teeth assessed by laser Doppler flowmeter. *Endod Dent Traumatol* 1988;**4**:265–8.

205. EDWALL B, GAZELIUS B, BERG JO, EDWALL L, HELLANDER K, OLGART L. Blood flow changes in the dental pulp of the cat and rat measured simultaneously by laser Doppler flowmetry and local I clearance. *Acta Physiol Scand* 1987;**131**:81–92.

206. OLGART L, GAZELIUS B, LINDH-STRÖMBERG U. Laser Doppler flowmetry in assessing vitality in luxated permanent teeth. *Int Endod J* 1988;**21**:300–6.

207. WILDER-SMITH PE. A new method for the non-invasive measurement of pulpal blood flow. *Int Endod J* 1988;**21**:307–12.

208. CONVERSE JM, RAPAPORT FT. The vascularization of skin autografts and homografts; experimental study in man. *Ann Surg* 1956;**143**:306–15.

209. CLEMMESEN T. The early circulation in split skin grafts. *Acta Chir Scand* 1962;**124**:11–8.

210. MARCKMANN A. Autologous skin grafts in the rat. Vital microscopic studies of microcirculation. *Angiology* 1966;**17**:475–82.

211. HALLER JA, BILLINGHAM RE. Studies of the origin of the vasculature in free skin grafts. *Ann Surg* 1967;**166**:896–901.

212. CLEMMESEN T. Experimental studies on the healing of free skin autografts. *Ugeskr Læger* 1967;**14**: (Suppl 11):1–74.

213. HINSHAW JR, MILLER ER. Histology of healing split-thickness, full-thickness autogenous skin grafts and donor sites. *Arch Surg* 1965;**91**:658–70.

214. ZAREM HA, ZWEIFACH BW, McGEHEE JM. Development of microcirculation in full thickness autogenous skin grafts in mice. *Am J Physiol* 1967;**212**:1081–5.

215. SOXMAN JA, NAZIF MM, BOUGUOT J. Pulpal pathology in relation to discoloration of primary anterior teeth. *ASDC J Dent Child* 1984;**51**:282–4.

216. CROLL TP, PASCON EA, LANGELAND K. Traumatically injured primary incisors: a clinical and histological study. *ASDC J Dent Child* 1987;**54**:401–22.

217. ANDREASEN JO, ANDREASEN FM. Root resorption following traumatic dental injuries. *Proc Finn Dent Soc* 1991;**88**:95–114.

218. KEREKES K, JACOBSEN I. Follow-up examination of endodontic treatment in traumatized juvenil incisors. *J Endod* 1980;**6**:744–8.

219. ANDREASEN JO. External root resorption: its implication in dental traumatology, paedodontics, periodontics, orthodontics and endodontics. *Int Endod J* 1985; **18**:109–18.

220. SONIS AL. Longitudinal study of discolored primary teeth and effect on succedaneous teeth. *J Pedodont* 1987;**11**:247–52.

221. COLL JA, JOSELL S, NASSOF S, SHELTON P, RICHARDS MA. An evaluation of pulpal therapy in primary incisors. *Pediatr Dent* 1988;**10**:178–84.

222. FLAITZ CM, BARR ES, HICKS MJ. Radiograhic evaluation of pulpal treatment for anterior primary teeth in a pediatric dentistry practice. *Pediatr Dent* 1987;**9**:171–2.

223. PRUHS RJ, OLEN GA, SHARMA PS. Relationship between formocresol pulpotomies on primary teeth and enamel defects on their permanent successors. *J Am Dent Assoc* 1977;**94**:698–700.

224. HOLAN G, TOPF J, FUKS AB. Effect of root canal infection and treatment of traumatized primary incisors on their permanent successors. *Endod Dent Traumatol* 1992;**8**:12–15.

225. LAWNIK D, TETSCH P. Spätfolgen nach Frontzahnverletzungen – Ergebnisse einer Nachuntersuchung. *Dtsch Zhnärztl Z* 1983;**38**:476–7.

226. POSUKIDIST, LEHMANN W. Die Prognose des traumatisierten Zahnes. *Dtsch Zahnärztl Z* 1983; **38**:478–9.

227. RAVN JJ. Dental traume epidemiologi i Danmark: en oversigt med enkelte nye oplysninger. *Tandlægebladet* 1989;**93**:393–6.

228. WEPNER F, BUKEL J. Problematik und Therapie der traumatischen Zahnluxation im Kindesalter. *Quintessenz* 1981;**32**:1541–7.

229. SMITH JW. Calcific metamorphosis: a treatment dilemma. *Oral Surg Oral Med Oral Pathol* 1982;**54**: 441–4.

230. RAVN JJ. Obliteration af tænder. En litteraturoversigt. *Tandlægebladet* 1982;**86**:183–7.

231. STRONER WF. Pulpal dystrophic calcification. *J Endod* 1984;**10**:202–4.

232. SCHINDLER WG, GULLICKSON DC. Rationale for the management of calcific metamorphosis secondary to traumatic injuries. *J Endod* 1988;**14**:408–12.

233. MOULE AJ, THOMAS RP. Cervical external root resorption following trauma – a case report. *Int Endod J* 1985;**18**:277–81.

234. ANDREASEN FM, ANDREASEN JO. Resorption and mineralization processes following root fracture of permanent incisors. *Endod Dent Traumatol* 1988;**4**: 202–14.

235. WALL WH. Universal polycarbonate fracture splint and its direct bonding potential. *Int J Oral Maxillofac Surg* 1986;**15**:418–21.

236. TURLEY PK, CRAWFORD LB, CARRINGTON KW. Traumatically intruded teeth. *Angle Orthod* 1987; **57**:234–44.

237. CUNHA RF, PAVARINI A, PERCINOTO C, LIMA JE. Pulp and periodontal reactions of immature permanent teeth in the dog to intrusive trauma. *Endod Dent Traumatol* 1995;**11**:100–4.

238. SHIBUE T, TANIGUCHI K, MOTOKAWA W. Pulp and root development after partial extrusion in immature rat molars: a histopathological study. *Endod Dent Traumatol* 1998;**14**:174–81.

239. Heling I, Slutzky-Goldberg I, Lustmann J, Ehrlich Y, Becker A. Bone-like tissue growth in the root canal of immature permanent teeth after traumatic injuries. *Endod Dent Traumatol* 2000;**16**:298–303.

240. Crona-Larsson G, Bjarnason S, Norén JG. Effect of luxation injuries on permanent teeth. *Endod Dent Traumatol* 1991;**7**:199–206.

241. Robertson A. *Pulp survival and hard tissue formation subsequent to dental trauma. A clinical and histological study of uncomplicated crown fractures and luxation injuries.* Thesis. Göteborg University, 1997.

242. Dumsha TC. Luxations injuries. *Dent Clin North Am* 1995;**39**:79–91.

243. Andreasen FM. Transient root resorption after trauma: the clinician's dilemma. *J Esthet Restor Dent* 2003; **15**:80–92.

244. Boyd KS. Transient apical breakdown following subluxation injury: a case report. *Endod Dent Traumatol* 1995;**11**:37–40.

245. Cohenca N, Karni S, Rotstein I. Transient apical breakdown following tooth luxation. *Dent Traumatol* 2003;**19**:289–91.

246. Robertson A, Andreasen FM, Bergenhholtz G, Andreasen JO, Norén JG. Incidence of pulp necrosis subsequent to pulp canal obliteration from trauma of permanent incisors. *J Endod* 1996;**22**: 557–60.

247. Çaliskan MK, Türkün M. Prognosis of permanent teeth with internal resorption: a clinical review. *Endod Dent Traumatol* 1997;**13**:75–81.

248. Hintze H, Wenzel A, Andreasen FM, Sewerin I. Digital subtraction radiography for assessment of simulated root resorption cavities. Performance of conventional and reverse contrast modes. *Endod Dent Traumatol* 1992;**8**:149–54.

249. Heithersay GS. Clinical, radiologic and histopathologic features of invasive cervical resorption. *Quintessence Int* 1999;**30**:27–37.

250. Heithersay GS. Invasive cervical resorption: an analysis of potential predisposing factors. *Quintessence Int* 1999;**30**:83–95.

251. Andreasen JO, Bakland L, Matras R, Andreasen FM. Traumatic intrusion of permanent teeth. Part 1. An epidemiological study of 216 intruded permanent teeth. *Dent Traumatol* 2006;**22**:83–9.

252. Andreasen JO, Bakland L, Andreasen FM. Traumatic intrusion of 140 permanent teeth. Part 2. A clinical study of the effect of preinjury and injury factors, such as sex, age, stage of root development, tooth location, and extent of injury including number of intruded teeth. *Dent Traumatol* 2006;**22**:90–8.

253. Andreasen JO, Bakland L, Andreasen FM. Traumatic intrusion of 140 permanent teeth. Part 3. A clinical study of the effect of treatment variables, such as treatment delay, method of repositioning, types of splint, length of splinting and antibiotics. *Dent Traumatol* 2006;**22**:99–111.

254. Andreasen FM, Sewerin I, Mandel U, Andreasen JO. Radiographic assessment of simulated resorption cavities. *Endod Dent Traumatol* 1987;**3**:21–7.

# 14

# Concussion and Subluxation

F. M. Andreasen & J. O. Andreasen

## Definitions

### Concussion

An injury to the tooth-supporting structures without abnormal loosening or displacement of the tooth, but with marked reaction to percussion (Fig.14.1).

### Subluxation (loosening)

An injury to the tooth-supporting structures with abnormal loosening, but without displacement (Fig. 14.2).

### Frequency

In a study from a larger trauma center, frequencies of 23% and 21% were found for concussion and subluxation respectively (6).

## Healing and pathology

In luxation injuries only minor damage has occurred in the periodontium. In the case of *concussion* the impact has resulted in bleeding and edema which makes the tooth sensitive to occlusal forces and to a percussion test. However, abnormal mobility is not present (Fig. 14.3).

In the case of *subluxation* some damage (rupture) to ligament fibers has occurred which makes the tooth mobile in horizontal direction and sometimes also with a small component in vertical direction (Fig. 14.3).

## Concussion

The patient complains that the tooth is tender to touch. Clinical examination reveals a marked reaction to percussion in horizontal or vertical direction (Fig. 14.3). The tooth shows, however, no abnormal mobility. There is no bleeding from the gingival sulcus. The tooth usually responds positively to sensibility tests.

## Subluxation

Subluxated teeth retain their normal position in the dental arch. However, the tooth is mobile in a horizontal direction and sensitive to percussion and occlusal forces. Hemorrhage from the gingival crevice is usually present, indicating damage to the periodontal tissue (Fig. 14.3). The tooth usually responds to sensibility tests.

## Radiographic findings

Usually no changes can be seen in the configuration of the periodontal ligament space. However, in cases with marked mobility (grade 3 including vertical mobility) a slight widening of the PDL space may be seen.

## Treatment

### Concussion/subluxation

Treatment may be confined to occlusal grinding of the opposing teeth and by repeated pulp tests during the follow-up period (see Appendix 3, p. 881, for follow-up schedule for the various types of luxation injuries) (Fig. 14.4). While splinting is not needed following these minor injuries, in the case of multiple tooth injuries these teeth may be included in the splint with no risk of damage to the periodontal ligament by the splinting procedure or splinting period.

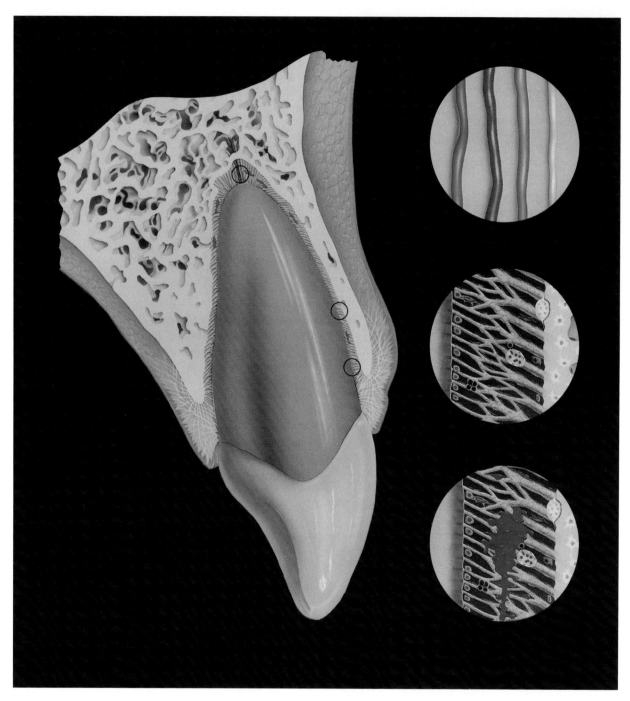

**Fig. 14.1** Mechanism and pathology of concussion injury. A frontal impact leads to hemorrhage and edema in the periodontal ligament.

## Follow-up

For follow-up schedule use 4 to 6 weeks. If clinical findings (including sensibility) tests and a radiographic examination show no abnormal findings controls can be terminated at this time.

## Complications

### Pulp necrosis

This event is very rare (1–5) (Figs 14.5 and 14.6).

### Root resorption

Surface resorption has been found in these trauma entities (1) (Figs 14.7 and 14.8).

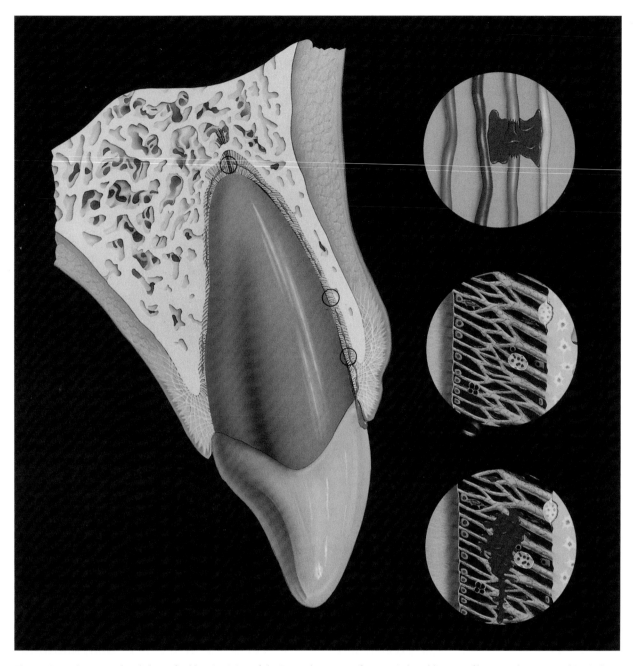

**Fig. 14.2** Mechanism and pathology of subluxation injury. If the impact has greater force, periodontal ligament fibers may be torn, resulting in loosening of the injured tooth.

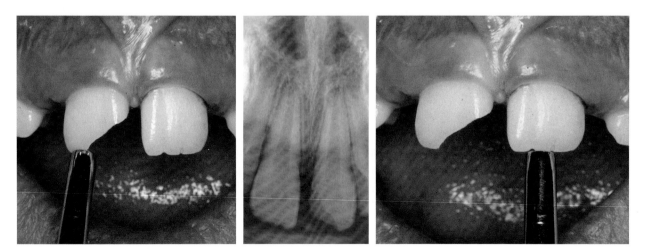

**Fig. 14.3** Clinical and radiographic features of concussion and subluxation. The right and left maxillary central incisors have received a blow and are tender to percussion. The right central incisor is firm in its socket (concussion), while the left central incisor is loose and with hemorrhage from the gingival sulcus (subluxation).

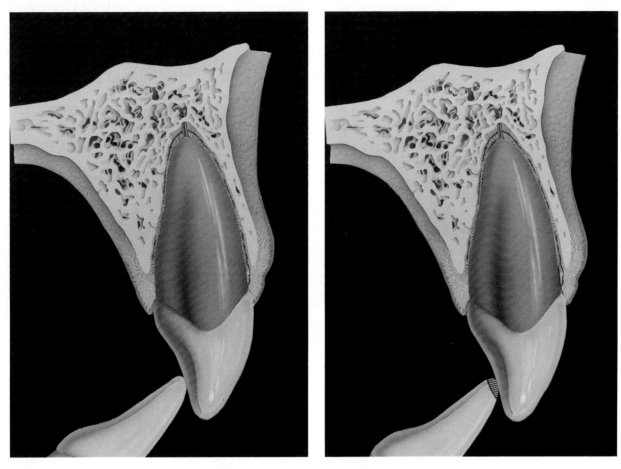

**Fig. 14.4** Treatment principles for concussion/subluxation. Relief of occlusal interference by selective grinding of opposing teeth may be necessary. In the case of severe loosening and/or multiple tooth injuries, teeth may be splinted. Otherwise, a soft diet is recommended for 14 days.

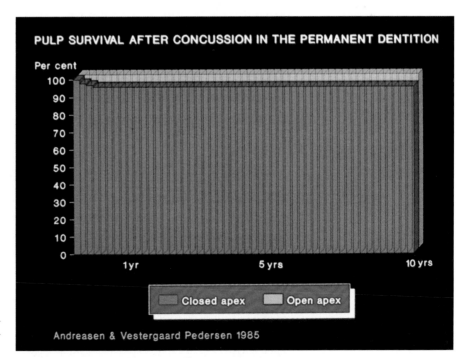

**Fig. 14.5** Pulp survival after concussion. From ANDREASEN & VESTER-GAARD PEDERSEN (1) 1985.

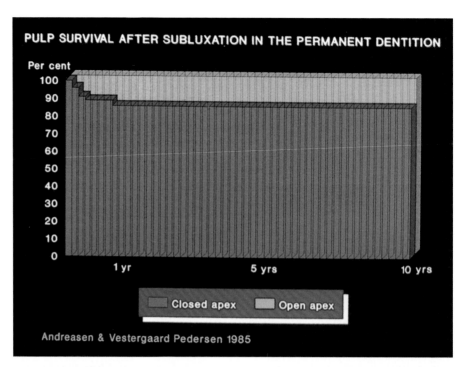

Fig. 14.6 Pulp healing after subluxation. From ANDREASEN & VESTERGAARD PEDERSEN (1) 1985.

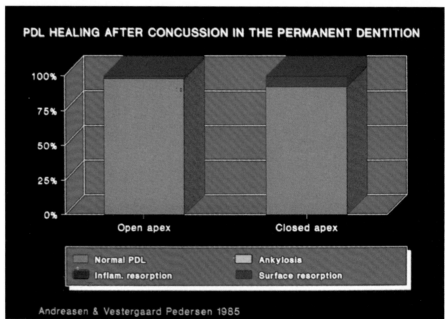

Fig. 14.7 Periodontal healing after concussion. From ANDREASEN & VESTERGAARD PEDERSEN (1) 1985.

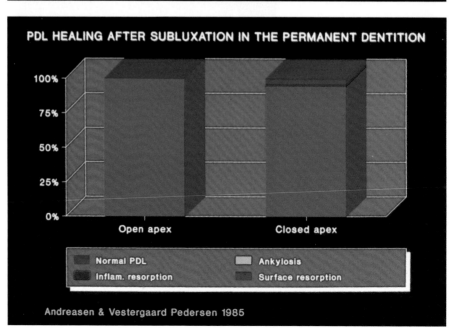

Fig. 14.8 Periodontal healing after subluxation. From ANDREASEN & VESTERGAARD PEDERSEN (1) 1985.

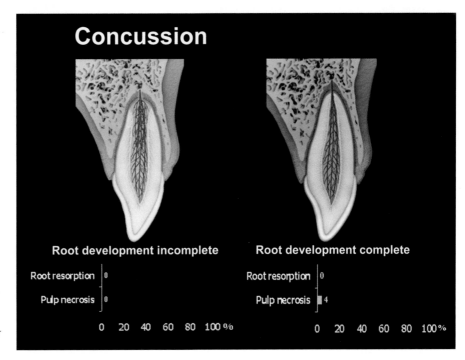

**Fig. 14.9** Predictors for healing after concussion.

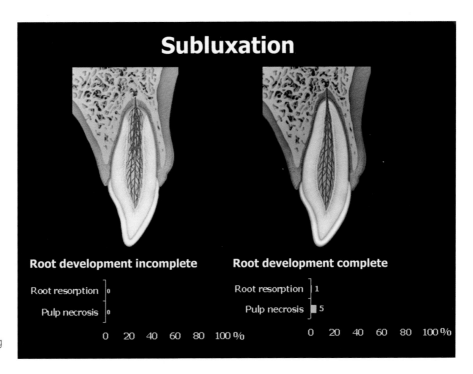

**Fig. 14.10** Predictors for healing after subluxation.

## Predictors for healing

Stage of root development and associated crown fracture have been found to be significantly related to the development of pulp necrosis following injury (1–3) (Figs 14.9 and 14.10).

**Table 14.1** Prevalence of external root resorption relation to concussion and subluxation. From ANDRŁASEN & VESTERGAARD PEDERSEN (1) 1985.

|  | No. of teeth | Surface resorption | Inflammatory resorption | Ankylosis |
|---|---|---|---|---|
| Concussion | 178 | 8 (4%) | 0 (0%) | 0 (0%) |
| Subluxation | 223 | 4 (2%) | 1 (0.5%) | 0 (0%) |

## Essentials

### Concussion and subluxation

(1) Relief of the occlusion on injured teeth and/or immobilization may be indicated, especially in the case of marked loosening. Otherwise, a soft diet for 14 days.
(2) Control the tooth radiographically and with sensibility testing.
(3) Follow-up period generally 4–6 weeks.

### Prognosis

Pulp necrosis: risk very limited.
Root resorption: Limited risk of surface resorption (Table 14.1).

## References

1. ANDREASEN FM, VESTERGAARD PEDERSEN B. Prognosis of luxated permanent teeth: the development of pulp necrosis. *Endod Dent Traumatol* 1985;**1**:207–20.
2. ANDREASEN FM. *Pulpal healing after luxation injuries and root fracture in the permanent dentition.* Thesis. Copenhagen University, 1995. ISBN 87-985538-0-1.
3. ROBERTSON A, ANDREASEN FM, ANDREASEN JO, NORÉN JG. Long-term prognosis of crown-fractured permanent incisors. The effect of stage of root development and associated luxation injury. *Int J Paediat Dent* 2000;**10**:191–9.
4. STÅLHANE I, HEDEGÅRD B. Traumatized permanent teeth in children aged 7–15 years. Part II. *Swed Dent J* 1975;**68**:157–9.
5. EKLUND G, STÅLHANE I, HEDEGÅRD B. Traumatized permanent teeth in children aged 7–15 years. III. A multivariate analysis of posttraumatic complications of subluxated and luxated teeth. *Swed Dent J* 1976;**69**:179–89.
6. BORUM MK, ANDREASEN JO. Therapeutic and economic implications of traumatic dental injuries in Denmark: an estimate based on 7549 patients treated at a major trauma centre. *Int J Paediat Dent* 2001;**11**:249–58.

# 15

# Extrusive Luxation and Lateral Luxation

F. M. Andreasen & J. O. Andreasen

## Definitions

### Extrusive luxation (peripheral dislocation, partial avulsion)

Partial displacement of the tooth out of its socket (Fig. 15.1).

### Lateral luxation

Displacement of the tooth in a direction other than axially. This is accompanied by comminution or fracture of the alveolar socket (Fig. 15.2).

### Frequency

The frequency of extrusive and lateral luxation has been found to be 7% and 11% among traumatized permanent teeth examined at a major trauma center (7).

## Healing and pathology

In these cases there is a complete rupture of the neurovascular supply to the pulp and severance of periodontal ligament fibers leading to extrusion. In case of lateral luxation the periodontal injury is accompanied by a fracture of the labial bone plate as well as contusion injury to the lingual cervical periodontal ligament.

In a recent study in rats the pulp response after extrusion was found to be separation of the odontoblast layer especially in the coronal part of the pulp; furthermore interstitial bleeding was found. After 4 and 8 weeks irregular dentin formation took place (8).

## Clinical findings

### Extrusion

Extruded teeth appear elongated and most often with lingual deviation of the crown, as the tooth is suspended only by the palatinal gingiva (Fig. 15.1). There is always bleeding from the periodontal ligament. The percussion sound is dull.

### Lateral luxation

The crowns of laterally luxated teeth are in most cases displaced lingually and are usually associated with fractures of the vestibular part of the socket wall (Fig. 15.2). Displacement of teeth after lateral luxation is normally evident by visual inspection. However, in case of marked inclination of maxillary teeth, it can be difficult to decide whether the trauma has caused minor abnormalities in tooth position. In such cases, occlusion should be checked. Due to the frequently locked position of the tooth in the alveolus, clinical findings revealed by percussion and mobility tests are identical with those found in intruded teeth (see Chapter 13, Table 13.1).

## Radiographic findings

*Extruded teeth* show an expanded periodontal space especially apically (Fig. 15.3). This will be evident in both occlusal and orthoradial exposures (Fig. 15.3).

Likewise, a *laterally luxated tooth* shows an increased periodontal space apically when the apex is displaced labially. However, this will usually be seen only in an occlusal or eccentric exposure. An orthoradial exposure will give little

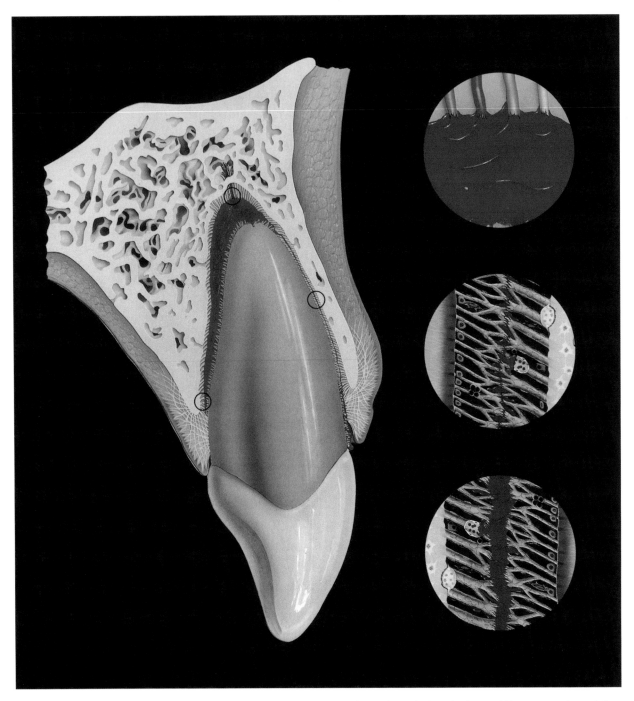

**Fig. 15.1** Pathogenesis of extrusive luxation. Oblique forces displace the tooth out of its socket. Only the palatal gingival fibers prevent the tooth from being avulsed. Both the PDL and the neurovascular supply to the pulp are ruptured.

or no evidence of displacement. The radiographic picture, which imitates extrusive luxation, is explained by the relation between the dislocation and direction of the central beam (1) (Fig. 15.4).

## Treatment

The treatment of *extruded* permanent teeth seen soon after injury consists of careful repositioning, whereby the coagu-

lum formed between the displaced root and socket wall will be slowly pressed out along the gingival crevice (Fig. 15.5). Administration of local anesthetic is generally not necessary. As the repositioned tooth often has a tendency to migrate incisally, a flexible splint should be applied for 2–3 weeks (see later) (Fig. 15.6).

In case of *lateral luxation*, repositioning is usually a very forceful and, therefore, a traumatogenic procedure (Figs 15.7 and 15.8). Prior to this procedure, it is necessary to anesthetize the area. An infraorbital regional block anesthesia on the appropriate side of the maxilla is the most effec-

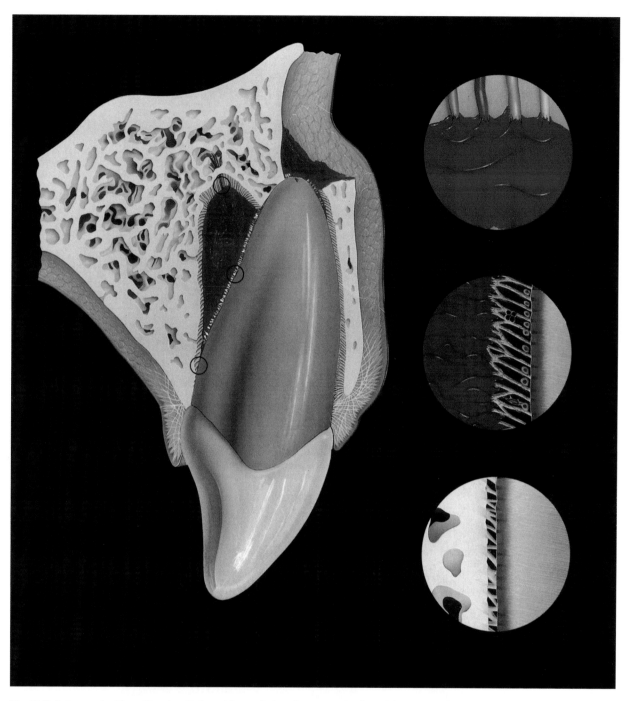

**Fig. 15.2** Pathogenesis of lateral luxation. Horizontal forces displace the crown palatally and the root apex facially. Apart from rupture of the PDL and the pulpal neurovascular supply, compression of the PDL is seen on the palatal aspect of the root.

tive. As indicated, this type of luxation is characterized by the forceful displacement of the root tip through the facial alveolar wall, which complicates the repositioning procedure. In order to dislodge the root tip from its bony lock, firm digital pressure in an incisal direction must first be applied immediately over the displaced root, which can be localized by palpating the corresponding bulge in the sulcular fold. Once the tooth is dislodged, it can be maneuvered apically into its correct position.

If manual repositioning is not possible, a forceps can be applied, whereby the tooth is first slightly extruded past the bony alveolar lock and then directed back into its correct position.

Once the tooth is repositioned, the labial and palatal bone plates should also be compressed, to ensure complete repositioning and to facilitate periodontal healing. Lacerated gingiva should then be re-adapted to the neck of the tooth and sutured. The tooth should be splinted in its normal position. A radiograph is then taken to verify repositioning and to register the level of the alveolar bone for later

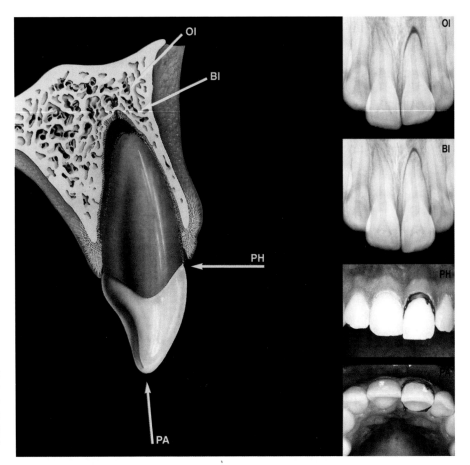

**Fig. 15.3** Clinical and radiographic features of extrusive luxation. The standard bisecting angle periapical radiographic technique is more useful than a steep occlusal exposure in revealing axial displacement. From ANDREASEN & ANDREASEN (1) 1985.

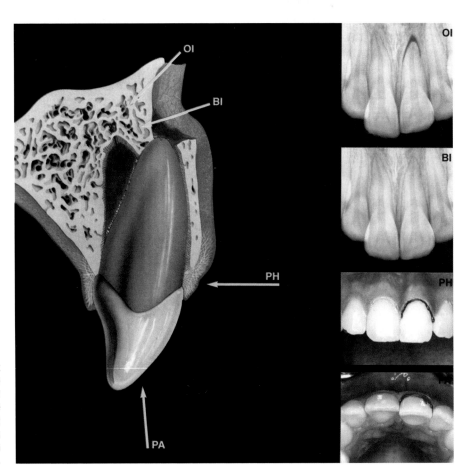

**Fig. 15.4** Clinical and radiographic features of lateral luxation. The steep occlusal radiographic exposure or an eccentric periapical bisecting angle exposure are more useful than an orthoradial bisecting technique in revealing lateral displacement. From ANDREASEN & ANDREASEN (1) 1985.

comparison. This is recommended in order to monitor eventual loss of marginal bone support in the follow-up period (see later).

If treatment of a laterally luxated or extruded permanent tooth is delayed (i.e. more than 3–4 days), it is usually found that the tooth is difficult to reposition. Recent studies seem to indicate that reduction procedures should be deferred and the tooth allowed to realign itself or that this should be accomplished orthodontically (2).

In young children, where the laterally luxated tooth does not interfere with occlusion, it might be indicated to await spontaneous repositioning (Fig. 15.9).

## Prognosis

Very few studies have been performed on the prognosis of extrusive and lateral luxation. In Tables 15.1 and 15.2 (see pages 422 and 423), the frequencies of complications such as pulp necrosis, pulp canal obliteration, root resorption and marginal breakdown are given. In the studies reported by the Copenhagen group (2, 4) and the Toronto group (5, 6) it should be noted that the latter group was confined to a pediatric population (children and adolescents).

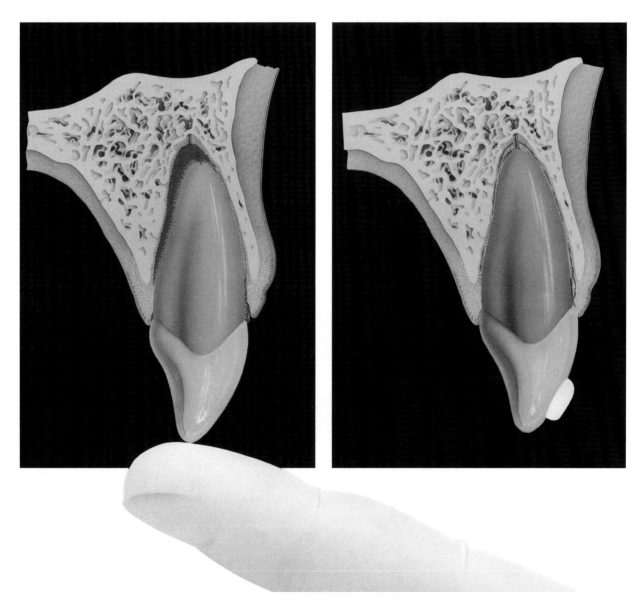

**Fig. 15.5** Treatment of extrusive luxation. The extruded tooth should be gently repositioned using axial finger pressure on the incisal edge and the tooth splinted.

**Fig. 15.6 Diagnosis and treatment of extrusive luxation**
This 17-year-old man has extruded the left central incisor and avulsed the lateral incisor, which could not be retrieved.

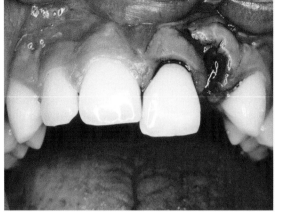
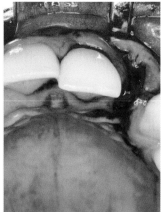

**Mobility and percussion test**
The tooth is very mobile and can be moved in horizontal and axial direction. The percussion test reveals slight tenderness and there is a dull percussion tone.

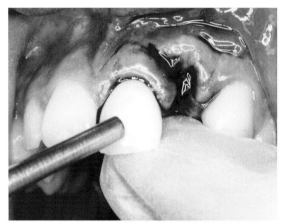
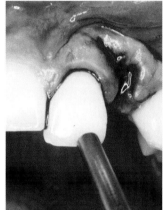

**Sensibility testing and radiographic examination**
The tooth does not respond to sensibility testing. The radiograph reveals coronal displacement of the tooth.

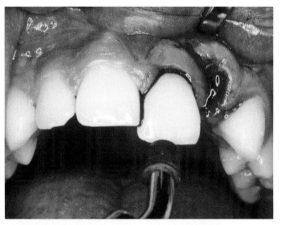
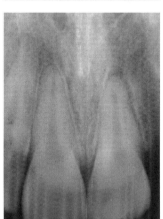

**Repositioning**
The tooth is gently pushed back into its socket. Thereafter the labial surfaces of both central incisors are etched in preparation for the splinting material.

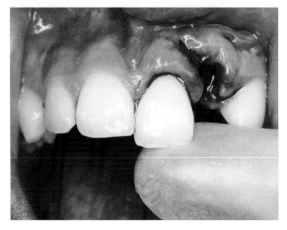
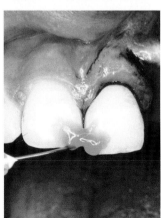

### Applying splinting material

After rinsing the labial surfaces with a water spray and drying with compressed air, the splinting material (Protemp®, Espe Corp.) is applied.

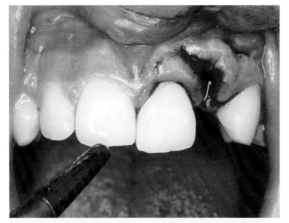
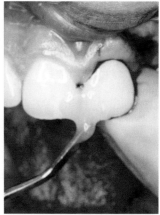

### Polishing the splint

The surface of the splint is smoothed with abrasive discs and contact with gingival removed with a straight scalpel blade.

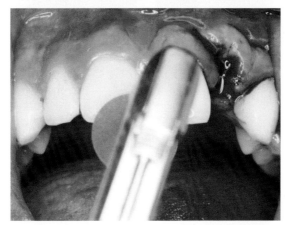
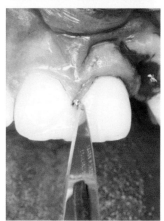

### The finished splint

Note that the splint allows optimal oral hygiene in the gingival region, which is the most likely port of entry for bacteria that may complicate periodontal and pulpal healing.

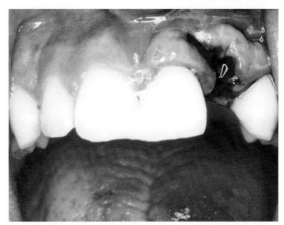
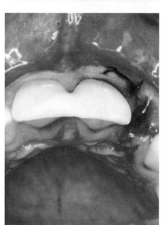

### Suturing the gingival wound

The gingival wound is closed with interrupted silk sutures. The final radiograph confirms optimal repositioning of the tooth.

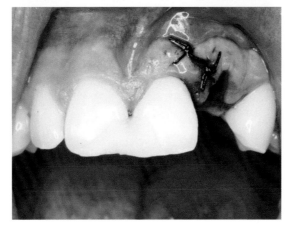
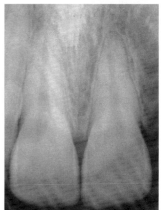

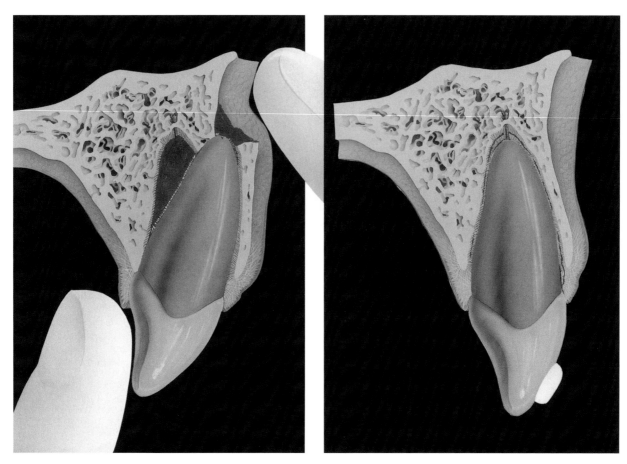

**Fig. 15.7** Treatment principles for extrusive luxation: repositioning and splinting.

## Pulp necrosis

### Extrusion

This complication appeared to be very dependent upon root development in the Copenhagen study, where immature root development had a superior healing potential compared to more mature root development (2, 4) (Table 15.1, Fig. 15.10).

### Lateral luxation

The same finding was made in regard to pulp necrosis (2, 4) (Table 15.2, Fig. 15.11).

## Pulp canal obliteration

### Extrusion

In cases where the pulp becomes revascularized, pulp canal obliteration was almost always a standard sequel to injury.

### Lateral luxation

The same finding was found as for extrusion.

## Root resorption (external)

### Extrusion

Surface resorption was quite common, inflammatory resorption rare. Ankylosis was not seen (2) (Fig. 15.12).

### Lateral luxation

The resorption pattern was quite similar to extrusions (Fig. 15.13). Ankylosis resorption was exceedingly rare and in these instances located to the cervical region, i.e. where the compression zones are located (2, 3) (Fig. 15.14).

Moreover, the frequent shortening of the root tips (i.e. surface resorption) appears to be related to the apical compression zone.

## Marginal bone loss

### Extrusion

As expected this trauma group showed no loss of marginal bone due to the limited nature of the injury (i.e. rupture of periodontal ligament) (Table 15.1).

**Fig. 15.8 Diagnosis and treatment of lateral luxation**
This 23-year-old man suffered a lateral luxation of the left central incisor.

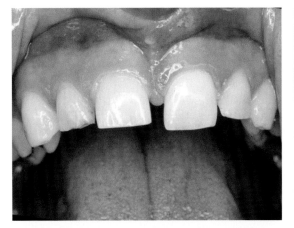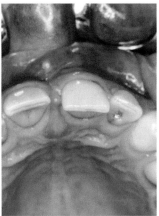

**Percussion test**
Percussion of the injured tooth reveals a high metallic sound.

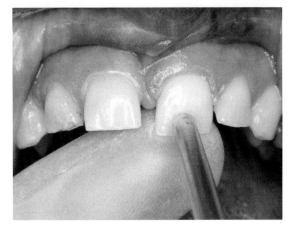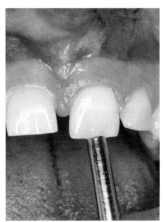

**Mobility and sensibility testing**
Mobility testing, using either digital pressure or alternating pressure of two instrument handles facially and orally, discloses no mobility of the injured tooth. There is no response to pulpal sensibility testing.

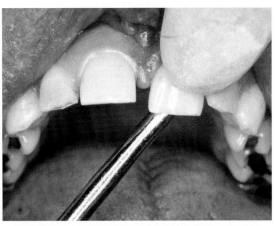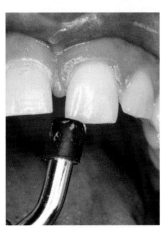

**Radiographic examination**
A steep occlusal radiographic exposure revealed, as expected, more displacement than the bisecting angle technique. A lateral radiograph reveals the associated fracture of the labial bone plate (arrow).

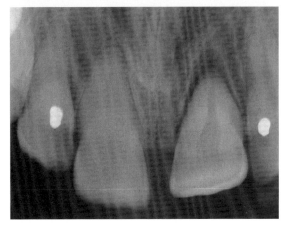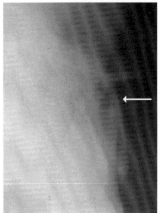

## Anesthesia

An infraorbital regional block is placed and supplemented with anesthesia of the nasopalatinal nerve.

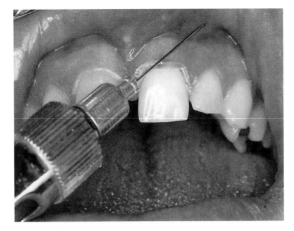
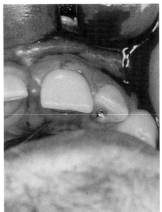

## Repositioning

The tooth is repositioned initially by forcing the displaced apex past the labial bone lock and thereby disengaging the root. Thereafter, axial pressure apically will bring the tooth back to its original position. It should be remembered that the palatal aspect of the marginal bone has also been displaced at the time of impact. This, too, must be repositioned with digital pressure to ensure optimal periodontal healing.

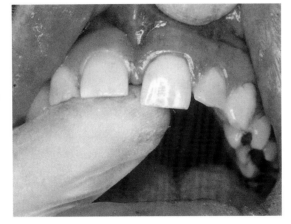
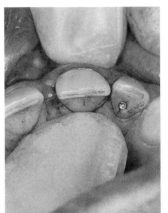

## Verifying repositioning and splinting with the acid-etch technique

Occlusion is checked and a radiograph taken to verify adequate repositioning. The incisal one-third of the labial aspect of the injured and adjacent teeth is acid-etched (30 seconds) with phosphoric acid gel.

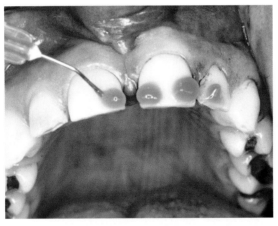
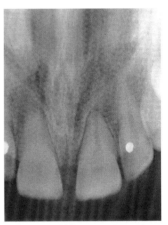

## Preparing the splinting material

The etchant is removed with a 20-second water spray. The labial enamel is dried with compressed air, revealing the matte, etched surface.

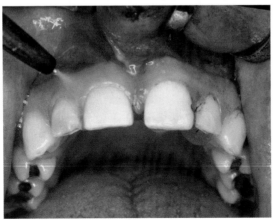
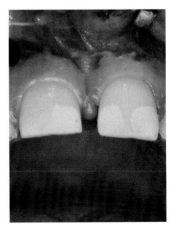

### Applying the splinting material

A temporary crown and bridge material (e.g. Protemp®) is then applied. Surplus material can be removed after polymerization using a straight scalpel blade or abrasive discs.

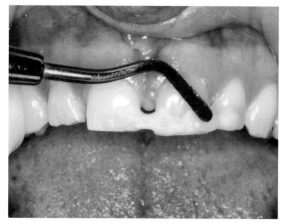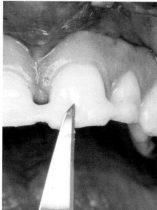

### Three weeks after injury

At this examination, a radiograph is taken to evaluate periodontal and pulpal healing. That is, neither periapical radiolucency nor breakdown of supporting marginal bone, as compared to the radiograph taken after repositioning.

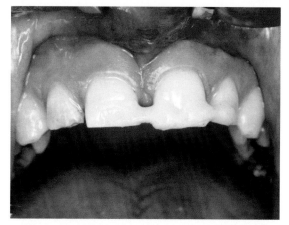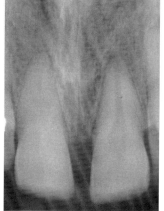

### Splint removal

The splint is removed using fissure burs, by reducing the splinting material interproximally and thereafter thinning the splint uniformly across its total span. Once thinned, the splint can be removed using a sharp explorer.

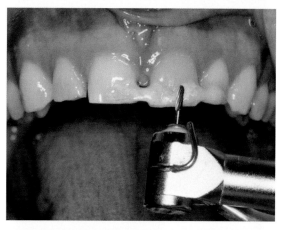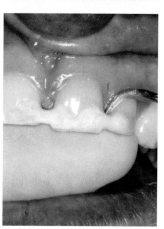

### Six months after injury

After 6 months, there is a slight sensibility reaction and normal radiographic conditions.

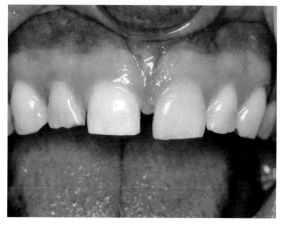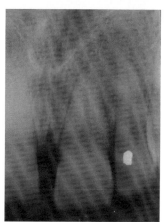

**Fig. 15.9 Non-repositioning of a laterally luxated central incisor which did not interfere with occlusion with spontaneous reposition.** Time of injury. Note the lingually displaced crown.

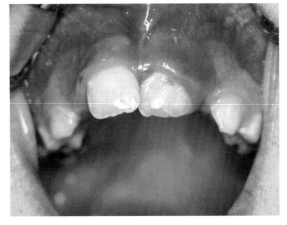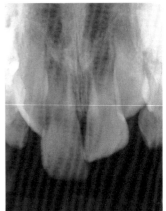

Axial clinical view and lateral radiograph

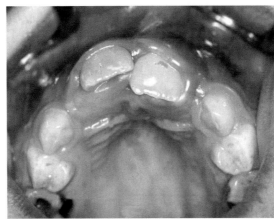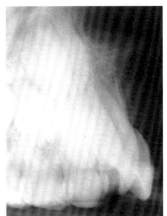

**Follow up** One year later, the tooth in its normal position. There is pulp canal obliteration.

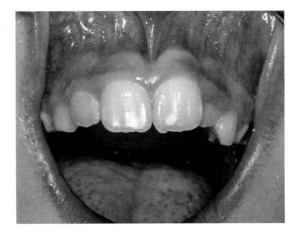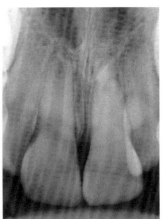

**Table 15.1** Pulp and periodontal healing complications following extrusive luxation.

| Author | Stage of root development | No. of teeth | Pulp necrosis | Pulp canal obliteration | Pulp survival | Root resorption | Marginal breakdown |
|---|---|---|---|---|---|---|---|
| Andreasen & Vestergaard Petersen (2) 1985, Andreasen (3) 1995 | Open apex | 34 | 3 (9%) | 20 (61%) | 10 (30%) | 4 (12%) | 3 (6%)** |
| | Closed apex | 20 | 11 (55%) | 4 (20%) | 15 (25%) | 4 (20%) | |
| Lee et al. (6)* 2003 | Open + closed apex | 54 | 23 (42%) | 19 (35%) | 12 (23%) | 3 (6%) | ? |

\*   Only children and adolescents.
\*\*  Open and closed apices.

**Table 15.2** Pulp and periodontal healing complications following lateral luxation.

| Author | Stage of root development | No. of teeth | Pulp necrosis | Pulp canal obliteration | Pulp survival | Root resorption | Marginal breakdown |
|---|---|---|---|---|---|---|---|
| Andreasen & Vestergaard Petersen (2) 1985, Andreasen (3) 1995 | Open apex | 34 | 3 (9%) | 24 (71%) | 7 (20%) | 3 (9%) | 9 (7%)** |
| | Closed apex | 88 | 68 (77%) | 10 (11%) | 10 (11%) | 34 (39%) | |
| Nikoui et al. (5)* 2003 | Open + closed apex | 58 | 23 (40%) | 23 (40%) | 12 (20%) | ? | ? |

\* Only children and adolescents.
\*\* Open and closed apices.

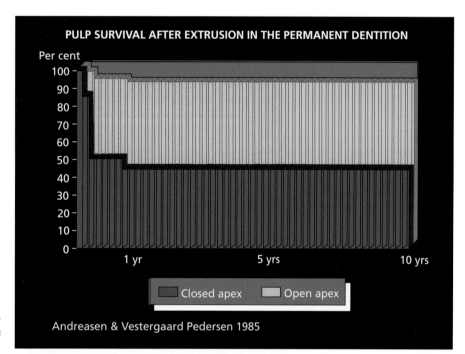

**Fig. 15.10** Pulpal healing after extrusive luxation. After ANDREASEN & VESTERGAARD PEDERSEN (2) 1985.

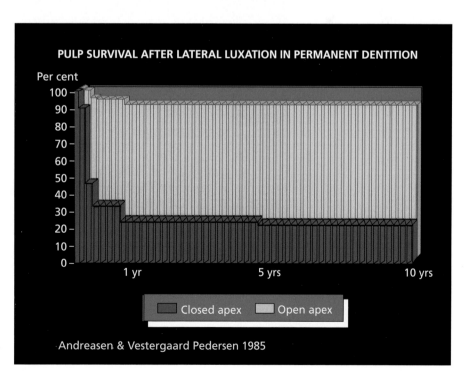

**Fig. 15.11** Pulpal healing after lateral luxation. After ANDREASEN & VESTERGAARD PEDERSEN (2) 1985.

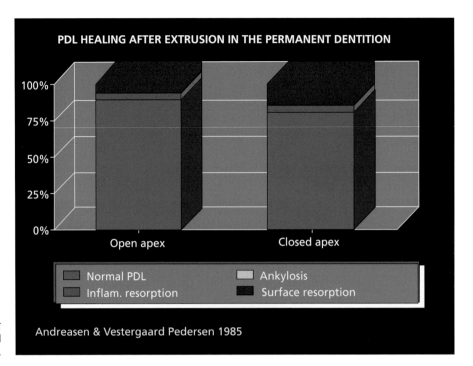

**Fig. 15.12** Periodontal healing after extrusive luxation. After ANDREASEN & VESTERGAARD PEDERSEN (2) 1985.

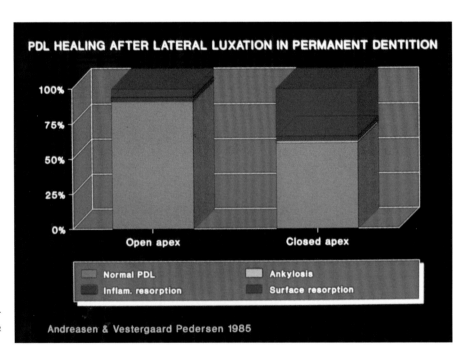

**Fig. 15.13** Periodontal healing after lateral luxation. After ANDREASEN & VESTERGAARD PEDERSEN (2) 1985.

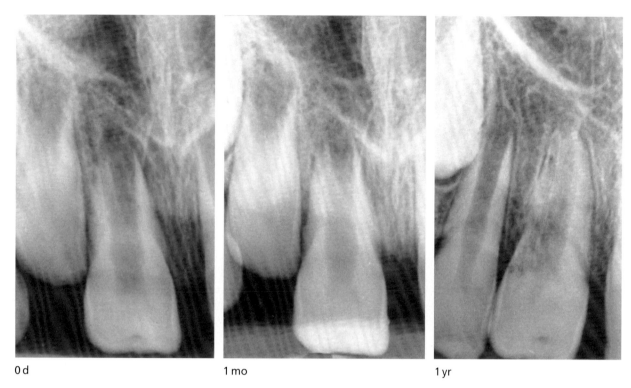

0 d                                    1 mo                                    1 yr

**Fig. 15.14** External replacement resorption of a central incisor as a sequel to lateral luxation. At the time of splint removal, one month after injury, there is no evidence of root resorption. At the one-year follow-up, ankylosis is evident distally.

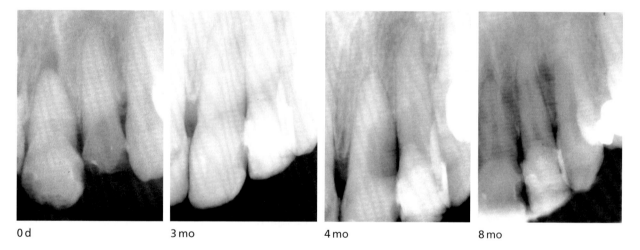

0 d                    3 mo                    4 mo                    8 mo

**Fig. 15.15** Transient marginal breakdown in a 46-year-old male who suffered lateral luxation of the left central incisor. Three months after reposition there is no sign of pathology. Four months after reposition a marked breakdown of bone is found between the central and the lateral incisor. Four months later the interdental bone has been reformed. Courtesy of Dr H LUND, Kolding, Denmark.

## Lateral luxation

In this trauma group loss of marginal bone was seen, which is explained by the compressive type of the injury in the cervical region (Table 15.2 and Fig. 15.15).

measuring the apical diameter (4). Moreover, it was found that increased age after completed root development was significantly related to pulp necrosis (2, 3). Figs 15.16 and 15.17 present the healing predictors for *extrusion* and *lateral luxation*.

## Predictors of healing

In a multivariate analysis, the only significant factors appeared to be the stage of root development (2, 3). The relation to root development could be further refined by

## Tooth survival

It appears from two clinical studies that excellent long-term survival can be expected for extrusions and lateral luxations (98% and 100% respectively) (5, 6).

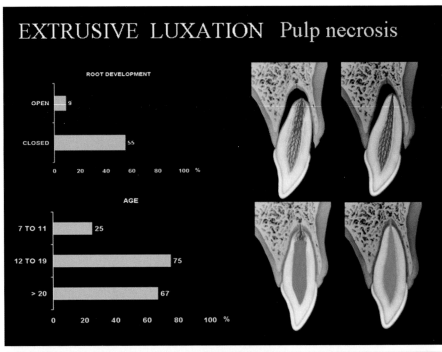

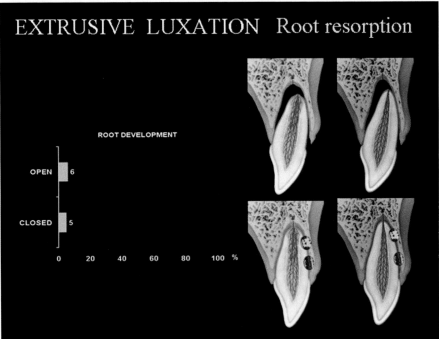

**Fig. 15.16** Predictors for healing outcome after extrusive luxation.

## Essentials

### Extrusive and lateral luxation

(1) Administer local anesthesia if forceful repositioning is anticipated (i.e. lateral luxation).

(2) Reposition the tooth into normal position (Figs 15.6 and 15.8). In case of delayed treatment, the teeth should be allowed to realign spontaneously into normal position or be moved orthodontically.

(3) Splint the tooth with an acid-etch/resin splint.

(4) Monitor the tooth radiographically.

(4) Splinting period:
　— Extrusion: 2–3 weeks.
　— Lateral luxation: 3 weeks. In case of marginal bone breakdown, extend fixation period to 6–8 weeks.

(5) Follow-up period: minimum 1 year.

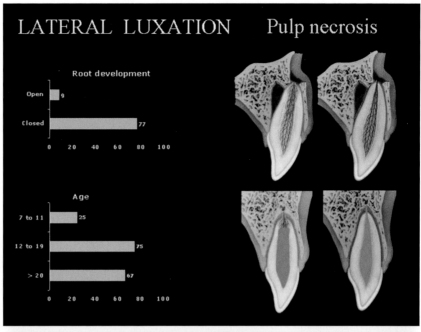

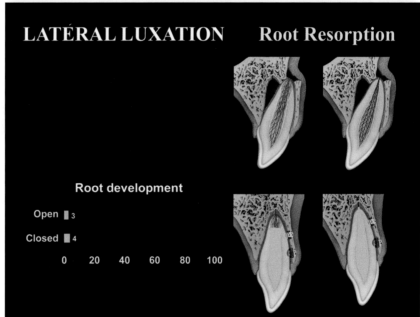

**Fig. 15.17** Predictors for healing outcome after lateral luxation.

## References

1. ANDREASEN FM, ANDREASEN JO. Diagnosis of luxation injuries. The importance of standardized clinical, radiographic and photographic techniques in clinical investigations. *Endodont Dent Traumatol* 1985;**1**:160–9.
2. ANDREASEN FM, VESTERGAARD PEDERSEN B. Prognosis of luxated permanent teeth – the development of pulp necrosis. *Endodont Dent Traumatol* 1985;**1**:207–20.
3. ANDREASEN FM. *Pulpal healing after luxation injuries and root fracture in the permanent dentition.* Thesis, Copenhagen University 1995. ISBN no. 87-985538-0-1.
4. ANDREASEN FM, YU Z, THOMSEN BL. The relationship between pulpal dimensions and the development of pulp necrosis after luxation injuries in the permanent dentition. *Endodont Dent Traumatol* 1986;**2**:90–8.

5. NIKOUI M, KENNY DJ, BARRETT EJ. Clinical outcomes for permanent incisor luxations in a pediatric population. III. Lateral luxations. *Dent Traumatol* 2003;**19**:280–5.
6. LEE R, BARRETT EJ, KENNY DJ. Clinical outcomes for permanent incisor luxations in a pediatric population. II. Extrusions. *Dent Traumatol* 2003;**19**:274–9.
7. BORUM MK, ANDREASEN JO. Therapeutic and economic implications of traumatic dental injuries in Denmark; an estimate based on 7549 patients treated at a major trauma centre. *Int J Paediat Dent* 2001;**11**:249–58.
8. SHIBUE T, TANIGUCHI K, MOTOKAWA W. Pulp and root development after partial extrusion in immature rat molars: a histopathological study. *Endodont Dent Traumatol* 1998;**14**:171–84.

# 16

# Intrusive Luxation

## J. O. Andreasen & F. M. Andreasen

## Definition

Intrusive luxation (intrusion) is displacement of the tooth into the alveolar bone along the axis of the tooth and is accompanied by comminution or fracture of the alveolar socket (Figs 16.1 and 16.2).

### Frequency

Intrusive luxations have been found to comprise 0.3–1.9% of the traumas affecting permanent teeth (1–5).

## Healing and pathology

An intrusion represents the most severe injury to the dentition through damage to the gingival attachment, contusion of the periodontal ligament and bone and damage to the Hertwig's epithelial root sheath (in the case of immature teeth). Moreover, the intrusive displacement of the tooth will force bacteria from the bacterial plaque covering the dental crown into the compromised wound site (Fig. 16.1). All of these events individually and combined have the potential of eliciting healing complications (see Chapter 2). It is, therefore, no wonder that intruded permanent teeth have a very grave long-term prognosis (20).

In regard to the histopathology changes after intrusion only a few experimental studies exist and studies have been made with rats (6, 7) and dogs (8–10), both models, which are not that comparable in relation to a human situation, due to significant differences in anatomy. In one study with dogs surgical repositioning was compared to spontaneous eruption. It was claimed that surgical repositioning showed more optimal healing but no histometric analysis was presented (10).

## Clinical findings

Due to their locked position in bone, most intruded teeth are not sensitive to percussion and are very firm in their socket (5). The extent of intrusion may vary from one millimeter to complete burial of the displaced tooth (5). The percussion test often elicits a high-pitched metallic sound, similar to an ankylosed tooth. This test is of great importance in determining whether erupting teeth are indeed intruded (5) (Fig. 16.1). A tooth which is completely buried in the alveolar process might be erroneously considered avulsed until a radiograph discloses the intruded position. Palpation of the alveolar process can often reveal the position of the displaced tooth.

If a permanent central incisor is completely intruded, it should be considered that the root apex is most likely forced

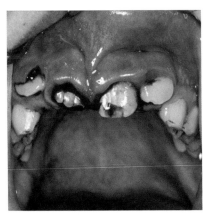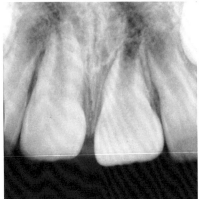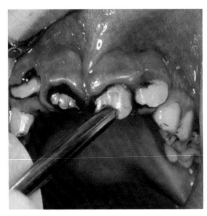

**Fig. 16.1** Intrusion of a tooth with incomplete root formation. The semi-erupted position of the tooth leaves doubt as to whether the tooth is under eruption or intruded from a more coronal position. A high percussion (ankylosis) tone, however, reveals the intrusion.

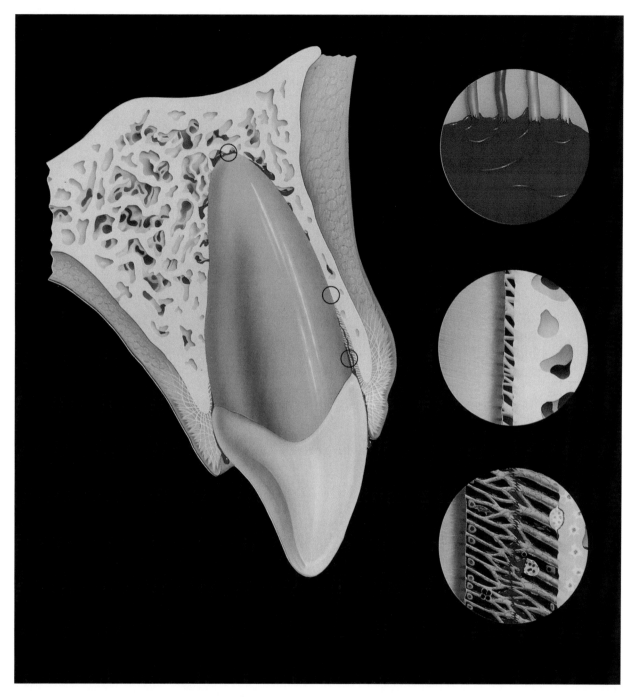

**Fig. 16.2** Pathogenesis of intrusion. Axial impact leads to extensive injury to the pulp and periodontium.

into the nasal cavity, resulting in bleeding from the nose. Examination of the floor of the nostril will reveal the protruding apex (Fig. 16.3).

## Radiographic findings

Following intrusive luxation, the periodontal ligament space will be partially or totally obliterated (5). However, it should be noted that in some cases of obvious displacement, a periodontal space of normal width can still be seen radiographically (5) (Fig. 16.4). In general, when the apex has been forced through the labial bone plate the intruded incisor will appear foreshortened when compared to the non-injured antimere (Fig. 16.5). Conversely an elongated tooth implies intrusion in the palatal direction (5).

A steep occlusal exposure gives a less reliable impression of the depth of intrusion compared to a conventional periapical (bisecting angle) exposure (Fig. 16.6). Another

**Fig. 16.3 Displacement of an intruded central incisor into the nasal cavity**
Clinical and radiographic condition. The tooth is completely intruded.

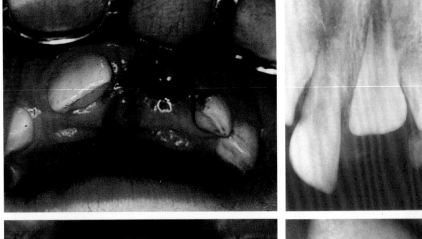

**Nasal inspection**
Inspection of the right nostril with a nasal speculum shows protrusion of the apex through the floor of the nose (arrow).

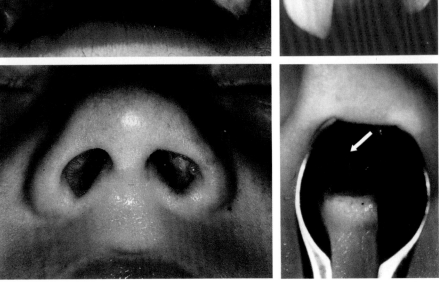

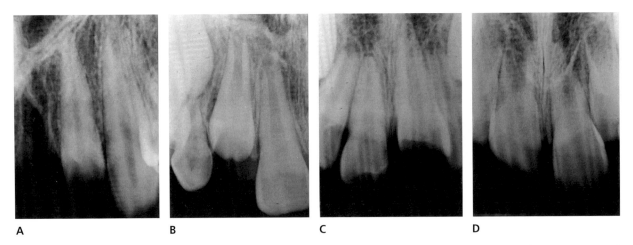

A                    B                    C                    D

**Fig. 16.4** Radiographic appearance of intrusions. A. Intrusive luxation of a lateral incisor. Note disappearance of the periodontal ligament space around the displaced tooth. B. Intruded lateral incisor Note that a periodontal space is present along most of the root surface. C and D. Intrusion of teeth with incomplete and complete root formation. Note the difference in position of the cemento-enamel junction compared with the adjacent tooth.

reliable finding in periapical exposures is the position of the cemento-enamel junction, which in erupted teeth is placed approximately one millimeter incisal to the bony crest (Fig. 16.7).

In the presence of an associated penetrating lip lesion, it is important to take a soft-tissue radiograph of the lip in order to diagnose embedded tooth fragments or other foreign bodies (Fig. 16.8) (see Chapter 21).

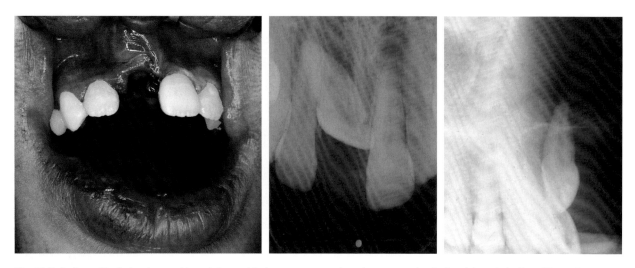

**Fig. 16.5** Radiographically foreshortened intruded central incisor appears on a lateral exposure to be displaced through the buccal bone plate.

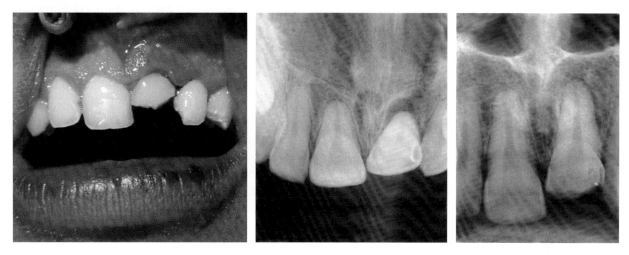

**Fig. 16.6** Radiographic appearance related to projection angle. A more steep exposure (i.e. an occlusal exposure) does not yield a reliable picture of the depth of intrusion compared to a periapical bisecting angle exposure.

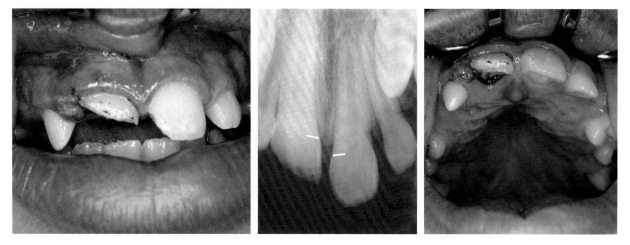

**Fig. 16.7** Slightly intruded permanent right central incisor. Note that the cemento-enamel border is positioned more apically than the non-injured antimere.

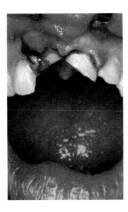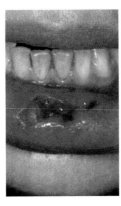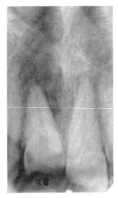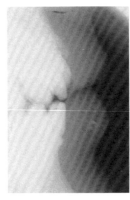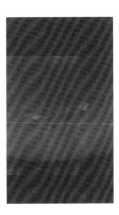

**Fig. 16.8** Diagnosis of foreign bodies in the lower lip in a case with combined intrusion injury and penetrating lip injury. Frontal and lateral radiographs disclose multiple foreign bodies in the lower lip.

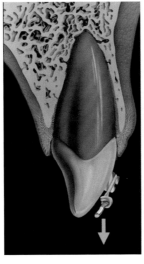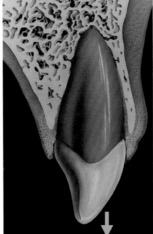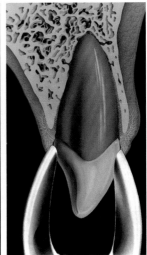

**Fig. 16.9** Treatment principles for intrusion: orthodontic extrusion, spontaneous eruption or surgical extrusion.

## Treatment

In the past, significant controversy has existed concerning the optimal treatment for intruded permanent teeth. (5, 11, 22) (Fig. 16.9). It has been found that intruded teeth with immature root formation may re-erupt spontaneously (11–14, 20, 21) and also in some cases with completed root formation (20–23). The advantage of this treatment philosophy has been that no additional damage due to active repositioning procedures is inflicted upon the already injured periodontium, a factor which should optimize marginal bone healing. This procedure has usually been confined to patients with immature root formation.

Realizing that spontaneous eruption can be unreliable, a second treatment philosophy has been to stimulate spontaneous re-eruption by orthodontically guided eruption (17).

Finally, surgical repositioning has been suggested, whereby the intruded tooth is brought back to its original position and splinted (11).

Today, no randomized study exists whereby the three treatment alternatives can be compared. However, in a large clinical retrospective study of 140 intruded teeth, the result of the three treatment models were compared with respect to pulp necrosis, root surface resorption and loss of marginal bone support.

The result of this study indicated that the stage of root development at the time of injury is the variable which dictates treatment alternative. In the case of immature root development, the treatment of choice appears to be anticipation of spontaneous eruption. However, it takes approximately 6 months for full eruption (ranges: 2–14 months) (21) (see below).

The general indication for orthodontic extrusion will be in cases with completed root formation. This strategy appears to result in slightly better bone healing. However, this treatment procedure implies significantly more treatment visits than surgical repositioning (21).

### Spontaneous re-eruption

This appears to be the treatment of choice for teeth with incomplete root formation. One prerequisite, however, is that the tooth is not totally intruded, i.e. including the incisal edge. If this is the case, the incisal edge must be exposed. Otherwise partial or total surgical repositioning should be carried out (21). To facilitate the re-eruption process, the

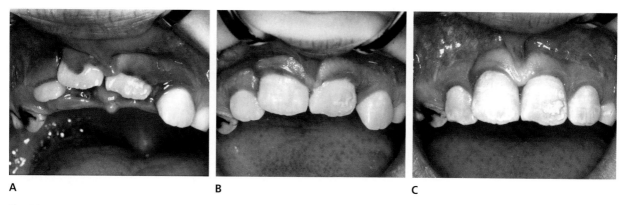

**Fig. 16.10** Spontaneous eruption of two intruded incisors. A. Clinical condition in a 7-year-old girl after an axial impact. B. Condition 6 weeks later, after onset of eruption. C. Follow-up 1 year after injury. Eruption is complete.

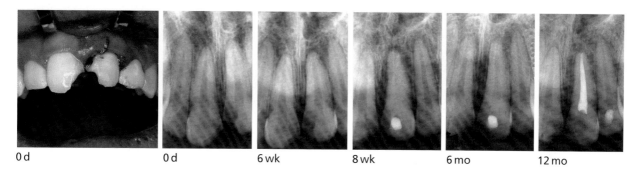

0 d                    0 d                    6 wk                    8 wk                    6 mo                    12 mo

**Fig. 16.11** Spontaneous eruption of an intruded left central incisor with mature root formation, and condition after 6 and 8 weeks and 6 and 12 months.

intruded tooth may be slightly loosened with forceps at the first visit (to release the mechanical grip of the bony walls on the root surface). Thereafter, re-eruption is awaited, which usually takes 6 months for completion (range = 2–14 months) (21) (Fig. 16.10).

If clinical and radiographic examination show no signs of re-eruption after one month, and particularly the percussion test shows signs of ankylosis, the tooth must be loosened with forceps and brought to occlusal height orthodontically. Throughout the eruption process, it is very important to monitor eventual signs of pulp necrosis and inflammatory root resorption. Suggested observation periods are listed in Appendix 3.

Spontaneous re-eruption has been found to take place up to the age of 17 years (Fig. 16.11). Beyond that age, active repositioning should be performed (21). However, in cases of completed root development, where there is a high risk of pulp necrosis and external root resorption, orthodontic extrusion is the treatment of choice (see below).

## Orthodontic extrusion

Ideally, orthodontic extrusion should be performed at a pace that keeps up with the repair of marginal bone. Furthermore, it is important that the tooth is sufficiently repositioned within 2–3 weeks to ensure access to the pulp chamber should endodontic treatment be necessary. In some cases a surgical exposure of the palatal crown surface

may enable access to the pulp. This is important, as external root resorption may be initiated by this time; and the only way to arrest this process is by endodontic therapy (see Chapter 22). This is also the reason for not awaiting spontaneous eruption in cases with completed root formation. As spontaneous re-eruption may take several months, root resorption can become quite advanced; and because of the semi-buried position of the tooth, there is no possibility of endodontic intervention.

Orthodontic movement of intruded permanent teeth can begin at the initial examination at the time of injury or some days later, when swelling has subsided (Fig. 16.12). The orthodontic appliances used for extrusion are similar to those used for extrusion of crown-root fractured teeth (see Chapter 24).

If the tooth has been completely intruded, it is essential that it is partially repositioned with a forceps after administration of local anesthesia so that half of the crown is exposed. This will hasten the final re-eruption and facilitate application of an orthodontic bracket on the labial surface. In some cases, it can be an advantage to luxate the tooth slightly prior to orthodontic extrusion. If this alternative is chosen, orthodontic extrusion should be postponed for a few days to avoid avulsion of the tooth upon activation of the appliance.

Compared to surgical repositioning, orthodontic extrusion appears to result in slightly improved marginal bone healing (21).

### Fig. 16.12 Orthodontic extrusion of an intruded incisor

Clinical and radiographic condition in a 22-year-old woman after an axial impact. Before application of orthodontic appliances the tooth may be slightly loosened with forceps.

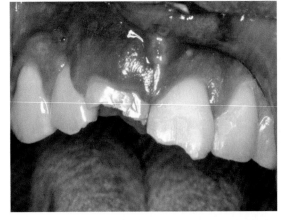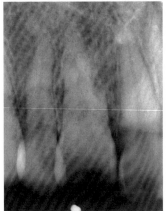

### Covering exposed dentin

The exposed dentin of both central incisors is covered with a hard-setting calcium hydroxide cement (e.g. Dycal®).

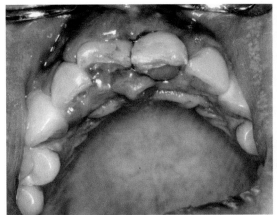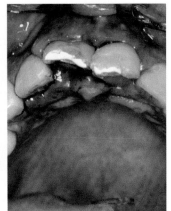

### Applying orthodontic traction

A 0.5 mm thick semi-rigid orthodontic wire is adapted to follow the curvature of the dental arch, including two adjacent teeth on either side of the intruded incisor. The orthodontic wire is bonded to the adjacent teeth using an acid-etch technique. In the area where elastic traction is exerted, a wire coil (e.g. 0.228 × 0.901 Elgiloy®) is placed in order to prevent slippage of the elastic.

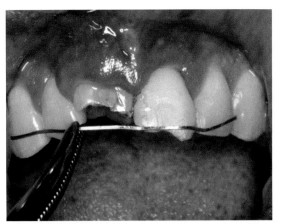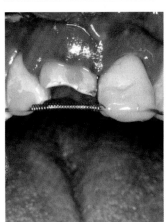

### Placing the bracket

The fractured incisal edge is covered with a temporary crown and bridge material. A bracket is placed on the labial surface.

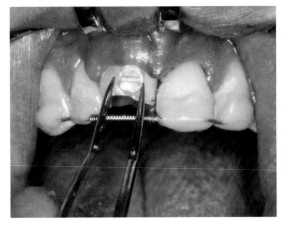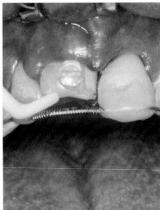

### Orthodontic traction

Elastic traction of 70–100 grams is activated. The direction of traction should extrude the tooth out of its socket in a purely axial direction. Elastic traction should wait for 4–6 days if loosening has been performed.

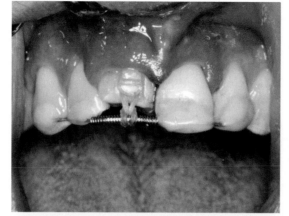
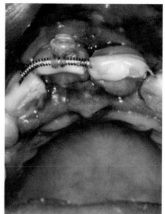

### Extrusion initiated

After approximately 10 days, osteoclastic activity around the intruded tooth has usually resulted in loosening; and extrusion can then take place. If extrusion has not yet begun after 10 days, a local anesthetic is administered and the tooth is luxated slightly with a forceps. After 2–3 weeks, a rubber dam is applied, the pulp extirpated and the root canal filled with calcium hydroxide paste.

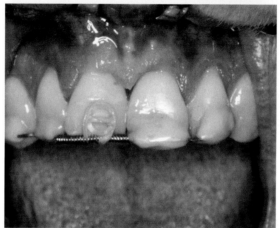
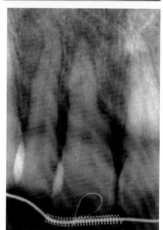

### Extrusion complete

After 4 weeks, the intruded tooth is extruded to its original position and retained in this position for 2–4 weeks. Thereafter, the orthodontic appliance can be removed.

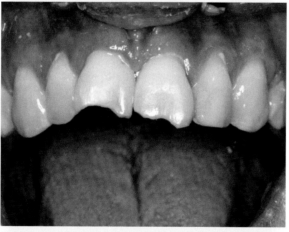
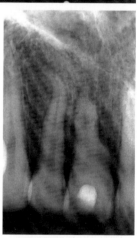

### Crown restoration

The fractured crowns are restored with composite resin.

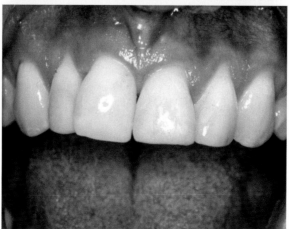
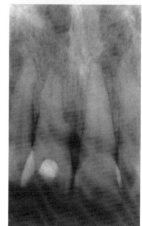

**Fig. 16.13** Surgical repositioning of an intruded left central incisor and repositioning and splinting of an extruded and root fractured right central incisor.

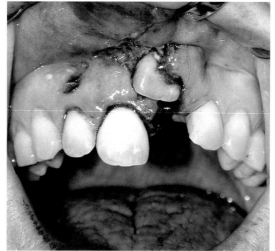
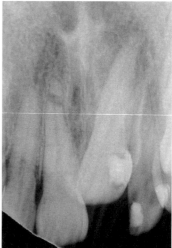

## Repositioning

After local anesthesia, the right central incisor is repositioned. The left central incisor is grasped proximally with forceps and repositioned. With finger pressure, the tooth is repositioned, as well as the displaced labial bone.

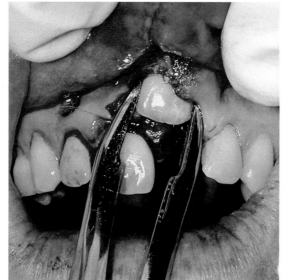
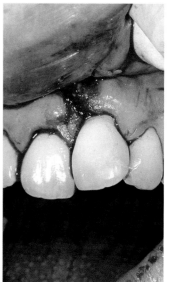

## Suturing and splinting

The lacerated gingiva is sutured. The incisal third of the labial enamel of all incisors is acid etched and splinting material applied.

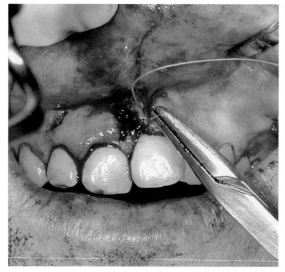
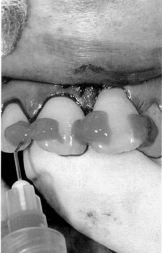

**Finishing the splint**
A Luxatemp® splint has been applied.

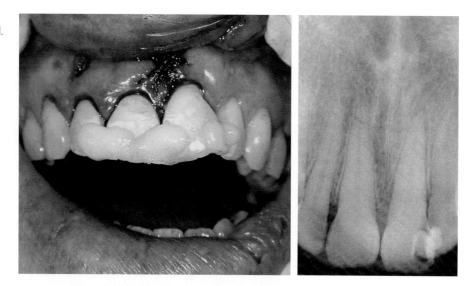

**Fig. 16.13** *Continued*

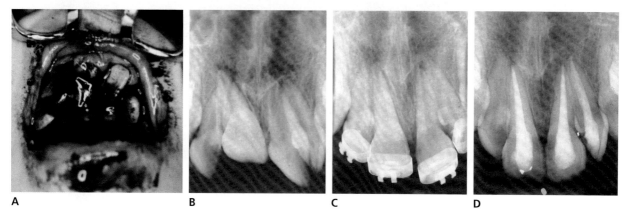

A                        B                          C                         D

**Fig. 16.14** Treatment of multiple severely displaced and intruded incisors. A, B and C. Multiple intrusions (three incisors) in a 10-year-old girl treated by surgical repositioning and splinting. D. Condition 6 months later. There is no evidence of root resorption.

## Surgical extrusion

This procedure implies immediate repositioning of the tooth into its normal position. After administration of local anesthesia, the tooth is grasped with a forceps (preferably proximally) and brought down into its normal position. Thereafter, the displaced labial and palatal bone is repositioned by finger pressure and gingival lacerations sutured (Fig. 16.13). A splint is applied and maintained for 6–8 weeks.

This procedure is primarily indicated in cases with *multiple intrusions* (Fig. 16.14) as well as in cases where the tooth is intruded more than *6 mm* (21). With multiple intrusions there may be difficulties in reaching stability after repositioning which must be taken into consideration when fabricating a splint, which has to be extended bilaterally to involve stable teeth.

## Treatment guidelines according to trauma scenario

In order to provide an evidence based treatment, certain pre-trauma and trauma factors must be incorporated in order to choose treatment alternative (i.e. spontaneous repositioning, orthodontic extrusion or surgical repositioning) (21).

Stage of root development (complete or incomplete) appears to be one of the strongest factors. In the case of incomplete root formation, the extent of intrusion becomes decisive. There is a cut-off at ages 12 years and >17 years with respect to choice of treatment; and whether there is one intruded tooth or multiple intrusions.

It should be noted that these treatment guidelines are only partially supported by a clinical study (21) (Fig. 16.15).

## Prognosis

A number of studies have been carried out on the long-term prognosis after intrusive luxation. All of these studies indicate that severe complications dominate the healing pattern (Table 16.1). Especially the frequent occurrence of pulp necrosis in teeth with immature root formation, external root resorption and loss of marginal bone are of concern, as these complications may lead to tooth loss (17, 18, 20, 21).

## Treatment Suggestions According to Trauma Scenario

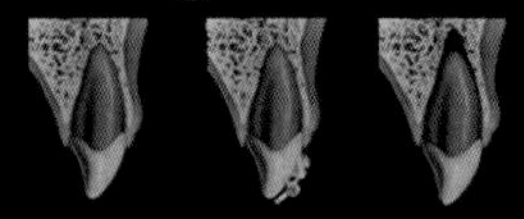

| | Age | | Reposition | | |
|---|---|---|---|---|---|
| | | | Spontaneous | Orthodontic | Surgical |
| 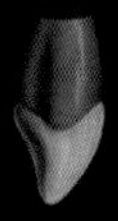 Root development incomplete | 6-11 years | Up to 7 mm | xxxx | | |
| | | More than 7 mm | xxxx | x | xx |
| 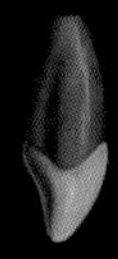 Root development complete | 12-17 years | Up to 7 mm | xxx | | |
| | | More than 7 mm | | x | xx |
| | More than 17 years | Up to 7 mm | | x | xx |
| | | More than 7 mm | | x | xx |

**XXXX**  Treatment procedure significantly the best
**XXX**   Treatment procedure has a tendency for better healing
**XX**    Treatment procedure practical to use in relation to the endodontic procedure and for simplicity of treatment
**X**     Treatment procedure acceptable

**Fig. 16.15** Treatment related to trauma scenario.

## Diagnosis of healing complications

### Pulp necrosis (PN)

It appears from Fig. 16.16 that PN is significantly related to stage of root development and can in most cases be diagnosed within 6 months after injury (6). However, in some cases a late diagnosis of PN is made due to the effect of partial pulp necrosis, whereby Hertwig's epithelial root sheath closes the root apex with hard tissue irrespective of necrotic root canal contents (see also Chapter 22) (Fig. 16.17).

### Root resorption (RR)

The most frequent type of root resorption appears to be inflammatory, followed by replacement resorption (ankylosis) and surface resorption (20).

In case of inflammatory root resorption, the resorption process can be arrested in the majority of cases by endodontic therapy (see Chapter 22, p. 632).

In approximately one-fourth of all cases with replacement resorption, the resorptive process appears to be transient.

From Fig. 16.18 it appears that the diagnosis RR is related to stage of root development; and that most cases can be diagnosed within the first year. While a relatively stable plateau of healing takes place up to 5 years after injury of immature teeth, new RR activity can be found up to 10 years after injury.

### Marginal bone loss

Marginal bone loss is a frequent complication and is related to stage of root development (Fig. 16.19).

Marginal bone loss may be transient in nature (Fig. 16.20). This phenomenon is further described in Chapter 13. Furthermore, bone loss is found on 'proximal' surfaces compared to distal in cases of multiple intrusions (20, 21) (Fig. 16.21).

The majority of marginal bone loss takes place in cases of incomplete root development within the first four years after injury; whereas teeth with completed root formation show a constant amount of bone loss throughout the observation period.

### Survival of intruded teeth

Two studies provide data which enables survival curves to be constructed. In both studies, long-term survival appears far from optimal (16, 18, 21).

It appears from Fig. 16.22 that there is rather constant loss of teeth throughout the observation period for teeth with incomplete and completed root formation. The choice of treatment procedure seems to favor spontaneous eruption and orthodontic repositioning (Fig. 16.23). Furthermore, approximately 30% are lost after 15 years irrespective of root development.

**Table 16.1** Clinical studies on prognosis of intrusion of permanent teeth.

| | No. of teeth | Age mean (range) | Tooth survival | Pulp necrosis | Root resorption | Loss of marginal bone |
|---|---|---|---|---|---|---|
| Andreasen (11) 1970 | 23 | | ? | 22 (96%) | 12 (52%) | 11 (48%) |
| Andreasen & Vestergaard Pedersen (12) 1985 | 61 | (6–67) | ? | 52 (85%) | 40 (66%) | 19 (31%) |
| Jacobsen (13, 14) 1983, 1991 | 40 | 8.0 (6–16) | 36 (90%) | 25 (63%) | ? | ? |
| Kinirons & Sutcliffe (15) 1991 | 29 | 9.5 (7–12) | 20 (69%) | ? | 11 (38%) | 7 (24%) |
| Ebeseleder et al. (16) 2000 | 58 | 11.1 (6–16) | 55 (95%) | 36 (64%) | 18 (31%) | 20 (34%) |
| Al-Badri et al. (17) 2002 | 61 | 9.3 (7.1–14) | 48 (79%) | ? | 36 (59%) | ? |
| Humphrey et al. (18) 2003 | 31 | 9.3 (6–18) | 26 (83%) | 14 (45%) | 25 (80%) | 12 (39%) |
| Chaushu et al. (19) 2004* | 31 | 8–11 | 28 (90%) | 26 (83%) | 13 (41%) | 2 (6%) |
| Andreasen et al. (20) 2005 | 140 | 15.6 (6–67) | 112 (80%) | 124 (88%) | 67 (48%) | 45 (32%) |

\* Including 22 case reports from the literature and all treated by orthodontic extrusion.

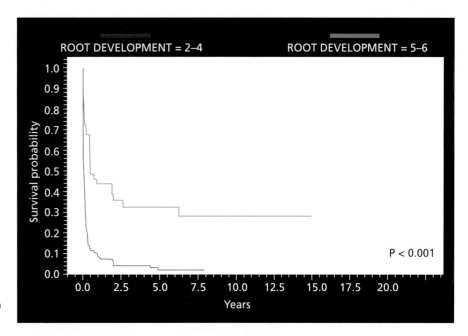

**Fig. 16.16** Pulp necrosis related to root development.

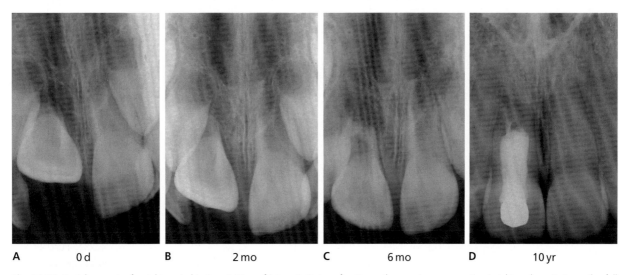

**Fig. 16.17** Partial necrosis of a right central incisor. A. Time of injury. B. Status after 2 months: spontaneous eruption is taking place. C. 6 months: full eruption and apical closure. The coronal part of the pulp has developed pulp. D. Status after 10 years.

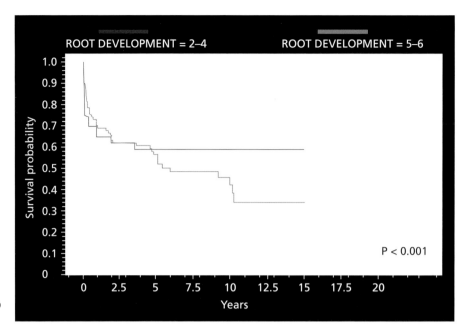

**Fig. 16.18** Root resorption related to root development.

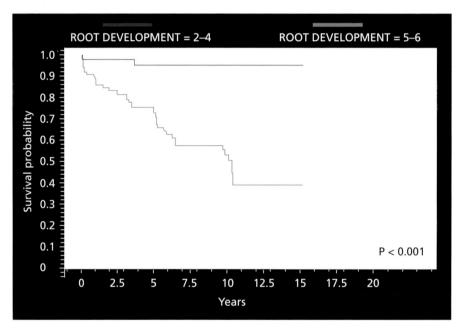

**Fig. 16.19** Marginal bone loss related to root development.

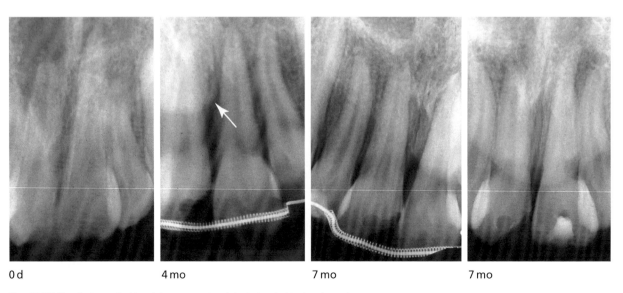

0 d               4 mo               7 mo               7 mo

**Fig. 16.20** Transient marginal breakdown around an intruded central incisor (arrow).

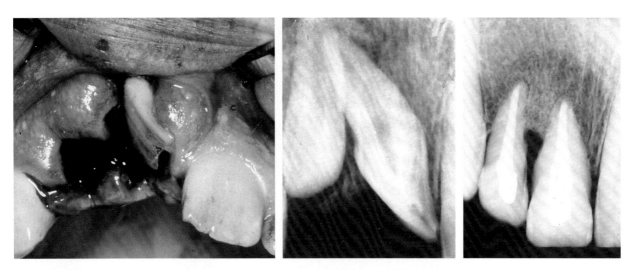

**Fig. 16.21** Multiple intrusions in a 16-year-old boy. More marginal bone loss is found 'proximally'.

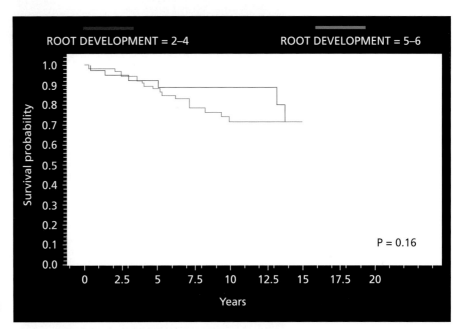

**Fig. 16.22** Tooth loss related to root development.

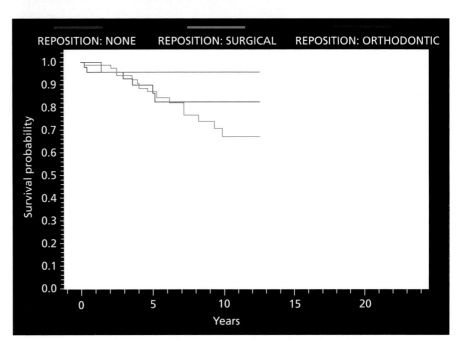

**Fig. 16.23** Tooth loss related to treatment procedure.

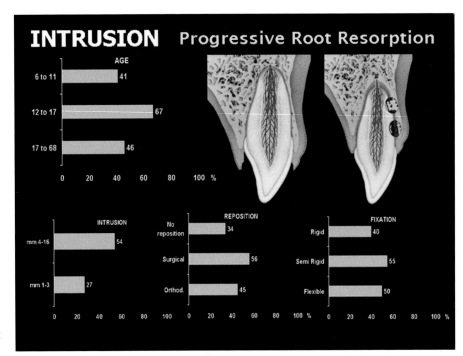

**Fig. 16.24** Predictors for root resorption.

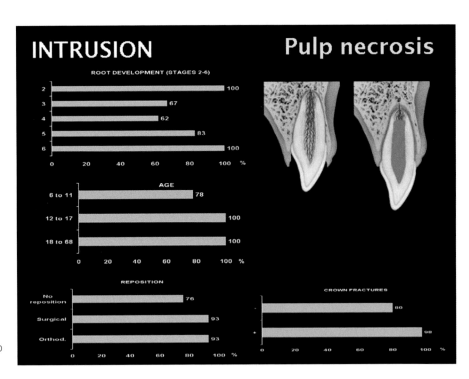

**Fig. 16.25** Predictors for pulp healing.

## Predictors for healing

Two recent studies have isolated a number of predictors for pulp necrosis, root surface resorption and loss of marginal bone support.

These predictors are shown in Figs 16.24 and 16.25. It appears that *stage of root development*, *extent of intrusion* and *method of repositioning* contained the greatest information about the risk of complications.

## Essentials

### Treatment alternatives

- *Spontaneous repositioning* should be anticipated in all teeth with incomplete root formation.
- *Surgical repositioning* is the treatment of choice in case of multiple intrusions and/or deep intrusions (i.e. >7 mm).
- *Orthodontic extrusion* is to be preferred over surgical repositioning due to slightly improved marginal bone healing.

However, this treatment alternative may complicate later endodontic intervention due to the position of the intruded tooth.

- *Suture* gingival lacerations.
- Conduct *radiographic controls* during the re-eruption phase.
- If signs of periapical radiolucency and/or inflammatory resorption are seen, *endodontic treatment* is indicated. In cases of completed root formation, prophylactic pulp extirpation is indicated with gutta-percha root filling and sealer.

# References

1. ANDREASEN JO, RAVN JJ. Epidemiology of traumatic dental injuries to primary and permanent teeth in a Danish population sample. *Int J Oral Surg* 1972;**1**:235–9.
2. GLENDOR U, HALLING A, ANDERSSON L, EILERT PETERSSON E. Incidence of traumatic tooth injuries in children and adolescents in the country of Västmanland, Sweden. *Swed Dent J* 1996;**20**:15–28.
3. BORSEN E, HOLM A-K. Traumatic dental injuries in a cohort of 16-year-olds in northern Sweden. *Endod Dent Traumatol* 1997;**13**:276–80.
4. SKAARE AB, JACOBSEN L. Dental injuries in Norwegians aged 7–18 years. *Dent Traumatol* 2003;**19**:67–71.
5. ANDREASEN JO, BAKLAND L, MATRAS R, ANDREASEN FM. Traumatic intrusion of permanent teeth. Part 1. An epidemiologic study of 216 intruded teeth. *Dent Traumatol* 2006;**22**:83–9.
6. MIYASHIN M, KATO J, TAKAGI Y. Experimental luxation injuries in immature rat teeth. *Endod Dent Traumatol* 1990;**6**:121–8.
7. MIYASHIN M, KATO J, TAKAGI Y. Tissue reaction after experimental luxation injuries in immature rat teeth. *Endod Dent Traumatol* 1991;**7**:26–35.
8. TURLEY PK, CRAWFORD LB, CARRINGTON KW. Traumatically intruded teeth. *Angle Orthod* 1987;**57**:234–44.
9. TURLEY PK, JOINER MW, HELLSTRÖM S. The effect of orthodontic extrusion on traumatically intruded teeth. *Am J Orthod* 1984;**85**:47–56.
10. CUNHA RF, PAVARINI A, PERCINOTO C, LIMA JE. Pulp and periodontal reactions of immature permanent teeth in the dog to intrusive trauma. *Endod Dent Traumatol* 1995;**11**:100–4.
11. ANDREASEN JO. Luxation of permanent teeth due to trauma. *Scand J Dent Res* 1970;**78**:273–86.
12. ANDREASEN FM, VESTERGAARD-PEDERSEN B. Prognosis of luxated permanent teeth – the development of pulp necrosis. *Endod Dent Traumatol* 1985;**207**:207–20.
13. JACOBSEN I. Clinical follow-up study of permanent incisors with intrusive luxation after acute trauma. *J Dent Res* 1983;**62**:486, abstract no. 37.
14. JACOBSEN I. Long-term prognosis of traumatized teeth in children and adolescents. In: Andreasen JO, Andreasen FM, Sjöström O, Eriksson B, eds. *Proceedings of the 2nd International Conference on Dental Trauma*. Stockholm: Bohusläningens Boktryckeri, 1991:44–52.
15. KINIRONS MJK, SUTCLIFFE J. Traumatically intruded permanent incisors: a study of treatment and outcome. *Br Dent J* 1991;**170**:144–6.
16. EBESELEDER KA, SANTIER G, GLOCKNER K, HULLA H, PERTL C, QUENHENBERGER F. An analysis of 58 traumatically intruded and surgically extruded permanent teeth. *Endod Dent Traumatol* 2000;**16**:34–9.
17. AL-BADRI S, KINIRONS M, COLE BOI, WELBURY RR. Factors afflicting resorption in traumatically intruded permanent incisors in children. *Dent Traumatol* 2002;**18**:73–6.
18. HUMPHREY JM, KENNY DJ, BARRETT EJ. Clinical outcomes for permanent incisor luxations in a pediatric population. I. Intrusions. *Dent Traumatol* 2003;**19**:266–73.
19. CHAUSHU S, SHAPIRO J, HELING J, BECKER A. Emergency orthodontic treatment after the traumatic intrusive luxation of maxillary incisors. *Am J Orthod Dentofacial Orthop* 2004;**126**:162–72.
20. ANDREASEN JO, BAKLAND L, ANDREASEN FM. Traumatic intrusion of permanent teeth. Part 2. A clinical study of the effect of preinjury and injury factors, such as sex, age, stage of root development, tooth location, and extent of injury including number of intruded teeth on 140 intruded permanent teeth. *Dent Traumatol* 2006;**22**:90–8.
21. ANDREASEN JO, BAKLAND L, ANDREASEN FM. Traumatic intrusion of permanent teeth. Part 3. A clinical study of the effect of treatment variables such as treatment delay, method of repositioning, type of splint, length of splinting and antibiotics on 140 teeth. *Dent Traumatol* 2006;**22**:99–111.
22. KINIRONS MJ. Treatment of traumatically intruded permanent incisor teeth in children. *Int J Paed Dent* 1998;**8**:165–8.
23. FARIA G, SILVA RAB, FIORI-JUNIOR M, NELSON-FILHO P. Re-eruption of traumatically intruded mature permanent incisor: case report. *Dent Traumatol* 2004;**20**:229–32.
24. OULIS C, VADIAKAS AG, SISKOS G. Management of intrusive luxation injuries. *Endod Dent Traumatol* 1996;**12**:113–19.

# 17
# Avulsions

J. O. Andreasen & F. M. Andreasen

## Terminology, frequency and etiology

*Tooth avulsion* (exarticulation, total luxation) implies total displacement of the tooth out of its socket (Figs 17.1 and 17.2).

Various statistics have shown that avulsion of teeth following traumatic injuries is relatively infrequent, ranging from 0.5 to 3% of traumatic injuries in the permanent dentition (125, 126). The main etiologic factors in the *permanent dentition* are fights and sports injuries (1, 127).

## Clinical findings

The maxillary central incisors are the most frequently avulsed teeth, while the lower jaw is seldom affected (6–8, 128, 129, 199–203).

Avulsion of teeth occurs most often in children from 7 to 9 years of age, when the permanent incisors are erupting (6–8, 199–203) (Fig. 17.1). At this age, the loosely structured periodontal ligament and low mineralized bone surrounding erupting teeth provide only minimal resistance to an extrusive force.

Most frequently, avulsion involves a single tooth; but multiple avulsions are occasionally encountered (6–8, 199–202). Other types of injuries are often associated with avulsions; among these, fractures of the alveolar socket wall and injuries to the lips are the most common (1). The level of the attachment apparatus of the avulsed tooth is essential when considering whether or not to replant the tooth. The presence of a ring of calculus or discoloration of the root surface is a good indicator (Fig. 17.3). Also, the contamination of the root surface should be registered, as this might influence healing. The circumstances related to extra-oral storage of the avulsed tooth should be noted such as extra-oral time and storage conditions; especially whether the tooth has been kept dry or under physiological conditions (Fig. 17.4).

## Radiographic findings

In cases where the avulsed tooth is found, radiographs should only be taken if the clinical examination arouses suspicion of bone fracture (Figs 17.5 and 17.6). Moreover in cases where the 'avulsed' tooth is not found there is an indication for radiographic examination since a fractured root may be left in the alveolus.

## Healing and pathology

The pathology of tooth replantation can be divided into pulpal and periodontal reactions. Both the pulp and the periodontal ligament suffer extensive damage during an extra-alveolar period with healing reactions almost entirely dependent upon the extra-alveolar period and extra-alveolar handling (Fig. 17.2).

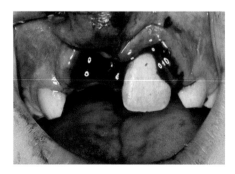
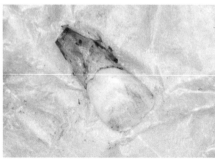

**Fig. 17.1** Avulsed central incisor in a 7-year-old boy. The tooth has been wrapped in paper for 60 minutes.

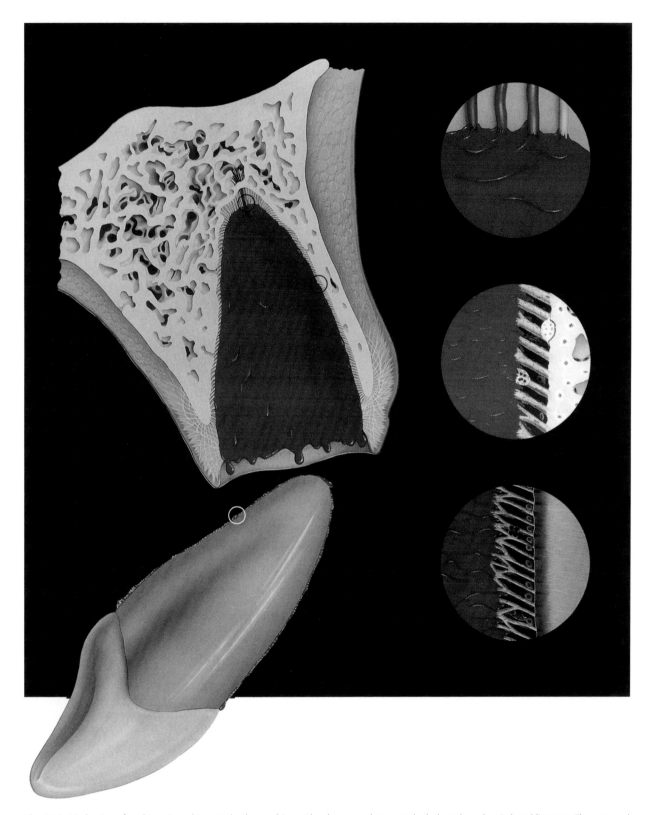

**Fig. 17.2** Mechanism of avulsion. Frontal impacts lead to avulsion with subsequent damage to both the pulp and periodontal ligament. The extra-oral time and environment determines the fate of the PDL and pulp after replantation.

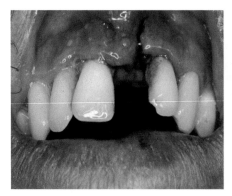
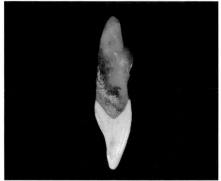

**Fig. 17.3** A ring of calculus on the root surface indicates the level of PDL attachment.

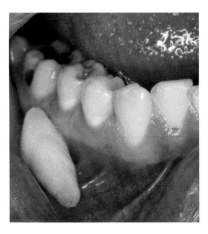
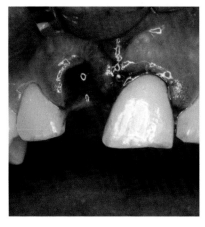
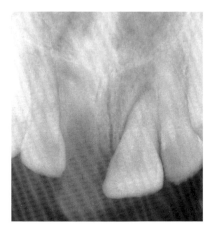

**Fig. 17.4** An avulsed central incisor is kept moist in saliva in the vestibulum.

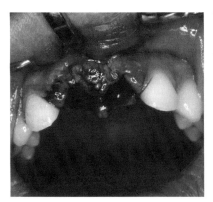
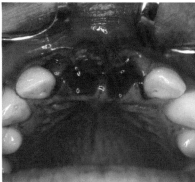
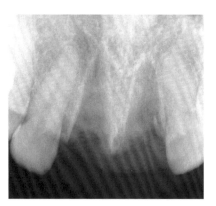

**Fig. 17.5** Contusion and fracture of the socket of two maxillary central incisors.

The healing reactions after replantation of teeth have been the subject of numerous experiments using mice (35), hamsters (36–42), rats (167–169, 309), guinea pigs (170), rabbits (27), cats (204–208), dogs (9–29, 130–137, 209–212, 306) and monkeys (17, 24, 31–34, 138–166, 213–226).

## Pulpal reactions

Studies on *pulp reactions* have mainly been performed in animals such as cats (204, 205), dogs (136, 137, 209–212)

and monkeys (225, 226). Experimental studies have disclosed various distinct pulpo-dentinal responses which can occur after immediate replantation and have been classified as follows (29) (Fig. 17.7):

(1) Regular tubular reparative dentin
(2) Irregular reparative dentin with diminished tubular structures
(3) Irregular reparative dentin with encapsulated cells (osteodentin)
(4) Irregular immature bone
(5) Regular lamellated bone or cementum

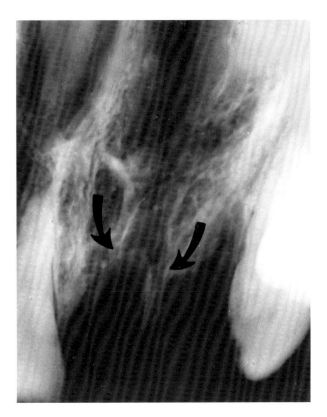

**Fig. 17.6** Radiograph illustrating an alveolar fracture (arrows) following avulsion of both central incisors.

(6) Internal resorption

(7) Pulp necrosis.

It is uncertain whether all of these reactions are encountered in humans; however, pulpal reactions observed in human patients after intentional replantation seem to support at least part of this classification (229).

Several comprehensive studies of pulp reactions of extracted and immediately replanted permanent premolars in human patients have been published (43, 227–229). Extensive pulpal changes could be observed as early as 3 days after replantation. The most severe damage was usually observed in the coronal part of the pulp. Signs of healing were seen within 2 weeks after replantation. Damaged coronal pulp tissue was gradually replaced by proliferating mesenchymal cells and capillaries (Figs 17.8 and 17.9). In the border zone between vital and necrotic tissue, neutrophils and round cells were present in some cases.

In the majority of cases with long observation periods, more advanced healing was found. This healing process led to the formation of a new cell layer along the dentinal wall in regions where the odontoblasts had been destroyed. The mesenchymal cells along the dentinal wall usually did not have processes extending into the dentinal tubules (Fig. 17.9). New hard tissue formation along the dentinal walls was noted after 17 days; but in most cases matrix formation started somewhat later. In the early stages of

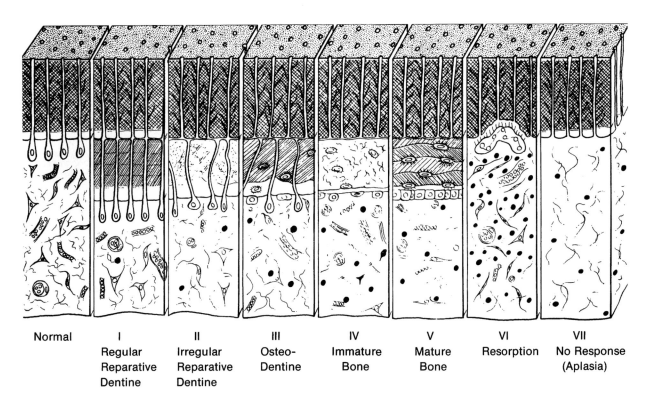

|  | I | II | III | IV | V | VI | VII |
|---|---|---|---|---|---|---|---|
| Normal | Regular Reparative Dentine | Irregular Reparative Dentine | Osteo-Dentine | Immature Bone | Mature Bone | Resorption | No Response (Aplasia) |

**Fig. 17.7** Schematic drawing illustrating the various pulp reactions following experimental replantation of incisors in dogs. From ANDERSON et al. (29) 1968.

**Fig. 17.8** A. Diagram illustrating initial pulp changes after replantation in humans. N = necrotic pulp tissue, M = mesenchymal cells, H = healing zone, P = preserved vital pulp tissue. M. Proliferating mesenchymal cells along the root canal wall at the level of necrotic and vital pulp tissue 10 days after replantation. ×410. C. Karyorrhexis and pyknosis in the coronal part of the pulp 3 days after replantation. ×200. From ÖHMAN (43) 1965.

A

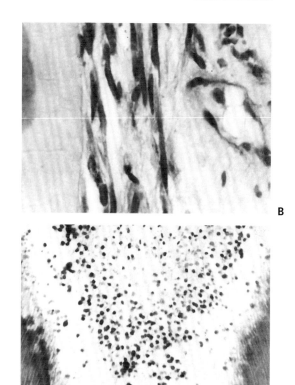

B

C

**Fig. 17.9** A. Diagram illustrating intermediate pulp changes after replantation in humans. New mesenchymal cells proliferate into the injured zones during the first months of the healing period. R = regenerated pulp tissue, P = preserved vital pulp tissue. B. The cells adjacent to the predentin in the apical part of the pulp appear to send no processes into the dentinal tubules (observation period = 17 days). ×430. C. Regenerated pulp cells are aligned nearly parallel with the long axis of the tooth. ×520. From ÖHMAN (43) 1965.

A

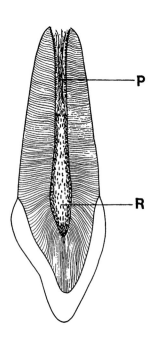

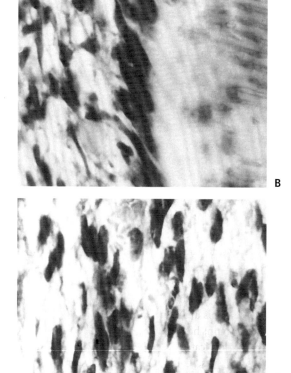

B

C

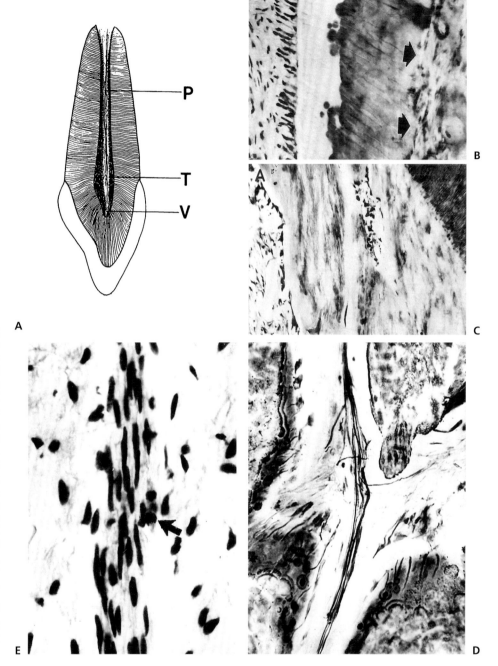

**Fig. 17.10** A. Diagram illustrating late pulp changes after replantation in humans. Extensive obliteration of the pulp chamber with hard tissue and strands of vital pulp tissue extending into the hard tissue. V = vital regenerated pulp tissue, T = newly formed hard tissue, P = preserved vital pulp tissue. B. Two phases of repair. First, irregular atubular matrix (arrows), second atubular dentin (observation period = 101 days). ×180. C. Irregular new hard tissue formation in an area with severe pulp damage (observation period = 158 days). ×125. D. Nerve fibers coursing through newly formed hard tissue in the pulp chamber (observation period = 360 days). Palmgren's silver stain. ×275. E. Nerve fibers with mitosis of Schwann cells (arrow) (observation period = 14 days). ×450. From ÖHMAN (43) 1965.

healing, a tissue was formed without dentinal tubules but with occasional cell inclusions (Fig. 17.10). Gradually, the cells along the pulp walls began to show similarities to odontoblasts with cytoplasmic processes within the newly formed matrix. This apparently corresponded to the degree of differentiation; however, in areas where new hard tissue formation indicated total primary destruction of the original odontoblasts, completely normal conditions were never found.

Severe primary pulpal damage was more often found in teeth with completed root formation than in those with an open apex, where the pulpal repair seemed also to be more rapid. Mitoses were seen in bands of Schwann cells 14 days after replantation (Fig. 17.10). Regenerating nerve fibers were observed after 1 month. In teeth with irregular hard tissue formation in the pulp chamber, bundles of nerve fibers passed between the trabeculae of hard tissue; separate fibers could be followed to the newly formed layer of irregular odontoblasts. However, neither the number nor the caliber of the nerve fibers reached normal levels. In microangiographic studies of the revascularization process after replantation of teeth in dogs, it was demonstrated that ingrowth of new vessels could be seen 4 days after replantation. After 10 days, vessels were seen in the apical half of the pulp and, after 30 days, in the entire pulp (136, 137).

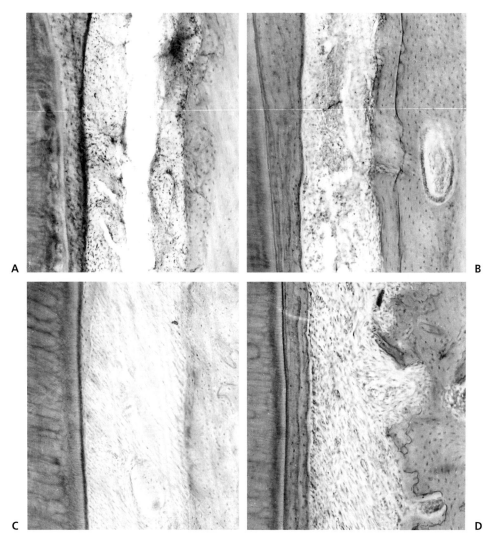

**Fig. 17.11** Healing sequence in the periodontal structures following experimental tooth replantations in dogs. A. Condition immediately after replantation. The line of separation is situated in the middle of the periodontal ligament. ×75. B. Three days later proliferating connective tissue cells invade the coagulum of the severed periodontal ligament. ×75. C. Two weeks later new collagenous fibers have bridged the periodontal space. ×75. D. Normal periodontal conditions 8 months after replantation. ×75.

## Periodontal healing reactions

The following healing sequence in the periodontal structures has been demonstrated after experimental immediate replantation in dogs (24, 33), monkeys (138, 162), and humans (230).

Immediately after replantation, a coagulum is found between the two parts of the severed periodontal ligament (Fig. 17.11A). The line of separation is most often situated in the middle of the periodontal ligament, although separation can occur at the insertion of Sharpey's fibers into cementum or alveolar bone. Proliferation of connective tissue cells soon occurs and, after 3 to 4 days, the gap in the periodontal ligament is obliterated by young connective tissue (Fig. 17.11B). After 1 week, the epithelium is reattached at the cementoenamel junction (138). This is of clinical importance because it may imply a reduced risk of gingival infection and/or reduced risk of bacterial invasion of either the root canal or periodontal ligament via the gingival pocket. Gingival collagen fibers are usually spliced, while the infrabony fibers are united in only a few areas at this time (138). The first superficial osteoclast attack can now be seen along the root surface (140).

After 2 weeks, the split line in the periodontal ligament is healed and collagen fibers are seen extending from the cementum surface to the alveolar bone (Fig. 17.11C). Resorption activity can now be recognized along the root surface (140).

Histologic examination of replanted human and animal teeth has revealed four different healing modalities in the periodontal ligament (44, 45, 147, 221, 222, 231).

### Healing with a normal periodontal ligament

Histologically, this is characterized by complete regeneration of the periodontal ligament (10, 24, 36, 44, 47, 48), which usually takes about 4 weeks to complete including the nerve supply (233, 306) (Fig. 17.12). This type of healing will only occur if the innermost cell layers along the root surface are vital (142, 215).

Radiographically, there is a normal periodontal ligament space without signs of root resorption (Fig. 17.13).

Clinically, the tooth is in a normal position with normal mobility and a normal percussion tone can be elicited.

This type of healing will probably never take place under clinical conditions (i.e. after tooth avulsion), as trauma will result in at least minimal injury to the innermost layer of the periodontal ligament, leading to surface resorption (see Chapter 2, p. 81).

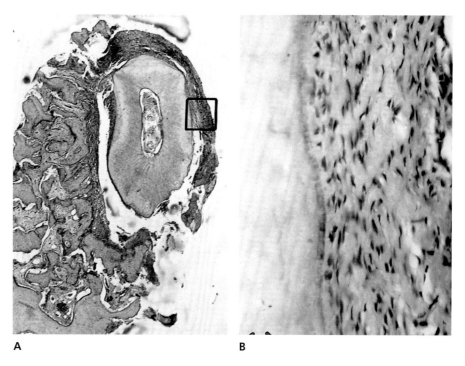

**Fig. 17.12** Healing with a normal periodontal ligament following replantation of a left lateral incisor. A. Apex removed 4 months after replantation. B. Normal periodontal ligament and cementum. ×12 and ×195. From ANDREASEN & HJÖRTING-HANSEN (44) 1966.

A

B

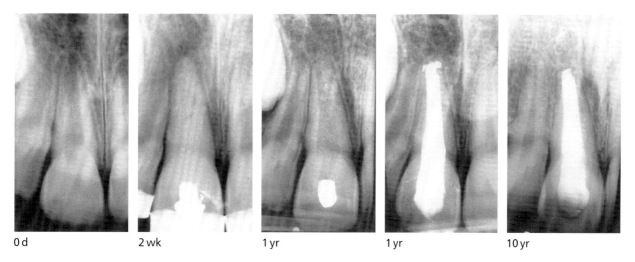

0 d          2 wk          1 yr          1 yr          10 yr

**Fig. 17.13** Periodontal ligament healing after replantation of right central incisor. From ANDREASEN et al. (202) 1995.

## Healing with surface resorption (repair-related resorption)

Histologically, this type of healing is characterized by localized areas along the root surface which show superficial resorption lacunae repaired by new cementum. This condition has been termed surface resorption, presumably representing localized areas of damage to the periodontal ligament or cementum which have been healed by periodontal ligament-derived cells (44, 140, 142, 146, 221, 222). In contrast to other types of resorption, surface resorption is not progressive and self-limiting and shows repair with new cementum (Fig. 17.14). Most resorption lacunae are superficial and confined to the cementum. In cases of deeper resorption cavities, however, healing occurs, but without restoration of the original outline of the root. It should be noted that resorption lacunae with similar morphology and location have been reported on non-traumatized root surfaces with a frequency as high as 90% of all teeth examined (49).

Due to their small size, surface resorptions are usually not disclosed radiographically. However, with ideal angulation of the central beam it is sometimes possible to recognize small excavations of the root surface with an adjacent periodontal ligament space of normal width (Fig. 17.15).

Clinically, the tooth is in a normal position and a normal percussion tone can be elicited.

## Healing with ankylosis (replacement resorption)

Histologically, ankylosis represents a fusion of the alveolar bone and the root surface and can be demonstrated 2 weeks

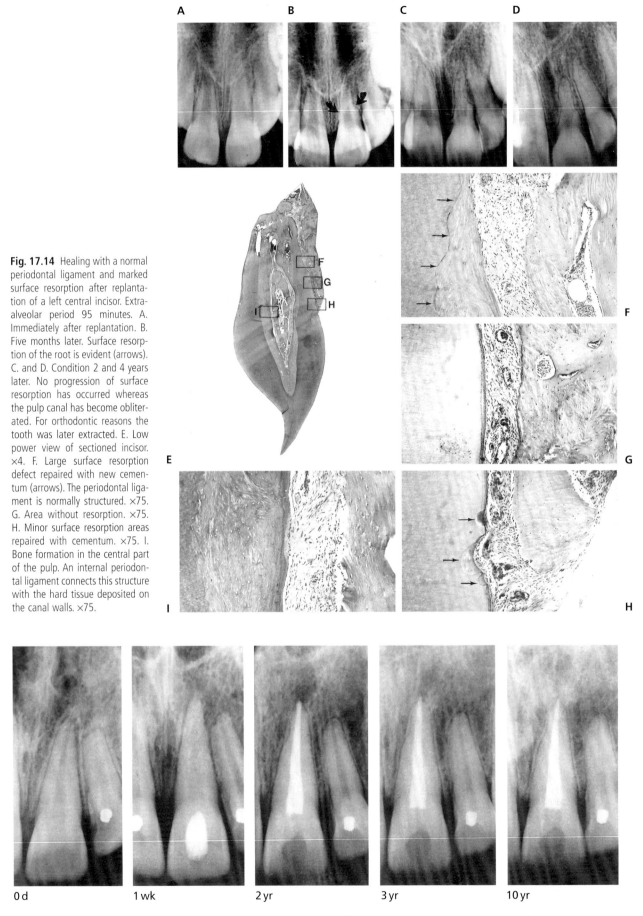

**Fig. 17.14** Healing with a normal periodontal ligament and marked surface resorption after replantation of a left central incisor. Extra-alveolar period 95 minutes. A. Immediately after replantation. B. Five months later. Surface resorption of the root is evident (arrows). C. and D. Condition 2 and 4 years later. No progression of surface resorption has occurred whereas the pulp canal has become obliterated. For orthodontic reasons the tooth was later extracted. E. Low power view of sectioned incisor. ×4. F. Large surface resorption defect repaired with new cementum (arrows). The periodontal ligament is normally structured. ×75. G. Area without resorption. ×75. H. Minor surface resorption areas repaired with cementum. ×75. I. Bone formation in the central part of the pulp. An internal periodontal ligament connects this structure with the hard tissue deposited on the canal walls. ×75.

0 d          1 wk          2 yr          3 yr          10 yr

**Fig. 17.15** Surface resorption of a replanted right central incisor. Note the superficial appearance on the root and sparse involvement on the lamina dura. The resorption cavity is stationary during the entire observation period. From ANDREASEN et al. (202) 1995.

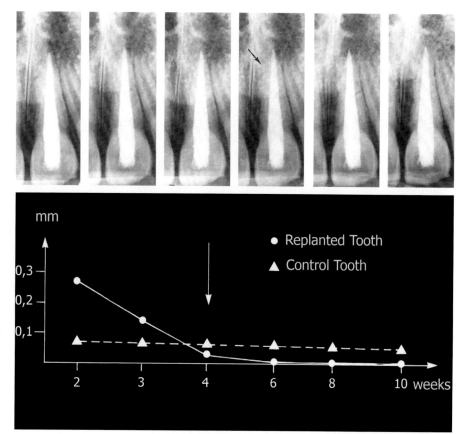

**Fig. 17.16** Mobility and permanent replacement resorption. Mobility values indicated that an ankylosis was established 4 weeks after replantation (lower arrow). Replacement resorption was first radiographically demonstrable 6 weeks after replantation (upper arrow). From ANDREASEN (171) 1975.

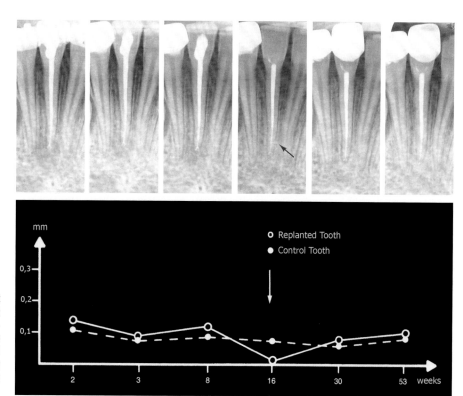

**Fig. 17.17** Transient replacement resorption. Mobility testing indicated an ankylosis 16 weeks after replantation. Ankylosis also demonstrable radiographically (arrow). A normal periodontal space was restored at later controls. From ANDREASEN (171) 1975.

after replantation (138, 311). The etiology of replacement resorption appears to be related to the absence of a vital periodontal ligament cover on the root surface (141–143, 216, 221, 231, 234, 311). Replacement resorption develops in two different directions, depending upon the extent of damage to the periodontal ligament cover of the root: either *progressive replacement resorption*, which gradually resorbs the entire root, or *transient replacement resorption*, in which a once-established ankylosis later disappears (144, 171) (Figs 17.16 and 17.17). *Progressive replacement resorption* is

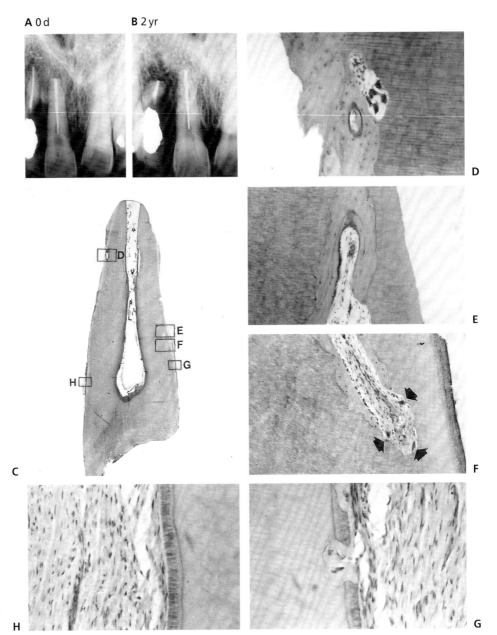

**A** 0 d   **B** 2 yr

**Fig. 17.18** Ankylosis (replacement resorption) after replantation of a right central incisor. A. Radiograph taken immediately after replantation. B. Condition at the time of extraction 2 years after injury. C. Low-power view of sectioned incisor. ×5. D. Bony union between root surface and surrounding alveolar bone. Note resorption lacunae with osteoclasts. ×75. E. and F. Replacement resorption with apposition of bone and active resorption (arrows). ×75. G. Surface resorption repaired with cellular cementum. ×195. H. Area with normal periodontal ligament. ×195. From ANDREASEN & HJÖRTING-HANSEN (44) 1966.

always elicited when the entire periodontal ligament is removed before replantation (143) or after extensive drying of the tooth before replantation (143, 146). It is assumed that the damaged periodontal ligament is repopulated from adjacent bone marrow cells, which have osteogenic potential and will consequently form an ankylosis (172). *Transient replacement resorption* is possibly related to areas of minor damage to the root surface. In these cases, the ankylosis is formed initially and later resorbed by adjacent areas of vital periodontal ligament. This theory is supported experimentally by research in which the effect of limited drying or limited removal of the periodontal ligament upon periodontal healing after replantation was studied (144).

Figure 17.18 demonstrates an initial phase of replacement resorption. The ankylosed root becomes part of the normal bone remodeling system and is gradually replaced by bone. After some time, little of the tooth substance remains. At this stage, the resorptive processes are usually intensified along the surface of the root canal filling, a phenomenon known as *tunneling resorption* (Fig. 17.19).

Radiographically, ankylosis is characterized by disappearance of the normal periodontal space and continuous replacement of root substance with bone (Fig. 17.20A–D).

Replacement resorption can first be recognized radiographically 2 months after replantation; however, in most cases 6 months or 1 year elapses (202) (Fig. 17.21).

Most cases can be diagnosed within 2 years, but it has been found that up to 10 years may elapse before radiographic diagnosis can be made (202) (Fig. 17.22). This problem of diagnosing ankylosis has also been verified in

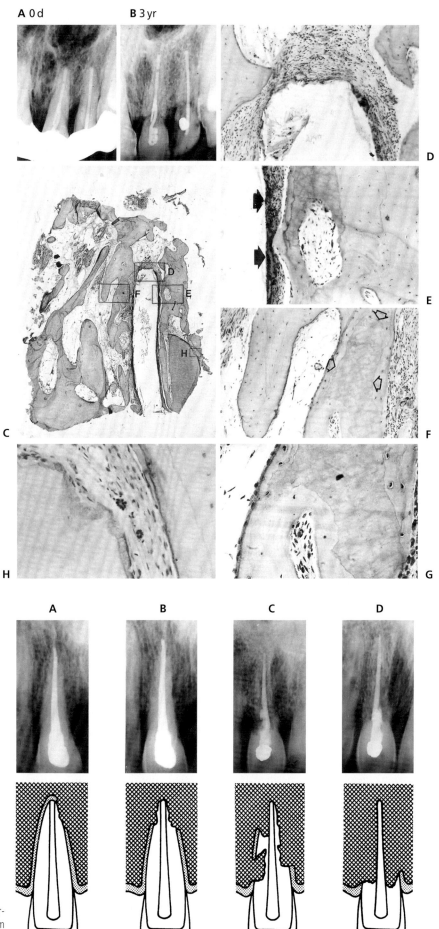

**A** 0 d

**B** 3 yr

**Fig. 17.19** Advanced ankylosis (replacement resorption) after replantation of upper left central and lateral incisors. A. Radiograph immediately after replantation. B. Condition at time of removal of the central incisor 3 years after replantation. C. Low power view of sectioned incisor. ×12. D. Apical part of root canal filling surrounded by bone and connective tissue. ×30. E. Haversian canal under remodeling. The walls consist of both dentin and bone. Note tunneling resorption along the root canal filling (arrows). ×30. F. Fragment of dentin incorporated in bone (arrows). ×30. G. Higher magnification of F. ×195. H. Area with normal cementum and periodontal tissue including epithelial rests of Mallassez. ×195. From ANDREASEN & HJÖRTING-HANSEN (44) 1966.

**Fig. 17.20** Schematic and radiographic appearance of replacement resorption. From ANDREASEN & HJÖRTING-HANSEN (6) 1966.

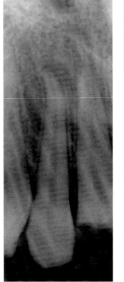 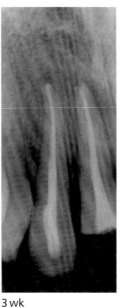 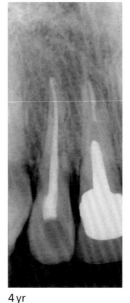 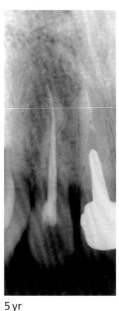

| 0 d | 2 wk | 3 wk | 4 yr | 5 yr |

**Fig. 17.21** Progression of replacement resorption is followed by tunneling inflammatory resorption along the root filling. From ANDREASEN et al. (202) 1995.

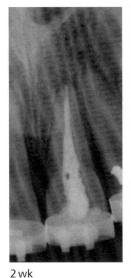 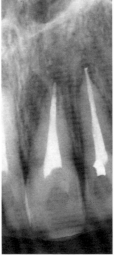 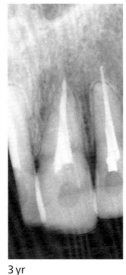 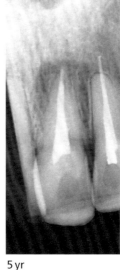 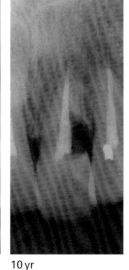

| 2 wk | 1 yr | 3 yr | 5 yr | 10 yr |

**Fig. 17.22** Late appearance of ankylosis. Resorption activity is suspected after 3 and 5 years and becomes manifest after 10 years. From ANDREASEN et al. (202) 1995.

experimental studies, where histologic findings were compared with radiography (235, 236).

Clinically, the ankylosed tooth is immobile and in children frequently in infraposition. The percussion tone is high, differing clearly from adjacent non-injured teeth. The percussion test can often reveal replacement resorption in its initial phases before it can be diagnosed radiographically (171, 202, 235).

Cases of transient replacement resorption can sometimes be demonstrated radiographically as small areas where the periodontal ligament space has disappeared (Fig. 17.17). Most often this type of ankylosis is demonstrated by its high percussion tone. Disappearance of the ankylosis, which

always happens within the first year, is followed by the return of a normal percussion tone (171).

## Healing with inflammatory resorption (infection-related resorption)

Histologically, inflammatory resorption is characterized by bowl-shaped resorption cavities in cementum and dentin associated with inflammatory changes in the adjacent periodontal tissue (44, 53–57, 139, 147) (Fig. 17.23). The inflammatory reaction in the periodontium consists of granulation tissue with numerous lymphocytes, plasma cells, and polymorphonuclear leukocytes. Adjacent to these

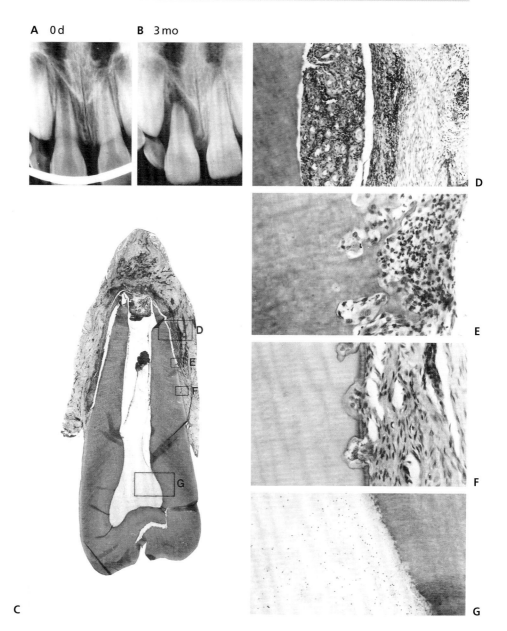

**A** 0d      **B** 3mo

**Fig. 17.23** Inflammatory resorption after replantation of a right central incisor. A. Radiograph taken immediately after replantation. B. Condition at time of removal 3 months later. C. Low power view of sectioned incisor. The pulp shows complete necrosis with autolysis. An intense inflammatory reaction is seen around the apical half of the root. ×7. D. Granulation tissue in relation to resorbed root surface. ×30. E. Area with active resorption. ×195. F. Surface resorption partly repaired with new cementum. ×195. G. Necrotic pulp tissue. ×30. From ANDREASEN & HJÖRTING-HANSEN (44) 1966.

areas, the root surface undergoes intense resorption with numerous Howship's lacunae and osteoclasts.

The pathogenesis of inflammatory resorption can be described as follows (139). Minor injuries to the periodontal ligament and/or cementum due to trauma or contamination with bacteria induce small resorption cavities on the root surface, presumably in the same manner as in surface resorption. If these resorption cavities expose dentinal tubules and the root canal contains infected necrotic tissue, toxins from these areas will penetrate along the dentinal tubules to the lateral periodontal tissues and provoke an inflammatory response. This in turn will intensify the resorption process which advances towards the root canal (44, 139). The resorption process can progress very rapidly, i.e. within a few months the entire root can be resorbed.

Inflammatory resorption is especially frequent and aggressive after replantation in patients from 6 to 10 years of age. The explanation for this is probably a combination of wide dentinal tubules and/or a thin protective cementum cover (6, 139). In older age groups, the resorption process follows a more protracted course.

It should be noted that replanted teeth can show simultaneous inflammatory and replacement resorption (Fig. 17.24). Moreover, if the resorption process is allowed to progress and involve large areas of the root surface, replacement resorption can take over once inflammatory resorption has been arrested by endodontic therapy.

Radiographically, inflammatory resorption is characterized by radiolucent bowl shaped cavitations along the root surface with corresponding excavations in the adjacent bone (Fig. 17.25). The first radiographic sign of inflammatory resorption can be demonstrated as early as 2 weeks after replantation and is usually first recognized at the cervical third of the root (6) (Fig. 17.25). As in the case of ankylosis, this resorption type is usually evident within the first 2 years after replantation.

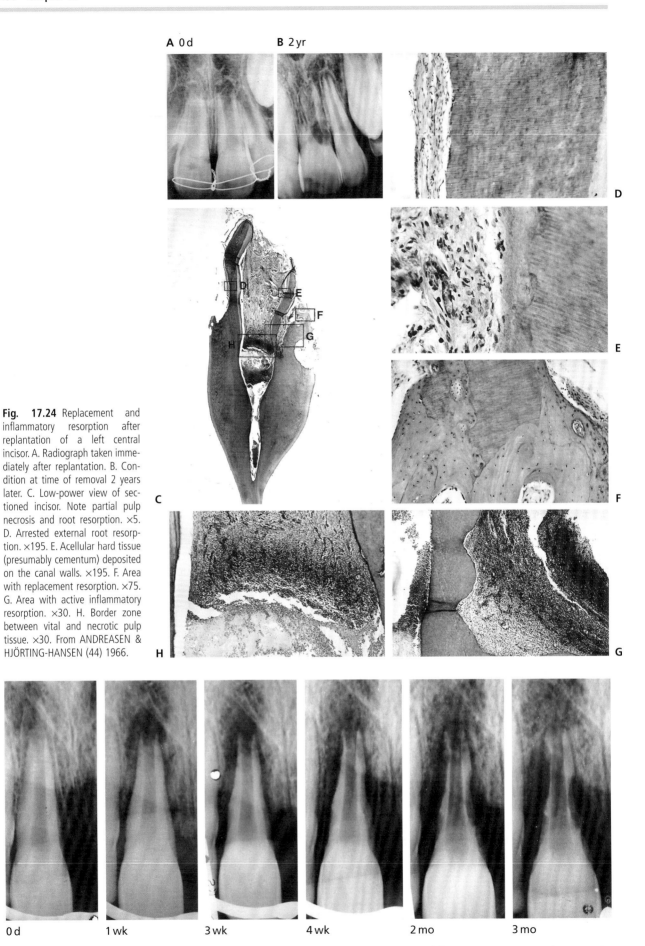

**A** 0 d    **B** 2 yr

**Fig. 17.24** Replacement and inflammatory resorption after replantation of a left central incisor. A. Radiograph taken immediately after replantation. B. Condition at time of removal 2 years later. C. Low-power view of sectioned incisor. Note partial pulp necrosis and root resorption. ×5. D. Arrested external root resorption. ×195. E. Acellular hard tissue (presumably cementum) deposited on the canal walls. ×195. F. Area with replacement resorption. ×75. G. Area with active inflammatory resorption. ×30. H. Border zone between vital and necrotic pulp tissue. ×30. From ANDREASEN & HJÖRTING-HANSEN (44) 1966.

0 d    1 wk    3 wk    4 wk    2 mo    3 mo

**Fig. 17.25** Inflammatory resorption of a replanted right central incisor. Note the excavating nature of the resorption process on the root and a corresponding marked resorption of the lamina dura. From ANDREASEN & HJÖRTING-HANSEN (6) 1966.

Clinically, the replanted tooth is loose and extruded. Moreover, the tooth is sensitive to percussion and the percussion tone is dull (compared with ankylosis).

## Treatment of the avulsed tooth

This issue has been the topic for several committees' attempts to create evidence based guidelines. With respect to avulsed teeth, this task is very difficult due to the paucity of clinically documented studies. The reader is referred to two published reviews by Barrett & Kenny (279) and Trope (304). The present guidelines are primarily based on an analysis of a series of experimental studies and a few clinical studies where enough data support the given procedures.

### At the site of accident

In some instances, a telephone call at the time of injury will precede the office visit. In these cases, the patient or an available adult should be instructed to replant the tooth immediately. In this way, the extra-alveolar period is decreased and the prognosis improved significantly. Replantation can be accomplished in the following manner.

If dirty, the tooth can be cleaned by simply rinsing it under running, cold tap water for 10 seconds and placing it immediately in its socket. This procedure has been found to decrease the extent of root resorption experimentally (310). If the replantation procedure cannot be performed at this time, the tooth can be stored in the patient's buccal vestibule. Animal experiments have shown that storage in milk or saliva has almost the same effect as storage in saline. However, long-term storage in tap water (i.e. more than 20 minutes) has an adverse effect on periodontal healing (146, 202). After replantation and en route to the dental office, the patient should be instructed to keep the tooth in place with either finger pressure or by biting on a handkerchief.

Avulsed teeth should always be replanted as soon as possible and if this is not possible a storage medium such as saliva, saline or milk should be used to store the replanted tooth until the dentist is visited. The patient should visit a dentist emergency service as soon as possible.

### At the clinic

The case history should include exact information on the time interval between injury and replantation as well as the conditions under which the tooth has been stored (e.g. saline, saliva, milk, tap water, or dry).

In this regard a commercial tissue culture medium (ViaSpan®) could be used for extra-oral storage. *In vitro* experiments have shown it to be effective even for several days of storage (238). In conditioned media it has been shown experimentally that teeth can be kept in storage for up to 96 hours and still present optimal healing (308). Another medium that has shown good effect is Propolis® (280). However, *in vivo* studies are still lacking that demonstrate the effectiveness. Moreover, commercial storage media are usually not available at the site of accident.

The avulsed tooth is examined for obvious contamination. The alveolus is also examined. As prognosis is significantly related to the length of the extra-alveolar period, pre-treatment radiographs can serve to extend this period and should, therefore, be taken prior to treatment only if there is suspicion of comminution or fracture of the socket wall.

Careful planning is of utmost importance for the success of replantation of avulsed teeth. The following conditions should be considered before replanting a permanent tooth:

(1) The avulsed tooth should be without advanced periodontal disease (Fig. 17.2).
(2) The alveolar socket should be reasonably intact in order to provide a seat for the avulsed tooth (Fig. 17.4).
(3) The extra-alveolar period should be considered, i.e. dry extra-oral periods exceeding 1 hour are usually associated with marked root resorption.
(4) The stage of root development should be considered.

While certain conditions, such as those listed above, might appear to contraindicate replantation of an avulsed incisor, it should be borne in mind that the time of injury is often not the time to make such decisions. Definitive treatment planning (e.g. orthodontic evaluation of a crowded dentition) can seldom be made in the heat of acute treatment. Furthermore, an extended extra-oral period – even dry storage – is not an absolute contraindication to replantation, as the root surface can be treated chemically to protract the resorption process in mature teeth (see later). In most situations, replantation of the avulsed tooth, even with a dubious prognosis, can be performed and the tooth considered as a temporary restoration until such time as definitive treatment planning, often following specialist consultation, can be carried out.

If replantation is decided upon, the following procedures are recommended (Fig. 17.26). The tooth is placed in saline. If visibly contaminated, the root surface is rinsed with a stream of saline from a syringe until visible contaminants have been washed away, including around the apical foramen. The alveolus is also rinsed with a flow of saline to remove the contaminated coagulum. No effort should be made to sterilize or mechanically cleanse the root surface, as such procedures will damage or destroy vital periodontal tissue and cementum (202).

In the case of a *closed apex*, the tooth is now replanted. In the case of an *open apex*, a pretreatment with tetracycline (solution or powder) may more than double the chance of revascularization (see Ch. 5, p. 193). However, it should be noted that these findings relate to animal experiments and have not yet been verified in humans.

The socket is then examined. If there is evidence of fracture, it is essential to reposition the fractured bone by inserting an instrument in the socket and then modeling the bone. Local anesthesia is usually not necessary unless gingival lacerations require suturing or the alveolar socket

### Fig. 17.26 Replantation of a tooth with completed root formation

Replantation of an avulsed maxillary right central incisor in a 19-year-old man. Radiographic examination shows no sign of fracture or contusion of the alveolar socket. The tooth was retrieved immediately after injury and kept moist in the oral cavity. Upon admission to the emergency service, the avulsed incisor was placed in physiologic saline.

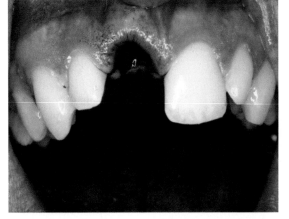 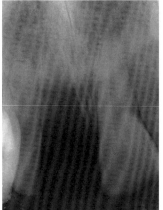

### Rinsing the tooth

The tooth is examined for fractures, position of the level of periodontal attachment and signs of contamination. The tooth is then rinsed with a stream of saline until all visible signs of contamination have been removed. If this is not effective, dirt is carefully removed using a gauze sponge soaked in saline. The coagulum in the alveolar socket is flushed out using a stream of saline.

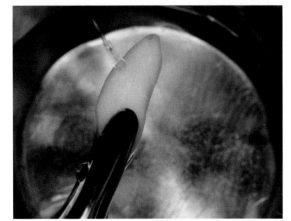 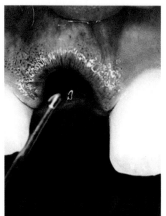

### Replanting the tooth

The tooth is grasped by the crown with forceps and partially replanted in its socket. Replantation is completed using gentle finger pressure. If any resistance is met, the tooth should be removed, placed again in saline and the socket inspected. A straight elevator is then inserted in the socket and an index finger is placed labially. Using lateral pressure, counterbalanced by the finger pressure, the socket wall is repositioned. Replantation can then proceed as described.

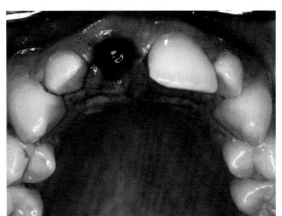 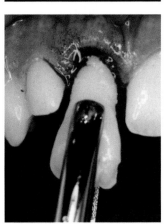

### Splinting

An acid-etch retained splint is applied. As soon after injury as possible, antibiotic therapy should be instituted. Suggested dosage: penicillin 1 million units immediately, thereafter 2–4 million units daily for 4 days. Good oral hygiene is absolutely necessary in the healing period. This includes brushing with a soft tooth brush and a 0.1% chlorhexidine mouth rinse.

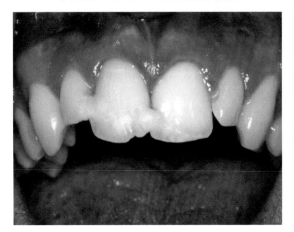 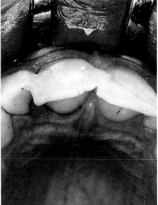

requires remodeling. The tooth is replanted using light digital pressure. It is important that only light pressure is used during the replantation procedure, as this will permit detection of resistance from displaced alveolar bone fragments that impede replantation. If resistance is met, the tooth should again be placed in saline while the alveolus is re-examined and any displaced bone fragments repositioned. Repositioning can then be completed. The replanted incisor should fit loosely in the alveolus in order to prevent further damage to the root surface.

Studies have shown that rigid splinting of replanted mature and autotransplanted immature teeth increases the extent of root resorption (147, 148, 173, 239–241, 303). Replanted teeth should, therefore, only be splinted for a minimal period of time. One week is normally sufficient to ensure adequate periodontal support, as gingival fibers in the cervical region are already healed by this time.

Proper repositioning can now be evaluated by the occlusion and the tooth splinted to adjacent incisors. An acid etch/resin splint is usually the method of choice. Finally, a radiograph is taken once the splint has been applied, to verify that the normal position of the tooth has been achieved.

When the splint is to be removed, it is important to remember that the replanted tooth is still rather loose. It is therefore important to remove the splinting material carefully, with finger support on the replanted tooth. Furthermore, if endodontic treatment is indicated, it should be carried out prior to splint removal (see suggestions in Ch. 22).

Tetanus prophylaxis is important, as most teeth have been in contact with soil, or the wound itself is soil-contaminated.

The value of antibiotic therapy is at this time questionable. Thus, experimental studies in monkeys have shown that systemic antibiotics may lessen the resorption attack on the root surface. However, pulpal healing is apparently not affected (226, 242). In a recent clinical study, no effect of antibiotics could be demonstrated in the frequency of pulpal or periodontal healing (200, 202). From animal experimentation, there seems to be an advantage of using *tetracycline* instead of *penicillin* (see Ch. 5, p. 188), assuming the patient is above 12 years of age (where the chance of discoloration of developing teeth is at a minimum).

In case of a closed apical foramen, endodontic treatment should always be performed prophylactically, as pulp necrosis can be anticipated. A long-debated question has been whether root canal treatment of incisors with mature root development (i.e. with the diameter of the apical foramen of less than 1.0 mm) should be performed before or after replantation, if survival of the pulp cannot be expected. Experimental studies in monkeys have shown that extra-oral root filling procedures as well as the root filling materials themselves apparently injure the periodontal ligament. This could be a result of seepage through the apical foramen or mechanical preparation of the root canal, which results in increased ankylosis apically when compared to non-endodontically treated teeth (149, 152). Thus, endodontic

treatment should be delayed for 1 week after replantation in order to prevent development of ankylosis and inflammatory resorption, as well as to allow splicing of periodontal ligament fibers which limits seepage of potentially harmful root filling materials into the traumatized periodontal ligament.

Where the apical foramen is wide open and replantation has been performed within 3 hours after injury, it is justifiable to await revascularization of the pulp (200, 243). In these cases, the topical application of doxycycline in a concentration of 1 mg in 20 ml physiologic saline has been shown to double the chance of revascularization in experiments in monkeys (312–314) (see Chapter 5).

Radiographic controls should be made 2 and 3 weeks after replantation, as the first evidence of root resorption and periapical osteitis can usually be seen at this time. If this occurs, endodontic therapy should be initiated immediately and calcium hydroxide introduced into the root canal to eliminate periapical inflammation and arrest root resorption (6, 45, 174, 244) (see Ch. 22, p. 621). The timing of the endodontic procedure when pulpal revascularization is absent is critical, as root resorption can proceed very rapidly in teeth with incomplete root formation (i.e. with a speed of up to 0.1 mm root substance loss per day) (Fig. 17.25).

In teeth with prolonged extra-alveolar periods, where the periodontal ligament can be assumed to be necrotic, it has been suggested that the root surface be treated with various substances, such as sodium fluoride (175), tetracycline, stannous fluoride (245, 246), citric acid (247, 248), hypochloric acid (161), calcium hydroxide (178), formalin (179), alcohol (180), diphosphonates (181), and indomethacin (249) in order to inhibit root resorption. However, apart from sodium fluoride, long-term resorption inhibition has not been demonstrated (see Chapter 5).

The incorporation of fluoride ions in the cementum layer has been found to yield a root surface resistant to resorption (175). Thus, in experiments with monkeys, a significant reduction in the amount of radiographically evident root resorption was seen in teeth treated with a fluoride solution (176). Based on these experiments, it has been suggested that mature teeth with prolonged dry extra-alveolar periods (i.e. greater than 1 hour) be placed in a fluoride solution (2.4% sodium fluoride phosphate acidulated at pH 5.5) for 20 minutes prior to replantation (Fig. 17.27). Prior to this, the necrotic periodontal ligament is removed e.g. with a scaler. After immersion in the fluoride solution, the root surface is rinsed with saline, the tooth replanted and then splinted for 6 weeks (177). The effect of this treatment seems to be a 50% reduction of the progression of root resorption of replanted human teeth (250).

Several attempts have been made to overcome the problem of ankylosis by placing different materials between the tooth and the socket, such as silicone grease and methyl methacrylate (methyl-2-cyanoacrylate) (178, 182, 183), absorbable surgical sponge (Gelfoam®, The Upjohn Co., Kalamazoo, USA) (184), venous tissue (160), fascia and cutaneous connective tissue (156). The general outcome of these experiments was that root resorption was either not prevented or that the teeth were exfoliated.

### Fig. 17.27 Replanting a tooth with an avital periodontal ligament

In this 21-year-old man, the tooth has been kept dry for 24 hours. Total and irreversible damage to the PDL and pulp can be expected. Furthermore, there is severe contusion of the alveolar socket. In this situation, delayed replantation (to allow healing of the socket), treatment of the root surface (to make it resistant to ankylosis) and endodontic therapy (to prevent inflammatory resorption) is the treatment of choice.

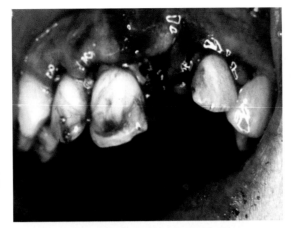
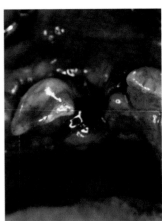

### Treatment of the root surface

The avulsed tooth in this case was kept dry in a refrigerator until healing of the contused socket has taken place. Prior to sodium fluoride treatment, the root surface is rinsed and scraped clean of the dead PDL and the pulp extirpated. The goal of therapy is to incorporate fluoride ions into the dentin and cementum in order to protract the resorption process.

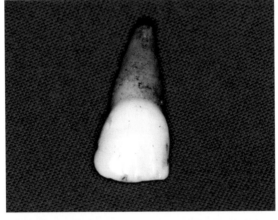
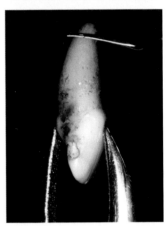

### Fluoride treatment of cementum and dentin

The pulp is extirpated and the root canal enlarged to provide access for the fluoride solution along the entire root canal. The tooth is then placed in a 2.4% solution of sodium fluoride (acidulated to pH = 5.5) for 20 minutes.

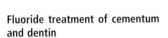
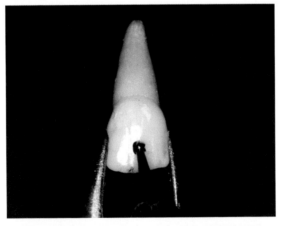
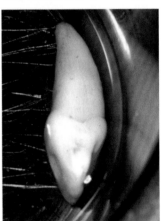

### Endodontic treatment

After rinsing in saline, the root canal is obturated with gutta-percha and a sealer.

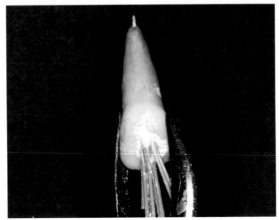
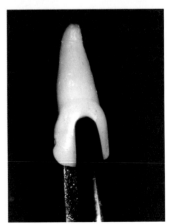

**Condition of the socket**
After 3 weeks, the socket area and the contused gingiva are healed.

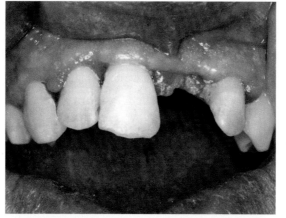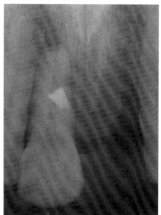

**Replanting the tooth**
The socket is evacuated with excavators and a surgical bur. The tooth is replanted after cleansing with saline to remove excess fluoride solution.

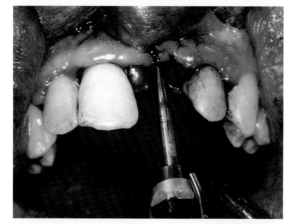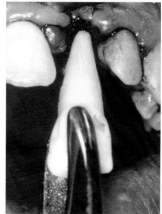

**Splinting**
The tooth is splinted for 6 weeks in order to create a solid ankylosis. In these cases, where no periodontal ligament exists, ankylosis is the only possible healing modality.

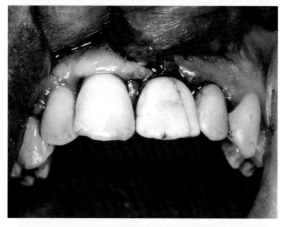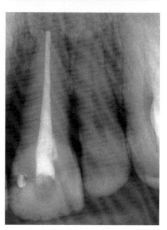

**Follow-up**
Radiographic follow-up over a 3-year period shows no progression of the ankylosis process.

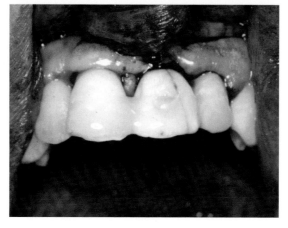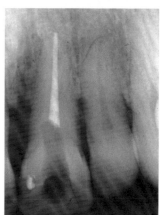

### Fig. 17.28 Apical resection and root extension with a ceramic implant

Pulp necrosis and arrested root formation in a 10-year-old child subsequent to trauma. The tooth is extracted with forceps having diamond grips. It is important that the forceps does not touch cementum after incision of the gingival fibers with a scalpel.

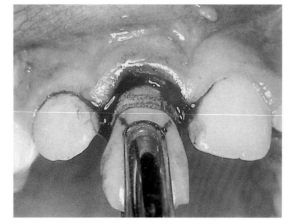 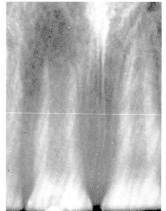

### Preparing the root for the implant

The apex is resected with a diamond disc to a level where there is no obvious resorption. The root canal is enlarged with a bur which matches the ceramic implant. The root canal is enlarged with a bur with internal cooling. During all tooth preparation the root is kept moist with saline.

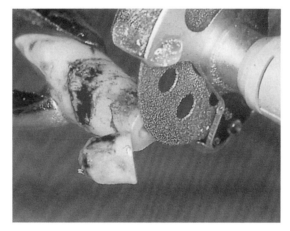 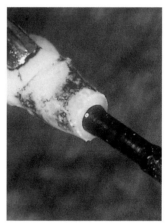

### Cementing the implant

After drying the cavity with a sterile pipe cleaner, an aluminium oxide or titanium implant which matches the dimension of the drill is cemented with Diaket®.

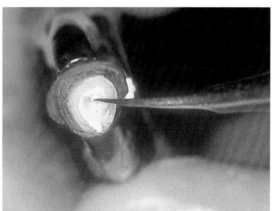 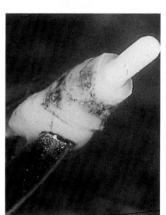

### Replanting the tooth

The base of the alveolus is enlarged with a drill to accommodate the root extension. After replantation, the tooth is splinted for 2 to 4 weeks. Subsequently, the crown should be opened palatally and filled to the level of the implant. The radiographic condition is shown 2 years after implantation. From KIRSCHNER et al. (253) 1980.

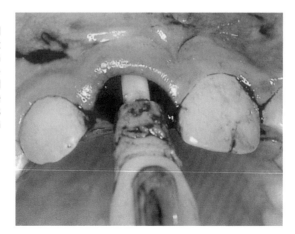 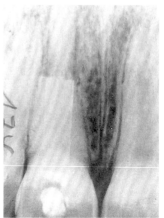

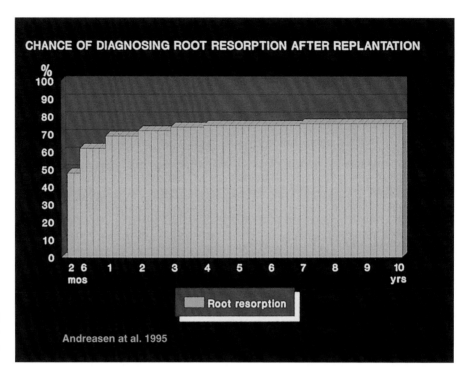

**Fig. 17.29** Chance of detection of root resorption with increasing observation period. From ANDREASEN et al. (202) 1995.

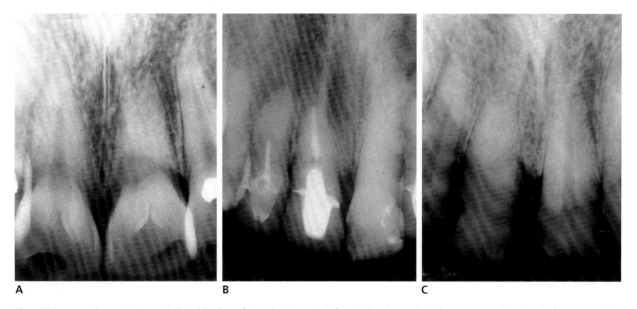

**A**  **B**  **C**

**Fig. 17.30** Cases demonstrating periodontal healing after replantation. A. Left central incisor replanted 13 years previously. B. Right central incisor replanted 37 years previously. C. Two central incisors replanted 40 years previously. From ANDREASEN & HJÖRTING-HANSEN (6) 1966.

To overcome the resorption problem, a number of procedures have been developed, e.g. replacement of the apical part of the root with a cast vitallium implant (68, 73, 78, 190). However, the results of these procedures have not been convincing. An attempt has been made to prolong the lifetime of replanted teeth by a replacement of the root tip with a ceramic implant (dense sintered aluminum oxide) or titanium (251–262) (Fig. 17.28). Before replantation, the apical half of the root is resected; the root canal is enlarged with special burs, whereafter a corresponding ceramic implant is cemented in place. Preliminary studies indicate that this procedure, as expected, does not prevent root resorption, but does tend to prolong the survival time of the replant (261, 262, 305).

## Follow-up procedures

Successive radiographic controls should be performed in the follow-up period in order to disclose root resorption (199) (see Appendix 3, p. 881). If not present within the first 2 years after injury, the risk of root resorption is significantly reduced, but can still occur (202) (Fig. 17.29).

The onset of resorption appears to be earlier in cases with crown damage, visible contamination and dry extra-alveolar time exceeding 15 minutes.

**Table 17.1** Long-term results of replantation of avulsed permanent teeth.

| Examiner | Observation period years (mean) | Age of patients (mean) | No. of teeth | Tooth survival % | PDL healing % | Pulp healing % | Gingival healing % |
|---|---|---|---|---|---|---|---|
| Lenstrup & Skieller (7, 8) 1957, 1959 | 0.2–5 | 5–18 | 47 | 57 | 4 | 9 | |
| Andreasen & Hjörting-Hansen (6) 1966 | 0.2–15 | 6–24 | 110 | 54 | 4 | 20 | 95 |
| Ravn & Helbo (69) 1966 | | 5–15 | 28 | | 4 | 4 | |
| Gröndahl et al. (187) 1974 | 2–5 | | 45 | 69 | 7 | 23 | 67 |
| Cvek et al. (188) 1974 | 2–6.5 | 6–17(11) | 38 | | | 50 | |
| Hörster et al. (128) 1976 | | | 38 | | | 26 | |
| Kemp et al. (127) 1977 | 0.1–10 | 10–15 | 71 | 61 | | 30 | |
| Ravn (129) 1977 | | 7–16 | 20 | | 5 | 20 | |
| Kock & Ullbro (263) 1982 | 1–9 | 7–17 | 55 | 65 | 4 | 27 | |
| Herforth (264) 1982 | 1–8(4.5) | 7–15 | 79 | 51 | 4 | 11 | |
| Jacobsen (265) 1986 | 1–14(5) | | 59 | 39 | 15 | 29 | |
| Gonda et al. (266) 1990 | 0.6–6.5 | (16) | 27 | 70 | 15 | 41 | |
| Mackie & Worthington (267) 1992 | 1–7 | 6–14(9) | 46 | 89 | | 46 | |
| Andreasen et al. (199–203) 1994, 1995 | 0.2–20(5.1) | 5–52(13.4) | 400 | 70 | 8 | 36 | 93 |
| Ebeseleder et al. (283) 1998 | (2.5) | | 112 | 21 | | | |
| Kinirons et al. (286) 1999 | | 6–16(9.8) | 84 | | | | |
| Schatz et al. (285) 1995 | (2.9) | 6–17 | 33 | | 27 | 25 | |
| Kinirons et al. (284) 2000 | 2.1–13.3(5.1) | 7.1–18(10.3) | 128 | | | 23 | |

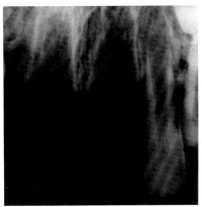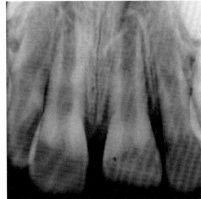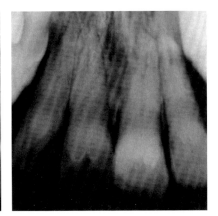

**Fig. 17.31** Pulpal healing in three replanted incisors after a long extra-alveolar period of 2 minutes dry and 88 minutes in saline in an 8-year-old boy. From ANDREASEN et al. (200) 1995.

## Prognosis

Replantation of teeth has been considered a temporary measure as many teeth succumb to root resorption. However, a number of cases have been reported where replanted teeth have been in service for 20 to 40 years with a normal periodontium, as revealed clinically (positive pulpal sensibility) and radiographically (6, 63–68, 186) (Fig. 17.30 and Table 17.1). Such reports demonstrate that replanted teeth, under certain conditions, can maintain their integrity and function.

## Tooth loss

Several studies have shown that teeth can function for 20 years or more after replantation (199, 263, 267) and that

tooth survival was significantly related to the stage of root development at the time of injury, being more favorable with increasing developmental maturity (199, 287) (Table 17.1).

## Pulp necrosis

In rare cases, revascularization of the pulp will occur in replanted teeth with completed root formation, provided that replantation is carried out immediately (6, 43). Pulps of teeth with *incomplete* root formation can become revascularized if replantation is carried out within 3 hours (6, 8, 9, 43, 63, 66, 79–85, 191–196, 200, 243, 268–270, 282) (Fig. 17.31). Pulpal sensibility tests are unreliable immediately after replantation. Functional repair of pulpal nerve fibers in human teeth is established approximately 36 days after replantation. At this time electrical stimuli can elicit

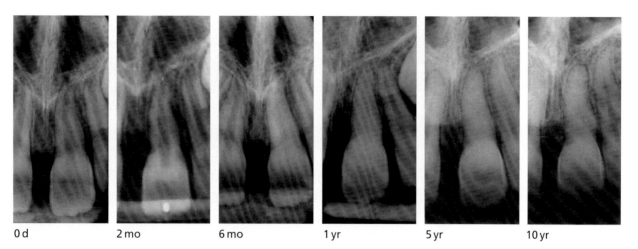

**Fig. 17.32** Pulp canal obliteration after replantation of a left central incisor. The canal obliteration becomes apparent after 6 months. From ANDREASEN et al. (200) 1995.

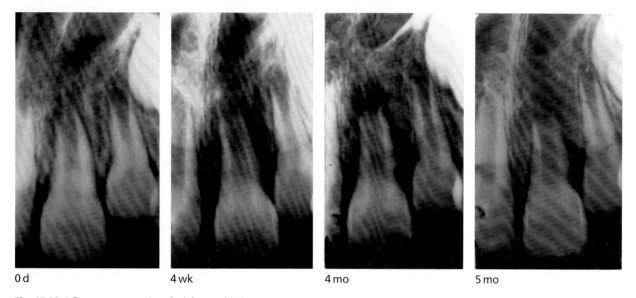

**Fig. 17.33** Inflammatory resorption of a left central incisor.

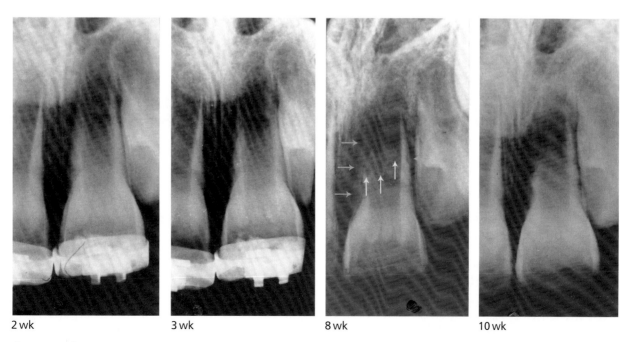

**Fig. 17.34** Inflammatory resorption in a replanted central incisor. Resorption is evident after 3 weeks. The resorption cavities appear as radiolucent areas within the root structure (white arrows). The mesial and distal part of the root also shows a resorption attack (gray arrows).

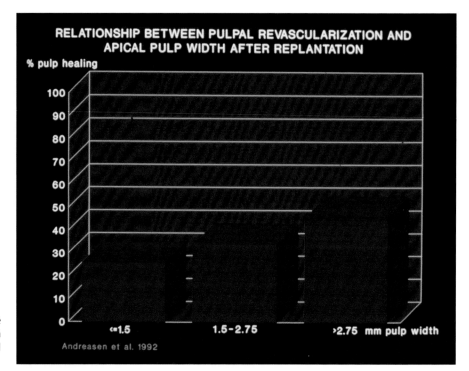

**Fig. 17.35** Relationship between size of foramen and pulp revascularization after replantation. From ANDREASEN et al. (200) 1995.

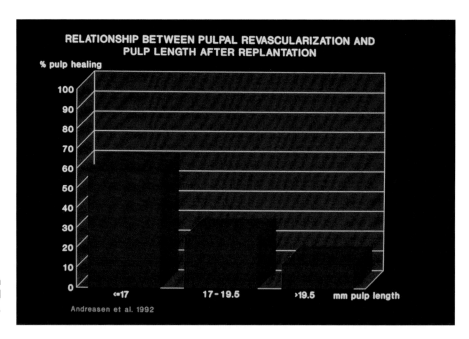

**Fig. 17.36** Relationship between length of the pulp canal and pulpal revascularization after replantation. From ANDREASEN et al. (200) 1995.

sensibility responses. With longer observation periods, an increasing number of teeth will respond (43, 200). In the absence of a reaction to electrical stimulation, it should be borne in mind that a decrease in the size of the coronal part of the pulp chamber or root canal on the radiograph is a more reliable sign of vital pulp tissue than thermal or electrical pulp testing (43) (Fig. 17.32).

The most significant predictors of pulpal healing appear to be the width and length of the root canal as well as the duration and type of extra-alveolar storage (200).

Pulp necrosis can usually be diagnosed after 2–4 weeks and normally shows up as a combined apical radiolucency and inflammatory resorption located to the midportion or cervical part of the root (200, 202) (Figs 17.33, 17.34).

### The width and length of the root canal

The relationship between the diameter of the apical foramen and the chance of pulpal revascularization apparently is

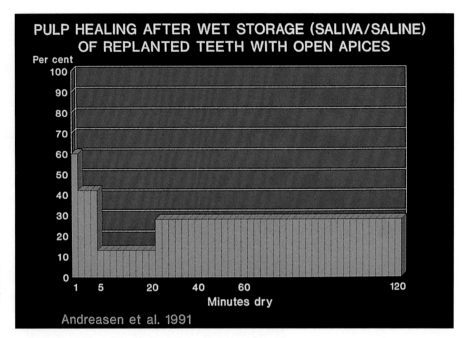

**Fig. 17.37** Relationship between pulpal healing of teeth with incomplete root formation and length of extra-alveolar wet storage. From ANDREASEN et al. (200) 1995.

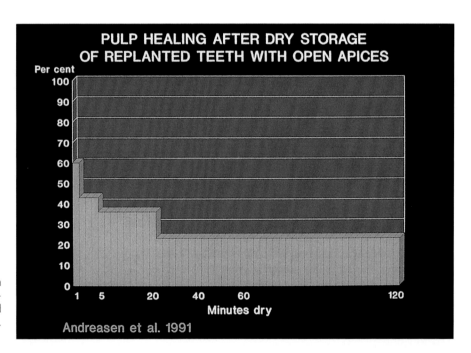

**Fig. 17.38** Relationship between pulpal healing of teeth with incomplete root formation and type and length of extra-alveolar dry storage. From ANDREASEN et al. (200) 1995.

an expression of the size of the contact area at the pulpo-periodontal interface (Fig. 17.35), whereas the length of the root canal probably reflects the time necessary to repopulate the ischemic pulp (200) (Fig. 17.36). With a favorable ratio (i.e. broad apical foramen and short root canal versus a narrow apical foramen and long root canal) the odds for an intervening pulpal infection are reduced (Fig. 17.36). A limiting factor in pulpal revascularization after replantation appears to be an apical diameter of less than 1.0 mm (200, 243) (Fig. 17.35). This size, however, is to a certain degree

arbitrary, as pulps in teeth with constricted apical foramina are usually extirpated prophylactically.

### Storage period and storage media

Another significant relationship which could be demonstrated in several clinical studies was the strong dependence between storage period and media and pulpal healing (200, 267). This is possibly due to the detrimental effect of cellular dehydration during dry storage on the apical portion of

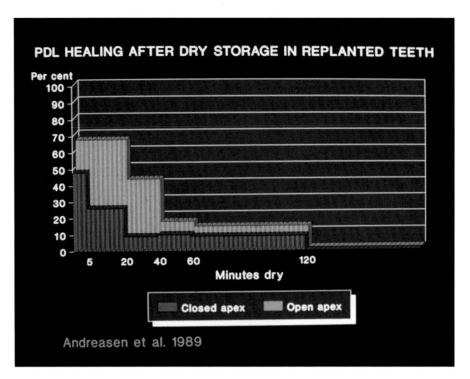

**Fig. 17.39** Relationship between PDL healing, length of extra-alveolar storage and stage of root development. From ANDREASEN et al. (202) 1995.

the pulp or by damage incurred by non-physiologic storage (e.g. prolonged tap water storage, chloramine, chlorhexidine and alcohol). The net result appears to be that with non-physiologic storage, the chances of pulpal revascularization are minimal; with storage in physiological media (e.g. saline, saliva or milk), there is only a weak relationship between the duration of storage and chances of pulpal revascularization (200, 267) (Fig. 17.37); in contrast, dry storage yields a constant and, with time, increasingly harmful effect on pulpal healing (Fig. 17.38). However, when compared to periodontal healing, this effect is less noticeable (200, 202).

In some cases where the Hertwig's epithelial root sheath has not survived, bony invasion of the root canal can take place, which might later lead to internal ankylosis (202) (Fig. 17.14F).

## Root resorption

Most replanted teeth demonstrate root resorption after a certain period of time. In the literature, the frequency of periodontal healing is usually around 20–25% (Table 17.1). However, a recent study following a series of public information campaigns showed a success rate of up to 36% after replantation (199).

A number of clinical factors have been shown to be associated with root resorption after replantation. Among these, the length and type of extra-alveolar storage (201), stage of root development and contamination of the root surface (201, 284). The type and length of storage has been found to be related to both the extent and progression of root resorption (203). Among these, the length of the dry extra-alveolar period seems to be the most crucial (6, 128, 171, 188, 189, 202, 203, 271–274, 285, 286) (Fig. 17.39). In a follow-up study of 400 teeth replanted after traumatic injury, 73% of the teeth replanted within 5 min demonstrated PDL healing; in contrast, PDL healing occurred in only 18% when the teeth were stored prior to replantation (202). These findings are in agreement with animal experiments (16, 28, 33, 70, 130, 146) assessing PDL vitality of extracted teeth allowed to dry out for varying periods (275–277).

## Storage media

Dry storage leads to cell necrosis and compromised healing (138, 146). Teeth prevented from drying will heal with a normal ligament (301) In most clinical cases, avulsed teeth have been stored either in the oral cavity or in other media, such as physiologic saline or tap water, before replantation. Tap water is detrimental to the cell viability (146, 188, 202) The reason for this is the low osmolality of tap water, resulting in quick cell death (291, 292) Experimental studies have indicated that the storage media more than the length of the extra-alveolar period determine prognosis. Milk and saline have been documented as good storage media in a number of experimental studies (238, 288–300). The positive effect of saliva for shorter storage periods have also been documented (146, 188, 289, 292).

Storage in saline or saliva did not significantly impair periodontal healing, while even short dry storage periods had an adverse effect (146, 272).

Although the above-mentioned experimental studies

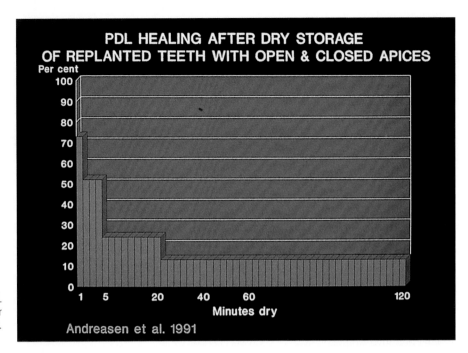

**Fig. 17.40** Relationship between PDL healing and length of extra-alveolar *dry* storage. From ANDREASEN et al. (202) 1995.

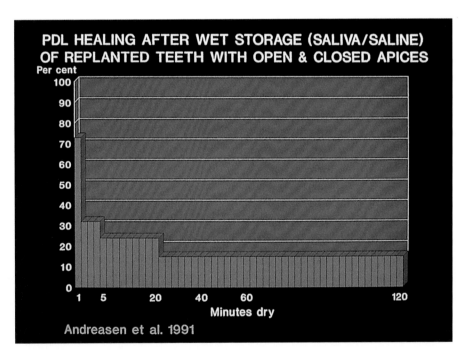

**Fig. 17.41** Relationship between PDL healing and length of extra-alveolar *wet* storage. From ANDREASEN et al. (202) 1995.

seem to stress the significance of the extra-alveolar period with these media, a less pronounced effect has been found in a larger clinical study (202, 203) (Figs 17.40 and 17.41). It should also be mentioned that successful cases have been reported after extra-alveolar periods of several hours (71, 72, 202).

## Stage of root development

In a clinical avulsion situation, the layer of PDL on the root can vary in thickness from a single cell layer to the full thickness of a periodontal ligament. Thus, the more mature the root formation the thinner is the PDL tissue layer. This could possibly explain the influence of root formation upon development of root resorption found in a recent clinical study (202). Thus, a thick periodontal ligament, which supposedly can tolerate a certain dry period before evaporation has killed the critical cell layers next to the cementum, showed less dependence upon dry storage (202, 221).

Among other factors influencing root resorption, experimental and human data have shown that the removal of the periodontal ligament prior to replantation is followed by extensive replacement resorption (25, 33, 48, 143). Consequently, this procedure, unless performed in relation to sodium fluoride treatment of the root surface is contraindicated (see p. 461).

## Splinting

Several clinical and experimental studies have shown that prolonged splinting (i.e. more than 10 days) leads to an increase in replacement resorption (286). Movement during healing promotes healing with less ankylosis (171, 303).

## Timing of pulp extirpation

In a recent clinical study, it was found that delayed pulp extirpation (i.e. after 20 days) resulted in acceleration of inflammatory resorption (286).

## Contamination of the root surface

Interesting studies have recently been published where the extent of contamination of the root surface prior to replantation and the cleansing procedure were found to be highly significant for subsequent PDL healing events (Tables 17.2 and 17.3). Using the results from two clinical studies (202, 284) and one experimental study (280) it seems reasonable to conclude that a short rinsing with tap water or saline is recommended.

**Table 17.2** Relationship between visible contamination of the root surface and cleansing procedures and subsequent root resorption. After KINIRONS et al. (284) 2000.

| Contamination | n | PDL resorption |
|---|---|---|
| None | 70 | 40 (57%) |
| Washed clean | 44 | 33 (75%) |
| Rubbed clean | 8 | 7 (88%) |
| Replanted but not clean p = 0.01 | 6 | 6 (100%) |

**Table 17.3** Relation between visible contamination and subsequent root resorption. After ANDREASEN et al. (202) 1995.

| Contamination | n | PDL resorption |
|---|---|---|
| No | 115 | 76 (64%) |
| Yes | 56 | 11 (81%) |
| p = 0.05 | | |

## Replacement resorption (ankylosis)

Ankylosis can usually be diagnosed clinically by a percussion test after 4–8 weeks, whereas radiographic evidence of root resorption usually requires a year (202). A mechanical device (Periotest®) which registers tooth mobility has also been shown to provide an early diagnosis of ankylosis (278).

A marked difference in the rate of progression of ankylosis is often seen in cases with similar extra-alveolar periods. This phenomenon might be related to differences in the initial damage to the root surface (6, 202, 203, 273), as well as the age of the patient and the type of endodontic treatment performed (203) (Fig. 17.42). Thus, if a tooth is replanted shortly after avulsion, the periodontal ligament is either re-established completely, or a few areas of ankylosis can arise (274). In the latter case, a long period will elapse before the process of replacement resorption results in total resorption of the root. Conversely, in teeth replanted with a long extra-alveolar period, an extensive ankylosis is formed which leads to rapid resorption of the root.

An alveolar fracture has been found to increase the chance of ankylosis (202) (Fig. 17.43).

If an ankylosis is established, its progression is also dependent upon the age of the patient, or rather the turnover rate of bone. Thus, replacement resorption is usually very aggressive in young individuals and runs a very protracted course in older patients (202, 203, 273).

A factor to be considered in young patients is that ankylosis can anchor the tooth in its position and thus disturb normal growth of the alveolar process. The result is a marked infraocclusion of the replanted tooth with migration and malocclusion of adjacent teeth (6, 55, 69, 129, 281) (Fig. 17.44). The treatment of choice in these cases is either decoronation or luxation with subsequent orthodontic extrusion (see Chapter 24, p. 700). Otherwise, later restorative procedures may be unnecessarily complicated by tooth migration and decreased height of the alveolar process (69). A review of treatment alternatives in cases with ankylosis and their relation to the growth of the young patient has recently been published (302).

In planning the decoronation of an ankylosed incisor, it is important to consider that ankylosed roots will ultimately be transformed to bone during the remodeling process. It is, therefore, not indicated to remove the root, as this will lead to a marked reduction in the height of the alveolar process. The treatment of choice is to remove the crown from the ankylosed and resorbed root and then remove the root filling. This technique is described in Chapter 24, p. 703.

In older patients an ankylosed tooth can be retained; the life-span of such a tooth can vary from 10 to 20 years, due to the slow remodeling rate of bone in older age groups.

## Inflammatory root resorption (infection-related root resorption)

Unless treated, inflammatory resorption can result in rapid loss of the replanted tooth, even as early as 3 months after

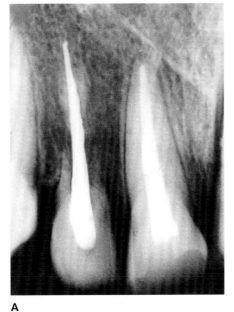 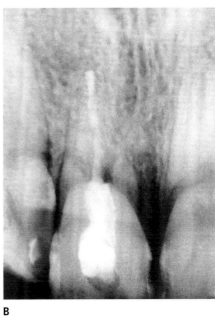

**Fig. 17.42** Difference in progression of replacement resorption after replantation. A. Marked replacement resorption of replanted right lateral incisor after 1¹/₂ years. B. Same degree of replacement resorption 9¹/₂ years after replantation of right central incisor. From ANDREASEN & HJÖRTING-HANSEN (6) 1966.

**A**    **B**

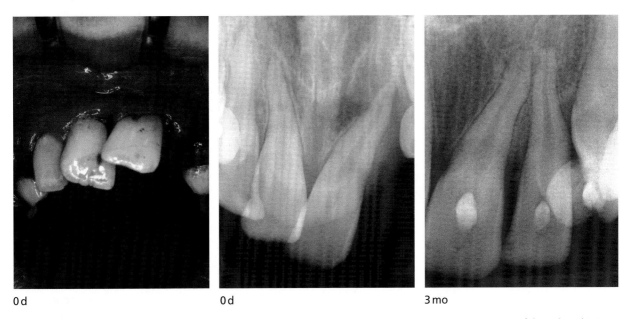

0 d                     0 d                     3 mo

**Fig. 17.43** The socket of the lateral incisor is involved in an alveolar fracture, leading to subsequent replacement resorption of the replanted incisor.

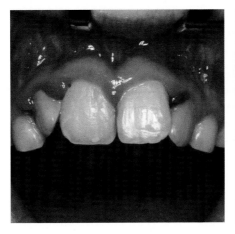 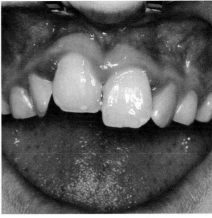

**Fig. 17.44** Progressive infraocclusion of an ankylosed replanted right central incisor. The replantation was carried out at the age of 7.

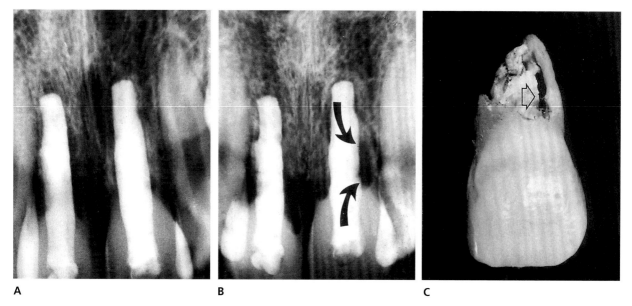

**Fig. 17.45** Left central incisor with simultaneous replacement and inflammatory resorption. A. Condition 2 years after replantation. Marked replacement resorption is evident. B. Three years after replantation. Replacement resorption has advanced to the root canal filling and inflammatory resorption is superimposed (arrows). C. The extracted tooth shows tunnelling resorption along root canal filling (arrow).

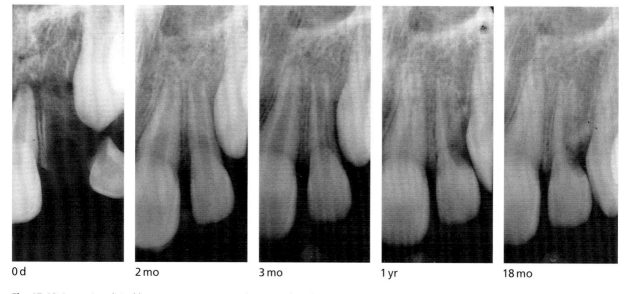

0 d          2 mo          3 mo          1 yr          18 mo

**Fig. 17.46** Resorption elicited by an erupting canine. Replantation of a left lateral incisor after extra-alveolar period of 90 minutes. Note marked root resorption apparently provoked by the erupting canine. The obliteration of the root canal shows that the pulp has survived replantation. From ANDREASEN et al. (201) 1995.

replantation (6) (Fig. 17.25). This type of resorption is, as mentioned before, related to the presence of an infected pulp. Thus, human and experimental data indicate that arrest of the resorptive processes can be achieved by appropriate endodontic therapy (6, 45, 149, 188, 202) (see Chapter 22, p. 632).

Replanted teeth can demonstrate simultaneous inflammatory and replacement resorption, a phenomenon possibly explained by superimposition of inflammatory resorption when replacement resorption exposes infected dentinal tubules or tubules leading to an infected necrotic pulp (Fig. 17.45).

## Resorption by erupting teeth

A special resorption phenomenon is encountered when a replanted tooth comes into contact with an erupting tooth, as when a lateral incisor lies close to the path of an erupting canine. Apparently, the pressure exerted by the follicle of the erupting tooth initiates or accelerates root resorption (202)

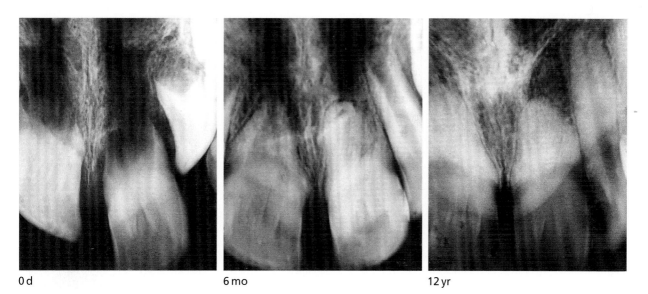

0 d        6 mo        12 yr

**Fig. 17.47** Continued root formation after replantation of a left central incisor.

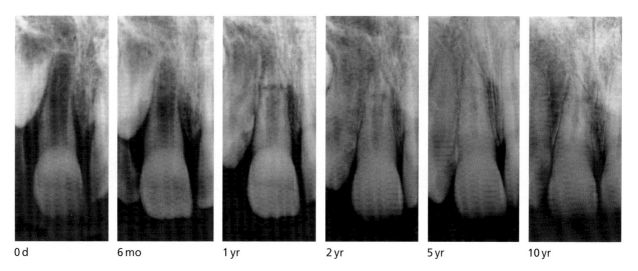

0 d    6 mo    1 yr    2 yr    5 yr    10 yr

**Fig. 17.48** Pulpal healing of a replanted maxillary right central incisor with full root and pulp canal obliteration after replantation. From ANDREASEN et al. (201) 1995.

(Fig. 17.46). A method to minimize the risk of resorption from the erupting tooth could be early removal of the primary predecessor in order to facilitate eruption, possibly in a direction away from the replanted tooth.

## Root development and disturbances in root growth

### Root growth

Continued root development can occur, especially if the pulp has become totally revascularized (Fig. 17.47).

However, root development can continue despite pulp necrosis (201) (Fig. 17.48). Most often, however, root development is partially or completely arrested and the root canal becomes obliterated (Fig. 17.49) or bone and PDL can invade the pulp chamber which in some cases can lead to an ankylosis (Fig. 17.50) (see also Chapter 22).

### Phantom roots

A rare complication to avulsion of immature permanent teeth is the formation of an abnormal root structure at the site of tooth loss (118–120, 194, 197, 198). The

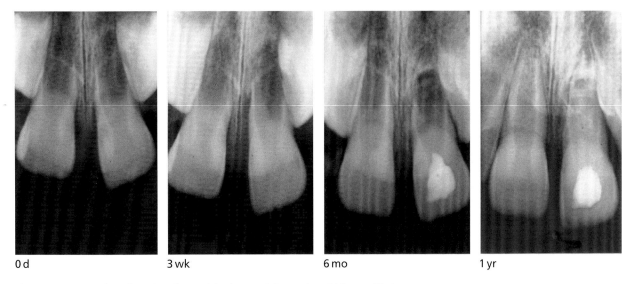

| | | | |
|---|---|---|---|
| 0 d | 3 wk | 6 mo | 1 yr |

**Fig. 17.49** Continued root formation after partial pulp necrosis in a replanted left central incisor.

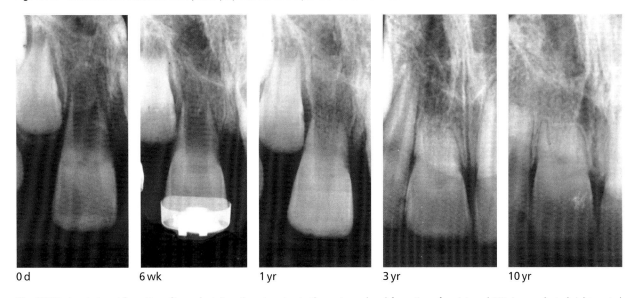

| | | | | |
|---|---|---|---|---|
| 0 d | 6 wk | 1 yr | 3 yr | 10 yr |

**Fig. 17.50** Arrested root formation after replantation. Bone invasion in the root canal and formation of an internal PDL in a replanted right central incisor. After 10 years infraocclusion was found apparently due to an internal ankylosis process. From ANDREASEN et al. (201) 1995.

explanation for this appears to be that pulp tissue and Hertwig's epithelial root sheath remain in the alveolar socket after avulsion. These tissues resume their formative function after injury. New dentin is formed by the odontoblasts, and the Hertwig's epithelial root sheath initiates root development (118) (Fig. 17.51). A parallel to this is the tooth-like structures occasionally formed when natal or neonatal teeth are extracted and the dental papilla is left *in situ* (121, 122).

## Gingival healing and loss of marginal attachment

Gingival healing is a common finding after replantation, irrespective of storage conditions (202) (Table 17.1). In cases where the trauma has elicited extensive alveolar damage, loss of marginal bone support may occur.

## Complications due to early loss of teeth

### Malformation in the developing dentition

If it is decided not to replant an avulsed permanent tooth, problems arise with regard to further treatment. The same applies to cases where extraction of the replanted tooth is necessary due to root resorption. If no treatment is instituted, a marked degree of spontaneous tooth migration is often seen (90–92, 129). Unfortunately, this drifting is often esthetically undesirable due to midline deviation. Therapy should therefore consist of either orthodontic space closure, prosthetic tooth replacement or autotransplantation or implantation to the site. These treatment solutions are described in Chapters 24–29.

### Predictors for pulpal and peridontal healing

The known predictors for pulpal healing appear in Fig. 17.52 (200) and for PDL healing in Fig. 17.53 (202).

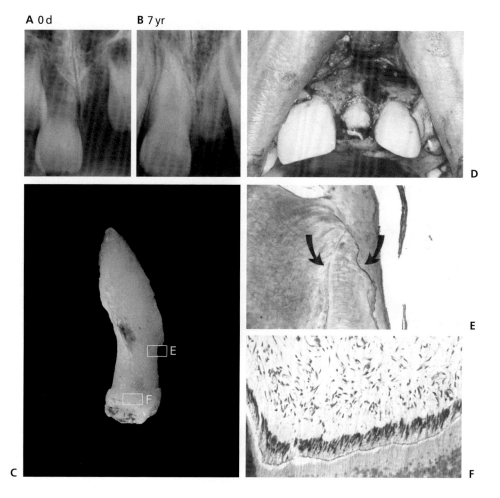

**A** 0 d　　**B** 7 yr

**Fig. 17.51** Root structure formed after avulsion of a permanent central incisor at the age of 7 years. A. Radiographic condition immediately after injury. B. At follow-up 3½ years later a root structure is found at the site of the avulsed tooth. C. The root is surgically removed. D. Low power view of sectioned incisor. ×5. E. Fragment of dentin (arrows) representing the apical area at time of injury which together with the pulp tissue and the Hertwig's epithelial root sheath has been left in the tooth socket after avulsion. ×75. F. Normal dentin and odontoblastic layer in the coronal part of the root structure. ×195. From RAVN (118) 1970.

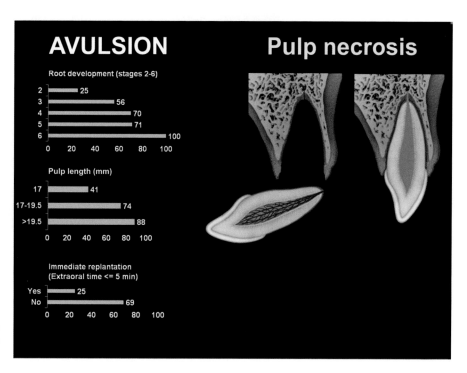

**Fig. 17.52** Predictors for pulp necrosis. From ANDREASEN et al. (200) 1995.

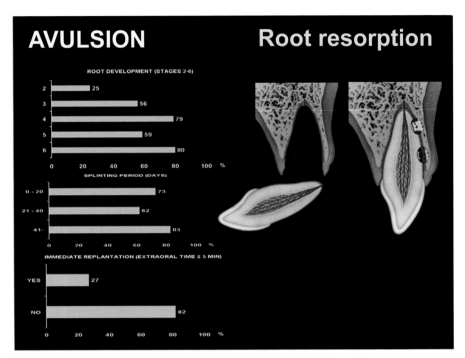

**Fig. 17.53** Predictors for root resorption. From ANDREASEN et al. (202) 1995.

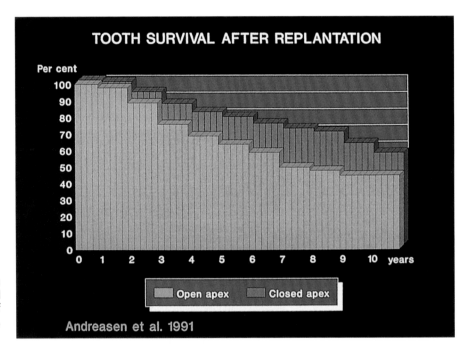

**Fig. 17.54** Life table analysis of tooth survival after 400 replantations related to root development stage at time of replantation. From ANDREASEN et al. (199) 1995.

## Tooth survival

In a large clinical study, it was found that over a 10-year period, approximately 50% of teeth with immature root formation survived, compared to 70% when root formation was complete (199) (Fig. 17.54). This finding has been supported by a study by Barrett and Kenny (287) 1997.

## Essentials

### Terminology

Complete avulsion (exarticulation)

## Frequency

Permanent dentition: 0.5–3% dental injuries

## Etiology

- Fall injuries
- Sports injuries
- Fight injuries

## Advice for the site of accident (e.g. telephone advice)

- Replant the tooth (primary teeth should however not be replanted.
- If contaminated rinse in tap water for 10 seconds.
- If not possible to replant store in patient's mouth (saliva), milk or saline.
- Visit a dental clinic as soon as possible.

## History

- Extra-alveolar period
- Condition under which the tooth has been preserved

## Clinical examination

- Condition of the avulsed tooth
- Condition of the alveolus

## Radiographic examination

Associated bone fractures

## Healing and pathology

### Repair of pulpal and periodontal structures

Root resorption, external:

(1) Surface resorption (repair-related resorption), related to minor areas of damage to the periodontal ligament upon the avulsed tooth.
(2) Ankylosis (replacement resorption), permanent or transient depending upon the initial extent of damage to the periodontal ligament upon the avulsed tooth.
(3) Inflammatory resorption (infection-related resorption), related to the presence of an infected root canal and associated damage to the root surface.

## Treatment of permanent teeth

### Indications for replantation

- The avulsed tooth should be without advanced periodontal disease.
- The alveolar socket should be reasonably intact in order to provide a seat for the avulsed tooth.

### Procedure for replantation of teeth with open or closed apices (Fig. 17.26)

(1) Immediate replantation by the patient should be encouraged. Rinsing for 10 seconds in cold water should be done before replantation. Otherwise the tooth should be stored in saline, saliva or milk.
(2) If obviously contaminated, cleanse the root surface and the apical foramen with a stream of saline (from a syringe). No attempt should be made to sterilize the root surface.
(3) In cases of immature root formation, the storage of the tooth for 5 minutes in a suspension of 1 mg doxycycline in 20 ml saline may double the chance of revascularization.
(4) Flush the coagulum from the socket with a flow of saline. Examine the alveolar socket. If there is a fracture of the socket wall, reposition the fracture with an instrument.
(5) *Closed apex*: replant the tooth in the socket using light digital pressure.
   *Open apex*: in these cases, pretreatment of the root with tetracycline may favor the chance of revascularization of the pulp. (a) The tooth is placed in a tetracycline solution for 5 min (doxycycline 10 mg/200 ml saline). (b) Alternatively, the root surface including the apex is powdered with Minocycline® (Arestin® Microspheres, Ora Pharma, Inc., 2005).
(6) Suture gingival lacerations.
(7) Apply a splint and maintain it for 7–10 days.
(8) Verify normal position of the replanted tooth radiographically.
(9) Provide tetanus prophylaxis and systemic antibiotic therapy. For children 12 years and younger: penicillin V at an appropriate dose for patient age and weight. For children older than 12 years of age, where there is little risk for tetracycline discoloration: tetracycline (doxycycline 2x per day for 7 days at appropriate dose for patient age and weight).
(10) In the case of mature teeth with a narrow apical foramen, endodontic therapy should be instituted 7–10 days after replantation and prior to splint removal (see Chapter 22, p. 620).
(11) When the apical foramen is wide open and the tooth replanted within 3 hours, revascularization of the pulp is possible.
(12) Control the tooth radiographically. If signs of inflammatory resorption appear, institute root canal treatment immediately (see Chapter 22, p. 632).
(13) Follow-up: minimum 1 year.

### Long extra-alveolar period

In cases with an extra-oral dry period of 60 min or more, treatment of the tooth with sodium fluoride should be considered.

(1) Remove the PDL and extirpate the pulp.
(2) Place the tooth for 20 min in a 2.4% sodium fluoride solution acidulated to a pH of 5.5.
(3) Root fill the tooth extra-orally.
(4) Remove the coagulum from the socket.
(5) Replant the tooth.
(6) Splint the tooth for 4 weeks.
(7) Follow-up: minimum 1 year.

## Treatment of root resorption

### Surface resorption

No treatment indicated.

## Replacement resorption

- Decoronation in cases with progressive infraocclusion of the ankylosed tooth and where residual alveolar growth is anticipated.
- Otherwise, preservation of the tooth in the interim before final treatment.

## Inflammatory resorption

Institute root canal therapy (see Chapter 22, p. 632).

## Prognosis

- Tooth survival: 21–89%
- PDL healing: 9–50%
- Pulp healing: 4–27%

## Complications after premature loss of permanent teeth

(1) Close the space orthodontically (see Chapter 24, p. 687).
(2) Maintain the space by means of autotransplantation, bridge/implant prosthetics or orthodontic closure (see Chapters 26–29).

# References

1. ANDREASEN JO. Etiology and pathogenesis of traumatic dental injuries. A clinical study of 1298 cases. *Scand J Dent Res* 1970;**78**:329–42.
2. GLENDOR U, HALLING A, ANDERSSON L, EILERT-PETERSSON E. Incidence of traumatic tooth injuries in children and adolescents in the county of Västmanland, Sweden. *Swed Dent J* 1996;**20**:15–28.
3. SUNDVALL-HAGLAND I. Olycksfallsskador på tänder och parodontium under barnaåren. In: Holst JJ, Nygaard Ostby B, Osvald O. *Nordisk Klinisk Odontologi.* Copenhagen: A/S Forlaget for Faglitteratur, Chapter 11, **III**:1–40.
4. GELBIER S. Injured anterior teeth in children. A preliminary discussion. *Br Dent J* 1967;**123**:331–5.
5. RAVN JJ, ROSSEN I. Hyppighed og fordeling af traumatiske beskadigelser af tænderne hos københavnske skolebørn 1967/68. *Tandlægebladet* 1969;**73**:1–9.
6. ANDREASEN JO, HJORTING-HANSEN E. Replantation of teeth. 1. Radiographic and clinical study of 110 human teeth replanted after accidental loss. *Acta Odontol Scand* 1966;**24**:263–86.
7. LENSTRUP K, SKIELLER V. Efterundersögelse af tænder replanteret efter exartikulation. *Tandlægebladet* 1957;**61**:570–83.
8. LENSTRUP K, SKIELLER V. A follow-up study of teeth replanted after accidental loss. *Acta Odontol Scand* 1959;**17**:503–9.
9. SANDERS E. Replantatie van tanden. *T Tandheelk* 1934;**41**:254–66.
10. SCHEFF J. Die Re-, Trans- und Implantation der Zähne. In: Scheff J. *Handbuch der Zahnheilkunde.* Vol. II, No. 2. Wien: Alfred Hölder, 1892:99–128.
11. LUNDQUIST GR. Histo-pathological studies of replanted teeth in dogs. In: Black AD. *Operative dentistry.* Vol. 4. Chicago: Medico-Dental Publishing Company, 1936:200–2.
12. SKILLEN WG, LUNDQUIST GR. A study of the replanted tooth in the dog. *J Dent Res* 1929;**9**:275–6.
13. SKILLEN WG, LUNDQUIST GR. Replanting dog teeth. *J Dent Res* 1934;**14**:177–8.
14. HATTYASY D. Replantationsversuche mit Zahnkeimen. *Dtsch Zahn Mund Kieferheilk* 1940;**9**:535–51.
15. WAITE DE. Animal studies on dental transplants. *Oral Surg Oral Med Oral Pathol* 1956;**9**:40–5.
16. KAQUELER JC, MASSLER M. Healing following tooth replantation. *J Dent Child* 1969;**36**:303–14.
17. SHERMAN P. Intentional replantation of teeth in dogs and monkeys. *J Dent Res* 1968;**47**:1066–71.
18. ROTHSCHILD DL, GOODMAN AA, BLAKEY KR. A histologic study of replanted and transplanted endodontically and nonendodontically treated teeth in dogs. *Oral Surg Oral Med Oral Pathol* 1969;**28**:871–6.
19. MITSCHERLICH A. Die Replantation und die Transplantation der Zähne. *Arch Klin Chir* 1863;**4**:375–417.
20. MENDEL-JOSEPH M, DASSONVILLE M. Recherches expérimentales sur le méchanisme de la consolidation dans la greffe dentaire. *Odontologie* 1906;**36**:99–112.
21. RÖMER KR. Ueber die Replantation von Zähnen. *Dtsch Monatschr Zahnheilk* 1901;**19**:297–306.
22. BÖDECKER CF, LEFKOWITZ W. Replantation of teeth. *Dent Items* 1935;**57**:675–92.
23. KNIGHT MK, GANS BJ, CALANDRA JC. The effect of root canal therapy on replanted teeth of dogs. A gross, roentgenographic, and histologic study. *Oral Surg Oral Med Oral Pathol* 1964;**18**:227–42.
24. HAMMER H. Der histologische Vorgang bei der Zahnreplantation. *Dtsch Zahn Mund Kieferheilk* 1934;**1**:115–36.
25. HAMMER H. Der histologische Vorgang bei der Zahnreplantation nach Vernichtung der Wurzelhaut. *Dtsch Zahn Mund Kieferheilk* 1937;**4**:179–87.
26. HAMMER H. Il reimpianto biologico dei denti. *Mondo Odontostomatol* 1967;**9**:291–302.
27. HOVINGA J. *Replantatie en transplantatie van tanden. Een experimenteel en klinisch onderzoek.* Amsterdam: Oosterbaan & Le Cointre N. V.-Goes, 1968.
28. ANDERSON AW, SHARAV Y, MASSLER M. Periodontal reattachment after tooth replantation. *Periodontics* 1968;**6**:161–7.
29. ANDERSON AW, SHARAV Y, MASSLER M. Reparative dentine formation and pulp morphology. *Oral Surg Oral Med Oral Pathol* 1968;**26**:837–47.
30. HOPPE W, BREMER H. Experimenteller Beitrag zur enossalen Implantation alloplastischen Materials im Kieferbereich. *Dtsch Zahnärztl Z* 1956;**11**:551–61.
31. WILKINSON FC. Some observations on the replantation and transplantation of teeth, with special reference to the pathohistology of the tissues of attachment. *Br Dent J* 1917;**38**:929–39.
32. ROSS WS. Apicectomy in the treatment of dead teeth. *Br Dent J* 1935;**58**:473–86.
33. LÖE H, WAERHAUG J. Experimental replantation of teeth in dogs and monkeys. *Arch Oral Biol* 1961;**3**:176–84.
34. SHULMAN LB, KALIS P, GOLDHABER P. Fluoride inhibition of tooth-replant root resorption in cebus monkeys. *J Oral Ther* 1968;**4**:331–7.

35. Grewe JM, Felts WJL. Autoradiographic investigation of tritiated thymidine incorporation into replanted and transplanted mouse mandibular incisors. *J Dent Res* 1968;**47**:108–14.

36. Meyers H, Nassimbene L, Alley J, Gehrig J, Flanagan VD. Replantation of teeth in the hamster. *Oral Surg Oral Med Oral Pathol* 1954;**7**:1116–29.

37. Meyers HI, Flanagan VD. A comparison of results obtained from transplantation and replantation experiments using Syrian hamster teeth. *Anat Rec* 1958;**130**:497–513.

38. Flanagan VD, Meyers HI. Long-range postoperative evaluation of survival of hamster second molars. *J Dent Res* 1958;**37**:37.

39. Flanagan VD, Meyers HI. The use of a semiliquid postoperative diet following reimplantation of hamster second molars. *J Dent Res* 1959;**38**:667.

40. Flanagan VD, Meyers HI. Postoperative antibiotic therapy used in association with hamster replantation procedures. *J Dent Res* 1960;**39**:726–7.

41. Sorg WR. Nerve regeneration in replanted hamster teeth. *J Dent Res* 1960;**39**:1222–31.

42. Costich ER, Hoek RB, Hayward JR. Replantation of molar teeth in the Syrian hamster. II. *J Dent Res* 1958;**37**:367.

43. Öhman A. Healing and sensitivity to pain in young replanted human teeth. An experimental, clinical and histological study. *Odontologisk Tidsskrift* 1965;**73**:165–228.

44. Andreasen JO, Hjörting-Hansen E. Replantation of teeth. II. Histological study of 22 replanted anterior teeth in humans. *Acta Odontol Scand* 1966;**24**: 287–306.

45. Andreasen JO. Treatment of fractured and avulsed teeth. *ASDC J Dent Child* 1971;**38**:29–48.

46. Hess W. Zur Frage der Replantation von Zahnkeimen. *Schweiz Monatschr Zahnheilk* 1943;**53**:672–7.

47. Silva IA, Lima ACP. Reimplantaçao dentária com preservaçao do periodonto. *An Fac Farm Odontol Sao Paulo* 1954;**12**:309–31.

48. Krömer H. Tannreplantasjon. En kirurgisk rotbehandlingsmetode. *Norske Tannlægeforenings Tidende* 1952;**62**:147–57.

49. Henry JL, Weinmann JP. The pattern of resorption and repair of human cementum. *J Am Dent Assoc* 1951;**42**:270–90.

50. Ciriello G. Impianti acrilici ed innesti dentarii nei tessuti mascellari a sostegno di protesi. *Riv Ital Stomatol* 1954;**9**:1087–143.

51. Langeland K. Om rotresorpsjoner i permanente tenner. *Norske Tannlægeforenings Tidende* 1958;**68**:237–47.

52. Messing JJ. Reimplantation of teeth. *Dent Practit Dent Rec* 1968;**18**:241–8.

53. Pindborg JJ, Hansen J. A case of replantation of an upper lateral incisor: A histologic study. *Oral Surg Oral Med Oral Pathol* 1951;**4**:661–7.

54. Lovel RW, Hopper FE. Tooth replantation: A case report with serial radiographs and histological examination. *Br Dent J* 1954; **97**:205–8.

55. Herbert WE. A case of complete dislocation of a tooth. *Br Dent J* 1958;**105**:137–8.

56. Deeb E, Prietto PP, McKenna RC. Reimplantation of luxated teeth in humans. *J South Calif Dent Assoc* 1965;**33**:194–206.

57. Rivas LA. Ergebnisse der Replantation nach Trauma im Frontzahnbereich bei Jugendlichen. *Dtsch Zahnärztl Z* 1968;**23**:484–9.

58. Dunker L. Über die Behandlung unfallgeschädigter Milchzähne. (Unter besonderer Berücksichtigung der Replantation). *Dtsch Zahndrztebl* 1967;**21**:174–80.

59. Sakellariou PL. Replantation of infected deciduous teeth: A contribution to the problem of their preservation until normal shedding. *Oral Surg Oral Med Oral Pathol* 1963;**16**:645–53.

60. Eisenberg MD. Reimplantation of a deciduous tooth. *Oral Surg Oral Med Oral Pathol* 1965;**19**:588–90.

61. Smellhaus S. Über die Replantation der Milchzähne. *Z Stomatol* 1925; **23**:52–7.

62. Cassardelli H. Zur Möglichkeit der Erhaltung unfallintrudierter Milchzähne. *Dtsch Stomatol* 1961;**11**:362–8.

63. Herbert WE. Three successful cases of replacement of teeth immediately following dislocation. *Br Dent* 1953;**94**:182–3.

64. Axhausen G. Ein Beitrag zur Zahnreplantation. *Zahnärztl Welt* 1948;**3**:130–2.

65. Jlg VK. Zur Theorie und Praxis der Replantation. *Dtsch Zahnärztl Z* 1951;**6**:585–94, 653–63.

66. Miller HM. Reimplanting human teeth. *Dent Surv* 1953;**29**:1439–42.

67. Kluge R. Indikation und Erfolgsaussichten bei Zahnrückpflanzung. *Zahnärztl Prax* 1957;**23**:1–2.

68. Sommer RF, Ostrander FD, Crowley MC. *Clinical endodontics. A manual of scientific endodontics.* 3 edn. Philadelphia: WB Saunders Company, 1966:445–88.

69. Ravn JJ, Helbo M. Replantation of akcidentelt eksarticulerede tinder. *Tandlægebladet* 1966;**70**: 805–15.

70. Flanagan VD, Meyers HI. Delayed reimplantation of second molars in the Syrian hamster. *Oral Surg Oral Med Oral Pathol* 1958;**11**:1179–88.

71. McCagie JNW. A case of re-implantation of teeth after five days. *Dent Practit Dent Rec* 1958;**8**:320–1.

72. Jonck LM. An investigation into certain aspects of transplantation and reimplantation of teeth in man. *Br J Oral Surg* 1966;**4**:137–46.

73. Ogus WI. Research report on the replant-implant of individual teeth. *Dent Dig* 1954;**60**:358–61.

74. Hammer H. Replantation and implantation of teeth. *Int Dent J* 1955;**5**:439–57.

75. Thonner KE. Vitalliumstift vid reimplantation av totalluxerade tinder. *Sverig Tandläkar Förbund Tidning* 1956;**48**:216–7.

76. Weiskopf J, Gehre G, Graichen K-H. Ein Beitrag zur Behandlung von Luxationen und Wurzelfrakturen im Frontzahngebiet. *Stoma (Heidelberg)* 1961;**14**: 100–13.

77. Ciriello G. Alcune considerazioni sulla tecnica del reimpianto dentario. *Riv Ital Stomatol* 1953;**8**: 764–99.

78. Orlay HG. Befestigung von lockeren Zähnen mit endodontischen Implantaten. *Schweiz Monatschr Zahnheilk* 1968;**78**:580–98.

79. ARCHER WH. Replantation of an accidentally extracted erupted partially formed mandibular second premolar. *Oral Surg Oral Med Oral Pathol* 1952;**5**:256–8.

80. LINDAHL B, MARTENSSON K. Replantation of a tooth. A case report. *Odontologisk Revy* 1960;**11**:325–30.

81. LJUNGDAHLL J, MÅRTENSSON K. Ett fall av multipla tandreplantationer. *Odontologisk Revy* 1955;**6**:222–32.

82. PÅLSSON F. Zur Frage der Replantation von Zahnkeimen. *Acta Odontol Scand* 1944;**5**:63–78.

83. HENNING FR. Reimplantation of luxated teeth. *Aust Dent J* 1965;**10**:306–12.

84. SWEDBERG Y. Replantation av accidentally luxerade tandanlag. *Svensk Tannläkar Tidning* 1966;**59**:649–54.

85. COOKE C, ROWBOTHAM TC. Treatment of injuries to anterior teeth. *Br Dent J* 1951;**91**:146–52.

86. ELLIS RG, DAVEY KV. *The classification and treatment of injuries to the teeth of children.* 5th edn. Chicago: Year Book Publishers Inc., 1970.

87. BENNET DT. Traumatised anterior teeth. VI. The class V injury. *Br Dent J* 1964;**116**:7–9.

88. ENGELHARDT JP. Die prothetische Versorgung des traumatisch geschädigten Jugendgebisses aus klinischer Sicht. *Zahnärztl Welt* 1968;**69**:264–70.

89. SEIDEL CM. Ortodontiska synpunkter beträffande terapien vid kronfraktur på framtänder hos barn i skolaldern. *Svensk Tannläkara Tidning* 1940;**33**:14–27.

90. PERSSON B. Bettortopediska synpunkter på behandlingen särskilt valet mellam konserverande terapi och extraktion i incisivområdet. In: Holst JJ, Nygaard Ostby B, Osvald O. *Nordisk Klinisk Odontologi.* Copenhagen: A/S Forlaget for Faglitteratur, 1964, Chapter 11, III:35–8.

91. PERSSON B. The traumatised front tooth. Orthodontic aspects. *Eur Orthodont Soc Trans* 1965;**41**:329–45.

92. BRUTSZT P. Die Selbstregelung der Zahnreihe nach dem Verlust des oberen mittleren Schneidezahnes im Wechselgebiss. *Schweiz Monatschr Zahnheilk* 1956;**66**:926–31.

93. HOTZ R. Die Bedeutung, Beurteilung und Behandlung beim Trauma im Frontzahngebiet vom Standpunkt des Kieferorthopäden. *Dtsch Zahnärztl Z* 1958;**13**:42–51, 401–16.

94. SCHMUTH GPF. Die Behandlung des traumatischen Zahnverlustes durch kieferorthopädische Massnahmen. *Zahnärztl Welt* 1967;**68**:15–9.

95. VETTER H. Zwei Fälle von frühzeitigem Frontzahnverlust durch Trauma und ihre Versorgung. *Fortschr Kieferorthop* 1954;**15**:90–101.

96. VOSS R. Problematik, Möglichkeiten und Grenzen des prothetischen Lückenschlusses im Frontzahnbereich bei Jugendlichen. *Fortschr Kieferorthop* 1969;**30**:89–101.

97. RINDERER L. Deux cas de traitement orthodontique après perte traumatique des deux incisives centrales. *Rev Stomatol (Paris);***61**:627–32.

98. REICHENBACH E. Unfallverletzungen im Kindesalter. *Dtsch Stomatol* 1954;**4**:33–42.

99. SCHULZE C. Über die Folgen des Verlustes oberer mittlerer Schneidezähne während der Gebissentwicklung. *Zahnärztl Rdsch* 1967;**76**:156–69.

100. ESCHLER J, SCHILLI W, WITT E. *Die traumatischen Verletzungen der Frontzähne bei J ugendlichen.* 3 edn. Heidelberg: Alfred Hüthig Verlag, 1972.

101. KIPP H. Traumatischer Zahnverlust bei kieferorthopädischen Krankheitsbildern. *Fortschr Kieferorthop* 1958;**19**:165–70.

102. RAVN JJ. *Ulykkesskadede fortænder på børn. Klassifikation og behandling.* Copenhagen: Odontologisk Forening, 1966.

103. LJUNDAHL L. Ett fall av korrektion efter trauma på överkäksincisiverna. *Odontologisk Revy* 1954;**5**: 212–7.

104. MAIER-MOHR I. Ober kieferorthopädische Massnahmen beim Verlust eines mittleren oberen Schneidezahnes. *Fortschr Kieferorthop* 1955;**16**:357–61.

105. FREUNTHALLER P. Möglichkeiten des Lückenschlusses durch orthodontische Massnahmen bei Frontzahnverlust. *Österr Z Stomatol* 1964;**61**:467–74.

106. HEDEGÅRD B. The traumatised front tooth. Some prosthetic aspects of therapeutic procedures. *Eur Orthod Soc Trans* 1965;**41**:347–51.

107. HECKMANN U. Die kieferorthopddische Therapie beim Frontzahnverlust im jugendlichen Alter. *Dtsch Zähnarztl Z* 1960;**15**:43–7.

108. ROSE JS. Early loss of teeth in children. *Br Dent J* 1966;**120**:275–80.

109. GRANATH L-E. Några synpunkter på behandlingen av traumatiserade incisiver på barn. *Odontologisk Revy* 1959;**10**:272–86.

110. BROGLIA ML, GUASTA G. Il problema terapeutico della lussazione totale traumatica degli incisivi permanenti nei pazienti di età pediatrica. *Minerva Stomatol* 1968;**17**:549–56.

111. BIOURGE A. Traumatismes violents des incisives supérieures dans le jeune age. *Rev Stomatol (Paris)* 1968;**69**:30–43.

112. HAUSSER E, BACKHAUS I, PELAEZ H, GREVE MR. Traitement orthodontique aprés traumatismes dento-alvéolaires. *Orthod Fr* 1967;**38**:382–3.

113. DRUSCH-NEUMANN D. Über die Lücken bei fehlenden Milchfrontzähnen. *Fortschr Kieferorthop* 1969;**30**:82–8.

114. ASH AS. Orthodontic significance of anomalies of tooth eruption. *Am J Orthod* 1957;**43**:559–76.

115. KORF SR. The eruption of permanent central incisors following premature loss of their antecedents. *ASDC J Dent Child* 1965;**32**:39–44.

116. BROGLIA ML, DANA F. Manifestazioni cliniche delle lesioni traumatishe accidentali della dentatura decidua. *Minerva Stomatol* 1967;**16**:623–35.

117. GYSEL C. Traumatologie et orthodontie. *Rev Fr Odontostomatol* 1962;**9**:1091–113.

118. RAVN JJ. Partiel roddannelse efter eksarticulation of permanent incisiv hos en 7-årig dreng. *Tandlægebladet* 1970;**74**:906–10.

119. LYSELL G, LYSELL L. A unique case of dilaceration. *Odontologisk Revy* 1969;**20**:43–6.

120. GIBSON ACL. Continued root development after traumatic avulsion of partly-formed permanent incisor. *Br Dent J* 1969;**126**:356–7.

121. SOUTHAM JC. Retained dentine papillae in the newborn. A clinical and histopathological study. *Br Dent J* 1968;**125**:534–8.

122. RYBA GE, KRAMER IRH. Continued growth of human dentine papillae following removal of the crowns of partly formed deciduous teeth. *Oral Surg Oral Med Oral Pathol* 1962;**15**:867–75.

123. ANDREASEN JO, SUNDSTRÖM B, RAVN JJ. The effect of traumatic injuries to primary teeth on their permanent successors. I. A clinical and histologic study of 117 injured permanent teeth. *Scand J Dent Res* 1971;**79**:219–83.

124. ANDREASEN JO, RAVN JJ. The effect of traumatic injuries to primary teeth on their permanent successors. II. A clinical and radiographic follow-up study of 213 teeth. *Scand J Dent Res* 1971;**79**:284–94.

125. HEDEGARD B, STÅLHANE I. A study of traumatized permanent teeth in children aged 7–15 years. Part 1. *Swed Dent J* 1973;**66**:431–50.

126. RAVN JJ. Dental injuries in Copenhagen schoolchildren, school years 1967–1972. *Community Dent Oral Epidemiol* 1974;**2**:231–45.

127. KEMP WB, GROSSMAN LI, PHILLIPS J. Evaluation of 71 replanted teeth. *J Endod* 1977;**3**:30–5.

128. HÖRSTER W, ALTFELD F, PLANKO D. Behandlungsergebnisse nach Replantation total luxierter Frontzähne. *Fortsch Kiefer Gesichtschir* 1976;**20**:127–9.

129. RAVN JJ. En redegörelse for behandlingen efter exarticulation of permanente incisiver i en skolebarnspopulation. *Tandlægebladet* 1977;**81**:563–9.

130. GROPER JN, BERNICK S. Histological study of the periodontium following replantation of teeth in the dog. *ASDC J Dent Child* 1970;**37**:25–35.

131. ANDERSON AW, MASSLER M. Periapical tissue reactions following root amputation in immediate tooth replants. *Israel J Dent Med* 1970;**19**:1–8.

132. MONSOUR FNT. Pulpal changes following the reimplantation of teeth in dogs. A histologic study. *Aust Dent J* 1971;**16**:227–231.

133. GOMBOS F, BUONAIUTO C, CARUSO F. Nuovi orientamenti sui reimpianti dentari studio clinico e sperimentale. *Mondo Odontostomatol* 1972;**4**:589–610.

134. SCHMID F, TRIADAN H, KOPPER W. Tierexperimentelle Untersuchungen zur Elektrostimulation der Pulpa nach Replantation. *Fortschrit Kiefer Gesichtschir* 1976;**20**:132–4.

135. WOEHRLE RR. Cementum regeneration in replanted teeth with differing pulp treatment. *J Dent Res* 1976;**55**:235–8.

136. SKOGLUND A, TRONSTAD L. A morphologic and enzyme histochemical study on the pulp of replanted and autotransplanted teeth in young dogs. *J Dent Res* 1978;**57**:IADR Abstract no. 478.

137. SKOGLUND A, TRONSTAD L, WALLENIUS K. A microangiographic study of vascular changes in replanted and autotransplanted teeth of young dogs. *Oral Surg Oral Med Oral Pathol* 1978;**45**:17–28.

138. ANDREASEN JO. A time-related study of root resorption activity after replantation of mature permanent incisors in monkeys. *Swed Dent J* 1980;**4**:101–10.

139. ANDREASEN JO. Relationship between surface- and inflammatory root resorption and changes in the pulp after replantation of permanent incisors in monkeys. *J Endod* 1981;**7**:294–301.

140. ANDREASEN JO. Analysis of topography of surface- and inflammatory root resorption after replantation of mature permanent incisors in monkeys. *Swed Dent J* 1980;**4**:135–44.

141. ANDREASEN JO, SCHWARTZ O, ANDREASEN FM. The effect of apicoectomy before replantation on periodontal and pulpal healing in monkeys. *Int J Oral Surg* 1985;**14**:176–83.

142. ANDREASEN JO. Relationship between cell damage in the periodontal ligament after replant or removal of the periodontal ligament. Periodontal healing after replantation of mature permanent incisors in monkeys. *Acta Odontol Scand* 1981;**39**:15–25.

143. ANDREASEN JO. Periodontal healing after replantation and autotransplantation of permanent incisors. Effect of injury to the alveolar or cemental part of the periodontal ligament in monkeys. *Int J Oral Surg* 1981;**10**:54–61.

144. ANDREASEN JO, KRISTERSON L. The effect of limited drying or removal of the periodontal ligament. Perodontal healing after replantation of mature permanent incisors in monkeys. *Acta Odontol Scand* 1981;**39**:1–13.

145. ANDREASEN JO, KRISTERSON L. Repair processes in the cervical region of replanted and transplanted teeth in monkeys. *Int J Oral Surg* 1981;**10**:128–36.

146. ANDREASEN JO. Effect of extra-alveolar period and storage media upon periodontal and pulpal healing after replantation of mature permanent incisors in monkeys. *Int J Oral Surg* 1981;**10**:43–53.

147. ANDREASEN JO. The effect of splinting upon periodontal healing after replantation of permanent incisors in monkeys. *Acta Odontol Scand* 1975;**33**:313–23.

148. ANDREASEN JO. The effect of excessive occlusal trauma upon periodontal healing after replantation of mature permanent incisors in monkeys. *Swed Dent J* 1981;**5**:115–22.

149. ANDREASEN JO. The effect of pulp extirpation or root canal treatment on periodontal healing after replantation of mature permanent incisors in monkeys. *J Endod* 1981;**7**:245–52.

150. ANDREASEN JO. The effect of removal of the coagulum in the alveolus before replantation upon periodontal and pulpal healing of mature permanent incisors in monkeys. *Int J Oral Surg* 1980;**9**:458–61.

151. ANDREASEN JO. Interrelation between alveolar bone and periodontal ligament repair after replantation of mature permanent incisors in monkeys. *J Periodontal Res* 1981;**16**:228–35.

152. ANDREASEN JO, KRISTERSON L. The effect of extra-alveolar root filling with calcium hydroxide on periodontal healing after replantation of permanent incisors in monkeys. *J Endod* 1981;**7**:349–54.

153. TRONSTAD L, ANDREASEN JO, HASSELGREN G, KRISTERSON L, RIIS I. pH changes in dental tissues after root canal filling with calcium hydroxide. *J Endod* 1981;**7**:17–22.

154. ANDREASEN JO, REINHOLDT J, RIIS I, DYBDAHL R, SÖDER PÖ, OTTESKOG P. Periodontal and pulpal healing of monkey incisors preserved in tissue culture before replantation. *Int J Oral Surg* 1978;**7**:104–12.

155. ANDREASEN JO. Delayed replantation after submucosal storage in order to prevent root resorption after replantation. An experimental study in monkeys. *Int J Oral Surg* 1980;**9**:394–403.

156. ANDREASEN JO, KRISTERSON L. Evaluation of different types of autotransplanted connective tissues as potential periodontal ligament substitutes. An experimental

replantation study in monkeys. *Int J Oral Surg* 1998;**10**:189–201.

157. HAMNER JE, REED OM, STANLEY HR. Reimplantation of teeth in the baboon. *J Am Dent Assoc* 1970;**81**: 662–70.

158. CASTELLI WA, NASJLETI CE, HUELKE DR, DIAZ-PEREZ R. Revascularization of the periodontium after tooth grafting in monkeys. *J Dent Res* 1971;**50**:414–21.

159. HURST RVV. Regeneration of periodontal and transseptal fibres after autografts in Rhesus monkeys. A qualitative approach. *J Dent Res* 1972;**51**: 1183–92.

160. KELLER EB, HAYWARD JR, NASJLETI CE, CASTELLI WA. Venous tissue replanted on roots of teeth in monkeys. *Oral Surg Oral Med Oral Pathol* 1972;**34**:352–63.

161. NORDENRAM Å, BANG G, ANNEROTH G. A histologic study of replanted teeth with superficially demineralised root surfaces in Java monkeys. *Scand J Dent Res* 1973;**81**:294–302.

162. NASJLETI CE, CAFFESSI RG, CASTELLI WA, HOKE JA. Healing after tooth reimplantation in monkeys. A radioautographic study. *Oral Surg Oral Med Oral Pathol* 1975;**39**:361–75.

163. NASJLETI CE, CASTELLI WA, BLANKENSHIP JR. The storage of teeth before reimplantation in monkeys. *Oral Surg Oral Med Oral Pathol* 1975;**39**:20–9.

164. BARBAKOW FH, AUSTIN JC, CLEATON-JONES PE. Experimental replantation of root-canal-filled and untreated teeth in the vervet monkey. *J Endod* 1977;**3**:89–93.

165. CAFFESSI RG, NASJLETI CE, CASTELLI WA. Long-term results after intentional tooth reimplantation in monkeys. *Oral Surg Oral Med Oral Pathol* 1977;**44**:666–78.

166. NASJLETI CE, CAFFESSI RG, CASTELLI WA. Replantation of mature teeth without endodontics in monkeys. *J Dent Res* 1978;**57**:650–8.

167. MANDELL ML, BERTRAM U. Calcitonin treatment for root resorption. *J Dent Res* 1970;**49**:182.

168. BJORVATN K, MASSLER M. Effect of fluorides on root resorption in replanted rat molars. *Acta Odontol Scand* 1971;**29**:17–29.

169. BJORVATN K, WEISS MB. Effect of topical application of fluoride, cortisone and tetracycline on replanted rat molars. *Fasset* 1971;**1**:27–31.

170. JOHANSEN JR. Reimplantation of mandibular incisors in the guinea pig: a histologic and autoradiographic study. *Acta Odontol Scand* 1970;**28**:633–60.

171. ANDREASEN JO. Periodontal healing after replantation of traumatically avulsed human teeth. Assessment by mobility testing and radiography. *Acta Odontol Scand* 1975;**33**:325–35.

172. LINE SE, POLSON AM, ZANDER HA. Relationship between periodontal injury, selective cell repopulation and ankylosis. *J Periodontol* 1974;**45**:725–30.

173. KRISTERSON L, ANDREASEN JO. The effect of splinting upon periodontal and pulpal healing after autotransplantation of mature and immature permanent incisors in monkeys. *Int J Oral Surg* 1983;**12**:239–49.

174. CVEK M. Treatment of non-vital permanent incisors with calcium hydroxide. II. Effect on external root resorption in luxated teeth compared with effect of root

filling with gutta percha. A follow-up. *Odontologisk Revy* 1973;**24**:343–54.

175. SHULMAN LB, GEDALIA I, FEINGOLD RM. Fluoride concentration in the root surfaces and alveolar bone of fluoride-immersed monkey incisors three weeks after replantation. *J Dent Res* 1973;**52**:1314–6.

176. SHULMAN LB, KALIS P, GOLDHABER P. Fluoride inhibition of tooth-replant root resorption in cebus monkeys. *J Oral Ther Pharm* 1968;**4**:331–7.

177. SHULMAN LB. Allogenic tooth transplantation. *J Oral Surg* 1972;**30**:395–409.

178. MINK JR, VAN SCHAIK M. Intentional avulsion and replantation of dog teeth with varied root surface treatment. *J Dent Res* 1968;**43**:48.

179. REEVE CM, SATHER AH, PARKER JA. Resorption pattern of replanted formalin-fixed teeth in dogs. *J Dent Res* 1964;**43**:825.

180. BUTCHER EO, VIDAIR RV. Periodontal fiber reattachment in replanted incisors of the monkey. *J Dent Res* 1955;**34**:569–76.

181. ROBINSON PJ, SHAPIRO IM. Effect of diphosphates on root resorption. *J Dent Res* 1976;**55**:166.

182. HODOSH M, POVAR M, SHKLAR G. The dental polymer implant concept. *J Prosthet Dent* 1969;**22**:371–80.

183. HUEBSCH RF. Implanting teeth with methyl-2-cyanoacrylate adhesive. *J Dent Res* 1967;**46**:337–9.

184. SHERMAN P. Intentional replantation of teeth in dogs and monkeys. *J Dent Res* 1968;**47**:1066–71.

185. MUELLER BH, WHITSETT BD. Management of an avulsed deciduous incisor. Report of a case. *Oral Surg Oral Med Oral Pathol* 1978;**46**:442–6.

186. BARRY GN. Replanted teeth still functioning after 42 years: report of a case. *J Am Dent Assoc* 1976;**92**: 412–3.

187. GRÖNDAHL H-G, KAHNBERG K-E, OLSSON G. *Traumatiserade tænder. En klinisk och röntgenologisk efterundersökning*. Göteborg: Tandläkar-Sällskaps Artikelserie no. 384 Årsbok, 1974:37–50.

188. CVEK M, GRANATH LE, HOLZENDER L. Treatment of nonvital permanent incisors with calcium hydroxide. III. Variation of occurrence of ankylosis of reimplanted teeth with duration of extra-alveolar period and storage environment. *Odontol Rev* 1974;**25**:43–56.

189. WEPNER F. Die Replantation der Frontzähne nach traumatischen Zahnverlust. *Österr Z Stomatol* 1976;**73**:275–82

190. HARNDT R, HOEFIG W. Replantation of traumatically avulsed teeth. *Quintessence Int* 1972;**3**:19–22.

191. TOSTI A. Reimplantation: report of a case. *Dent Dig* 1970;**76**:98–100.

192. ADATIA AK. Odontogenesis following replantation of erupted maxillary central incisor. *Dent Pract* 1971;**21**:153–5.

193. PORTEOUS JR. Vital reimplantation of a maxillary central incisor tooth: report of a case. *ASDC J Dent Child* 1972;**39**:429–31.

194. BARKER BCW, MAYNE JR. Some unusual cases of apexification subsequent to trauma. *Oral Surg Oral Med Oral Pathol* 1975;**39**:144–50.

195. ECKSTEIN A. Reimplantation of permanent front teeth with incomplete root growth. *Fortschr Kiefer Gesichtschir* 1976;**20**:125–7.

196. MEYER-BARDOWICKS J. Eine Zahnreplantation mit Erhaltung der Pulpavitalität. *Quintessenz* 1977;**28**: 39–42.

197. BURLEY MA, REECE RD. Root formation following traumatic loss of an immature incisor: a case report. *Br Dent J* 1976;**141**:315–6.

198. OLIET S. Apexogenesis associated with replantation. A case history. *Dent Clin North Am* 1974;**18**:457–64.

199. ANDREASEN JO, BORUM M, JACOBSEN HL, ANDREASEN FM. Replantation of 400 traumatically avulsed permanent incisors. I. Diagnosis of healing complications. *Endod Dent Traumatol* 1995;**11**: 51–8.

200. ANDREASEN JO, BORUM M, JACOBSEN HL, ANDREASEN FM. Replantation of 400 avulsed permanent incisors. II. Factors related to pulp healing. *Endod Dent Traumatol* 1995;**11**:59–68.

201. ANDREASEN JO, BORUM M, ANDREASEN FM. Replantation of 400 avulsed permanent incisors. III. Factors related to root growth after replantation. *Endod Dent Traumatol* 1995;**11**:69–75.

202. ANDREASEN JO, BORUM M, JACOBSEN HL, ANDREASEN FM. Replantation of 400 avulsed permanent incisors. IV. Factors related to periodontal ligament healing. *Endod Dent Traumatol* 1995;**11**:76–89.

203. ANDREASEN JO, BORUM M, ANDREASEN FM. Progression of root resorption after replantation of 400 avulsed human incisors. In: Davidovitch Z. ed. *The biological mechanisms of tooth eruption, resorption and replacement by implants.* Boston: Harvard Society for the Advancement of Orthodontics, 1994:577–82.

204. KVINNSLAND I, HEYERAAS KJ. Dentin and osteodentin matrix formation in apicoectomized replanted incisors in cats. *Acta Odontol Scand* 1989;**47**:41–52.

205. KVINNSLAND I, HEYERAAS KJ. Cell renewal and ground substance formation in replanted cat teeth. *Acta Odontol Scand* 1990;**48**:203–15.

206. HOLLAND GR, ROBINSON PP. Pulp re-innervation in reimplanted canine teeth of the cat. *Arch Oral Biol* 1987;**32**:593–7.

207. LOESCHER AR, ROBINSON PP. Characteristics of periodontal mechanoreceptors supplying reimplanted canine teeth in cats. *Arch Oral Biol* 1991;**36**:33–40.

208. ROBINSON PP. An electrophysiological study of the reinnervation of reimplanted and autotransplanted teeth in the cat. *Arch Oral Biol* 1983;**28**:1139–47.

209. SKOGLUND A, TRONSTAD L, WALLENIUS K. A microangiographic study of vascular changes in replanted and autotransplanted teeth of young dogs. *Oral Surg Oral Med Oral Patol* 1978;**45**:17–28.

210. SKOGLUND A. Vascular changes in replanted and autotransplanted apicoectomized mature teeth of dogs. *Int J Oral Surg* 1981;**10**:100–10.

211. SKOGLUND A. Pulpal changes in replanted and autotransplanted apicectomized mature teeth of dogs. *Int J Oral Surg* 1981;**10**:111–21.

212. SKOGLUND A, HASSELGREN G, TRONSTAD L. Oxidoreductase activity in the pulp of replanted and autotransplanted teeth in young dogs. *Oral Surg Oral Med Oral Pathol* 1981;**52**:205–9.

213. KIRSCHNER H, MICHEL G. Mikromorphologische Untersuchungen der Nervregeneration im heilenden Desmodont bei Java-Makaken (Cynomolgus). *Dtsch Zahnärztl Z* 1982;**37**:929–36.

214. DURR DP, SVEEN OB. Influence of apicoectomy on the pulps of replanted monkey teeth. *Pediatr Dent* 1986;**8**:129–33.

215. LINDSKOG S, BLOMLÖF L, HAMMERSTRÖM L. Mitoses and microorganisms in the periodontal membrane after storage in milk or saliva. *Scand J Dent Res* 1983;**91**:465–72.

216. LINDSKOG S, PIERCE A, BLOMLÖF L, HAMMERSTRÖM L. The role of the necrotic periodontal membrane in cementum resorption and ankylosis. *Endod Dent Traumatol* 1985;**1**:96–101.

217. LINDSKOG S, BLOMLÖF L, HAMMARSTRÖM L. Cellular colonization of denuded root surfaces in vivo: cell morphology in dentin resorption and cementum repair. *Clin Periodontol* 1987;**14**:390–5.

218. LINDSKOG S, BLOMLÖF L, HAMMERSTRÖM L. Dentin resorption in replanted monkey incisors. Morphology of dentinoclast spreading in vivo. *J Clin Periodontol* 1988;**15**:365–70.

219. ANNEROTH G, LUNDQUIST G, NORDENRAM Å, SÖDER P-O. Re- and allotransplantation of teeth – an experimental study in monkeys. *Int J Oral Maxillofac Surg* 1988;**17**:54–7.

220. NASJLETI CE. Effect of fibronectin on healing of replanted teeth in monkeys: A histologic and autoradiographic study. *Oral Surg Oral Med Oral Pathol* 1987;**63**:291–9.

221. ANDREASEN JO. Experimental dental traumatology: development of a model for external root resorption. *Endod Dent Traumatol* 1987;**3**:269–87.

222. ANDERSSON L, JONSSON BG, HAMMARSTRÖM L, BLOMLÖF L, ANDREASEN JO, LINDSKOG S. Evaluation of statistics and desirable experimental design of a histomorphometrical method for studies of root resorption. *Endod Dent Traumatol* 1987;**3**: 288–95.

223. KRISTERSON L, ANDREASEN JO. Influence of root development on periodontal and pulpal healing after replantation of incisors in monkeys. *Int J Oral Surg* 1984;**13**:313–23.

224. KRISTERSON L, ANDREASEN JO. Autotransplantation and replantation of tooth germs in monkeys. Effect of damage to the dental follicle and position of transplant in the alveolus. *Int J Oral Surg* 1984;**13**:324–33.

225. CVEK M, CLEATON-JONES P, AUSTIN J, LOWNIE J, KLING M, FATTI P. Pulp revascularization in reimplanted immature monkey incisors – predictability and the effect of antibiotic systemic prophylaxis. *Endod Dent Traumatol* 1990;**6**:157–69.

226. CVEK M, CLEATON-JONES P, AUSTIN J, KLING M, LOWNIE J, FATTI P. Effect of topical application of doxycycline on pulp revascularization and peridontal healing in reimplanted monkey incisors. *Endod Dent Traumatol* 1990;**6**:170–6.

227. BREIVIK M, KVAM E. Evaluation of histological criteria applied for decription of reactions in replanted human premolars. *Scand J Dent Res* 1977;**85**:392–5.

228. BREIVIK M. Human odontoblast response to teeth replantation. *Eur J Orthod* 1981;**3**:95–108.

229. BREIVIK M, KVAM E. Secondary dentin in replanted

teeth – a histometric study. *Endod Dent Traumatol* 1990;**6**:150–2.

230. BREIVIK M, KVAM E. Histometric study of root resorption on human premolars following experimental replantation. *Scand J Dent Res* 1987;**95**:273–80.

231. ANDREASEN JO, ANDREASEN FM. Root resorption following traumatic dental injuries. *Proc Finn Dent Soc* 1991;**88**:95–114.

232. HACKER W, FISCHBACH H. Spätergebnisse nach 35 Zahnreplantationen im Frontzahnbereich. *Dtsch Zahnärztl Z* 1983;**38**:466–9.

233. MANDEL U, VIIDIK A. Effect of splinting on the mechanical and histological properties of the healing periodontal ligament after experimental extrusive luxation in the vervet monkey (*Cercopithecus aethiops*). *Arch Oral Biol* 1989;**34**:209–17.

234. HAMMERSTRÖM L, BLOMLÖF L, LINDSKOG S. Dynamics of dentoalveolar ankylosis and associated root resorption. *Endod Dent Traumatol* 1989;**5**:163–75.

235. ANDERSSON L, BLOMLÖF L, LINDSKOG S, FEIGLIN B, HAMMARSTRÖM L. Tooth ankylosis. Clinical, radiographic and histological assessments. *Int J Oral Surg* 1984;**13**:423–31.

236. STENVIK A, BEYER-OLSEN EMS, ÅBYHOLM F, HÅNÆS HR, GERNER NW. Validity of the radiographic assessment of ankylosis. Evaluation of long-term reactions in 10 monkey incisors. *Acta Odontol Scand* 1990;**48**:265–69.

237. SCHMITZ R, DONATH K. Morphologische Veränderungen an traumatisierten Zähnen. Eine klinische and patho-histologische Studie. *Dtsch Zahnärztl Z* 1983;**38**:462–5.

238. HILTZ J, TROPE M. Vitality of human lip fibroblasts in milk, Hanks balanced salt solution and Viaspan storage media. *Endod Dent Traumatol* 1991;**7**:69–72.

239. MORLEY RS, MALLOY R, HURST RVV, JAMES R. Analysis of functional splinting upon autologously reimplanted teeth. *Dent Res* 1978;**57**:IADR Abstract no.593.

240. NASJLETI CE, CASTELLI WA, CAFFESSE RG. The effects of different splinting times on replantation of teeth in monkeys. *Oral Surg Oral Med Oral Pathol* 1982;**53**:557–66.

241. ANDERSSON L, LINDSKOG S, BLOMLÖF L, HEDSTRÖM K-G, HAMMARSTRÖM L. Effect of masticatory stimulation on dentoalveolar ankylosis after experimental tooth replantation. *Endod Dent Traumatol* 1985;**1**:13–6.

242. HAMMARSTRÖM L, BLOMLÖF L, FEIGLIN B, ANDERSSON L, LINDSKOG S. Replantation of teeth and antibiotic treatment. *Endod Dent Traumatol* 1986;**2**:51–7.

243. KLING M, CVEK M, MEJARE I. Rate and predictability of pulp revascularization in therapeutically reimplanted permanent incisors. *Endod Dent Traumatol* 1986;**2**:83–9.

244. HAMMARSTRÖM L, BLOMLÖF L, FEIGLIN B, LINDSKOG S. Effect of calcium hydroxide treatment on periodontal repair and root resorption. *Endod Dent Traumatol* 1986;**2**:184–9.

245. BJORVATN K, SELVIG KA, KLINGE B. Effect of tetracycline and SnF on root resorption in replanted incisors in dogs. *Scand J Dent Res* 1989;**97**:477–82.

246. SELVIG KA, BJORVATN K, CLAFFEY N. Effect of stannous flouride and tetracycline on repair after delayed replantation of root-planed teeth in dogs. *Acta Odontol Scand* 1990;**48**:107–12.

247. KLINGE B, NILVÉUS R, SELVIG KA. The effect of citric acid on repair after delayed tooth replantation in dogs. *Acta Odontol Scand* 1984;**42**:351–9.

248. ZERVAS PI, AMBRIANIDIS T, KARABOUTA-VULGAROPUOLOU I. The effect of citric acid treatment on periodontal healing after replantation of permanent teeth. *Int Endod J* 1991;**24**:317–25.

249. WALSH JS, FEY MR, OMNELL LM. The effects of indomethacin on resorption and ankylosis in replanted teeth. *ASDC J Dent Child* 1987;**54**:261–6.

250. COCCIA CT. A clinical investigation of root resorption rates in reimplanted young permanent incisors: A five-year study. *J Endod* 1980;**6**:413–20.

251. KIRSCHNER H, BOLZ U, ENOMOTO S, HOTTEMANN RW, MEINEL W, STURM J. Eine neue Methode kombinierter auto-alloplastischer Zahnreplantation mit partieller $Al_2O_3$ – Keramikwurzel. *Dtsch Zahnärztl Z* 1978;**33**:549.

252. BOLZ U, HÖTTEMANN RW, KIRSCHNER H, STURM J. Indications for the clinical use of combined auto-alloplastic tooth reimplantation with aluminium oxide ($Al_2O_3$) ceramic. In: Heimke G, ed. *Dental implants. Materials and systems.* München, Wien: Carl Hanser Verlag 1980:81–8.

253. KIRSCHNER H, BOLZ U, HOTTEMANN RW, STURM J. Autoplastic tooth reimplantation with partial ceramic roots made of $Al_2O_3$. In: Heimke G, ed. *Dental implants. Materials and systems.* München, Wien: Carl Hanser Verlag 1980:55–62.

254. BURK W, BRINKMANN E. Indikation und Anwendung des auto-alloplastischen Replantationsverfahrens nach Kirschner. Vorläufiger Bericht. *Zahnärztl Prax* 1980;**31**:347–55.

255. KIRSCHNER H. Chirurgische Zahnerhaltung. Experimente mit Aluminiumoxid-Keramik. *Dtsch Zahnärztl Z* 1981;**36**:274–85.

256. BRINKMANN E. Indikation und Anwendung der chirurgischen Zahnerhaltung. Zahnärztl Mitt 1982;**72**:1–12.

257. BRINKMANN E. Die Einzelzahnlücke aus implantologischer Sicht. *Zahnärztl Prax* 1982;**7**:286–91.

258. HERFORTH A. Zur Stabilisierung gelockerter Zähne durch transdentale Fixation. *Dtsch Zahnärztl Z* 1983;**38**:129–30.

259. KIRSCHNER H. Chirurgische Zahnerhaltung. Experimente mit Aluminiumoxid-Keramik. *Dtsch Zahnärztl Z* 1981;**36**:274–85.

260. KIRSCHNER H. *Atlas der chirurgischen Zahnerhaltung.* München: Hanser Verlag, 1987.

261. NENTWIG GH. Geschlossene keramische Implantate zur Reintegration traumatisch geschädigter bleibender Zähne. *Fortschr Zahnärztl Implantol* 1985;**1**:272–6.

262. NENTWIG GH, BERBECARIU C, SALLER S. Zur Prognose des replantierten Zahnes nach schweren Luxationsverletzungen. *Dtsch Zahnärztl Z* 1987;**42**:205–7.

263. KOCH G, ULLBRO C. Klinisk funktionstid hos 55 exartikulerade och replanterade tænder. *Tannläkartidningen* 1982;**74**:18–25.

264. HERFORTH A. *Traumatische Schädigungen der Frontzähne bei Kindern und, Jugendlichen im Alter von 7*

*bis 15 Jahren*. Berlin: Quintessenz Verlag GmbH, 1982.

265. JACOBSEN I. Long term evaluation, prognosis and subsequent management of traumatic tooth injuries. In: Gutmann JL, Harrison JW, eds. *Proceedings of the International Conference on Oral Trauma*. Chicago: American Association of Endodontists Endowment & Memorial Foundation, 1986:129–34.

266. GONDA F, NAGASE M, CHEN R-B, YAKATA H, NAKAJIMA T. Replantation: an analysis of 29 teeth. *Oral Surg Oral Med Oral Pathol* 1990;**70**:650–5.

267. MACKIE IC, WORTHINGTON HV. An investigation of replantation of traumatically avulsed permanent incisor teeth. *Br Dent J* 1992;**172**:17–20.

268. FUSS Z. Successful self-replantation of avulsed tooth with 42-year follow-up. *Endod Dent Traumatol* 1985;**1**:120–2.

269. JOHNSON WT, GOODRICH JL, JAMES GA. Replantation of avulsed teeth with immature root development. *Oral Surg Oral Med Oral Pathol* 1985;**60**:420–7.

270. KRENKEL C, GRUNERT I. Replantierte nicht endodontisch behandelte Frontzähne mit offenem Foramen Apicale. *Zahnärztl Prax* 1986;**37**:290–8.

271. ANDREASEN JO, SCHWARTZ O. The effect of saline storage before replantation upon dry damage of the periodontal ligament. *Endod Dent Traumatol* 1986;**2**:67–70.

272. MATSSON L, ANDREASEN JO, CVEK M, GRANATH L. Ankylosis of experimentally reimplanted teeth related to extra-alveolar period and storage environment. *Pediatr Dent* 1982;**4**:327–9.

273. ANDERSSON L, BODIN I, SÖRENSEN S. Progression of root resorption following replantation of human teeth after extended extraoral storage. *Endod Dent Traumatol* 1989;**5**:38–47.

274. ANDERSSON L, BODIN I. Avulsed human teeth replanted within 15 minutes – a long-term clinical follow-up study. *Endod Dent Traumatol* 1990;**6**:37–42.

275. HAMMARSTRÖM L, PIERCE A, BLOMLÖF L, FEIGLIN B, LINDSKOG S. Tooth avulsion and replantation – a review. *Endod Dent Traumatol* 1986;**2**:1–8.

276. MODÉER T, DAHLLOF G, OTTESKOG P. Effect of drying on human periodontal ligament repair *in vitro*. *J Int Assoc Dent Child* 1984;**15**:15–20.

277. ZIMMERMANN M, NENTWIG G-H. Überlebensrate desmodontaler Zellen in Abhängigkeit von der ekstraoralen Austrocknung. *Schweiz Monatsschr Zahnmed* 1989;**99**:1007–10.

278. CORNELIUS CP, EHRENFELD M, UMBACH T. Replantationsergebnisse nach traumatischer Zahnluxation. *Dtsch Zahnärztl Z* 1987;**42**:211–5.

279. BARRETT EJ, KENNY DJ. Avulsed permanent teeth: a review of the literature and treatment guidelines. *Endod Dent Traumatol* 1997;**13**:153–63.

280. MARTIN MP, PILEGGI R. A quantitative analysis of Propolis: a promising new storage media following avulsion. *Dent Traumatol* 2004;**20**:85–9.

281. KAWANAMI M, ANDREASEN JO, BORUM MK, SCHOU S, HJØRTING-HANSEN E, KATO H. Infraposition of ankylosed permanent maxillary incisors after replantation related to age and sex. *Endod Dent Traumatol* 1999;**15**:50–6.

282. KRENKEL C, GRUNERT I. Replantierte nicht endodontisch behandelte Frontzähne mit offenem Foramen apicale. *Zahnärztliche Praxis* 1986;**8**:290–8.

283. EBESELEDER KA, FRIEHS S, RUDA C, PERTL C, GLOCKNER K, HULLA H. A study of replanted permanent teeth in different age groups. *Endod Dent Traumatol* 1998;**14**:274–8.

284. KINIRONS MJ, GREGG TA, WELBURY RR, COLE BOI. Variations in the presenting and treatment features in reimplanted permanent incisors in children and their effect on the prevalence of root resorption. *Brit Dent J* 2000;**189**:263–6.

285. SCHATZ JP, HAUSHERR C, JOHO JP. A retrospective clinical and radiologic study of teeth re-implanted following traumatic avulsion. *Endod Dent Traumatol* 1995;**11**:235–9.

286. KINIRONS MJ, BOYD DH, GREGG TA. Inflammatory and replacement resorption in reimplanted permanent incisor teeth: a study of the characteristics of 84 teeth. *Endod Dent Traumatol* 1999;**15**:269–72.

287. BARRETT EJ, KENNY DJ. Survival of avulsed permanent maxillary incisors in children following delayed replantation. *Endod Dent Traumatol* 1997;**13**:269–75.

288. BLOMLÖF L, LINDSKOG S, ANDERSSON L, HEDSTROM KG, HAMMARSTRÖM L. Storage of experimentally avulsed teeth in milk prior to replantation. *J Dent Res* 1983;**62**:912–6.

289. BLOMLÖF L. Storage of human periodontal ligament cells in a combination of different media. *J Dent Res* 1981;**60**:1904–6.

290. BLOMLÖF L, LINDSKOG S, HAMMARSTRÖM L. Periodontal healing of exarticulated monkey teeth stored in milk or saliva. *Scand J Dent Res* 1981;**89**:251–9.

291. BLOMLÖF L, OTTESKOG P, HAMMARSTRÖM L. Effect of storage in media with different ion strengths and osmolalities on human periodontal ligament cells. *Scand J Dent Res* 1981;**89**:180–7.

292. BLOMLÖF L. Milk and saliva as possible storage media for traumatically exarticulated teeth prior to replantation. *Swed Dent J Suppl* 1981;**8**:1–6.

293. BLOMLÖF L, LINDSKOG S, HEDSTRÖM KG, HAMMARSTRÖM L. Vitality of periodontal ligament cells after storage of monkey teeth in milk or saliva. *Scand J Dent Res* 1980;**88**:441–5.

294. BLOMLÖF L, OTTESKOG P. Viability of human periodontal ligament cells after storage in milk or saliva. *Scand J Dent Res* 1980;**88**:436–40.

295. NORDENVALL KJ. Milk as storage medium for exarticulated teeth: report of case. *ASDC J Dent Child* 1992;**59**:150–5.

296. ASHKENAZI M, SARNAT H, KEILA S. *In vitro* viability, mitogenicity and clonogenic capacity of periodontal ligament cells after storage in six different media. *Endod Dent Traumatol* 1999;**15**:149–56.

297. TROPE M, FRIEDMAN S. Periodontal healing of replanted dog teeth stored in Viaspan, milk and Hank's balanced salt solution. *Endod Dent Traumatol* 1992;**8**:183–8.

298. KENNY DJ, BARRETT EJ. Pre-replantation storage of avulsed teeth: fact and fiction. *J Calif Dent Assoc* 2001;**29**:275–81.

299. LEKIC PC, KENNY DJ, BARRETT EJ. The influence of storage conditions on the clonogenic capacity of

periodontal ligament cells: implications for tooth replantation. *Int Endod J* 1998;**31**:137–40.

300. LAYUG ML, BARRETT EJ, KENNY DJ. Interim storage of avulsed permanent teeth. *J Can Dent Assoc* 1998;**64**:357–63, 365–9.

301. BLOMLÖF L, ANDERSSON L, LINDSKOG S, HEDSTROM KG, HAMMARSTRÖM L. Periodontal healing of replanted monkey teeth prevented from drying. *Acta Odontol Scand* 1983;**41**:117–23.

302. ANDERSSON L, MALMGREN B. The problem of dentoalveolar ankylosis and subsequent replacement resorption in the growing patient. *Aust Endod J* 1999;**25**:57–61.

303. ANDERSSON L, LINDSKOG S, BLOMLÖF L, HEDSTRÖM KG, HAMMARSTRÖM L. Effect of masticatory stimulation on dentoalveolar ankylosis after experimental tooth replantation. *Endod Dent Traumatol* 1985;**1**:13–16.

304. TROPE M. Clinical management of the avulsed tooth. *Dent Clin North Am* 1995;**39**:93–112.

305. POHL Y, FILIPPI A, TEKIN U, KIRSCHNER H. Periodontal healing after intentional autoalloplastic reimplantation of injured immature upper front teeth. *J Clin Periodontol* 2000;**27**:198–204.

306. YAMADA H, MAEDA T, HANADA K, TAKANO Y. Re-innervation in the canine periodontal ligament of replanted teeth using an antibody to protein gene products 9.5: an immunohistochemical study. *Endod Dent Traumatol* 1999;**15**:221–34.

307. DONALDSON M, KINIRONS MJ. Factors affecting the onset of resorption in avulsed and replanted incisor teeth in children. *Dent Traumatol* 2001;**17**:205–9.

308. HUPP JG, MESAROS SV, AUKHIL I, TROPE M. Periodontal ligament vitality and histologic healing of teeth stored for extended periods before transplantation. *Endod Dent Traumatol* 1998;**14**:79–83.

309. NISHIOKA M, SHIIYA T, UENO K, SUDA H. Tooth replantation in germ-free and conventional rats. *Endod Dent Traumatol* 1998;**14**:163–73.

310. WEINSTEIN FM, WORSAAE N, ANDREASEN JO. The effect on periodontal and pulpal tissues of various cleansing procedures prior to replantation of extracted teeth. An experimental study in monkeys. *Acta Odontol Scand* 1981;**39**:251–5.

311. ANDREASEN JO. Analysis of pathogenesis and topography of replacement resorption (ankylosis) after replantation of mature permanent incisors in monkeys. *Swed Dent J* 1980;**4**:231–40.

312. CVEK M, CLEATON-JONES P, AUSTIN J, KLING M, LOWNIE J, FATTI P. Effect of topical application of doxycycline on pulp revascularization and periodontal healing in reimplanted monkey incisors. *Endod Dent Traumatol* 1990;**6**:170–6.

313. RITTER ALS, RITTER AV, MURRAH V, SIGURDSSON A, TROPE M. Pulp revascularization of replanted immature dog teeth after treatment with minocycline and doxycycline assessed by laser Doppler flowmetry, radiography and histology. *Dent Traumatol* 2004;**20**:75–84.

314. YANPISET K, TROPE M. Pulp revascularization of replanted immature dog teeth after different treatment methods. *Endod Dent Traumatol* 2000;**16**:211–17.

# 18

# Injuries to the Supporting Bone

J. O. Andreasen

## Terminology, frequency and etiology

Injuries to the supporting bone can be divided into the following types (Fig. 18.1):

(1) *Comminution of the alveolar socket:* Crushing of the alveolar socket, associated with intrusive or lateral luxation.
(2) *Fracture of the alveolar socket wall:* A fracture confined to the facial or lingual socket wall.
(3) *Fracture of the alveolar process:* A fracture of the alveolar process which may or may not involve alveolar sockets.
(4) *Fracture of mandible or maxilla (jaw fracture)* A fracture involving the base of the mandible or maxilla and usually also the alveolar process. The fracture may or may not involve alveolar sockets.

The primary etiologic factors are fights and automobile accidents (1, 2). Thus, after automobile accidents, alveolar fractures result from direct impact against the steering wheel or other interior structures (2, 3, 76).

In infants, where only the incisors have erupted, lack of support in the lateral regions can imply that forceful occlusion resulting from impact to the chin can result in fracture of the anterior portion of the alveolar process (Fig. 18.2).

## Clinical findings

Clinical features and treatment of comminution of the alveolar socket have already been described in connection with luxation injuries (see Chapter 13, p. 372).

Fractures of the *alveolar socket wall* are primarily seen in the upper incisor region, where the fracture usually involves several teeth (1). Among associated dental injuries, luxation with dislocation and avulsion are the most common (Fig. 18.3). Palpation usually discloses the fracture site. Abnormal mobility of the socket wall is demonstrated when the mobility of involved teeth is tested.

Fractures of the *alveolar process* usually affect older age groups. A common location is the anterior region, but the canine and premolar regions can also be involved. The fracture line may be positioned beyond the apices, but in most cases involves the alveolar socket. In these cases concomitant dental injuries, such as extrusive or lateral luxations as well as root fractures, are common findings (1–6).

Fracture of the alveolar process is usually easy to diagnose due to displacement and the mobility of the fragment (Fig. 18.4). Typically, when mobility of a single tooth is tested, adjacent teeth move with it. Furthermore, the percussion tone of the teeth in the fragment differs clearly from adjacent teeth in that the former yield a dull sound.

Approximately one-half of all jaw fractures involve teeth in the fracture line (Fig. 18.5), and most of these are found in the mandible (8) (see p. 496).

The location of *jaw fractures* is significantly related to the state of the dentition (11). Of the tooth-bearing areas, the lower third molar region is most often involved; the mandibular canine, incisor and premolar regions follow with decreasing frequency (12, 13). The presence of a marginal periodontal bone defect also appears to be related to the location of a fracture line (85). In children, developing permanent teeth in the line of fracture are usually seen in the mandibular canine and incisor regions (14, 15).

Clinically, there is displacement of fragments and disturbance of occlusion (Fig. 18.5). Palpation with a finger placed over the alveolar process can disclose a step in the bony contours. In the absence of dislocation, bimanual manipulation of the jaws will usually reveal mobility between the fragments, often with accompanying crepitus. Pain provoked by movement of the mandible or maxilla, or upon palpation, is also a positive sign of fracture.

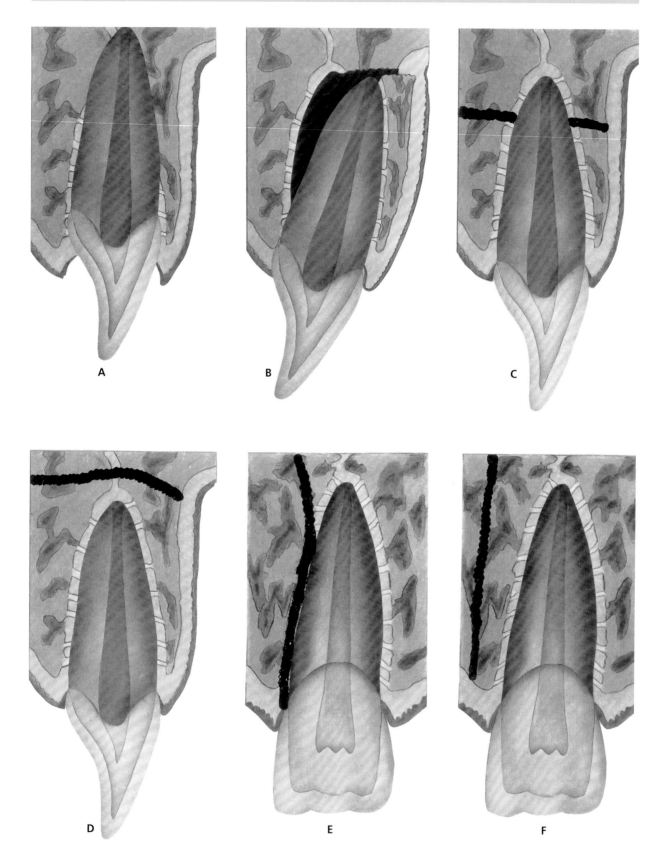

**Fig. 18.1** Injuries to the supporting bone. A. Comminution of alveolar socket. B. Fractures of the facial or lingual alveolar socket wall. C and D. Fractures of the alveolar process with (C) and without (D) involvement of the socket. E and F. Fractures of the mandible or maxilla (jaw fractures) with and without involvement of the socket.

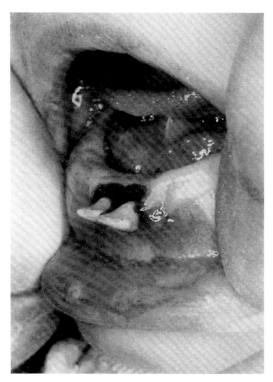
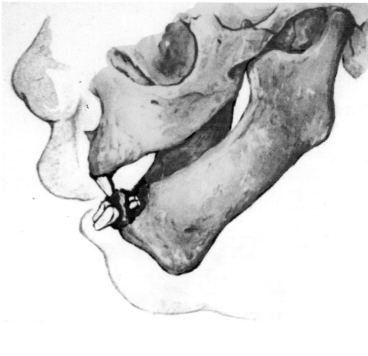

**Fig. 18.2** Pathogenesis of fractures of the mandibular alveolar process in infants. The energy from impact to the chin area is transmitted exclusively to the incisor region due to the lack of lateral tooth support. From MÜLLER (4) 1969.

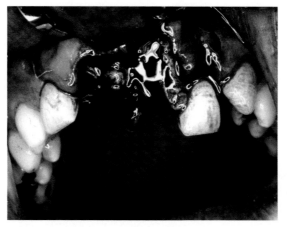
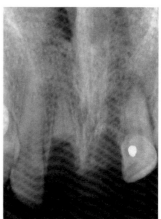

**Fig. 18.3** Contusion and gingival laceration of the facial socket wall following avulsion of both central incisors.

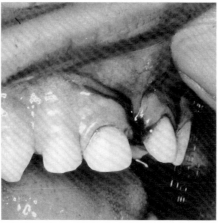
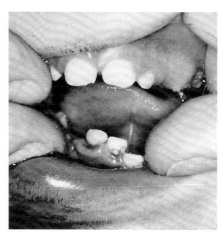

**Fig. 18.4** A. Facial displacement of alveolar fracture affecting left incisors in a 2-year-old boy. B. Lingual displacement of alveolar fracture, involving right incisors in a 1¹/₂-year-old child.

A

B

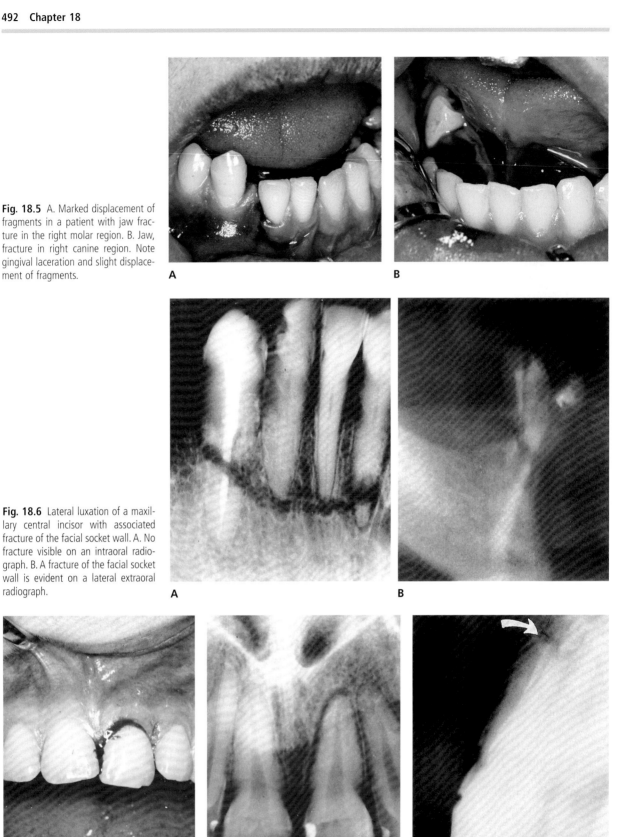

**Fig. 18.5** A. Marked displacement of fragments in a patient with jaw fracture in the right molar region. B. Jaw, fracture in right canine region. Note gingival laceration and slight displacement of fragments.

A                                    B

**Fig. 18.6** Lateral luxation of a maxillary central incisor with associated fracture of the facial socket wall. A. No fracture visible on an intraoral radiograph. B. A fracture of the facial socket wall is evident on a lateral extraoral radiograph.

A                                    B

**Fig. 18.7** Dislocation of mandibular alveolar fragment clearly demonstrated by the extraoral lateral radiographic technique (arrow).

## Radiographic findings

Intraoral radiographs of the socket wall seldom reveal the line of fracture; but a laterally exposed extraoral radiograph will usually disclose the fracture's location (Fig. 18.6). In fractures involving the alveolar process, a distinct fracture line is usually visible in intraoral as well as extraoral radiographs (Figs 18.6–18.8). Fracture lines may be positioned at all levels, from the marginal bone to the root apex (Fig.

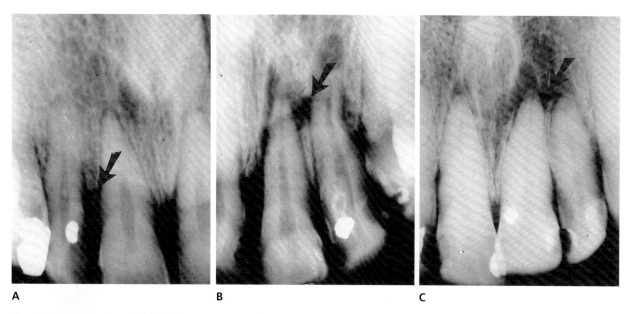

A          B          C

**Fig. 18.8** Various locations of alveolar fractures. A. Fracture line passing through the marginal part of the interdental septum (arrow). B. Alveolar fracture traversing the septal bone close to the midportion of the root (arrow). Note the marked extrusive luxation of involved teeth. C. Alveolar fracture located close to the apices (arrow).

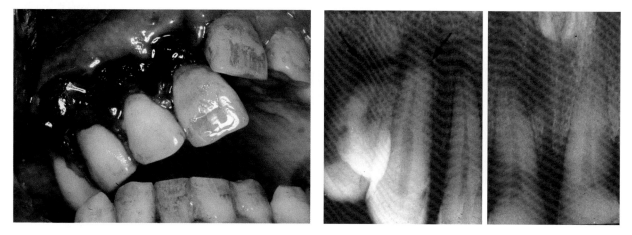

**Fig. 18.9** Fracture of the right maxillary alveolar process. Radiograph taken after reduction reveals the fracture line. Note the associated root fracture of upper first premolar. The alveolar fracture mimics a root fracture in the canine region.

18.8). Despite strong clinical evidence of a fracture, they are often very difficult to visualize radiographically (Figs 18.9 and 18.10). When fracture lines traverse interdental septa, extrusive luxation and root fractures are often concomitant findings. Fractures involving the most apical portion of the root are quite common, but are often overlooked, especially in the lower anterior region. On the other hand, alveolar fracture lines transversing the apices may simulate root fractures. Careful examination of the radiographs (e.g. continuity of root surfaces and root canals) will usually reveal a superimposed fracture line and intact teeth (Fig. 18.9). Moreover, superimposed alveolar fracture lines will change position in relation to height along the root surface when the angulation of the central beam is altered (Fig. 18.11).

Radiographic examination of mandibular or maxillary fractures with tooth involvement should include extraoral as well as intraoral exposures. Generally, extraoral radiographs,

especially panoramic exposures, are valuable in determining the course and position of fracture lines (84, 85) (Fig. 18.12), while intraoral radiographs can reveal the relationship between the fracture line and involved teeth. This is especially important in cases of maxillary fractures, which can be difficult to diagnose from extraoral radiographs due to superimposition of many anatomical structures (Fig. 18.13).

The fracture usually follows the midline of the septum or the contours of the alveolar socket; but a combination of these routes can sometimes be seen (Fig. 18.14). Fractures of the body of the mandible do not always run parallel with the long axis of the teeth, but obliquely downwards and posterior towards the base of the mandible (13, 16) (Fig. 18.15).

Fractures generally follow the path of least resistance (Figs 18.14 and 18.16). Thus, at the angle of the mandible, the position of the lower third molar generally determines the course of the fracture line (13, 114).

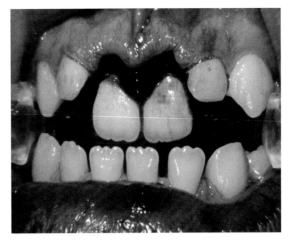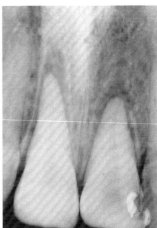

**Fig. 18.10** Alveolar fracture confined to the central incisor region. Although clinically obvious at the time of injury, there is no clear radiographic evidence of bone fracture.

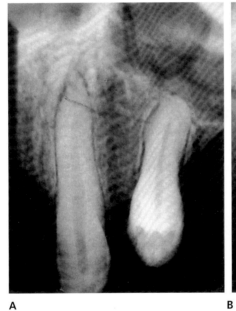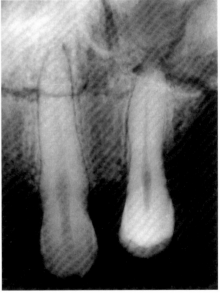

**Fig. 18.11** Alveolar fracture in the canine and premolar regions. A. In the canine region the fracture line simulates a root fracture. B. By altering angulation of the central beam, the superimposed fracture line changes position, thus ruling out a root fracture.

A                                    B

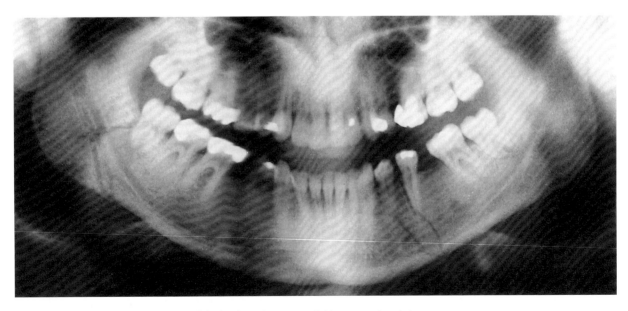

**Fig. 18.12** Fracture lines in the premolar and third molar regions as revealed by panoramic technique.

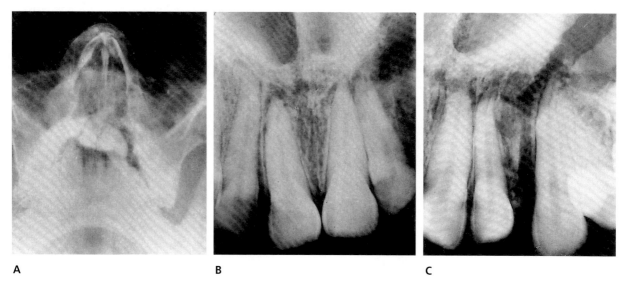

**A**                          **B**                          **C**

**Fig. 18.13** Fracture of the maxilla involving incisors, premolars, and molars. A. Only few details are depicted on extraoral radiograph. B. and C. Intraoral radiographs reveal the relationship between involved teeth and fracture lines.

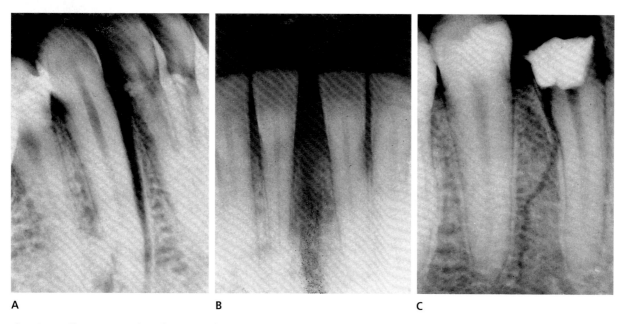

**A**                          **B**                          **C**

**Fig. 18.14** Different courses of jaw fracture line following the periodontal ligament space. A. Jaw fracture passing through the periodontal ligament. B. Jaw fracture passing through the middle of the interdental septum. C. Combination of periodontal and septal involvement.

It should be remembered that two lines will be seen radiographically if the central beam is not parallel to the plane of fracture, as the fracture lines of both outer and inner cortical bone plates will be depicted (114) (Figs 18.17 and 18.18).

## Pathology

Most fractures of the supporting bone represent a complex injury where there is damage not only to supporting bone but also to the pulp, periodontal ligament and the gingiva (Fig. 18.19). Due to this multiplicity of involved tissues, various types of healing complications can occur, such as loss of supporting bone, root resorption and pulp necrosis.

Adequate knowledge of bony repair after fracture is necessary in order to appreciate the role teeth play in these events. As relatively little information exists on the healing events after jaw fractures, most of our present knowledge is derived from clinical and experimental findings from fractures of the shaft of long bones (18, 19, 20–44) and a few studies in dogs (22–25). The following description of fracture healing is therefore based upon the latter material. Special implications for bone healing in the jaws will be discussed later in this chapter.

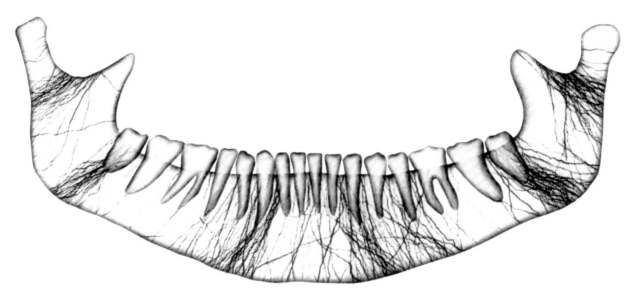

**Fig. 18.15** Location and course of fracture lines in 225 patients with mandibular fractures due to fights. The course of the fracture lines was determined from panoramic radiographs. Note that the majority of the fracture lines are situated in the so-called weak areas of the mandible, the subcondylar, third molar, and canine regions. Fractures of the body of the mandible usually run obliquely downwards and backwards to the base of the mandible. From OIKARINEN & MALMSTRÖM (13) 1969.

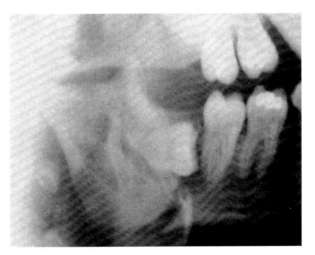 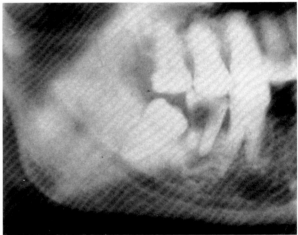

**Fig. 18.16** Fracture lines in the lower third molar region following the line of least resistance as determined by impacted third molars.

The events immediately following fracture include extravasation and clotting of blood exuding from injured vessels. The normal vascular supply to the fracture site is compromised and necrosis of osteocytes is seen in adjacent areas. Organization of the blood clot by formation of granulation tissue begins within the first 24 hours after injury. Its primary function is removal of necrotic or damaged tissue components. The granulation tissue becomes dense connective tissue in which cartilage and fibrocartilage develop, forming a cuff of fibrocartilaginous callus around the fracture site and thereby closes the gap between the fracture edges.

New bone originating from the deeper layers of the periosteum and endosteum is formed some distance from the fracture site. Immature bone then invades the fibrocartilaginous callus and ultimately unites the two fragments,

whereupon mineralization of the callus takes place. At the same time, resorptive and remodeling processes make the bone structure on either side of the fracture less dense, a change often observed in follow-up radiographs (26). Subsequently, reorganization of the bony callus occurs, and the immature fibrillar bone is replaced by mature lamellated bone. Eventually, functional reconstruction takes place, i.e. internal reconstruction and resorption of excess bone.

It is presumed that the above-mentioned healing processes also apply to jaw fractures. The presence of a cartilaginous callus has, however, been questioned. In a study of experimental jaw fractures in dogs, no evidence of cartilage formation was found (22), whereas other investigators have found occasional islands of cartilage in animal experiments (23–25, 33, 35) and in human material (26). Finally, it has been shown that mobility of the jaw fragments influences

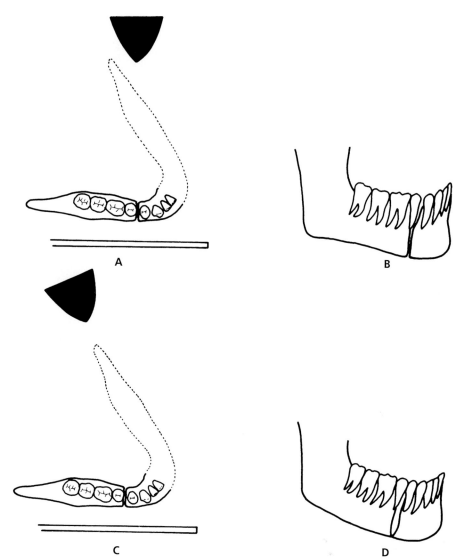

**Fig. 18.17** Diagrams illustrating the difference in the radiographic appearance of a single fracture line depending on the angle of the central beam. A and B. Central beam parallel to the fracture plane results in a single fracture line. C and D. A more posterior exposure results in projection of the fracture of the outer and inner cortical bone plate as separate lines.

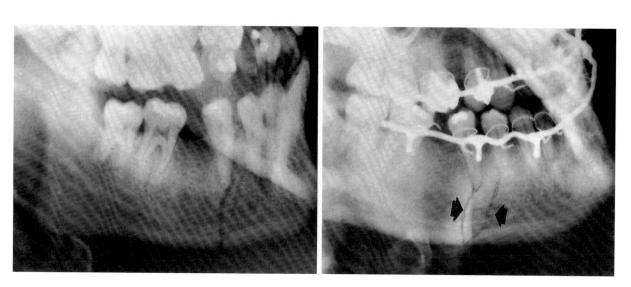

**Fig. 18.18** Radiographs illustrating change in position of the fracture lines when the angle of the central beam is altered. A. Central ray almost parallel to the fracture plane. B. A change in the projection angle results in two distinct fracture lines (arrows).

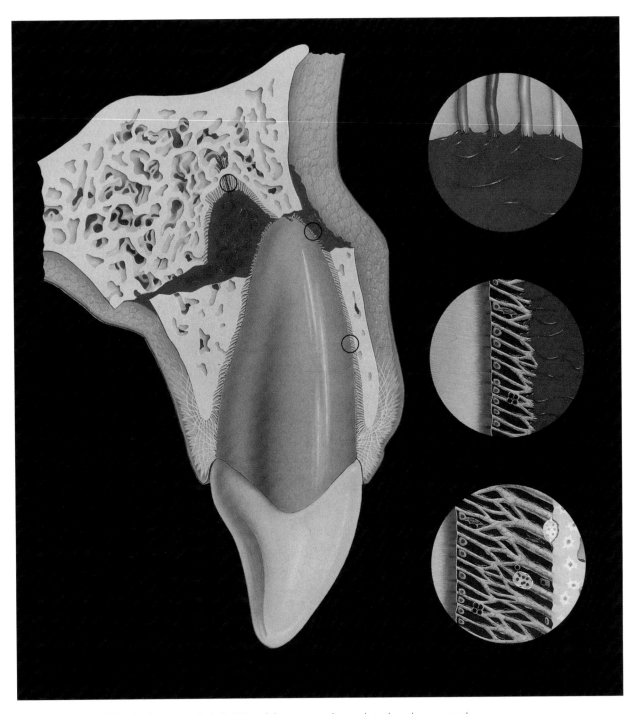

**Fig. 18.19** Fracture of the alveolar process. Both the PDL and the neurovascular supply to the pulp are severed.

the rate of bony callus formation. When fragments are mobile, more time elapses before bony bridging is seen as compared to immobilized fractures (24).

The influence of the presence of teeth upon fracture healing has been elucidated primarily by animal experiments (22, 28–31). Experimental jaw fractures in dogs, with teeth present along the fracture line, have revealed formation of granulation tissue which resorbs the interdental bone and adjacent root surfaces (22). Examination of human teeth located along the fracture line, however, has shown evidence of repair of resorption areas (45, 46).

Figs 18.20 and 18.21 show the early histologic healing events following fracture of the vestibular socket wall and alveolar process.

## Treatment

### Fractures of the socket wall

Fractures of the socket wall are usually associated with dislocation of teeth. Thus, the first step after administration of

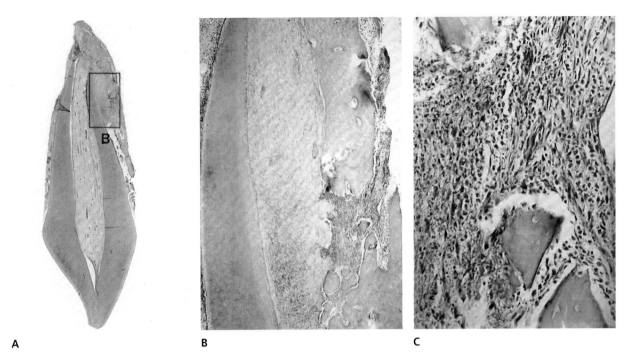

**Fig. 18.20** Early histologic changes following fracture of the facial socket wall in a 1¹/₂-year-old child. A. Low-power view of sectioned incisor, removed 5 days after injury. ×5. B and C. Higher magnification of the fracture area. The blood clot has been organized by granulation tissue. ×30 and ×195.

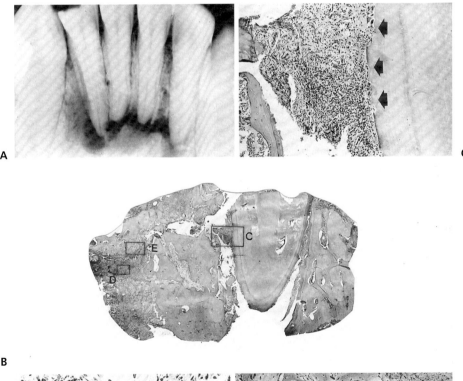

**Fig. 18.21** Healing events following a fracture of the alveolar process in the mandibular incisor region. A. Radiograph taken at time of injury. B. Surgical specimen including apex of left lateral incisor removed 18 days after trauma. ×10. C. Superficial resorption of the mesial aspect of the root (arrows). ×30. D. Remnants of coagulum. ×195. E. Developing young immature bone bridging the fracture line. ×75.

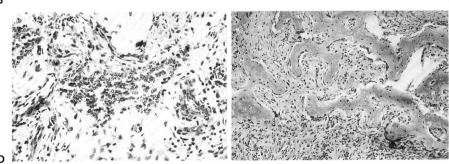

local anesthesia is to reposition the displaced teeth. Reduction in these cases is similar to that after lateral luxation (see Chapter 15, p. 418); that is, by disengaging the apices from the vestibular bone plate. This is done by simultaneous digital pressure in an incisal direction over the apical area and in a facial direction at the lingual aspect of the crown. This maneuver will usually free the apices and permit repositioning of the fragment. The socket wall is repositioned at the same time. In case of open comminuted fractures, it may be necessary to remove loose fragments which are not adherent to the periosteum. Clinical experience has shown that, despite removal of the entire vestibular bone plate, there is still enough structural support to ensure adequate stability of the teeth. After reduction of displaced teeth and bone fractures, lacerations of soft tissues should be sutured. Although it is tempting to suture immediately, suturing of soft tissue wounds should be left to last, as suturing early in the treatment procedure limits access for repositioning procedures. Splinting is carried out according to the principles outlined in Chapter 32.

Due to rapid bony healing in children, most fractures of the alveolar socket wall involving the primary dentition do not require splinting. In these cases, the parents should be instructed to restrict nourishment to a soft diet during the first 2 weeks after injury.

## Fractures of the alveolar process

Treatment of fractures of the alveolar process includes reduction and immobilization (4, 6, 47–50, 76–77) (Fig. 18.22). After administration of local anesthesia, the alveolar fragment is repositioned with digital pressure. In this type of fracture, apices of involved teeth can often be locked in position by the vestibular bone plate. Reduction in these cases follows the principles mentioned under fractures of the alveolar socket wall.

Splinting of alveolar fractures can be achieved by means of an acid-etch/resin splint or arch bars. Intermaxillary fixation is not required provided that a stable splint is used (Fig. 18.22). A fixation period of 4 weeks is usually recommended. However, due to more rapid healing in children, this period can be reduced to 3 weeks.

Teeth in a loose alveolar fragment might be doomed to extraction due to marginal or periapical inflammation. However, these extractions should generally be postponed until bony healing has stabilized the fragment (Fig. 18.23), otherwise the entire alveolar fragment might be inadvertently removed with the teeth. Again, regarding treatment sequence, associated soft tissue lacerations should be sutured last in order to allow access for intraoral manipulation.

Treatment of alveolar fractures in children offers special problems due to lack of sufficient teeth for splinting procedures. In most cases where the fragment can be reduced into a stable position, one can omit the splinting procedure. In such cases, nourishment should be restricted to soft or liquid foods. Alternatively, an acrylic splint fastened with per-

mandibular wires can be a solution (see Chapter 19).

## Fractures of the mandible or maxilla

Jaw fracture and especially mandibular fracture are often combined with dental injuries (118).

The management of fractures of the mandible or maxilla involves many procedures beyond the scope of this book. In this regard, only teeth involved in the fracture area will be considered. The reader is otherwise referred to standard textbooks on this subject (53, 86, 87).

Treatment of jaw fractures in children with developing teeth in the line of fracture follows the given general principles, i.e. exact repositioning and usually intermaxillary fixation. A review survey article has been published by Hard and von Arx (119). It is important that developing permanent teeth in the fracture line be preserved. The only exception would be in cases of infection along the fracture line being maintained by infected tooth germs (54, 55, 120). Moreover, in case of open reduction, screws should be place at a distance from developing teeth (120–122) (see Chapter 20).

Treatment of jaw fractures in adults with teeth in the fracture line is a controversial issue (68) and has been the subject of a review article (88). Particularly prior to the antibiotic era, it was customary to extract all teeth in the fracture line. However, studies have shown that this approach does not reduce the frequency of complications, which has gradually led to more conservative treatment.

### Teeth in the line of fracture

In the past, a number of clinical studies have appeared concerning the effect of various factors related to healing complications when teeth were involved in the line of fracture (56–63, 68–74, 78–82, 123, 150). However, all of these studies are retrospective, implying a possible bias in the evaluation of extraction therapy and the use of antibiotics. The resultant conclusions should therefore be regarded with extreme caution. In the following, a survey of factors related to fracture healing complications is presented.

The presence of teeth in the fracture line apparently represents an increased risk for infection compared to a fracture where no teeth are involved (68, 89).

### *Type of teeth involved*

The type of tooth involved also appears to be of importance. Thus, multirooted teeth appear to enhance the risk of complications compared to single-rooted teeth (68, 70) (Table 18.1).

### Fig. 18.22 Treatment of an alveolar fracture

This 21-year-old woman suffered a fracture of the maxillary alveolar process including the lateral and central incisors.

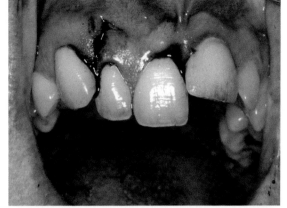 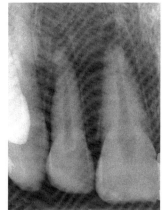

### Anesthetizing the traumatized region

An infraorbital block and infiltration to the incisive canal are necessary prior to repositioning.

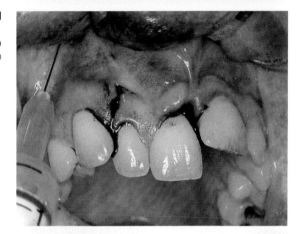 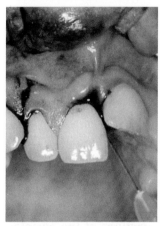

### Repositioning

With firm finger pressure to the apical region, the apices are disengaged. If this is not possible, the fragment must be moved in a coronal and palatal direction with the help of a forceps.

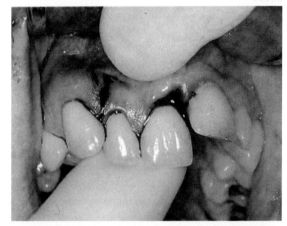 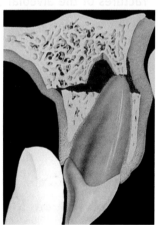

### Verifying repositioning

Occlusion is checked and a radiograph taken to verify adequate repositioning.

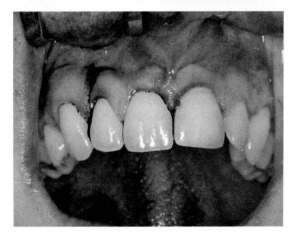 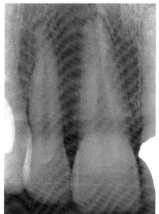

## Splinting

The incisal one-third of the labial aspect of injured and adjacent teeth are acid-etched (30 seconds) with phosphoric acid gel. The etchant is removed with a 20-second water spray. The labial enamel is dried with compressed air, revealing the mat, etched surface, whereafter the splinting material is applied. During polymerization of the splinting material, the patient occludes in order to ensure correct repositioning of the alveolar segment.

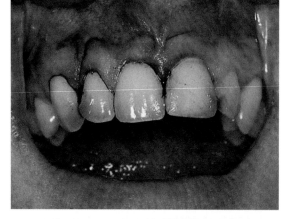 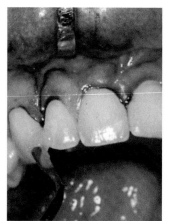

## Finished splint

The splint does not contact the gingiva so that optimal oral hygiene can be maintained.

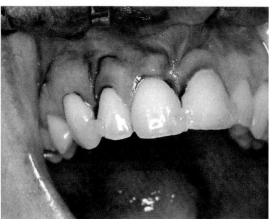 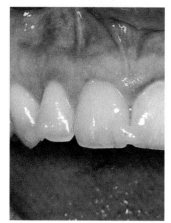

## Removing the splint

After 4 weeks the splint is removed with a scaler or fissure bur.

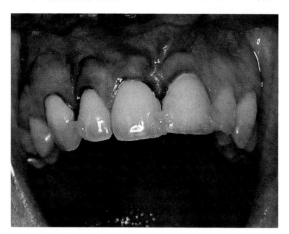 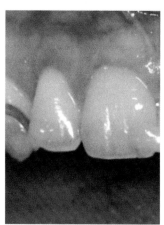

## Controlling pulpal sensitivity

Pulpal revascularization is monitored after 3 months. Due to a lack of response to pulp testing as well as a slight apical radiolucency, pulp necrosis is suspected.

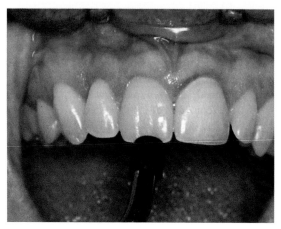 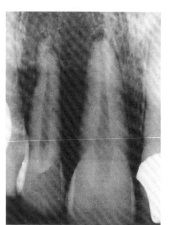

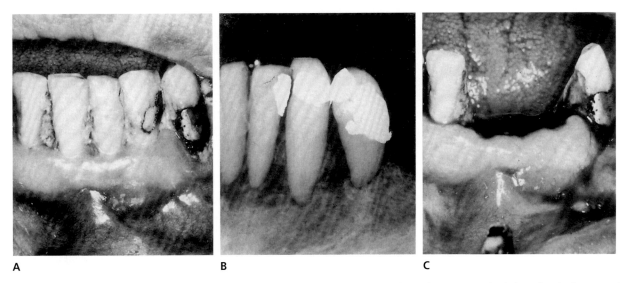

**A**    **B**    **C**

**Fig. 18.23** A and B. Alveolar fracture in left incisor and canine region associated with marginal periodontitis. It was decided to splint the fracture and postpone extraction of lower incisors for 6 weeks. C. Lower incisors extracted without damage to the alveolar process.

**Table 18.1** Frequency of complicated fracture healing in adults with teeth preserved along the fracture line.

| Examiner | No. of cases | No. of complications (inflammation) |
|---|---|---|
| Götte (57) 1959 | 178** | 30 (17%) |
| Andrä & Sonnenburg (56) 1966 | 264** | 40 (15%) |
| Andrä & Sonnenburg (56) 1966 | 139*+ | 7 (5%) |
| Müller (68) 1968 | 118++ | 23 (19%) |
| Neal et al. (79) 1978 | 132* | 39 (29%) |
| Rink & Stoehr (91) 1978 | 99* | 13 (13%) |
| Kahnberg & Ridell (81) 1979 | 132* | 10 (8%) |
| Choung et al. (89) 1983 | 152** | 4 (3%) |
| de Amaratunga (92) 1987 | 124** | 6 (5%) |
| Gerbino et al. (124) 1997 | 78 | 8 (10%) |
| Krenkel & Grunert (152) 1986 | 36 | 0 (0%) |
| Marker et al. (123) 1994 | 57*++ | 2 (4%) |
| Rubin et al. (125) 1990 | 69*++ | 16 (23%) |
| Ellis (150) 2002 | 258 | (19.5%) |

\* antibiotics given in all cases; \*\* antibiotics given in some cases; + single-rooted teeth; ++ multi-rooted teeth.

## Eruption status

The most frequent tooth involved in jaw fractures appears to be the third molar. The eruption status of this tooth (especially semi-erupted) appears to be significantly related to the occurrence of healing complications. Thus, complications are usually only seen with semi-erupted mandibular third molars; whereas fully erupted or impacted third molars rarely develop complications along the line of fracture (91) (Fig. 18.24).

## Extraction of teeth

In general, no beneficial effect has been demonstrated following the extraction of teeth in the line of fracture. In fact, a few studies have shown an increased morbidity (57–59, 79, 124) but most studies no effect of extraction (56, 77, 78, 89, 90, 92, 113, 125, 126, 150). However, none of the cited

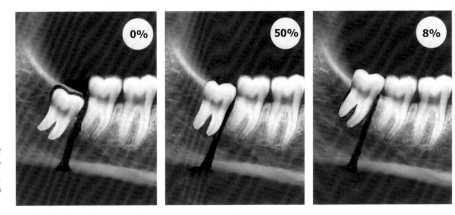

**Fig. 18.24** The infection risk in the fracture bone is strongly related to the eruption status of the third molar. The frequency is indicated according to RINK & STOEHR (91) 1978.

studies were designed as randomized investigations with respect to extraction of teeth in the line of fracture. Only one randomized study has been published dealing with the effect of extracting the third molar. In this study it was found that only removal of semiimpacted molars had en advantage in avoiding fracture healing complications (91) (Fig. 18.24). Furthermore, there was no difference in the complication rate of completely impacted teeth, whether open or closed repositioning (114).

### Effect of antibiotics

In cases of conservatively or surgically treated mandibular fractures, prospective randomized studies have shown that antibiotic treatment given from 30 min before surgery and up to 1 day afterwards significantly decreased the frequency of infection (93–95, 126, 127). However, an increase in antibiotic coverage for more than 1 day did not decrease the rate of infection (94, 95, 127, 128).

The effect of antibiotics on infection in the line of fracture in dentulous parts of the jaws is presently a subject of debate. If teeth are present in the line of fracture, there is an uncertain (56, 57) or no value of antibiotic therapy (91), whereas one study showed a positive effect (60).

If teeth were extracted, the rate of infection was unaffected by antibiotic therapy in one investigation (91) and found to be reduced in another (56). In one study, it was found that a positive effect was only related to multirooted teeth (68).

### Delay in treatment

Delay in treatment seems to play a questionable role in the frequency of healing complications. In case of alveolar fractures, treatment delay appears to be related to pulp necrosis and root resorption (6). Concerning jaw fractures, four studies showed no significant difference between immediate and delayed treatment (126, 154–156). One study showed a preference for healing for cases treated within 3 days (153), whereas another study indicated that treatment between 3 and 5 days after injury was optimal, with the lowest rate of complications (97). In conclusion, there is presently no strong evidence for either acute or delayed treatment of mandibular fractures in order to minimize healing complications; new studies, including a number of cases treated on an acute basis, are needed (157).

### Type of splinting

An increase in the rate of infection was found following rigid internal fixation (i.e. surgical repositioning and osteosynthesis using wire or plates) in fractures with teeth in the fracture line compared to similar fractures treated by closed reduction and conventional intermaxillary fixation (98–100).

Another factor which influences fracture healing is rigid arch bar fixation compared to a flexible wire splint. By eliminating movement of the fragments, seepage of saliva along the fracture line is prevented, which thus decreases the possibility of secondary infection (57). Finally, interdental wiring in jaw fractures does not appear to lead to adverse effects in the periodontium (138).

In conclusion, teeth present in the line of fracture should generally be preserved, as they can later serve as functional units. Moreover, their removal may further traumatize the fracture site and lead to dislocation of the fragment (59, 101). Exceptions to this approach would be teeth with crown-root fractures, semi erupted third molars and teeth with severe marginal or apical breakdown whose fate is already compromised. Teeth with pulp necrosis and apical breakdown can possibly be saved by endodontic therapy. This also applies to teeth with complicated crown and root fractures. Treatment of these injuries follows principles outlined in previous chapters. However, root canal treatment must necessarily be postponed until the intermaxillary fixation has been removed. When pulp exposures due to crown fractures are present, pulp extirpation should be carried out and the root canal provisionally sealed until removal of the intermaxillary fixation allows completion of therapy. Root fractured teeth are stabilized with splints.

If inflammation occurs, the treatment of choice is antibiotic therapy, possibly together with extraction of teeth involved in the inflammatory process, or endodontic therapy if pulp necrosis has developed.

## Prognosis

### Fractures of the socket wall

The immediate course of healing after fracture of the socket wall is usually uneventful; however, later follow-ups can reveal resorption of roots of involved teeth. These events are described for laterally luxated teeth (see Chapter 15, p. 411).

### Fractures of the alveolar process

The healing events of alveolar fractures in the permanent dentition are in most cases uneventful; however, in rare cases, sequestration of bone and/or involved teeth can occur (Fig. 18.25). Careful follow-up is mandatory in order to register later pulp necrosis and periapical inflammation (5, 6). Such complications are rather frequent and apparently related to the time interval between injury and fixation (Fig. 18.26). Thus, teeth splinted within 1 hour after injury develop pulp necrosis less frequently than teeth splinted after longer intervals (6).

Apart from pulp necrosis, pulp canal obliteration, root resorption (Table 18.2 and Figs 18.27 and 18.28) and loss of supporting bone (Fig. 18.29) are common complications (6).

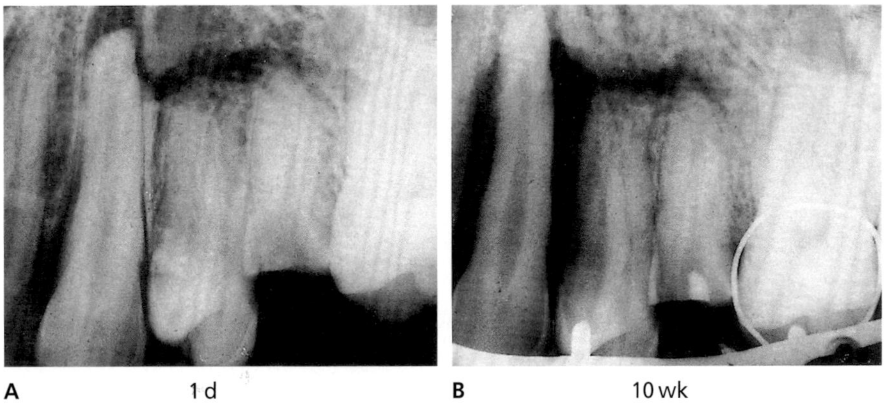

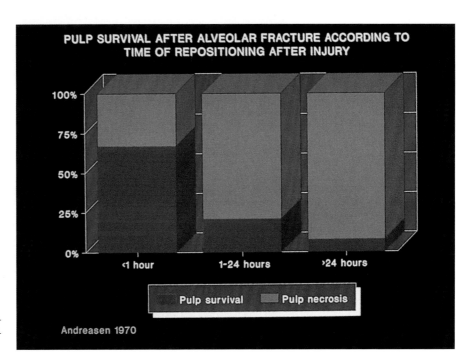

**Fig. 18.25** Persistent infection in the fracture line of an alveolar fracture involving canine and premolars. A. Condition immediately after injury. B. Radiograph 10 weeks later reveals marked bone destruction in the fracture area.

A            1 d

B            10 wk

**Fig. 18.26** Pulpal healing after alveolar fracture in the permanent dentition. From ANDREASEN (6) 1970.

PULP SURVIVAL AFTER ALVEOLAR FRACTURE ACCORDING TO TIME OF REPOSITIONING AFTER INJURY

Pulp survival    Pulp necrosis

Andreasen 1970

Concerning the prognosis of alveolar fractures in the primary dentition, it has been found that root development of preserved primary teeth is often arrested (51).

## Fractures of the mandible or maxilla in children

### Inflammation at the line of fracture

Fractures of the mandible or maxilla in children with developing teeth along the fracture line are seldom complicated by inflammation. It appears from the studies listed in Table 18.3 that frequencies of complications were found to range from 10 to 18%. The clinical picture of inflammation in the fracture area is characterized by swelling and abscess formation. Draining fistulae may also develop, as well as immediate or protracted sequestration of involved tooth germs (65).

When inflammation does occur, antibiotic therapy is the treatment of choice. Surgical removal of involved teeth may be indicated if radiographs reveal infected tooth germs in the fracture area (64–67). In such cases, osteolytic changes will be found in the fracture area, with disappearance of distinct outlines of the dental crypts of the involved teeth. It is conjectured from animal experiments (27) and human data (65) that infected tooth germs in these cases are responsible for protracted inflammation.

### Disturbances in the developing dentition

Another problem which should be considered when treating jaw fractures in children is odontogenic disturbances in involved developing teeth (see Chapter 20, p. 544).

**Table 18.2** Frequency of late dental complications following fractures of the alveolar process.

| | No. of cases | No. of involved teeth | Frequency of pulp necrosis | Frequency of pulp canal obliteration | Frequency of progressive root resorption | Frequency of loss of marginal supporting bone |
|---|---|---|---|---|---|---|
| Andreasen (6) 1970 | 29 | 71 | 75% | 15% | 11% | 13% |
| Krenkel & Grunert (152) 1986 | 23 | 73 | 63% | 11% | 6% | 6% |

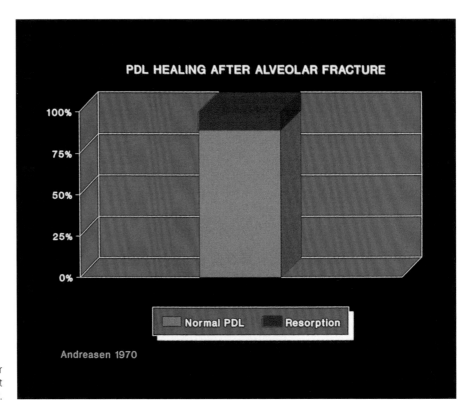

**Fig. 18.27** Periodontal healing after alveolar fracture in the permanent dentition. From ANDREASEN (6) 1970.

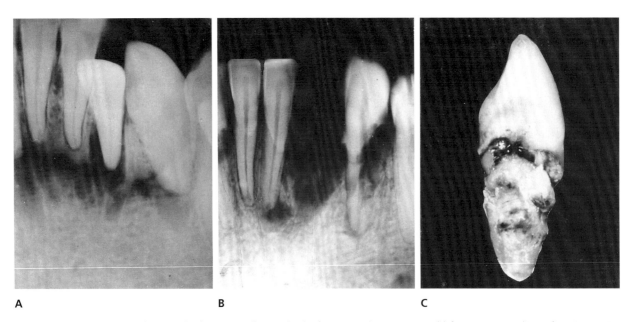

A                    B                    C

**Fig. 18.28** Root resorption and periapical inflammation after an alveolar fracture involving incisors and left canine. A. Condition after injury. B. Re-examination 3 years after injury reveals periapical inflammation as well as inflammatory root resorption. C. Clinical view of extracted canine. Marked resorption areas present on root surface. From ANDREASEN (6) 1970.

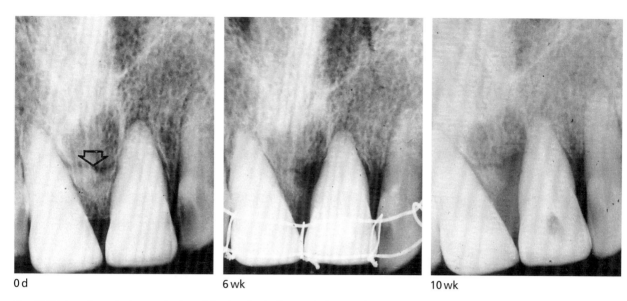

0 d  6 wk  10 wk

**Fig. 18.29** Loss of marginal supporting bone following alveolar fracture in the central incisor region. Horizontal fracture line is evident on radiograph taken at time of injury (arrow). At follow-up, loss of marginal supporting bone is evident around left central incisor. From ANDREASEN (6) 1970.

**Table 18.3** Frequency of complicated fracture healing in children with developing permanent teeth involved in the fracture line.

| Examiner | No. of cases | No. of complications (inflammation) |
|---|---|---|
| Lenstrup (14) 1955 | 22 | 4 (18%) |
| Taatz (64) 1962 | 29 | 3 (10%) |
| Koenig et al. (139) 1994 | 30 | 0 (0%) |

# Fractures of the mandible or maxilla in adults

## Fibrous union

In a recent study of 714 mandibular fractures, fibrous union was found in 27 patients (3.8%); and was apparently related to the presence of teeth in the fracture line. However, a more detailed analysis of this material revealed no relation to fracture sites where teeth had been removed or maintained (145).

## Inflammation at the line of fracture

Studies of jaw fractures in adults have shown that the frequency of inflammatory complications along the line of fracture when teeth are preserved ranges from 3 to 29% (Table 18.1, Fig. 18.30). A tooth positioned along the line of fracture can be the source of inflammation due to pulp necrosis from compromised circulation to the pulpal tissues or already established infection in the pulp which can spread to the fracture site (Fig. 18.31). This finding is supported by the finding that pulp necrosis in involved teeth is common

when a fracture directly involves the apical region (69, 82). Infection can also occur along the denuded root surface when a fracture directly involves the alveolar socket (26).

## Pulpal healing and pulp necrosis

Teeth preserved along a fracture line should be carefully followed in order to detect later pulp necrosis (58, 69, 74, 81, 102, 140, 142) (Table 18.4). In interpreting pulpal sensibility of involved teeth, one should remember that reactions may be temporarily decreased and later return to normal (75, 81, 103). It has been found that pulp necrosis is primarily associated with the relationship of the apices of involved teeth to the fracture line (69, 82, 83, 102). Thus, if the apex is exposed by the fracture line, the risk of pulp necrosis is increased (81, 141, 146) (Fig. 18.31). Moreover, fractures treated more than 48 hours after injury show an increased incidence of later pulp necrosis (69, 82, 102). Finally, the use of open repositioning and plates (compared to closed repositioning and intermaxillary fixation) resulted in significantly more pulp necrosis, also in adjacent teeth (147).

In the follow-up period, obliteration of the root canal is often seen in teeth involved in the fracture, and especially in individuals below 20 years of age (102) (Figs 18.32 and 18.33).

## PDL healing and root resorption

Root resorption following jaw fractures is a rare finding and has been found to affect up to 4% of the teeth involved in the fracture line (69, 81, 87, 140–142) (Table 18.4).

No difference was found in mobility of teeth involved in jaw fractures, whether with conservative or surgical repositioning (148).

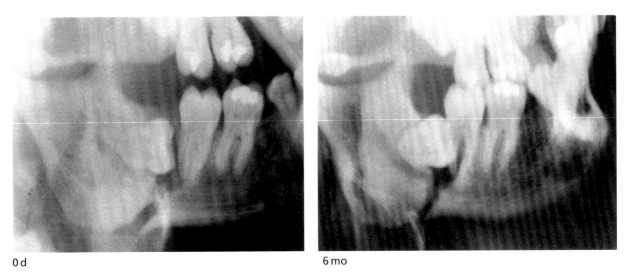

0 d                                                    6 mo

**Fig. 18.30** Radiograph illustrating delayed fracture healing due to inflammation maintained by an impacted third molar. Six months later, bone healing has not occurred.

**Fig. 18.31** Pulp necrosis and incomplete healing of marginal periodontium following jaw fracture in the canine region. Note that the fracture line involves the apex of the canine. Follow-up examination after 6 months revealed incomplete healing of the marginal periodontium as well as pulp necrosis with periapical involvement. From ROED-PETERSEN & ANDREASEN (69) 1970.

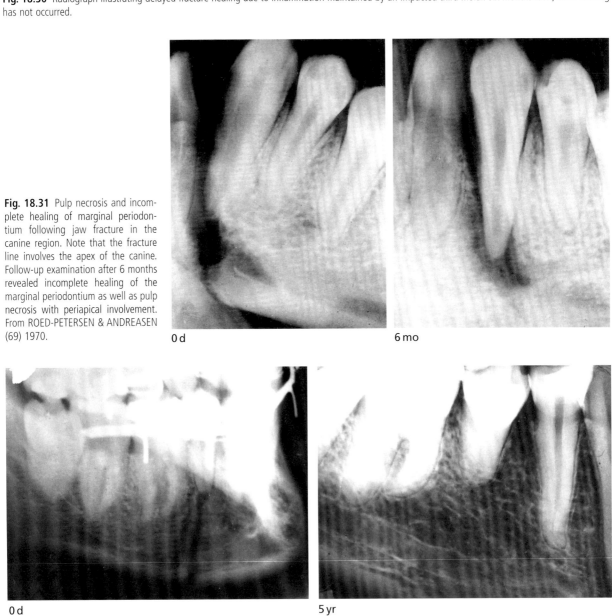

0 d                                                    6 mo

0 d                                                    5 yr

**Fig. 18.32** Obliteration of pulp canal in a second premolar following jaw fracture. The fracture line involves the apical area. At follow-up a marked pulp canal obliteration is evident. From ROED-PETERSEN & ANDREASEN (69) 1970.

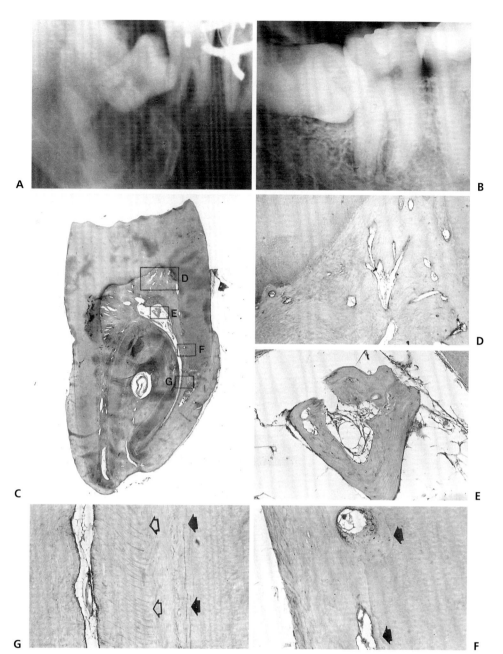

**Fig. 18.33** Obliteration of the pulp canal secondary to a jaw fracture. A. Time of injury – the jaw fracture involves the third molar region. B. Six years later, marked pulp canal obliteration of the third molar is evident. C. Low power view of sectioned molar. ×3. D. Coronal part of the pulp completely occluded with hard tissue. ×30. E. Islands of bone in the middle of the pulp. ×75. F. Apposition of hard tissue following initial resorption of the canal walls (arrows). ×75. G. Normal dentin deposited after formation of atubular dentin immediately after injury (arrows). ×75.

**Table 18.4** Frequency of late dental complications following jaw fractures.

| Examiner | No. of cases | No. of involved teeth | Frequency of pulp necrosis | Frequency of pulp canal obliteration | Frequency of progressive root resorption | Frequency of loss of marginal supporting bone |
|---|---|---|---|---|---|---|
| Roed-Petersen & Andreasen (69) 1970 | 68 | 110 | 25% | 5% | 0% | 12% |
| Ridell & Astrand (82) 1971 | 84 | 142 | 5% | 2% | 1% | 11% |
| Kahnberg & Ridell (81) 1979 | 132 | 185 | 14% | – | 3% | 12% |
| Krenkel & Grunert (140) 1987 | 21 | 50 | 23% | 2% | 2% | 2% |
| Oikarinen et al. (141) 1990 | 45 | 47 | 38% | 24% | 4% | 18% |
| Berg & Pape (142) 1992 | 41 | 59 | 22% | | 5% | 12% |
| Thaller & Mabourakh (143) 1994 | 142 | | 9% | | | |

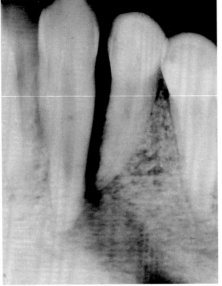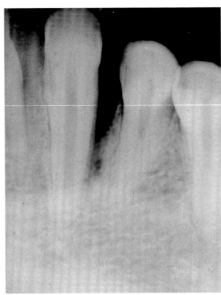

**Fig. 18.34** Incomplete healing of marginal periodontium following jaw fracture in the canine region. 4 years later – deep pocket formation and loss of supporting bone is found. From ROED-PETERSEN & ANDREASEN (69) 1970.

0 d                                    4 yr

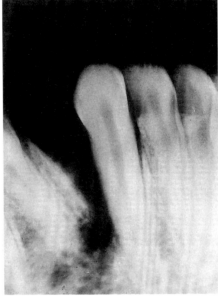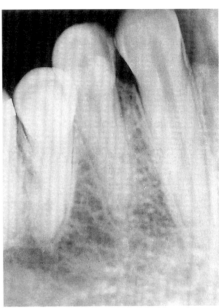

**Fig. 18.35** Complete healing of the periodontium despite extensive dislocation of fragments and exposed cementum of a lower right canine. From ROED-PETERSEN & ANDREASEN (69) 1970.

0 d                                    3 yr

## Gingival healing and loss of marginal attachment

Generally speaking periodontal healing is the usual event after a jaw fracture involving interdental bone (149).

In case of arch bar fixation (i.e. Sauer's, Schuchardt's or Erich's arch bar), no significant difference in periodontal health after splinting has been found in a clinical situation (105). Experimentally, a mild periodontitis has been observed during the splinting period (106–108). However, these inflammatory changes appear to be reversed following splint removal (109, 110, 138).

The dental septum and gingiva involved in jaw fractures appear to possess a good healing potential. Complications, such as loss of interdental bone and pocketing, are rare (111).

Loss of marginal bone can be recorded at later follow-up examinations (69, 82, 102). This is found especially among involved canines. Incomplete reduction of displaced fragments appears to be the main cause of loss of marginal bone support (Fig. 18.34), while optimal repositioning will ensure complete periodontal repair (69, 81) (Fig. 18.35). However, a slight long-term increase in mobility of teeth along the line of fracture has been reported (102, 112).

## Essentials

### Terminology (Fig. 18.1)

- Comminution of alveolar socket
- Fracture of alveolar socket wall
- Fracture of alveolar process
- Fracture of mandible or maxilla (jaw fracture)

### Frequency

- Permanent dentition: 16% of dental injuries
- Primary dentition: 7% of dental injuries

### Etiology

- Fight injuries
- Automobile accidents

### History

- Symptoms

### Clinical examination

- Palpation of facial skeleton
- Mobility of fragments
- Dislocation of fragments
- Reaction to sensibility tests

### Radiographic examination

- Dislocation of fragments
- Relation between bone fracture and marginal and apical periodontium

### Pathology

- Fracture healing
- Superficial root resorption

### Treatment (Fig. 18.22)

(1) Administer local or general anesthesia.
(2) Reposition displaced fragments.
(3) Teeth in jaw fracture lines should generally be preserved unless severe inflammatory changes of marginal or apical origin are present. Teeth with periapical inflammation can be maintained if antibacterial medication is placed in the root canal. Semierupted third molars should, as a rule, be removed.
(4) Apply fixation (acid-etch/resin splint). In the primary dentition, a direct splinting method with acrylic may be used. In cases where the fragment can be reduced into a stable position, one may refrain from splinting. In such cases, the patient should be instructed to restrict nourishment to soft food.
(5) Check reduction radiographically.
(6) Antibiotic therapy may be indicated in the treatment of jaw fractures.
(7) Control the involved teeth radiographically and with sensibility tests.
(8) Immobilize for 4 weeks.
(9) Follow-up period minimum one year.

### Prognosis for permanent teeth involved in fractures of the alveolar process

- Pulp necrosis: 75%
- Pulp canal obliteration: 15%
- Progressive root resorption: 11%
- Loss of marginal bone support: 13%

### Prognosis for permanent teeth involved in fractures of the maxilla or the mandible

- Infection in the fracture line: 5–29%
- Pulp necrosis: 5–38%
- Pulp canal obliteration: 2–24%
- Progressive root resorption: 0–4%
- Loss of marginal bone support: 11–18%

### Treatment of pulp necrosis

See Chapter 22.

### Treatment of root resorption

See Chapter 22.

### Treatment of inflammation in the fracture line

(1) Antibiotic therapy
(2) Extraction or endodontic therapy of involved permanent teeth if they sustain inflammation

## References

1. ANDREASEN JO. Etiology and pathogenesis of traumatic dental injuries. A clinical study of 1,298 cases. *Scand J Dent Res* 1970;**7**:329–42.
2. HUELKE DF, HARGER JH. Maxillofacial injuries: their nature and mechanisms of production. *J Oral Surg* 1969;**27**:451–60.
3. HAGAN EH, HUELKE DF. An analysis of 319 case reports of mandibular fractures. *J Oral Surg* 1961;**19**:93–104.
4. MÜLLER W. Diagnostik und Therapie der Alveolarfortsatzfrakturen in der zahnärzlichen Praxis. *Dtsch Zahnärztekalender* 1969;**28**:20–34.

5. FREIHOFER HPM. Ergebnisse der Behandlung vom Alveolarfortsatzfrakturen. *Schweiz Monatsschr Zahnheilkd* 1969;**79**:623–9.

6. ANDREASEN JO. Fractures of the alveolar process of the jaw. A clinical and radiographic follow-up study. *Scand J Dent Res* 1970;**78**:263–72.

7. GEHRE G. Ein Beitrag zur Therapie der Alveolarfortsatzfrakturen unter besonderer Berücksichtigung des Krankengutes der Leipziger Universitätsklinik der Jahre 1955–1966. *Dtsch Stomatol* 1962;**12**:97–104.

8. ENGHOFF A, SIEMSSEN SO. Kaebefrakturer gennem 10 år. *Tandlaegebladet* 1956;**60**:851–84.

9. GISCHLER E, LOCHE R. Beitrag zur Häufigkeit der Frakturen im Bereich der Kiefer-und Gesichtsschädelknochen. *Dtsch Zahnärztl Z* 1962;**17**:649–55.

10. NEUNER O. Zur Entstehung und Verhütung der Bruchspaltostitis bei Unterkieferfrakturen. *Zahnärztl Welt* 1963;**64**:66–78.

11. HUELKE DF, BURDI AR, EYMAN CE. Mandibular fractures as related to the site of trauma and the state of dentition. *J Dent Res* 1961;**40**:1262–74.

12. FUHR K, SETZ D. Nachuntersuchungen über Zähne, die zum Bruchspalt in Beziehung stehen. *Dtsch Zahnärztl Z* 1963;**18**:638–43.

13. OIKARINEN VJ, MALMSTRÖM M. Jaw fractures. A roentgenological and statistical analysis of 1284 cases including a special study of the fracture lines in the mandible drawn from orthopantomograms in 660 cases. *Suomi Hammaslääk Toim* 1969;**65**:95–111.

14. LENSTRUP K. On injury by fractures of the jaws to teeth in course of formation. *Acta Odontol Scand* 1955;**13**:181–202.

15. VELGOS S, STANKO V, PREVRATILOVA D. Kieferfrakturen bei Kindern. *Dtsch Stomatol* 1969;**19**:481–6.

16. UENO T, OKA T, MIYAGAWA Y, KOBAYASHI Y. Clinical and experimental studies of the location and lines of mandibular fractures. *Bull Tokyo Med Dent Univ* 1957;**4**:245–51.

17. OLECH E. Fracture lines in mandible. Comparison of radiographic and anatomic findings. *Oral Surg Oral Med Oral Pathol* 1955;**8**:582–90.

18. URIST MR, JOHNSON RW. Calcification and ossification IV. The healing of fractures in man under clinical conditions. *J Bone Joint Surg* 1943;**25**: 375–426.

19. MCLEAN FC, URIST MR. *Bone. An introduction to the physiology of skeletal tissue.* Chicago: University of Chicago Press, 1961:200–14.

20. SPRINTZ R. Healing of subcondylar fracture of the mandible after ablation of the lateral pterygoid in rats. *J Dent Res* 1969;**48**:1097–8.

21. MESSER EJ, HAYES DE, BOYNE PJ. Use of intraosseous metal appliances in fixation of mandibular fractures. *J Oral Surg* 1967;**25**:493–502.

22. GREVE K. *Der Heilverlauf von einfachen und komplizierten Unterkieferfrakturen mit besonderer Berücksichtigung des Mandibularkanals und der Zähne. Eine tierexperimentelle und histologische Studie.* Deutsche Zahnheilkunde No. 67. Leipzig: Georg Thieme Verlag, 1927:1–64.

23. GRIMSON KS. Healing of fractures of the mandible and zygoma. *J Am Dent Assoc* 193;**24**:1458–69.

24. RICHMAN PT, LASKIN DM. The healing of experimentally produced fractures of the zygomaticomaxillary complex. *Oral Surg Oral Med Oral Pathol* 1964;**17**:701–11.

25. HORNOVA J, MALY F. Die Heilung der durch verschiedene Mechanismen und in verschiedenen Bedingungen entstandenen Knochendefekte. *Schr Med Fac Med Brun* 1967;**40**:177–85.

26. KRAMER IRH. The structure of bone and the processes of bone repair. In: Rowe NL, Killey HC. eds. *Fractures of the facial skeleton.* London: E & S Livingstone, 1968:615–25.

27. PASCHKE H. Experimentelle Untersuchungen über den Heilverlauf von Unterkieferfrakturen. *Zahnärztl Rdsch* 1931;**40**:2172–5.

28. SARNAT BG, SCHOUR I. Effect of experimental fracture on bone, dentin, and enamel. Study of the mandible and the incisor in the rat. *Arch Surg* 1944;**49**:23–38.

29. BENCZE J. Zahnkeimläsionen infolge Kieferfrakturen im Tierversuch. *Stoma* 1967;**20**:165–73.

30. SCHAFER H. Über die Kallusbildung nach Unterkieferfrakturen. *Schweiz Monatsschr Zahnheilkd* 1923;**33**:567–624.

31. SKLANS S, TAYLOR RG, SHKLAR G. Effect of diphenylhydantoin sodium on healing of experimentally produced fractures in rabbit mandibles. *J Oral Surg* 1967;**25**:310–19.

32. FRY WK, WARD T. *The dental treatment of maxillo facial injuries.* Oxford: Blackwell Scientific Publications, 1956:72–92.

33. BONNETTE GH. Experimental fractures of the mandible. *J Oral Surg* 1969;**27**:568–71.

34. HOFFER O. Indagine sperimentale sul processo evolutivo di guarigione delle ferite ossee (Con particulate reguardo alla traumatologia del condilo). *Minerva Stomatol* 1969;**18**:1–6.

35. KANEKO Y. Experimental studies on vascular changes in fracture and osteomyelitis. Part I. Vascular changes in mandibular fracture and healing. *Bull Tokyo Dent Coll* 1968;**9**:123–46.

36. SZABÒ C, TARSOLY E. Kompresszios osteosynthesis gyogyeredményei a kutya mandibulâjân. *Fogorv Szle* 1967;**60**:915.

37. GILHUUS-MOE O. *Fractures of the mandibular condyle in the growth period.* Thesis. Oslo Universitetsforlaget, 1969.

38. BOYNE PJ. Osseous healing after oblique osteotomy of the mandibular ramus. *J Oral Surg* 1966;**24**: 125–33.

39. BOYNE PJ. Osseous repair and mandibular growth after subcondylar fractures. *J Oral Surg* 1967;**25**:300–9.

40. YRASTORZA JA, KRUGER GO. Polyurethane polymer in the healing of experimentally fractured mandibles. *Oral Surg Oral Med Oral Surg* 1963;**16**:978–84.

41. CLARK HB Jr, HAYES PA. A study of the comparative effects of 'rigid' and 'semirigid' fixation on the healing of fractures of the mandible in dogs. *J Bone Joint Surg* 1963;**45-A**:731–41.

42. LIGHTERMAN I, FARRELL J. Mandibular fractures treated with plastic polymers. *Arch Surg* 1963;**87**:868–76.

43. Fries R. Die stabile Osteosynthese von Unterkieferfrakturen unter besonderer Berücksichtigung der offenen axialer Markdrahtung. II Teil. *Öst Z Stomatol* 1969;**66**:298–319.

44. Hunsuck EE. Vascular changes in bone repair. *Oral Surg Oral Med Oral Pathol* 1969;**27**:572–4.

45. Wannenmacher E. Ein Beitrag zur pathologischen Histologie der Pulpa. (Die Veränderungen der Pulpen von Zähnen, welche im Bereiche von Kieferfrakturen standen). *Dtsch Monatsschr Zahnheilk* 1927;**45**:12–38.

46. Reichardt P. *Untersuchungen an Zähnen, welche im Bereich von Kieferfrakturen standen, mit besonderer Berücksichtigung des Zementmantels.* Thesis. Tübingen: Verlag Franz Pietzcker, 1933.

47. Bataille R, Kolf J. Les fractures alvéolaires de la région incisive et leur traitement. *Actual Odontostomatol (Paris)* 1957;**40**:543–59.

48. Alexandre E, Marie J-L. A propos du traitement des traumatismes dentaires antérieurs avec fracture du rebord alvéolaire. *Rev Stomatol* 1967;**68**:399–406.

49. Kupfer SR. Fracture of the maxillary alveolus. *Oral Surg Oral Med Oral Pathol* 1954;**7**:830–6.

50. Fliege H, Heuser H, Warnke M. Beitrag zur Behandlung stark dislozierter Alveolarfortsatzbrücke. *Dtsch Zahn Mund Kieferheilk* 1937;**4**:545–52.

51. Müller W, Taatz H. Therapie und Spätergebnisse der Alveolarfortsatzfrakturen des Unterkiefers im Säuglings- und Kleinkindesalter. *Dtsch Zahnärztl Z* 1965;**20**:1190–6.

52. Pfeifer G. Freihändige Kunststoffschienung bei Alveolarfortsatzfrakturen und Luxationen im Milchgebiss. *Fortschr Kiefer Gesichtschir* 1959;**5**:328–32.

53. Rowe NL, Killey HC. *Fractures of the facial skeleton.* London: E & S Livingstone, 1968.

54. Bencze J. Zahnkeimschäden imfolge Kieferfrakturen in der Jugend. *Stoma* 1964;**17**:330–5.

55. Bencze J. Spätergebnisse nach im Kindesalter erlittenen Unterkieferbrüchen. *Acta Chir Acad Sci Hung* 1964;**5**:95–104.

56. Andrä A, Sonnenburg I. Die Bruchspaltostitis als Komplikation bei Unterkieferbrüchen in Beziehung zum primär vitalen Zahn am oder im Bruchspalt. *Dtsch Stomatol* 1966;**16**:336–44.

57. Götte H. Die Belassung von Zähnen im Bruchspalt in Abhängigkeit von der Art des Kieferbruchverbandes. *Fortschr Kiefer Gesichtschir* 1959;**5**:333–8.

58. Schönberger A. Behandlung der Zähne im Bruchspalt. *Fortschr Kiefer Gesichtschir* 1956;**2**:108–11.

59. Wilkie CA, Diecidue AA, Simses RJ. Management of teeth in the line of mandibular fracture. *J Oral Surg* 1953;**11**:227–30.

60. Heidsieck C. Über die Behandlungsergebnisse bei Unterkieferfrakturen. *Dtsch Stomatol* 1954;**4**:271–4.

61. Déchaume M, Crépy C, Régnier J-M. Conduite a tenir au sujet des dents en rapport avec les foyers de fracture des maxillaires. *Rev Stomatol* 1957;**58**:512–19.

62. Krömer H. Teeth in the line of fracture: A conception of the problem based on a review of 690 jaw fractures. *Br Dent J* 1953;**95**:43–6.

63. Herrmann M, Grasser H-H, Beisiegel I. Die Kieferbrücke and der Zahn-, Mund- und Kieferklinik in Mainz von 1949–1959. *Dtsch Zahnärztl Z* 1960;**15**:657–64.

64. Taatz H. Untersuchungen über Ursachen und Häufigkeit exogener Zahnkeimschäden. *Dtsch Zahn Mund Kieferheilk* 1962;**37**:468–84.

65. Taatz H. Spätschäden nach Kieferbrüchen im Kindesalter. *Fortschr Kieferorthop* 1954;**15**:174–84.

66. Fischer H-G. *Traumata im jugendlichen Kieferbereich, Heilergebnisse und ihr Einfluss auf die Keime der bleibenden Zähne.* Thesis. Leipzig, 1951.

67. Friederichs W. Kieferbrücke im Kindesalter und seltene Zysten. *Dtsch Zahnärztl Wschr* 1940;**43**:508–10.

68. Müller W. Häufigkeit und Prophylaxe der Bruchspaltostitiden im Zeitalter der Antibiotika. *Stomatol* 1968;**31**:1107.

69. Roed-Petersen B, Andreasen JO. Prognosis of permanent teeth involved in jaw fractures. A clinical and radiographic follow-up study. *Scand J Dent Res* 1970;**78**:343–52.

70. Müller W. Zur Frage des Versuchs der Erhaltung der im Bruchspalt stehenden Zähne unter antibiotischem Schutz. Dtsch *Zahn Mund Kieferheilk* 1964;**41**:360–70.

71. Weiskopf J. Zahnärztlich-orthopädische Methoden der Frakturversorgung. *Dtsch Stomatol* 1961;**11**:682–97.

72. Brachmann F. Penicillinbehandlung bei der Kieferbruchversorgung. *Zahnärztl Welt* 1951;**6**:231.

73. Schönberger A. Über das Schicksal im Bruchspalt belassener Zähne. *Dtsch Stomatol* 1955;**5**:19–29.

74. Rottke B, Kark U. Zur Frage der Extraktion in Bruchspalt stehender Zähne. *Ost Z Stomatol* 1969;**66**:465–9.

75. Kolarow D, Siskova S, Darvodelska M. The problem of electrical excitability of teeth in mandibular fractures. *Stomatologiya (Sofia)* 1966;**48**:238–44.

76. Müller W. Die Frakturen des Alveolarfortsatzes. *Dtsch Stomatol* 1972;**22**:135–48.

77. Bernstein L, Keyes KS. Dental and alveolar fractures. *Otolaryngol Clin North Am* 1972;**5**:273–81.

78. Hamill JP, Owsley JQ, Kauffman RR, Blackfield HM. The treatment of fractures of the mandible. *Calif Med J* 1964;**101**:184–7.

79. Neal DC, Wagner WF, Alpert B. Morbidity associated with teeth in the line of mandibular fractures. *J Oral Surg* 1978;**36**:859–62.

80. Schneider SS, Stern M. Teeth in the line of mandibular fractures. *J Oral Surg* 1971;**29**:107–9.

81. Kahnberg K-E, Ridell A. Prognosis of teeth involved in the line of mandibular fractures. *Int J Oral Surg* 1979;**8**:163–72.

82. Ridell A, Astrand P. Conservative treatment of teeth involved by mandibular fractures. *Swed Dent J* 1971;**64**:623–32.

83. Jirava E. Contribution to diagnostics of teeth in fragile fissures in fractures of body of the lower jaw. *Ceskoslovenska Stomatol* 1973;**73**:102–6.

84. Matteson SR, Tyndall DA. Pantomographic radiology. Part II. Pantomography of trauma and inflammation of the jaws. *Dent Radiography Photography* 1983;**56**:21–48.

85. Krekeler G, Petsch K, Flesch-Gorlas M. Der Frakturverlauf im parodontalen Bereich. *Dtsch Zahnärztl Z* 1983;**38**:355–7.

86. Rowe NL, Williams JL. *Maxillofacial injuries.* Edinburgh: Churchill Livingstone, 1985: Vols 1 and 2.

87. FONSECA RJ, WALKER RV. eds. *Oral and maxillofacial trauma*. Philadelphia: WB Saunders, 1991: Vols 1 and 2.

88. SHETTY V, FREYMILLER E. Teeth in the line of fracture: a review. *J Oral Maxillofac Surg* 1989;**47**:1303–6.

89. CHOUNG R, DONOFF RB, GURALNICK WC. A retrospective analysis of 327 mandibular fractures. *J Oral Maxillofac Surg* 1983;**41**:305–9.

90. GÜNTER M, GUNDLACH KKH, SCHWIPPER V. Der Zahn im Bruchspalt. *Dtsch Zahnärztl Z* 1983;**38**:346–8.

91. RINK B, STOEHR K. Weisheitzähne im Bruchspalt. *Stomatol DDR* 1978;**28**:307–10.

92. DE AMARATUNGA NA. The effect of teeth in the line of mandibular fractures on healing. *J Oral Maxillofac Surg* 1987;**45**:312–14.

93. ZALLEN RD, CURRY JT. A study of antibiotic usage in compound mandibular fractures. *J Oral Surg* 1975;**33**:431–4.

94. ADERHOLD L, JUNG H, FRENKEL G. Untersuchungen über den Wert einer Antibiotika-Prophylaxe bei Kiefer-Gesichtsverletzungen – eine prospektive Studie. *Dtsch Zahnärztl Z* 1983;**38**:402–6.

95. GERLACH KL, PAPE HD. Untersuchungen zur Antibiotikaprophylaxe bei der operativen Behandlung von Unterkieferfrakturen. *Dtsch Z Mund Kiefer Gesichtschir* 1988;**12**:497–500.

96. EICHE H, SELLE G. Zur Problematik des Zahnes am Bruchspalt. Eine retrospektive Untersuchung. *Dtsch Zahnärztl Z* 1983;**38**:352–4.

97. WAGNER WF, NEAL DC, ALPERT B. Morbidity associated with extraoral open reduction of mandibular fractures. *J Oral Surg* 1979;**37**:97–100.

98. HÖLTJE W-J, LUHR H-G, HOLTFRETER M. Untersuchungen über infektionsbedingte Komplikationen nach konservativer oder operativer Versorgung von Unterkieferfrakturen. *Fortschr Kiefer Gesichtschir* 1975;**19**:122–5.

99. JOOS U, SCHILLI W, NIEDERDELLMANN H, SCHEIBE B. Komplikationen und verzögerte Bruchheilung bei Kieferfrakturen. *Dtsch Zahnärztl Z* 1983;**38**:387–8.

100. STOLL P, NIEDERDELLMANN H, SAUTER R. Zahnbeteiligung bei Unterkieferfrakturen. *Dtsch Zahnärztl Z* 1983;**38**:349–51.

101. KAHNBERG K-E. Extraction of teeth involved in the line of mandibular fractures. I. Indications for extraction based on a follow-up study of 185 mandibular fractures. *Swed Dent J* 1979;**3**:27–32.

102. OIKARINEN K, LAHTI J, RAUSTIA AM. Prognosis of permanent teeth in the line of mandibular fractures. *Endod Dent Traumatol* 1990;**6**:177–82.

103. POLLMANN L. Längsschnittuntersuchungen der Sensibilität nach Kieferwinkelfrakturen. *Dtsch Zahnärztl Z* 1093;**38**:4825.

104. ROED-PETERSEN B, MORTENSEN H. Periodontal status after fixation with Sauer's and Schuchardt's arch bars in jaw fractures. *Int J Oral Surg* 1972;**1**:43–7.

105. ROED-PETERSEN B, MORTENSEN H. Arch bar fixation of fractures in dentulous jaws: a comparative study of Sauer's and Erich's bar. *Danish Med Bull* 1973;**20**:164–8.

106. BIENENGRABER V, SONNENBURG I, WILKEN J. Klinische und tierexperimentelle Untersuchungen über den Einfluss von Drahtschienenverbänden auf das marginale Parodontium. *Dtsch Stomatol* 1973;**23**:86–94.

107. NGASSAPA DN, FREIHOFERH-PM, MALTHA JC. The reaction of the periodontium to different types of splints. (I). Clinical aspects. *Int J Oral Maxillofac Surg* 1986;**15**:240–9.

108. NGASSAPA DN, MALTHA JC, FREIHOFER H-PM. The reaction of the periodontium to different types of splints. (II). Histological aspects. *Int J Oral Maxillofac Surg* 1986;**15**:250–8.

109. HÄRLE F, KREKELER G. Die Reaktion des Parodontiums auf die Drahtligaturenschiene (Stout-Obwegeser). *Dtsch Zahnärztl Z* 1977;**32**:814–16.

110. FRÖHLICH M, GABLER K. Der Einfluss von Kieferbruchshienenverbänden auf das Parodont. *Stomatol DDR* 1981;**31**:238–47.

111. SCHMITZ R, HÖLTJE W, CORDES V. Vergleichende Untersuchungen über die Regeneration des parodontalen Gewebes nach Unfallverletzungen und Osteotomien des Alveolarfort satzes. *Dtsch Zahnärztl Z* 1973;**28**:219–23.

112. HOFFMEISTER B. Die parodontale Reaktion im Bruchspalt stehender Zähne bei Unterkieferfrakturen. *Dtsch Zahnärztl Z* 1985;**40**:32–6.

113. BERGGREN RB, LEHR HB. Mandibular fractures: a review of 185 fractures in 111 patients. *J Trauma* 1967;**7**:357–66.

114. SAFDAR N, MEECHAN JG. Relationsship between fractures of the mandibular angle and the presence an state of eruption of the lower third molar. *Oral Surg Oral Med Oral Pathol Oral Radiol Endod* 1995;**79**:680–4.

115. FREITAG V, LANDAU H. Das Setzen experimentelle Frakturen am Unterkiefer des Hundes. *Dtsch Z Mund Kiefer Gesichts Chir* 1986;**10**:357–60.

116. FREITAG V, LANDAU H. Healing of dentate or edentulous mandibular fractures treated with rigid or semirigid plate fixation – an experimental study in dogs. *J Cran Maxillofac Surg* 1996;**24**:83–7.

117. FREITAG V, LANDAU H. Histological findings in the alveolar sockets and tooth roots after experimental mandibular fractures in dogs. *J Cran Maxillofac Surg* 1997;**25**:203–11.

118. IGNATIUS ET, OIKARINEN KS, SILVENNOINEN U. Frequency and type of dental traumas in mandibular body and condyle fractures. *Endod Dent Traumatol* 1992;**8**:235–40.

119. HARD N, VON ARX T. Fractures de la machoire inférieure de l'enfant. Fréquence, classification, concept thérapeutique. *Rev Mens Suisse Odonto-Stomatol* 1989;**99**:807–16.

120. PERKO M, PEPERSACK W. Spätergebnisse der Osteosynthesebehandlung bei Kieferfrakturen im Kindesalter. *Fortschr Kiefer Gesichts Chir* 1975;**19**:206–8.

121. NIXON F, LOWEY MN. Failed eruption of the permanent canine following open reduction of a mandibular fracture in a child. *Br Dent J* 1990;**168**:204–5.

122. JONES KM, BAUER BS, PENSLER JM. Treatment of mandibular fractures in children. *Ann Plast Surg* 1989;**23**:280–3.

123. MARKER P, ECKERDAL A, SMITH-SIVERTSEN C. Incompletely erupted third molars in the line of mandibular fractures. A retrospective analysis of 57 cases. *Oral Surg Oral Med Oral Pathol* 1994;**78**:426–31.

124. GERBINO G, TARELLO F, FASOLIS M, DE GIOANNI PP. Rigid fixation with teeth in the line of mandibular fractures. *Int J Oral Maxillofac Surg* 1997;**26**:182–6.

125. RUBIN MM, KOLL TJ, SADOFF RS. Morbidity associated with incompletely erupted third molars in the line of mandibular fractures. *J Oral Maxillofac Surg* 1990;**48**:1045–7.

126. CHOLE RA, YEE J. Antibiotic prophylaxis for facial fractures. *Arch Otolaryngol Head Neck Surg* 1987;**113**:1055–7.

127. ABUBAKER AO, ROLLERT MK. Postoperative antibiotic prophylaxis in mandibular fractures: a preliminary randomized double-blind, and placebo-controlled clinical study. *J Oral Maxillofac Surg* 2001;**59**: 1415–19.

128. ANDREASEN JO, JENSEN SS, SCHWARTZ O, HILLERUP S. A systematic review of prophylactic antibiotics in the surgical treatment of maxillofacial injuries. *J Oral Maxillofac Surg* 2006;**64**:1664–8.

129. CAWOOD JI. Small plate osteosynthesis of mandibular fractures. *Br J Oral Maxillofac Surg* 1985;**23**:77–91.

130. NAKAMURA S, TAKENOSHITA Y, OKA M. Complications of miniplates osteosynthesis for mandibular fractures. *J Oral Maxillofac Surg* 1994;**52**:233–8.

131. FROST DE, EL-ATTAR A, MOOS KF. Evaluation of metacarpal bone plates in the mandibular fracture. *Br J Oral Surg* 1983;**21**:214–21.

132. RENTON TF, WIESENFELD D. Mandibular fracture osteosynthesis: a comparison of three techniques. *Br J Oral Maxillofac Surg* 1996;**34**:166–73.

133. STONE IE, DODSON TB, BAYS RA. Risk factors for infection following operative treatment of mandibular fractures: a multivariate analysis. *Plast Reconstr Surg* 1993;**91**:64–8.

134. MOULTON-BARRETT R, RUBINSTEIN AJ, SALZHAUER MA, et al. Complications of mandibular fractures. *Ann Plast Surg* 1998;**41**:258–63.

135. CHOLE RA, YEE J. Antibiotic prophylaxis for facial fractures. A prospective, randomized clinical trial. *Arch Otolaryngol Head Neck Surg* 1987;**113**:1055–7.

136. SMITH WP. Delayed miniplate osteosynthesis for mandibular fractures. *Br J Oral Maxillofac Surg* 1991;**29**:73–6.

137. HERMUND NU, HILLERUP S, SCHWARTZ O, ANDREASEN JO. Effect of early or delayed treatment upon healing of jaw fractures. *Dent Traumatol* 2006. In press.

138. THOR A, ANDERSSON L. Interdental wiring in jaw fractures: effects on teeth and surrounding tissue after a one-year follow-up. *Br J Oral Maxillofac Surg* 2001;**39**:398–401.

139. KOENIG WR, OLSSON AB, PENSLER JM. The fate of developing teeth in facial trauma: tooth buds in the line of mandibular fractures in children. *Ann Plast Surg* 1994;**32**:503–5.

140. KRENKEL C, GRUNERT I. Der Zahn im und am Bruchspalt bei Unterkieferfrakturen versorgt mit Silicadraht-Klebeschienen. *Dtsch Z Mund Kiefer Gesichts Chir* 1987;**11**:208–10.

141. OIKARINEN K, LAHTI J, RAUSTIA AM. Prognosis of permanent teeth in the line of mandibular fractures. *Endod Dent Traumatol* 1990;**6**: 177–82.

142. BERG S, PAPE H-D. Teeth in the fracture line. *Int J Oral Maxillofac Surg* 1992;**21**:145–6.

143. THALLER SR, MABOURAKH S. Teeth located in the line of mandibular fracture. *J Craniofac Surg* 1994;**5**:16–21.

144. HAUG RH, SCHWIMMER A. fibrous union of the mandible: a review of 27 patients. *J Oral Maxillofac Surg* 1994;**52**:832–9.

145. KOHN MW. Discussion: fibrous union of the mandible: a review of 27 patients. *J Oral Maxillofac Surg* 1994;**52**:839.

146. KAMBOOZIA AH, PUNNIA-MOORTHY A. The fate of teeth in the mandibular fracture lines. A clinical and radiographic follow-up study. *Int J Oral Maxillofac Surg* 1993;**22**:97–101.

147. STOLL P, NIEDERDELLMANN H, SAUTER R. Zahnbeteiligung bei Unterkieferfrakturen. *Dtsch Zahnärztl Z* 1983;**8**:349–51.

148. HOFFMEISTER B. Die parodontale Reaction im Bruchspalt stehender Zähne bei Unterkieferfrakturen. *Dtsch Zahnärztl Z* 1985;**40**:32–6.

149. SCHMITZ VR, HÖLTJE W, CORDES V. Vergleichende Untersuchungen über die Regeneration des parodontalen Gewebes nach Unfallverletzungen und Osteotomien des Alveolarfortsatzes. *Dtsch Zahnärztl Z* 1973;**28**:219–23.

150. ELLIS E 3rd. Outcomes of patients with teeth in line of mandibular angle fractures treated with stable internal fixation. *J Oral Maxillofac Surg.* 2002;**60**:863–5, 866 (discussion).

151. ELLIS E. Outcome of patients with teeth in the line of mandibular angle fractures treated with stable internal fixation. *J Oral Maxillofac Surg* 2002;**60**:863–5.

152. KRENKEL C, GRUNERT I. Alveolarfortsatz- und Kieferfrakturen – eine Indication für Silicadraht-Klebeschienen. *Dtsch Z Mund Kiefer Gesichts Chir* 1986;**10**:458–63.

153. MALONEY PL, WELCH TB, DOKU MC. Early immobilization of mandibular fractures: a retrospective study. *J Oral Maxillofac Surg* 1991;**49**:698–702.

154. TERRIS DJ, LALAKEA L, TUFFO KM, SHINN JB. Mandible fracture repair: specific indications for new techniques. *Otolaryngol Head Neck Surg* 1994;**III**:751–7.

155. KAUFMAN MS, MARCIANI RD, THOMSON SF, HINES WP. Treatment of facial fractures in neurologically injured patients. *J Oral Maxillofac Surg* 1984;**42**:250–2.

156. MOULTON-BARRET R, RUBENSTEIN AJ, SALZHAUER MA, BROWN M, ANGULO J, ALSTER C, COLLINS W, KLINE S, DAVIS C, THALLER SR. Complications of mandibular fractures. *Ann Plast Surg* 1998;**41**:258–63.

157. HERMUND NU, HILLERUP S, KOFOD T, SCHWARTZ O, ANDREASEN JO. Effect of early or delayed treatment upon healing of mandibular fractures: a systematic literature review. *Dent Traumatol* 2006. In press.

# 19

# Injuries to the Primary Dentition

M. T. Flores, G. Holan, M. Borum & J. O. Andreasen

## Introduction

This chapter describes the specific characteristics of injuries to the primary dentition, the exclusive reaction patterns of primary teeth to trauma and explains the rationale of the approach to treatment and how it is different from that for permanent teeth.

The major shortcoming of the topic of traumatic injuries to the primary teeth is lack of scientific data. Thus, in many publications, the description of outcomes of injuries to primary teeth is based on opinions and beliefs rather than evidence. In addition, suggested treatment protocols are supported mainly by empirical treatment and anecdotal case reports rather than well-controlled research studies.

Three factors have a major influence on the selection of treatment for injured primary teeth:

(1) The relatively short period primary teeth are in function in the child's mouth. The maxillary primary central incisors, which are involved more than any other tooth in traumatic injuries, usually serve the child no longer than six years.

(2) The close proximity of the root of the primary tooth to its developing permanent successor (Figs 19.1 and 19.2). This implies that damage to the permanent tooth may be inflicted not only when the primary teeth are injured,

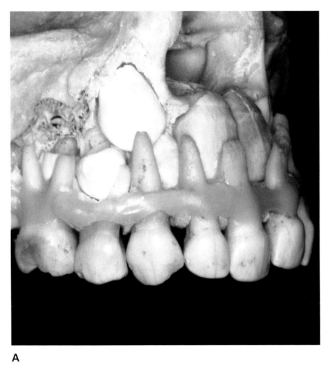

A

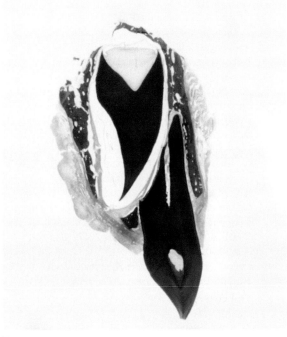

B

**Fig. 19.1** Anatomic relationship between the two dentitions. A. The maxilla in the skull of a 3-year-old child. B. The intimate facial-oral relationship is shown between the primary central incisor and the permanent successor in a histologic section. From ANDREASEN (1) 1976.

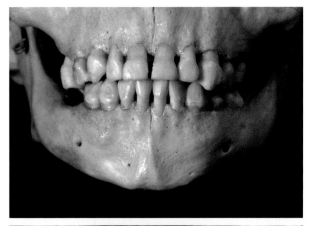

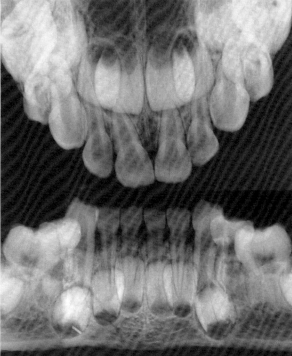

**Fig. 19.2** Skull of 3-year-old individual with a full set of primary teeth. The radiographs illustrate the vertical closeness of the two dentition.

but also later as a result of the treatment rendered. This must be considered as an important factor when weighing the cost and benefit of various treatment options for injured primary teeth. The option that has the least likelihood to have a deleterious effect on the permanent tooth should be considered as the treatment of choice. If no damage is expected to the permanent tooth, a conservative approach should be adopted and attempts made to save injured primary teeth. In some cases, however, extraction is the only reasonable option leaving the child with a missing tooth for several years. Several consequences of early loss of primary incisors are mentioned in the dental literature. However, most lack scientific support.

(3) The difficulty of gaining the child's compliance. Traumatic injuries to the primary teeth occur more often in very young children before they have mastered walking

skills and later running skills. These children are too young to understand what is required, and most of them are defiant and cannot cooperate during examination and implementation of treatment. However, safe use of sedative agents is an integral part of the regular services provided by pediatric dentists in many countries. Thus, lack of child cooperation should not be considered an argument against conservative treatment of injured primary teeth. Moreover, the need to cope with the child's behavior cannot be ignored even if extraction is the treatment of choice.

Consequently, the objectives of trauma management in the primary dentition are:

- To comfort the child and parents in the acute state.
- To avoid inducing dental fear and anxiety in young children who may be experiencing their first dental problem. This implies being very conservative in choice of treatment, partly by ensuring sufficient pain control and in some cases proper premedication with a tranquilizing drug before necessary intervention.
- To minimize the risk of further damage to the permanent teeth:
  — by limiting the number of acute extractions (which may lead to loss of facial alveolar bone in the area as well as damage to the gubernacular cord (see Chapter 2))
  — by following the traumatized dentition with appropriate control intervals to detect and treat any symptoms of infection in the area as early as possible.

There are many ways in which an injured primary tooth may transmit damage to the permanent successor.

The direct displacement of a primary incisor toward the developing permanent tooth germ may result in a significant injury (Fig. 19.3). An ensuing infection caused by invasion of bacteria into the injury site may be another threat to the developing successor (Fig. 19.4). Finally both extraction and attempt to reposition a displaced primary tooth may compromise development of the permanent successor, depending upon the technique used.

Disturbances in permanent tooth germs are latent complications that may be seen following all types of primary tooth injuries especially intrusion, avulsion, and alveolar bone fracture. This topic is presented in Chapter 20.

A series of animal experiments has been carried out to estimate the risk of the above mentioned factors (1–6). The general treatment concepts are primarily based on the results of these studies as well as a few clinical studies in humans (7–14, 49).

## Epidemiology and etiology

Injuries to the primary dentition are common and occur with a significantly higher annual incidence than in the permanent dentition (15–17). Especially between 18 to 30 months, children are very prone to accidents (Fig. 19.5)

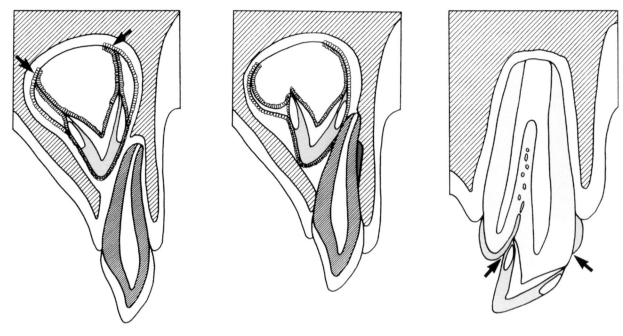

**Fig. 19.3** Intrusion of a primary tooth into the follicle of the permanent successor. All odontogenic tissue becomes involved and a crown dilaceration is the result.

**Fig. 19.4 Acute infection following intrusion**
This 3-year-old boy suffered intrusion of two central incisors. As the root tips were displaced away from the developing tooth germs, spontaneous eruption was anticipated.

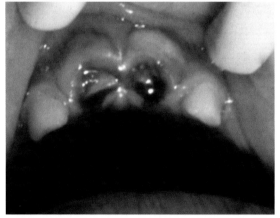
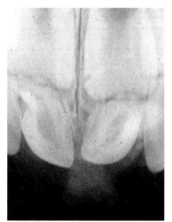

**Follow-up, 2 weeks after injury**
Acute infection with swelling and pus formation around the displaced incisors has developed.

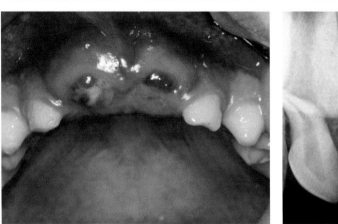

(15–26). This is possibly related to poor motor coordination and sometimes due to the child's inability to evaluate potential risks. As falls are the predominant etiology for dental injuries in young age groups, the trauma incidence is usually equally high in both sexes (15–17) (Fig. 19.5). It is not until early school age (coinciding with the eruption of permanent teeth) that boys become more prone to dental trauma (15–17).

Several studies have shown that one out of three children has suffered a traumatic dental injury by age 5 (15–17,

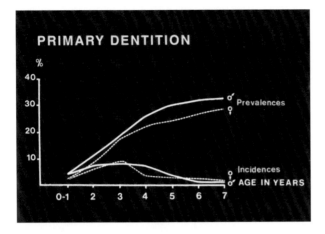

**Fig. 19.5** Trauma incidence in the primary dentition. Among annual trauma incidences (i.e. the number of new injuries suffered during a year), peak incidences in the primary dentition are found at 2–3 years of age, when motor coordination is developing and the children start moving around on their own. After ANDREASEN & RAVN (15) 1972.

27–30). For further information concerning the epidemiology and etiology of dental trauma, the reader is referred to Chapter 8.

In some countries, traumatic dental injuries are often not presented as an emergency because parents usually do not seek treatment for the child immediately (31–33). In a US study of 487 dental trauma visits seen at children's hospital during a 3-year period, 69% occurred after regular office hours. The emergency visit was the first contact with a dentist for 80% of children 3.5 years old and younger (24). This naturally may present a psychological impact upon the child, a condition that is discussed in Chapter 7.

## Self-inflicted oro-dental injuries

Although rare, case reports of self-mutilation injuries in children have been published, some of them related to Leigh disease and Lesch-Nyhan syndrome. In these cases, lacerations of oral and perioral areas are associated with early eruption of primary teeth (34–42). The baby self-inflicts wounds by biting the surrounding soft tissues such as the tongue, cheeks and lips. It seems to be a painless condition and appears with increasing severity when the primary dentition becomes complete.

## Battered child syndrome

The physical abuse which may lead to injuries of the teeth and soft tissues is described in Chapter 8.

## Pathogenesis

One difference between injuries in the primary and permanent dentition appears to be the difference in the mechanical properties of the supporting periodontium. In primary dentition, the surrounding bone is less dense and less mineralized, which implies that a tooth hit by a traumatic impact can easily be displaced instead of fractured (43). In

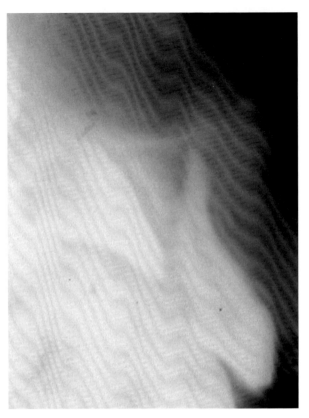

**Fig. 19.6** Intrusion of a primary incisor. It has penetrated the labial bone plate.

a follow-up study from Denmark, up to 98% of the injured primary teeth suffered a type of luxation injury, whereas only 10% showed crown or crown-root fractures (44). This difference in the trauma pattern favoring luxations rather than fractures has been found to be typical for the primary dentition (16, 17).

Due to the direction of impact in falls against the ground, floor or furniture, frontal trauma is quite frequent, resulting in lateral luxations with oral displacement of the crown. Consequently, the apical part of the root will almost inevitably penetrate (or fracture) the thin labial bone plate (Fig. 19.6). In falls in which the impact has an axial component, the teeth will be intruded due to the labial curvature of the root; the intrusion will usually result in an axial and labial displacement in which the apex penetrates the labial bone plate (Fig 19.6). In some cases the impact direction may have a strong oral component, typically when the child falls with an object in the mouth (e.g. pacifier or toy). In these cases the apex of an injured tooth may be forced into the follicle of the permanent successor, sometimes resulting in a severe injury to the developing permanent tooth germ (see Chapter 20). However, it is important to emphasize that direct involvement of the permanent tooth germ in the injury is not restricted to cases of oral displacement of the apical part of the primary incisor into the follicle. If the displacement is large enough, the coronal part of an intruded or laterally luxated primary incisor can also be forced against the underlying tooth germ, causing displacement of the germ and squeezing of the epithelial root sheet, with the

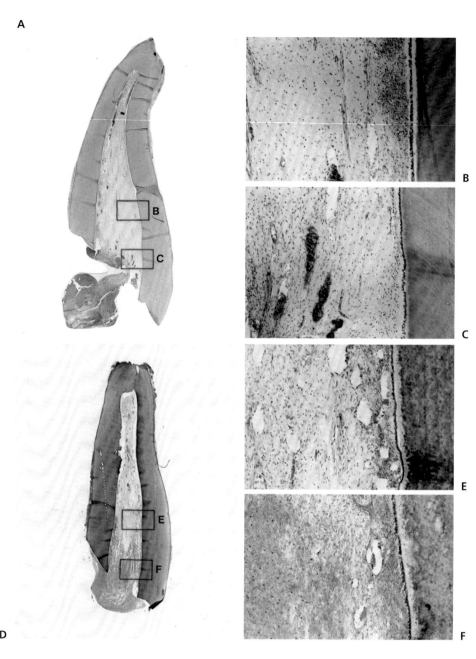

**Fig. 19.7** Early pulp reactions following complicated crown fractures in maxillary primary incisors. A. Low power view of incisor removed 19 hours after injury. Moderate inflammatory changes are present in the coronal part of the pulp while the apical part shows only minor changes, such as hyperemia and perivascular bleeding. ×9. B. Hyperemia and perivascular bleeding. ×75. C. Moderate inflammatory changes. ×75. D. Low power view of incisor removed 41 hours after injury. Marked inflammatory changes are present in the coronal part of the pulp and spread of the inflammation apically is evident. ×9. E. Moderate inflammation. ×75. F. Marked inflammatory changes. ×75.

latter resulting in malformation of the crown or arrested root formation of the successor (1, 45).

## Healing and pathology

Most luxations represent a combined injury to the pulp and periodontium. However, the pathology of luxation injuries of primary teeth has received little attention. At present, no specific changes can be ascribed to the periodontal ligament after luxation injury, whereas pulp changes have been reported in a few studies.

## Pulp

### Crown fractures with pulp exposure

Histologically, exposed pulp tissue in complicated crown fractures is quickly covered by a layer of fibrin. Eventually the superficial part of the pulp shows capillary budding, numerous leukocytes and proliferation of histiocytes (Fig. 19.7A–C). This inflammation spreads apically with increasing observation periods (Fig. 19.7D–F).

## Luxation injuries

Changes seen in the pulp soon after injury include edema and disorganization of the odontoblast layer as well as nuclear pyknosis of pulp cells (Fig. 19.8).

Histologic evidence of pulp necrosis, including nuclear pyknosis and disappearance of odontoblasts and stromal elements can be seen by 6 days after injury (Fig. 19.8). This reponse is related to either partial or total rupture of the pulpal neurovascular supply. The later events of pulpal healing after luxation injury are presently unknown.

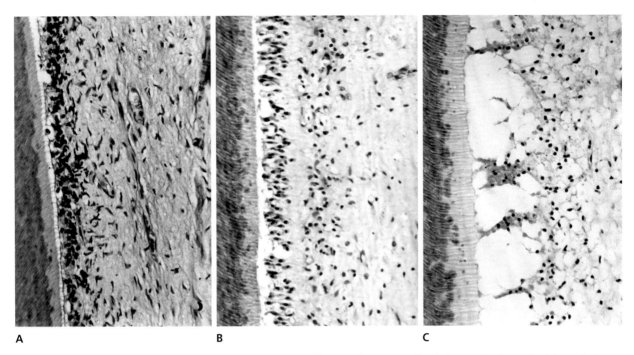

**Fig. 19.8** Early pulp changes at various time intervals following intrusive luxation of primary maxillary incisors. A. Two hours after injury, pulpal structures – including the odontoblasts – are without significant change, apart from edema. ×195. B. After 13 hours nuclear pyknosis and disintegration of odontoblast layer is evident. ×195. C. Six days after injury, only pyknotic nuclei are seen within a stroma of autolyzed pulp tissue. ×195.

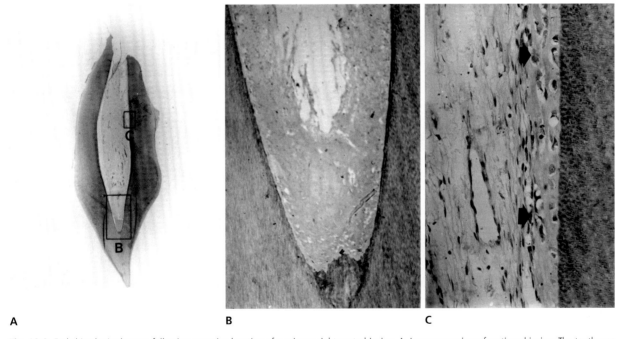

**Fig. 19.9** Early histologic changes following extrusive luxation of a primary right central incisor. A. Low-power view of sectioned incisor. The tooth was extracted 4 weeks after injury. ×6. B. Complete necrosis of the coronal part of the pulp. ×30. C. More apically, formation of new hard tissue with numerous cell inclusions (arrows). ×195.

If the pulp survives or becomes revascularized, a number of regressive pulp changes can occur, such as hyalinization and deposition of amorphous, diffuse calcifications. Furthermore, the injury usually interferes with normal dentin formation. This interference is apparently related to a number of clinical factors, among which the stage of root formation and the type of luxation injury seem to be decisive (46, 47).

In teeth with incomplete root development, a distinct incremental line usually indicates arrest of normal tubular dentin formation at the time of injury. Most of the dentinal tubules stop at this line, while the original predentin layer is often preserved.

After a certain period, apposition of new hard tissue is resumed, but without the normal tubular structure (Fig. 19.9). This tissue often contains cell inclusions which main-

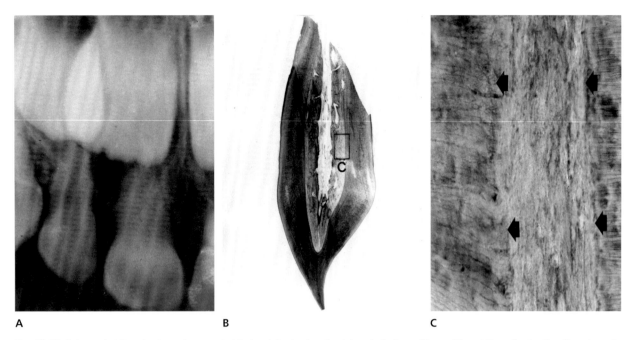

**Fig. 19.10** Pulp canal obliteration in a primary central incisor following luxation injury. A. Radiographic condition at time of extraction. No pulp cavity is discernible. B. Low power view of sectioned specimen. Obliteration of the pulp canal is evident. ×10. C. Note atubular dentin deposited immediately after trauma followed by a return to tubular dentin (arrows). ×75.

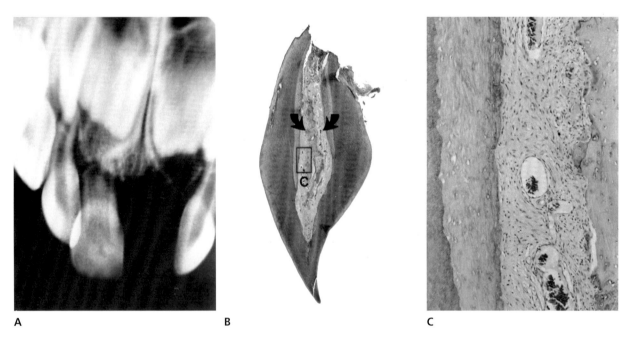

**Fig. 19.11** Bone invasion in the pulp after trauma in a primary incisor. A. Radiographic exposure. Note the two longitudinal radiopaque stripes in the root canal. B. Histopathologic section showing incomplete ring of calcified tissue in the pulp canal surrounded by non-inflamed pulp tissue. C. Note that odontoblasts are not seen along the root dentin and the irregular secondary dentin.

tain their tubular connections with dentin formed before the injury, as well as vascular inclusions. This hard tissue formation often continues to the point of total obliteration of the root canal (Fig. 19.10).

Although the calcified cellular formed in response to the injury may resemble bone and cementum, it lacks the cellular organization characteristic of these tissues. Due to its tendency to convert to tubular dentin, the repair tissue has been termed cellular dentin.

Furthermore tube-like mineralization in the dental pulp of traumatized primary incisors has been described (Fig. 19.11) (48). This phenomenon is possibly analogous to the ingrowth of bone into the pulp cavity of injured permanent teeth (see Chapters 2 and 22).

## PDL healing

These events have so far not been reported.

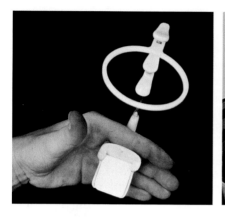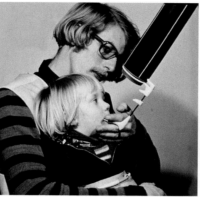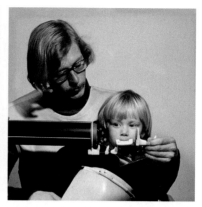

**Fig. 19.12** Radiographic examination of a young child. A parent can assist in stabilizing the child during the examination. The parent and child are furnished with lead aprons. One arm is used to hold the child, while the other holds the filmholder and stabilizes the child's head against the parent's chest.

## Clinical and radiographic findings and treatment of various injury types

### Examination

#### Extraoral examination

The child must be checked for facial asymmetry (indicating jaw fractures), swelling of the lips, skin lacerations and cuts, and scars (indicating previous injuries). Bleeding from the nostrils and subcutaneous hemorrhage near the nostrils may indicate fracture of the alveolar bone. Limited ability of mouth opening may indicate damage to the temporomandibular joint. Sensitivity of facial bones when palpated may point to underlying jaw fractures.

A laceration or hematoma located at the chin should draw attention to a possible fracture of the mandible at the symphysis or condyle (50). Fractures of molar teeth resulting from sudden impact of the mandibular teeth against their maxillary antagonists should also be looked for after traumatic injuries to the chin (51, 52, 73).

#### Intraoral examination

Intraoral tissues must be carefully examined. The surrounding soft tissues (lips, oral mucosa, attached and free gingivae and frenum) should be checked for lacerations and hematomas caused by recent injuries or fistulae, which may be the result of old injuries. Submucosal hemorrhage in the upper lip may result from a direct impact or fracture of the labial bone plate. Similarly, submucosal hemorrhage under the tongue should raise the suspicion of fracture of the mandible. Midline fracture in the mental suture area appears in children under one year of age.

Signs of bleeding from the sulcus surrounding the injured tooth indicate damage to the periodontal ligament.

Palpation of the gingivae and the vestibule may reveal a fluctuant hematoma above a displaced tooth and sometimes a displaced root can be felt.

#### Tooth mobility

An injured tooth can present increased mobility in the horizontal as well as vertical plane. Increased mobility is a sign of injury to the periodontal ligament. It appears in subluxation, root fracture, extrusive luxations and associated infection. Sometimes the patient seeks treatment several days after the trauma due to tooth mobility caused by an infection. In cases of crown-root fractures the coronal fragments will present increased mobility. If mobility of a segment of teeth is observed, fracture of the alveolar bone should be suspected (see Chapter 18).

#### Tooth alignment

Changes in tooth alignment can be seen following luxation injuries. In case of doubt, parents should be asked about the original tooth alignment. Extrusion or lateral luxation may result in occlusal interference.

Pulp vitality testing by electric or thermal methods has not been proven to be valid in the primary dentition.

### Radiographic examination

The general features of radiographic examination of primary tooth injuries have been described in Chapter 9. Radiographs are an important adjunct to the clinical examination, providing valuable information that may affect the decision regarding treatment of the injured primary tooth. It shows the degree of development of the primary tooth and its permanent successor and the relationship between the two. Furthermore, physiologic and pathologic root resorption and the position of displaced primary teeth can be seen. An acceptable radiograph appears to be the occlusal exposure due to the fact that neither the child nor relatives can position the film in an optimal position (periapical exposure) (Fig. 19.12).

In the radiographic examination it is important to consider the relation between the injured primary tooth and the permanent successor. In this regard a very simple rule exists: if the tooth appears foreshortened compared with its

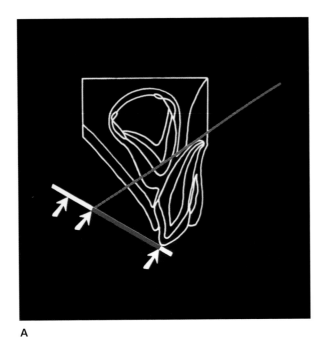

A

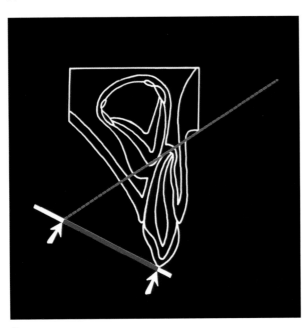

B

**Fig. 19.13** Schematic illustration of the geometric relationship between an intruded primary incisor and the developing tooth germ and the resultant radiographic image. A. If the primary tooth is *away* from the developing tooth germ, the radiographic image will be *foreshortened*. B. If the primary tooth is intruded *into* the developing tooth germ, the radiographic image will be *elongated*.

non-injured antimere, this indicates a labial displacement of the root with a minimal risk for the permanent successor. On the other hand, if a displaced primary tooth radiographically appears elongated, this tooth has most likely been intruded into the follicle of the permanent tooth and must be removed (Fig 19.13). Another important feature is to evaluate the position of the mineralized part of the permanent tooth in the follicle. In case of displacement an

asymmetry will be seen compared to a non-injured antimere (Fig. 19.14).

These guidelines can only be applied when the central beam is oriented exactly at the midline between the two incisors to be compared. Apart from this, lateral projections can be of assistance in determining the direction of dislocation of the displaced tooth as well as its relationship to the nasal floor and labial alveolar bone (Fig. 19.15) (see Chapter 9). If there is doubt about the position of a displaced primary incisor in relation to the nasal floor, a lateral exposure can be of value (Fig 19.15).

## Treatment regimens

The overall principle of treatment is not to take any risk with regard to the permanent successor which usually implies a very conservative approach.

Acute treatment can often be restricted to dealing with conditions causing marked symptoms, such as crown fractures with pulp exposure and repositioning or removing displaced teeth with occlusal interference (55) or which have invaded the follicle of the permanent successor.

As most dental injuries occur during early childhood, when the child is not able to communicate or express pain intensity, the use of topical anesthetics, local anesthesia and sedation should be considered. It has been demonstrated that from birth the child can experience pain which may cause prolonged behavioral consequences if not alleviated immediately (56). In more complicated tooth injuries, such as those affecting the alveolar bone as intrusion, lateral luxation and alveolar fractures, prescription of non-steroidal anti-inflammatory drugs could be indicated if the child is in pain before further examination and treatment (see also Chapter 6).

In addition, use of analgesics may improve the quality of care when pain is anticipated, such as application of a local anesthesia. The administration of a single dose of analgesic one hour before injection and the use of topical anesthetic will reduce the discomfort of a local anesthetic (56).

Apart from advising the parents to administer adequate pain control, adequate hygiene procedures and a soft diet to the child's liking must be reviewed.

In the following pages, each type of trauma will be described as it presents clinically and radiographically, along with currently recommended treatment (22, 44, 57–59). However, most of the recommended treatment procedures have minimal evidence supporting their value (60, 61).

## Crown fractures

Crown fractures cause relatively few symptoms. Exposure of the pulp is rare due to the minute dimension of the crown (Fig. 19.16).

### Radiography

This will normally show the relation of the fracture to the pulp.

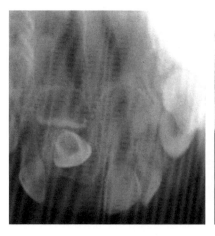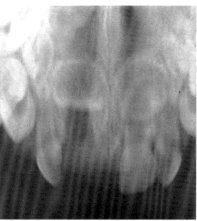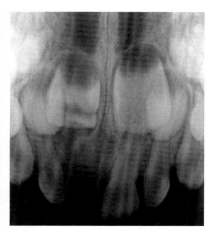

**Fig. 19.14** Radiographic demonstration of displacement of the developing permanent tooth germ following intrusion of the primary incisor. The distance between the incisal edge and mineralization front of the involved developing tooth germ is shorter than the same distance in the non-involved tooth germ, implying luxation of the involved tooth germ. Although the displaced primary tooth was removed, a slight dilaceration of the permanent crown developed.

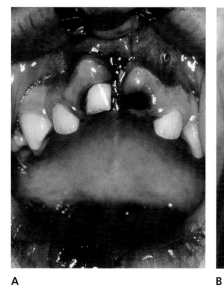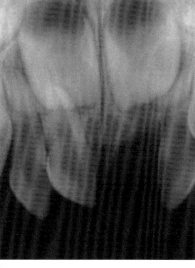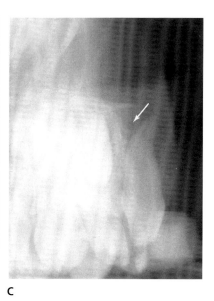

A    B    C

**Fig. 19.15** Radiographic demonstration of the direction of displacement in a case of intrusive luxation of a primary central incisor. A. Clinical condition. B. Right central incisor appears shorter than right lateral incisor due to displacement in apico-labial direction of the former. C. Lateral radiograph reveals the relationship between the apex of the displaced tooth and the permanent tooth germ as well as the direction of dislocation. Note that the apex of the primary tooth has been forced through the facial bone plate (arrow).

### Treatment

In cases of uncomplicated fractures with sharp fracture edges, an abrasive disc or bur can be used to smooth the fractures. If the parents demand an esthetic solution, and the patient can comply, the crown can be repaired with composite resin.

Complicated crown fracture is a difficult emergency to deal with if there is lack of cooperation from the child and because the treatment (pulpotomy) is technique-sensitive. The treatment options are partial pulpotomy with calcium hydroxide or pulpotomy with formocresol or zinc oxide eugenol (62, 63). It seems that the outcome is as good between the choices available, supporting the indication for a conservative approach to treat these injuries. In one clinical study, the success rate of pulpotomy was 76% (64). In another clinical study, pulpotomies (using formocresol) and pulpectomy (using zinc oxide eugenol) were compared and found to have success rates of 86% and 78% respectively (65). A disturbing finding concerning pulpectomy was, however, that the majority of cases showed incomplete resorption of the zinc oxide eugenol dressing, a fact which may leave zinc oxide particles in the gingival area (65). This procedure can therefore not be recommended.

Mineral trioxide aggregate (MTA) has recently been proposed for pulpotomy (66, 67, 75) but long-term clinical studies are needed before recommending its general use.

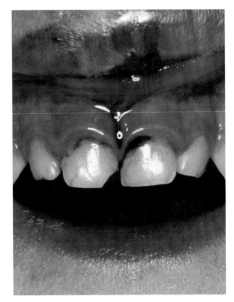
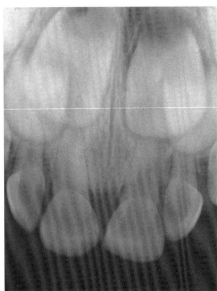

**Fig. 19.16** Uncomplicated crown fracture of a right central incisor and subluxation of both central incisors in a 2-year-old girl.

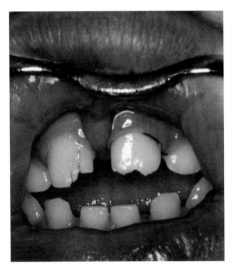
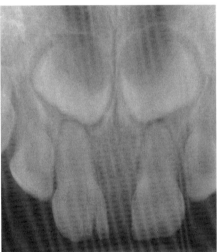

**Fig. 19.17** Mesial crown-root fracture of a right central incisor and an uncomplicated (enamel) fracture of the left central incisor.

## Crown-root fractures

Crown-root fractures are rare and the crown fragment is usually kept *in situ* by the gingival and periodontal fibers. Because of mobility during mastication there might be transitory pain (Fig. 19.17).

### Radiography

In laterally positioned fractures the extent in relation to the gingival margin can be seen.

### Treatment

Extraction is usually the treatment of choice.

## Root fractures

The crown fragment appears loosened and usually displaced in a coronal and oral direction.

### Radiography

The fracture is usually located mid-root or in the apical third.

### Treatment

Root fractures with minimal displacement of the coronal fragment can be left untreated and will resorb at the expected time (Fig. 19.18). When the coronal fragment is very loose the extruded coronal fragment should be extracted to prevent the child inhaling it. The apical fragment can be left for physiological resorption (Fig. 19.19) (58, 61). If the child is able to cope and the coronal fragment is not displaced, a wire-composite splint has been suggested for 3 weeks. However, the value of such a treatment seems questionable.

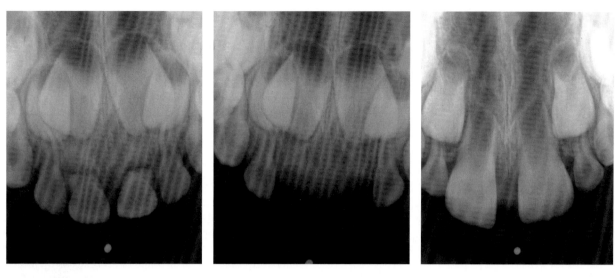

**Fig. 19.18** Normal physiologic resorption after root fracture of both primary central incisors in a 4-year-old child. Note apparently normal physiologic resorption of the traumatized incisors.

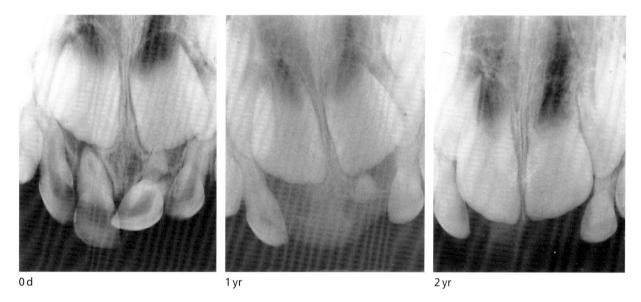

0 d                                    1 yr                                    2 yr

**Fig. 19.19** Lateral luxation of a right central incisor and root fracture of left central incisor in a 5-year-old child. The right incisor was extracted, as was the coronal portion of the left central incisor. Condition after 1 year. After 2 years, both permanent central incisors are erupting and the apex of the left primary incisor has been resorbed.

## Concussion and subluxation

### Clinical findings

In concussion the tooth is sensitive to percussion (performed with a finger tip). In subluxation the tooth appears loosened and may be bleeding from the gingival crevice. It is not possible to diagnose concussion or even subluxation if examination is performed several days after injury.

### Radiography

The teeth appear *in situ* in their socket.

### Treatment

These injuries require no acute treatment apart from instructing the parents to maintain good oral hygiene to prevent bacterial contamination through the periodontal ligament. Application of chlorhexidine to the tooth-gingival junction twice a day for 7 days can be recommended.

## Extrusion

### Clinical findings

The tooth appears elongated and with the crown usually displaced in lingual direction and there is usually a marked loosening of the tooth.

### Radiography

A marked apical periodontal ligament space is seen.

## Treatment

Extruded primary teeth can be repositioned and stabilized for a short period if the child is seen soon after the injury. If a blood clot has already become organized in the alveolar socket and repositioning is no longer applicable, the tooth can be left for spontaneous alignment or extracted depending on the degree of extrusion and mobility.

## Lateral luxation

### Clinical findings

The crown is usually tilted in the oral direction and the tooth firm in its displaced position (Fig. 19.20). Most of these luxations result from a frontal impact that causes a tilting of the tooth with the crown displaced in lingual direction and the apex with a labial bone plate displaced in labial direction. In rare cases, in which the child has fallen with an object in the mouth, the opposite displacement direction can be found. These cases may represent a danger to the permanent successor as the apex of the primary tooth may have invaded the follicle. These teeth should either be repositioned or extracted.

### Treatment

In some cases of lateral luxation there might be occlusal interference. In these cases, after the use of local anesthesia, the tooth is repositioned by combined labial and palatal pressure (Fig 19.20). If necessary and possible, a splint can be used for 2–3 weeks.

Because of the common anterior open bite in young children most lateral luxated primary teeth have no occlusal interference and can be left without treatment, and spontaneous repositioning influenced by physiologic forces of the tongue can usually be expected within 3 months (Fig. 19.21). However, in a follow-up study, 5% of laterally luxated primary teeth were not fully repositioned after 1 year (44).

To treat lateral luxations with no open bite which cannot be respositioned, grind the incisal edges of the upper and lower teeth or temporarily add composite to the occlusal surface of the molars to create an artificial anterior open bite.

## Intrusion

### Clinical findings

In the primary dentition, the apices of intruded teeth will usually be driven through the thin vestibular bone, the direction probably being determined by the direction of the impact and the labial curvature of the root. This usually results in marked swelling of the upper lip due to hematoma.

The degree of intrusion cannot always be assessed by measuring the length of the clinical crown as the gingiva may be enlarged due to swelling. The degree of intrusion and re-eruption are determined by the distance between the incisal edge of the intruded tooth and the horizontal line connecting the incisal edges of two adjacent non-injured teeth.

For later comparison, the degree of dislocation should be recorded in millimeters (i.e. the distance between the incisal edge of the intruded incisor and the non-intruded adjacent tooth), with the direction of dislocation indicated as well. Especially in the primary dentition, it is of great importance to determine whether the apex is dislocated facially or orally because in the latter case, the permanent successors can be directly involved (see Fig. 19.14).

In some cases the tooth has disappeared completely into the socket and can often be palpated labially.

### Radiography

An occlusal radiograph is indicated and will normally show the position of the displaced tooth and its relation to the permanent successor. If there is doubt about this question a lateral exposure can be of value (see Fig. 19.15). A lateral extraoral exposure has traditionally been recommended to assess the relations between the intruded primary incisor and its permanent successor. A recent study addressed the value of lateral exposures in determining the relative position between the root apex of the intruded primary tooth and the labial surface of its permanent successor (68). It was found that in the majority of cases the contribution of the lateral extraoral radiograph to the assessment of the relation between the root of an intruded primary incisor and its permanent successor was limited. Thus diagnostic value was low when more than one incisor was intruded, when lateral incisors were intruded, and often due to overlap of anatomical structures. The relations are obvious when the root of the intruded primary incisor has been pushed labially accompanied by fracture of the labial bone plate. In these cases, however, the lateral extraoral radiograph is unnecessary as clinical signs and a periapical radiograph are sufficient to determine the relationship (68).

### Treatment

The treatment of intruded teeth is still being debated. The essential problem is the prevention of injuries transferred to the developing permanent teeth. In experimental studies in monkeys, in which primary incisors were intentionally intruded toward the permanent successor, it appeared that extraction of the intruded primary incisor histologically resulted in minor damage to the reduced enamel epithelium of the permanent successor compared to when the intruded primary incisor was preserved (1). However, in a similar macroscopic study, it was found that the frequency and extent of the macroscopic enamel defects were almost identical in the two groups (2).

Clinical studies have also demonstrated only small and insignificant differences in the extent and frequency of developmental disturbances in the permanent dentition when preservation or extraction of the intruded primary incisor was compared (8–14).

In conclusion, when the outcome appears identical, conservative measures instead of surgical seem appropriate to recommend at least until further studies have proved otherwise.

**Fig. 19.20 Repositioning of a laterally luxated primary central incisor**
This 4-year-old boy suffered a lateral luxation of the left maxillary primary central incisor. Repositioning is indicated due to occlusal interference.

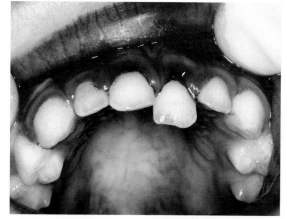 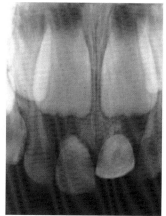

**Treatment evaluation**
Due to interference with occlusion and the distance between the apex of the primary tooth and the permanent tooth germ, repositioning is indicated.

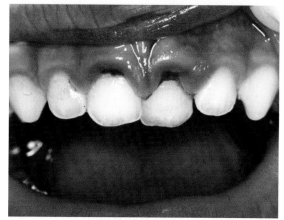 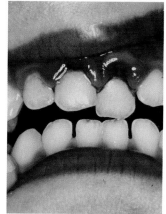

**Repositioning**
After application of a local anesthetic, the tooth is repositioned with combined labial and palatal pressure.

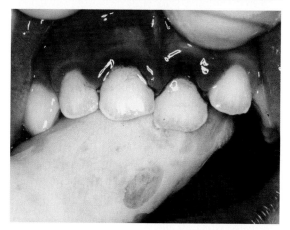 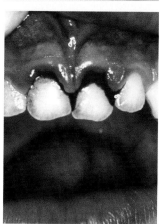

**Postoperative condition**
The tooth has been adequately repositioned, as revealed both clinically and radiographically.

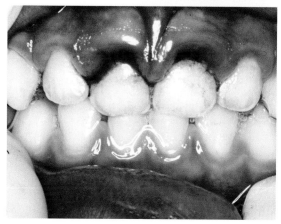 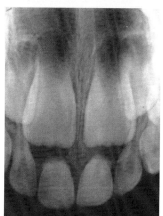

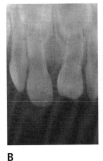
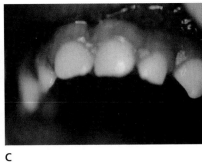
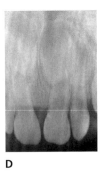

A                    B                    C                    D

**Fig. 19.21** Spontaneous reposition of a lateral luxated primary incisor in a 1.4-year-old boy. A. Lateral luxation of a left central incisor. B. The tooth appears foreshortened in the radiographic examination compared with the contralateral. Spontaneous repositioning is therefore anticipated. C and D. At follow-up, 2 months after injury there is spontaneous realignment.

In the few cases where the intruded primary incisor has been displaced into the follicle, surgical removal is indicated. In this context, it is important to consider that a proper surgical technique be employed so as to avoid further injury to the developing dentition. Elevators should never be used due to the risk of their entering the follicular space. Moreover, it is necessary that the intruded incisor be grasped proximally with narrow forceps and removed with the root pointing in a labial direction. These precautions are necessary to avoid collision with the developing tooth germ. Finally, once the tooth has been removed, the palatal and facial bone plates should be repositioned with slight digital pressure. The open wound should then be sutured (Fig. 19.22).

In general, spontaneous eruption should be awaited, which normally takes place within 3 months (44) (Fig. 19.23). However, in a recent study, one out of four intruded teeth were not fully erupted one year after trauma and no decisive factor could be identified to explain the lack of realignment (44).

During the re-eruption phase of intruded primary teeth, there is a risk of acute inflammation around the displaced tooth. This is manifested clinically as swelling and hyperemia of the gingiva, sometimes with abscess formation and oozing of pus from the gingival crevice (Fig. 19.4). There is a rise in temperature and complaint of pain from the traumatized region. In these cases, immediate extraction and antibiotic therapy are essential to prevent the spread of inflammation to the permanent tooth germ.

In rare cases an intruded primary incisor becomes ankylosed in an intruded position. In most cases this will only imply a slight delay in shedding of the tooth.

In conclusion the optimal therapy for most intruded primary teeth appears to be to wait for spontaneous eruption.

## Avulsion

### Clinical findings

The tooth appears missing in the dental arch. The clinical appearance resembles that of complete intrusion or root fracture with loss of the coronal fragment. Before making the diagnosis of a primary tooth avulsion, alternative trauma scenarios should be explored:

- Was the primary tooth actually avulsed; has it been found?
- Is there a possibility that the tooth is deeply intruded? (Take a radiograph)
- Has the tooth been inhaled? Have there been any coughing or breathing problems subsequent to the injury? (Refer for chest X-ray)
- Even if there is no intention to replant the avulsed primary incisor, the tooth must be found to ensure that it has not been aspirated (69). If the tooth is not found, the child should be referred to a pediatrician for further examination.

### Radiography

This should be performed to verify an empty socket and rule out that the missing tooth is totally intruded.

### Treatment

Though several reports have been published on replantation of avulsed teeth (70–72), this practice cannot be recommended until further evidence suggests that the permanent successor will not be involved, because replantation of a primary tooth may displace a coagulum into the follicle of the permanent incisor. Furthermore, a periapical inflammation subsequent to the pulp necrosis in the replanted primary tooth may cause mineralization disturbances in the permanent dentition. The space created by loss of a maxillary primary incisor can be restored for esthetic purposes by fixed appliances (Fig. 19.24). However, special attention should in these cases be paid to a possible interference with the physiologic expansion of the maxilla.

## Fractures of the alveolar process

### Clinical findings

In this situation an entire fragment of the jaw is involved. This happens typically when a severe frontal impact hits the mandible or the maxilla. Displacement may vary according to direction of the impact, usually being frontal in the

### Fig. 19.22 Intrusion, severe follicle invasion

This 1-year-old boy sustained an axial impact, resulting in complete intrusion of the central incisor. Note the displacement of the permanent tooth germ in the follicle. Removal of the primary incisor is mandatory.

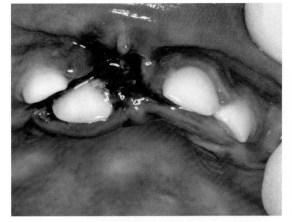
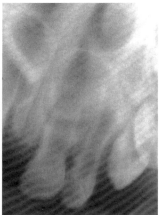

### Removing the displaced tooth

Using sedation and local anesthesia, the tooth is grasped proximally with forceps and removed in a labial direction. The fractured and displaced palatal bone is repositioned with digital pressure, and a suture placed to close the entrance to the socket.

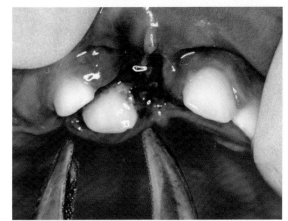
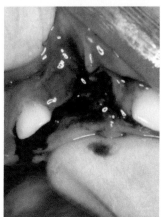

### Follow-up

At examination 1 week later, a slight change in the position of the tooth germ is seen.

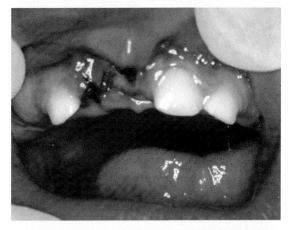
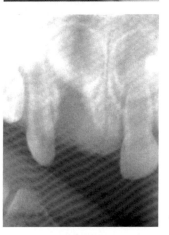

### Disturbance in eruption

At the age of 6 years, it is evident that a crown dilaceration has developed.

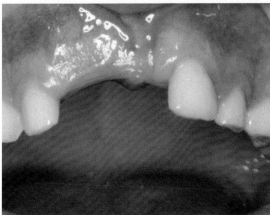
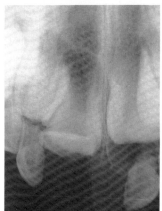

**Fig. 19.23 Spontaneous reeruption of an intruded primary incisor**
This 2-year-old boy suffered an intrusion of the right central incisor. The foreshortened appearance of the intruded tooth implies labial displacement. Spontaneous re-eruption is therefore anticipated.

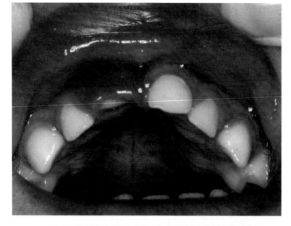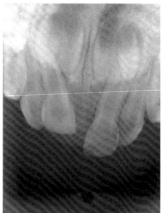

**Follow-up, 2 months after injury**
The tooth has erupted approximately 2 mm coronally.

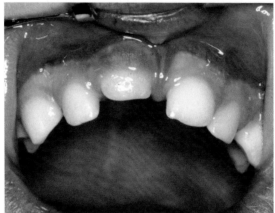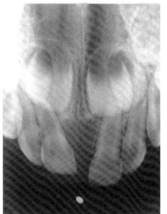

**Follow-up, 3 months after injury**
The tooth lacks 1 mm for complete eruption.

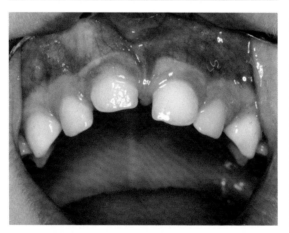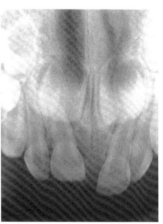

**Follow-up, 1 year after injury**
The tooth is in normal position. Crown color is normal, and the radiographs show no sign of pathology.

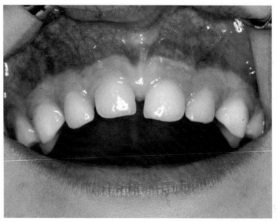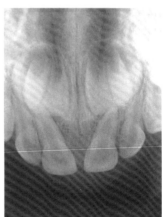

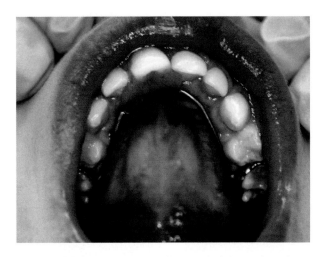

**Fig. 19.24** Lost primary incisor replacement with a prosthetic device anchored to the primary molars.

maxilla and sometimes the result of a fall with an object in mouth in the mandible. In these cases the fragment tilts in labial direction (Fig. 19.25).

### Radiography

This will reveal the topography of the horizontal fracture line to the apices of the primary teeth and their permanent successors. A lateral radiograph may also give valuable information about the relation between the two dentitions (Fig. 19.25).

### Treatment

Reposition is essential to normalize occlusion. General anesthesia is often indicated. The treatment of this trauma entity is described in Chapter 18.

## Fractures secondary to chin trauma

When there has been an impact to the chin, multiple crown and crown-root fractures may occur in the molar regions (51, 52, 73). The treatment depends on the extent and severity of the fractures. While minor enamel fractures can be left without treatment, composite restoration should be considered for fractures with dentin exposure to prevent the development of caries. Stainless steel crowns should be used to cover primary molars with large fractures extending slightly below the gingival margins. Pulpotomy can be performed if the fracture involves the pulp. Extraction is the treatment of choice for other more severe fractures in which the tooth is not restorable. In these cases space maintenance must be considered.

## Complications in the primary dentition

As with the permanent dentition, a series of pulp and periodontal complications may occur especially in relation to the more severe luxation injuries. In regard to diagnosis of healing the chosen observation periods appears to be of significance (44, 74). Most complications can be diagnosed between 6 weeks and 8 months.

## Pulp healing complications

The status of the pulp is mainly evaluated from color changes of the crown and radiographic changes as electrometric pulp testing is not reliable in young children due to lack of cooperation. In the following section, the validity of these findings will be discussed.

### Color changes

Color changes are frequent following luxation injuries. In one study of 545 injured primary incisors, more than half of the teeth present at follow-up showed discoloration during the follow-up period (44).

**Gray** discoloration can be transient or permanent, and the latter occurs in about half of the cases (44, 49, 78). **Transient gray** discoloration is often followed by permanent yellow discoloration (Fig. 19.26). **Permanent gray** discoloration is often associated with pulp necrosis.

However, gray coloration alone is not enough to establish this diagnosis, which requires radiographic findings (periapical radiolucency or signs of root resorption).

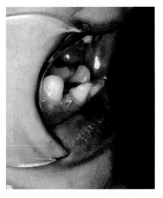 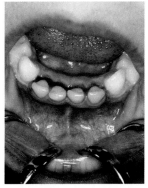 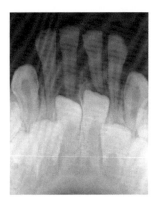 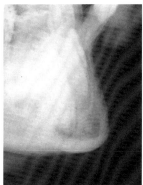

**Fig. 19.25** Alveolar fracture comprising all primary incisors in a 5-year-old boy.

**Fig. 19.26 Clinical and radiographic follow-up after primary tooth injury**
Reversal of coronal discoloration of a subluxated primary incisor.

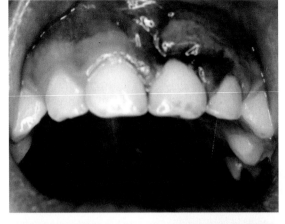 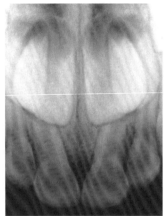

**Follow-up, 3 weeks after injury**
Intense reddish brown discoloration is seen.

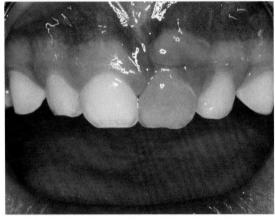 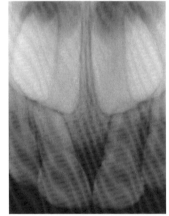

**Follow-up, 1 year after injury**
The color has changed to yellow, and the radiographs demonstrate pulp canal obliteration.

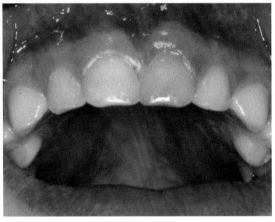 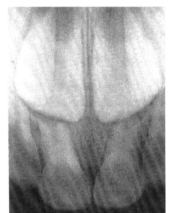

The question naturally occurs about the histological status of teeth in which gray discoloration is the only sequel after trauma. In two clinical and radiographic studies, it was found that it was not possible to relate color changes to the histological status of the pulp (47, 76) whereas the opposite was found in another study (77).

In clinical studies, it has been shown that the majority of discolored primary teeth do not develop radiographic or clinical signs of infection and are exfoliated at the expected time (49, 79–83). Thus, the presence of discoloration alone is not an indication for treatment, but an adequate follow-up schedule should be maintained in order to detect any additional symptoms.

### Radiographic findings

A periapical radiolucency may develop after 3 weeks. Another radiographic sign is arrested root development and lack of pulp canal obliteration (i.e. the width of the root canal does not change after injury). This is considered a sign of pulp necrosis and should lead to either extraction or endodontic treatment of the tooth (see p. 536). In the evaluation of radiographs it should be considered that during the initial phases of eruption of the permanent successor an enlargement of the follicle of the permanent successor takes place that may imitate a periapical radiolucency related to a pulp necrosis of the primary incisor (Fig. 19.27). In one

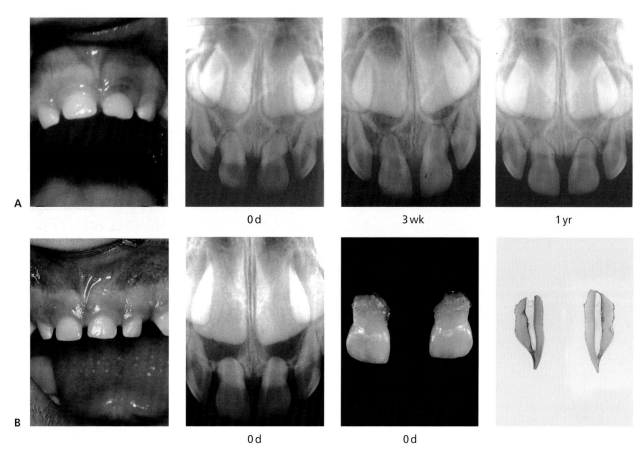

**Fig. 19.27** An expanding follicle simulates apical pathology of both primary central incisors subsequent to a luxation injury. A. The patient suffered a subluxation injury of the left central incisor at the age of 4. At the one-year control, apical rarefication/expansion of both follicles was found in the central incisor region. B. A month after this control, the patient suffered a new injury where both incisors became subluxated. At that time both incisors were extracted but showed normal histologic pulp conditions.

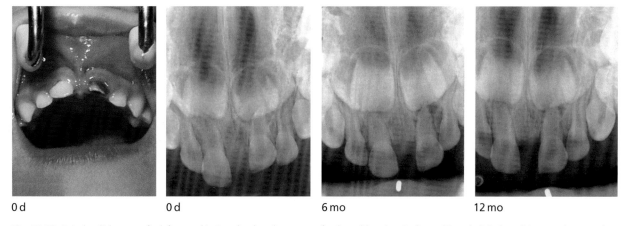

**Fig. 19.28** Apical radiolucency of a left central incisor developed one year after lateral luxation. Radiographic and clinical condition are shown at time of injury and after 6 and 12 months.

study this phenomenon appeared in 72% of follow-up cases of primary teeth showing dark discoloration. In the 26% control teeth the same feature was seen. At present there is no valid explanation for this phenomenon (49).

### Other findings

In rare cases, a fistula or an abscess almost always indicates pulp infection.

### Pulp necrosis

Pulp necrosis is seen with almost the same frequency in the primary as in the permanent dentition after similar types of luxation (43, 44, 80) and can usually be diagnosed 6–8 weeks after trauma (Fig. 19.28). In a multivariate analysis, the decisive factors in the primary dentition were the *age* of the patient (with the lowest frequency of necrosis in the very young patients), the *extent of displacement* as well as the *extent of loosening* of the luxated tooth, and finally – as in the permanent dentition – the presence of a *crown fracture* (44).

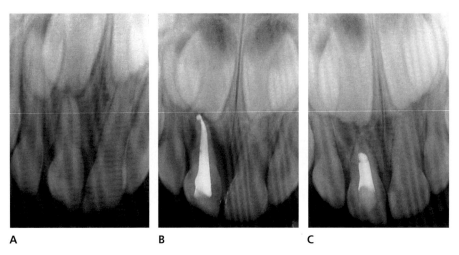

**Fig. 19.29** Endodontic treatment of primary central incisor with pulp necrosis. A. Radiograph taken two days after luxation of the maxillary right central incisor in a 4 year-old girl. B. Radiograph taken immediately after completion of endodontic treatment 4 weeks after the injury. Note the external root resorption and the expansion of the periodontal ligament space. C. Radiograph taken 12 months after the endodontic treatment. Note the resorption of the filling material from the root canal, the accelerated resorption of the root canal and the expansion of the dental follicle of the permanent successor. Clinically the tooth is asymptomatic.

Pulp necrosis is evident when conclusive clinical symptoms are present, including development of a fistula or acute inflammation with swelling and abscess formation. But in the absence of these signs pulp necrosis may very well be present.

The diagnosis of pulp necrosis of primary teeth is based primarily on gray color changes of the crown and radiographic evidence of a periapical rarefaction and/or lack of root formation. A therapeutic problem is whether, during the observation period, pulp necrosis may inflict damage to the permanent tooth germ. Admittedly, there is a long-term effect of pulp necrosis and chronic periapical inflammation upon permanent successors (see Chapters 2 and 20). However, an experimental study in monkeys has shown that pulp necrosis and periapical inflammation of primary incisors of only 6 weeks' duration do not lead to developmental disturbance of the permanent succesors (3). Thus, a short observation period appears to be justified, thereby facilitating a diagnosis of pulp necrosis.

### Methodology of root canal treatment of traumatized primary incisors

The tooth is isolated with a rubber dam without a clamp, the pulp chamber is exposed from the palatal aspect of the crown using a #330 tungsten bur on a high-speed hand piece with water spray. Local anesthesia is not used if the pulp is considered to be necrotic. If the patient complains of pain during insertion of the broach, local anesthetic is injected directly into the root canal. The pulp is removed, root canal cleaned, washed with hydrogen peroxide and saline and dried with paper points. A resorbable paste is used to fill the root canal with a spiral lentulo on a slow-speed hand piece, and the tooth is restored with a composite resin using the acid-etch technique. A postoperative radiograph is taken to assess the extent of root filling (Fig. 19.29).

### Results of treatment

In a recent study of endodontic treatment of primary teeth with pulp necrosis a combination of an initial calcium hydroxide dressing and later obliteration with zinc oxide eugenol was used (53). A success rate of only 64% was found, a finding that can hardly support the general use of this treatment procedure, especially considering the resources used in teeth that are going to be shed in the foreseeable future.

An important issue is whether endodontic treatment *per se* may induce developmental disturbances in the permanent dentition (53, 65, 84). Considering the effect of endodontic treatment on permanent successors, one clinical study found that root filling of primary teeth with zinc oxide eugenol resulted in 60% disturbance in enamel formation in the permanent successors compared with 21% in a non-treated group. However, the enamel disturbances were usually minimal in both groups (84).

Finally, a recent study has shown no difference in the long-term outcome for both the primary teeth and their permanent successors, whether mere observation therapy or root canal treatment of dark-gray discolored asymptomatic primary incisors was performed (83).

### Predictors for pulp necrosis

In a recent multivariate analysis on the long-term prognosis of injuries to primary teeth it was found that older age, presence of *dislocation* and *mobility* were predictors for pulp necrosis (44).

Finally it should be considered that re-eruption of luxated teeth occurs irrespective of whether pulp necrosis develops. Thus, a recent study on the fate of re-erupted intruded primary teeth showed that almost half of the cases erupted with a necrotic pulp (44).

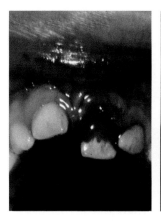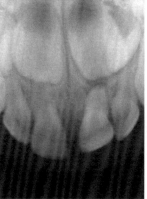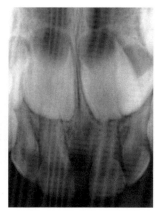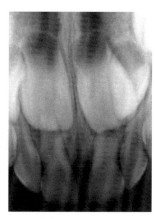

**Fig. 19.30** Pulp canal obliteration subsequent to lateral luxation of a primary central incisor.

### Pulp canal obliteration

Pulp canal obliteration is a frequent complication, especially after luxation injuries in the younger age groups before physiologic root resorption is radiographically evident (usually around the age of 4–5 years (44, 74, 82)). Even though there is a close relationship with yellow discoloration of the crown, radiographic evidence of pulp canal obliteration can often be seen in teeth with normal color and even in initially gray discolored teeth (Figs 19.26 and 19.30). In some cases, pulp canal obliteration was the only evidence of a previous trauma when seen on radiographs in coincidence with acute examination of a new injury.

Secondary pulp necrosis can occur in teeth with pulp canal obliteration; and frequencies of 0–13% have been reported (44, 79, 80). It is reasonable to assume that when a secondary necrosis occurs, it is related to a new trauma as an obliterated pulp has less healing potential due to the narrow pulp canal.

## External root resorption

This phenomenon is divided into physiologic root resorption and pathologic root resorption (20, 44).

### Pathologic root resorption

#### External root resorption
This entity can be divided into *repair related resorption* (surface resorption), *infection related resorption* (inflammatory resorption) and *replacement resorption* (ankylosis). In a long-term study of 387 traumatized primary incisors repair-related resorption was found to be extremely rare (1%). Inflammatory resorption was found in 10% and was frequently related to intrusion and lateral luxation (44). In a recent study of discolored primary teeth after trauma, the frequency of inflammatory resorption was found in 11% of the cases (49).

Finally, ankylosis was very rare, only affecting 3% of the luxated teeth, with a preference for intruded teeth (44). In case of ankylosis, spontaneous resorption by the erupting permanent successor was found to take place in most cases (Fig. 19.31).

In conclusion, external root resorption patterns seem to follow that of permanent teeth, although at a much lower rate (see Chapter 13). This can possibly be explained by the softer bone structure, which allows tooth displacement with less trauma to the root surface.

## Internal root resorption

This phenomenon is extremely rare; only two studies found internal root resorption in 2% of the cases (44, 49) (Fig. 19.32).

In conclusion external or internal root resorption does not appear to be a significant problem in the management of primary tooth injuries. In case of inflammatory resorption either endodontic treatment or extraction should be performed. In case of replacement resorption, spontaneous shedding, although delayed, can be expected.

## Essentials

### Epidemiology

Children at the age of 6 worldwide have a trauma experience to the primary dentition of 20–40%.

### Pathogenesis

Because of anatomical conditions and the common direction of traumatic impacts, primary teeth are usually displaced away from the permanent successor.

### Examination procedure

By clinical and radiographic means an exact position of the displaced primary incisor in the jaw in relation to the permanent successor should be made.

### Treatment principles

The important factor is to safeguard the development of the permanent successor and to avoid inducing dental fear and anxiety in children.

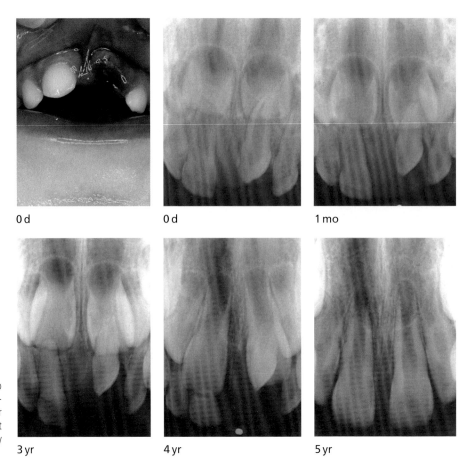

0 d        0 d        1 mo

**Fig. 19.31** Ankylosis subsequent to intrusion of a central incisor in a 2-year-old girl. The intruded incisor became ankylosed, but the permanent incisor was able to shed the primary tooth.

3 yr        4 yr        5 yr

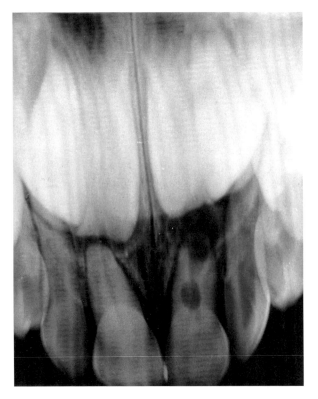

**Fig. 19.32** Internal root canal resorption subsequent to a luxation injury.

## Enamel and enamel-dentin fractures

These fractures can be treated by grinding sharp edges or restoring with composite.

## Complicated crown fracture

If the child can cooperate, partial pulpotomy can be performed with due consideration to the degree of physiological resorption of the involved tooth. Otherwise, extraction must be performed.

## Crown-root fracture

Extraction of the tooth is usually the treatment of choice.

## Root fracture

If the coronal fragment is not displaced the tooth can be left *in situ*. If the crown fragment is very mobile and displaced, the coronal fragment should be extracted to prevent the child from swallowing or inhaling the loose fragment; the apical fragment is left for physiological resorption.

## Alveolar fracture

Reposition the displaced segment and splint it to adjacent teeth for up to 4 weeks. General anesthesia is often necessary.

## Concussion and subluxation

No active treatment indicated. Careful oral hygiene is required, with a follow-up after 8 weeks.

## Extrusion

Depending on the extent of injury, the tooth may be repositioned and if possible splinted for 3 weeks.

If the tooth has suffered a severe extrusion, extraction is usually indicated to prevent the child from swallowing or inhaling the tooth.

Follow-up: minimum 1 year.

## Lateral luxation

- Lateral luxated teeth should generally be allowed to realign spontaneously. However, if a lateral luxated tooth interferes with occlusion, repositioning should be attempted. After the use of local anesthesia, the tooth is repositioned.
- Clinical and radiographic follow-up after 1 and 2 months.
- Follow-up: minimum 1 year.

## Intrusive luxation

- Intruded primary teeth should generally be allowed to realign spontaneously. If a radiographic examination reveals that an intruded tooth has been forced into the follicle of the permanent tooth germ, extraction of the primary tooth is indicated.
- If a conservative approach is chosen, the intruded tooth should be re-examined clinically and radiographically after 1 and 2 months to monitor healing.
- Follow-up: minimum 1 year.
- If the influence of trauma on the permanent successor must be evaluated, an additional follow-up examination is indicated at the age of 6.

## Avulsion

- A radiographic examination is essential to ensure that the missing tooth is not intruded.
- Avulsed primary teeth should not be replanted.

## Fractures of the alveolar process

Reposition the displaced segment and splint it to adjacent teeth for up to 4 weeks. General anesthesia is often necessary.

## Fractures secondary to chin injuries

If crown and crown-root fractures occur in the molar region, treatement will depend on the extent and severity of injuries.

## Complications in the primary dentition

There in no need for root canal treatment in dark gray discolored teeth when no other clinical or radiographic symptoms are present.

## Instructions to parents

- The affected area should be kept clean by brushing the child's teeth carefully after each meal with a soft toothbrush.
- Chlorhexidine should be applied topically twice a day for one week.
- The use of pacifiers and nursing bottles should be restricted.
- Dental care should be sought if new symptoms occur (e.g. fever, swelling, prolonged loosening or pain).

## References

1. ANDREASEN JO. The influence of traumatic intrusion of primary teeth on their permanent successors. A radiographic and histologic study in monkeys. *Int J Oral Surg* 1976;**5**:207–19.
2. THYLSTRUP A, ANDREASEN JO. The influence of traumatic intrusion of primary teeth on their permanent successors in monkeys. A macroscopic, polarized light and scanning electron microscopic study. *J Oral Pathol* 1977;**6**:296–306.
3. ANDREASEN JO, RIIS I. Influence of pulp necrosis and periapical inflammation of primary teeth and their permanent successors. Combined macroscopic and histological study in monkeys. *Int J Oral Surg* 1978;**7**:178–87.
4. WINTER GB, KRAMER IRH. Changes in periodontal membrane, bone and permanent teeth following experimental pulpal injury in deciduous molar teeth of monkeys (Macaca iris). *Arch Oral Biol* 1972;**17**:1771–9.
5. VALDERHAUG J. A histologic study of experimental induced periapical inflammation in primary teeth in monkeys. *Int J Oral Surg* 1974;**3**:111–23.
6. VALDERHAUG J. Periapical inflammation in primary teeth and its effect on the permanent succesors. *Int J Oral Surg* 1974;**3**:171–82.
7. ANDO S, SANKA Y, NAKASHIMO T, SHINBO K, KIYOKAWA K, OSHIMA S, AIZAWA K. Studies on the consecutive survey of succedaneous and permanent dentition in the Japanese children. Part 3. Effects of periapical osteitis in the deciduous predecessors and the surface malformation of their permanent successors. *J Nihon Univ Sch Dent* 1966;**8**:21–41.
8. ANDREASEN JO, RAVN JJ. The effect of traumatic injuries to primary teeth on their permanent successors. II. A clinical and radiographic follow-up study of 213 teeth. *Scand J Dent Res* 1971;**79**:284–94.
9. ANDREASEN JO, SUNDSTRÖM B, RAVN JJ. The effect of traumatic injuries to primary teeth on their permanent successors. I. A clinical and histologic study of 117 injured permanent teeth. *Scand J Dent Res* 1971;**79**:219–83.
10. VON ARX T. Traumatology in the deciduous dentition (I). The clinical and therapeutic aspects. *Schweiz Monatsschr Zahnmed* 1990;**100**:1194–208.

11. von Arx T. Deciduous tooth intrusions and the odontogenesis of the permanent teeth. Developmental disorders of the permanent teeth following intrusion injuries to the deciduous teeth. *Schweiz Monatsschr Zahnmed* 1995;**105**:11–17.

12. Sleiter R, von Arx T. Posttraumatiche Entwichlungsstörungen bleibender Zähne nach Milchzahntrauma: eine retrospective Studie. *Schweiz Monatschr Zahnmed* 2002;**112**:214–19.

13. Selliseth N-E. The significance of traumatized primary incisors on the development and eruption of permanent teeth. *Eur Orthod Dent Soc* 1970;**46**:443–59.

14. Ravn JJ. Sequelae of acute mechanical trauma in the primary dentition. *ASDC J Dent Child* 1968;**35**:281–9.

15. Andreasen JO, Ravn JJ. Epidemiology of traumatic dental injuries to primary and permanent teeth in a Danish population sample. *Int J Oral Surg* 1972;**1**:235–9.

16. Glendor U, Halling A, Andersson L, Eilert-Petersson E. Incidence of traumatic tooth injuries in children and adolescents in the county of Västmanland, Sweden. *Swed Dent J* 1996;**20**:15–28.

17. Glendor U. On dental trauma in children and adolescents. Incidence, risk, treatment, time and costs. *Swed Dent J Suppl* 2000;**140**:1–52.

18. Belcheva AB, Ilieva EL, Veleganova VK. Comparative investigation of the traumatic injuries' prevalence of primary and permanent incisors at children aged 3 to 14. *Folia Med (Plovdiv)* 2003;**45**:43–5.

19. Bijella MF, Yared FN, Bijella VT, Lopes ES. Occurrence of primary incisor traumatism in Brazilian children: a house-by-house survey. *ASDC J Dent Child* 1990;**57**:424–7.

20. Borum MK, Andreasen JO. Therapeutic and economic implications of traumatic dental injuries in Denmark: an estimate based on 7549 patients treated at a major trauma centre. *Int J Paediatr Dent* 2001;**11**:249–58.

21. Cunha RF, Pugliesi DM, Mello Vieira AE. Oral trauma in Brazilian patients aged 0–3 years. *Dent Traumatol* 2001;**17**:210–12.

22. Fried I, Erickson P, Schwartz S, Keenan K. Subluxation injuries of maxillary primary anterior teeth: epidemiology and prognosis of 207 traumatized teeth. *Pediatr Dent* 1996;**18**:145–51.

23. Llarena del Rosario ME, Acosta AV, Garcia-Godoy F. Traumatic injuries to primary teeth in Mexico City children. *Endod Dent Traumatol* 1992;**8**:213–14.

24. Lombardi S, Sheller B, Williams BJ. Diagnosis and treatment of dental trauma in a children's hospital. *Pediatr Dent* 1998;**20**:112–20.

25. Nelson LP, Shusterman S. Emergency management of oral trauma in children. *Curr Opin Pediatr* 1997;**9**:242–5.

26. Cardoso M, Carvalho Rocha MJ. Traumatized primary teeth in children assisted at the Federal University of Santa Catarina, Brazil. *Dent Traumatol* 2002;**18**:129–33.

27. Garcia-Goday F, Morban-Laucher F, Corominas LR, Franjul RA, Noyola M. Traumatic dental injuries in preschoolchildren from Santo Domingo. *Community Dent Oral Epidemiol* 1983;**11**:127–30.

28. Yagot KH, Nazhat NY, Kuder SA. Traumatic dental injuries in nursery schoolchildren from Baghdad, Iraq. *Community Dent Oral Epidemiol* 1988;**16**:292–3.

29. Kramer PF, Zembruski C, Ferreira SH, Feldens CA. Traumatic dental injuries in Brazilian preschool children. *Dent Traumatol* 2003;**19**:299–303.

30. Al-Moyed J, Murray JJ, Maguire A. Prevalence of dental trauma in 5–6 and 12–14-years-old boys in Riyadh, Saudi Arabia. *Dent Traumatol* 2001;**17**:153–8.

31. Gabris K, Tarjan I, Rozsa N. Dental trauma in children presenting for treatment at the Department of Dentistry for Children and Orthodontics, Budapest, 1985–1999. *Dent Traumatol* 2001;**17**:103–8.

32. Osuji OO. Traumatised primary teeth in Nigerian children attending University Hospital: the consequences of delays in seeking treatment. *Int Dent J* 1996;**46**:165–70.

33. Rai SB, Munshi AK. Traumatic injuries to the anterior teeth among South Kanara school children – a prevalence study. *J Indian Soc Pedod Prev Dent* 1998;**16**:44–51.

34. Thompson CC, Park RI, Prescott GH. Oral manifestations of the congenital insensitivity-to-pain syndrome. *Oral Surg Oral Med Oral Pathol* 1980;**50**:220–5.

35. Steadman RH, McIntosh G, Gross BD. Lesch-Nyhan syndrome. *J Oral Maxillofac Surg* 1982;**40**:750–2.

36. Goho C. Neonatal sublingual traumatic ulceration (Riga-Fede disease): reports of cases. *ASDC J Dent Child* 1996;**63**:362–4.

37. Davila JM, Aslani MB, Wentworth E. Oral appliance attached to a bubble helmet for prevention of self-inflicted injury. *ASDC J Dent Child* 1996;**63**:131–4.

38. Rashid N, Yusuf H. Oral self-mutilation by a 17-month-old child with Lesch-Nyhan syndrome. *Int J Paediatr Dent* 1997;**7**:115–17.

39. Baghdadi ZD. Riga-Fede disease: report of a case and review. *J Clin Pediatr Dent* 2001;**25**:209–13.

40. Terzioglu A, Bingul F, Aslan G. Lingual traumatic ulceration (Riga-Fede disease). *J Oral Maxillofac Surg* 2002;**60**:478.

41. Lee JH, Berkowitz RJ, Choi BJ. Oral self-mutilation in the Lesch-Nyhan syndrome. *ASDC J Dent Child* 2002;**69**:12, 66–9.

42. Medina AC, Sogbe R, Gomez-Rey AM, Mata M. Factitial oral lesions in an autistic paediatric patient. *Int J Paediatr Dent* 2003;**13**:130–7.

43. Ravn JJ. Sequelae of acute mechanical traumata in the primary dentition. A clinical study. *ASDC J Dent Child* 1968;**35**:281–9.

44. Borum MK, Andreasen JO. Sequelae of trauma to primary maxillary incisors. I. Complications in the primary dentition. *Endod Dent Traumatol* 1998;**14**:31–44.

45. Borum, MK. *Traumer i det primære tandsæt: Komplikationer i det primære tandsæt og i blandingstandsættet*. Thesis, Copenhagen University, 1994.

46. Robertson A, Lundgren T, Andreasen T, Dietz W, Hoyer I, Norén JG. Pulp calcifications in traumatized primary incisors. A morphologic and inductive analysis study. *Eur J Oral Sci* 1997;**105**:196–206.

47. Croll TP, Pascon EA, Langeland K. Traumatically injured primary incisors: a clinical and histologic study. *ASDC J Dent Child* 1987;**54**:401–22.

48. Holan G. Tube-like mineralizations in the dental pulp of traumatized primary incisors. *Endod Dent Traumatol* 1998;**14**:279–84.

49. HOLAN G. Development of clinical and radiographic signs associated with dark discolored primary incisors following traumatic injuries: a prospective controlled study. *Dent Traumatol* 2004;**20**:276–87.

50. MYALL RW, SANDOR GK, GREGORY CE. Are you overlooking fractures of the mandibular condyle? *Pediatrics* 1987;**79**:639–41.

51. MARECHAUX SC. Chin trauma as a cause of primary molar fracture: report of case. *ASDC J Dent Child* 1985;**52**:452–4.

52. HOLAN G. Traumatic injuries to the chin: a survey in a paediatric dental practice. *Int J Paediatr Dent* 1998;**8**:143–8.

53. ROCHA MJC, CARDOSA M. Federal University of Santa Catarina. Endodontic treatment of traumatized primary teeth – part 2. *Dent Traumatol* 2004;**20**:314–26.

54. BERDE CB, SETHNA NF. Analgesics for the treatment of pain in children. *N Engl J Med* 2002;**347**:1094–103.

55. ANDREASEN JO, ANDREASEN FM, SKEIE A, HJÖRTING-HANSEN E, SCHWARTZ O. Effect of treatment delay upon pulp and periodontal healing of traumatic dental injuries – a review article. *Dent Traumatol* 2002;**18**:116–28.

56. HALLONSTEN AL, VEERKAMP J, RÖLLING I. Pain, pain control and sedation in children and adolescents. In: Koch G, Poulsen S. eds. *Pediatric dentistry. A clinical approach.* Copenhagen: Munksgaard, 2001:147–12.

57. DIAB M, ELBADRAWY HE. Intrusion injuries of primary incisors. Part I: Review and management. *Quintessence Int* 2000;**31**:327–34.

58. HARDING AM, CAMP JH. Traumatic injuries in the preschool child. *Dent Clin North Am* 1995;**39**:817–35.

59. WILSON CF. DIY guide to primary tooth trauma repair. *Tex Dent J* 1997;**114**:43–7.

60. FLORES MT. Traumatic injuries in the primary dentition. *Dent Traumatol* 2002;**18**:287–98.

61. FLORES MT, ANDREASEN JO, BAKLAND LK, FEIGLIN B, GUTMANN JL, OIKARINEN K, FORD TR, SIGURDSSON A, TROPE M, VANN WF, Jr. Guidelines for the evaluation and management of traumatic dental injuries. *Dent Traumatol* 2001;**17**:1–4.

62. KUPIETZKY A, HOLAN G. Treatment of crown fractures with pulp exposure in primary incisors. *Pediatr Dent* 2003;**25**:241–7.

63. RAM D, HOLAN G. Partial pulpotomy in a traumatized primary incisor with pulp exposure: case report. *Pediatr Dent* 1994;**16**:44–8.

64. FLAITZ CM, BARR ES, HICKS MJ. Radiographic evaluation of pulpal therapy for primary anterior teeth. *ASDC J Dent Child* 1989;**56**:182–5.

65. COLL JA, JOSELL S, NASSOF S, SHELTON P, RICHARDS MA. An evaluation of pulpal therapy in primary incisors. *Pediatr Dent* 1988;**10**:178–84.

66. AGAMY HA, BAKRY NS, MOUNIR MM, AVERY DR. Comparison of mineral trioxide aggregate and formocresol as pulp-capping agents in pulpotomized primary teeth. *Pediatr Dent* 2004;**26**:302–9.

67. HOLAN G, EIDELMAN E, FUKS AB. Long-term evaluation of pulptomy in primary molars using mineral trioxide aggregate or formocresol as dressing materials. *Pediatr Dent* 2005;**27**:129–36.

68. HOLAN G, RAM D, FUKS AB. The diagnostic value of lateral extraoral radiography for intruded maxillary primary incisors. *Pediatr Dent* 2002;**24**:38–41.

69. HOLAN G, RAM D. Aspiration of an avulsed primary incisor. A case report. *Int J Paediatr Dent* 2000;**10**:150–2.

70. FILIPPI A, POHL Y, KIRSCHNER H. Replantation of avulsed primary anterior teeth: treatment and limitations. *ASDC J Dent Child* 1997;**64**:272–5.

71. GATEWOOD JC, THORNTON JB. Successful replantation and splinting of a maxillary segment fracture in the primary dentition. *Pediatr Dent* 1995;**17**:124–6.

72. KAWASHIMA Z, PINEDA FR. Replanting avulsed primary teeth. *J Am Dent Assoc* 1992;**123**:90–1, 94.

73. SASAKI H, OGAWA T, KAWAGUCHI M, SOBUE S, OOSHIMA T. Multiple fractures of primary molars caused by injuries to the chin: report of two cases. *Endod Dent Traumatol* 2000;**16**:43–6.

74. CARDOSO M, ROCHA MJC. Federal University of Santa Catarina follow-up management routine for traumatized teeth – part I. *Dent Traumatol* 2004;**20**:307–13.

75. SALAKO N, JOSEPH B, RITWIK P, SALONEN J, JOHN P, JUNAID TA. Comparison of bioactive glass, mineral trioxide aggregate, ferric sulfate, and formocresol as pulpotomy agents in rat molar. *Dent Traumatol* 2003;**19**:314–20.

76. SOXMAN JA, NAZIF MM, BOUQUOT J. Pulpal pathology in relation to discoloration of primary anterior teeth. *ASCD J Dent Child* 1984;**51**:282–4.

77. HOLAN G, FUKS AB. The diagnosis value of coronal dark-gray discoloration in primary teeth following traumatic injuries. *Pediatr Dent* 1996;**18**:224–7.

78. AGUILO L, GANDIA JL. Transient red discoloration; report of case. *ASDC J Dent Child* 1998;**65**:346–8, 356.

79. JACOBSEN I, SANGNES G. Traumatized primary anterior teeth. Prognosis related to calcific reactions in the pulp cavity. *Acta Odontol Scand* 1978;**36**:199–204.

80. SCHRÖDER U, WENNBERG E, GRANATH LE, MÖLLER H. Traumatized primary incisors – follow-up program based on frequency of periapical osteitis related to tooth color. *Swed Dent J* 1977;**1**:95–8.

81. SONIS AL. Longitudinal study of discolored primary teeth and effect on succedaneous teeth. *J Pedod* 1987;**11**:247–52.

82. HOLAN G, RAM D. Sequelae and prognosis of intruded primary incisors: a retrospective study. *Pediatr Dent* 1999;**21**:242–7.

83. HOLAN G. Long-term effect of different treatment modalities for traumatized primary incisors presenting dark coronal discoloration with no other signs of injury. *Dent Traumatol* 2006;**22**:14–17.

84. HOLAN G, TOPF J, FUKS AB. Effect of root canal infection and treatment of traumatized primary incisors and their permanent successors. *Endod Dent Traumatol* 1992;**8**:12–15.

# 20
# Injuries to Developing Teeth

## J. O. Andreasen & M. T. Flores

## Terminology, frequency and etiology

Traumatic injuries to developing teeth can influence their further growth and maturation, usually leaving a child with a permanent and often readily visible deformity. Especially when the injury occurs during initial stages of development, enamel formation can be seriously disturbed due to interference with a number of stages in ameloblastic development, i.e., the morphogenetic, organizing, formative and maturation stages (1, 2).

The close relationship between the apices of primary teeth and the developing permanent successors explains why injuries to primary teeth are easily transmitted to the permanent dentition (Figs 20.1 and 20.2). Likewise, bone fractures located in areas containing developing tooth germs can interfere with further odontogenesis (181, 183). Also, the force of the impact may cause an underlying crown fracture of the unerupted permanent incisor (184)

The nature of these injuries has been studied clinically in humans (1, 2, 120–123, 130, 131, 157–162) and experimentally in animals (3–12, 124–129). Thus, anatomic and histological deviations due to injuries to developing teeth can be classified as follows (1):

- White or yellow-brown discoloration of enamel
- White or yellow-brown discoloration of enamel with circular enamel hypoplasia
- Crown dilaceration
- Odontoma-like malformation
- Root duplication
- Vestibular root angulation
- Lateral root angulation or dilaceration
- Partial or complete arrest of root formation
- Sequestration of permanent tooth germs
- Disturbance in eruption.

In this classification, the term *dilaceration* describes an abrupt deviation of the long axis of the crown or root portion of the tooth. This deviation originates from a traumatic non-axial displacement of already formed hard tissue in relation to the developing soft tissue (1).

The term *angulation* denotes a curvature of the root resulting from a gradual change in the direction of root development without evidence of abrupt displacement of the tooth germ during odontogenesis (1).

The prevalence of such disturbances, secondary to dental injuries in the primary dentition, ranges from 12 to 69%, according to the studies listed in Table 20.1. Considering the frequency of traumatic injuries to primary teeth (see Chapter 8, p. 224), it is apparent that enamel hypoplasia of traumatic origin must be rather common. In a clinical study, it was estimated that 10% of all enamel hypoplasias affecting anterior teeth in schoolchildren in Copenhagen were related to trauma in the primary dentition (121). The type of *dental trauma* sustained apparently determines the type and degree of developmental disturbance. Avulsion and intrusive luxation represent injuries with very high frequencies of developmental disturbance, while subluxation and extrusion represent low-risk groups (Table 20.2) (2, 16, 123, 130, 131, 158, 162, 181, 186, 202). Furthermore, the age at the time of injury is of major importance; thus, fewer complications are seen in individuals over 4 years of age than in individuals in the younger age groups (2) (Table 20.3).

According to the studies listed in Table 20.4, the frequency of developmental disturbances due to *jaw fractures* ranges from 19 to 68%. Furthermore, the frequency of developmental disturbances has been found to be related to fragment displacement at the time of injury (132). Treatment of jaw fractures by osteosynthesis has also been shown to increase damage to developing teeth (135) (Fig. 20.3).

Oral surgical procedures can also induce dental malformations. Thus, patients operated for cleft palate show a very high frequency of enamel defects in the primary as well as the permanent dentitions. Histologic findings in these cases indicate that the surgical trauma could be a contributing factor (22, 23). Exodontia has also been recorded among surgical etiologic factors. Due to the close relationship between the developing crowns of the permanent premolars and the roots of their primary predecessors, developing premolars are especially prone to disturbances in enamel and dentin formation resulting from extraction of primary

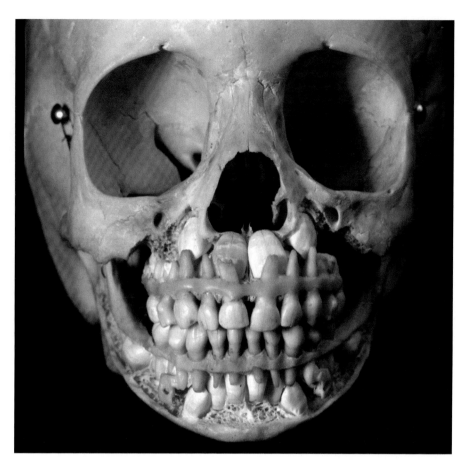

**Fig. 20.1** Skull of a 5-year-old child revealing the relationship between primary and permanent teeth.

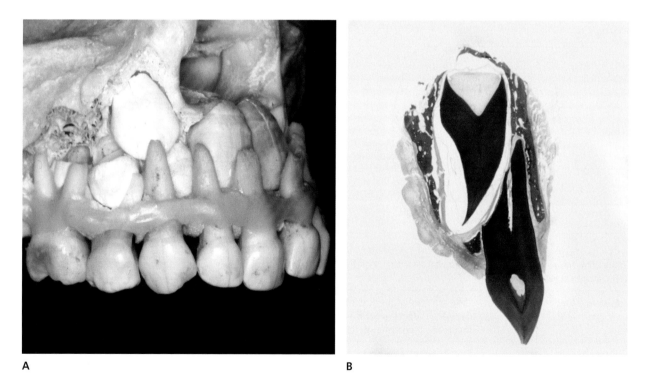

A                                                                B

**Fig. 20.2** A. Anatomic relationship between the primary incisor and its permanent successor in a human skull. Note that both central and lateral primary incisors are in close relation to the permanent central incisor. B. Histologic relationship between a primary incisor and its permanent successor. Note that most of the resorbing primary root is separated from the permanent tooth germ by only a thin layer of soft tissue. From ANDREASEN (127) 1976.

**Table 20.1** Frequency of disturbances in development of permanent teeth after traumatic injuries to the primary dentition.

| Examiner | No. of teeth involved | No. of teeth with developmental disturbances |
|---|---|---|
| Zelnner (13) 1956 | 26 | 3 (12%) |
| Schreiber (14) 1959 | 42 | 8 (19%) |
| Taatz (15) 1962 | 33 | 7 (21%) |
| Ravn (17) 1968 | 90 | 51 (57%) |
| Lind et al. (120) 1970 | 72 | 36 (50%) |
| Selliseth (16) 1970 | 128 | 88 (69%) |
| Andreasen & Ravn (2) 1971 | 213 | 88 (41%) |
| Andreasen & Ravn (121) 1973 | 147 | 85 (58%) |
| Mehnert (122) 1974 | 28 | 10 (36%) |
| Watzek & Skoda (123) 1976 | 77 | 39 (51%) |
| Brin et al. (157) 1984 | 56 | 72 (47%) |
| Morgantini et al. (160) 1986 | 60 | 15 (25%) |
| Ben Bassat et al. (159) 1985 | 414 | 190 (46%) |
| Ishikawa et al. (185) 1990 | 126 | 72 (57%) |
| von Arx (162) 1991 | 144 | 33 (23%) |
| von Arx (187) 1993 | 255 | 59 (23%) |
| Sleiter & von Arx (186) 2002 | 74 | 24 (32%) |

**Table 20.2** Frequency of disturbances in development of permanent teeth according to type of injury to the primary dentition. From ANDREASEN & RAVN (2) 1971.

| Type of injury | No. of teeth | No. of teeth with disturbances in development |
|---|---|---|
| Subluxation | 45 | 12 (27%) |
| Extrusive luxation | 76 | 26 (34%) |
| Avulsion | 27 | 14 (52%) |
| Intrusive luxation | 36 | 25 (69%) |

**Table 20.3** Frequency of developmental disturbances of permanent teeth related to the age at which injury to the primary dentition occurred. From ANDREASEN & RAVN (2) 1971.

| Age (years) | No. of teeth | No. of teeth with disturbances in development |
|---|---|---|
| 0–2 | 62 | 39 (63%) |
| 3–4 | 43 | 23 (53%) |
| 5–6 | 88 | 21 (24%) |
| 7–9 | 20 | 5 (25%) |

**Table 20.4** Frequency of developmental disturbances among permanent teeth involved in jaw fractures.

| Examiner | No. of teeth involved | No. of teeth with developmental disturbances |
|---|---|---|
| Fischer (18) 1951 | 12 | 7 (58%) |
| Lenstrup (19) 1955 | 22 | 15 (68%) |
| Taatz (15) 1962 | 29 | 14 (48%) |
| Bencze (20, 21) 1964 | 10 | 5 (50%) |
| Ideberg & Persson (132) 1971 | 100 | 19 (19%) |
| Ridell & Åstrand (133) 1971 | 170 | 6 (35%) |
| Ranta & Ylipaavalniemi (134) 1973 | 37 | 19 (51%) |
| Perko & Pepersack (135) 1975 | 35 | 16 (46%) |

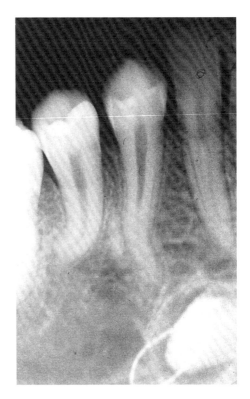

**Fig. 20.3** A 14-year-old patient with an impacted mandibular permanent canine due to osteosynthesis at the age of 5. From PERKO & PEPERSACK (135) 1975.

molars (24) (Fig. 20.4). Also root canal infection can influence enamel formation of the permanent successor (186) (see also Chapters 2 and 19).

Evaluation of the full extent of complications following injuries sustained in early childhood must await complete eruption of all involved permanent teeth, a problem which should be considered in the case of legal action or insurance claims. However, most serious sequelae (i.e. disturbances in tooth morphology) can usually be diagnosed radiographically within the first year after trauma (2).

Injuries which occur very early can also interfere with the development of the primary dentition (188). Thus, a study of prematurely born and intubated infants revealed enamel hypoplasias affecting the primary dentition in 18–80% of the children (163–165, 188), usually on the left side of the maxilla corresponding to the customary placement of the tube (164, 165, 188) (Fig. 20.5). A later autopsy study has supported the theory that compression of the alveolar process during endotracheal intubation in neonates is the causative factor which can elicit these disturbances in primary tooth development (166, 167) (Fig. 20.6).

Finally, it should be borne in mind that a number of other pathological conditions may result in enamel hypoplasia (e.g. fluorine, rickets, hypoparathyroidism, exanthematous fevers, severe infections and metabolic disturbances such as celiac disease and acidosis). However, these are unfortunately not entirely pathognomonic, but often overlapping in their expression. A classification system for developmental defects of enamel (DDE index) has been developed (168)

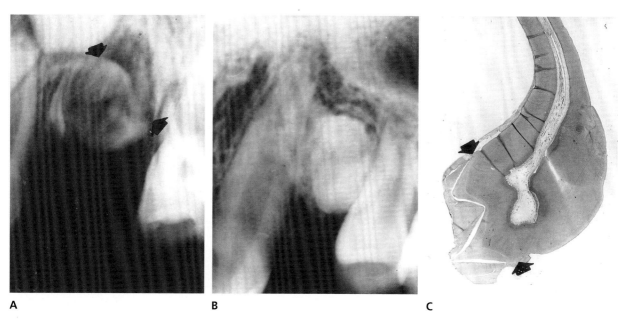

**A**        **B**        **C**

**Fig. 20.4** Crown dilaceration and impaction of a first premolar following extraction of the first primary molar. A. Radiograph taken immediately after extraction of the primary molar at the age of 4 years. The permanent tooth germ appears to be dislocated (arrows). B. Radiograph at the age of 14 years. As the first premolar was impacted, it was decided the tooth be removed. C. Low power view of sectioned premolar. Slight crown dilaceration is seen (arrows). ×5.

**Fig. 20.5** Enamel hypoplasias caused by a laryngoscopy and/or prolonged endotracheal intubation. The enamel defects are usually located on the left side of the maxilla due to the selective pressure in this area by the laryngoscope. From SEOW et al. (164) 1984.

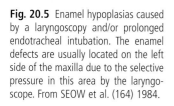

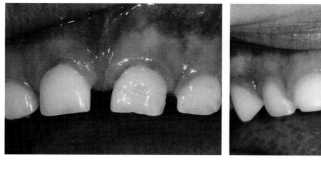

**Fig. 20.6** Dilaceration of primary tooth germ due to endotracheal intubation. This 3-day-old child was intubated postpartum due to respiratory distress but died after 3 days. A. At necropsy the unaffected part of the alveolar process shows a normal primary incisor tooth germ. B. Sections from the deformed alveolar ridge where the tube has rested shows disruption of the tooth germ with deviation of the long axis and a resultant cystic space around the enamel matrix. From BOICE et al. (166) 1976.

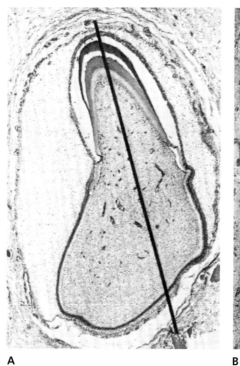

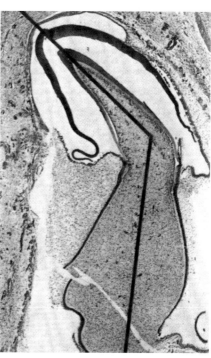

**A**                    **B**

## Fig. 20.7 Discoloration and morphologic changes secondary to injuries to the primary dentition

From ANDREASEN et al. (1) 1971. A. Slight white enamel discolorations involving both central incisors. B. Slight white and yellow-brown staining of the enamel of both central incisors.

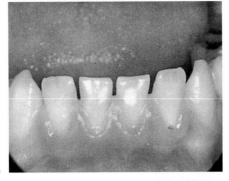
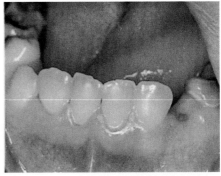

## Marked color changes and enamel hypoplasia

C. Marked color changes of permanent left central and lateral incisors associated with distal inclination of the crown of the central incisor. D. Yellow-brown enamel changes of central incisor associated with a cavity in the enamel surface.

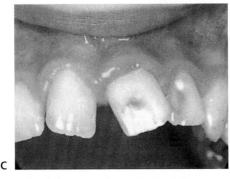
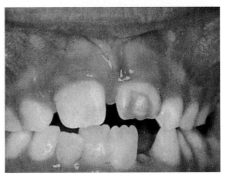

## Yellow-brown discoloration and circular enamel hypoplasia

E. Slight circular enamel hypoplasia apical to a yellow-brown discoloration of enamel with an external cavity in a central incisor (arrow). F. Same changes as in E; note the same positional relationship between hypoplasia and area of discoloration (arrows).

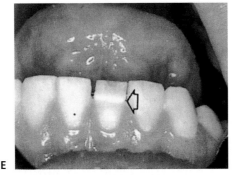
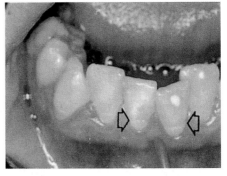

## Severe malformation

G, H. Severe disturbances in development of three permanent incisors. Right central incisor is partly impacted due to malformation, left central incisor shows marked color changes. A horizontal enamel hypoplasia is especially evident in H (see also Fig. 20.14 which shows the condition after orthodontic realignment of the right central incisor).

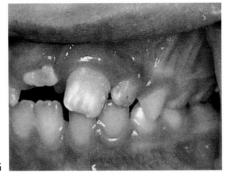
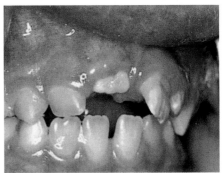

which, to a certain degree, incorporates some of the pathological features for various developmental disturbances and has been used in multifactorial analysis of enamel defects (169–171).

# Clinical, radiographic and pathologic findings

Pathologic changes in permanent tooth germs have been studied experimentally in intrusions of primary teeth in monkeys (127) and in rat molars (189). Immediate changes consisted of contusion and displacement of the reduced enamel epithelium and slight displacement of the hard dental tissue in relation to the Hertwig's epithelial root sheath (see Chapter 2, p. 69). After 6 weeks, metaplasia of the reduced enamel epithelium into a thin stratified squamous epithelium took place. In most cases, changes in morphology of the dentin and/or enamel matrices were seen (see Chapter 2, p. 65).

Developmental disturbances of human teeth caused by trauma have been studied in humans (1) and can be divided into the following types:

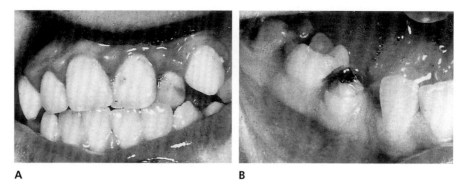

**Fig. 20.8** A. Enamel discolorations affecting left central and lateral incisors following a fracture of the maxilla at the age of 4 years. B. Disturbed enamel formation following a jaw fracture at the age of 3 years. Defective enamel covering the occlusal surface of the lower first premolar. From LENSTRUP (19) 1955.

**A**

**B**

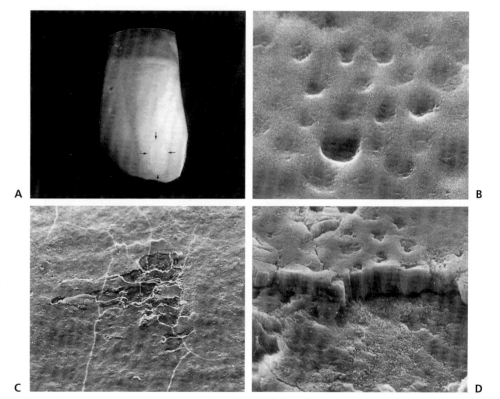

**Fig. 20.9** A. Maxillary right permanent central monkey incisor 6 weeks after traumatic intrusion of the primary incisor. Note the circumscribed white discoloration of the enamel (arrows). B. Scanning electron micrograph of the adjacent non-affected enamel. The pits indicate arrest of matrix formation. ×3300. C. General view of white enamel discoloration showing rupture of the enamel surface. ×110. The enclosed area is shown at a higher magnification in D. ×2400. From THYLSTRUP & ANDREASEN (129) 1977.

**A**

**B**

**C**

**D**

## White or yellow-brown discolorations of enamel

These lesions appear as sharply demarcated, stained enamel opacities, most often located on the facial surface of the crown; their extent varies from small spots to large fields (1, 2, 13, 14, 17, 25–38, 121, 136, 159) (Fig. 20.7A–C). These color changes are usually not associated with clinically detectable defects in the enamel surface; however, some cases can present such defects (1) (Fig. 20.7D). In this context, it should be mentioned that white enamel discolorations with a diameter of less than 0.5 mm are frequent in teeth without a history of trauma (121, 169, 172).

The frequency of these lesions has been reported to be 23% following injuries to the primary dentition (2), commonly affecting maxillary incisors, with the age of patients at the time of injury ranging from 2 to 7 years. The stage of

development of the permanent tooth germ at the time of injury may vary (159). No specific type of injury is especially related to this group of lesions.

Similar disturbances in enamel formation may be seen in developing teeth involved in jaw fractures (19, 20) (Fig. 20.8). For the sake of completeness, it should be mentioned that color changes with or without a defect in the enamel surface may occur as a sequel to periapical inflammation of primary teeth, (15, 40–45, 137–141) giving rise to so-called Turner teeth.

The nature of white enamel discolorations has been studied by means of microradiography and polarized light microscopy, as well as transmission and scanning electron microscopy (Figs 20.9, 20.10 and 12.11). Findings from these investigations indicate that the trauma interferes with enamel mineralization, while matrix formation is apparently not involved (1, 129) (Fig. 20.10). An experimental study in

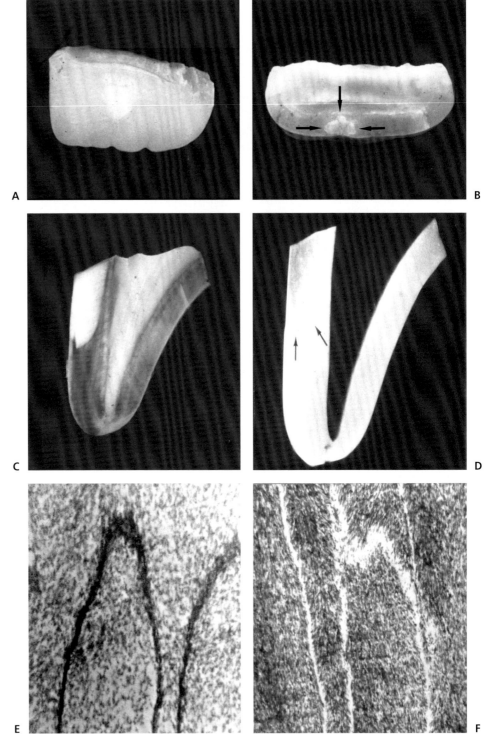

**Fig. 20.10** White enamel discoloration affecting the left central permanent incisor secondary to a dental injury at the age of 1$^1$/$_2$ years. A. Macroscopic frontal view of specimen consisting of the incisal part of the crown. B. Axial view of the fracture surface; note the extension of the white lesion (arrows). C. Ground section of the specimen photographed in incident light. ×15. D. A microradiograph of the same section reveals that the clinical white area is less mineralized (arrows) than surrounding non-involved enamel. ×15. E. Electron micrographs of decalcified non-involved enamel. The black areas represent organic material. ×8,000. F. Electron micrograph of clinical white area; note that this area contains an increased amount of organic stroma. ×8,000. From ANDREASEN et al. (1) 1971.

monkeys indicated that these areas develop corresponding to areas where trauma has altered the reduced enamel epithelium into a flattened stratified squamous epithelium (see Chapter 2, p. 69) (127).

Radiographic examination prior to tooth eruption will usually not reveal defective mineralization. Consequently, these disturbances can only be diagnosed clinically after complete eruption (2).

## White or yellow-brown discoloration of enamel with circular enamel hypoplasia

These lesions are a more severe manifestation of trauma sustained during the formative stages of the permanent tooth germ (1, 2, 29, 46–48, 121, 128, 185, 190, 191). The typical finding in this group, which distinguishes these lesions from those in the first group, is a narrow horizontal groove which

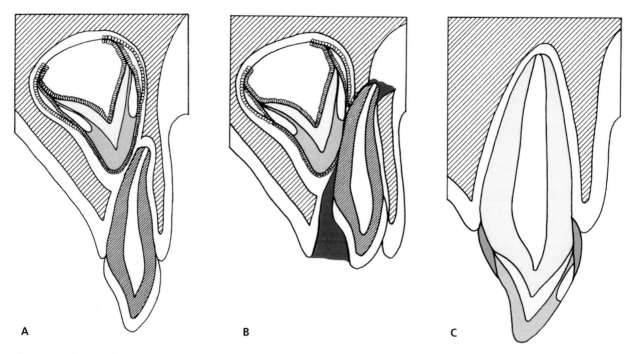

**Fig. 20.11** Schematic drawing illustrating the mechanism of white or yellow-brown discolorations of enamel. A. Condition before injury. B. Primary incisor intruded through the labial socket wall resulting in moderate damage to the reduced enamel epithelium of the permanent successor. C. As a result, enamel maturation is arrested in the area with affected enamel epithelium, creating a white or yellow-brown enamel discoloration.

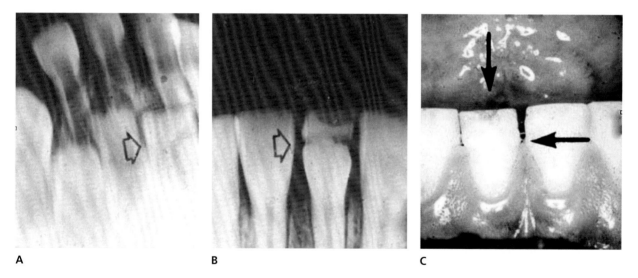

**Fig. 20.12** Discoloration and circular enamel hypoplasia of a permanent incisor following injury to the primary dentition. A. Slight intrusive luxation of left central primary incisor at the age of 1 year. Note the degree of mineralization of the permanent incisor (arrow). B. and C. Radiographic and clinical condition at the age of 12 years. Note mineralization disturbances of the incisal edge as well as the circular hypoplasia related to the part of the tooth formed at time of injury (arrow). From ANDREASEN et al. (1) 1971.

encircles the crown cervical to the discolored areas (Fig. 20.7E–H). In some cases, an external defect is found centrally in the coronally placed white or yellow-brown lesions (Fig. 20.7E).

The frequency of this type of change has been reported to be 12% following injuries to the primary dentition (2). Maxillary central incisors are usually involved; the age at the time of injury is usually 2 years. The stage of development of the permanent tooth germ varies from half to complete crown

formation at the time of injury. As a rule, the injury to the primary tooth is either avulsion, extrusive or intrusive luxation (1).

Radiographic examination of these teeth reveals a transverse radiolucent line at the level of indentation and usually a radiolucent area corresponding to the coronally placed enamel defect (Fig. 20.12). This type of developmental disturbance can usually be diagnosed before eruption (2).

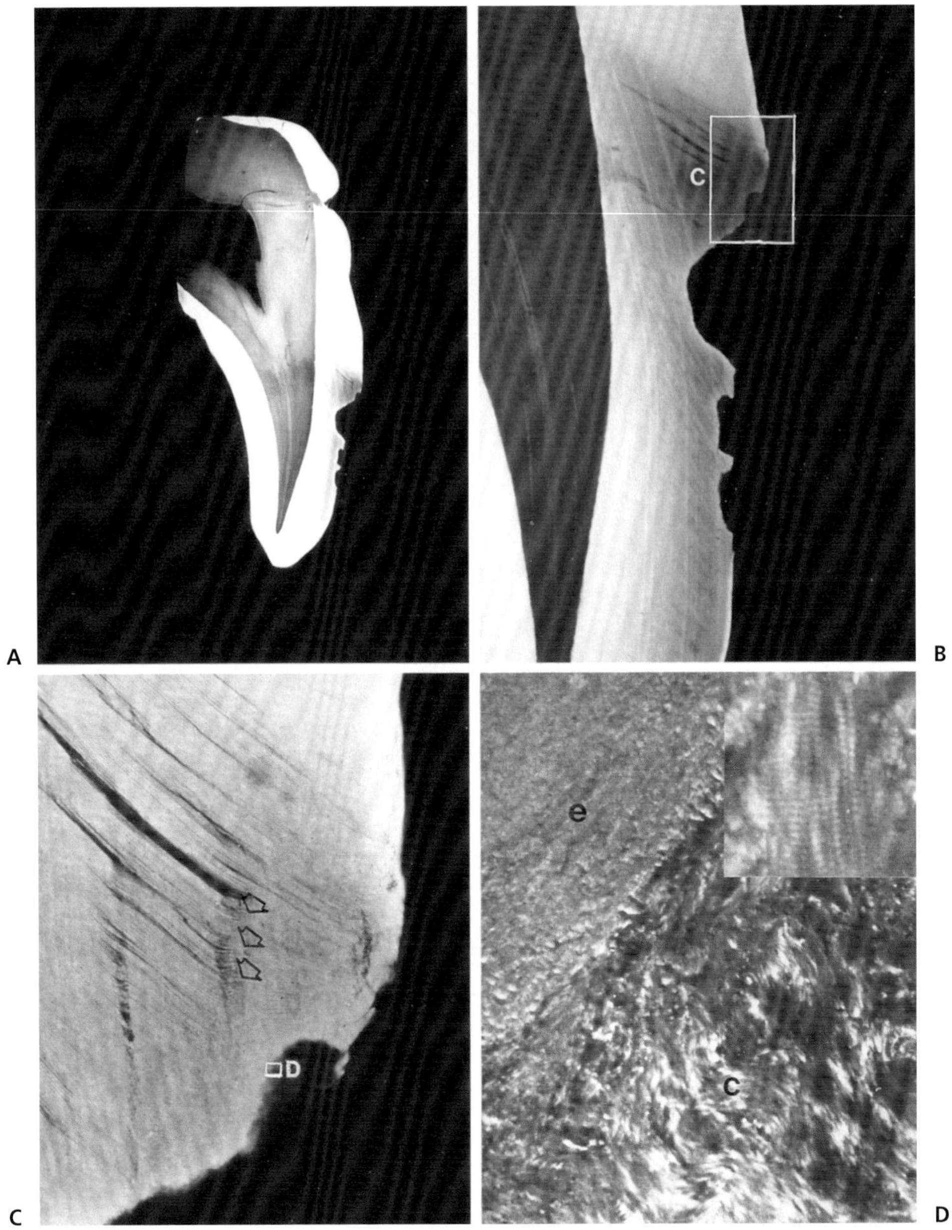

Fig.    20.13 Microradiographic and electron microscopic findings in a permanent central incisor with crown dilaceration and a yellow-brown enamel discoloration. The patient sustained intrusion of the primary incisor at the age of 2 years. A. Microradiograph of ground section. B. Higher magnification of the enamel defect. Note the radiolucency in this area, indicating a decrease in mineral content. C. Note angulation of enamel prisms (arrows), possibly the result of a direct trauma sustained during matrix formation. The scalloped external surface possibly indicates resorption before deposition of new hard tissue. D. Electron micrograph showing transition between the injured enamel in the cavity (e) and cementum-like tissue (c) deposited in the defect. ×10000. Insert, in upper right corner, a higher magnification of the cementum-like tissue showing cross-banded fibers (collagen). ×20000. From ANDREASEN et al. (1) 1971.

It should be noted that the enamel changes are confined to the site of coronal mineralization at the time of injury (Fig. 20.13). Although the pathogenesis of color changes in enamel has not yet been completely clarified, it is assumed that the displaced primary tooth traumatizes tissue adjacent to the permanent tooth germ and possibly the odontogenic epithelium, thereby interfering with final mineralization of enamel. The configuration of the resulting hypomineralized area closely coincides with the outline of normal progressive 'secondary' mineralization. The lesions are usually white; however, blood breakdown products in the traumatized area can seep into areas of mineralization during further enamel formation. This could explain why yellow-brown areas are located exclusively apical to the white lesions (1) (Fig. 20.7 B). Surface defects in the enamel most probably reflect direct injury to the enamel matrix before mineralization has been completed (Figs 20.13 and 20.14).

Experiments in monkeys have shown that circular enamel hypoplasia represents localized damage to the ameloblasts in their formative stages due to traumatic displacement of already formed hard tissue in relation to the developing soft tissues (127) (Figs 20.15 and 20.16).

## Crown dilaceration

These malformations are due to traumatic non-axial displacement of already formed hard tissue in relation to the developing soft tissues (1, 2, 17, 27, 31, 49–77, 142–145, 161, 162, 178). Three per cent of the injuries to primary teeth result in this type of malformation (2).

Due to their close contact to the primary incisors, crown-dilacerated teeth are usually maxillary or mandibular central incisors (1, 192–194). Approximately half of these teeth become impacted, whereas the remaining erupt normally or

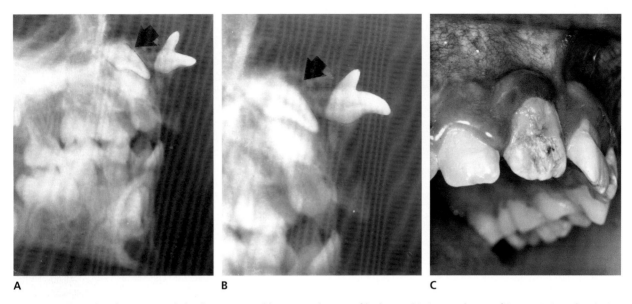

**Fig. 20.14** Severe disturbances in tooth development caused by intrusive luxation of both central incisors at the age of 3 years. A. Lateral projection showing displaced primary incisors (arrow). B. Enlarged view of A. Note that one of the displaced teeth (the right central incisor) faces the facial surface of the permanent tooth germ (arrow). C. Clinical view after surgical exposure and orthodontic realignment of right permanent central incisor. Note the hypoplastic enamel corresponding to previous trauma region (see also Fig. 20.7, G and H). From ANDREASEN et al. (1) 1971.

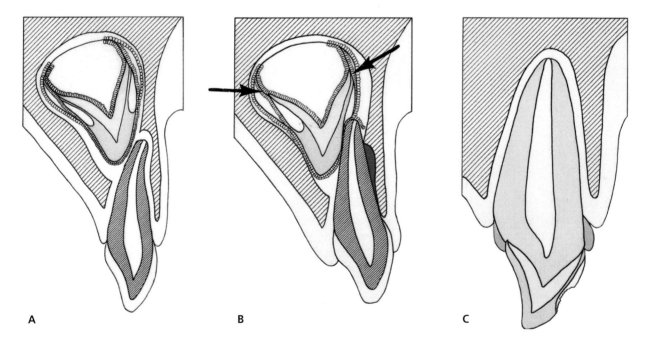

**Fig. 20.15** Schematic drawing illustrating the possible mechanism of enamel discoloration and circular enamel hypoplasia. A. Condition before injury. B. Slight axial dislocation of the already formed part of the tooth in relation to the remaining tooth germ. C. While enamel formation is resumed apical to the site of dislocation from the intact cervical loops, no further enamel formation occurs coronal to this level. Thus, a horizontal indentation is created between enamel formed before and after injury. From ANDREASEN et al. (1) 1971.

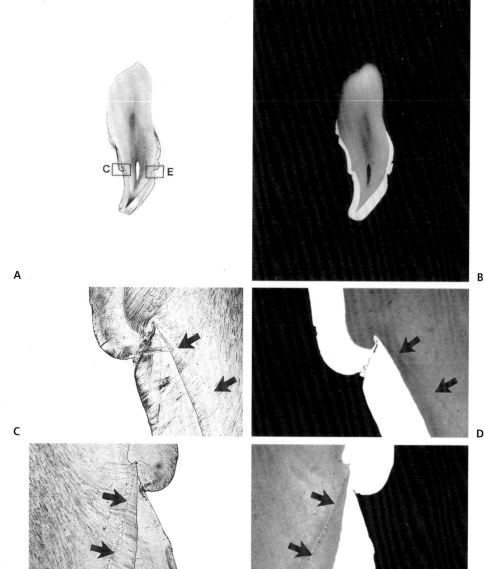

**Fig. 20.16** Yellow-brown discoloration of enamel and circular enamel hypoplasia of a maxillary lateral incisor as a result of avulsion of the primary predecessor at the age of 3 years. A. Ground section of extracted incisor. ×3. B. Microradiograph of the same section. ×3. C. and D. Higher magnification of lingual surface of the crown. Note a slight axial displacement and the calcio-traumatic line in the dentin revealing disturbance in dentin formation immediately after injury (arrows). ×30. E. and F. Higher magnification of facial surface of the crown. The same findings are present in this area as described above. ×30. From ANDREASEN et al. (1) 1971.

in facio- or linguo-version. Injury to the primary dentition usually occurs at the age of 2 years, with a range of from less than 1 year to 5 years. Most often the injury occurs at a time when up to half the crown has been formed, a finding possibly related to the anatomy of the developing tooth germ which allows tilting of the tooth germ within its socket. The trauma to the primary dentition which can result in crown dilaceration is usually avulsion or intrusion (1).

The pathology of crown-dilacerated teeth supports the theory of displacement of the enamel epithelium and the mineralized portion of the tooth in relation to the dental papilla and cervical loops (1, 73–77) (Figs 20.17 to 20.19). This results in the loss of enamel on a part of the facial surface of the crown. On the lingual aspect, a cone of hard tissue is formed which projects into the root canal, while the lingual cervical loop forms an enamel-covered cusp (1). A

pathogenesis of displacement of the non-mineralized portion of the tooth in the socket is supported by radiographic findings immediately after injury where a tilting of the tooth germ can be seen (see Chapter 19, p. 531).

The deviation of the coronal portion varies according to the tooth's location. Maxillary incisors usually show lingual deviation, while lower incisors are usually inclined facially (1).

Radiographically, unerupted crown-dilacerated teeth are seen as foreshortened coronally.

## Odontoma-like malformations

These malformations are rare sequelae to injuries in the primary dentition. Reported cases are confined primarily to

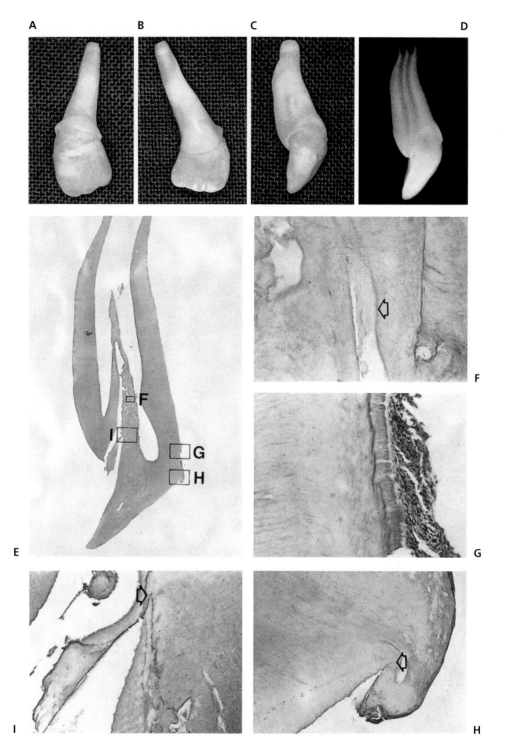

**Fig. 20.17** Clinical, radiographic, and histologic features of a crown dilacerated maxillary central incisor. The patient sustained intrusive luxation of the corresponding primary incisor at the age of $2^{1}/_{2}$ years. A to C. Clinical appearance of extracted incisor. Note area on the facial surface of the crown without enamel and the white and yellow-brown discoloration of the enamel. D. A radiograph discloses an internal cone of hard tissue. E. Low power view of sectioned incisor. ×4. F. Internal hard tissue cone consisting of enamel matrix (arrow) and dentin. ×195. G. Enamel-free crown area covered with cementum. ×195. H and I. Dilaceration area facially and lingually. Arrows indicate the margins of hard tissue formed at the time of injury. ×75. From ANDREASEN et al. (1) 1971.

maxillary incisors (1, 29, 35, 51, 55, 68, 78–81, 161, 162, 201). The age at the time of injury ranges from less than 1 year to 3 years. The type of injury affecting the primary dentition appears to be intrusive luxation or avulsion (1) (Fig. 20.20). The histology and radiology of these cases show a conglomerate of hard tissue, having the morphology of a complex odontoma or separate tooth elements (Figs 20.21 to 20.23). Experimental evidence supports the theory that these malformations occur during early phases of odontogenesis and affect the morphogenetic stages of ameloblastic

development (4, 5, 10, 82) (Figs 20.22 and 20.23). The traumatic origin of these malformations is further supported by the observation that similar changes have been reported after ritual extractions of primary canines in peoples in Africa (83) (Fig. 20.24), as well as sequelae to extraction of primary molars due to pulpal complications (24).

Radiographically there is a radio-opaque mass with little resemblance to a tooth germ. Sometimes, however, a relatively normal root may be seen (Fig. 20.22). Fig. 20.25 illustrates the possible mechanism of formation.

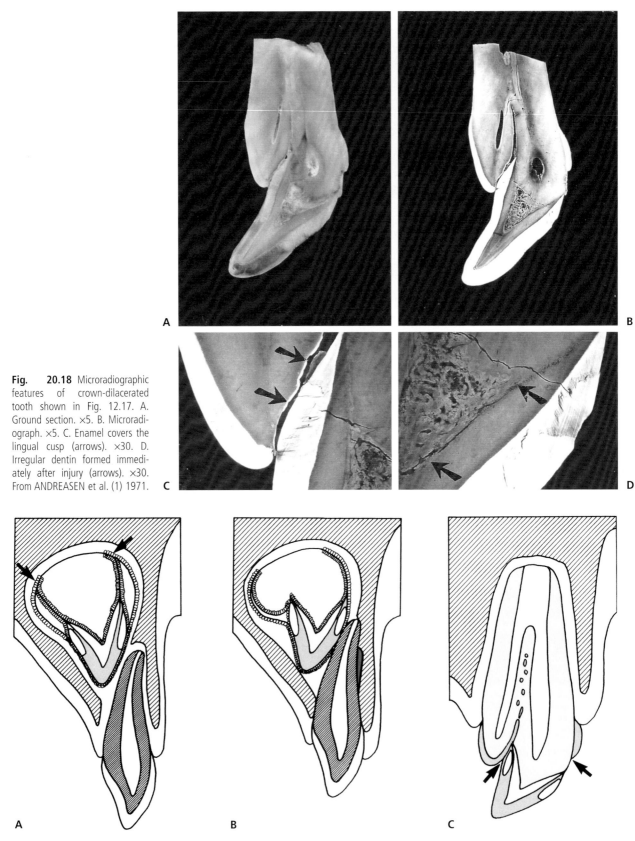

**Fig. 20.18** Microradiographic features of crown-dilacerated tooth shown in Fig. 12.17. A. Ground section. ×5. B. Microradiograph. ×5. C. Enamel covers the lingual cusp (arrows). ×30. D. Irregular dentin formed immediately after injury (arrows). ×30. From ANDREASEN et al. (1) 1971.

**Fig. 20.19** Schematic drawing illustrating the possible mechanism of crown dilaceration. A. Condition before injury (arrows indicate the cervical loops). B and C. Non-axial dislocation of the already formed part of the tooth in relation to the dental papilla, inner and outer dental epithelium and the cervical loops. Facially, the stretched inner enamel epithelium is able to induce differentiation of new odontoblasts, but its enamel forming capacity is not expressed. Consequently, a horizontal band of dentin will be left without enamel facially. The facial cervical loop has either not been injured or has been completely regenerated, thus explaining normal amelogenesis apical to the trauma site (arrow). On the lingual aspect of the crown, the displaced inner enamel epithelium and ameloblasts form a cone of hard tissue projecting into the pulp canal. Presumably the ameloblasts stripped from their matrix proliferate and induce dentin as well as enamel matrix formation. The presumably intact lingual cervical loop forms an enamel-covered cusp (arrow). From ANDREASEN et al. (1) 1971.

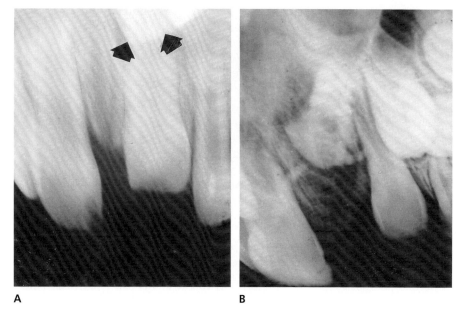

**Fig. 20.20** Odontoma-like malformation of permanent tooth germ due to intrusive luxation of primary left central incisor at the age of 2 years. A. Condition at time of injury. Note the outline of the calcified portion of the permanent tooth germ (arrows). B. Radiograph taken at the age of 8 years. An odontoma-like malformation is found at the site of the central incisor. From ANDREASEN et al. (1) 1971.

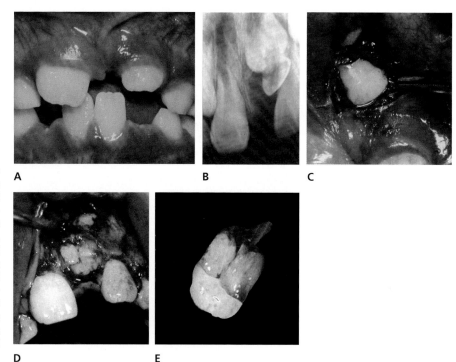

**Fig. 20.21** Odontoma-like malformation of a permanent tooth germ due to intrusive luxation of primary left central incisor at the age of 8 months. A. Clinical condition at the age of 8 years. The left central incisor has not erupted. B. The radiograph reveals intrusion and ankylosis of the primary incisor. An odontoma-like malformation is found at the site of the central incisor. C. Surgical removal of the ankylosed primary tooth. D. and E. Surgical removal of the permanent incisor which shows severe malformation. Frontal view of removed odontoma.

## Root duplication

This is a rare occurrence, seen following intrusive luxation of primary teeth (1, 84, 85, 173, 192). This complication is usually the result of an injury at the time when half or less than half of the crown is formed (1) (Fig. 20.26). The pathology of these cases indicates that a traumatic division of the cervical loop occurs at the time of injury, resulting in the formation of two separate roots (84) (Fig. 20.27).

Radiographically, a mesial and distal root can be demonstrated which extends from a partially formed crown (Figs 20.26 and 20.27).

## Vestibular root angulation

This developmental disturbance appears as a marked curvature confined to the root as a result of an injury sustained at the age of 2 to 5 years (1, 25, 30, 31, 71, 75, 86–96). The malformed tooth is usually impacted and the crown palpable in the labial sulcus. The only teeth demonstrating this malformation are maxillary central incisors. The injuries to the primary dentition consist of intrusive luxation and avulsion (1).

The histopathologic findings in these cases consist of a thickening of cementum in the area of angulation, but with

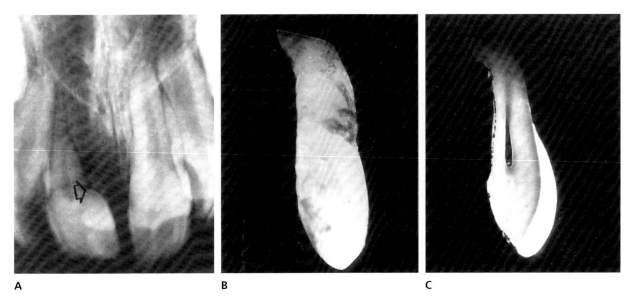

**Fig. 20.22** Development of a separate tooth element following intrusive luxation of primary incisors at the age of 3 years. A. Radiographic condition at the age of 8 years. Note the small tooth element in the central incisor region (arrow). B. Lateral view of removed odontoma. C. Microradiograph reveals an enamel layer covering part of the tooth element. From ANDREASEN et al. (1) 1971.

**Fig. 20.23** Odontoma-like malformation of a permanent lateral incisor following avulsion of the primary lateral incisor at the age of 2 years. A. Left central incisor shows a marked crown dilaceration (arrow). B. Radiograph revealing odontoma-like malformation of left lateral incisor (arrow). C. Low power view of sectioned lateral incisor. ×7. D. Apical part of the odontoma bears similarities to a normal root. Note intact odontoblast layer. ×75. E. Odontoma-like enamel inclusions – most of the enamel was lost during demineralization. ×75. F. Reduced enamel epithelium. ×195. G and H. Preserved enamel matrix. ×75. From ANDREASEN et al. (1) 1971.

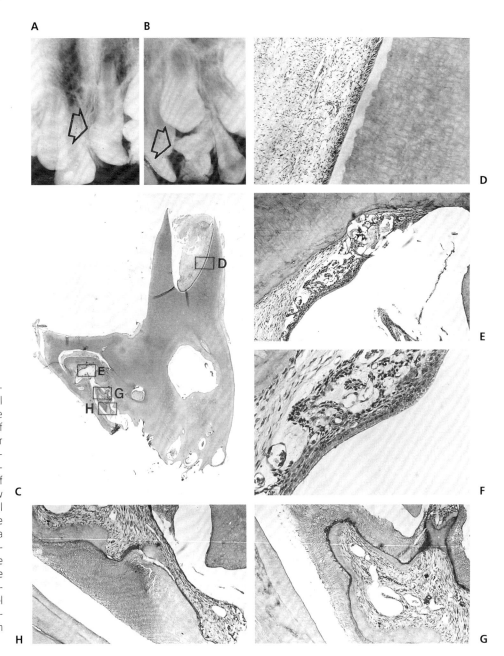

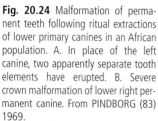

**Fig. 20.24** Malformation of permanent teeth following ritual extractions of lower primary canines in an African population. A. In place of the left canine, two apparently separate tooth elements have erupted. B. Severe crown malformation of lower right permanent canine. From PINDBORG (83) 1969.

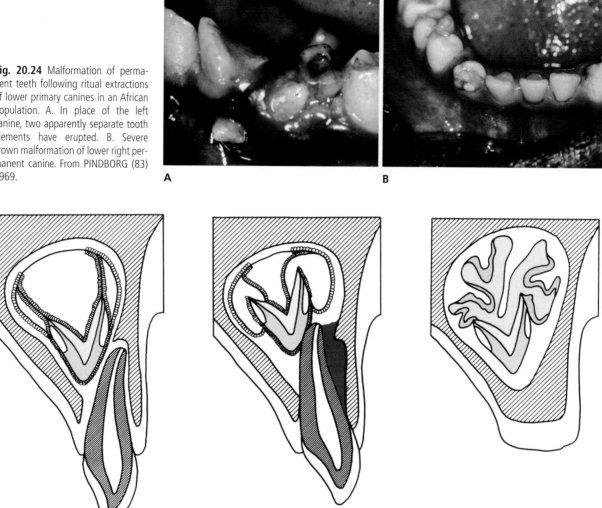

A   B   C

**Fig. 20.25** Schematic drawing illustrating possible mechanism for odontoma-like malformation. A. Condition before injury. B. Axial dislocation of the primary incisor with extensive damage to the permanent tooth germ. C. Formation of an odontoma-like malformation.

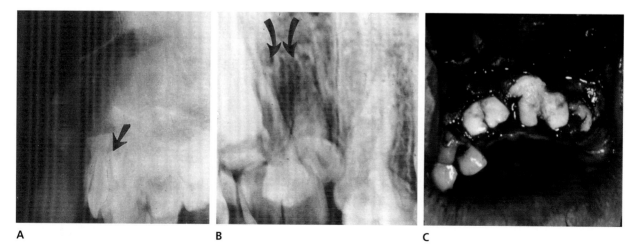

A   B   C

**Fig. 20.26** Root duplication of 2 central incisors following intrusive luxation of both primary incisors at the age of 2 years. A. Lateral radiograph at time of injury. Note the displaced primary incisors (arrow). B. Radiograph taken at the age of 9 years. The root is divided into a mesial and distal portion in both incisors (arrows). C. After surgical exposure, abnormal root development is evident as well as vertical fractures of the crown of both central incisors (arrows), presumably a result of the previous injury.

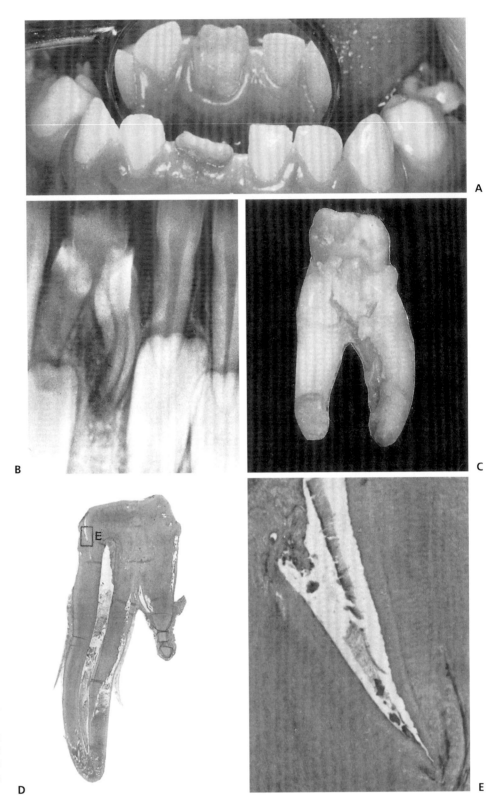

**Fig. 20.27** Histologic features of root duplication of a right permanent central incisor due to an injury sustained at the age of 6 months. A. Clinical appearance. B. Radiograph showing root division. C. Frontal aspect of the extracted tooth. D. Low power view of sectioned incisor. E. Higher magnification of D indicates that the incisal part of the crown has been intruded. The cleft is lined with enamel. The dentinal tubules are compressed at the bottom of the cleft. From EDLUND (84) 1964.

no sign of acute traumatic changes in the hard tissue formed (1, 75, 87) (Fig. 20.28). The loss of a primary incisor can present an obstacle in the eruption of the developing tooth, forcing it to change its path of eruption in a labial direction (Figs 20.28, 20.29). Presumably Hertwig's epithelial root sheath remains in position despite the impact and thereby creates a curvature of the root (1). It should be mentioned,

however, that the traumatic origin of this malformation has been questioned. Thus, in a study of 29 teeth, Stewart (146) found no history of trauma. Moreover, this type of malformation was 6 times more frequent in girls than in boys. According to Stewart, the most likely explanation for facial root angulation was ectopic development of the tooth germ (146).

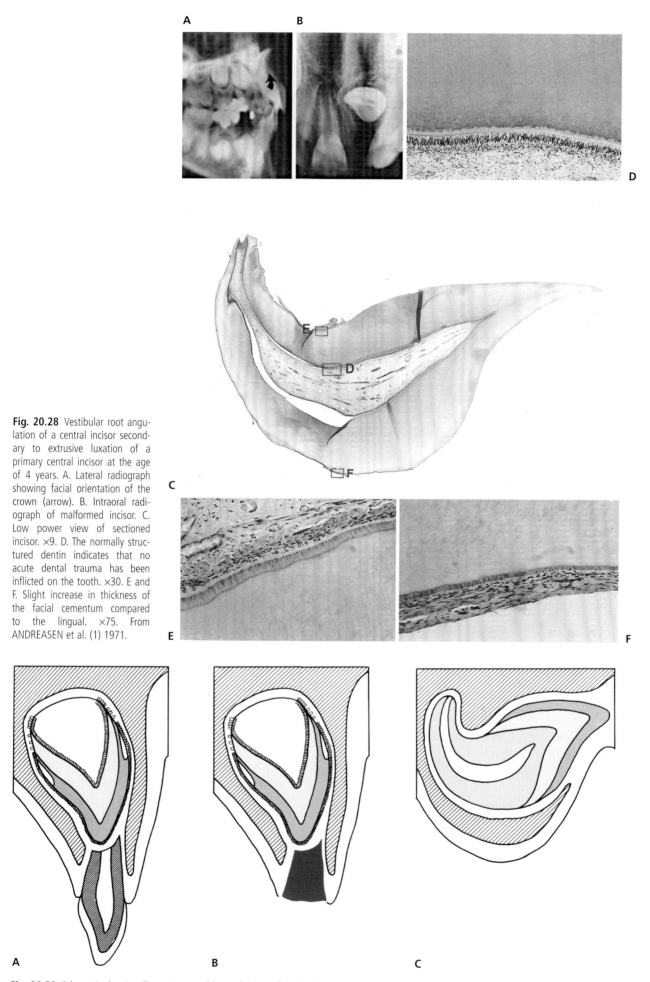

**Fig. 20.28** Vestibular root angulation of a central incisor secondary to extrusive luxation of a primary central incisor at the age of 4 years. A. Lateral radiograph showing facial orientation of the crown (arrow). B. Intraoral radiograph of malformed incisor. C. Low power view of sectioned incisor. ×9. D. The normally structured dentin indicates that no acute dental trauma has been inflicted on the tooth. ×30. E and F. Slight increase in thickness of the facial cementum compared to the lingual. ×75. From ANDREASEN et al. (1) 1971.

**Fig. 20.29** Schematic drawing illustrating possible mechanism of vestibular root angulation. A. Condition before injury. B. Primary incisor lost at an early age. C. Possibly due to formation of scar tissue along the path of eruption, the developing tooth changes its position facially.

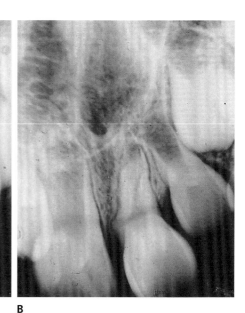

**Fig. 20.30** Lateral root angulation as a result of avulsion of left primary lateral and central incisors at the age of 5 years. A. Condition after injury. Note that root development of the central incisors has just started. B. Radiograph taken at the age of 7 years reveals angulation between the root and crown portion. From ANDREASEN et al. (1) 1971.

**A**                    **B**

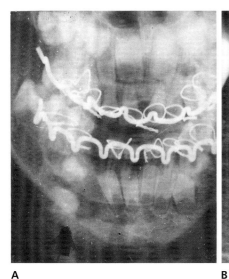
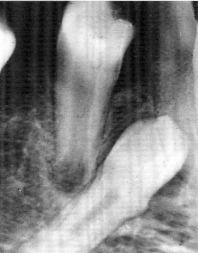
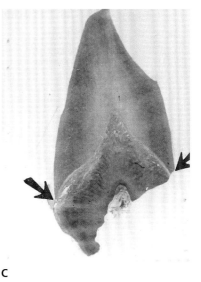

**A**                    **B**                    **C**

**Fig. 20.31** Slight root dilaceration and impaction of a right canine after jaw fracture sustained at the age of 5 years. A. Radiograph taken 5 days after the injury. Note displacement of the developing canine (arrow). B. Condition 9 years later. Note that the impacted and dislocated canine shows slight root dilaceration. C. Histologic examination of the coronal part of the canine. The dilaceration is clearly visible (arrows). From LENSTRUP (19) 1955.

Radiographically a root-angulated tooth appears fore-shortened. Lateral projections can more precisely localize the position of the tooth within the jaw (Fig. 20.28).

## Lateral root angulation or dilaceration

These changes appear as a mesial or distal bending confined to the root of the tooth (29, 30, 52, 55, 71, 77, 78, 86, 94, 98, 147, 161, 195, 201) (Fig. 20.30). They are seen in 1% of cases with injury to the primary dentition, usually avulsion. The injury usually occurs at age 2 to 7 years and usually affects the maxillary incisors. In contrast to vestibular angulation, most teeth with lateral root angulation or dilaceration erupt spontaneously (1). Similar malformations have been seen in developing teeth involved in jaw fractures (15, 18–21, 99, 100, 148) (Fig. 20.31).

The pathogenesis of these lesions is not fully understood, but histologic studies have shown that displacement apparently occurs between the mineralized root portion and the developing soft tissues (19, 77) (Fig. 20.31).

## Partial or complete arrest of root formation

This is a rare complication among injuries in the primary dentition, affecting 2% of involved permanent teeth (1, 2, 29, 69, 71, 86, 101–107, 161, 162, 195, 196) (Figs 20.32–20.37). The injury to the primary dentition usually occurs between 5 and 7 years of age and normally affects maxillary incisors. The injury sustained is usually avulsion of the primary incisors (1). A number of teeth with this type of root malformation remain impacted, while others erupt precociously and are often exfoliated due to inadequate peri-

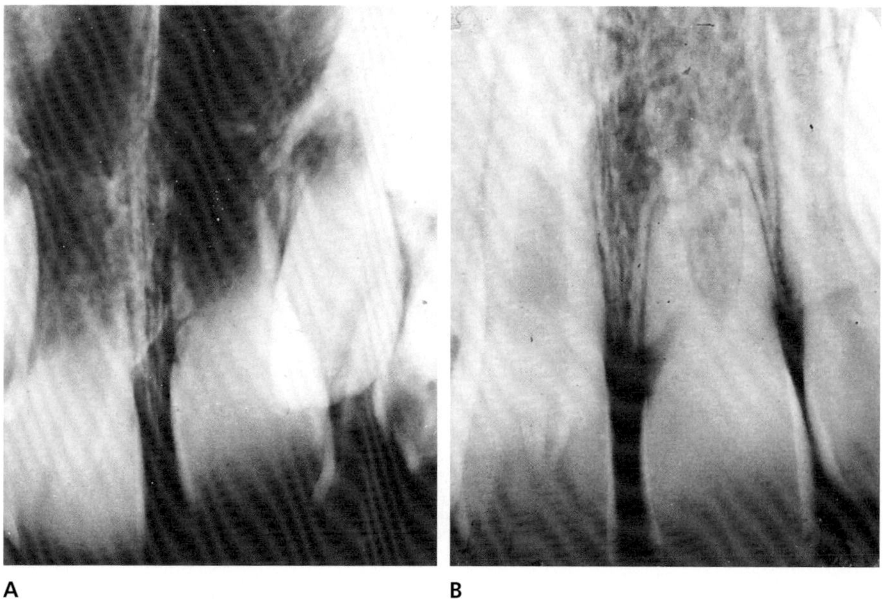

**Fig. 20.32** Complete arrest of root formation following avulsion of a left primary central incisor at the age of 5 years. A. Radiograph at time of injury. B. Condition at the age of 7 years. Note complete arrest of root development, invasion of bone into the root canal and development of an internal periodontal ligament. From ANDREASEN et al. (1) 1971.

A

B

A

B

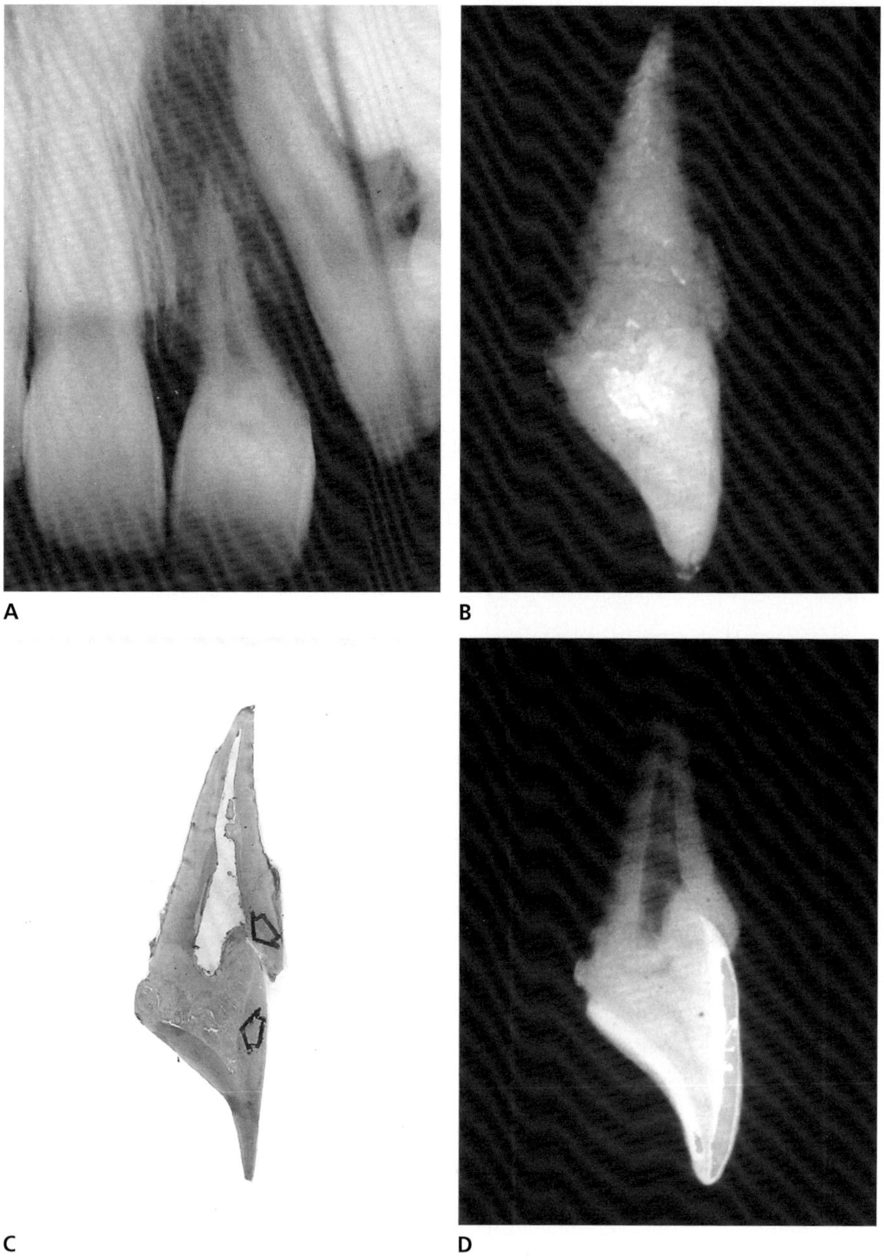

**Fig. 20.33** Partial arrest of root formation of an upper left central incisor. The patient sustained an injury to the primary dentition at the age of 5 years. A. Radiographic examination at the age of 8 years shows a secondary pulp necrosis and a periapical radiolucency. Pulp necrosis was possibly induced by bacterial invasion through the poorly mineralized tissue formed immediately following injury. B. Mesial view of extracted incisor. C. Low power view of sectioned incisor. A slight dilaceration and a marked calcio-traumatic line with poorly mineralized tissue (arrows) indicate that an acute injury has occurred during odontogenesis. ×3. D. Microradiograph of the sectioned tooth. From ANDREASEN et al. (1) 1971.

C

D

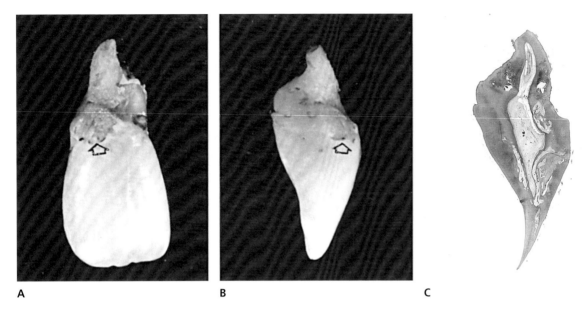

A                              B                              C

**Fig. 20.34** Partial arrest of root formation of a right central incisor. The patient sustained luxation injury of both primary central incisors at the age of 5 years. A and B. Frontal and lateral views of extracted incisor. A small resorption cavity is evident cervically (arrows) possibly inflicted by previous surgical exposure of the impacted tooth. C. Low-power view of sectioned incisor. Apart from peripheral root resorption there is no evidence of acute injury. ×5. From ANDREASEN et al. (1) 1971.

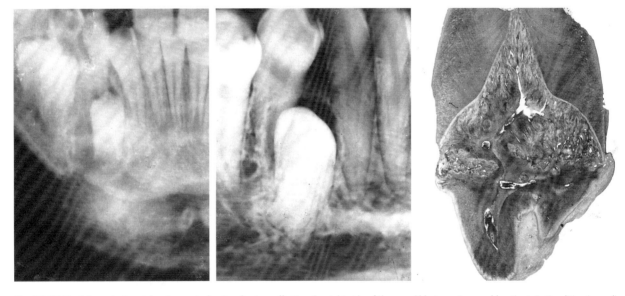

**Fig. 20.35** Partial arrest of root development after jaw fracture affecting the right side of the mandible in an 8-year-old patient. A. Condition immediately after injury. B. Six years later. The canine is impacted with a partial arrest of root development. C. Histologic examination of the removed canine. Note sharp demarcation between pre- and post-traumatic hard tissue formation. ×8. From LENSTRUP (19) 1955.

odontal support. Similar root abnormalities have been found in developing teeth involved in jaw fractures (15, 18, 19, 99, 108–111).

The histopathology of root malformation varies. Some cases show diminutive root development without evidence of a previous acute traumatic episode during hard tissue deposition (1, 106, 107) (Fig. 20.33). Scar tissue developing after premature loss of the primary predecessor has been thought to prevent normal eruption and also to interfere with root formation (1). In other instances, a typical calciotraumatic line, separating hard tissue formed before and after injury, is seen (1, 19, 103, 112) (Figs 20.34 and 20.35). In these cases, the trauma has

apparently directly injured Hertwig's epithelial root sheath, thus compromising normal root development (Fig. 20.36).

Radiographic examination reveals typical foreshortening of the root. Root resorption may also be seen with this type of root abnormality (19, 108, 111) (Fig. 20.37).

## Sequestration of permanent tooth germs – dentigerous cyst

This is exceedingly rare after injuries to the primary dentition (71, 92, 161) (Figs 20.38 and 20.39). Infection can complicate healing of jaw fractures. In these instances, swelling, suppuration and fistula formation are typical clinical

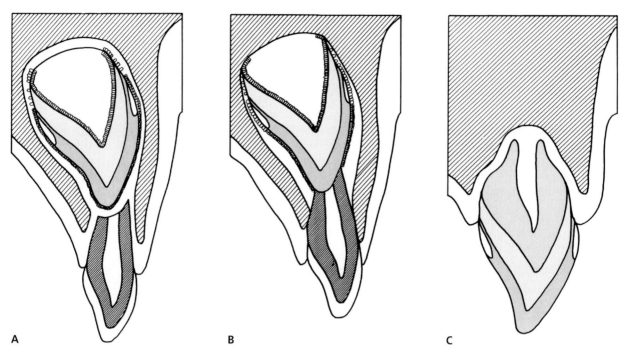

**Fig. 20.36** Schematic drawing illustrating mechanism of partial arrest of root formation. A. Condition before injury. B. The impact from the intruded primary incisor is transmitted to the permanent incisor with subsequent damage to the Hertwig's epithelial root sheath. C. Partial arrest of root formation.

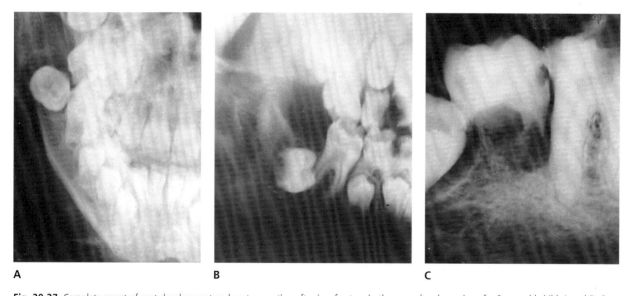

**Fig. 20.37** Complete arrest of root development and root resorption after jaw fracture in the second molar region of a 9-year-old child. A and B. Condition immediately after trauma. The developing second molar is displaced. C. Condition 7 years later. The second molar has erupted; however, there is a complete arrest of root development and root resorption. From LENSTRUP (19) 1955.

features, sometimes leading to spontaneous sequestration of involved tooth germs (18, 100, 111, 113) (Fig. 20.39). Clinical cases have reported swelling of the maxilla, retained darkened primary incisors and absence of the permanent incisor. It has been hypothesized that chronic periapical inflammation of injured primary incisors may stimulate proliferation of the reduced enamel epithelium of the adjacent developing tooth germ, leading to a follicular cyst (182, 197, 198).

Radiographic examination discloses osteolytic changes around the tooth germ, including disappearance of the outline of the dental crypt and expanded cortical alveolar bone (Figs 20.38 and 20.39).

## Disturbances in eruption

Disturbances in permanent tooth eruption may occur after trauma to the primary dentition and it is suggested that this is related to abnormal changes in the connective tissue overlying the tooth germ (149). The eruption of succeeding permanent incisors is generally delayed for about 1 year after premature loss of primary incisors (114, 115),

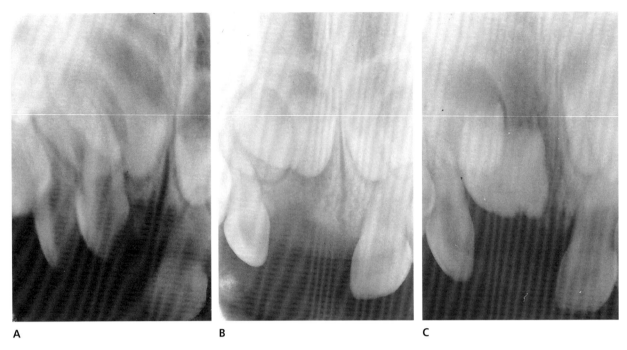

**Fig. 20.38** Sequestration of a permanent central incisor tooth germ in a 1¹/₂-year-old child. A. Radiographic examination at the time of injury reveals intrusion of the right primary central incisor. The primary incisor was removed 2 weeks later due to acute inflammation and a labial abscess. B. A chronic fistula appeared in the region 2 months later. Antibiotic therapy was instituted and the fistula disappeared. However, upon withdrawal of antibiotics, the fistula returned. C. Radiographic condition after 6 months. Note the osteolytic changes around the permanent tooth germ. At this time, the tooth germ was removed. Courtesy of Dr. H. ECHERBOM, Luleå, Sweden.

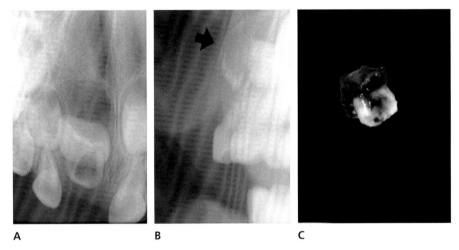

**Fig. 20.39** Sequestration of a permanent cental incisor tooth germ in a 4-year-old child. The girl fell from her cradle at the age of 6 month and expirienced another fall at the age of 2 years. A. Radiographic examination at the time she sought treatment (4 year old) reveals osteolytic changes around the permanent tooth germ. B. The lateral radiograph discloses an expansion of the cortical alveolar bone and a large radiolucency area surrounding the tooth grem. Note the expanded bone causing upper lip deformity. C. The central incisor was removed under general anesthesia. The removed tooth was included in a dentigerous cyst.

whereas premature eruption of permanent successors is rare (69, 71). Early loss of primary incisors (avulsion or extraction) leads to space loss only in rare instances (158, 162, 199). However, ectopic eruption of permanent successors has been seen, possibly due to lack of eruption guidance otherwise offered by the primary dentition (158). These teeth often erupt labially (162). Impaction is very common among teeth with malformations confined to either the crown or root (1, 116, 195). When the permanent tooth does erupt, it is often in facio- or linguoversion (114, 115, 150).

## Treatment

Minor white or yellow-brown discolorations of enamel seldom require treatment. However, if the enamel changes are esthetically disturbing, recently developed techniques for enamel microabrasion have been suggested (174–177) (Fig. 20.40). This implies application of an 18% hydrochloric acid-pumice paste to the isolated enamel surfaces for a series of, for example, 6–8 sequential 5-sec rubbing applications

**Fig. 20.40 Microabrasion of a tooth with superficial enamel discoloration**

A central incisor with multicolored superficial enamel defects is shown on the left. Immediately after enamel microabrasion (right), the discoloration is eliminated. Courtesy of Dr. T. P. CROLL, Doyletown, USA.

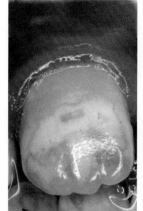 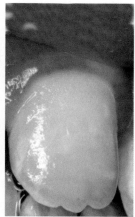

**Microabrasion of trauma-induced enamel discolorations**

The enamel changes consist of opaque white and yellow color changes.

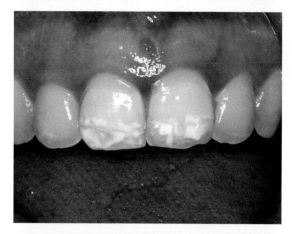 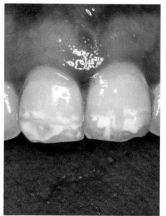

**Enamel abrasion**

Both central incisors are isolated with a rubber dam and enamel abrasion carried out with hydrochloric acid pumice mixture, a mandrel tip and a hand applicator.

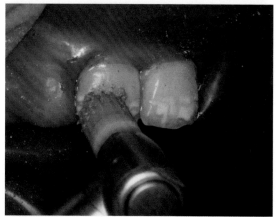 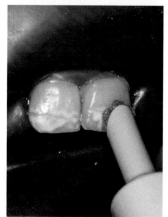

**Condition after enamel abrasion**

The enamel changes are markedly accentuated compared to the status before enamel abrasion.

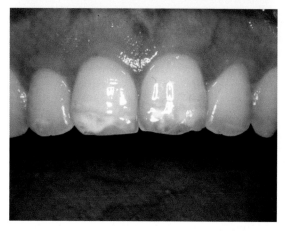 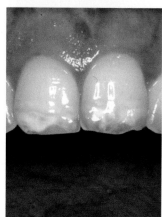

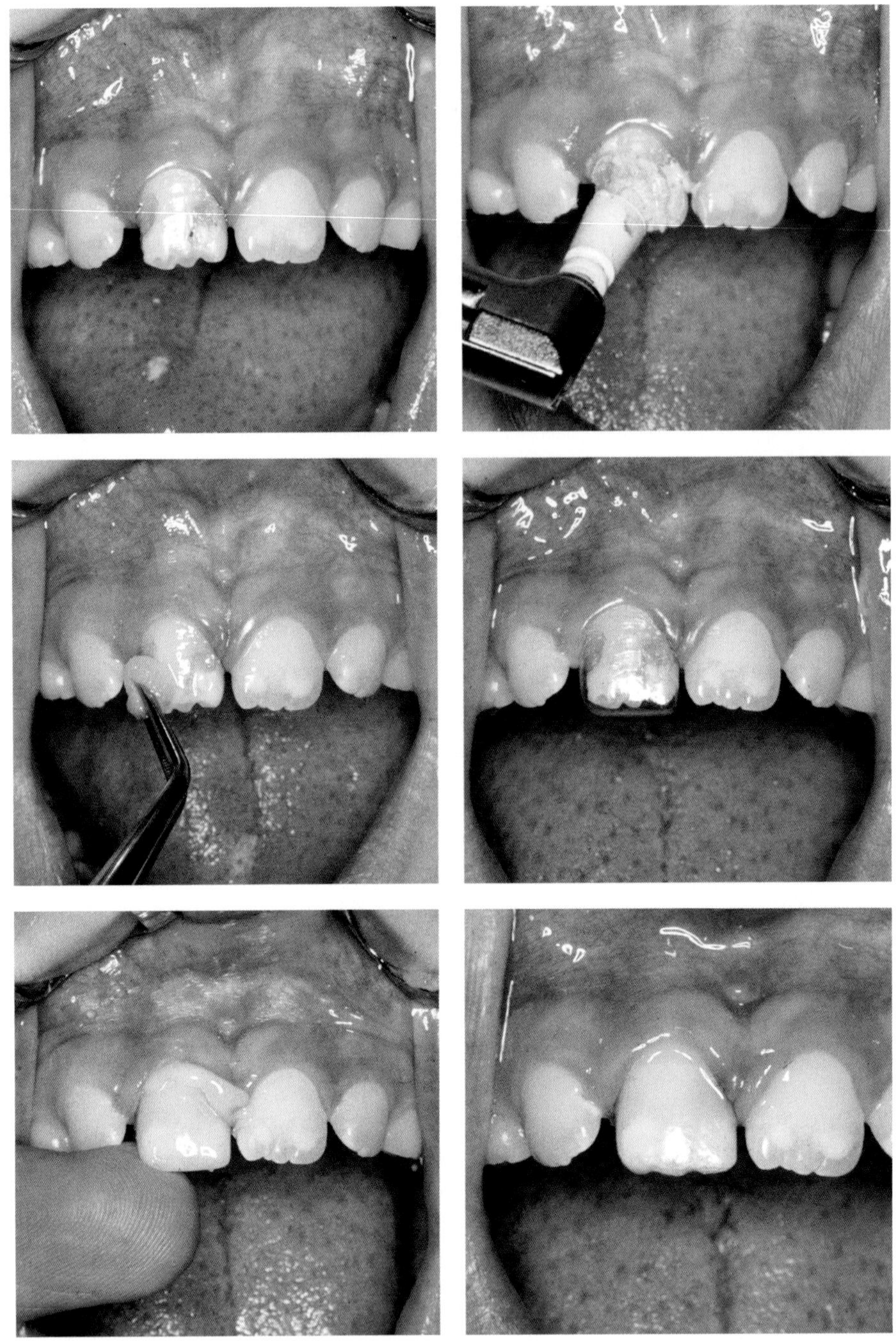

**Fig. 20.41** Restoration of a right central incisor with yellow-brown discolored enamel with composite resin. A. Clinical condition. B. Cleansing the enamel with pumice followed by a bur. C. Etching the enamel. D and E. A celluloid crown form is used as a matrix for the composite resin. F. The finished restoration.

with 10-sec interim water rinsings. This treatment is followed by a 4-min application of 2% sodium fluoride gel and polishing with abrasives when necessary.

It has been found experimentally on extracted teeth with intact enamel surfaces, that such a procedure removes 12 μm enamel initially and 26 μm with successive applications (177), but that the amount of enamel which was lost was clinically undetectable (175). Unfortunately most enamel discolorations due to trauma penetrate the entire enamel thickness (1) (Figs 20.10, 20.13 and 20.19). This fact explains why this technique does not work satisfactorily in trauma-related enamel discoloration and may sometimes even accentuate these discolorations (Fig. 20.40).

Treatment of white or yellow-brown discoloration of enamel with circular enamel hypoplasia implies removal of the discolored enamel with a bur, etching with an acid conditioner and restoration with a composite resin (151–156) (Fig. 20.41).

When discoloration and enamel defects occupy most of the labial surface, a porcelain jacket crown or laminate veneer can be indicated (117, 118).

Crown dilacerated teeth often erupt spontaneously into normal position. In some cases, surgical exposure of the crown is necessary (Fig. 20.42). Because of the severity of the malposition, surgical exposure sometimes must be supplemented with orthodontic realignment (178, 179) (Chapter 24, p. 694).

When the tooth has erupted to the level such that the dilacerated area is free of the gingiva, restorative therapy should be instituted, as the central lumen of the 'internal

**Fig. 20.42 Surgical and restorative treatment of a crown-dilacerated incisor**

The patient sustained an intrusion injury of both right primary incisors at the age of 1 year. These teeth were later removed due to pulp necrosis. The radiographic examination shows crown dilaceration of the right central incisor and enamel hypoplasia of the right lateral incisor.

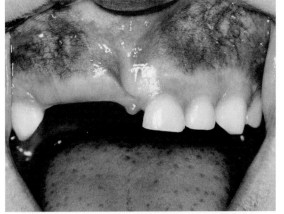
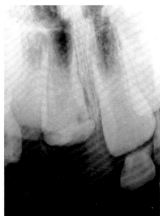

**Clinical and radiographic condition at the age of 7 years**

Eruption of the right central incisor has not taken place. Surgical exposure was therefore planned.

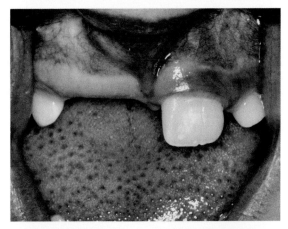
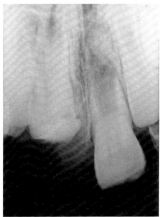

**Surgical exposure of the malformed incisors**

After administration of a local anesthesia both incisors were surgically exposed.

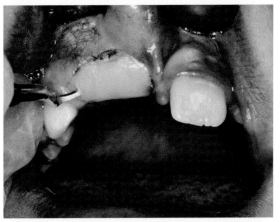
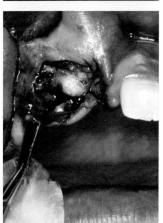

**Condition after exposure**

Two weeks after surgical exposure a new gingival collar has been formed.

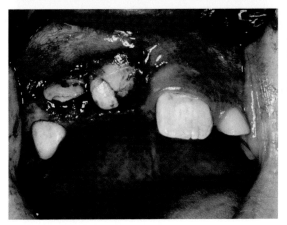
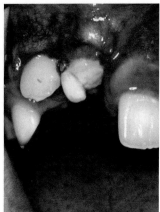

### Condition 4 months later

The incisors have further erupted and are now ready for restoration.

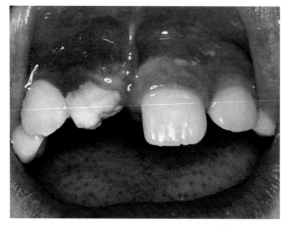
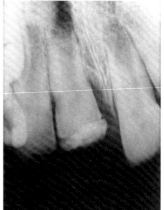

### Removing the dilacerated crown portion

After a local anesthesia the dilacerated crown portion is removed and the exposed dentin is covered with a hard-setting calcium hydroxide cement.

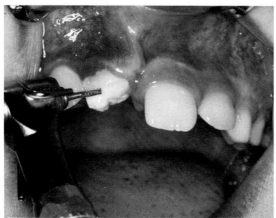
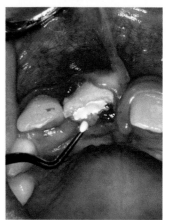

### Temporary restoration

The incisor is temporarily restored. Due to problems with moisture control the tooth was initially restored with a steel crown and later with a temporary crown and bridge material.

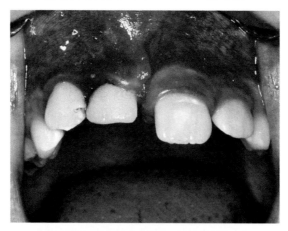
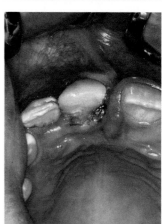

### Restoration with composite resin

As an interim restoration both incisors were restored with composite resin.

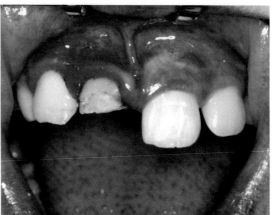
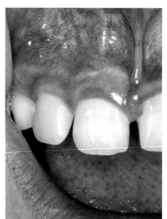

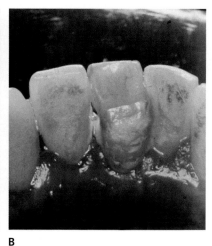
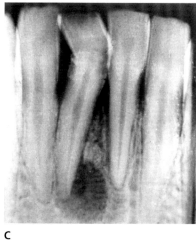

A          B          C

**Fig. 20.43** Pulp necrosis and periapical inflammation following crown dilaceration of a central incisor. A and B. Frontal and lingual view of involved incisor. C. Radiographic demonstration of pulp necrosis and periapical inflammation.

root' constitutes a pathway for bacteria into the pulp. Thus, a number of these teeth have been found to develop pulp necrosis and periapical inflammation after eruption without any evidence of decay (1, 74, 76, 136) (Fig. 20.43). It is therefore important to remove the dilacerated part of the crown as soon as possible. A temporary crown can then be placed until eruption is complete, when an acid-etch/composite resin restoration, a veneer or a cast restoration can be made (Fig. 20.42).

Malformed impacted teeth, e.g., odontoma-like malformations, teeth with root duplication, root dilaceration or angulation should generally be removed. However, future treatment needs (i.e. dental implants) might indicate their preservation in order to maintain the alveolar ridge at an acceptable height. A possible exception is vestibular root angulation. Provided there is adequate space, such teeth can be realigned by surgical exposure followed by orthodontic intervention (29, 86, 91, 119, 136) (see Chapter 24, p. 694). An alternative therapy can be extraction of the malformed tooth, resection of the angulated root portion and insertion of an apical implant (200).

Although rare, chronic periapical inflammation of injured primary teeth may lead to dentigerous cysts and spontaneous sequestration of the tooth germ. If not, they should be removed surgically (137).

In some cases, premature loss of primary teeth can lead to disturbance in eruption. Apparently the tooth germ is not able to penetrate the mucosa covering the alveolar process. In these cases, excision of the tissue overlying the incisal edge will result in rapid eruption of the impacted tooth (149, 180) (Fig. 20.44). If the teeth are impacted with their crowns inclined facially and above the mucogingival junction, it is important to know that a wide incision of nonfunctional mucosa can give rise to retraction of the gingiva. Furthermore, the gingiva is nonkeratinized and prone to periodontal disease (149) (Fig. 20.45). While this finding has been questioned in a case report (180), it is recommended that a smaller incision be made, preferably only in the functional gingiva. When the permanent tooth erupts it is often in facio- or linguoversion (Figs 20.45 and 20.46).

## Essentials

### Terminology

- White or yellow-brown discoloration of enamel
- White or yellow-brown discoloration of enamel and circular enamel hypoplasia
- Crown dilaceration
- Odontoma-like malformation
- Root duplication
- Vestibular root angulation
- Lateral root angulation or dilaceration
- Partial or complete arrest of root formation
- Sequestration of permanent tooth germ
- Disturbance in eruption

### Frequency

- Injuries to primary teeth: 12–69% of involved permanent teeth
- Jaw fractures: 19–68% of involved permanent teeth

### Pathology

- Disturbances in mineralization and morphology

### Treatment

#### Yellow-brown discoloration of enamel with or without enamel hypoplasia

- Enamel microabrasion (Fig. 20.40)
- Composite resin restoration (Fig. 20.41)
- Porcelain-fused-to-gold restoration
- Porcelain jacket crown

#### Crown dilaceration (Fig. 20.42)

- Surgical exposure and possibly orthodontic realignment
- Removal of dilacerated part of the crown
- Temporary crown until root formation is completed
- Semi- or permanent restoration

### Fig. 20.44 Surgical exposure of impacted permanent incisors

This 1-year-old girl suffered avulsion of all primary incisors due to a fall.

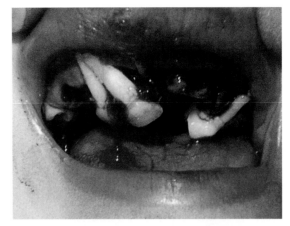
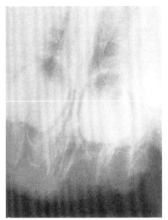

### Condition at the age of 10

There is no sign of eruption in spite of advanced root development. The incisal edges of the impacted incisors can be palpated.

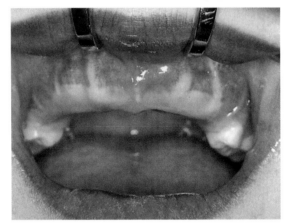
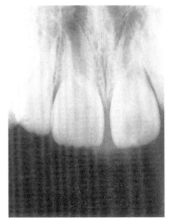

### Exposing the incisors

After administration of a local anesthesia the mucosa overlaying the incisal edges is removed with a surgical blade.

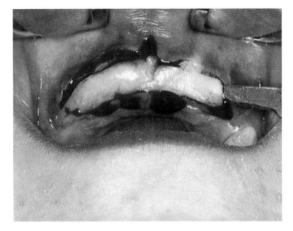
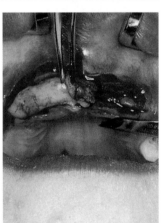

### Condition 6 months after exposure

The incisors are now fully erupted.

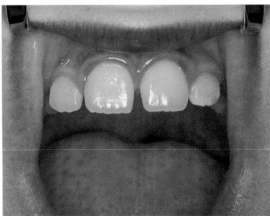
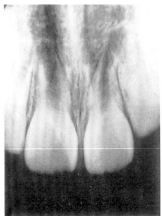

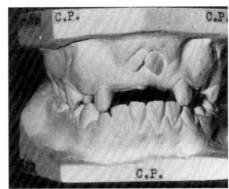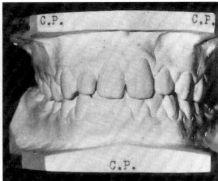

**Fig. 20.45** Gingival retraction and enlarged gingival cuffs in a patient where both central incisors were exposed above the muco-gingival junction. From DIBIASE (149) 1971.

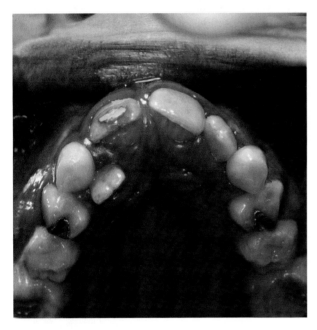

Fig 20.46 Permanent lateral incisor erupted in linguoversion.

### Vestibular root angulation

• Combined surgical and orthodontic realignment

### Other malformations

• Extraction is usually the treatment of choice

### Disturbance in eruption (Fig. 20.44)

• Surgical exposure

## References

1. ANDREASEN JO, SÜNDSTRÖM B, RAVN JJ. The effect of traumatic injuries to primary teeth on their permanent successors. 1. A clinical and histologic study of 117 injured permanent teeth. *Scand J Dent Res* 1971;**79**:219–83.
2. ANDREASEN JO, RAVN JJ. The effect of traumatic injuries to primary teeth on their permanent successors. II. A clinical and radiographic follow-up study of 213 injured teeth. *Scand J Dent Res* 1971;**79**:284–94.
3. SARNAT BG, SCHOUR I. Effect of experimental fracture on bone, dentin and enamel. Study of the mandible and the incisor in the rat. *Arch Surg* 1944;**49**:23–38.
4. SANTONÉ P. Über die Folgen von umschriebenen, traumatischen Verletzungen in Geweben der Zahnanlage. Dtsch *Zahn Mund Kieferheilk* 1937;**4**:323–37, 602–14.
5. LEVY BA. Effects of experimental trauma on developing first molar teeth in rats. *J Dent Res* 1968;**47**:323–7.
6. SCHUUR I. The effect of tooth injury on other teeth. I. The effect of a fracture confined to one or two incisors and their investing tissues upon the other incisors in the rat. *J Physiol Zool* 1934;**7**:304–29.
7. ADLOFF P. Experimentelle Untersuchungen zur Regeneration des Gebisses. *Dtsch Monatschr Zahnheilk* 1920;**38**:385–412.
8. SHAPIRO HH, LEFKOWITZ W, BODECKER CF. Role of the dental papilla in early tooth formation. Part I – Roentgenographic study. *J Dent Res* 1942;**21**:391–4.
9. LEFKOWITZ W, BODECKER CF, SHAPIRO HH. Experimental papillectomy. Part II: Histological study. (Preliminary report). *J Dent Res* 1944;**23**:345–61.
10. BRAUER W. Mechanisch erzeugte Entwicklungsstörungen des Zahnkeimes. ('Experimentelle Zahnkeimmissbildungen'.) *Dtsch Monatschr Zahnheilk* 1928;**46**:737–51.
11. BENCZE J. Zahnkeimläsionen infolge Kieferfrakturen im Tierversuch. *Stoma (Heidelberg)* 1967;**20**:165–73.
12. GREWE JM, FELTS WJL. The consequences of mandibular incisor extraction in the young mouse I. Histologic aspects. *J Dent Res* 1969;**48**:583–9.
13. ZELLNER R. Schmelzmissbildungen am permanenten Gebiss nach Milchzahnluxation. *Zahnärztl Prax* 1956;**7**:1–2.
14. SCHREIBER CK. The effect of trauma on the anterior deciduous teeth. *Br Dent J* 1959;**106**:340–3.
15. TAATZ H. Untersuchungen über Ursachen und Häufigkeit exogener Zahnkeimschäden. Dtsch *Zahn Mund Kieferheilk* 1962;**37**:468–84.
16. SELLISETH N-E. The significance of traumatised primary incisors on the development and eruption of permanent teeth. *Eur Orthodont Dent Soc* 1970;**46**:443–59.
17. RAVN JJ. Sequelae of acute mechanical traumata in the primary dentition. *ASDC J Dent Child* 1968;**35**:281–9.

18. FISCHER H-G. Traumata im jugendlichen Kieferbereich – Heilergebnisse und ihr Einfluss auf die Keime der bleibenden Zähne. Thesis, Leipzig, 1951.

19. LENSTRUP K. On injury by fractures of the jaws to teeth in course of formation. *Acta Odontol Scand* 1955;**13**:181–202.

20. BENCZE J. Spätergebnisse nach im Kindesalter erlittenen Unterkieferbrücken. *Acta Chir Acad Sci Hung* 1964;**5**:95–104.

21. BENCZE J. Zahnkeimschäden infolge Kieferfrakturen in der Jugend. *Stoma (Heidelberg)* 1964;**17**:330–5.

22. DIXON DA. Defects of structure and formation of the teeth in persons with cleft palate and the effect of reparative surgery on the dental tissues. *Oral Surg Oral Med Oral Pathol* 1968;**25**:435–46.

23. MINK JR. Relationship of hypoplastic teeth and surgical trauma in cleft repair. *J Dent Res* 1959;**38**:652–3.

24. WILLIAMSON JJ. Trauma during exodontia. An aetiologic factor in hypoplastic premolars. *Br Dent J* 1966;**121**:284–9.

25. ELLIS RG, DAVEY KV. *The classification and treatment of injuries to the teeth of children*. 5th edn. Chicago: Year Book Publishers Inc., 1970.

26. RADKOVEC F. Les dents de Turner. 8 congrés dentaire international, Section 3. Paris **1931**:210–21.

27. BENNET DT. Traumatised anterior teeth. *Br Dent J* 1964;**116**:52–5.

28. SZYMANSKA-JACHIMCZAK I. Wplyw ostrych mechanicznych urazów zebów mlecznych na znieksztalcenia koron zebow stalych w okresie ich wczesnego rozwoju. *Czas Stomatol* 1960;**13**:9–21.

29. HOTZ R. Die Bedeutung, Beurteilung und Behandlung beim Trauma im Frontzahngebiet vom Standpunkt des Kieferorthopäden. *Dtsch Zahnärztl Z* 1958;**13**:42–51.

30. BJÖRK A. Störningar i tandutvecklingen som följd av trauma. *Svensk Tandläkar Tidning* 1943;**36**:470–85.

31. MACGREGOR SA. Management of injuries to deciduous incisors. *J Canad Dent Assoc* 1969;**35**:26–34.

32. BRUSZT P. Die Beeinflussbarkeit der Schmelzoberfläche bleibender Zähne durch Traumen der Milchzähne in frühester Jugend. *Dtsch Zahnärztl Z* 1956;**11**:190–2.

33. PAPILLON-LÉAGE, VILLENEUVE. Dystrophie de cause locale. *Rev Stomatol (Paris)* 1951;**52**:320–5.

34. MONICA WS. Anaplasia. Report of a case. *Oral Surg Oral Med Oral Pathol* 1960;**13**:581–3.

35. SCHINDLER J. Über traumatische Schädigungen des Zahnkeimes und ihre Folgen. *Schweiz Monatschr Zahnheilk* 1943;**53**:697–702.

36. SCHEUER O. Ein Beitrag zur Kenntnis von Infraktionen der Zähne. *Österr Ung Vjschr Zahnheilk* 1914;**30**:303–7.

37. DECHAUME M. Dystrophies et malpositions dentaires et maxillaires d'origine traumatique. *Rev Stomatol (Paris)* 1935;**37**:87–102.

38. ANDERSON BG. Developmental enamel defects. Clinical descriptions and classification. *Am J Dis Child* 1942;**63**:154–63.

39. PERINT EJ. A case of local hypoplasia of the second upper premolar due to trauma. *Dent Practit Dent Rec* 1952;**2**:51.

40. BAUER WH. Effect of periapical processes of deciduous teeth on the buds of permanent teeth. Pathological-clinical study. *Am J Orthod* 1946;**32**:232–41.

41. BINNS WH, ESCOBAR A. Defects in permanent teeth following pulp exposure of primary teeth. *ASDC J Dent Child* 1967;**34**:4–14.

42. MCCORMICK J, FILOSTRAT DJ. Injury to the teeth of succession by abscess of the temporary teeth. *ASDC J Dent Child* 1967;**34**:501–4.

43. MORNINGSTAR CH. Effect of infection of the deciduous molar on the permanent tooth germ. *J Am Dent Assoc* 1937;**24**:786–91.

44. KAPLAN NL, ZACH L, GOLDSMITH ED. Effects of pulpal exposure in the primary dentition of the succedaneous teeth. *ASDC J Dent Child* 1967;**34**:237–42.

45. MATSUMIYA S. Experimental pathological study on the effect of treatment of infected root canals in the deciduous tooth on growth of the permanent tooth germ. *Int Dent J* 1968;**18**:546–59.

46. VIA WF. Enamel defects induced by trauma during tooth formation. *Oral Surg Oral Med Oral Pathol* 1968;**25**:49–54.

47. FECHNER F. Frühkindliche Frontzahntraumen und ihre Folgen. *Zahnärztl Prax* 1965;**16**:221.

48. POWERS DF. Enamel dysplasia due to trauma. *Dent Surv* 1962;**38**:43–6.

49. WEDL C. Ueber Knickungen und Drehungen an den Kronen und Wurzeln der Zähne. *Dtsch Vjschr Zahnheilk* 1867;**7**:247–53.

50. M'QUILLEN JH. Dilaceration, or flexion of the crown of a left superior central incisor. *Dent Cosmos* 1874;**16**:80–3.

51. PECKERT. Ein Fall von Zahnmissbildung durch Trauma. *Korresp Bl Zahnärzte* 1912, **41**:58–61.

52. DECHAUME M. Dystrophies dentaires d'origine traumatique. *Presse Med* 1933;**41**:1832.

53. KOWARSKY M. Zur Kauistik der traumatischen Affektion der *Zähne. Z Stomatol* 1934;**32**:1082–7.

54. MERLE-BÉRAL J. Malformation et anomalie dentaires. *Rev Stomatol (Paris)* 1936;**38**:844–8.

55. ASCHER F. Unfallfolgen während der Kleinkinderzeit in der Betrachtung als kieferorthopädisches Problem. *Zahnärztl Welt* 1949;**4**:283–8.

56. ASCHER F. Folgen nach Unfällen während der Kleinkinderzeit. Zahn- Mund- und Kieferheilkunde in Vorträgen. No. 9. München: Carl Hanser Verlag, 1952:107–16.

57. GUSTAFSON G, SUNDBERG S. Dens in dente. *Br Dent J* 1950;**88**:111–22.

58. CHEMIN. Anomalie de forme par traumatisme. *Rev Stomatol (Paris)* 1951;**52**:325–7.

59. BOYLE PE. *Kronfeld's histopathology of the teeth and their surrounding structures*. 4th edn. Philadelphia: Lea & Febiger, 1956:452–3.

60. JACHNO R, LISKA K. PriIspvek k traumatickému poskozeni zubnick zdrodku. *Cs Stomatol* 1967;**67**:285–92.

61. PFEIFER H. Erhaltung traumatisch geschädigter Zähne. *Dtsch Zahnärztl Z* 1969;**24**:263–7.

62. GLENN FB, STANLEY HR. Dilaceration of a mandibular permanent incisor. Report of a case. *Oral Surg Oral Med Oral Pathol* 1952;**13**:1249–52.

63. BODENHOFF J. Dilaceratio dentis. *Tandlaegebladet* 1963;**67**:710–17.

64. MICHANOWICZ AE. Somatopsychic trauma as a result of a dilacerated crown. *ASDC J Dent Child* 1963;**30**: 150–2.

65. BOHATKA L. Dilaceratio dentis. *Fogorv Szle* 1969;**62**:43–8.

66. KLUGE R. Auswirkung einer zweimaligen Traumatisierung auf einen unteren Frontzahn. *Dtsch Zahnärztl Z* 1964;**19**:800–8.

67. GERLING K. Ein Fall von Pfählungsverletzung bleibender Frontzahnkeime. *Dtsch Stomatol* 1965;**15**:273–7.

68. GAGLIANI N. Malposizioni e malformazioni dentarie conseguenti a trauma in dentatura decidua. *Dent Cadm (Milano)* 1967;**35**:1393–409.

69. GYSEL C. Traumatologie et orthodontie. *Rev Fr Odontostomatol* 1962;**9**:1091–113.

70. SCHROETER. Formanomalie und Retention eines Zahnes, bedingt durch Trauma im Entwicklungsstadium. *Zahnärztl Rdsch* 1925;**34**:175.

71. BROGLIA ML, DANA F. Manifestazioni cliniche delle lesioni traumatiche accidentali della dentatura decidua. *Minerva Stomatol* 1967;**16**:623–35.

72. TOMES JA. *System of dental surgery.* London: John Churchill, 1859:240–1.

73. RUSHTON MA. Partial duplication following injury to developing incisors. *Br Dent J* 1958;**104**:9–12.

74. ZILKENS K. Beiträge zur traumatischen Zahnschädigung. In: Wannenmacher E. *Ein Querschnitt der deutschen Wissenschaftlichen Zahnheilkunde.* No. 33. Leipzig: Verlag von Hermann Meusser, 1938:43–70.

75. ARWILL T. Histopathologic studies of traumatized teeth. *Odontologisk Tidsskrift* 1962;**70**:91–117.

76. CASTALDI CR. Traumatic injury to unerupted incisors following a blow to the primary teeth. *J Canad Dent Assoc* 1959;**25**:752–62.

77. TAATZ H, TAATZ H. Feingewebliche Studien an permanenten Frontzähnen nach traumatischer Schädigung während der Keimentwicklung. *Dtsch Zahnärztl Z* 1961;**16**:995–1002.

78. BRUSZT P. Durch Traumen verursachte Entwicklungsstörungen bei Schneidezähnen. *Z Stomatol* 1936;**34**:1056–77.

79. RODDA JC. Gross maldevelopment of a permanent tooth caused by trauma to its deciduous predecessor. *N Z Dent J* 1960;**56**:24–5.

80. GIUSTINA C. Su di un caso di malformazione dentaria d'origine traumatica. *Minerva Stomatol* 1954;**3**:190–5.

81. HITCHIN AD. Traumatic odontome. *Br Dent J* 1969;**126**:260–5.

82. GLASSTONE S. The development of halved tooth germs. A study of experimental embryology. *J Anat* 1952;**86**:12–5.

83. PINDBORG JJ. Dental mutilation and associated abnormalities in Uganda. *Am J Physiol Anthrop* 1969;**31**:383–9.

84. EDLUND K. Complete root duplication of a lower permanent incisor caused by traumatic injury. Case report. *Odontol Rev* 1964;**15**:299–306.

85. ARWILL T, ÅSTRAND P. Dilaceration av 2+. Ett intressant fall. *Odontologisk Tidsskrift* 1968;**76**:427–49.

86. ESCHLER J. *Die traumatischen Verletzungen der Frontzähne bei Jugendlichen.* 2nd edn. Heidelberg: Alfred Hilthig Verlag, 1966:87.

87. TRIEBSCH E. Durchbruchsstörungen nach Zahnkeimschüdigung und traumatischem Milchzahnverlust. *Fortschr Kieferorthop* 1958;**19**:170–9.

88. WUNSCHHEIM GV. Frakturen, Infraktionen und Knickungen der Zähne. *Österr Ung Vjaschr Zahnheilk* 1904;**20**:45–102.

89. GRADY R. An everted crown. *Dent Cosmos* 1889;**31**: 911–12.

90. SMITH JM. A case of dilaceration. *Dent Cosmos* 1930;**72**:667.

91. HERRING H, KRUSE H. Über die Dilaceration von Zähnen. *Zahnärztl Welt* 1961;**62**:33–7.

92. ALEYT G. Milchzahnintrusionen und mögliche Folgen an den oberen permanenten Schneidezähnen. *Dtsch Stomatol* 1969;**19**:459–64.

93. BROGLIA ML, RE G. Malformazioni dentarie secondarie a traumatismo dei germi permanenti. *Minerva Stomatol* 1959;**8**:520–6.

94. RECKOW JF v. Das intraorale Röntgenbild und seine klinische Auswertung. Zahn-, Mund- und Kieferheilkunde in Forträgen. No. 16. Zahnärztliche Röntgenologie in diagnostischer und therapeutischer Anwendung. München: Carl Hanser Verlag, 1955:9–30.

95. BORGMANN H. Das akute Trauma im Milchgebiss. *Dtsch Zahnärztl Z* 1959;**14**:325–31.

96. EULER H. *Die Anomalien, Fehlbildungen und Verstümmelungen der menschlichen Zähne.* München-Berlin: JF Lehmanns Verlag, 1939:125–41.

97. MEYER W. Der verbogene obere mittlere Schneidezahn. *Zahnärztl Welt* 1955;**10**:406–7.

98. TAATZ H. *Verletzungen der Milchzähne und ihre Behandlung. In Reichenbach, E. Zahnärztliche Fortbildung.* No. 16. *Kinderzahnheilkunde im Vorschulalter.* Leipzig: Johan Ambrosius Barth, 1967:363–86.

99. FUHR K, SETZ D. *Über die Folgen von Zahnkeimschädigungen durch Kieferfrakturen.* Dtsch Zahnärztl Z 1963;**18**:482–6.

100. TAATZ H. Spätschäden nach Kieferbrüchen im Kindesalter. *Fortschr Kieferorthop* 1954;**15**:174–84.

101. BECKMANN K, BECKMANN P. Wurzelverkümmerung durch Trauma. *Quintessenz Zahnärztl Lit* 1967;**18**:79.

102. BALL JS. A sequel to trauma involving the deciduous incisors. *Br Dent J* 1965;**118**:394–5.

103. FIELD GS. Case of repair after injury to developing permanent incisors. *N Z Dent J* 1931;**24**:125.

104. SCHMELZ H. Über die Bedeutung traumatisch geschädigter Zahnkeime für den kieferorthopädischen Behandlungsplan. *Zahnärztl Welt* 1957;**58**:327–30.

105. FREY JS. Dilaceration. *Oral Surg Oral Med Oral Pathol* 1966;**21**:321–2.

106. MEYER W. Ein Beitrag zur traumatischen Schädigung von Zahnkeimen. *Dtsch Monatschr Zahnheilk* 1924;**42**:497–510.

107. WALLENIUS B, GRÄNSE KA. Eruption disturbances: two cases with different etiology. *Odontologisk Revy* 1954;**5**:297–310.

108. CARMICHAEL AF, NIXON GS. Two interesting cases of root resorption. *Dent Rec* 1954;**74**:258–60.

109. PARFITT GJ. Maxillofacial injuries in children and their sequelae. *Dent Rec* 1946;**66**:159–68.

110. HALL SR, IRANPOUR B. The effect of trauma on normal

tooth development. Report of two cases. *ASDC J Dent Child* 1968;**35**:291–5.

111. FRANKL Z. Über die Folgen von Zahnkeimschädigungen durch Kieferfrakturen. *Dtsch Zahnärztl Z* 1963;**18**:1225–7.

112. BERGER B, FISCHER C-H. Frontzahntrauma und Zahnentwicklung. *Dtsch Zahn Mund Kieferheilk* 1967;**49**:319–27.

113. FRIEDERICHS W. Kieferbrüche im Kindesalter und seltene Zysten. *Dtsch Zahnärztl Wochenschr* 1940;**43**:508–10.

114. ASH AS. Orthodontic significance of anomalies of tooth eruption. *Am J Orthod* 1957;**43**:559–76.

115. KORF SR. The eruption of permanent central incisors following premature loss of their antecedents. *ASDC J Dent Child* 1965;**32**:39–44.

116. BROGLIA ML. Considerazioni su un caso di intrusione traumatica di un dente deciduo causa di ritenzione del correspondente permanente. *Minerva Stomatol* 1959;**8**:811–3.

117. FADDEN LE. The restoration of hypoplastic young anterior teeth. *ASDC J Dent Child* 1951;**18**:21–30.

118. MAGNUSSON B. Några synpunkter på unga permanenta tander med emaljhypoplasier. *Svensk Tandläkar Tidskrift* 1960;**53**:53–72.

119. SCHULZE C. Über die Folgen des Verlustes oberer mittlerer Schneidezähne während der Gebissentwicklung. *Zahnärztl Rdsch* 1967;**76**:156–69.

120. LIND V, WALLIN H, EGERMARK-ERIKSSON I, BERNHOLD M. Indirekta traumaskador. Kliniska skador på permanenta incisiver som följd av trauma mot temporära incisiver. *Sverig Tandläkar Förbund Tidning* 1970;**62**:738–56.

121. ANDREASEN JO, RAVN JJ. Enamel changes in permanent teeth after trauma to their primary predecessors. *Scand J Dent Res* 1973;**81**:203–9.

122. MEHNERT H. Untersuchungen über die Auswirkungen von Milschzahnverletzungen auf das bleibende Gebiss. *Österr Z Stomatol* 1974;**71**:407–13.

123. WATZEK G, SKODA J. Milchzahntraumen und ihre Bedeutung für die bleibenden Zähne. *Zahn Mund Kieferheilk* 1976;**64**:126–33.

124. BIENENGRABER V, SOBKOWIAK E-M. Tierexperimentelle Untersuchungen zur Frage des indirekten Milschzahntraumas. *Z Exper Chir* 1971;**4**:174–80.

125. CUTRIGHT DE. The reaction of permanent tooth buds to injury. *Oral Surg Oral Med Oral Pathol* 1971;**32**:832–9.

126. FREDÉN H, HEMDEN G, INGERVALL B. Traumatic injuries to enamel formation in rat incisors. *Scand J Dent Res* 1975;**83**:135–44.

127. ANDREASEN JO. The influence of traumatic intrusion of primary teeth on their permanent successors. A radiographic and histologic study in monkeys. *Int J Oral Surg* 1976;**5**:207–19.

128. SUCKLING GW, CUTRESS TW. Traumatically induced defects of enamel in permanent teeth in sheep. *J Dent Res* 1977;**56**:1429.

129. THYLSTRUP A, ANDREASEN JO. The influence of traumatic intrusion of primary teeth on their permanent successors in monkeys. A macroscopic, polarized light

and scanning electron microscopic study. *J Oral Pathol* 1977;**6**:296–306.

130. RAVN JJ. Developmental disturbances in permanent teeth after exarticulation of their primary predecessors. *Scand J Dent Res* 1976;**83**:131–41.

131. RAVN JJ. Developmental disturbances in permanent teeth after intrusion of their primary predecessors. *Scand J Dent Res* 1976;**84**:137–46.

132. IDEBERG M, PERSSON B. Development of permanent tooth germs involved in mandibular fractures in children. *J Dent Res* 1971;**50**:721.

133. RIDELL A, ÅSTRAND P. Conservative treatment of teeth involved by mandibular fractures. *Swed Dent J* 1971;**64**:623–32.

134. RANTA R, YLIPAAVALNIEMI P. The effect of jaw fractures in children on the development of permanent teeth and the occlusion. *Proc Finn Dent Soc* 1973;**69**:99–104.

135. PERKO M, PEPERSACK W. Spätergebnisse der Osteosynthesebehandlung bei Kieferfrakturen im Kindesalter. *Fortschr Kiefer Gesichtschir* 1975;**19**:206–8.

136. VAN GOOL AV. Injury to the permanent tooth germ after trauma to the deciduous predecessor. *Oral Surg Oral Med Oral Pathol* 1973;**35**:2–12.

137. ANDO S, SANKA Y, NAKASHIMAT, SHINBO K, KIYOKAWAK, OSHIMA S, ÀIZAWA K. Studies on the consecutive survey of succedaneous and permanent dentition in the Japanese children. Part 3. Effects of periapical osteitis in the deciduous predecessors on the surface malformation of their permanent successors. *J Nihon Univ Sch Dent* 1966;**8**:21–41.

138. WINTER GB, KRAMER IRH. Changes in periodontal membrane, bone and permanent teeth following experimental pulpal injury in deciduous molar teeth of monkeys (*Macaca irus*). *Arch Oral Biol* 1972;**17**:1771–9.

139. VALDERHAUG J. A histologic study of experimentally induced periapical inflammation in primary teeth in monkeys. *Int J Oral Surg* 1974;**3**:111–23.

140. VALDERHAUG J. Periapical inflammation in primary teeth and its effect on the permanent successors. *Int J Oral Surg* 1974;**3**:171–82.

141. MÖLLER E. En efterundersögelse af patienter med paradentale ostitter i mälketandsättet med henblik på mineralisationsforstyrrelser i det blivende tandsät.3 (Autoreferat) *Tandlaegebladet* 1957;**61**:135–7.

142. TAYLOR RMS. Dilaceration of incisor tooth crowns. Report of two cases. *N Z Dent Y* 1970;**66**:71–9.

143. VAN DEN HUL H. Het gevolg van trauma op een tandkiem. *Ned T Tandhelk* 1972;**79**:75–80.

144. EDLER R. Dilaceration of upper central and lateral incisors. A case report. *Br Dent J* 1973;**134**:331–2.

145. EDMONSON HD, CRABB JJ. Dilaceration of both upper central incisor teeth: a case report. *J Dent* 1975;**3**:223–4.

146. STEWART DJ. Dilacerate unerupted maxillary central incisors. *Br Dent J* 1978;**145**:229–33.

147. KVAM E. Et tilfelle av misdannelse av roten på den maxilläre lateral. *Norske Tannlaegeforenings Tidende* 1971;**81**:289–92.

148. LORBER CG. Einige Untersuchungen zur Pathobiologie unfallgeschädigter Zähne. *Schweiz Monatschr Zahnheilk* 1973;**83**:989–1014.

149. DiBiase DD. Mucous membrane and delayed eruption. *Dent Practit* 1971;**21**:241–50.

150. Haavikko K, Rantanen L. A follow-up study of injuries to permanent and primary teeth in children. *Proc Finn Dent Soc* 1976;**72**:152–62.

151. Ulvestad M, Kerekes K, Danmo C. Kompositkronen. En ny type semipermanent krone. *Norske Tannlageforenings Tidende* 1973;**83**:281–4.

152. Oppenheim MN, Ward GT. The restoration of fractured incisors using a pit and fissure sealant and composite material. *J Am Dent Assoc* 1974;**89**: 365–8.

153. Crabb JJ. The restoration of hypoplastic anterior teeth using an acid-etched technique. *J Dent* 1975;**3**:121–4.

154. Koch G, Paulander J. Klinisk uppföljning av compositrestaureringar utförda med emaljetsningsmetodik. *Swed Dent J* 1976;**69**:191–6.

155. Jordan RE, Suzuki M, Gwinnett AJ, Hunter JK. Restoration of fractured and hypoplastic incisors by the acid etch resin technique; a three-year report. *J Am Dent Assoc* 1977;**95**:795–803.

156. Mink JR, McEvoy SA. Acid etch and enamel bond composite restoration of permanent anterior teeth affected by enamel hypoplasia. *J Am Dent Assoc* 1977;**94**:305–7.

157. Brin I, Ben-Bassat Y, Fuks A, Zilberman Y. Trauma to the primary incisors and its effect on the permanent successors. *Pediatr Dent* 1984;**6**:78–82.

158. Brin I, Ben Bassat Y, Zilbermany, Fuks A. Effect of trauma to the primary incisors on the alignment of their permanent successors in Israelis. *Comm Dent Oral Epidemiol* 1988;**16**:104–6.

159. Ben Bassat Y, Brin I, Fuks A, Zilberman Y. Effect of trauma to the primary incisors on permanent successors in different developmental stages. *Pediatr Dent* 1985;**7**:37–40.

160. Morgantini J, Maréchaux SC, Joho JP. Traumatismes dentaires chez l'enfant en âge préscolaire et répercussions sur les dents permanentes. *Schweiz Monatsschr Zahnmed* 1986;**96**:432–40.

161. Zilberman Y, Ben Bassat Y, Lustmann J. Effect of trauma to primary incisors on root development of their permanent successors. *Pediatr Dent* 1986;**8**:289–93.

162. von Arx T. Traumatologie im Milchgebiss (II). Langzeitergebnisse sowie Auswirkungen auf das Milchgebiss and die bleibende Dentition. *Schweiz Monatsschr Zahnmed* 1991;**101**:57–69.

163. Moylan FMB, Seldin EB, Shannon DC, Todres ID. Defective primary dentition in survivors of neonatal mechanical ventilation. *J Pediatr* 1980;**96**:106–8.

164. Seow WK, Brown JP, Tudehope DI, O'Callaghan M. Developmental defects in the primary dentition of low birthweight infants: adverse effects of laryngoscopy and prolonged endotracheal intubation. *Pediatric Dent* 1984;**6**:28–31.

165. Angelos GM, Smith DR, Jorgenson R, Sweeney EA. Oral complications associated with neonatal oral tracheal intubation: a critical review. *Pediatr Dent* 1989;**11**:133–140.

166. Boice JB, Krous HF, Foley JM. Gingival and dental complications of orotracheal intubation. *J Am Med Assoc* 1976;**236**:957–5.

167. Wetzel RC. Defective dentition following mechanical ventilation. *J Pediatr* 1980;**96**:334.

168. Ainamo J, Cutress TW. An epidemiological index of developmental defects of dental enamel (DDE Index). *Int Dent J* 1982;**3**:159–67.

169. Suckling GW, Brown RH, Herbison GP. The prevalence of developmental defects of enamel in 696 nine-year-old New Zealand children participating in a health and development study. *Com Dent Health* 1985;**2**:303–13.

170. Dummer PHM, Kingdon A, Kingdon R. Prevalence of enamel developmental defects in a group of 11- and 12-year-old children in South Wales. *Com Dent Oral Epidemiol* 1986;**14**:119–22.

171. Clarkson J, O'Mullane D. A modified DDE Index for use in epidemiological studies of enamel defects. *J Dent Res* 1989;**68**:445–50.

172. Holm A-K, Andersson R. Enamel mineralization disturbances in 12-year-old children with known early exposure to fluorides. *Com Dent Oral Epidemiol* 1982;**10**:335–9.

173. Kaufman AY, Keila S, Wasersprung D, Dayan D. Developmental anomaly of permanent teeth related to traumatic injury. *Endod Dent Traumatol* 1990;**6**: 183–8.

174. Croll TP, Cavanaugh RR. Enamel color modification by controlled hydrochloric acid-pumice abrasion. I. Technique and examples. *Quintessence Int* 1986;**17**: 81–7.

175. Croll TP, Cavanaugh RR. Enamel color modification by controlled hydrochloric acid-pumice abrasion. II. Further examples. *Quintessence Int* 1986;**17**:157–64.

176. Croll TP, Cavanaugh RR. Hydrochloric acid-pumice enamel surface abrasion for color modification: results after six months. *Quintessence Int* 1986;**17**:335–41.

177. Waggoner WF, Johnston WM, Schumann S, Schikowski E. Microabrasion of human enamel in vitro using hydrochloric acid and pumice. *Pediatr Dent* 1989;**11**:319–23.

178. van Gool AV. Lésions des germes définitifs suite à des traumatismes de la dentition de lait. *Rev Belge Med Dent* 1986;**41**:96–9.

179. ben Bassat Y, Brin I, Zilberman Y. Effects of trauma to the primary incisors on their permanent successors: multidisciplinary treatment. *ASDC J Dent Child* 1989;**56**:112–6.

180. Lundberg M, Wennström JL. Development of gingiva following surgical exposure of a facially positioned unerupted incisor. *J Periodontol* 1988;**59**:652–5.

181. Kaufman AY, Keila S, Wasersprung D, Dayan D. Developmental anomaly of permanent teeth related to traumatic injury. *Endod Dent Traumatol* 1990;**6**:183–8.

182. Naclerio H, Simoes WA, Zindel D, Chilvarquer I, Aparecida TA. Dentigerous cyst associated with an upper permanent central incisor: case report and literature review. *J Clin Pediatr Dent* 2002;**26**:187–92.

183. Calderon S, Kaplan I, Gal G. Developmental arrest of tooth bud after correction of mandibular fracture. *Endod Dent Traumatol* 1995;**11**:105–7.

184. Abbott PV, Gregory PJ. Complicated crown fracture of an unerupted permanent tooth – a case report. *Endod Dent Traumatol* 1998;**14**:48–56.

185. Ishikawa M, Satoh K, Miyashin M. A clinical study of traumatic injuries to deciduous teeth. (3). The influence on their permanent successors. *Shoni Shikagaku Zasshi* 1990;**28**:397–406.

186. Sleiter R, von Arx T. Developmental disorders of permanent teeth after injuries of their primary predecessors. A retrospective study. *Schweiz Monatsschr Zahnmed* 2002;**112**:214–19.

187. von Arx T. Developmental disturbances of permanent teeth following trauma to the primary dentition. *Aust Dent J* 1993;**38**:1–10.

188. Seow WK, Perham S, Young WG, Daley T. Dilaceration of a primary maxillary incisor associated with neonatal laryngoscopy. *Pediatr Dent* 1990;**12**:321–4.

189. Taniguchi K, Okanura K, Hayashi M, Funakoshi T, Motokoma W. The effect of mechanical trauma on the tooth germ of rat molars at various developmental stages: a histopathological study. *Endod Dent Traumatol* 1999:**15**:17–25.

190. Morfis AS. Enamel hypoplasia of a maxillary central incisor. *Endod Dent Traumatol* 1989;**5**:204–6.

191. von Arx T. Deciduous tooth intrusions and the odontogenesis of the permanent teeth. Developmental disorders of the permanent teeth following intrusion injuries to the deciduous teeth. *Schweiz Monatsschr Zahnmed* 1995;**105**:11–17.

192. Prabhakar AR, Reddy VV, Bassappa N. Duplication and dilaceration of a crown with hypercementosis of the root following trauma: a case report. *Quintessence Int* 1998;**29**:655–7.

193. Maragakis MG. Crown dilaceration of permanent incisors following trauma to their primary predecessors. *J Clin Pediatr Dent* 1995;**20**:49–52.

194. Chadwick SM, Millett D. Dilaceration of a permanent mandibular incisor. A case report. *Br J Orthod* 1995;**22**:279–81.

195. Kamat SS, Kumar GS, Raghunath V, Rekha KP. Permanent maxillary central incisor impaction: report of two cases. *Quintessence Int* 2003;**34**:50–2.

196. Nagatani S, Mathieu GP. Partially arrested root formation in a permanent maxillary central incisor subsequent to trauma to the primary dentition. *Endod Dent Traumatol* 1994;**10**:23–6.

197. Killian CM, Leventhal PH, Tamaroff JL. Dentigerous cyst associated with trauma to a primary incisor: a case report. *Quintessence Int* 1992;**23**:683–6.

198. Seddon RP, Fung DE, Barnard KM, Smith PB. Dentigerous cysts involving permanent incisors: four case reports. *Int J Paediatr Dent* 1992;**2**:105–11.

199. Brin I, ben Bassat Y, Zilberman Y, Fuks A. Effect of trauma to the primary incisors on the alignment of their permanent successors in Israelis. *Com Dent Oral Epidemiol* 1988;**16**:104–8.

200. Filippi A, Pohl u, Tekin U. Transplantation of displaced and dilacerated anterior teeth. *Endod Dent Traumatol* 1998;**14**:93–98.

201. Diab M, ElBadrawy HE. Intrusion injuries of primary incisors. Part III: Effects on the permanent successors. *Quintessence Int* 2000;**31**:377–84.

202. Odersjö ML, Koch G. Developmental disturbances in permanent successors after intrusion to maxillary peimary teeth. *Eur J Paediatric Dent* 2001;**4**:165–72.

203. Ogunyinka A. Localized enamel hypoplasia: a case report. *Dent Update* 1996;**23**:64, 68.

204. Ben Bassat Y, Brin I, Zilberman Y. Effects of trauma to the primary incisors on their permanent successors: multidisciplinary treatment. *ASDC J Dent Child* 1989;**56**:112–16.

# 21
# Soft Tissue Injuries

L. Andersson & J. O. Andreasen

## Terminology, frequency and etiology

A large number of dental traumas are associated with injuries to the lip, gingiva and oral mucosa. One third of all patients treated for oral injuries in dental emergency settings and more than half of all patients treated in a hospital emergency setting are associated with soft tissue injury (1–4).

The dentition is shielded by the lips covering the teeth in case of impact to the lips (Fig. 21.1). Trauma energy will be absorbed in the soft tissue resulting in less severe tooth injuries. However, this will result in various types of soft tissue trauma depending on the direction of force, shape and size of object, and energy (see Chapter 8).

Moreover, when a patient is subjected to trauma, the teeth may also cause injury to the surrounding soft tissue, most commonly penetrating into the lips but sometimes also the cheeks and tongue. When teeth are dislocated the gingiva will sometimes be lacerated.

Incorrect primary treatment may result in unesthetic scarring (Fig. 21.2).

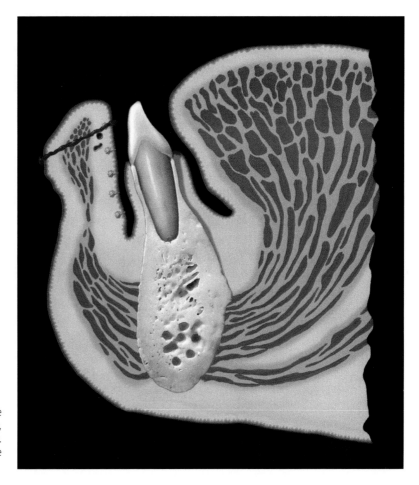

**Fig. 21.1** Section through a human lower lip in the midline. Note the composite structure of the lip, with musculature, salivary glands and hair follicles. Most of the musculature is oriented parallel to the vermilion border.

**Fig. 21.2 Scarring subsequent to a penetrating wound in the lower lip**
A 3-cm wide laceration of the cutaneous and mucosal aspects of the lower lip in a 9-year-old girl. Suturing of the cutaneous aspect of the wound was the only treatment provided.

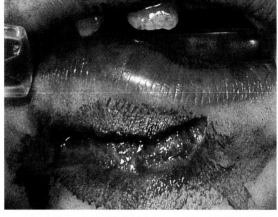 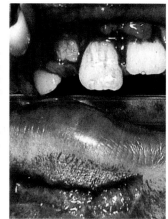

**Condition after 1 week**
Note saliva seepage and non-closure of the wound.

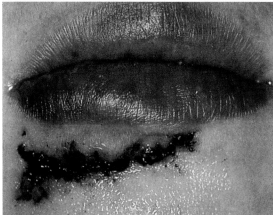 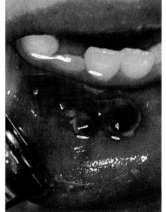

**Follow-up**
Healing has resulted in extreme scarring of the skin, whereas the wound on the mucosa is hardly noticeable.

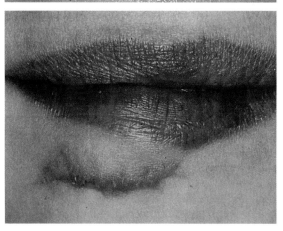 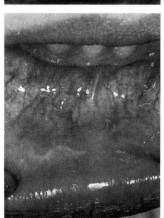

## Types of soft tissue trauma

Soft tissue injuries are usually classified into the following groups and their characteristics are described below. They can be seen extraorally (skin) as well as intraorally (gingiva and oral mucosa).

### Abrasion

An abrasion is a superficial wound produced by rubbing and scraping of the skin or mucosa leaving a raw, bleeding surface (Fig. 21.3). This injury is usually seen on knees and elbows in children and in the oral region the lips, chin, cheek or tip of the nose are frequently affected. The friction between the object and the surface of the soft tissue removes the epithelial layer and papillary layer of the dermis, and the reticular layer of the dermis is exposed. Superficial abrasions can be quite painful because terminal nerve endings are exposed.

### Contusion

A contusion is a bruise usually produced by impact with a blunt object and not accompanied by a break in the skin or mucosa but usually causing subcutaneous or submucosal hemorrhage in the tissue (Figs 21.4. and 21.5). Contusions may also be caused by the disrupting effect of fractured bone in maxillofacial injuries. Contusions may therefore indicate an underlying bone fracture.

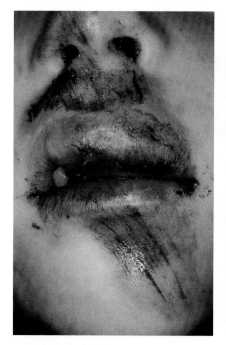

**Fig. 21.3** Abrasion of the upper and lower lip.

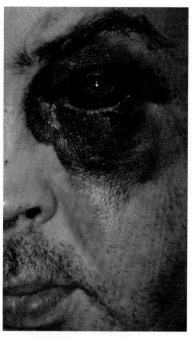

**Fig. 21.4** Periorbital hematoma indicating contusion injury after road traffic accident. Clinical and radiographical examination revealed underlying bone fracture.

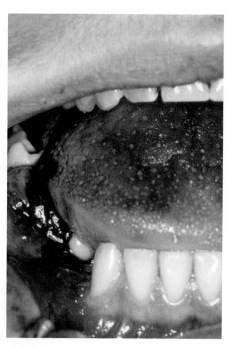

**Fig. 21.5** Hematoma of soft tissue in right premolar region. Perimandibular hematoma is strongly indicative of mandibular fracture and radiographic examination revealed a mandibular fracture.

## Laceration

A laceration is a shallow or deep wound in the skin or mucosa resulting from a tear and is usually produced by a sharp object or by teeth penetrating into the soft tissue (Figs 21.6 and 21.7). Laceration involves epithelial and subepithelial tissues and if deeper may disrupt blood vessels, nerves, muscles and involve salivary glands. The most frequent lacerations in the oral region caused by trauma are seen in lips, oral mucosa and gingiva. More seldom the tongue is involved.

## Avulsion

Avulsion (tissue loss) injuries are rare but seen with bite injuries or deep abrasions (Fig. 21.8). These are complex injuries from a treatment point of view in the emergency phase because a decision has to be made whether to excise and primary close the defect with flaps or grafts (large defects) or wait for spontaneous healing (small defects).

## Emergency management

After the diagnosis has been established, the extent and contamination of the lesion is examined. Ascertainment of the extent of tissue damage demands thorough exploration after administration of local anesthesia. Soft tissue injuries are often seen together with dental injuries and bone fractures. A systematic approach is recommended. If the soft tissue injuries are sutured first, before intraoral treatment of teeth and bone fractures, the sutures will most likely make the tissue rupture when later intraoral manipulation is taking place. This will also result in the tissue margins being more difficult to close in a second suturing. For this reason it is important to plan the emergency treatment so that intraoral treatment is performed first, and extraoral suturing of lips after the intraoral treatment. This is in contrast to the examination procedure where we start with extraoral examination before we perform intraoral examination. A golden rule: '*Examine from outside towards inside – treat from inside towards outside*' may help one to remember the examination and treatment sequences.

Local anesthetics should be used to allow manipulation of the tissue without pain. Topical anesthetics are preferable, and recent reports have indicated that those containing a combination of prilocaine/lidocaine are effective in reducing pain from needle stick injury, so that it may be possible to close minor lacerations without injection (70).

There are four major steps in the emergency management of soft tissue injuries: *cleansing, debridement, hemostasis* and *closure* (5). One of the aims of wound cleansing is to remove or neutralize microorganisms, which contaminate the wound surface, in order to prevent infection. Wound detergents reduce the bioburden (6). However, the fact remains that almost all common wound disinfectants have been shown to have a detrimental effect upon wound

**Fig. 21.6** (Left) Laceration of lip after road traffic accident.

**Fig. 21.7** (Right) Intraoral laceration of the upper lip. The blood around the anterior teeth originated from this laceration and not from any dental injuries.

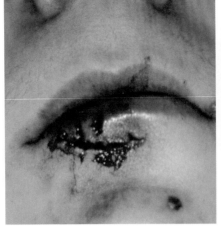 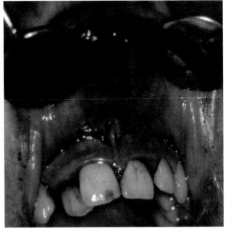

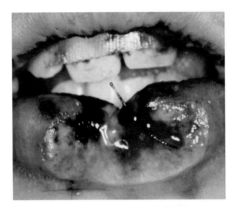 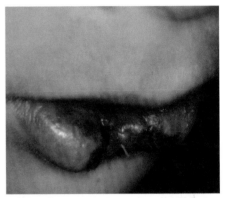

**Fig. 21.8** Avulsion injury of lower lip. Note the loss of soft tissue. Nevertheless this was left for spontaneous healing without flaps or grafts. Note the final result one year after trauma. A normal contour of the lip is seen. Scar tissue is seen centrally in a circular area at the vermilion border with a 9 mm diameter.

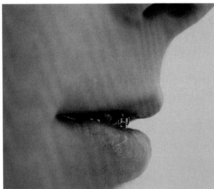 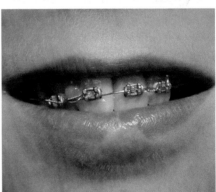

healing (7). Physiologic saline or Ringers solution appear to be without a harmful effect upon cells in the wound. Even water can be used for rinsing. The volume of fluid seems to be more important than if saline or water is used (8).

The presence of foreign bodies in the wound significantly increases the risk of infection (9) and retards healing, even in wounds free of infection (10) (see Chapter 1, p. 42). Foreign bodies also contribute to extensive scarring and tattooing of tissues. This finding emphasizes the importance of adequate removal of all foreign particles prior to suturing.

## Abrasion

It is important to remove all dirt, gravel, asphalt and other foreign bodies to avoid future permanent tattoo and scarring in the skin (Fig. 21.9). This is very time consuming but extremely important (Fig. 21.10). There is only one chance to clean the abrasion properly and that is during the emergency phase. After administration of local anesthesia, the wound and surroundings are thoroughly rinsed and washed with saline. A scrub brush, gauze swabs or even a soft toothbrush may be used. If the contamination is severe a mild

**Fig. 21.9 Cleansing of a skin wound containing asphalt particles**

A, B. In order to adequately cleanse the abrasions, a topical anesthetic is necessary. In this case, a lidocain spray was used. Note that the nostrils are held closed to reduce discomfort from the spray entering the nose. C. Washing the wounds. The lips are washed with surgical sponges or gauze swabs soaked in a wound detergent.

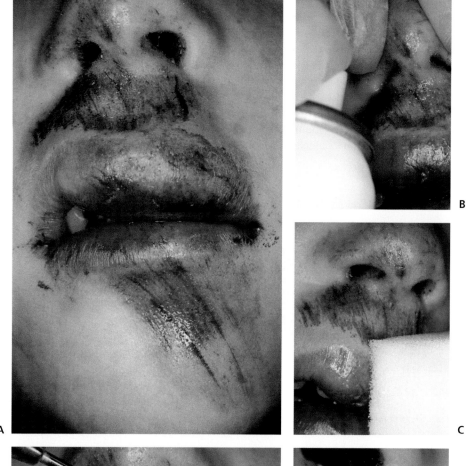

A

B

C

**Removing asphalt particles**

D and E. The impacted foreign bodies cannot be adequately removed by scrubbing or washing; but should be removed with a small excavator or a surgical blade held perpendicular to the direction of the abrasions.

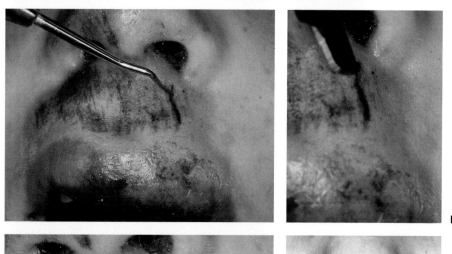

D

E

**Cleaned wound and follow-up**

F and G. Two weeks after injury, the soft tissue wounds have healed without scarring.

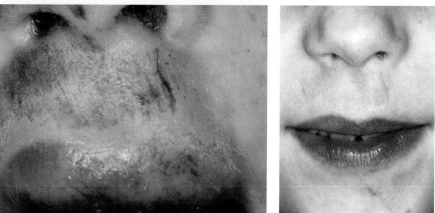

F

G

soapy solution may be used (Fig. 21.9). Thereafter, all foreign bodies are removed with a small excavator or a surgical blade which is placed perpendicular to the cutaneous surface in order to prevent it from cutting into the tissue. Finally irrigation with saline should be performed. The wound is usually left open without any applications but may be covered with a bandage. The patient should avoid excessive sunlight during the first 6 months to decrease risk of permanent hyperpigmentation. Intraoral abrasions do not have to be treated but limited to removal of any foreign bodies.

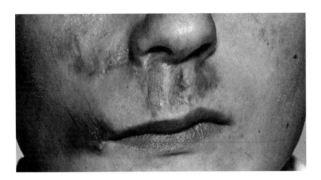

**Fig. 21.10** Extensive asphalt tattoo. The patient suffered an injury years earlier. Inadequate wound debridement resulted in extensive asphalt tattooing. Courtesy of Dr. S. BOLUND, University Hospital, Copenhagen.

## Contusion

Swelling and bruising may indicate a deeper injury; usually only bleeding but sometimes bone fractures are the causes of contusions (Figs 21.4 and 21.5). Radiographic examination is therefore indicated. Care should be taken to extend the clinical examination also to indirect trauma related areas such as palpation and radiographic examination of the condyles when a bruise is seen in the chin region. Make sure that there is no ongoing bleeding if the swelling is located in a sensitive area for the airways such as the floor of the mouth or the tongue. No treatment is necessary for contusions when the injury is limited to soft tissue injury.

## Laceration

The possibility of contamination of the wound requires inspection for foreign bodies or tooth fragments. In deeper wounds, clinical inspection should be supplemented with a radiographic examination which can reveal at least some of the contaminating foreign bodies.

The removal of foreign bodies in facial and oral tissues after laceration is known to be a difficult and time-consuming procedure (11). A syringe with saline under high pressure, a scrub brush or gauze swabs soaked in saline can be used to remove foreign bodies. If this is not effective, a surgical scalpel blade or a small spoon excavator may be

**Fig. 21.11 Treatment of horizontal gingival laceration with tissue displacement in the permanent dentition**
Due to an impact the gingiva has been lacerated and displaced whereas the central incisors are left intact.

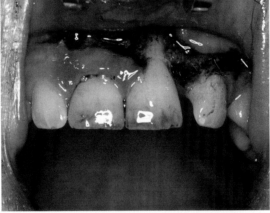
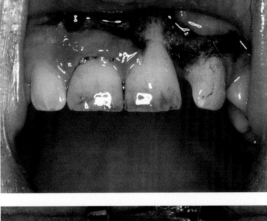
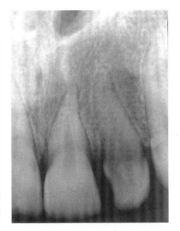

**The displaced attached gingiva is repositioned and sutured**
Postoperatively a scan is seen midroot in the left incisor region

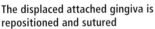
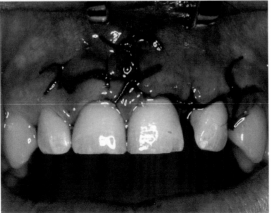
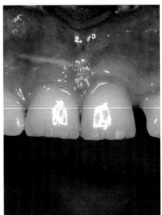

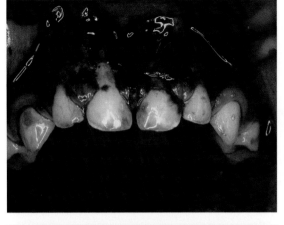
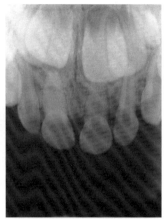

**Fig. 21.12 Treatment of a gingival laceration with exposure of bone in the primary dentition**
Due to a fall against an object, the gingiva has been displaced into the labial sulcus and bone is exposed whereas the incisors are left intact.

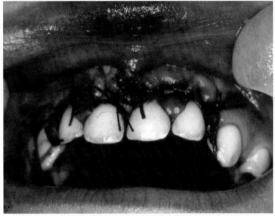
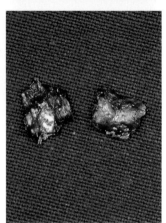

**Repositioning and suturing of the gingiva**
The condition immediately after gingival repositioning and suturing. Loose labial bone fragments have been removed.

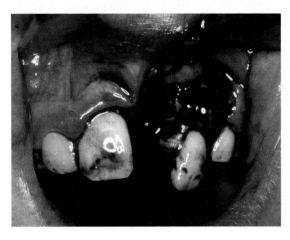
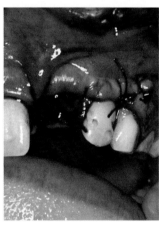

**Fig. 21.13** Gingival tissue loss. The central incisor has been avulsed and lost. There is tissue loss with exposure of labial bone. A flap is raised and the periosteum incised, whereby it is possible to cover the denuded bone.

used. Complete removal of all foreign bodies is important, to prevent infection and also to prevent disfiguring scarring or tattooing in the skin.

Devitalized soft tissue serves to enhance infection by at least three mechanisms: first, as a culture medium that can promote bacterial growth; second, by inhibiting leukocyte migration, phagocytosis and subsequent bacterial kill; and third, by limiting leukocyte function due to the anaerobic environment within devitalized tissue (i.e. low oxygen tension impairs killing of bacteria) (9, 12, 13) (see Chapter 1). However, the maxillofacial region has a rich blood supply. For this reason debridement should be kept to a minimum. However, severely contused and ischemic tissue should be removed in order to facilitate healing (14, 15).

## Gingival and vestibular lacerations

After administration of a local anesthetic, the wound is cleansed with saline, and foreign bodies removed. The lacerated gingiva is brought back into normal position, implying that displaced teeth have been repositioned (Figs 21.11 and 21.12). After repositioning of the gingiva, the necessary numbers of thin sutures are placed to prevent displacement of tissue. A minimum number of sutures should be used. The patient is then placed on an oral hygiene regimen using 0.1% chlorhexidine for 4–5 days, whereafter the sutures are removed. In cases of loss of gingival tissue, a gingivoplasty should be performed whereby flaps are elongated by placement of periosteal incision (Fig. 21.13). If tissue loss has occurred in the region of erupting teeth, it is important to

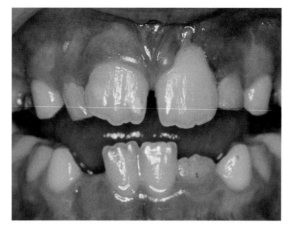
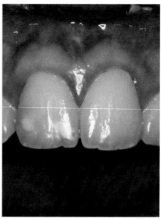

**Fig. 21.14** Gingival loss in an erupting permanent central incisor. In erupting teeth, gingival displacement or tissue loss should be assessed in relation to the position of the cemento-enamel junction. In this case of a 12-year-old boy, trauma resulted in tissue loss not extending beyond the cemento-enamel junction of the left central incisor. At a follow-up examination 5 years later, there is almost complete gingival symmetry.

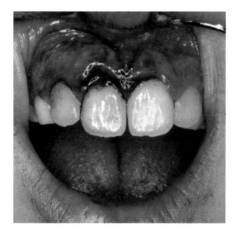
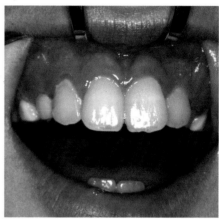

**Fig. 21.15** Gingival laceration with spontaneous regeneration. The marginal gingiva in this 9-year-old girl was displaced apically and not repositioned. At the 1-month follow-up examination, normal gingival relations could be observed.

consider whether tissue loss has exposed the cemento-enamel junction. If this is not the case, further eruption and physiologic gingival retraction will normalize the clinical appearance with time (Fig. 21.14). With minor displacements, gingival regeneration amounting to approximately 1 mm will usually occur (68) (Fig. 21.15).

A trauma force parallel to the front of the maxilla or the mandible will result in complete displacement of the labial mucosa into the sulcus area (67) (Fig. 21.16). Vestibular laceration with denuding of soft tissue from the bone is sometimes accompanied by severe contamination (Fig. 21.17). Wound cleansing and removal of all foreign bodies is very important before closure with sutures. Wound closure and primary healing is the main objective in these injuries and should aim at covering of bone. Later wound dehiscence with exposure of sequestred bone is sometimes seen and secondary healing with the loss of a thin superficial layer of the exposed bone will take place over a long time (Fig. 21.18). In that case daily rinsing is necessary to keep the area clean and support healing. The scarring from this secondary healing can be accepted because it is intraorally located and does not have any esthetic consequences for the patient.

## Lip lacerations

In cases of a frontal impact, the labial surfaces of protruding incisors may act as a bayonet, resulting in a sagittal split of the lip (Fig. 21.19). Because of the circumferential orientation of the orbicularis oris muscles, these wounds will usually gape, with initially intense arterial bleeding due to the rich vasculature in the region. Hemorrhage is usually soon spontaneously arrested due to vasoconstriction and coagulation but with manipulation of tissue bleeding may start again. Sometimes electrocoagulation may be necessary but it should be borne in mind that extensive use of electrocoagulation in the lip should be avoided.

If the direction of impact is more vertical, parallel to the axis of either the maxillary or mandibular incisors, the incisal edges may penetrate the entire thickness of the lip. When the incisal edges hit the impacting object, fracture of the crown usually occurs.

To find foreign bodies a thorough exploration of the laceration is important. Radiographic examination adds to the information and may show a variety of typical foreign bodies, such as tooth fragments, calculus, gravel, glass and fragments of paint (Fig. 21.20). However, other typical foreign bodies such as cloth and wood cannot be seen (69).

The radiographic technique consists of placing a dental film between the lip and the alveolar process. In cases of a wide lesion, orientation of images is facilitated by placing a small metal indicator (e.g. a piece of lead foil) in the midline of the vermilion border in order to locate possible foreign bodies. The exposure should be made at a low kilovoltage (to increase contrast), and the exposure time should be kept at the lowest value to be able to reveal particles with low radiographic contrast. If the intraoral film discloses foreign

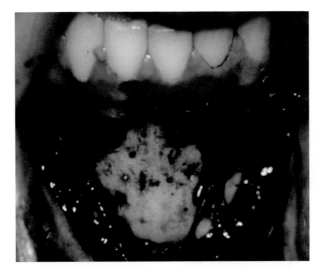

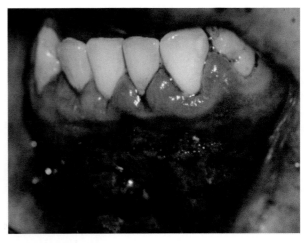

**Fig. 21.16** Vestibular laceration in the mandibular front region. This laceration was caused by a bicycle accident with degloving of the lower lip and vestibular tissue from the alveolar bone.

**Fig. 21.17** Severely contaminated vestibular laceration. This was caused by a football player falling on the chin in the grass resulting in degloving of the soft tissue from the bone. All soil and foreign bodies have to be removed before closure can take place.

**Fig. 21.18** Vestibular laceration with exposed bone. In spite of meticulous cleaning and closure and suturing in the emergency phase this laceration opened up and bone was exposed 2 weeks after trauma. This exposure was treated by daily rinsing by the patient and weekly follow up visits with irrigations at the clinic. A superficial sequestration was seen after 3 weeks. Completed healing is seen 7 weeks after trauma.

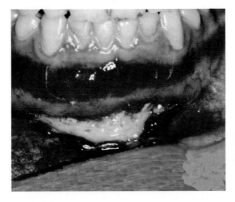

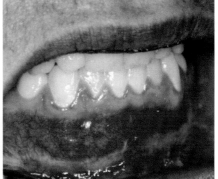

**Fig. 21.19** Split lip due to a frontal impact. This patient was hit in the face with a bottle, resulting in a split lip and lateral luxation of the right central incisor. The vermilion border is sutured first, whereafter the rest of the laceration is closed with interrupted sutures (e.g. Prolene® 6.0).

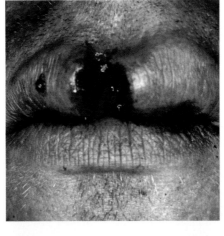

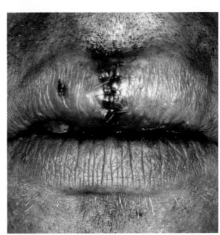

**Fig. 21.20** Radiographic appearance of typical foreign bodies. From left to right, the following types of foreign body are seen: tooth fragment, composite resin filling material, gravel, glass and paint. The different objects vary in radio-opacity.

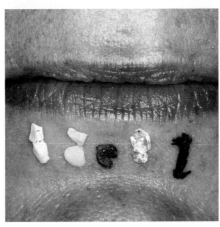

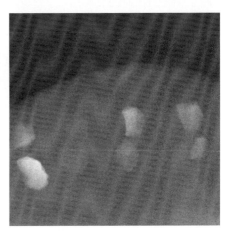

### Fig. 21.21 Penetrating lip lesion with embedded foreign body

This 8-year-old boy fell against a staircase, whereby the maxillary incisors penetrated the prolabium of the lower lip. Parallel lesions are found corresponding to each penetrating incisor.

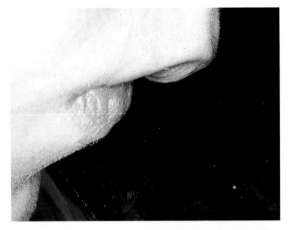
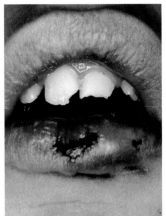

### Radiographic investigation

A dental film was placed between the lip and the dental arch. Exposure time is 1/4 of that for conventional dental radiographs. A large occlusal film is placed on the cheek and a lateral exposure taken using half the normal exposure time.

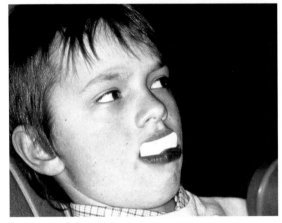
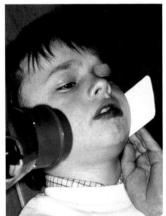

### Radiographic demonstration of multiple foreign bodies in the lower lip

Orthoradial and lateral exposures show multiple fragments in lower lip. The lateral exposure could demonstrate that the fragments are equally distributed from the cutaneous to the mucosal aspect of the lip.

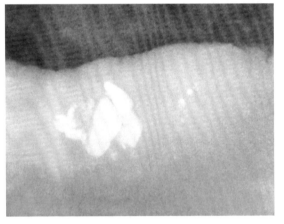
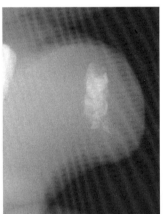

### Retrieved dental fragments

The lip lesion is sutured after removal of tooth fragments, foreign bodies such as tooth fragments, plaque, calculus, and fragments from the impacting object usually become trapped within the lip.

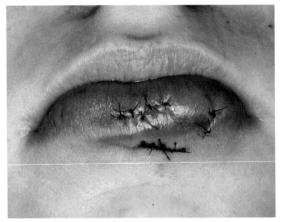
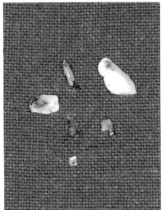

bodies, a lateral exposure may verify their position in a sagittal plane (Fig. 21.21).

In the case of narrow penetrating wounds, a special technique of opening up the wound, as illustrated in Fig. 21.22, is recommended. Management of a broad penetrating lip lesion is seen in Fig. 21.23. Treatment starts by cleansing the wound and surrounding tissue. The wound edges are elevated and foreign bodies are found and retrieved. It is essential to consider that foreign bodies are usually contained within a small sac within the wound. When all fragments that have been registered on radiographs have been retrieved, the wound is debrided for contused muscle and salivary gland tissue. The anatomy of the wound should be respected. Never excise wounds to make long straight scars which invariably are more visible. Thereafter the wound is carefully rinsed with saline; and a check is made to ensure that bleeding has been arrested.

When suturing the lip special attention must be paid to carefully approximate the transition of skin to mucosa (vermilion border) as any inaccuracy in wound closure will be very esthetically apparent. A minimum of sutures should be used, as deep sutures in contaminated wounds have been shown to increase the risk of infection (9). In penetrating lesions the mucosal side of the wound is first sutured so that no saliva can enter the wound (Fig. 21.23). A few resorbable 5.0 sutures are placed in the musculature to reduce tension on the cutaneous sutures. Thereafter, the cutaneous part of the wound is closed with 6.0 sutures. Magnifying lenses, e.g. ordinary spectacles with $4 \times$ loupes can be used to ensure meticulous suturing. Intracutaneous sutures may be used for cutaneous closure in estehtically sensitive areas (Fig. 21.24). Adhesive tape/strips may be used in addition to relieve tension (Fig. 21.25).

## Tongue lacerations

Other than in patients suffering from epilepsy, tongue lesions due to trauma are rare. In the former instance, bite lesions may occur along the lateral part of the tongue during seizures. Furthermore, following an impact to the chin with the tongue protruding, a wound may be caused by incisor penetration through the apex of the tongue.

A wound located on the dorsal surface of the tongue should always be examined for a ventral counterpart (Fig. 21.26). If there are concomitant crown fractures, fragments may be located within the wound. These fragments can be revealed by a radiographic examination (see above).

Treatment principles include cleansing of the wound, removal of foreign bodies and suturing of the dorsal and ventral aspects of the lesion. After administration of anesthesia (local, regional or general), foreign bodies are retrieved, the wound cleansed with saline, and the wound entrances sutured tightly (Fig. 21.26). Deep lacerations in the tongue will increase the risk of postoperative bleeding and some of these patients should be observed postoperatively so that continuing deep bleeding in the tongue and floor of the mouth with life threatening occlusion of airways can be prevented.

## Avulsion of tissue

Tissue loss may be seen intra- and extraorally. In case of loss of gingival tissue, a gingivoplasty should be performed whereby flaps are elongated by the placement of periosteal incisions (Fig. 21.13).

Tissue losses on the skin side are complex injuries from a treatment point of view in the emergency phase. There is a high risk for extensive scar contraction resulting in esthetic failure if not properly handled by an experienced specialist. Minor injuries in young individuals may be left for secondary healing and possible later reconstruction (Fig. 21.8). With larger avulsion injuries secondary healing should be avoided due to excessive scar formation and local flaps or skin grafts should be used in the early treatment of these cases (16–18).

Tissue losses are sometimes seen with animal bites to the face and are usually caused by dogs (19–21). Because of contamination from the dog's saliva the main concern is infection. Copious irrigation by saline and debridement should be performed. Antibiotics should always be administered regardless of duration. Rabies vaccine should be considered depending on the status of the dog. Ideally the animal should be caught and observed. Fluorescine antibody test should be performed to see if the animal has rabies. The incubation period of rabies is 2–8 weeks in humans and the patient can be treated within this period with a rabies vaccination protocol.

## Wound closure materials and principles

The management of facial soft tissue wounds is not a well-documented area and wound healing often leads to scarring (69). Sutures and tapes/strips are the traditional methods for closure of wounds in the skin of the face. Strips can be used together with sutures to relieve tension (Fig. 21.25). Strips can also be used alone to close small superficial wounds. Tissue adhesives e.g. cyanoacrylate or fibrine glue, have been used in emergency rooms (22–25). The advantage is that the closure procedure can be performed in less time and with less pain as compared to suturing. There are some reports comparing tissue adhesive and sutures in pediatric facial lacerations (23, 26, 27). The results showed comparable esthetic results between tissue adhesives and suturing. However it should be borne in mind that lip lacerations were excluded from these studies. There may also be problems associated with this location, such as the child licking or biting off the glue. Moreover, a statistically significant increase in wound dehiscence has been found with tissue adhesives (28). Further studies are needed to learn more about the indications for tissue adhesives in lip injuries before they are generally applied (29, 30).

A general principle in wound treatment is the approximation of wound edges in order to reduce the distance for the wound healing module and thereby increase the speed of healing. This principle has, unfortunately, not been supported by animal experiments in which sutures were used to approximate wound edges (27, 30–35). The explanation for

### Fig. 21.22 Treatment of narrow penetrating lip lesion

This 27-year-old man fell, causing the right central incisor to penetrate the lower lip and fracture. A radiograph shows that multiple tooth fragments are buried in the lip.

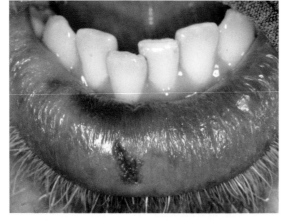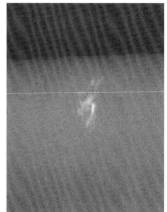

### Removing foreign bodies from the lip

After administration of local anesthesia the narrow penetrating wound is opened using a pincette. When the pincette is open, a rectangular wound is formed whereby two sides of the wound become clearly visible. Foreign bodies are removed and the wound cleansed with saline.

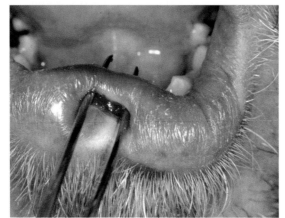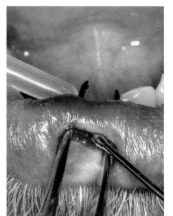

### Repeating the cleansing procedure

The pincette is turned 90° and the procedure is repeated.

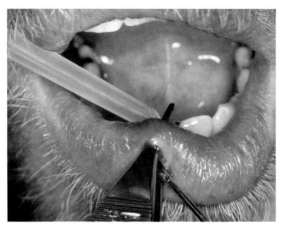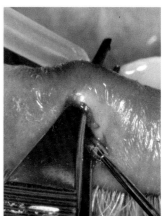

### Suturing the wound

The wound is sutured with interrupted 6.0 silk sutures. A radiograph shows that all fragments have been removed.

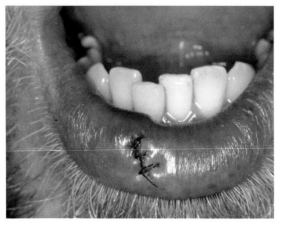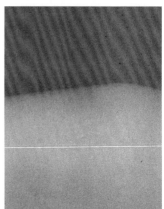

### Fig. 21.23 Treatment of a broad penetrating lip lesion

Penetrating lesion of the upper lip in a 66-year-old woman due to a fall. Clinical appearance 4 hours after injury.

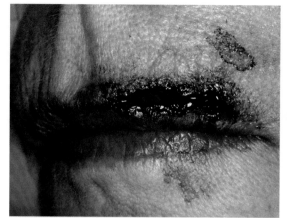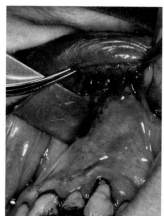

### Dental injuries

The crown of the left central and lateral incisors and canine have been fractured while the lateral incisor and canine have been intruded. Soft tissue radiographs demonstrate multiple foreign bodies in the upper lip.

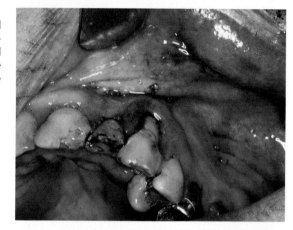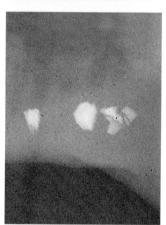

### Wound cleansing

The cutaneous and mucosal aspects of the wounds are cleansed with a surgical detergent followed by saline.

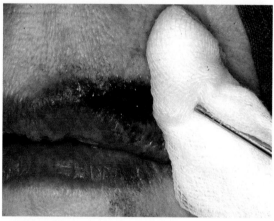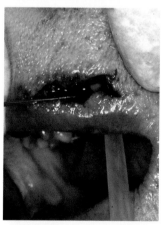

### Removal of foreign bodies

All radiographically demonstrated tooth fragments are located and removed.

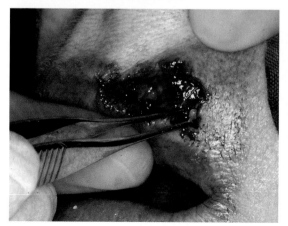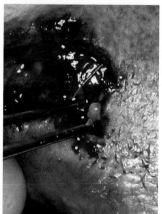

### Wound debridement
Traumatized salivary glands are excised in order to promote rapid healing.

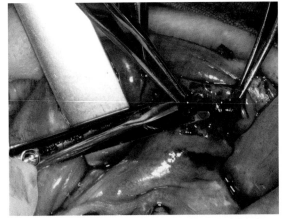
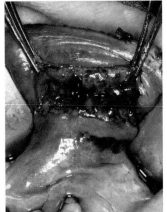

### Wound closure
The oral wound is closed with interrupted 4.0 silk sutures.

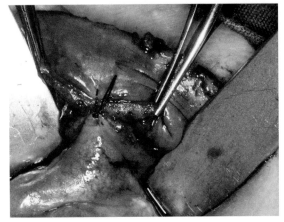
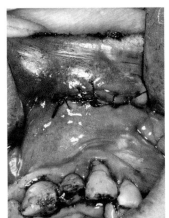

### Repeated cleansing of the cutaneous wound
The cutaneous aspect of the wound is cleansed with saline to minimize contamination from closure of the mucosal wound.

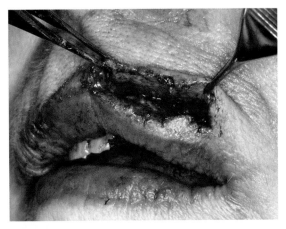
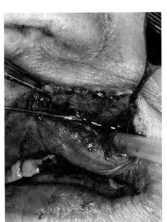

### Buried sutures
As a matter of principle, buried sutures should be kept to a minimum number; and, when indicated, be resorbed over a short period of time (e.g. Vicryl® sutures). The point of entry of the needle should be remote from the oral and cutaneous wound surfaces in order to place the knot (i.e. the most infection-prone part of the suture) far from the wound edges; that is, at approximately one-half the total thickness of the lip.

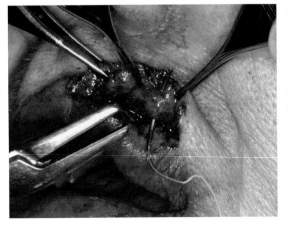
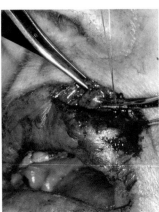

**Assessing cutaneous wound closure**

After closing the muscular tissue, the cutaneous part of the wound is evaluated. It is important that after muscular approximation, the wound edges can be approximated without tension. If this is not possible, approximation of the muscular part of the wound must be revised.

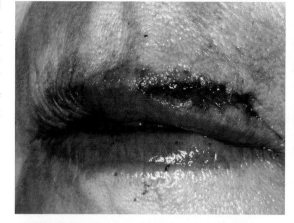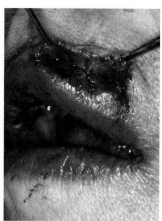

**Suturing the cutaneous wound**

Wound closure is principally begun at the vermilion border. In cases where the wound is parallel to the vermilion border, the first suture is placed at a site where irregularities of the wound edge ensure an anatomically correct closure. The wound is closed with fine, monofilament interrupted sutures (Prolene® 6.0), under magnification (i.e. using spectacles with a 2 or 4 × magnification).

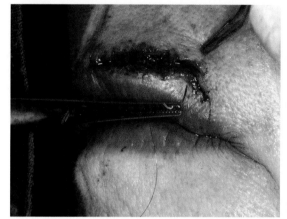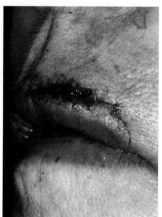

**Suturing completed**

The wound is now fully closed and antibiotics administered (i.e. penicillin, × 4, for 2 days in doses according to weight).

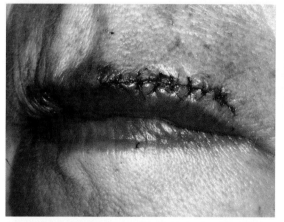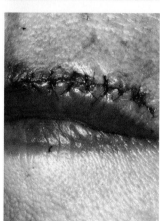

**Healing 6 weeks after injury**

There is a minimum of scarring.

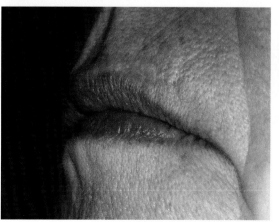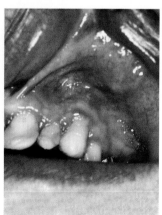

these findings could be that, as well as approximating the wound edges, suturing also induces ischemia of wound edges and acts as a wick, leading bacteria into the wound. Thus, the placement of just a single suture, however, significantly decreases the number of bacteria needed to cause wound infection (32) (see Chapter 1).

The tissue response to various types of sutures in the oral mucosa has been studied extensively in animals (36–42) and in humans (43, 44), and a vigorous inflammatory reaction around the sutures could be demonstrated. The general findings in these experimental studies have been that silk and catgut sutures (plain or chromic) elicited a very intense clinical and histological inflammatory reaction after 3, 5 and 7 days; whereas polyglycolic acid showed considerably less clinical and histological reaction (42).

The greatest part of the inflammatory reaction is probably related to the presence of bacteria within the interstices of multifilament suture materials (34, 37–40). Thus the impregnation of multifilament sutures with antibiotics has been shown to decrease the resultant tissue response (40). A further finding has been that monofilament sutures (e.g. nylon) display a significant reduction of adverse reactions compared to multifilament sutures, a finding possibly related to a reduced wick effect of monofilament sutures (41–45).

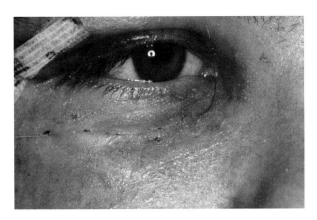

**Fig. 21.24** Intracutaneous suture of an infraorbital soft tissue wound. Note the excellent adaptation of tissue without stitch marks 5 days after suturing.

Monofilament suture material has been developed from a very inert and tissue compatible biomaterial made of polytetrafluoroethylene (PTFE). A comparison between the tissue response in oral mucosa between this material and silk sutures shows definitively less tissue response in the former (46).

Finally, it should be borne in mind that it has been shown experimentally that there is an increased risk of infection with both increased suture diameter and submucosal/subcutaneous suture length (9).

The essential lesson of all these experiments in suturing and subsequent wound healing is therefore that suturing is still the best overall method to use intra- and extraorally, using a minimal number of sutures with a small diameter, preferably monofilament and, finally, instituting early suture removal (i.e. after 3–4 days in oral tissues), eventually in two stages, i.e. 3 and 6 days.

The choice of sutures varies with the surgeon. There is an ongoing development to use synthetic absorbable sutures in the mucosa such as polyglycolic acid (Dexon®) polyglactic acid (Vicryl®) or polydioxanone (PDS®). Although absorbable sutures can also be used for skin closure, many surgeons prefer non-absorbable sutures such as nylon (Dermalon®, Ethilon®), polypropylene (Prolene®) or polybutester (Novofil®) for skin closure. Tape/strips may be used for skin closure in addition to sutures to relieve tension or used as an alternative to sutures for closing shallow, small wounds. The use of tissue adhesives/glue in the perioral region is not yet sufficiently evidence based.

## Antibiotic prophylaxis

It is surprising that the benefit of antibiotic therapy in oral soft tissue injuries has only been sparsely documented. Due to their pathogenesis, almost all of these injuries can be considered contaminated with microorganisms and sometimes with foreign bodies. Based on this assumption, it has been proposed that the surgical treatment of mucosal and cutaneous wounds should always be supported by prophylactic antibiotic coverage (47). However, clinical evidence for the

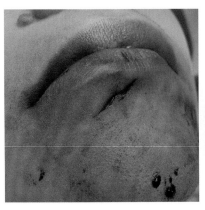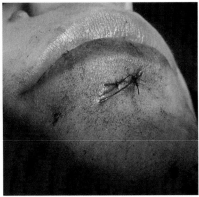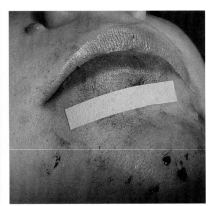

**Fig. 21.25** Laceration of the lower lip. This laceration was closed by intracutaneous suturing. To relieve tension two supplementary separate sutures were placed at the angles of the Z shaped laceration. To cover the sutured wound and to further relieve tension a tape was finally placed.

### Fig. 21.26 Treatment of a penetrating tongue lesion

This 10 year-old girl suffered a penetrating tongue lesion. Note the parallel lacerations on the dorsal and ventral surfaces of the tongue.

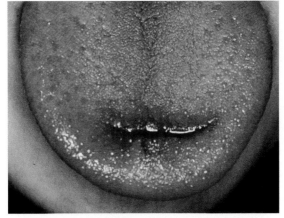
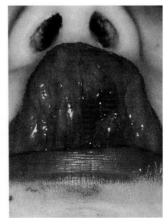

### Radiographic examination

A dental film is placed under the extended tongue and exposed at $\frac{1}{4}$ the normal exposure time. The exposure demonstrated several tooth fragments embedded within the tongue.

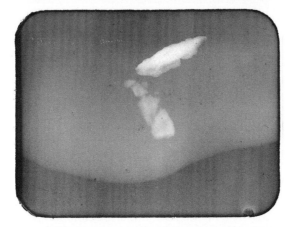
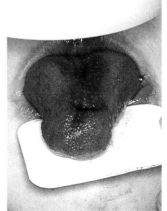

### Removal of tooth fragments

After administration of regional anesthestic, all tooth fragments were retrieved. It is important that all radiographically demonstrated fragments are also retrieved in order to prevent infection and/or scar formation.

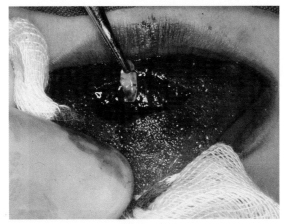
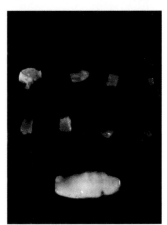

### Suturing the tongue wound

After all foreign bodies have been removed, the wound is cleansed and sutured on the dorsal and ventral surfaces.

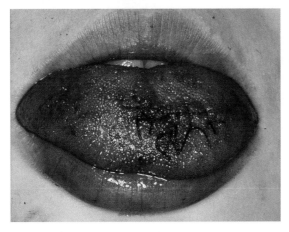
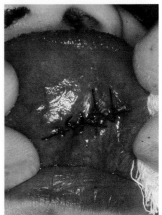

**Table 21.1** Effect of systematic antibiotic treatment subsequent to various combinations of cutaneous and oral mucosal wounds. After GOLDBERG (48) 1965.

| Type of lesion | Antibiotic treatment | No. of cases | Frequency of infection | Probability level* |
|---|---|---|---|---|
| Mucosal wounds | − | 32 | 4 (13%) | 0.66 |
| | + | 17 | 2 (12%) | |
| Mucosal and penetrating wounds (penetrating lesions) | − | 33 | 11 (33%) | 0.16 |
| | + | 24 | 4 (17%) | |

\* Probability level based on Fisher's exact test.

**Table 21.2** Effect of systemic antibiotic treatment subsequent to various combinations of facial cutaneous and oral mucosal wounds. After PATERSON et al. (49) 1970.

| Type of lesion | Antibiotic treatment | No. of cases | Frequency of infection | Probability level* |
|---|---|---|---|---|
| Mucosal wounds | − | 23 | 0 (0%) | 1.0 |
| | + | 12 | 0 (0%) | |
| Cutaneous wounds | − | 85 | 2 (2%) | 0.06 |
| | + | 51 | 6 (12%) | |
| Mucosal and cutaneous wounds | − | 21 | 0 (0%) | 1.0 |
| | + | 23 | 0 (0%) | |
| Mucosal and penetrating wounds (penetrating lesions) | − | 24 | 3 (13%) | 0.08 |
| | + | 48 | 15 (31%) | |

\* Probability level based on Fisher's exact test.

benefit of this treatment is presently tenuous (48–52) (Table 21.1). Thus, no effect of antibiotic therapy could be shown on the rate of infection in cutaneous and/or mucosal wounds. In penetrating wounds to the oral cavity, conflicting results have been reported (48, 49) (Table 21.2).

Based on these findings it seems reasonable – until further studies are presented – to restrict the prophylactic use of antibiotics in soft tissue wounds to the following situations:

- When the wound is heavily contaminated and wound debridement is not optimal (e.g. impacted foreign bodies or otherwise compromised wound cleansing).
- When wound debridement has been delayed (i.e. more than 24 hours) (41).
- Penetrating lesions through the full substance of the lip (5).
- When open reduction of jaw fractures is part of the treatment. In these situations, the benefit of short-term antibiotic coverage preceding and following osteosynthesis has been documented (47, 53–55) (see also Chapter 18). This relationship is in contrast to the lack of effect of antibiotic treatment in relation to 'clean' orthognathic surgery (56–59).
- When the general defense system of the patient is compromised (e.g. insulin dependent diabetes, alcohol abuse, immunocompromised patients, patients with prosthetic cardiac valves, cardiac surgical reconstructions, valvar dysfunction or malformations, or history of endocarditis (5).
- Human or animal bite wounds (60–62).

If prophylactic antibiotic coverage is decided upon, early institution is very important. Thus, experimental studies have shown that the first 3 hours after trauma are critical; i.e. to obtain an optimal effect from the antibiotics, they should be administered within this period (see Chapter 1).

If delayed, contaminating bacteria may multiply and invade the wound (12–14). Antibiotics should therefore be administered before surgery and maintained for 24 hours (63). Prolonged administration does not optimize healing (64–66), and has a serious effect upon the ecology of the oral microflora. The antibiotic of first choice is penicillin (phenoxymethyl penicillin). The dosage (adults) should be: 2 million units (= 1.2 g) orally at once followed by 2 million units (1.2 g) 3 times for 1 day. For children the dosage is given in relation to body weight. If the patient is allergic to penicillin, clindamycin should be administered. The dosage (adults) should be: 600 mg orally at once followed by 300 mg 3 times for 1 day. In children the dosage is 15 mg/kg body weight given 3 times for 1 day.

## Tetanus prophylaxis

Tetanus prophylaxis should always be considered in the case of contaminated wounds. In a previously immunized patient (i.e. longer than 10 years previous to injury), a dose of 0.5 ml tetanus toxoid should be given (booster injection). In unimmunized patients, passive immunization should be provided.

## Essentials

### Type of soft tissue lesion

- Abrasion
- Laceration
- Contusion (including hematoma)
- Tissue loss (avulsion)

## General treatment principles

- Contusions need not be treated but may indicate an underlying bone fracture.
- Abrasions and lacerations should be thoroughly cleansed and all foreign bodies removed.
- Larger avulsion injuries should be treated by specialists.

## Gingival lacerations (Figs 21.11–21.14)

- Rinse the wound and surroundings with a wound detergent.
- Reposition displaced gingiva.
- Place a few fine sutures (4.0 or 5.0 Vicryl®, Dexon® or PDS®).
- Instruct in good oral hygiene including daily mouth rinse with 0.1% chlorhexidine.
- Remove sutures after 4–5 days.

## Lip lacerations

Establish whether the injury is a penetrating wound of the lip or a laceration of the vermilion border (split-lip lesion).

### Penetrating lip wounds (Figs 21.22 and 21.23)

- Administer antibiotics if indicated (see Antibiotic prophylaxis).
- Take a radiograph of the lip with decreased exposure time.
- Use regional anesthesia.
- Rinse the wound and surroundings with a wound detergent.
- Remove foreign bodies and contused muscle and salivary gland tissue.
- Suture the labial mucosa (4.0 or 5.0 Vicryl®, Dexon®, PDS®).
- Rinse the wound again with saline.
- Suture the cutaneous wound with fine sutures (6.0 nylon or Prolene®). Take special consideration of the vermilion border.
- Remove sutures after 4–5 days.

### Split lip wounds (Fig. 21.19)

Use the same procedure as for penetrating lip lesions. However, in this case a few buried resorbable sutures are indicated (e.g. Dexon® 4.0/5.0).

## Tongue lacerations

Examine whether the injury is a penetrating wound or a lesion of the lateral border.

### Penetrating tongue wounds (Fig. 21.26)

- Administer antibiotics if indicated (see Antibiotic prophylaxis).
- Take a radiograph of the tongue with decreased exposure time.
- Use a regional or general anesthesia.

- Rinse the wound with saline.
- Remove foreign bodies.
- Rinse the wound again with saline.
- Suture the mucosal wounds.
- Remove sutures after 4–5 days.

### Lateral tongue border wounds

After administration of a regional anesthetic the wound is rinsed and sutured. Buried resorbable sutures are sometimes indicated in order to approximate the wound edges and relieve tension on the mucosal sutures.

## References

1. ANDREASEN JO. Etiology and pathogenesis of traumatic dental injuries. *Scand J Dent Res* 1970;**78**:329–42.
2. GALEA H. An investigation of dental injuries treated in an acute care general hospital. *J Am Dent Assoc* 1984;**10**:434–8.
3. O'NEIL DW, CLARKE MV, LOWE JW, HARRINGTON MS. Oral trauma in children: a hospital survey. *Oral Surg Oral Med Oral Pathol* 1989;**68**:691–6.
4. PETERSSON EE, ANDERSSON L, SÖRENSEN S. Traumatic oral vs non-oral injuries. An epidemiological study during one year in a Swedish county. *Swed Dent J* 1997;**21**:55–68.
5. PETERSON L, ELLIS E, HUPP J, TUCKER M. *Contemporary oral and maxillofacial surgery.* 4th edn. St Louis: Mosby, 2003.
6. LINDFORS J. A comparison of an antimicrobial wound cleanser to normal saline in reduction of bioburden and its effect on wound healing. *Ostomy Wound Manag* 2004;**50**:28–41.
7. BRÅNEMARK P-J, EKHOLM L, ALBREKTSSON B, LINDSTRÖM J, LUNDBORG G, LUNDSKOG J, Tissue injuries caused by wound disinfectants. *J Bone Joint Surg* 1967;**49A**:48–62.
8. VALENTE JH, FORTI RJ, FREUNDLICH LF, ZANDIEH SO, CRAIN EF. Wound irrigation in children: saline solution or tap water? *Ann Emerg Med* 2003;**41**:609–16.
9. EDLICH RF, RODEHEAVER G, THACKER JG. EDGERTON MT. Technical factors in wound management. In: Hunt TK, Dunphy JE. eds. *Fundamentals of wound management.* New York: Appleton-Century-Crofts, 1979:364–545.
10. FORRESTER JC. Sutures and wound repair. In: Hunt TK. ed. *Wound healing and wound infection. Theory and surgical practice.* New York: Appleton-Century-Crofts, 1980:194–207.
11. OSBON DB, Early treatment of soft tissue injuries of the face. *J Oral Surg* 1969;**27**:480–7.
12. BURKE JF. Infection. In: Hunt TK, Dunphy JE. eds. *Fundamentals of wound management.* New York: Appleton-Century-Crofts, 1979:171–240.
13. EDLICH RF, KENNEY JG, MORGAN RE, et al. Antimicrobial treatment of minor soft tissue lacerations: A critical review. *Emerg Med Clin North Am* 1986;**4**:561–80.
14. EDLICH R, RODEHEAVER GT, THACKER JC. Technical factors in the prevention of wound infections. In: Howard RJ, Simmons RL. eds. *Surgical infectious diseases.* New York: Appleton-Century-Crofts, 1982:449–72.

15. HAURY B, RODEHEAVER G, VENSKO J, EDGERTON MT, EDLICH RF. Debridement: An essential component of traumatic wound care. In: Hunt TK. ed. W*ound healing and wound infection. Theory and surgical practice*. New York: Appleton-Century-Crofts, 1980:229–41.

16. HERFORD AS. Early repair of avulsive facial wounds secondary to trauma using interpolation flaps. *J Oral Maxillofac Surg* 2004;**62**:959–65.

17. CLARK N, BIRELY B, MANSON PN, SLEZAK S, KOLK CV, ROBERTSON B, CRAWLEY W. High-energy ballistic and avulsive facial injuries: classification, patterns, and an algorithm for primary reconstruction. *Plas Reconstr Surg* 1996;**98**:583–601.

18. KOZAK J, VOSKA P. Experience with the treatment of facial gunshot injuries. *Acta Chir Plast* 1997;**39**:48–52.

19. RHEE ST, COLVILLE C, BUCHMAN SR. Conservative management of large avulsion of the lip and local landmarks. *Pediatr Emerg Care* 2004;**20**:40–2.

20. MILLER TA. Wound contraction as treatment of dog bite avulsions of the lip. *Ann Plast Surg* 1987;**19**: 42–5.

21. HALLOCK GC. Dog bites of the face with tissue loss. *J Cranio Maxillofacial Trauma*. 1996;**2**:49–55.

22. DE BLANCO LP. Lip suture with isobuthyl cyanoacrylate. *Endod Dent Traumatol* 1994;**10**:15–18.

23. BRUNS TB, SIMON HK, MCLARIO DJ. Laceration repair using tissue adhesive in a children's emergency department. *Pediatrics* 1996;**98**:673–5.

24. OSMOND MH, QUINN JV, SUTCLIFFE T, JARMUSKE M, KLASSEN TP. A randomized, clinical trial comparing butylcyanoacrylate with octylcyanoacrylate in the management of selected pediatric facial lacerations. *Acad Emerg Med* 1999;**6**:171–7.

25. SIMON HK, ZEMPSKY WT, BRUNS TB, SULLIVAN KM. Lacerations against Langer's lines: to glue or suture? *J Emerg Med* 1998;**16**:185–9.

26. QUINN J, WELLS G, SUTCLIFFE T, JARMUSKE M, MAW J, STIELL I, JOHNS P. Tissue adhesive versus suture wound repair at 1 year randomized clinical trial correlating early, 3-month, and 1-year cosmetic outcome. *Ann Emerg Med* 1998;**32**:645–9.

27. HOLGER JS, WANDERSEE SE, HALE DB. Cosmetic outcome of facial lacerations repaired with tissue adhesive, absorbable and non-absorbable sutures. *Am J Emerg Med* 2004;**22**:254–7.

28. FARION K, OSMOND MH, HARTLING L. Tissue adhesives for traumatic lacerations in children and adults. *Cochrane Database of Systematic Reviews*, 2002(3).

29. SMITH J, MACONOCHIE I. Should we glue lip lacerations in children? *Arch Dis Child* 2003;**88**:83–4.

30. COULTHARD P, WOTHINGTON H, ESPOSITO M, ELST M, WAES OJ. Tissue adhesive for closure of surgical incisions. *Cochrane Database of Systematic Reviews*, 2004(2).

31. BRUNIUS U. Wound healing impairment from sutures. *Acta Chir Scand* 1968; Supplement 395.

32. FORRESTER JC, ZEDERFELDT BH, HUNT TK. The tapeclosed wound – a bioengineering analysis. *J Surg Res* 1969;**9**:537–42.

33. CONOLLY WB, HUNT TK, ZEDERFELDT B, CAFFERATA HT, DUNPHY JE. Clinical comparison of surgical wounds closed by suture and adhesive tapes. *Ann J Surg* 1969;**11**:318–22.

34. ELEK SD. Experimental staphylococcal infections in the skin of man. *Ann NY Acad Sci* 1956;**65**:85–90.

35. EDLICH RF, RODEHAVER G, GOLDEN GT, EDGERTON MT. The biology of infections: Sutures, tapes and bacteria. In: Hunt TK. ed. *Wound healing and wound infection. Theory and surgical practice*. New York: Appleton-Century-Crofts 1980:214–28.

36. BERGENHOLZ A, ISAKSSON B. Tissue reactions in the oral mucosa to catgut, silk, and mersilene sutures. *Odontol Rev* 1967;**18**:237–50.

37. LILLY GE. Reaction of oral tissues to suture materials. *Oral Surg Oral Med Oral Pathol* 1968;**26**:28–33.

38. LILLY GE, ARMSTRONG JH, SALEM JE, CUTCHER JL. Reaction of oral tissues to suture materials. Part II. *Oral Surg Oral Med Oral Pathol* 1968;**26**:592–9.

39. LILLY GE, SALEM JE, ARMSTRONG JH, CUTCHER JL. Reaction of oral tissues to suture materials. Part III. *Oral Surg Oral Med Oral Pathol* 1969;**28**:432–8.

40. LILLY GE, CUTHER JL, JONES JC, ARMSTRONG JH. Reaction of oral tissues to suture materials. Part IV. *Oral Surg Oral Med Oral Pathol* 1972;**33**:152–7.

41. KACLOVA J, JANOUSKOVA M. Etude experimental sur la reáction des tissus de la cavite buccale aux differents materiaux de suture en chirurgie. *Med Hyg (Geneve)* 1965;**23**:1239.

42. CASTELLI WA, NASJLETI CE, CAFFESSE RE, DIAZ-PEREZ R. Gingival response to silk, cotton, and nylon suture materials. *Oral Surg Oral Med Oral Pathol* 1978;**45**:179–85.

43. WALLACE WR, MAXWELL GR, CAVALARIS CJ. Comparison of polyglycolic-polylactic acid suture to black silk, chromic, and plain catgut in human oral tissues. *J Oral Surg* 1970;**28**:739–46.

44. RACEY GL, WALLACE WR, CAVALARIS CJ, MARQUARD JV. Comparison of a polyglycolic-polylactic acid suture to black silk and plain catgut in human oral tissues. *J Oral Surg* 1978;**36**:766–70.

45. POWERS MP, BERTZ JB, FONSECA RJ. Management of soft tissue injuries. In: Fonesca RL, Walker RV. eds. *Oral and maxillofacial trauma*. Philadelphia: WB Saunders Company, 1996:16–50.

46. RIVERA-HIDALGO F, CUNDIFF EJ, WILLIAMS FE, MCQUADE MG. Tissue reaction to silk and Goretex sutures in dogs. *J Dent Res* 1991;**71**:(Spec Issue):508.

47. ZALLEN RD, BLACK SL. Antibiotic therapy in oral and maxillofacial surgery. *J Oral Surg* 1976;**34**:349–51.

48. GOLDBERG MH. Antibiotics and oral and oral-cutaneous lacerations. *J Oral Surg* 1965;**23**:117–22.

49. PATERSON JA, CARDO VA, STRATIGOS GT. An examination of antibiotic prophylaxis in oral and maxillofacial surgery. *J Oral Surg* 1970;**28**:753–9.

50. GUGLIEMO BJ, HOHN DC, KOO PJ, HUNT TK, SWEET RL, CONTE JE. Antibiotic prophylaxis in surgical procedures. A critical analysis of the literature. *Arch Surg* 1983; **11**:43–55.

51. CUMMINGS P, DEL BECCARO MA. Antibiotics to prevent infection of simple wounds: a meta-analysis of randomized studies. *Am J Emerg Med* 1995;**13**: 396–400.

52. VERSCHUUR H, WEVER WD W, BRUIJN AD A, BENTHEM PVP. Antibiotic prophylaxis in clean and clean-contaminated ear surgery. *Cochrane Database of Systematic Reviews*, 2004(3).

53. ZALLEN RD. A study of antibiotic usage in compound mandibular fractures. *J Oral Surg* 1975;**33**:431–4.

54. ADERHOLD L, LJUNG H, FRENKEL G. Untersuchungen uber den Wert einer Antibiotica-prophylaxe bei Kiefer-Gesichtsverletzungen eine prospektive Studie. *Dtsch Zahnärztl Z* 1983;**38**:402–6.

55. GERLACH KL, PAPE HD. Untersuchungen zur Antibiotica-prophylaxe bei der operativen Behandlung von Unterkieferfrakturen. *Dtsch Z Mund Kiefer Gesichtschir* 1988;**12**:497–500.

56. ZALLEN RD, STRADER RJ. The use of prophylactic antibiotics in extraoral procedures for mandibular prognathism. *J Oral Surg* 1971;**29**:178–9.

57. YRASTORZA JA. Indication for antibiotics in orthognatic surgery. *J Oral Surg* 1976;**34**:514–6.

58. PETERSON LJ, BOOTH DF. Efficacy of antibiotic prophylaxis in intraoral orthognathic surgery. *J Oral Surg* 1976;**34**:1088–91.

59. MARTIS C, KARABOUTA I. Infection after orthognathic surgery, with and without preventive antibiotics. *Int J Oral Surg* 1984;**13**:490–4.

60. ZACKOWSKI D, LEHMAN JA JR, TANTRI MD. Management of dog bite avulsions of the lip vermilion. *Pediatr Emerg Care* 1986;**2**:85–7.

61. VENTER TH. Human bites of the face. Early surgical management. *S Afr Med J* 1988;**74**:277–9.

62. MEDEIROS I, SACONATO H. Antibiotic prophylaxis for mammalian bites. *Cochrane Database of Systematic Reviews*, 2001(2).

63. BECKERS H, KUHNLE T, DIETRICH H-G. Einfluss prophylactisher Antibiose auf infectiöse Komplikationen nach Dysgnathioperationen. *Fortscher Kiefer Gesichthir* 1984;**29**:118–9.

64. BURKE JF. Preventive antibiotics in surgery. *Postgrad Med J* 1975;**58**:65–8.

65. CONOVER MA, KABAN LB, MULLIKEN JB. Antibiotic prophylaxis for major maxillocraniofacial surgery. *J Oral Maxillofacial Surg* 1985;**43**:865–70.

66. RUGGLES JE. Antibiotic prophylaxis in intraoral orthognathic surgery. *J Oral Maxillofac Surg* 1984;**42**: 797–801.

67. SHOCKLEDGE RR, MACKIE IC. Oral soft tissue trauma: gingival degloving. *Endod Dent Traumatol* 1996;**11**: 109–111.

68. MONEFELDT I, ZACHRISSON BU. Adjustment of clinical crown height by gingivectomy following orthodontic space closure. *Angle Orthod* 1977; **47**: 256–64.

69. OIKARINEN KS, NIEMINEN TM, MAKARAINEN H, PHYTINEN J. Visibility of foreign bodies in soft tissue in plain radiographs, computed tomography, magnetic resonance imaging and ultrasound. *Int J Maxillofac Surg* 1993;**22**:119–24.

70. ALMELH M, ANDERSSON L, BEBEHANI E. Reduction of pain from needlestick in the oral mucosa by topical anesthetics: a comparative study between lidocaine/prilocaine and benzocaine. *J Clin Dent* 2006. In press.

# 22

# Endodontic Management and the Use of Calcium Hydroxide in Traumatized Permanent Teeth

## M. Cvek

The majority of accidents affect children and adolescents, often when root development of the injured teeth is not completed. In the following, the treatment of young permanent teeth with the use of calcium hydroxide will be addressed and an attempt made to give a clinically oriented description. Within the last decade a new endodontic material, mineral trioxide aggregate (MTA), has been introduced for the treatment of injured teeth. The properties and clinical use of this material are presented in Chapter 23.

## Crown fractures with dentin exposure

### Healing and pathology

Crown fractures involving dentin result in exposure of dentinal tubules to the oral environment. Exposure of dentin, as such, causes only insignificant changes in the pulp which may resolve and the exposed dentinal tubules be sealed off by formation of secondary dentin (1). However, if deeply exposed dentin is left unprotected, bacteria and their components in dental plaque on the fracture surface may penetrate the tubules and cause inflammation in the underlying pulp (2–5) (Figs 22.1 and 22.2). Judging from experimental studies, the subsequent reparative or degenerative changes depend on the time that has elapsed since injury and the distance between the fracture surface and pulp. In young permanent teeth, wide dentinal tubules may be an additional factor (Fig. 22.3). If irritation is eliminated by treatment of the exposed dentin, localized inflammation in the pulp may resolve, with damaged tissue being replaced by reparative dentin (6, 134, 135).

When deeply exposed dentin is left unprotected over a longer period of time, the pulp may in some cases become necrotic and the crown discolored. However, a more fre-

quent cause of pulp necrosis in crown-fractured teeth is probably impaired blood circulation in the pulp due to a concomitant luxation injury (see Chapter 10).

### Treatment

A crown fracture is usually an isolated injury and the crown can be restored at the first visit, normally with a resin composite material and dental bonding techniques. Treatment procedures are described in detail in Chapter 25.

Modern dentin bonding systems have been reported to increase the bonding strength of composite restorations, reduce microleakage, decrease permeability of dentin and possess an antibacterial effect (136–139, 141–150, 289, 290). The occasional occurrence of pulp inflammation has been explained by various factors, but poor bonding, which permits microleakage and penetration of bacteria into the pulp seems to be the most common. It has, therefore, been recommended that in the case of deep carious lesions, the pulp should be protected, e.g. by the lining of the deepest part of the cavity before a dentin bonding agent is placed over the rest of the dentin. This strategy should also be valid for crown-fractured teeth with deeply exposed dentin (145, 150). The value of lining with calcium hydroxide preparations beneath permanent restorations has been questioned (291). However, in cases where the color of the pulp can be seen through a very thin dentin layer or when a deep fracture is left untreated over a couple of days, it may be advisable that the dentin be initially treated with calcium hydroxide and the crown temporarily restored for about 2–3 weeks (Fig. 22.4). In such teeth, treatment with calcium hydroxide may remove bacteria from the fracture surface and give an eventually inflamed pulp a chance to recover and seal off the exposed dentinal tubules by deposition of reparative dentin (7, 151, 152). Moreover, calcium hydrox-

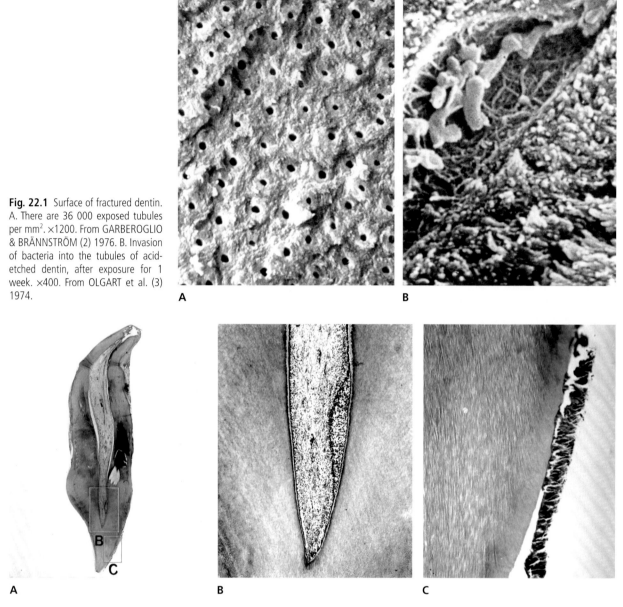

**Fig. 22.1** Surface of fractured dentin. A. There are 36 000 exposed tubules per mm². ×1200. From GARBEROGLIO & BRÄNNSTRÖM (2) 1976. B. Invasion of bacteria into the tubules of acid-etched dentin, after exposure for 1 week. ×400. From OLGART et al. (3) 1974.

**Fig. 22.2** Early changes in the pulp of a primary incisor 3 days after an uncomplicated crown fracture. A. Low power view. ×3. B. Displacement of odontoblasts and slight infiltration of leukocytes corresponding to the fracture surface. ×30. C. Bacterial accumulation along the fracture surface. ×75.

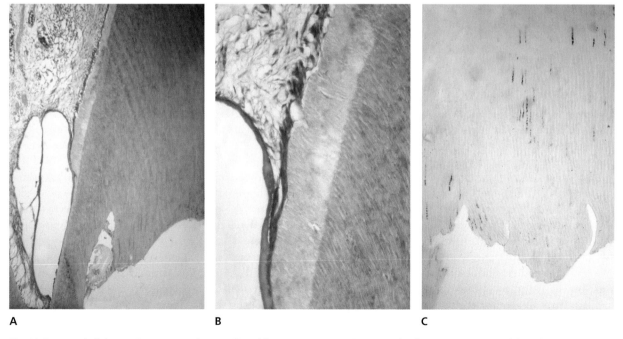

**Fig. 22.3** Late pulpal changes in an untreated uncomplicated fracture. A primary incisor 4 months after injury. A. Necrosis of the pulp tissue subjacent to the fracture surface. ×32. B. Formation of reparative dentin at a distance from the fracture surface. ×60. C. Penetration of bacteria through the dentin, from fracture surface towards the pulp, Brown & Brenn bacterial stain. ×200.

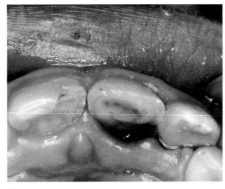 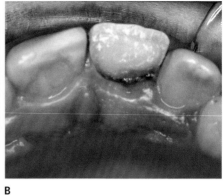

**Fig. 22.4** Treatment of exposed dentin and affected pulp. A. Appearance of fracture after the crown-root fragment has been removed and the surface cleansed 3 days after injury. A hyperemic pulp can be seen through the thin dentin, probably due to irritation from plaque between the fragments. B. Four weeks after treatment with calcium hydroxide; the red discoloration has disappeared.

**A**

**B**

ide significantly decreases the permeability of dentin to penetration by bacterial components into the pulp, which may provide additional pulp protection under a subsequent restoration (7, 151, 152).

If, for some reason, crown restoration cannot be performed immediately, e.g. due to incorporation in a splint, the pulpo-dentinal complex should be protected. Before the splint is adapted, the exposed dentin may be covered with hard-setting calcium hydroxide compound or glass ionomer cement (see Chapter 10, p. 288).

## Prognosis

Restoration of a fractured crown with resin composites and dental bonding techniques can be regarded as an effective tooth repair. However, it should be noted that bacterial leakage has been demonstrated in the gaps between composites and dentinal walls in experimental cervical cavities (152, 153). But most uncomplicated fractures do not involve the cervical area; and, according to clinical studies, the risk of later pulpal damage seems to be minimal (154, 155, 220) (see Chapter 10, p. 301).

## Crown fractures with pulp exposure

### Healing and pathology

A crown fracture through the pulp chamber causes laceration and exposure of the pulp to the oral environment. Healing does not occur spontaneously and untreated exposures ultimately lead to pulp necrosis, a process in which bacteria are the dominant factor (8). The early changes in the pulp are hemorrhage and local inflammation, caused by breakdown products from lacerated tissue and bacterial toxins (9, 10). The fibrin clot that forms over the wound surface resolves after a couple of days. The subsequent changes can either be proliferative, such as a pulp polyp, or destructive, such as abscess formation or pulp necrosis.

During the first days after injury, a fresh wound or proliferative changes, i.e. formation of granulation tissue at the exposure site, seem to be most common (Fig. 22.5). In studies of patients aged 7 to 16 years, seen 12 hours or more after injury, hyperplasia was a typical pulpal reaction seen in crown-fractured incisors, regardless of the extent of the exposure (11, 156). Similar observations have been made in multi-rooted human teeth when the pulp was exposed by removal of the crown and left untreated for 2 weeks (12). These findings have also been supported by experimental studies in which pulps of monkey incisors were exposed by either crown fracture or grinding. In these experiments, pulpal changes were characterized by a proliferative response, invariably associated with only superficial inflammation, extending not more than 2 mm from the exposure site (13, 14) (Fig. 22.5).

A proliferative response of the pulp is probably favored by an exposure which permits salivary rinsing and prevents impaction of contaminated debris, as occurs in caries or experimentally induced cavities (13, 157).

Necrosis of an exposed pulp is a rare occurrence. A common etiological factor seems to be plaque and contaminated debris that are permitted to accumulate over the exposure, which may allow bacteria to settle into injured or necrotized pulp tissue (Fig. 22.6). Thus, in monkey incisors in which the coronal cavities were left open for 7 days after pulpotomy, impaction of contaminated food debris caused deep abscesses in the underlying pulp (13).

### Treatment

The aim of treatment should be the preservation of a vital, non-inflamed pulp, biologically walled off by a continuous hard tissue barrier. In most cases, this can be achieved by pulp capping or pulpotomy (293). When these treatment alternatives are not possible, the pulp must be extirpated and the root canal filled with an adequate root filling material. Indications for these forms of treatment are discussed later in connection with endodontic procedures. Some factors, however, such as maturity of the tooth, concomitant luxation injury, age of the patient as well as the effect of surgical procedures and choice of wound dressing, must also be considered.

The maturity of the tooth is of utmost importance in the choice of treatment. It is generally agreed that the exposed vital pulp should be maintained in young teeth with incomplete root formation; while it can be removed in mature

**Fig. 22.5 Clinical appearance of pulp exposures at various observation periods**

Four hours after injury hemorrhage is the predominant finding. After 2 days (right), granulation tissue is formed at the exposure site.

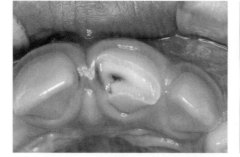
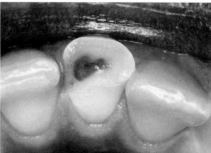

**Clinical appearance**

One week after injury (left): hyperplasia of the pulp. Three months after injury (right): a polyp has been formed and is covered with plaque.

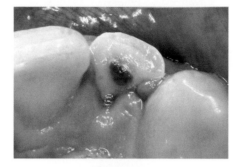
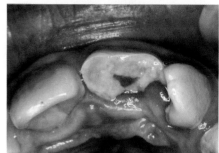

**Histologic appearance**

Pulp reactions to experimental exposure in monkey incisors. After 2 days (left), the exposed surface is covered with fibrin, under which a limited pulp proliferation can be seen with moderate infiltration of inflammatory cells to a depth of 1.4 mm. ×90. After 1 week (right), there is proliferation of the pulp through the exposure and moderate inflammation in the proliferated tissue and a mild infiltration of inflammatory cells in the pulp to a depth of 0.4 mm. ×32. From CVEK et al. (13) 1982.

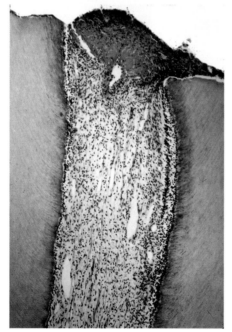
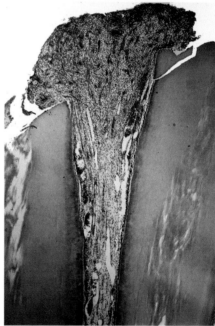

**Fig. 22.6** Necrosis of the pulp at the exposure site. A. Necrosis of the pulp tissue in a tooth in which the exposure was only covered with a surgical packing for 2 weeks. B. Necrosis of the pulp at the exposure site 4 weeks after injury. The tooth was initially restored with a temporary crown, seated with temporary cement which was lost after 3 weeks.

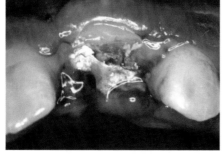
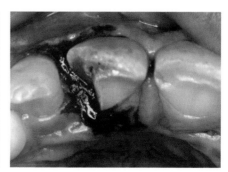

A

B

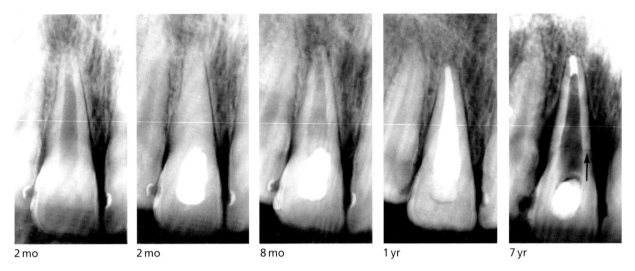

| 2 mo | 2 mo | 8 mo | 1 yr | 7 yr |

**Fig. 22.7** Spontaneous root fracture due to thin dentinal walls after pulp necrosis at an early stage of root development and over ambitious reaming. Permanent incisor treated with calcium hydroxide and root filled with gutta-percha. Cervical fracture of the thin dentinal walls (arrow) occurred during chewing 6 years later.

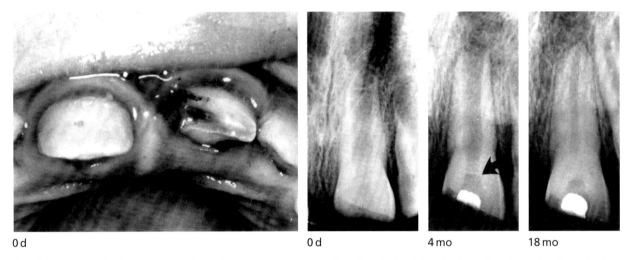

| 0 d | 0 d | 4 mo | 18 mo |

**Fig. 22.8** Treatment of pulp exposure in a slightly dislocated immature incisor. Formation of a hard tissue barrier in the pulp, continued root development and diminishing of the pulp subsequent to partial pulpotomy.

teeth where constriction of the apical foramen allows adequate obturation of the root canal. However, maturation of a tooth is not complete with constriction of the apical foramen. Removal of the pulp in children and adolescents deprives the tooth of physiologic dentin apposition which, together with mechanical cleansing, leaves thin dentinal walls, which may increase the risk of later cervical root fractures, a problem that should be considered in treatment planning (15, 16, 221) (Fig. 22.7).

A concomitant luxation injury compromises the nutritional supply to the pulp and, in principle, contraindicates conservative treatment. However, in luxated immature teeth the chance of pulp survival is considerable and conservative treatment may allow further root development (17, 18) (Fig. 22.8). Treatment should therefore be determined considering severity of the periodontal injury and maturity of the tooth.

The effect of age is controversial. Experimentally, an inferior response to injury and treatment has been observed in pulps of old rats compared to young ones (9, 10). Yet, successful treatment of pulp exposure due to either trauma or caries in older patients has repeatedly been reported (19, 22). For various reasons, degenerative changes in the pulp undoubtedly increase with age. Thus, removal of the pulp could be a more successful procedure, although no age limit can be set for either pulp preservation or removal. However, conservative treatment, i.e. capping or pulpotomy, should not be performed if degenerative or inflammatory changes are anticipated, e.g. in teeth with reduced pulpal lumen due to trauma or age, or in periodontally involved teeth in adults (23–26).

Surgical pulp procedures invariably cause further injury to the remaining pulp and should be kept to a minimum. Various instruments have been recommended for pulpal

**Fig. 22.9 Effect of pulp amputation technique upon the pulp**
The effect of cutting with an abrasive diamond instrument in a high speed contra-angle hand piece; no tissue damage below the wound surface. ×25 and 100. From GRANATH & HAGMAN (31) 1971.

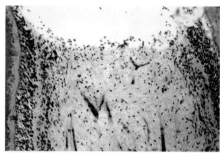
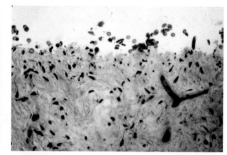

**Effect of calcium hydroxide on the pulp**
Left: Formation of liquefaction necrosis (L) close to calcium hydroxide. Coagulation necrosis (C) close to the vital pulp is colored yellow. ×75. Right: formation of hard tissue 17 days after capping; layer of necrotic tissue (N) and dark stained band of necrotic and later calcified tissue (C) and osteoid-like tissue (O) with lining cells. ×75. From SCHRÖDER & GRANATH (35) 1971.

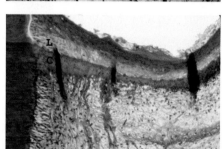
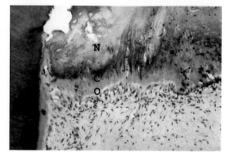

**Formation of a hard tissue barrier**
A completely formed hard tissue barrier after capping with calcium hydroxide paste (Calasept®). ×25. Right: formation of hard tissue barrier without visible intermediate layer of necrosis after capping with hard-setting calcium hydroxide compound (Dycal®). ×25. From BRÄNNSTRÖM et al. (39) 1979.

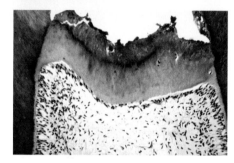
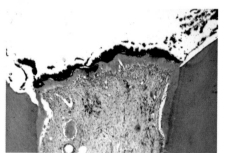

amputation, such as spoon excavators, slowly rotating round burs and high-speed abrasive diamonds. Of these, the spoon excavator, successfully used in molars, has proven unsuitable in young incisors (27). Slowly rotating instruments are known to inflict significant injury to the remaining pulp, limiting the chance of survival (28–30). However, it has been shown that injury to the underlying tissue is minimal when abrasive diamond is used at high speed to remove part of the pulp, provided that the bur and tissues are adequately cooled (31) (Fig. 22.9). If effective cooling is not possible, e.g. when the amputation site is deep in the root canal, a round bur at low speed should be used in order to avoid overheating the pulp.

The commonly used wound dressing is calcium hydroxide. This material has been widely used for the treatment of accidentally exposed pulps since the first histological studies appeared decades ago (32, 33, 158). Calcium hydroxide has been the subject of extensive experimental research and several explanations have been offered for its effect on the vital pulp (159). When placed over the vital pulp, pure calcium hydroxide causes a superficial tissue necrosis, approximately 1–1.5 mm in depth (34). This necrosis consists of several layers, including a layer of firm coagulation necrosis in close contact with vital tissue, which seems not to be appreciably affected (35). Based on observations in experiments with sound human teeth, it has been suggested

that it is neither calcium hydroxide nor its components, but the low-grade irritation from coagulation necrosis that induces defensive reactions in the pulp, resulting in formation of a demarcating hard-tissue barrier (35, 36, 160). The underlying tissue seems to react to this irritation by producing collagen that is subsequently mineralized, while the coagulated tissue is calcified, which is later followed by differentiation of dentin (Fig. 22.9). This hypothesis of a low-grade irritation that is not strong enough to destroy the pulp tissue but is sufficient to elicit defensive reactions was strongly supported by findings of the formation of hard tissue barriers after only 10 minutes' treatment with calcium hydroxide or capping with cyanoacrylate, a material possessing none of the calcium or hydroxyl ions that are thought to be responsible for induction of hard tissue (160) (Fig. 22.10).

Cyanoacrylate is degradable in a biological environment and it is probable that some released substance(s) may exert just enough irritation to elicit defensive reactions in the pulp leading to formation of a hard tissue barrier (161). Similar results have been reported in experiments with light-cured composite, zinc phosphate and silicate cements (162, 195). On the other hand, when a biologically inert material, such as Teflon, has been brought into contact with pulpal tissue no hard tissue formation could be found in relation to this material (160, 163). Thus, the role of calcium hydroxide

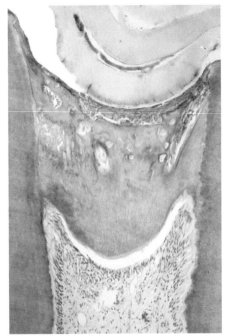
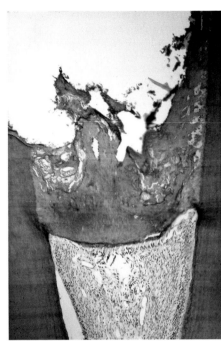

**A**                                    **B**

**Fig. 22.10** Response of monkey incisor to capping with cyanoacrylate or 10 minutes dressing with calcium hydroxide. A. Formation of hard tissue barrier 3 months after the pulp was treated with calcium hydroxide for 10 minutes, then washed away, and the pulpal wound covered with several sterile Teflon discs sealed in place with IRM®. ×50. B. Formation of hard tissue barrier 3 months after the pulp was covered with cyanoacrylate. ×40. Note that hard tissue barriers are not continuous and include vascular tunnels (arrow). From CVEK et al. (160) 1987.

appears to be limited to its chemical effect that is able to elicit defensive processes in the pulp by exerting a low-grade irritation, either through the induction of coagulation necrosis or directly on the pulp tissue without a visible necrosis when hard-setting compounds are used (37, 164–167) (Figs 22.9 and 22.10). Accordingly, formation of the hard tissue barrier itself can be regarded as a defensive, probably stereotypic, reaction of the pulp to a non-specific low-grade irritant (168).

During the course of time, various materials have been tested for pulpal dressing (161, 169). Indeed, in the absence of bacteria, healing of the pulp with or without formation of hard tissue was observed after capping with various materials, such as cyanoacrylate, zinc-phosphate, tricalcium phosphate or silicate cements and various composite materials. The results, obtained mostly in experimental animals such as monkeys, dogs and rats, were not always unanimous. Comprehensive, long-term clinical studies would be desirable before recommending some drugs for routine clinical use (162, 170–172, 293, 294).

Calcium hydroxide seems to be a suitable and well-tested pulp dressing which repeatedly gives predictable results in the form of a non-inflamed pulp under a well-formed hard-tissue barrier. However, it should be stressed that calcium hydroxide as such has no beneficial effect on healing of a chronically inflamed pulp (38). In clinical terms, this means that the compound should be placed against vital pulp tissue with intact vascularity in teeth which respond to sensibility testing. Internal dentin resorption and dystrophic calcifications, reported to occur after dressing of the pulp with calcium hydroxide, seem to be related to the presence of an extra-pulpal blood clot or to the damage caused by operative procedures (29, 39–44). Thus, when an extra-pulpal blood clot was not allowed to form and a gentle amputation

technique was used for amputation, these changes were not observed clinically or histologically (11, 36, 156, 173–175).

## Pulp capping

Capping of the pulp is indicated when a small exposure can be treated shortly after injury which, according to experimental studies, seems to mean within 24 hours (167, 176, 177). Pulp capping implies that the pulpal wound caused by the injury is covered with calcium hydroxide. It is thought that, in small exposures treated soon after injury, the mechanical damage and inflammation in the pulp cannot be deeper than the necrotizing effect of calcium hydroxide. Thus, the effect actually is exerted on healthy pulp tissue, while bacteria on the dentin fracture and the wound surfaces are eliminated by the action of calcium hydroxide. Accordingly, the primary contamination of the pulp should not be critical for healing. However, pulp healing may be threatened by later contamination due to microleakage of defective restorations, since all calcium hydroxide compounds gradually lose their antibacterial property. Furthermore, the hard tissue barriers may include structural defects which may increase their permeability and, in the case of 'tunnel' formation, due to vascular inclusions, offer a direct contact with underlying pulp tissue (160, 162, 178–183) (Fig. 22.10).

### *Treatment procedure*

The fracture surface and pulpal wound are washed with saline. When bleeding has ceased, the exposed pulp is covered with a soft- or a hard-setting calcium hydroxide compound. If the pulp is covered with a soft calcium hydroxide compound, the exposed dentin should be protected with glass ionomer cement or a hard-setting calcium

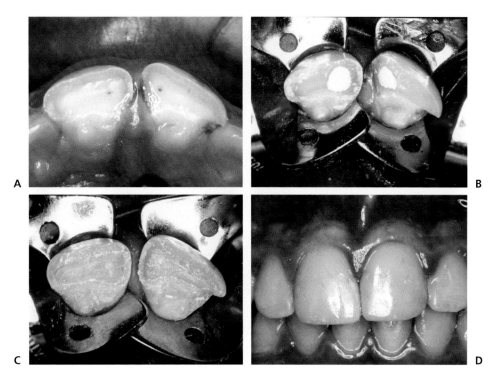

**Fig. 22.11** Treatment of a complicated crown fracture with pulp capping. A. Fractured incisor with a small pulp exposure 4 hours after injury. Note the good vascularity of the exposed pulp. B and C. After isolation with a rubber dam, the exposed pulp is covered with a soft calcium hydroxide compound (Calasept®) which together with the remaining dentin is covered with hard-setting calcium hydroxide cement. D. The tooth is restored with a composite.

hydroxide liner before the crown is restored (Fig. 22.11). If the definitive restoration of the crown must be postponed, a temporary crown restoration should be placed with a material that does not allow microleakage, e.g. zinc oxide-eugenol or polycarboxylate cement (184, 185).

## Pulpotomy

Pulpotomy involves removal of damaged and inflamed tissue to the level of a clinically healthy pulp, followed by a calcium hydroxide dressing. Depending on the size of the exposure and time elapsed since injury, different levels of pulpal amputation have been recommended, i.e. partial or deep pulpotomy (11, 45). It has been shown, however, that neither exposure size nor time interval between injury and treatment are critical for healing when only superficial layers of the pulp are removed (11, 156, 173). Thus, in teeth showing vital and/or hyperplasic pulp tissue at the exposure, only superficial layers of the pulp and surrounding dentin should be removed; i.e. a partial pulpotomy can be performed in immature as well as mature teeth.

### Treatment procedure

Pulpotomy should be performed with a diamond bur, of a size corresponding to the exposure, in a high speed contra-angle handpiece (Fig. 22.12). Effective cooling is essential. To avoid injury to the pulp due to insufficient cooling, the tooth and cutting instrument should be flushed continuously with water or saline by means of a syringe or the turbine spray. Furthermore cutting should be performed intermittently for brief periods and without unnecessary pressure.

The level of amputation should be about 2 mm below the exposure site. This level is deep enough to remove inflamed tissue and provide an adequate cavity for both the dressing and the sealing material. The pulpal wound is then rinsed with saline until bleeding has ceased. The wound surface is covered with calcium hydroxide and adapted with cotton pellets using light pressure, whereby the water from the paste is also removed. The surplus of calcium hydroxide is then easily removed with an excavator. The coronal cavity is closed with a tight-sealing material, e.g. zinc oxide-eugenol cement. However, as eugenol may interfere with polymerization of composites, it should be covered with a liner or glass ionomer cement before restoration with composites, especially if the crown is restored immediately after pulpotomy. Alternatively, the cavity can be sealed with Prader's zinc-sulphate cement (186). This material does not interfere with polymerization, but possesses sealing properties equal to those of zinc oxide-eugenol cement (184).

The advantage of partial pulpotomy lies in the minimal injury to the pulp and undisturbed physiologic apposition of dentin, especially in the critical cervical area of the tooth. The limited loss of crown substance offers continued opportunity for sensitivity testing and, in most cases, a post in the root canal will not be required for crown restoration. Compared with pulp capping, this procedure implies better wound control and, by sealing off the cavity with a material which does not allow microleakage, provides effective protection for the pulp. Most probably, this is one of the reasons for the high rate of healing reported after this type of treatment (11, 156, 173, 294, 295) (Figs 22.13 and 22.14). The frequency of failures is low and, judged from clinical observations, depends on factors, such as misjudged pulp diagnosis, overheating pulp at the time of treatment and poor restoration of the crown, which allows microleakage and

**Fig. 22.12 Treatment of a complicated crown fracture with partial pulpotomy**
A complicated crown fracture of an immature incisor 2 days after injury.

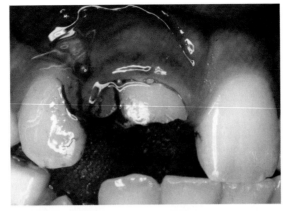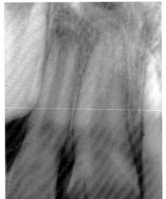

### Clinical condition
After the crown fragments were removed a large pulp exposure is found.

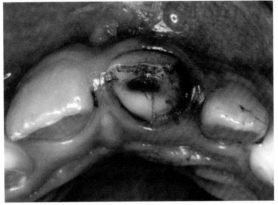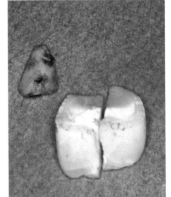

### Isolation with a rubber dam
After administration of a local anesthesia, the tooth is isolated with a rubber dam and washed with saline. A diamond bur is chosen for the pulpotomy.

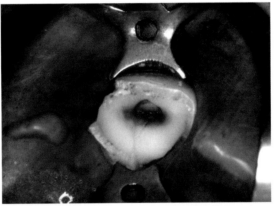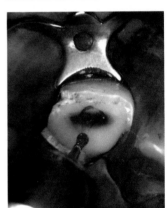

### Pulpotomy
The pulpotomy is carried out to a depth of 1.5–2.0 mm. The cutting of the pulp and surrounding dentin is performed using a high-speed turbine. This is done intermittently, with brief cutting periods and continuous gushing with the water spray from the turbine, eventually supplemented with extra saline from a syringe.

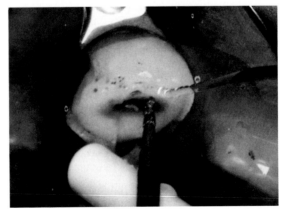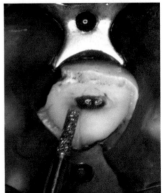

## Cavity preparation
The cavity should be boxlike, with a slight undercut in dentin.

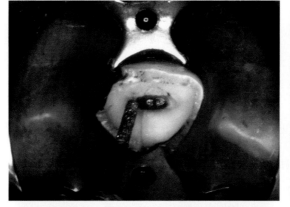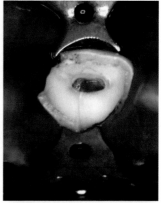

## Applying the dressing material
Hemostasis is awaited, and usually takes place within a couple of minutes. Otherwise a slight pressure can be applied with a cotton pellet soaked in saline or an anaesthetic solution with vasoconstrictor. After complete arrest of bleeding, calcium hydroxide paste (e.g. Calasept©) is placed over the pulpal wound.

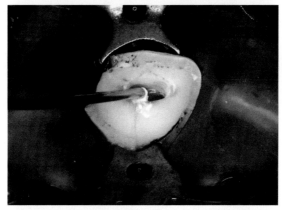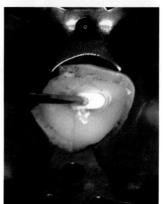

## Compressing the dressing material
The material is compressed slightly with a dry cotton pellet to adapt the material to the wound surface. After surplus dressing material is removed, the amputation cavity is sealed with zinc-eugenol cement. In cases where the tooth is immediately restored, the cavity is sealed with a hard-setting calcium hydroxide compound, or zinc phosphate cement can be used.

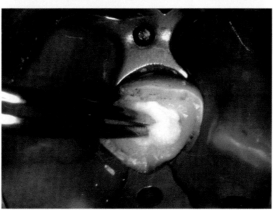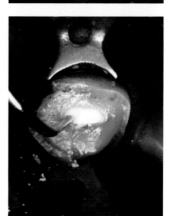

## Restoration
The tooth has been restored during the same sitting with composite resin and a dentin bonding agent.

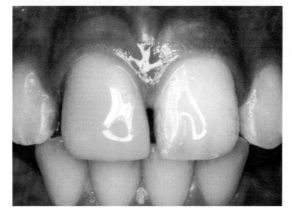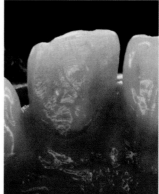

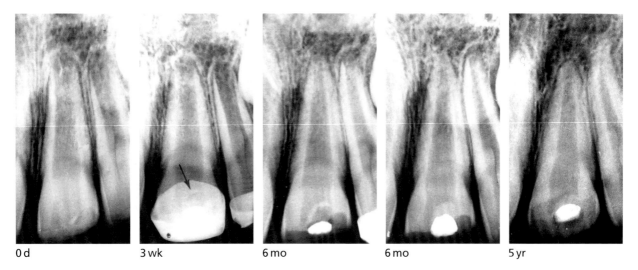

| 0 d | 3 wk | 6 mo | 6 mo | 5 yr |

**Fig. 22.13** Radiographic demonstration of healing after partial pulpotomy in an incisor with immature root. The tooth was treated 3 hours after injury. Note initial formation of hard tissue after 3 weeks (arrow) and completed barrier after 6 months. A control after 5 years shows healing and completed root development.

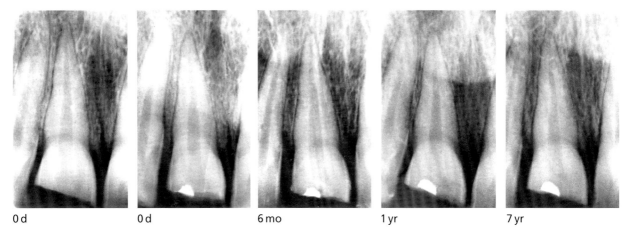

| 0 d | 0 d | 6 mo | 1 yr | 7 yr |

**Fig. 22.14** Radiographic demonstration of healing after partial pulpotomy in an incisor with completed root formation. The tooth was treated 12 hours after injury. Formation of a hard tissue barrier is present after 6 months and healing is evident 7 years after treatment.

penetration of the bacteria into the pulp (Fig. 22.15). It has been suggested that, after capping of pulp exposures close to the cervical area of anterior teeth, formation of hard tissue may compromise the blood supply to the coronal part of the pulp tissue, causing its degeneration (23). However, this phenomenon appears to be rare (187). Thus, in a comprehensive clinical study, no adverse effects could be observed after partial pulpotomy treatment of proximal exposures in crown-root fractured teeth (156) (Fig. 22.16).

When necrotic tissue or obviously impaired vascularity is present at the exposure site of immature teeth, the pulp should be amputated to a level at which fresh bleeding tissue is found, i.e. a cervical or deep pulpotomy should be performed (Fig. 22.17). Due to problems with adequate cooling of the diamond at high speed at that level, a round carbide bur at low speed should be used. In mature teeth, a pulpectomy is the treatment of choice.

## Pulpectomy

Pulpectomy, i.e. removal of the entire pulp to the level of 1–2 mm from the apical foramen, is performed in mature teeth when conservative pulp treatment is not indicated (46, 47). After removal of the pulp, the root canal is cleansed chemomechanically and obturated with gutta-percha points and a suitable sealer. There are, however, instances when interim dressing with calcium hydroxide is the treatment of choice, i.e. when periapical healing and closure of the apical foramen with hard tissue is desired before obturation, or when adequate treatment is not possible due to the presence of splints (48, 49). In the latter instance, it is difficult to adapt a rubber dam and access to the root canal can be limited. In such cases, calcium hydroxide can be used as an interim dressing and treatment continued once the splint has been removed.

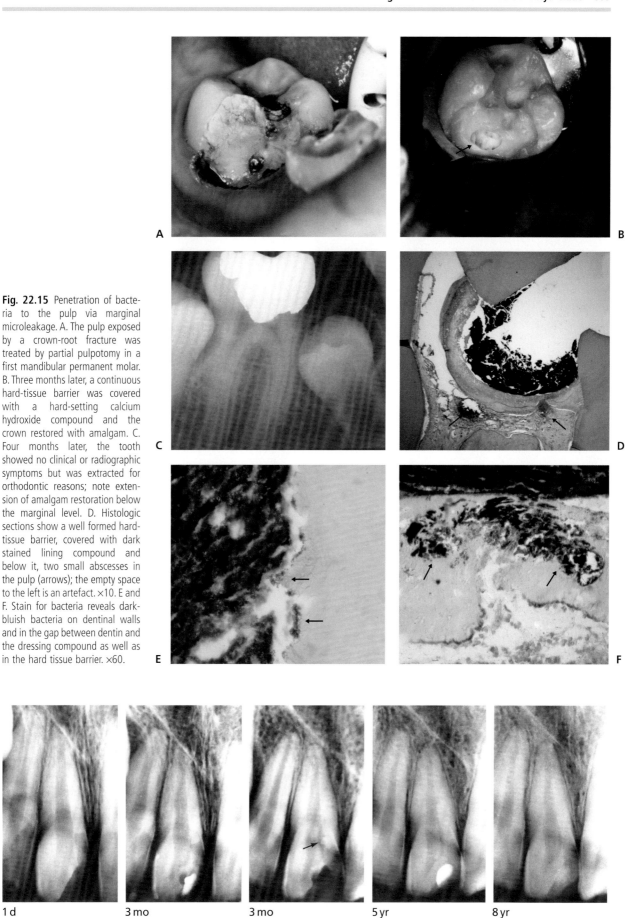

**Fig. 22.15** Penetration of bacteria to the pulp via marginal microleakage. A. The pulp exposed by a crown-root fracture was treated by partial pulpotomy in a first mandibular permanent molar. B. Three months later, a continuous hard-tissue barrier was covered with a hard-setting calcium hydroxide compound and the crown restored with amalgam. C. Four months later, the tooth showed no clinical or radiographic symptoms but was extracted for orthodontic reasons; note extension of amalgam restoration below the marginal level. D. Histologic sections show a well formed hard-tissue barrier, covered with dark stained lining compound and below it, two small abscesses in the pulp (arrows); the empty space to the left is an artefact. ×10. E and F. Stain for bacteria reveals dark-bluish bacteria on dentinal walls and in the gap between dentin and the dressing compound as well as in the hard tissue barrier. ×60.

1 d          3 mo          3 mo          5 yr          8 yr

**Fig. 22.16** A crown-root fractured incisor with a proximal exposure of the pulp, treated 24 hours after injury with a partial pulpotomy. A loose fragment was removed 3 months later (arrow). There is formation of a hard tissue barrier but no further constriction of the coronal pulp.

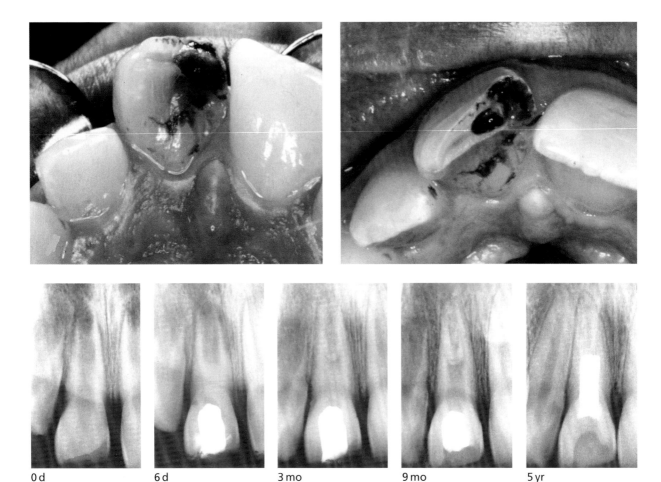

0 d　　　　　　6 d　　　　　　3 mo　　　　　9 mo　　　　　5 yr

**Fig. 22.17** Deep pulpotomy in an incisor with crown fracture and impaired pulpal vascularity. Vital and bleeding pulp tissue was found in the middle of the root canal. Three and 9 months after a deep pulpotomy, formation of a hard-tissue barrier can be seen deep in the root canal. A 5-year control of the subsequent root canal filling with gutta-percha shows completed root development.

## Clinical evaluation of pulp healing

Only histological techniques can verify pulpal healing, i.e. a non-inflamed pulp walled off by a continuous hard tissue barrier. However, a fairly adequate evaluation can be made according to the following criteria:

(1) No clinical symptoms
(2) No radiographically demonstrable intraradicular or periradicular pathological changes
(3) Continued root development in immature teeth
(4) Radiographically observed (and eventually clinically verified) continuous hard tissue barrier
(5) Positive sensitivity to electrical stimulation
(6) Follow-up for at least 3 years.

These criteria apply both to pulp capping and pulpotomy, with the exception of sensitivity testing which usually is not possible if the amputation site was placed in the root canal. In the pulps of teeth treated with partial pulpotomy and judged to be healed according to these criteria, no or only insignificant pathologic changes were found in the histologically examined pulps (174, 175).

A hard tissue barrier that appears continuous in radiographs may be discontinuous when examined histologically. On the other hand, it has been found that teeth which demonstrate a clinically continuous barrier usually contain non-inflamed pulps (30, 50, 174). Clinical exploration by probing can therefore be used as a criterion when pulp healing is evaluated, but is not compulsory (156). It is important to consider that a continuous hard tissue barrier and positive sensitivity do not exclude chronic pulpal inflammation which may persist in an asymptomatic tooth (Fig. 22.15). Thus, the follow-up period should be extended. In a comprehensive long-term clinical study of permanent incisors treated with partial pulpotomy, all failures occurred within 26 months after treatment (156). The teeth that were judged as healed at the 3-year control remained healed 10–15 years thereafter, indicating that a 3-year follow-up should be considered adequate.

Pulp canal obliteration and pulp necrosis are rather frequent long-term complications after a cervical or deep pulpotomy. This procedure is therefore regarded as a temporary treatment to be followed by pulpectomy once root formation is complete (169). Furthermore, the treatment may cause a loss of tooth substance in the cervical area to such an extent that a full crown restoration with anchorage in the root canal is often required to prevent a root fracture.

## Prognosis

The frequency of healing after pulp capping, partial or cervical pulpotomy treatments varies from 72–96% (11, 50–53, 156, 157, 173, 188–190, 295, 296). Results in more comprehensive clinical studies are shown in Table 22.1. The reported frequency of success after pulpectomy and filling of the root canal with various materials varies from 80–96% (54–57, 191).

## Root fractures

### Healing and pathology

Pulp necrosis with subsequent periradicular involvement occurs with a relatively low frequency, in about 25% of root-fractured teeth (see Chapter 12). It is a characteristic of a root fracture that only the coronal fragment is dislocated and that pulpal circulation in the apical fragment is not severely disturbed. Thus, when pulp necrosis does occur, it normally takes place only in the coronal fragment, while in the apical fragment the pulp remains vital (58, 59, 191–194, 298–302). However, if the coronal fragment is left untreated, the bacteria from its necrotic pulp may spread and cause inflammation and necrosis of the pulp in the apical fragment as well.

### Diagnosis of pulp necrosis

Clinical symptoms, such as changes in crown color and pulp sensibility are interpreted in the same way as in other traumatically injured teeth. The first radiographic sign of pulp necrosis is often a progressive widening of the space between the two fragments, later followed by pathologic changes in the adjacent periradicular bone, seen as a widened and diffusely outlined periodontal space or radiolucency, usually present within 3 months after injury (192, 193) (Fig. 22.18). If the tooth is not splinted, these changes can make the coronal fragment loose and tender to percussion.

Internal surface or tunneling resorption seem to be a part of healing processes and normally do not require endodontic intervention (193, 194) (see Chapter 12, p. 346). On the other hand, external inflammatory root resorption indicates necrotic and infected pulp tissue (60).

**Table 22.1** Healing frequencies after treatment of the exposed pulp in crown fractured teeth.

| Examiner | No of teeth | Healing |
|---|---|---|
| **Pulp capping** | | |
| Kozlowska (51) 1960 | 53 | 38 (72%) |
| Ravn (52) 1982 | 84 | 74 (88%) |
| Fuks et al. (188) 1982 | 38 | 31 (81%) |
| **Partial pulpotomy** | | |
| Cvek (11) 1978 | 60 | 58 (96%) |
| Fuks et al. (173) 1987 | 63 | 59 (94%) |
| Cvek (156) 1993 | 178 | 169 (95%) |
| **Cervical pulpotomy** | | |
| Hallet & Porteous (53) 1963 | 93 | 67 (72%) |
| Gelbier & Winter (189) 1988 | 175 | 139 (79%) |

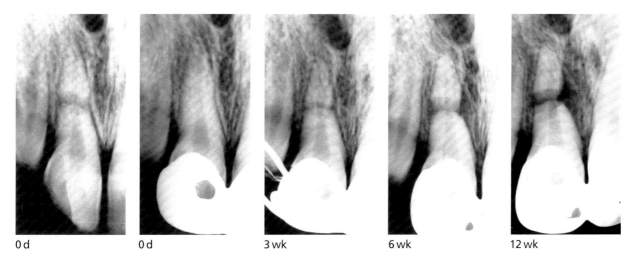

| 0 d | 0 d | 3 wk | 6 wk | 12 wk |

**Fig. 22.18** Radiographic signs of pulp necrosis after root fracture. Note progressive widening of the space between fragments, appearance of radiolucency in the adjacent alveolar bone.

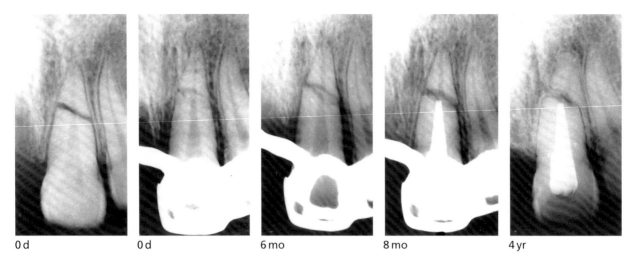

0 d          0 d          6 mo          8 mo          4 yr

**Fig. 22.19** Endodontic treatment of the coronal fragment of a root fractured incisor with gutta-percha. Condition is shown before and after repositioning of the coronal fragment at the time of injury. After 6 weeks, a slightly widened space between the fragments and radiolucency in the adjacent alveolar bone indicate pulp necrosis in the coronal fragment. The tapered root canal in the fragment permitted an adequate filling with gutta-percha.

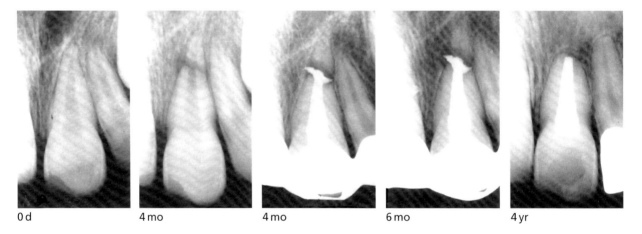

0 d          4 mo          4 mo          6 mo          4 yr

**Fig. 22.20** Difficulties in root canal obturation of the coronal fragment after root fracture. After 4 months there is a widening of the space between the fragments and a radiolucency adjacent to the fracture. After antibacterial treatment, the coronal root canal was obturated and gutta-percha became extruded into the fracture site. After six months the space between the fragments as well as the adjacent radiolucency have increased whereafter the apical fragment was removed. At the 4-year control, periapical healing is evident.

## Treatment procedure

Endodontic treatment in teeth with a fracture involving the *cervical* part of the root has been shown to be of a poor value (301). When coronal fragment in a mature tooth should, for some reason, be removed and the length of the apical fragment is judged to be able to support a prosthetic crown, the root canal can be filled with gutta-percha and the fragment extruded orthodontically into the desired position (see Chapter 24, p. 687).

Conservative endodontic treatment of teeth with fracture in the *middle* or *apical* part of the root can be divided into treatment of the coronal fragment alone or both fragments (61–64, 302). If these treatments are unsuccessful, surgical removal of the apical fragment can be indicated.

The choice of treatment depends on radiographic findings, such as periradicular changes, width of the pulp lumen and separation between the two fragments, as well as on the clinical finding of pulp vitality in the apical fragment at the time of treatment (i.e., pulp canal obliteration). The location of the fracture in the middle or apical part of the root does not affect the choice of treatment.

Root canal treatment of the coronal fragment alone is indicated for teeth which do not show pathologic changes periapically and in which bleeding and/or sensitivity to probing at the fracture site indicate a vital pulp in the apical fragment. This is the case in the majority of root fractured teeth with pulpal complications. The coronal fragment may be filled with gutta-percha immediately after chemomechanical cleaning if the anatomy of the root canal permits adequate obturation (Fig. 22.19). This is especially true for teeth with fracture in the apical part of the root, where the root canal is usually narrow. When the root canal is wide, as in very young teeth or in fractures in the middle of the root, it can be difficult to achieve satisfactory cleansing and adequate obturation with gutta-percha (Fig. 22.20). The coronal

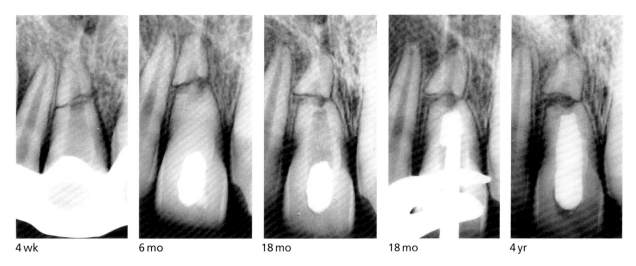

**Fig. 22.21** Treatment of the coronal fragment of a root fractured incisor with a wide pulpal lumen 4 weeks after injury with calcium hydroxide. After 18 months, periradicular healing has taken place and a hard tissue barrier has formed apically in the coronal fragment, against which an adequate root filling with gutta-percha can be performed.

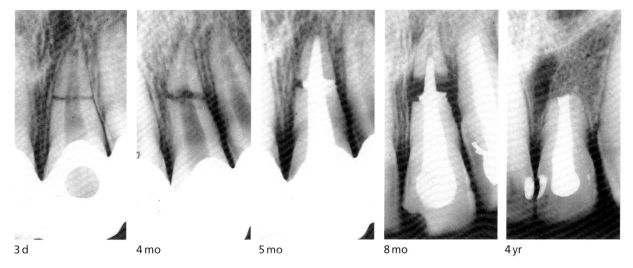

**Fig. 22.22** Root canal treatment of both fragments of a root fractured incisor. Note the widening of the space between fragments and the adjacent radiolucency 4 months after injury. The root canal in both fragments was filled with gutta-percha which was extruded into the space between the two fragments. After 8 months, the space between the fragments and adjacent radiolucency increased and the apical fragment was therefore removed. Periradicular healing can be seen 4 years later.

fragment can instead be treated initially with calcium hydroxide and filled with gutta-percha after a hard tissue barrier has formed apically in the coronal fragment and periradicular healing has taken place (Fig. 22.21). Clinical procedures and the effect of calcium hydroxide are discussed later in connection with treatment of non-vital immature teeth.

Root canal treatment of both fragments can be performed when the entire pulp is necrotic. The treatment is complicated, as it is difficult to avoid impacting necrotic tissue and filling debris between the fragments during mechanical cleansing as well as overfilling with gutta-percha (Fig. 22.22). This could explain the poor prognosis of this type of treatment. However, once the root fracture has healed, leaving no empty space between the fragments, this type of

treatment may have a better prognosis, in the case of a late secondary pulp necrosis (Fig. 22.23).

Root canal treatment of the coronal fragment and surgical removal of the apical fragment is indicated in teeth in which the apical fragment with necrotic pulp is not accessible for treatment or when prognosis is poor due to a wide space between the two fragments (Figs 22.22 and 22.24), as well as in teeth in which either of the first two treatments has not been successful (Figs 22.20 and 22.22).

In the case of a concomitant crown fracture, the exposed dentin is covered with hard-setting calcium hydroxide or glass ionomer cement, followed by a layer of composite material. The final restoration of the crown is performed after splint removal, i.e. periodontal healing has taken place.

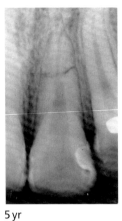 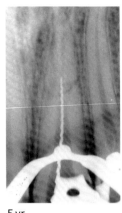 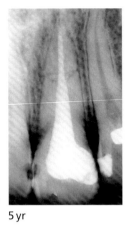 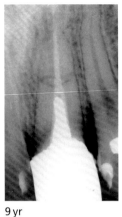

3 yr          5 yr          5 yr          5 yr          9 yr

**Fig. 22.23** Treatment of a tooth with healed root fracture and subsequent pulpitis due to a carious lesion. Three years after injury the root fracture appears healed. Two years later, a deep carious lesion was filled temporarily. Due to symptoms of pulpitis endodontic treatment was instituted. Note that there was no gutta-percha pressed between fragments at the time of filling and no periradicular changes 4 years later (i.e. 9 years after injury).

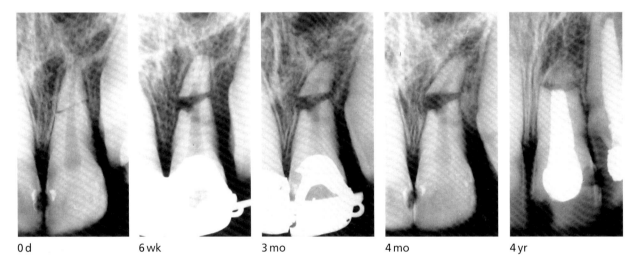

0 d          6 wk          3 mo          4 mo          4 yr

**Fig. 22.24** Endodontic treatment of the coronal fragment and simultaneous surgical removal of the apical fragment. Displacement of the apical fragment made endodontic treatment of both fragments impossible.

An exposed pulp is treated by pulp capping or partial pulpotomy, provided that vital and fresh bleeding tissue is found at the exposure site (302) (Fig. 22.25). Root canal treatment is instituted later in the event of pulp necrosis.

## Prognosis

Successful conservative treatment of root-fractured teeth with partial or total pulp necrosis has been described and reported in a number of publications (61–66, 191, 192). In a recent study, types of conservative endodontic treatment were evaluated in 98 teeth with a fracture in the middle or apical part of the root (302). It was found that frequency of healing was minimal (0%) in teeth in which the root canal in both fragments was filled with gutta-percha. The failures were judged to be due to extrusion of filling material and necrotic debris in between the fragments, resulting in persistent radiolucency in adjacent tissues. In teeth treated by filling with gutta-percha of the root canal in only the coronal

fragment, healing occurred in 76% of teeth. However, the majority of fractures were in the apical part of the root, where the root canal is narrow and could be obturated without overfilling (Fig. 22.19). In teeth in which the coronal fragment was filled with gutta-percha and the apical fragment was removed surgically, healing was seen in 68%. This type of treatment is an arduous procedure, especially for children and adolescents, and should, therefore, be avoided. But, it has a reasonable prognosis and may be considered in exceptional cases, provided the coronal fragment can support the crown during function. Periodontal healing with formation of a hard tissue barrier apically in the coronal fragment, treated by calcium hydroxide and subsequent obturation with gutta-percha, was found in 86% of 65 teeth, 4 years after the last treatment. Furthermore, in most teeth with vital tissue in the apical fragment at the time of treatment, the pulpal lumen became obliterated by the formation of hard tissue (65, 192) (Figs 22.19 and 22.21).

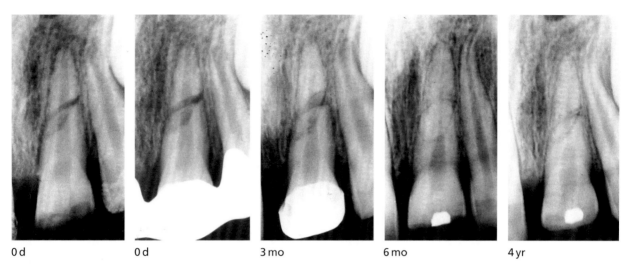

0 d          0 d          3 mo          6 mo          4 yr

**Fig. 22.25** Treatment of an incisor with concomitant complicated crown and root fracture. A partial pulpotomy was performed and the tooth splinted. At the final control, a hard tissue barrier is seen in the coronal fragment as well as a connective tissue healing of the root fracture.

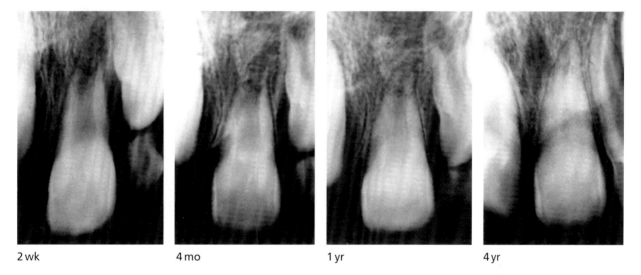

2 wk          4 mo          1 yr          4 yr

**Fig. 22.26** Continued root development after replantation of an immature incisor. The tooth was replanted after 30 min dry storage. From KLING et al. (203) 1986.

## Luxated or avulsed and replanted teeth

### Healing and pathology

When a tooth is forcefully displaced in its alveolus, vessels at the apical foramen can be compressed, lacerated or severed. Subsequent reactions in the pulp depend on the degree and duration of circulatory disturbances, the stage of root development and eventual bacterial contamination of the affected tissues. In general, the risk of pulp necrosis increases with increasing stages of root development and severity of the luxation injury (67–69, 196–200) (see Chapters 2, and 13).

A sudden, complete break in pulpal circulation leads to infarction and coagulation necrosis of the pulp. In mature teeth and in the absence of bacteria, such tissue may persist without clinical symptoms or obvious radiographic change for long periods of time. The infarcted tissue can be also revascularized, i.e. replaced by ingrowth of mesenchymal tissues. This is followed by deposition of hard tissue along the canal walls and, sometimes, continued root development (Fig. 22.26). These processes are described in detail in Chapter 2. However, the necrotic pulp most often becomes contaminated by micro-organisms from the oral cavity, with subsequent periapical involvement (70–74, 200).

In clinical and experimental studies of immature replanted teeth, the frequency of complete pulp revascularization was found to be rather low (75, 200–203). In all teeth in which revascularization did not occur, a periapical radiolucency and/or inflammatory root resorption developed, i.e. changes known to be related to the presence of micro-organisms in the pulpal lumen. In experimental studies designed to imitate clinical conditions, the presence of

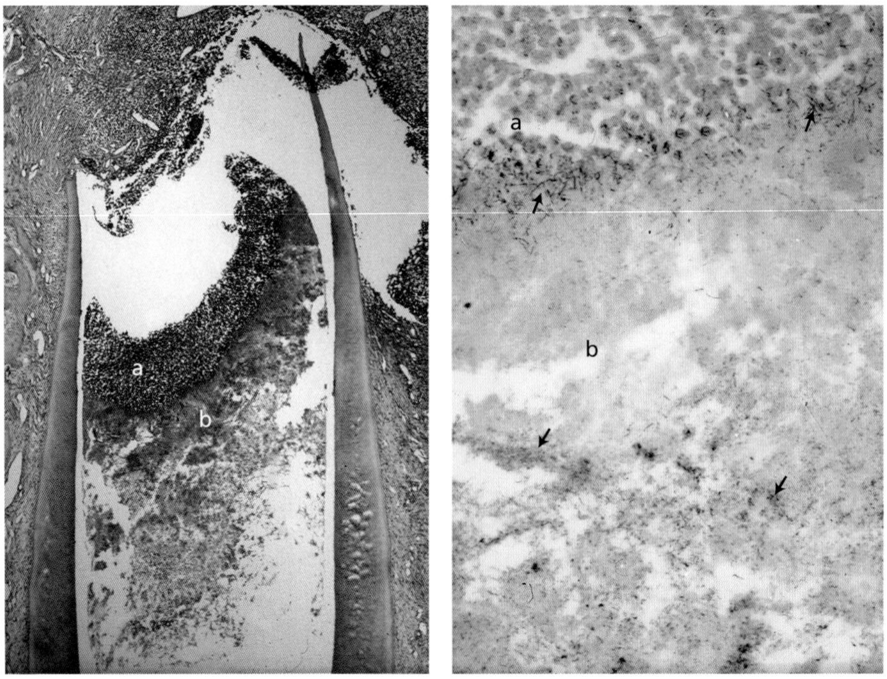

**Fig. 22.27** Presence of a contaminated blood clot in the pulpal lumen of a replanted immature monkey incisor. A. Apical area of the tooth; abscess formation at the apical foramen (a) and beneath it a blood clot (b). ×15. B. Enlarged view of the area between dense accumulation of leukocytes (a) and blood clot (b) shows heavy contamination of the blood clot with micro-organisms (arrows), Brown & Brenn bacterial stain. ×140. From CVEK et al. (201) 1990.

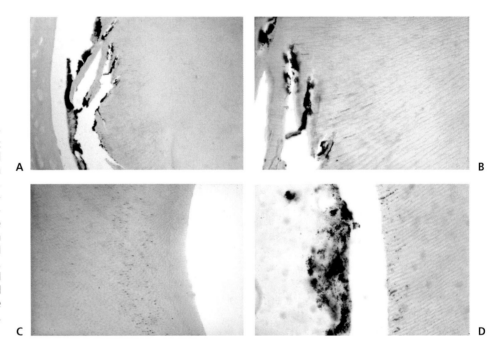

**Fig. 22.28** Pathway of micro-organisms via cervical root damage to the pulpal lumen. A and B. Crushed cementum and dentin in the cervical area of the tooth, formation of plaque and penetration of micro-organisms into dentinal tubules, which could be followed in serial sections through the dentinal wall into the pulpal lumen. ×30 and 140. C and D. Micro-organisms in the dentinal wall close to the pulpal lumen and formation of colonies in the necrotic pulp. From CVEK et al. (201) 1990.

micro-organisms was the predominant reason for the absence of complete revascularization (200). Two particular sources of contamination were demonstrated. One was the presence of blood clots harboring bacteria in the apical area of the pulpal lumen, most probably contaminated during the extra-alveolar period (Fig. 22.27). The other source of contamination was mechanically damaged cervical root surfaces through which bacteria from dental plaque could penetrate into the necrotic pulp tissue (Fig. 22.28).

Systemic treatment with doxycycline had no effect on the frequency of pulp revascularization or presence of bacteria in the pulpal lumen (201). On the other hand, when avulsed teeth were treated topically with doxycycline for 5 minutes before replantation, the frequency of revascularization was significantly increased and the presence of bacteria in the pulpal lumen decreased (201). This effect seems to be due to elimination of bacteria from the root surface, while contamination via dentinal tubules from mechanical damage on the root surface cervically was not affected (303, 304).

Regarding luxated teeth, the pathways for bacterial invasion to the damaged pulp tissue are still obscure. One pathway appears to be invasion of bacteria from mechani-

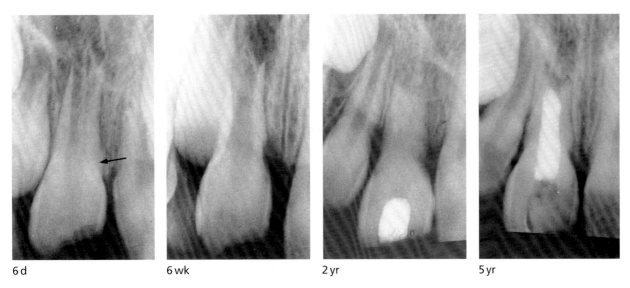

6 d                 6 wk                 2 yr                 5 yr

**Fig. 22.29** Effect of the impact of marginal bone on the root surface of intruded incisor. The arrow points to the area of impact. Six weeks later there is resorption of the root surface and periapical radiolucency. After calcium hydroxide treatment and filling of the root canal with gutta-percha, root resorption is arrested and periapical healing evident 5 years after injury.

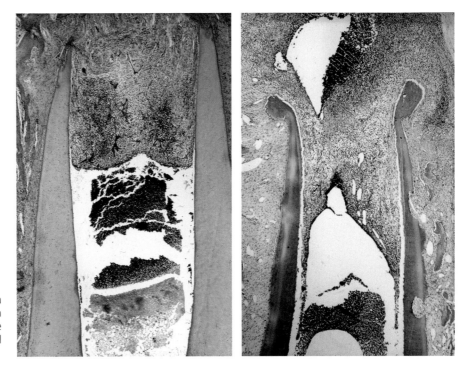

**Fig. 22.30** Presence of vital tissue in the apical portion of the pulpal lumen in replanted immature incisors, despite presence of abscesses in the pulpal lumen and periapically. ×20.

cal damage on the cervical root surface that can be inflicted by e.g. the fulcrum effect of marginal bone at the time of luxation (305) (Fig. 22.29). It is also conceivable that bacteria may originate from a contaminated blood clot along the root surface. Anachoretic contamination of the pulp by blood-borne bacteria appears less likely in healthy individuals, although it cannot be excluded. Thus it has been shown that the damaged dental tissues can be contaminated when severe septicemia is experimentally introduced by repeated intravenous injections of a bacterial suspension (204).

In most experimentally replanted immature teeth with necrotic and contaminated pulps, vital pulp tissue and sometimes formation of new hard tissues can be seen in the apical portion of the pulpal lumen, despite adjacent inflammation and abscess formation either in the root canal or periapically (200, 201) (Fig. 22.30). In some teeth, formation of dentin can even be seen, indicating that a part of the original pulp has survived, probably due to the diffusion of nutrients from periapical tissues (205) (Fig. 22.31).

The presence of vital tissue in the apical part of the pulpal lumen is important from a therapeutic point of view, as this may ensure a more rapid formation of a hard-tissue barrier and sometimes continued root development after treatment

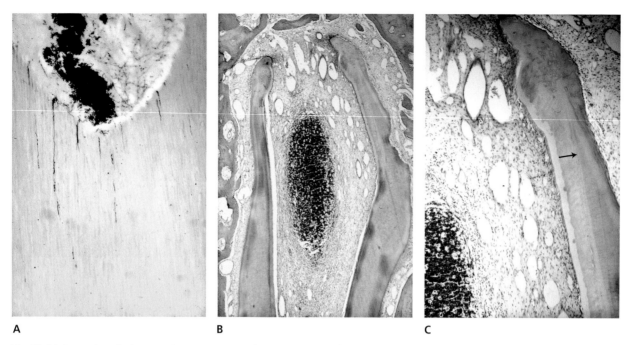

A                              B                              C

**Fig. 22.31** Penetration of micro-organisms into necrotic pulp. A. Immature monkey incisor replanted after 30 min storage in saliva foramen, penetration of micro-organisms through dentinal tubules of coronal dentin into the pulpal lumen; bacterial colonies are seen in the necrotized pulp, Brown & Brenn bacterial stain. ×100. B. Abscess formation in apical area. ×15. C. Formation of dentin is seen. The arrow indicates the line between pre- and post-traumatically formed dentin. ×33. From CVEK et al. (201) 1990.

of non-vital immature teeth with calcium hydroxide (76–78).

## Diagnosis of pulp necrosis

Acute clinical symptoms, such as pain or swelling, are seldom present in the early post-traumatic period. However, the tooth may become loose and tender to percussion (198). Clinical diagnosis of pulpal status and decision on endodontic treatment should be based on evaluation of coronal color changes, sensibility testing and radiographic findings including disturbances in root development of immature teeth. Regarding clinical decision making, there is no difference between the various types of injuries, with the exception of severely intruded or replanted mature teeth. In these teeth no healing of the pulp can be expected and the root canal treatment should therefore be instituted, irrespective of clinical findings, 1–2 weeks after injury in order to prevent inflammatory root resorption.

Discoloration of the crown subsequent to trauma has been described as pink, yellow, brown and gray or a combination of these (68). A color change to pink or reddish seen within 2–3 days after injury indicates intrapulpal bleeding, which may resolve and the crown may regain its natural color 2–3 weeks later (68, 79, 80, 207, 208). Persistent discoloration, especially with a shift to gray, indicates necrosis and probably bacterial contamination of the pulp (81, 208) (see Chapter 9).

Sensibility of the pulp can be checked in different ways; but the usual method is electrical stimulation (see Chapter 9, p. 258). There is, however, no correlation between the sensibility threshold and the histological condition of the pulp (82, 83). Erupting non-injured teeth, for example, may not respond to electrical stimulation; and injured teeth which do not respond to testing immediately after injury may regain their sensitivity, sometimes months or years after injury (84–86, 206–212). Furthermore, a negative response is sometimes found in teeth in which the pulpal lumen has been reduced by hard tissue formation (87, 88, 209). Electrical sensibility testing should therefore be regarded only as a diagnostic aid; a negative response alone should not be considered the sole indication for endodontic treatment, whereas a positive response is a relatively safe sign of pulpal innervation. The test should be correctly performed, as a positive response may be elicited by contact of the electrode with gingiva or a moist crown surface (209) (see Chapter 9, p. 264). However, an alternative test of pulp vitality is possible by using the laser Doppler technique (211, 212, 306) (see Chapter 9, p. 267).

Radiographic findings, such as a widened and diffusely outlined periodontal space, radiolucency and/or external inflammatory root resorption can normally be seen within 2–8 weeks after injury. However, periapical radiolucency may appear later (206, 207) (Figs 22.32–22.34).

Inflammatory changes of periradicular tissues are clearly related to the presence of bacteria in the pulpal lumen (60, 74, 200, 213). However, it has been recently reported that in about 10% of extruded or laterally luxated mature permanent teeth periapical radiolucency may spontaneously heal and be followed by pulp canal obliteration (206, 208). This finding points out the intricacy of healing processes after traumatic injuries, which are still not understood in full

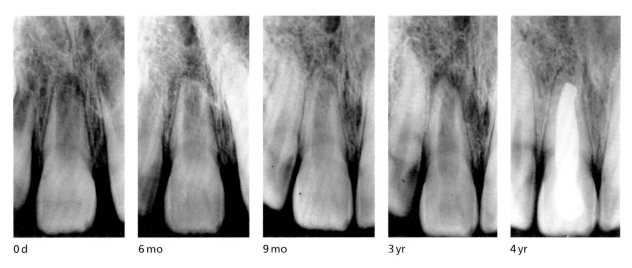

**Fig. 22.32** Arrested root development after a luxation injury. There is formation of hard tissue apically but none in the rest of pulpal lumen, indicating necrosis of the underlying pulp. Periapical radiolucency is seen 3 years after injury. Periapical healing is evident 4 years after treatment with calcium hydroxide and following obturation with gutta-percha.

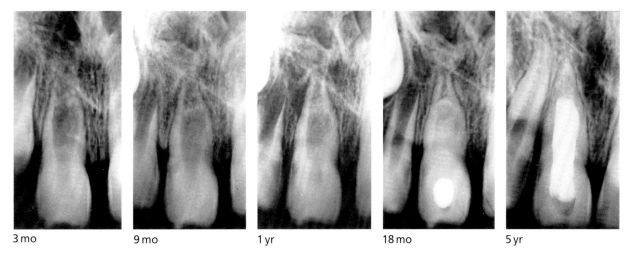

**Fig. 22.33** Minor disturbance in root development of a luxated incisor. There is formation of irregular hard tissue in the apical area, followed by further root development. Note the absence of hard tissue formation in the rest of pulpal lumen, indicating pulp necrosis. Periapical radiolucency was noted 1 year after injury. Periradicular healing is evident 5 years after root canal treatment with calcium hydroxide and subsequent filling with gutta-percha.

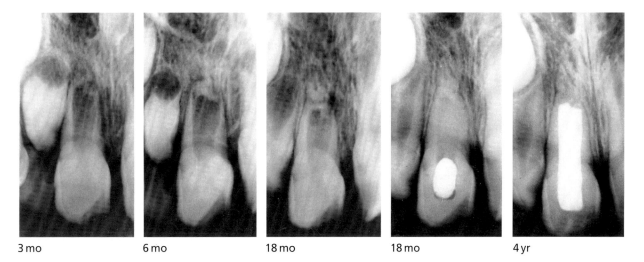

**Fig. 22.34** Disturbance in root development and formation of a root tip. There is formation of hard tissue apically but none in the rest of pulpal lumen, indicating necrosis of the remaining pulp. Formation of separate root tip as well as periradicular radiolucency was noted 18 months after injury. Healing is evident after root canal treatment with calcium hydroxide and subsequent filling with gutta-percha, 4 years after the endodontic treatment.

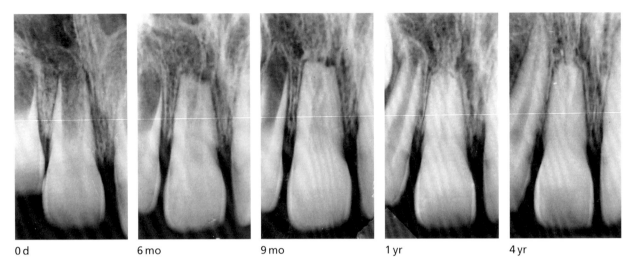

**Fig. 22.35** Arrested root development after a luxation injury. The pulpal lumen is successively diminished by formation of hard tissue, indicating presence of vital tissue.

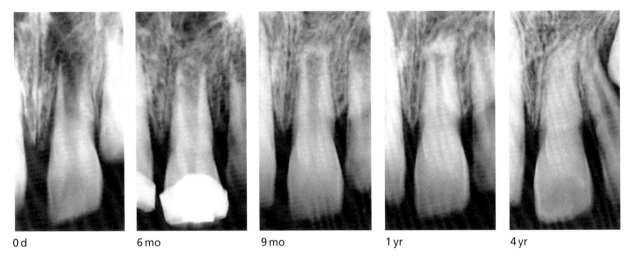

**Fig. 22.36** Disturbance in root development of an immature incisor after a luxation injury. Note successive diminution of the pulpal lumen by formation of hard tissue.

detail, and emphasises the need for further research. Clinical implications, however, seem to be minor. Considering the low frequency of this phenomenon and maturity of the involved teeth, the risk of a false diagnosis or a negative consequence of the root canal treatment in these teeth appears minimal. On the other hand, expectation that healing will occur may neglect a risk of inflammatory root resorption. However, guidelines for a more conservative approach are presented in Chapter 13, p. 383.

Disturbed or arrested root development is frequently seen after luxation injuries to immature teeth and is usually followed by obliteration of the pulpal lumen, indicating the presence of vital pulp tissue (Figs 22.35 and 22.36). Barrier-like formation of hard tissue apically, with or without continued root development, may also occur when the coronal pulp is necrotic. However, sooner or later it becomes bacterially contaminated with acute or chronic periapical inflammation as a result. Thus, absence of any hard tissue formation in the rest of the pulp cavity in these teeth, indi-

cating no cell activity, is a strong indication of a coronal pulp necrosis (Figs 22.32–22.34). In these teeth, endodontic intervention should therefore be considered before the appearance of radiographic periapical changes.

In general, the decision to perform endodontic treatment should be based on an evaluation of clinical and radiographic findings as well as history and information gained from a comparison between radiographs at the time of injury and subsequent controls.

Replanted immature teeth, in which revascularization can be expected to occur, should not be treated endodontically until signs of periapical lesions or external inflammatory root resorption are observed. This implies close radiographic follow-up, as root resorption in immature teeth may progress very rapidly. Controls at 3, 6 and 8 weeks after injury will normally disclose these changes.

In replanted mature teeth it is advisable to postpone endodontic treatment until 1–2 weeks after replantation and just prior to splint removal, to avoid further damage to the

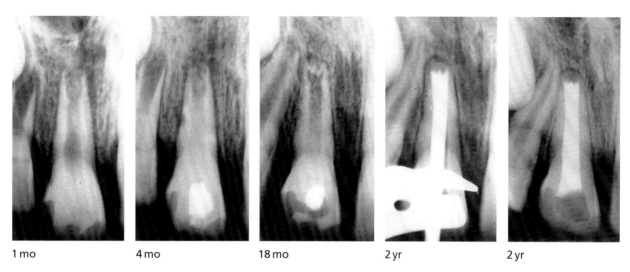

1 mo          4 mo          18 mo          2 yr          2 yr

**Fig. 22.37** Treatment of a non-vital immature tooth with calcium hydroxide. Periapical healing and apical closure with hard tissue was present after 18 months and the tooth was permanently filled with gutta-percha. A master point with a heat-softened tip was placed against the hard tissue barrier and, thereafter, the root canal was obturated with additional points, using lateral condensation.

periodontal ligament by the endodontic procedures. During early stages of periodontal healing, it is easy to expel drugs and filling materials into the periodontal space and, if calcium hydroxide is used, it may be expelled to the periapical area and cause necrosis of living cells on the root surface apically with ankylosis as a result (214).

## Treatment of immature teeth

Wide or funnel-shaped root canals make endodontic treatment in immature teeth difficult. The difficulties lie in removing all necrotic tissue from the dentinal walls and achieving adequate obturation of the root canal. A number of treatment procedures have been described; but it was not until calcium hydroxide was introduced that favorable results could be obtained. Since then, numerous clinical and histological investigations have been carried out; and calcium hydroxide is today the most commonly used root canal dressing for the treatment of immature non-vital teeth (88–92, 307–311).

### The effect of calcium hydroxide

The purpose of calcium hydroxide treatment is to achieve healing of periradicular tissues, including arrest of inflammatory root resorption and formation of a hard tissue barrier apically, against which an adequate root filling can be placed (Fig. 22.37). In clinical and experimental studies, this has been shown to occur with a high predictability (93–102, 215–237, 307–311) (Table 22.2).

These favorable results depend on several properties of the calcium hydroxide, all related to its high pH = 12.5 (223). One property is its strong antibacterial effect (103, 105, 215–230, 312). Thus, *in vitro*, 99.9% of bacteria from the common root canal flora were killed within a few minutes

**Table 22.2** Frequency of periapical healing in non-vital teeth after root canal treatment with calcium hydroxide.

| Examiner | Number of teeth | Healing |
|---|---|---|
| **Immature teeth** | | |
| Kerekes et al. (94) 1980 | 66 | 62 (94%) |
| Mackie et al. (217) 1988 | 112 | 108 (96%) |
| Cvek (221) 1992 | 328 | 314 (96%) |
| **Mature teeth** | | |
| Vernieks & Masser (106) 1978 | 78 | 62 (79%) |
| Kerekes et al. (94) 1980 | 27 | 26 (96%) |
| Caliskan & Sen (332) 1996 | 172 | 139 (81%) |
| Cvek (221) 1992 | 441 | 414 (94%) |

upon direct contact with calcium hydroxide (224), *Enterococcus faecalis* apparently being the only resistant strain. In contact with calcium hydroxide, bacteria are killed at pH 12.5 but not at pH 11.5. Resistance of *E. faecalis* to short exposure to calcium hydroxide has been confirmed *in vitro* experiments with contaminated dentin, but findings as to its resistance to a longer exposure have not been unanimous. In one study, the bacteria survived a 10-day exposure while in another they were killed after 24 hours (227, 230). In clinical studies, however, *E. faecalis* do not seem to cause endodontic problems. Thus, from infected root canals very few bacteria could be cultivated after 1–4 weeks' dressing with calcium hydroxide and, among these, the presence of *E. faecalis* was rare (105, 224, 227).

Another property of calcium hydroxide is its capacity to dissolve necrotic pulp remnants, rendering root canal walls clean (221, 228, 313). Hence, no difference in the debridement effect was found when the root canal dressing with calcium hydroxide was compared with ultrasonic instrumentation (233). This is important for the treatment of immature teeth, in which the thin dentinal walls do not permit intensive reaming.

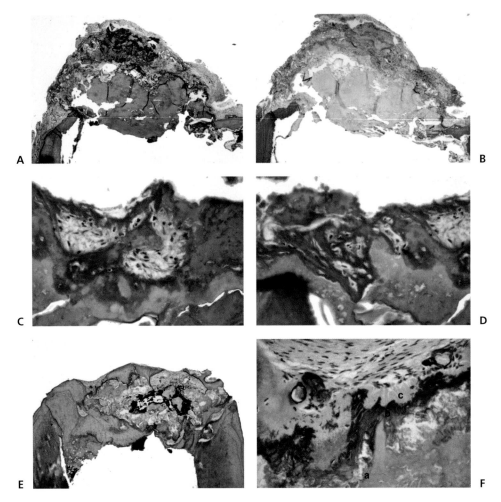

**Fig. 22.38** Development of hard tissue apically in a non-vital immature incisor treated with calcium hydroxide. A. Histologic section through the apical area of a non-vital immature incisor, treated with calcium hydroxide and extracted a week later. Light blue stained amorphous formation across the apical opening; haematoxylin-eosin stain. ×10. B. In a following section, stained with a polychrome stain, the same formation is stained yellow, indicating coagulation necrosis. ×10. C. In a similar section from a tooth, extracted 3 weeks after treatment, red colored collagen is seen appositioned on the coagulated tissue. ×40. D. In another tooth, extracted after 3 months, appositioned of cementum- or bone-like tissue is evident on the brown-yellowish colored, coagulated and probably calcified tissue. ×40. E. An irregular hard-tissue barrier with inclusions of soft tissue and empty space; dark stained gutta-percha, intruded into a hollow place in the barrier caused no adverse reactions. ×10. F. In larger magnification, although haphazardly arranged, hard tissue layers similar to those formed in the pulp can be seen, with a difference that instead of dentin a cementum-like tissue is formed: a. Remnants of coagulated tissue, b. A darkly stained band of dystrophically calcified tissue, c. A layer of cementum-like hard tissue.

Findings regarding the ability of calcium hydroxide to induce ectopic bone have not been convincing (234, 236). However, elimination of bacteria from the root canal makes healing of the surrounding vital tissue and the formation of an apical hard tissue barrier possible. When in contact with vital tissue in the apical area, calcium hydroxide seems to cause tissue reactions similar to those in the coronal pulp (Fig. 22.38). Thus, layers of the hard tissue in an apical barrier are similar to those formed after pulpotomy or pulp capping, the only difference being that a reparative or cementum-like hard tissue is formed instead of dentin, indicating involvement of periapical tissues in the barrier formation (95, 102, 232). These tissue layers can be arranged very irregularly and often include islands of soft connective tissue, probably a result of placing calcium hydroxide against lacerated tissue (Fig. 22.38). An apical barrier can be formed around the apex of the tooth, over the apical foramen or in the root canal. The location of the barrier seems to depend on the level at which calcium

hydroxide has been brought into contact with vital tissue (Fig. 22.39).

The ability of periodontal tissues to respond with hard-tissue formation in contact with calcium hydroxide does not seem to be related to the maturity of the tooth, the time of treatment after injury, or the location on the root surface. Thus, after repeated dressings, formation of the hard tissue can be seen apically in mature teeth (106, 309) (Fig. 22.40), in root perforations (90, 107, 108, 237–239) (Fig. 22.41), at the fracture site in the coronal fragment of root fractured teeth (65, 192, 302) (Fig. 22.42), after unsuccessful apicoectomy or periapical curettage (108, 240) and in teeth in which the root development ceased years prior to treatment (Fig. 22.43).

In immature teeth, continued root development or formation of a separate part of the root may occasionally occur, probably due to the survival of a part of pulp tissue and/or the Hertwig's epithelial root sheath (76–78) (Figs 22.34 and 22.44).

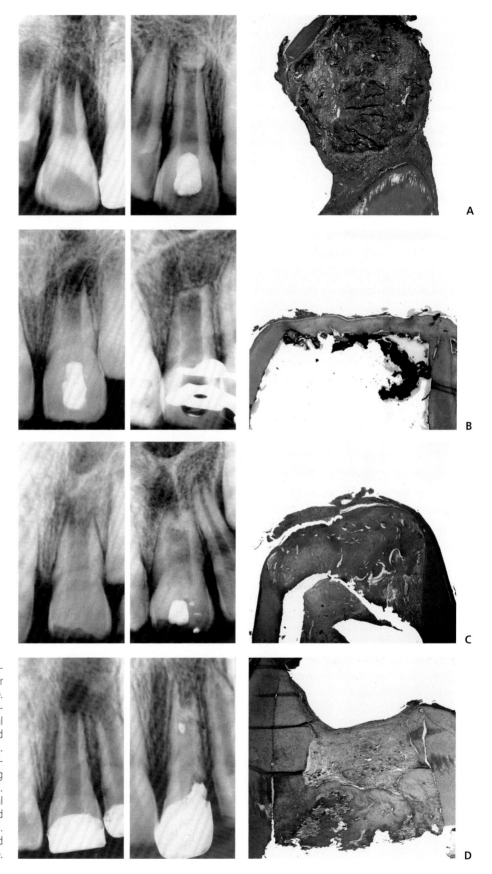

**Fig. 22.39** Different levels of formation of the hard tissue barrier after treatment with calcium hydroxide. Radiographs were taken before treatment and after completed apical closure. The teeth were extracted because of cervical root fractures. A. Formation of hard tissue in the periapical area as a result of overfilling with calcium hydroxide. ×10. B and C. Barriers formed across the apical foramen. ×20. D. Formation of hard tissue barrier within the root canal. ×20. In all cases, newly formed hard tissue was found to be cementum-like.

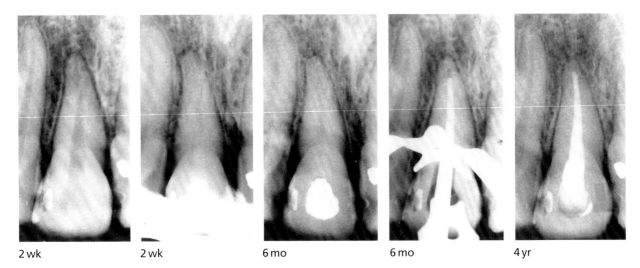

2 wk        2 wk        6 mo        6 mo        4 yr

**Fig. 22.40** Treatment of a mature permanent incisor with calcium hydroxide. Periapical healing and closure apically with hard tissue was found after 6 months and the root canal was filled with gutta-percha. Periapical healing is seen at a 4-year control.

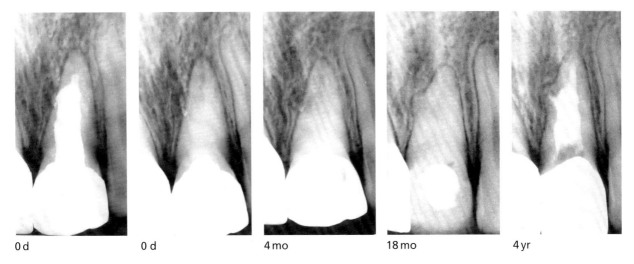

0 d        0 d        4 mo        18 mo        4 yr

**Fig. 22.41** Treatment of accidental root perforation with calcium hydroxide. A radiolucency adjacent to perforation was found 2 years after gutta-percha filling. The tooth was initially treated by a cervical pulpotomy because of a pulp exposure and a root perforation occurred at the time of removing the hard tissue barrier in connection with pulpectomy. The root canal was treated with calcium hydroxide; the initial formation of hard tissue was seen after 4 months and the perforation was completely sealed with hard tissue at 18 months. The control 4 years after subsequent filling with gutta-percha shows periodontal healing.

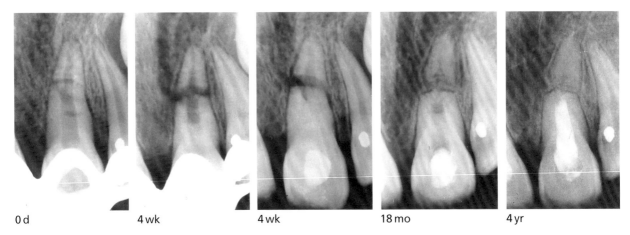

0 d        4 wk        4 wk        18 mo        4 yr

**Fig. 22.42** Root fracture and treatment of the non-vital coronal fragment with calcium hydroxide. Four weeks after injury there is widening of the space between fragments and adjacent radiolucency. The coronal fragment was treated with calcium hydroxide and 1$^1/_2$ years later, periradicular healing and apical closure with hard tissue of the coronal fragment was observed. Four years after filling with gutta-percha, periradicular healing is evident. From CVEK (65) 1974.

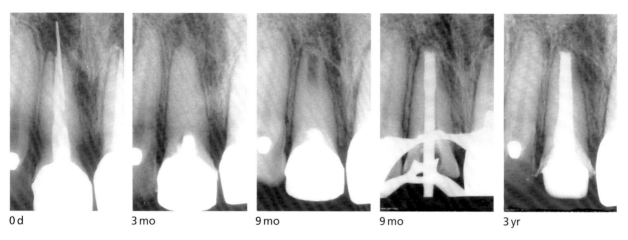

**Fig. 22.43** Late endodontic treatment of an incisor with arrested root development. Control 4 years after previous treatment shows incomplete root canal obturation and a broken file left in the canal with associated periapical radiolucency. After removal of the root filling and the file, the root canal was filled with calcium hydroxide. Nine months later, periapical healing and formation of apical hard tissue barrier was found, against which adequate obturation with gutta-percha was performed. Periapical healing is evident 3 years later.

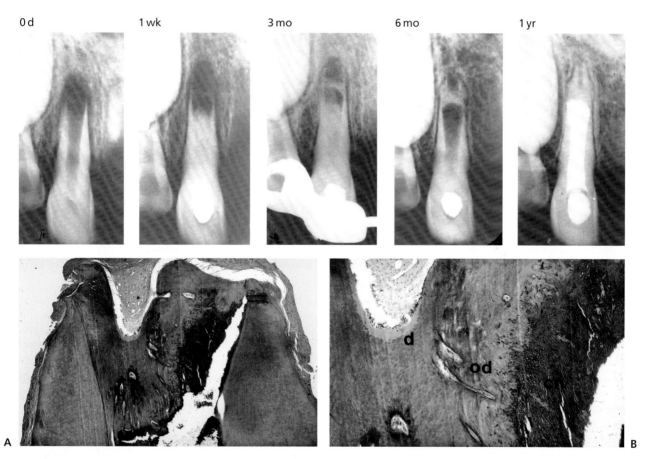

**Fig. 22.44** Continued root development after treatment of an incisor with partial pulp necrosis. Note the level of calcium hydroxide in the root canal, indicating the presence of some vital tissue in the apical portion. Formation of a hard-tissue barrier and continued root development can be seen at controls 6 and 12 months after initial treatment. A and B. Histologic section of a similarly treated tooth, extracted due to cervical root fracture. Close to the calcium hydroxide is a darkly stained area of necrotic and later calcified tissue (cn), followed by a layer of bone-like tissue (od), and above it dentin and predentin with lining odontoblasts (d). ×20 and 40.

## Timing of endodontic procedure after replantation

This is a delicate treatment problem as the endodontic procedure should ideally prevent development of inflammatory resorption or treat this condition at a stage where it is limited (337). At the same time PDL healing should be sufficiently advanced that the use of substances such as calcium hydroxide cannot interfere with the healing process and cause apical ankylosis due to its high pH (336). Combining results from an experimental (338) and a clinical study (339) the optimal time for pulp extirpation appears to be 7–14 days after replantation. Naturally the tooth needs to be

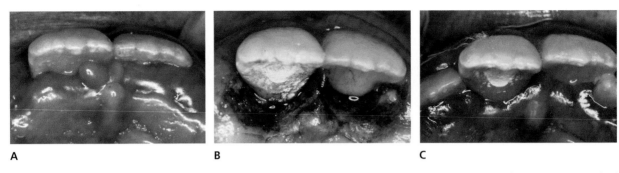

**A**　　　　　　　　**B**　　　　　　　　**C**

**Fig. 22.45** Surgical excision of gingiva in order to allow endodontic treatment in a partially erupted incisor. A. Condition before treatment. B. A palatal gingivectomy and root canal treatment were performed at the same visit. C. Condition 6 weeks later.

splinted or stabilized during the procedure as PDL healing is not complete at this time (140). This naturally implies that pulp extirpation is performed as a prophylaxis against root resorption (e.g. in the case of root canal closed teeth or teeth with incomplete root formation, or such a long extraoral storage that pulp revascularization is not likely (see Chapter 17)). In established inflammatory resorption an experimental study in dogs has shown that long term placement of calcium hydroxide (i.e. 2 months) led to more optimal healing than 1 week's treatment (328).

## Technical procedure

Permanent teeth can be injured before they have erupted completely or by being intruded, with subsequent development of pulp necrosis. In such cases, a palatal gingivectomy may be necessary to allow adaptation of a rubber dam and provide access into the root canal (Fig. 22.45).

In partially erupted or splinted teeth, adaptation of a rubber dam can be difficult. As leakage may occur, solutions that can damage oral tissues should not be used for disinfection (Fig. 22.46). A satisfactory effect can be achieved if the crown is cleaned with water-mixed pumice using a rubber cup and, after a rubber dam is adapted, the crown is washed with a mild disinfectant, e.g. a solution of chlorhexidine in 96% ethyl alcohol (109).

When access to the root canal has been gained and necrotic pulp tissue removed, an effective chemo-mechanical cleansing of the root canal is necessary because necrotic tissue remnants always remain along the dentinal walls. In immature teeth, this is a difficult procedure because of wide root canals and inadequacy of files or reamers (110, 111). Canal cleansing should be performed by careful, methodical filing of the dentinal walls, using lateral pressure and vertical movements. Only moderate pressure should be used, in order to avoid weakening of the root canal walls in the cervical area, as well as to avoid fracture of the fragile dentinal walls in the apical region, which may impair periapical healing (112). It is important to consider that the vital tissue present in the apical part of the pulpal lumen should not be removed, as this tissue may improve the quality and speed of apical bridging or provide further root development, depending on the type and differentiation of the cells involved. During cleansing, the canal should be repeatedly flushed with 0.5% sodium hypochlorite (113, 114, 241, 242).

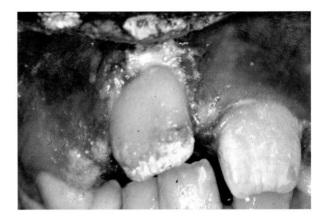

**Fig. 22.46** Damage of the soft tissues due to the leakage of 30% hydrogen peroxide. Hydrogen peroxide was used for disinfection in the case of a poorly adapted rubber dam on an infrapositioned incisor.

After cleansing, the root canal is filled with calcium hydroxide with a spiral. In immature teeth with wide root canals, a syringe with a special cannula may be used (Fig. 22.47). After filling, the calcium hydroxide dressing is compressed slightly towards the apex with a cotton pellet in order to ensure contact with the vital tissue apically; thereafter the access cavity is sealed with zinc oxide-eugenol cement. The root canal can be filled with calcium hydroxide immediately after chemo-mechanical cleansing (105, 224–226). Calcium hydroxide that is eventually pressed through the apical foramen during filling is readily resorbed by periapical tissues (115). However, necrotic and infected pulp tissue remnants pressed into the periapical space may cause an acute exacerbation of a chronic periapical inflammation (116) (Fig. 22.48).

The addition to calcium hydroxide of toxic antibacterial drugs, such as camphorated parachlorophenol, does not seem to be justified (111, 114, 117, 224), nor does the mixing of calcium hydroxide with corticosteroids or antibiotics (243).

After being filled with calcium hydroxide, the teeth should be controlled at 3- to 6-month intervals. Intermediary replacements of calcium hydroxide did not appear in an experimental study in monkeys to advance the apexification (332); however, in a clinical study it was found that frequent change of calcium hydroxide (ie. more than 5 months between shifts compared to less than 5 months) resulted in more rapid formation of an apical barrier (333).

**Fig. 22.47 Filling of the root canal with calcium hydroxide**
A palatal opening is made wide enough to allow adequate mechanical cleansing of the root canal.

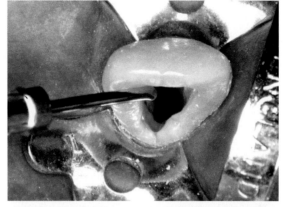
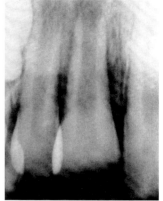

**Filling the root canal**
After completed cleansing, the cannula is introduced in the root canal close to the apical area and then slowly withdrawn while pressing calcium hydroxide out of the syringe.

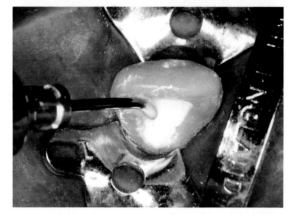
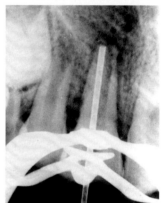

**Compressing calcium hydroxide**
The paste is then pressed lightly towards the apex with a dry cotton pellet to ensure apical contact with vital tissue. Filling and condensing of calcium hydroxide is repeated until the root canal assumes same radiodensity as surrounding dentin.

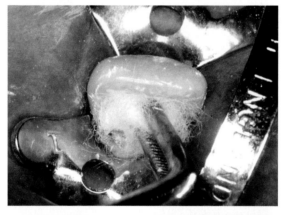
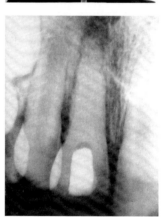

**Sealing the access cavity**
After the excess of the paste is removed, the coronal cavity is sealed of with zinc oxide-eugenol cement. One year after root canal treatment, periapical healing and formation of the apical hard-tissue barrier is seen.

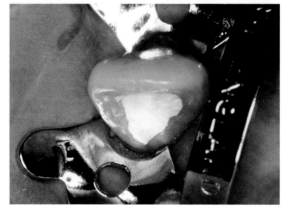
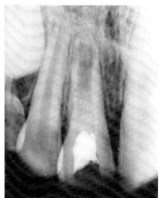

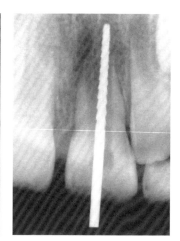

**Fig. 22.48** Effect of over-instrumentation. Over-ambitious cleansing in an immature incisor resulting in exacerbation of periapical inflammation 3 days after treatment.

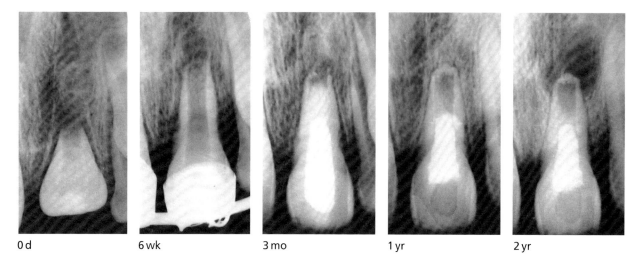

0 d            6 wk           3 mo           1 yr            2 yr

**Fig. 22.49** Reccurrence of periapical inflammation. Periapical radiolucency and inflammatory root resorption were evident 6 weeks after injury. The root canal was treated with calcium hydroxide and a complete apical closure was observed 12 months later. Note the absence of calcium hydroxide above sealing material, pressed into the root canal at a previous treatment. Thereafter, the patient was not available for control and when seen again after 2 years, new periapical radiolucency has developed.

If periapical healing does not occur, the root canal should be retreated. In the root canal, calcium hydroxide is dissolved and eventually forms compounds with different ions available from the vital tissue present at the apical foramen, resulting in the fall of the calcium hydroxide level in the root canal. In immature teeth, this appears to be an ongoing process that continues until the apical foramen is closed with a hard-tissue barrier. In the presence of a large periapical radiolucency, formation of hard tissue could be often seen first after repeated filling. It is conceivable that to achieve the effect of calcium hydroxide, presence of cells capable of hard tissue formation is necessary, which may take place after resolution of periapical destruction. When left empty, the root canal can become re-infected and new periapical radiolucency can occur, most probably due to leakage from an inadequate coronal seal (Fig. 22.49). These teeth can sometimes be successfully retreated with calcium hydroxide (Fig. 22.50). However, if bacteria have settled in the newly-formed hard tissue apically, this may be difficult and apical surgery may be necessary. Thus, when the level of calcium hydroxide falls in the cervical part of the root canal,

it should be refilled, in order to assure further formation of the hard-tissue barrier.

Permanent obturation with gutta-percha and a sealer is performed when radiographic and clinical examination demonstrates periapical healing and the root canal closed apically with a hard-tissue barrier. Depending on the width of apical foramen and size of the periapical lesion, this may take 6 to 18 months after initial treatment (93, 106, 218–221, 310). The apical barriers have proven in clinical and histological investigations to be quite resistant to pressure exerted during condensation of gutta-percha (93, 95). However, a thin barrier can be damaged or broken and gutta-percha expelled into the periapical space if excessive pressure is used (Fig. 22.51). A gentle obturation technique is therefore recommended (118). Experience has shown that the following procedure gives satisfactory results (314). The tip of a gutta-percha master point, i.e. the largest point that can easily reach the apical barrier, is warmed by passing it once through an alcohol flame. The point is then immediately introduced into the root canal and gently but steadily pressed against the apical barrier. To achieve the desired

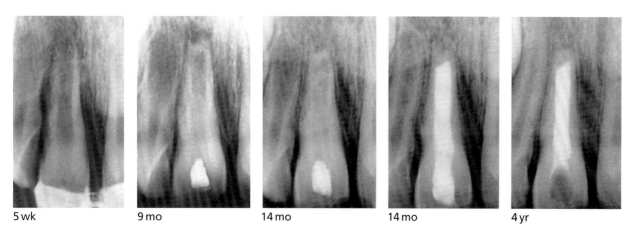

5 wk  9 mo  14 mo  14 mo  4 yr

**Fig. 22.50** Retreatment of periapical inflammation. Five weeks after injury there is widened and diffusely outlined periodontal space periapically and inflammatory root resorption. Nine months after treatment with calcium hydroxide, there is arrest of inflammatory resorption, hard tissue formation apically and periapically radiolucency. Note the inadequate coronal seal. Periapical healing could be seen 5 months after retreatment with calcium hydroxide. Condition 4 years after obturation of the root canal with gutta-percha. From CVEK (221) 1992.

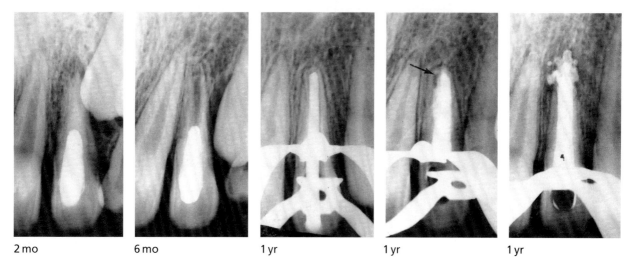

2 mo  6 mo  1 yr  1 yr  1 yr

**Fig. 22.51** Disruption of the apical hard tissue barrier due to forceful obturation of the root canal. During filling of the canal with gutta-percha, an attempt was made to fill a void in the root canal (arrow). The pressure applied resulted in the rupture of the thin hard tissue barrier and overfilling.

results, i.e. the apical part of the root canal filled and the gutta-percha point well-adapted to the barrier, only the tip of the gutta-percha point should be softened and the rest of it should remain stiff (Fig. 22.52). Once the gutta-percha has cooled in the root canal and a control radiograph is taken, the root canal can be obturated by lateral condensation of additional points which have been dipped into resin-chloroform, or by using an endodontic sealer. The other possibilities for adequate obturation of wide root canals include methods using thermo-plasticized gutta-percha and vertical condensation.

## Prognosis

Successful treatment with calcium hydroxide, i.e. periapical healing and formation of a hard-tissue barrier, has been reported to occur in 79–96% of the treated teeth (92–94, 216–222, 307–311). The results obtained in more comprehensive studies are shown in Table 22.2.

In a long-term study of calcium hydroxide treated incisors, periapical healing was observed in 92% of 589 teeth, 4 years after permanent filling of the root canal with gutta-percha (221). No difference was found between immature and mature teeth, indicating that the prognosis of root filling in immature teeth was not impaired by their wide root canals and often irregular hard tissue barriers containing inclusions of soft tissue. On the other hand, long-term tooth survival of immature teeth was seriously threatened by the occurrence of 'spontaneous' cervical root fractures. It is commonly known that root-filled teeth are more prone to be fractured than vital teeth and believed that desiccation of dentin and loss of dentin during reaming of root canal could be reasons for fracture (315, 316) (Fig. 22.7).

In immature teeth cervical fractures were found to be clearly related to the stage of root development. Frequency of cervical fractures fell gradually from 77% in 26 teeth with the lowest degree of root development, to 2% in 362 mature teeth (Fig. 22.54), which indicated that in young immature

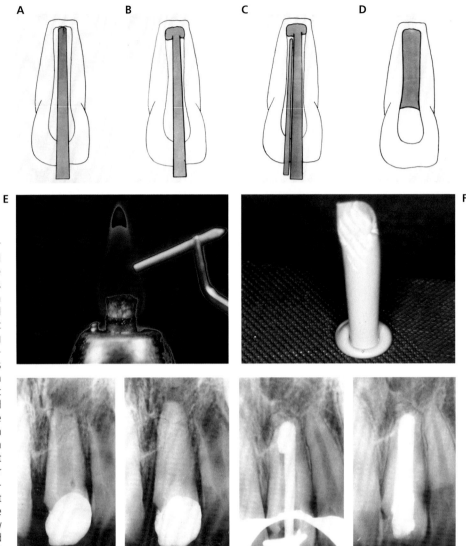

**Fig. 22.52** Clinical procedures for filling the canal with partially heated gutta-percha. A. Selection of a suitable master point. B. The tip of the point is softened by passing it once through ethanol flame and then introduced into the root canal and pressed against the apical barrier. C. Subsequent filling using lateral condensation. D. Completed filling. E. The tip of the point is softened by passing it once through ethanol flame. Only the tip of the point should be softened and the rest should remain stiff if the desired effect is to be achieved. F. The effect of pressing a partially softened point against a firm surface. G–J. Obturation of the root canal in non-vital immature incisor after treatment with calcium hydroxide. The softened tip of a master point was pressed against the hard tissue barrier and the root canal completely obturated by additional points, dipped in resin-chloroform, and using lateral condensation.

incisors the thin dentinal walls, left behind after the pulpal death, could be the reason for their occurrence (221) (Figs 22.53 and 22.54). This view was further supported by finding a significant relationship between fractures and defects left after arrested inflammatory resorption in the root, increasing susceptibility for a fracture especially in teeth with more advanced root development (221).

A similar phenomenon has been earlier observed in experiments with immature dog teeth (15). However, findings in *in vitro* experiments with animal and human dentin, suggested that calcium hydroxide, especially used in long-term therapies, may, due to denaturation and dissolution of its protein contents, increase the brittleness of dentin and risk of cervical root fractures (317, 318). Furthermore it was found in *in vitro* experiments, that sodium hypochlorite (3 or 5%), possesses a similar effect on hardness and brittleness of dentin (318, 319). It appears logical to assume that such effects would be more expressed in immature teeth, with

thin or weakened dentinal walls than in mature teeth (Fig. 22.7). Thus, it is conceivable that the high frequency of fractures could be the result of several, concomitantly involved factors in the treatment of the young immature teeth. Further experimental and clinical studies seem to be necessary before the reason or reasons for fractures could be clarified and the clinical procedures adapted. Hopefully, using new techniques for strengthening roots of immature teeth, the frequency of cervical fractures may be reduced (320–322). This technique is described in Chapter 23. In any case, much is gained if a young, immature incisor can be kept as space maintainer during the periods of maxillary growth (Fig. 22.55).

Finally, it should be mentioned that reappearance of periapical changes in teeth filled with gutta-percha can often be resolved by the re-treatment with calcium hydroxide and subsequent refilling of the root canal (334) (Fig. 22.56).

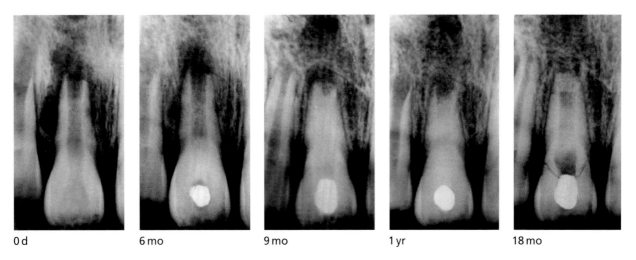

0 d          6 mo          9 mo          1 yr          18 mo

**Fig. 22.53** Cervical root fracture after successful endodontic treatment of an incisor with immature root development. A minor trauma caused the cervical root fracture 18 months after initial treatment.

**Fig. 22.54** Frequency of cervical root fractures. Frequencies of cervical fractures in 759 luxated, non-vital maxillary incisors, after calcium hydroxide treatment and 4 years observation following gutta-percha filling, distributed according to the stage of root development. From CVEK (221) 1992.

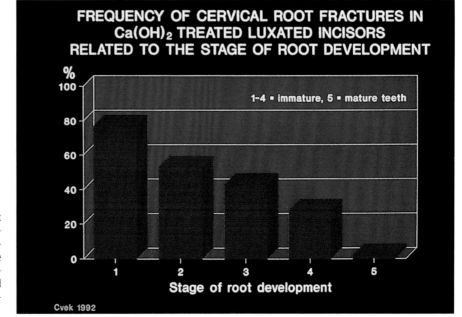

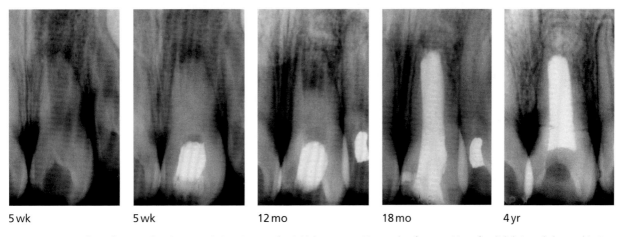

5 wk          5 wk          12 mo          18 mo          4 yr

**Fig. 22.55** Cervical root fracture of an immature incisor 6 years after initial treatment. Five weeks after reposition of a slightly intruded central incisor a periapical radiolucency indicates pulp necrosis. 12 months after treatment with calcium hydroxide periapical healing and formation of the apical hard-tissue barrier is seen. The tooth is root filled with gutta-percha 18 months after initial treatment. A cervical root fracture is seen 4 years later, caused by biting into a piece of chocolate. Note root development of the lateral, neighboring incisor.

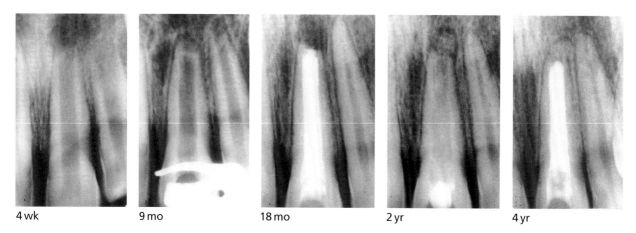

4 wk      9 mo      18 mo      2 yr      4 yr

**Fig. 22.56** Treatment of secondary periapical inflammation. After initial treatment with calcium hydroxide and root filling with gutta-percha, a new periapical radiolucency developed 18 months after late treatment. Gutta-percha was removed and root canal treated again with calcium hydroxide. Six months later, there is formation of new hard tissue barrier at the apical foramen and a diminished radiolucency. Periapical healing is seen at the 4-year control of new obturation of the root canal with gutta-percha.

## Treatment of mature teeth

Treatment of non-vital traumatized mature teeth is the same as for the teeth with pulp necrosis of other etiology. Commonly accepted endodontic procedures, drugs and filling materials can be used (244, 245). However, high frequencies of healing have been reported if the root canals have been dressed with calcium hydroxide prior to filling with gutta-percha (94, 106, 221, 309, 332). Dressing with calcium hydroxide before obturation with gutta-percha can therefore be recommended for routine use in teeth with infected root canals and periapical lesions.

## Prognosis

Periapical healing after treatment and obturation of the root canal with various filling materials has been reported in various clinical studies to range from 76 to 91% (54, 57, 245, 332). Periapical healing, after initial dressing with calcium hydroxide and subsequent filling with gutta-percha, was found in 92–96% of the treated teeth (94, 106, 221, 309).

## External inflammatory root resorption

### Pathology

External root resorption in luxated or replanted teeth has been described as surface, inflammatory or replacement resorption, of which only inflammatory resorption is related to a necrotic and infected pulp (60, 119, 200–202, 221). When dentinal tubules are exposed by the resorption of damaged tissues on the root surface, bacteria and toxins from the root canal may via dentinal tubules diffuse to the adjacent periodontal tissues causing inflammation and progressive root resorption (Fig. 22.57). This resorption seems to be more frequent and rapid in immature teeth, most probably due to the thin dentinal walls and wide tubules (5, 85). Whether systemic antibiotics may prevent the occurrence of inflammatory resorption in replanted teeth is controversial (203, 323–326.) To judge from the clinical experience, systemic antibiotics for 7–10 days do not prevent inflammatory resorption after treatment has been completed. However, once bacteria have settled in the necrotic pulp, the arrest or healing of inflammatory resorption depends only on removal of bacteria from pulpal lumen and adjacent dentin tubules by endodontic therapy.

## Diagnosis and treatment

Radiographically, external inflammatory root resorption is characterized by a progressive loss of tooth substance associated with a persistent or progressive radiolucency in the adjacent alveolar bone (Fig. 22.58). The critical period for onset of these changes seems to be about 2–8 weeks after injury (see Chapter 2 and Chapter 17, p. 457). It is important that endodontic therapy is instituted as soon as clinical and radiographic signs of pulp necrosis and inflammatory resorption are evident.

Endodontic treatment of teeth with inflammatory root resorption is identical to treatment of other non-vital traumatized teeth. In principle, the choice of antibacterial drugs or filling materials are of minor importance, as the effect on healing depends upon effective removal of the necrotic pulp and bacteria from the pulpal lumen (120, 327). However, dressing the root canal with calcium hydroxide before filling with inert gutta-percha has been shown to give a high frequency of healing (120, 221, 328). It may therefore be preferable to use in teeth in which periodontal healing and formation of reparative hard tissue in resorption lesions is desirable (Figs 22.58–22.60).

The effect of calcium hydroxide upon the arrest and healing of inflammatory root resorption is not clearly understood. Elimination of bacteria from the root canal and dentinal tubules appears to be the main factor. It has also

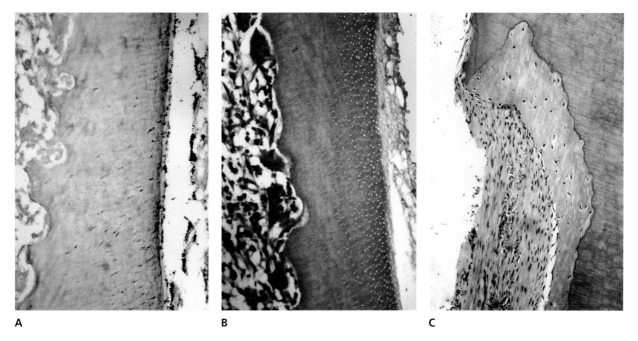

**Fig. 22.57** Histologic appearance of inflammatory root resorption. A. Penetration of bacteria through dentinal tubules, from the contaminated pulpal lumen towards the periodontium, Brown & Brenn bacterial stain. ×100. B. Bacteria and their toxins cause accumulation of leukocytes. As these cannot reach bacteria in the tubules, osteoclasts are stimulated to resorb dentin. ×100. C. If bacteria are removed from the root canal, resorption lesions can be repaired by cementum-like tissue. ×80.

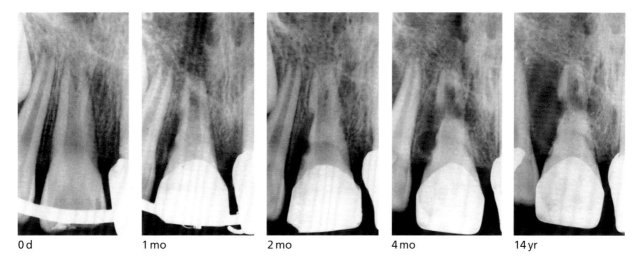

**Fig. 22.58** Radiographic appearance of external inflammatory root resorption. There is a progressive loss of root substance associated with increasing radiolucency in the adjacent alveolar bone.

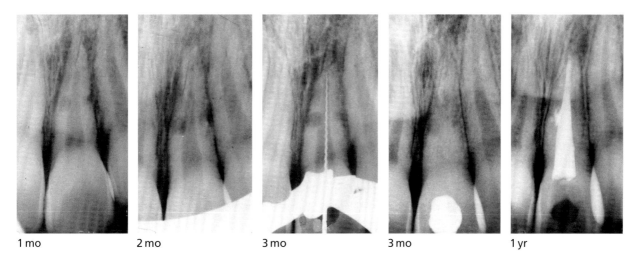

**Fig. 22.59** Treatment of inflammatory root resorption which has perforated to the root canal. Three months after injury, the root canal was treated with calcium hydroxide and after 1 year, a gutta-percha filling was inserted. Note that the filling material has been forced into the resorption defect, but was not displaced into the periodontal space.

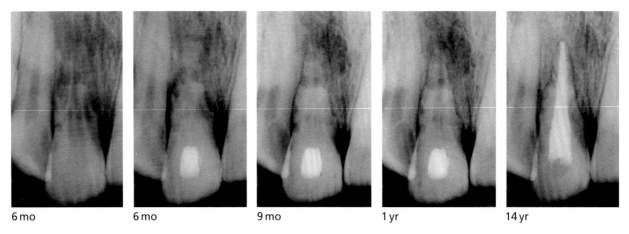

6 mo                   6 mo                   9 mo                   1 yr                   14 yr

**Fig. 22.60** Treatment of inflammatory root resorption. Six months after luxation extensive inflammatory resorption cavities are seen and, in some places, only very thin dentinal walls seem to have remained. The root canal was filled with calcium hydroxide. After 9 months, there is arrest of resorption and periodontal healing. At the 1-year control of the gutta-percha filling, deposition of hard tissue into the resorption cavities is evident.

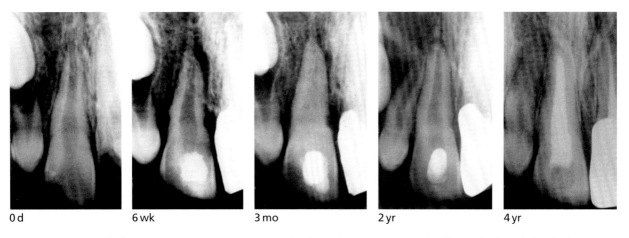

0 d                    6 wk                   3 mo                   2 yr                   4 yr

**Fig. 22.61** Treatment of inflammatory root resorption apparent 6 weeks after replantation. Two years after filling with calcium hydroxide, there is periradicular healing and arrest of root resorption. At a 4-year control, there is repair of resorption lesions.

been reported that calcium hydroxide from the root canal may raise the pH at the root surface to such a level that the tissue along the resorption cavity, including the resorbing cells, can be damaged (246). But this effect appears to be of short duration; and the repair of the experimental lesions in the root surface by deposition of new hard tissue has been observed soon after (247, 248). It is conceivable that hydroxyl ions passing through the dentinal tubules denature or precipitate its protein contents, whereby further release of hydroxyl ions towards the periodontium is prevented or reduced to harmless concentrations.

## Follow-up and prognosis

Radiographically, healing is characterized by the arrest of the resorption process and reestablishment of the periodontal space, bordered by a lamina dura. Arrest and healing may occur irrespective of the extent of resorption and the amount of root substance lost (Figs 22.59–22.63). Arrest of inflammatory resorption may usually leave a defect on the

root surface which, however, can be diminished by the successive apposition of new hard tissue and the resorption lesion wholly repaired (Fig. 22.61). In the cervical area of the root, such a defect may become a site of minor resistance leading to a cervical root fracture, especially in teeth with early stages of root development (221) (Figs 22.62 and 22.63).

In replanted teeth, ankylosis can often develop at sites of previously arrested inflammatory resorption (Fig. 22. 64). It has been suggested that short-lasting or repeated release of calcium hydroxide from the root canal may contribute to occurrence of ankylosis by damaging periodontal cells (248–250). This assumption, however, is in conflict with clinical studies of luxated teeth, in which the damaging effect of hydroxide release should be the same as in replanted teeth; and very high frequencies of arrest and healing of inflammatory resorption were found after treatment with calcium hydroxide (120, 221). In these studies, ankylosis was rare and seen only after severe intrusive luxations. This seems to indicate that initial periodontal injury, inflicted by injury or desiccation, rather than calcium hydroxide should

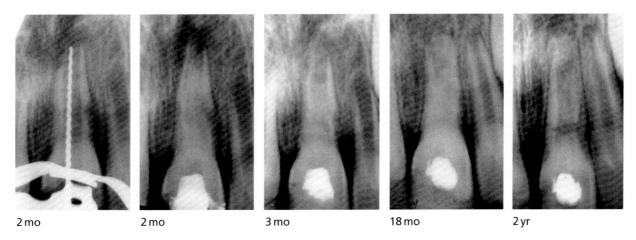

2 mo        2 mo        3 mo        18 mo        2 yr

**Fig. 22.62** Arrest of inflammatory root resorption after calcium hydroxide treatment. After 18 months there is periapical healing and arrest of root resorption. Six months later, a cervical root fracture has occurred through the resorption defect. From CVEK (221) 1992.

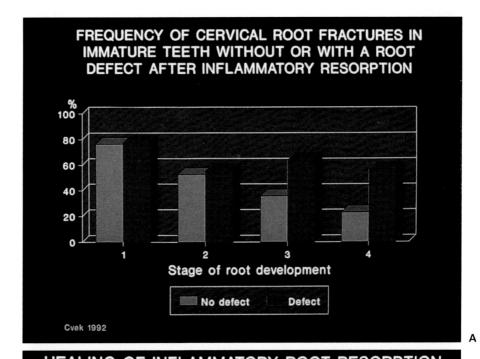

A

**Fig. 22.63** A. Relationship between cervical root fractures and presence of defects and inflammatory root resorption. Fractures in 397 non-vital immature incisors, following calcium hydroxide treatment and an observation period of 4 years after filling with gutta-percha. The material is distributed according to the presence of resorption defects in the cervical area of the root as well as the stage of root development. From CVEK (221) 1992. B. Healing of inflammatory root resorption after luxation injuries. The frequency of root resorption arrest and healing as well as the occurrence of ankylosis in 187 luxated non-vital permanent incisors, treated with calcium hydroxide. From CVEK (221) 1992.

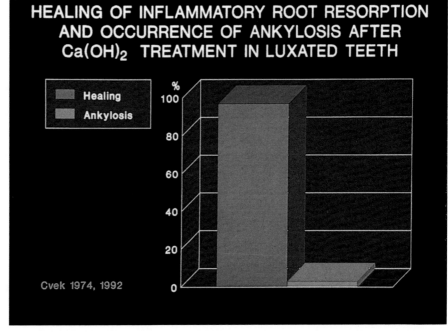

B

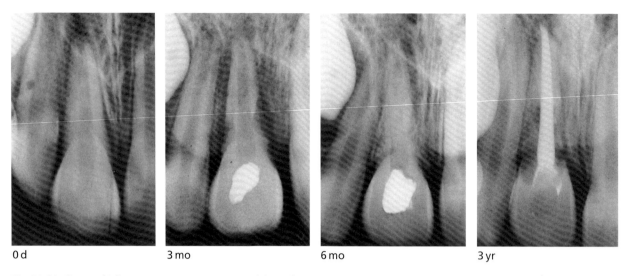

0 d                3 mo                6 mo                3 yr

**Fig. 22.64** Change of inflammatory root resorption into ankylosis after treatment with calcium hydroxide. The tooth was replanted after 60 min dry storage. Three months after replantation there is inflammatory root resorption with associated radiolucency in the adjacent alveolar bone and the tooth was treated with calcium hydroxide. Six months after treatment there is periradicular healing with development of replacement resorption, i.e. dentoalveolar ankylosis.

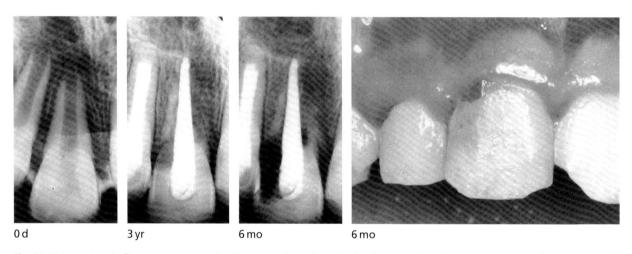

0 d                3 yr                6 mo                6 mo

**Fig. 22.65** Late external inflammatory root resorption. Three years after replantation there is progressive replacement resorption. At the 6-month control, marked inflammatory root resorption is found cervically. Clinically, a pink discoloration of the crown and perforating granulation tissue is seen close to the gingival margin.

be blamed for the occurrence of ankylosis, subsequent to healing of inflammatory resorption (Fig. 22.63).

## Late external inflammatory root resorption

### Pathology

Progressive external resorption associated with inflammatory changes in surrounding tissue, may occur years after injury and is, as a rule, located near the cemento-enamel junction (251, 252). It is primarily found in replanted and ankylosed teeth in infraposition, but may also occur in luxated, mostly intruded, teeth. In its advanced stages, resorption may undermine the crown and become clinically

evident as a pink spot below the cervical enamel, in both vital and root-filled teeth (Fig. 22.65). The etiology is obscure. One conceivable factor could be the presence of bacteria in the gingival crevice and their penetration into dentinal tubules, exposed by active or poorly repaired resorption (251, 253). This may cause inflammation in the area and elicit a progressive root resorption, sometimes interfering with the ankylosing processes (Figs 22.65 and 22.66).

### Treatment

Cervical root resorption can be treated in several ways. If esthetic considerations are of minor importance and the resorption cavity does not extend below the cervical bone

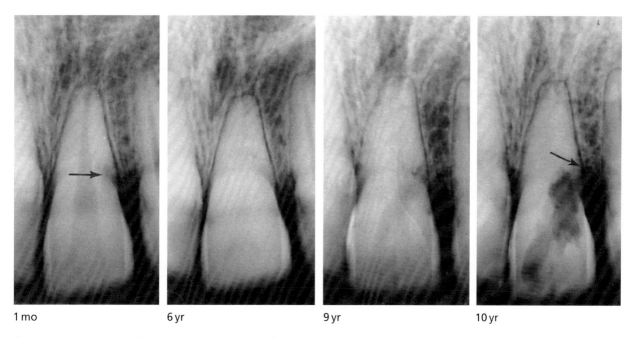

1 mo           6 yr           9 yr           10 yr

**Fig. 22.66** Late progression of external root resorption. A small external root resorption cavity (arrow) is seen 1 month after a luxation injury. At the 6-year control, the pulpal lumen has been diminished by hard tissue and the external resorption apparently arrested. Controls 9 and 10 years after injury show a rapid progression of external root resorption and the reduced level of marginal bone (arrow).

**Fig. 22.67** Treatment of a late external root resorption in a vital incisor. A and B. Cervical resorption seen 6 years after subluxation. C. Appearance of resorption after elevation of a flap. D. Preparation of the resorption cavity disclosed no connection with the pulpal lumen. Dentin was covered with calcium hydroxide and the cavity restored. E and F. Radiographic and clinical status 10 years after treatment.

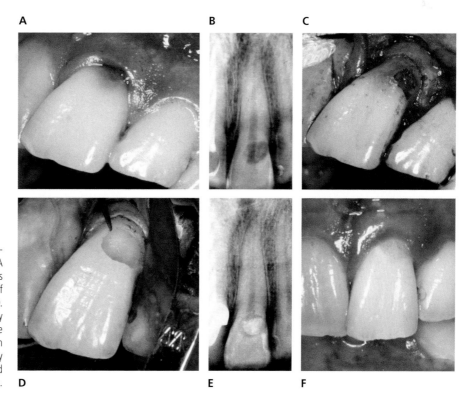

margin, a gingivectomy with subsequent filling of the resorption cavity with a dentin bonded composite or glass ionomer cement is the method of choice (254–256). If esthetic considerations are important, a gingival flap can be raised and the same restoration as above performed (121, 255) (Fig. 22.67). In cases where the cervical resorption

defect extends below the alveolar crest, orthodontic or surgical extrusion can be considered before cavity restoration (256–259). In cases where the cervical resorption is related to ankylosis, the choice is either to accept the condition or to remove the crown and leave the ankylosed root to bony replacement (260) (see Chapter 24, p. 700).

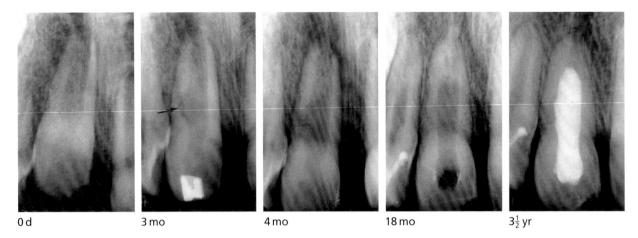

| 0 d | 3 mo | 4 mo | 18 mo | 3½ yr |

**Fig. 22.68** Internal inflammatory root canal resorption after intrusive luxation of a central incisor. Three and 4 months after injury, an inflammatory internal resorption with communication to the periodontium has developed cervically (arrow). After 18 months' treatment with calcium hydroxide, there is apical closure with hard tissue and communication with periodontium was no longer found. A control 3½ years after filling of the root canal with gutta-percha shows periradicular healing.

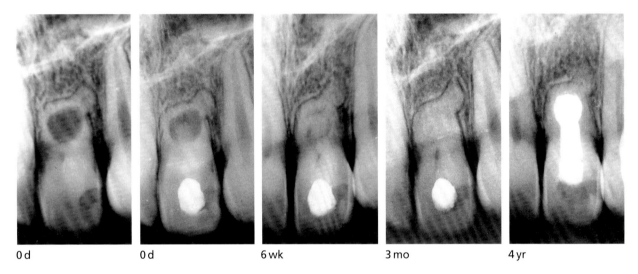

| 0 d | 0 d | 6 wk | 3 mo | 4 yr |

**Fig. 22.69** Treatment of internal inflammatory root canal resorption in a crown dilacerated incisor with calcium hydroxide. Repeated filling with calcium hydroxide was done at 3-week intervals. Note that the calcium hydroxide has step-wise filled the entire resorption cavity, indicating absence of soft tissue in the lesion. At the control 4 years after filling with gutta-percha there are normal periradicular conditions.

## Root canal resorption (internal resorption)

### Pathology

Root canal resorption is related to the amount of vital tissue in the pulpal lumen. It is often seen in root-fractured, but seldom in only luxated teeth (194, 208). The processes have been described as *transient or progressive surface* or *tunneling resorption. Surface resorption* is seen radiographically as a limited loss of hard tissue, usually at the fracture site or near the apical foramen in luxated teeth. *Tunneling resorption* is characterized by the loss of root substance behind the predentin border which slowly progresses in a coronal direction, followed by obliteration of both resorption lesions and the pulpal lumen (194). Although the triggering mechanisms have not been assessed, these changes can possibly be looked upon as a part of healing processes in which resorption of damaged or altered tissue is necessary before repair can take place (see Chapter 2, p. 84). Thus, endodontic treatment is not indicated unless other changes occur, such as periradicular inflammatory changes.

Progressive internal resorption is a late and rare complication that usually occurs in the cervical area of the root canal in luxated teeth (Figs 22.68 and 22.69). It is characterized radiographically by the progressive loss of root substance with no hard tissue formation in the resorption cavity. The process seems to be elicited by irritation from bacteria or its components in dentinal tubules, originating from a mechanical damage, dilaceration or cracks in the cervical area of the root or by metaplasia of pulp to bone (261–263).

Occasionally, progressive dentin resorption may also occur in root-filled teeth. A conceivable reason for this could be presence of bacteria in the root canal and communica-

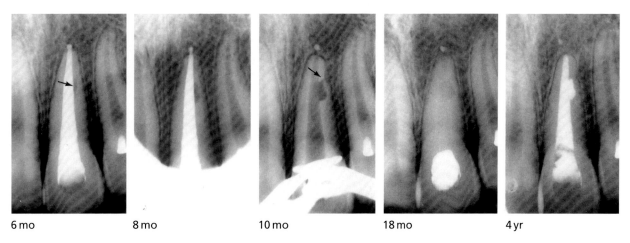

6 mo          8 mo          10 mo          18 mo          4 yr

**Fig. 22.70** Internal root canal resorption in a luxated and root filled central incisor. At controls 6, 8 and 10 months after filling of the root canal with gutta-percha, a progressive internal root canal is seen in relation to an accessory root canal in the apical area of the tooth (arrow). The root canal was treated with calcium hydroxide and after 18 months filled with gutta-percha. There is no extrusion of the filling material into the periodontal space through the previous accessory canal.

tion with the periodontium via an accessory canal, from which soft tissue may proliferate into the root canal and resorb contaminated dentin (Fig. 22.70).

## Treatment

Endodontic treatment of teeth with progressive, internal root resorption is complicated by the difficulty in removing tissue from a resorption cavity. Soft tissue remnants may impede healing if communication exists with the periodontium. However, soft tissue in the lesion can be dissolved by means of repeated filling with calcium hydroxide at 2- to 3-week intervals. If treatment with calcium hydroxide is maintained for a couple of months, communication with the periodontium may be closed by apposition of hard tissue and thus overfilling with gutta-percha can be avoided (Figs 22.68–22.70).

## Pulp necrosis following pulp canal obliteration

### Pathology

Pulp canal obliteration by progressive hard tissue formation is relatively common after luxation injuries. The hard tissue varies histologically depending on the origin and differentiation of cells involved in its production (see Chapter 2, p. 84). Formation of hard tissue can be followed radiographically as it assumes typical morphologic patterns. There may be ingrowth of bone and periodontal tissue into the root canal, usually after pulp revascularization in replanted or luxated teeth (Fig. 22.71) or the pulpal lumen may be diminished by excessive, irregular hard tissue formation (Fig. 22.72). These changes are only seen in young teeth with incomplete root formation, resulting in cessation of further root development. In these teeth neither prophylactic nor therapeutic endodontic treatment can be recom-

mended because of apparent problems of a mechanical nature as the irregular arrangement of hard tissue prevents effective canal cleansing.

In most canal obliterated teeth, the new hard tissue is deposited regularly along dentinal walls and the pulpal lumen diminishes gradually until only a narrow root canal remains which may or may not be seen in the radiographs (Fig. 22.73). In these instances, periapical radiolucency has been reported to occur in 13–16% of teeth with traumatically-induced pulp canal obliteration, during observation periods of up to 20 years (88, 122). According to clinical experience, occurrence of periapical lesions can in most cases be related to caries, inadequate crown restorations or new trauma (Figs 22.74 and 22.75). In other teeth with apparently intact crowns the pathogenesis can be difficult to define. An additional minor injury may cause ischemic necrosis of a pulp due to rupture of the few existing blood vessels. However, the access of bacteria to the pulpal lumen remains to be explained.

The progressive diminishing of the pulpal lumen by formation of hard tissue represents a challenge for endodontic therapy (264, 329). Opinions vary as to whether a prophylactic endodontic treatment should be instituted as soon as the onset of pulp canal obliteration has been diagnosed (123–125, 264, 265). In teeth with normal periradicular conditions, there seem to be only two logical justifications for endodontic intervention. One is on the premise of ongoing degenerative changes leading to necrosis of the pulp, and the second is on the premise that ongoing obliteration will make the root canal inaccessible for a later endodontic treatment. However, when the pulps from prophylactically treated teeth with reduced pulpal lumen were examined histologically, changes were characterized by an increase of collagen content and a varying decrease in the number of cells, i.e. changes which do not seem to warrant endodontic intervention (126).

In another study, the accessibility for mechanical treatment was investigated in 54 obliterated incisors treated for

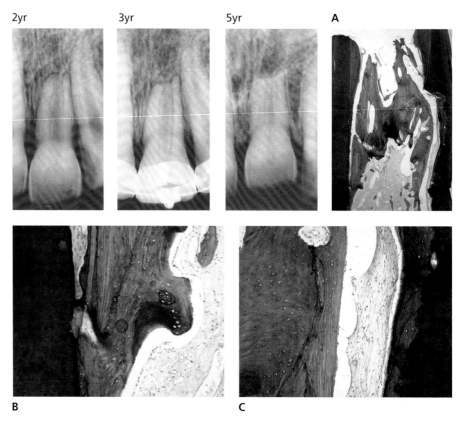

**Fig. 22.71** Radiographic and histologic appearance of bony ingrowth into the pulpal lumen. There is increasing infraposition of the tooth at 2 and 5 year controls after injury. Histologic appearance of bone ingrowth into pulpal lumen of an intruded and subsequently infrapositioned incisor, 3 years after injury. A. Low power view of the extracted tooth. Note ingrowth of the bone into the root canal. ×3. B. Internal ankylosis. ×40. C. Internal periodontal ligament. ×40.

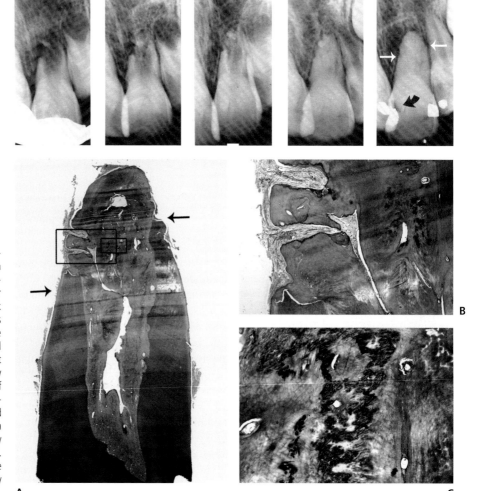

**Fig. 22.72** Irregular hard tissue formation in the pulpal lumen of a luxated immature incisor with subsequent pulp necrosis. Six years after injury, a deep carious lesion (black arrow) and a periapical radiolucency is seen. A. Low power view of the extracted tooth. Note arrested normal root development, according to extent of development at time of injury (arrows), and irregular formation of hard tissue in the pulpal lumen containing islands of soft, inflamed and necrotic tissue. ×7. B. Connection between necrotic pulp and chronically inflamed periodontal space. ×10. C. Areas of dystrophically calcified tissue are surrounded by the irregularly formed dentin. ×50.

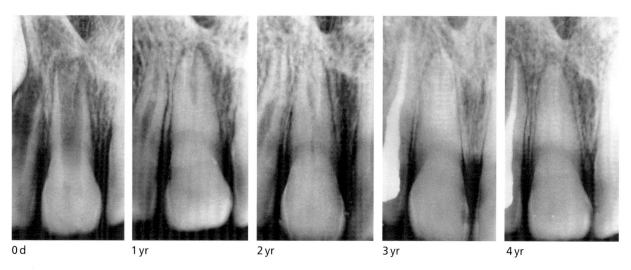

0 d 1 yr 2 yr 3 yr 4 yr

**Fig. 22.73** Radiographic appearance of the gradually diminished pulpal lumen by apposition of hard tissue on dentinal walls. A luxated incisor at the time of injury and 1, 2, 3 and 4 years afterwards.

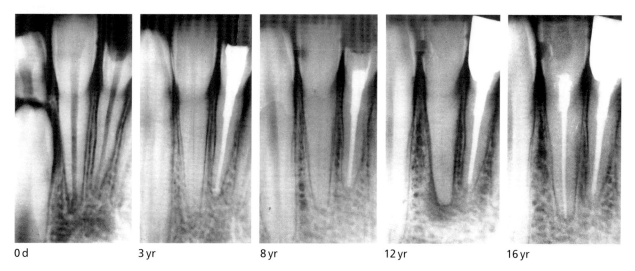

0 d 3 yr 8 yr 12 yr 16 yr

**Fig. 22.74** An incisor with reduced pulpal lumen and pulp necrosis due to a deep carious lesion. Periapical healing can be seen 4 years after root canal treatment. From CVEK et al. (134) 1982.

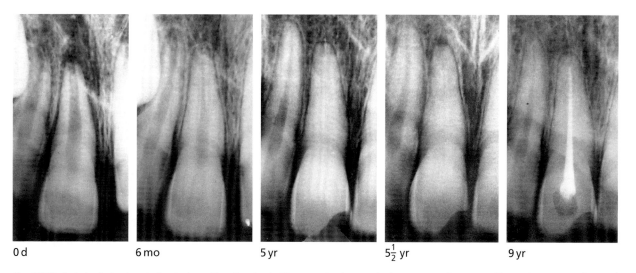

0 d 6 mo 5 yr $5\frac{1}{2}$ yr 9 yr

**Fig. 22.75** Endodontic treatment of an incisor with reduced pulpal lumen and pulp necrosis due to a secondary trauma. The tooth was crown fractured in a new injury 5 years after the initial injury. Root canal treatment was performed at this time. Six months later, periapical radiolucency has developed. At the 4-year control after root canal treatment (9 years after initial injury), periapical healing is evident.

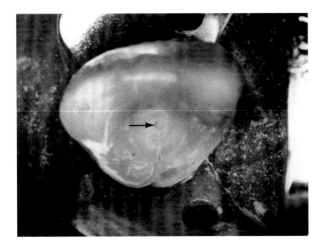

**Fig. 22.76** Preparation for root canal treatment of an incisor with an obliterated pulpal lumen. An area of discolored dentin (arrow) indicates the location of the obliterated root canal.

periapical lesions (127). The root canal could be found in all teeth but one, although no or only a hairline canal was visible in preoperative radiographs. During treatment, fracture of a file or perforation of the root occurred in 10 teeth; but in only 5 of these teeth a complication resulted in a failure. Periapical healing was seen in 80% of 55 teeth, 4 years after treatment. Thus, considering the low frequency of late periapical osteitis and relative accessibility of these teeth for endodontic treatment (including surgical retrograde filling techniques), routine endodontic intervention in teeth with ongoing obliteration of the root canal does not seem justified. However, such prophylactic endodontic treatment intervention could be considered in crown-fractured teeth in which a post in the root canal is necessary for future restoration.

## Treatment

Mechanical preparation of an obliterated root canal requires patience and cannot be forced. Just locating the root canal may take more than one appointment. A cavity is prepared through the oral surface to the level of the cervical part of the root. Control radiographs taken after injury may be of help with respect to the level in the root at which the canal can be expected. After the access cavity has been rinsed, the canal is patiently sought with the thinnest file. If the canal cannot be found, the cavity is prepared a step further and the search continued. Sometimes, a change in the color of dentin in the center of the root will indicate the position of the canal (Fig. 22.76). The use of a contrast medium, e.g. 10% potassium iodine, can sometimes disclose a root canal which could not be seen in earlier radiographs (128). A cotton pellet is soaked in the contrast medium and placed in the cavity, which is then sealed with zinc oxide-eugenol cement, supplied with firm pressure for 10 seconds to facilitate penetration of the contrast medium into the root canal (Fig. 22.77). Thereafter, at least two radiographs are taken at different angulations in order to establish the position of the root canal. An operating microscope, which can magnify the

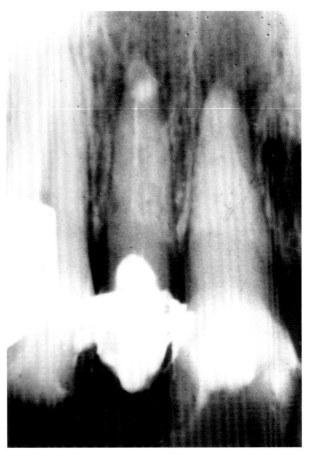

**Fig. 22.77** Use of 10% potassium iodide as contrast medium for disclosing the root canal. In a lateral incisor, the contrast is seen in the root canal that was not visible radiographically prior to treatment. From HASSELGREN & STRÖMBERG (128) 1976.

base of the cavity, may also help in locating the root canal (266).

When the entrance to the canal has been found, further reaming should be performed step by step, carefully and without unnecessary pressure, in order to avoid fracture of the file. It is important that the thinnest file be used to track the root canal all the way to the apical foramen (Fig. 22.78). A too early change to a larger file may lead to a false route or may complicate further treatment by pressing dentin debris in the root canal. To avoid obturation of the canal with dissolved dentin, solutions capable of dissolving hard tissue should not be used at an early stage of treatment. However after the root canal has been reamed to the apical area, ethylene diamine tetra-acetic acid can be used to facilitate widening of the canal. It is not necessary to remove all hard tissue formed after injury; just enough to assure an adequate root canal filling with gutta-percha and a sealer (Fig. 22.78).

## Prognosis

The prognosis for successful endodontic treatment of incisors with pulp canal obliteration, pulp necrosis and periapical involvement has been found to be 80% (127).

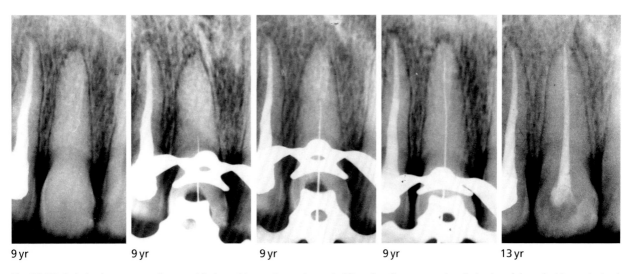

9 yr          9 yr          9 yr          9 yr          13 yr

**Fig. 22.78** Endodontic treatment of a central incisor with complete pulp canal obliteration. Note progressive diminution of the pulpal lumen by hard tissue after a luxation injury. Periapical radiolucency developed 9 years after injury. The root canal was found and carefully reamed using the finest files. Periapical healing is evident 4 years after root canal filling with gutta-percha. From CVEK et al. (127) 1982.

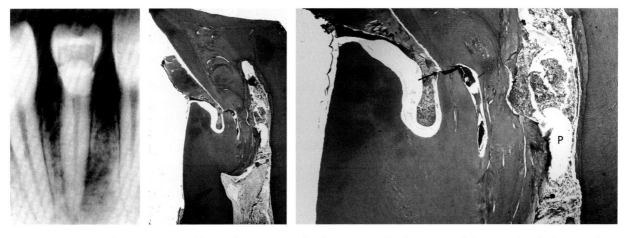

**Fig. 22.79** Periapical radiolucency in crown-dilacerated incisor 18 months after eruption. A histologic section of the extracted tooth shows a pathway via the dilaceration for bacterial penetration to the pulp canal (P) resulting in a pulp necrosis (arrow). ×2.5 and 15.

## Crown malformations

### Pathology

Impact from a displaced primary incisor can be the cause of mineralization disturbances in developing permanent successors, which later may assume various morphologic deviations (129–131) (Figs 22.79 and 22.80) (see also Chapter 20, p. 542). Soft tissue inclusions in hypomineralized dentin and malformations in dilacerated teeth may serve as pathways for rapid bacterial penetration, from plaque or a carious lesion, towards the pulp (Fig. 22.79).

Inflammation and subsequent necrosis of the pulp may occur already during or soon after eruption, when hypomineralized dentin or the dilacerated part of the crown or root comes into contact with the oral environment (132, 133) (Fig. 22.79).

### Treatment

To avoid involvement of the pulp and ensure further root development, it is important that defects in the crown, especially those in which hypomineralized dentin is not covered with enamel, are treated as soon as possible after eruption. Hypoplastic lesions should be cleaned, eventually treated with calcium hydroxide, and thereafter restored e.g., with glass ionomer cement and/or composite resin (Fig. 22.80).

In crown-dilacerated teeth, there is always a fissure present, according to the site of dilaceration, through which bacteria can enter the invaginated part of the tooth. This fissure should be enlarged, the bottom carefully cleaned and thereafter the cavity restored with a composite material (Fig. 22.81).

Non-vital teeth can be treated by conventional endodontic procedures if the root canal is accessible for treatment

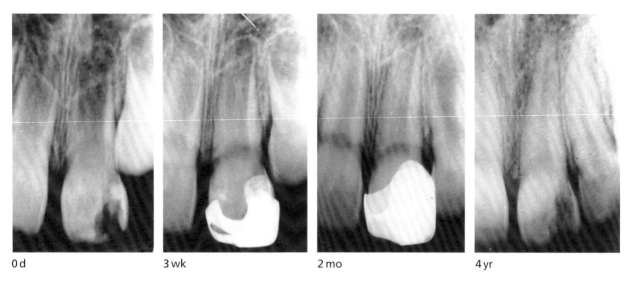

0 d                      3 wk                     2 mo                     4 yr

**Fig. 22.80** Treatment of permanent incisor with external enamel and dentin hypoplasia, due to the impact from luxated predecessor. Large hypomineralized area in the crown of a newly erupted incisor. The external hypoplasia was treated with calcium hydroxide and temporarily restored with a stainless steel crown. Four years after subsequent restoration with a composite material, root formation is complete.

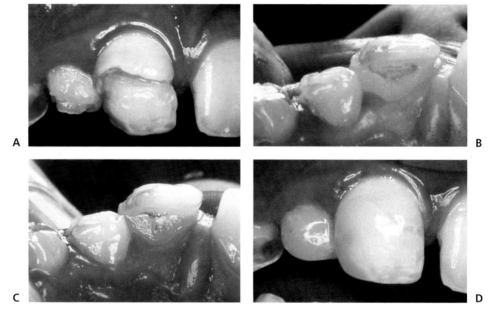

**Fig. 22.81** Restoration of malformed crowns of two permanent incisors. A and B. Dilacerated crown of central incisor and hypoplastic crown of the lateral incisor. C. Preparation of the palatal fissure. D. The hypoplastic areas and the base of the palatal cavity were covered with hard setting calcium hydroxide and the crowns restored with a composite using an acid-etch technique.

and the root sufficiently developed to support an eventual crown restoration (Fig. 22.82).

## Discoloration of non-vital teeth

Discoloration of the crown caused by intrapulpal bleeding is a relatively common sequel to luxation injuries. A pink discoloration that occurs shortly after the injury, i.e. within 2–3 days, can be reversible (68, 79, 80, 207, 208). Extravasated blood can be resorbed, tissue damage repaired and the crown can regain its natural color. On the other hand, a persistent or later appearing discoloration, especially with a shade of grey, indicates irreversable changes, i.e. necrosis of the pulp.

Discoloration of the crown may occur and persist without radiographic changes. However, for esthetic reasons, a severe discoloration can *per se* be considered an indication for endodontic treatment, in order to make bleaching of the crown or other treatment solutions possible (267).

### Pathology

In traumatized teeth, a persistent discoloration of the clinical crown has been ascribed to hemorrhage and/or decomposition of pulp tissue and presence of bacteria in the pulpal chamber. After lysis of extravasated erythrocytes in a necrotic pulp, the released hemoglobin breaks down to variously colored substances, such as hematoidin, hematoporphyrin and hemosiderin which, after diffusion into the

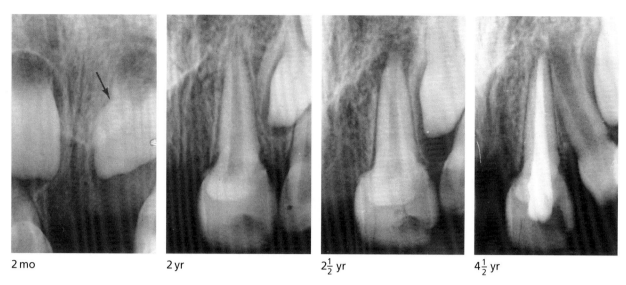

| 2 mo | 2 yr | $2\frac{1}{2}$ yr | $4\frac{1}{2}$ yr |

**Fig. 22.82** Endodontic treatment of malformed permanent incisor with pulp necrosis. Cervical dilaceration of the tooth (arrow) was noted 2 months after the intrusive luxation of primary incisor which later was removed. Six months after eruption of permanent incisor, periapical radiolucency was observed. After root canal treatment, periapical healing has taken place.

dental tubules, cause discoloration of dentin. In the event of infection, bacteria produce hydrogen sulphide which may combine with iron from hemoglobin and form iron sulphide, a black compound that further enhances discoloration (267, 268). The treatment of discoloration is described in Chapter 33.

## Essentials

### Crown fractures with pulp exposure

The exposed pulp can be treated with capping, partial pulpotomy, cervical pulpotomy or pulpectomy.

### Pulp capping (Fig. 22.11)

Indicated in mature and immature teeth when exposure is minimal and can be treated soon after injury; i.e. within 24 hours.

(1) Isolate with rubber dam and wash with saline.
(2) Cover the exposed pulp with calcium hydroxide and the exposed dentin with a liner. When using a hard-setting calcium hydroxide, both pulp and dentin are covered with the compound.
(3) Restore the crown with a composite using acid-etch technique or another type of restoration, e.g. porcelain laminate veneer.
(4) If immediate restoration is not possible, restore the tooth temporarily, with a glass ionomer cement or a temporary crown cemented with zinc oxide-eugenol cement. If the tooth is incorporated in a splint, cover the fracture surface with glass ionomer cement before the splint is adapted.

(5) Follow-up: clinical and radiographic controls after 6 months, 1 year and annually for a minimum of 3 years.

*Prognosis*: pulp healing in 71–88%.

### Partial pulpotomy (Fig. 22.12)

Indicated in mature and immature teeth showing vital pulp tissue at the exposure site, irrespective of its size and interval between injury and treatment. When the pulp is necrotic or demonstrates impaired vascularity, consider cervical pulpotomy in immature or pulpectomy in mature teeth.

(1) Administer local anesthesia.
(2) Isolate with a rubber dam and wash with a mild disinfectant.
(3) Amputate the pulp together with surrounding dentin to a depth of about 2 mm below the exposure site with a diamond bur in high-speed contra-angle hand-piece, using a continuous water spray. Cut intermittently, for brief periods and without unnecessary pressure.
(4) Await hemostasis.
(5) Cover the wound with calcium hydroxide and seal the cavity. If the crown is to be immediately restored with a composite material, seal the coronal cavity with zinc sulphate cement according to Prader (186) (consists of two parts: part a: zinc oxide 300 g; part b: zinc sulphate 150 g, boric acid 1 g and distilled water 120 ml; mix parts a. and b. to a paste consistency). If the crown is restored temporarily, seal the cavity with zinc oxide-eugenol cement.
(6) Follow-up: clinical and radiographic controls after 6 months, 1 year and annually for at least 3 years.

*Prognosis*: pulp healing in 94–96%.

## Cervical pulpotomy (Fig. 22.17)

Indicated for immature teeth when necrotic tissue or obviously impaired vascularity is seen at the exposure site.

(1) Administer local anesthesia.
(2) Isolate with a rubber dam and wash with a mild disinfectant.
(3) Amputate the pulp to a level at which fresh bleeding is encountered, usually in the cervical region. Due to problems of inadequate cooling of a diamond bur run at high speed, a round bur at low speed should be used.
(4) Await hemostasis.
(5) Cover the pulp with calcium hydroxide and seal the coronal cavity. If the crown is restored immediately with a composite resin, seal the cavity with Prader's sulphate cement, otherwise with zinc oxide-eugenol cement.
(6) Follow-up: clinical and radiographic controls after 6 months, 1 year and annually to completion of root development. Consider then eventual further endodontic or prosthetic treatment.

*Prognosis*: pulp healing in 72–79%.

## Pulpectomy

Indicated in mature teeth when necrotic tissue or impaired pulp vascularity is seen at the exposure site, or when extensive loss of crown substance indicates restoration with a post in the root canal.

(1) Administer local anesthesia.
(2) Isolate with a rubber dam and wash with a mild disinfectant.
(3) Amputate the pulp 1–2 mm from the apical foramen.
(4) Clean the root canal mechanically while constantly flushing with saline or 0.5% sodium hypochlorite solution.
(5) Obturate the root canal with gutta-percha, using resin-chloroform, chloropercha or another sealer.
(6) Follow-up: clinical and radiographic controls after 6 months, 1 year and annually for a minimum of 4 years.

*Prognosis*: periapical healing in 90%.

## Root fractured teeth

Root canal treatment of coronal fragment is performed when the pulp in the apical fragment is vital.

(1) When the anatomy of the root canal permits adequate obturation, i.e. a narrow or tapering root canal, it may be treated and filled conventionally with gutta-percha and a sealer.
(2) When the root canal and/or the space between the fragments are wide, the initial treatment is with calcium hydroxide in order to induce formation of a hard tissue barrier at the fracture site of coronal fragment before filling with gutta-percha. (For more specific procedures, see treatment of non-vital immature teeth.)

Root canal treatment of both fragments is performed when the pulp is necrotic in both fragments and the space between the fragments is narrow.

Root canal treatment of coronal fragment and surgical removal of apical fragment is performed when the root canal in a non-vital apical fragment is not accessible for treatment.

*Prognosis*:

- Filling with gutta-percha of both fragments: no healing
- Filling of only coronal fragment with gutta-percha: healing in 76%
- Filling of coronal fragment with gutta-percha and removal of apical fragment, healing in 68%
- Treatment of coronal fragment with calcium hydroxide and following filling with gutta-percha: healing in 86%.

## Luxated or replanted teeth with pulp necrosis

### Immature permanent teeth (Fig. 22.47)

(1) Isolate with a rubber dam and wash with a disinfectant.
(2) Establish access to the root canal.
(3) Remove necrotic pulp with a barbed broach; clean the walls of the root canal using large files and a copious flow of 0.5% sodium hypochlorite solution.
(4) Fill the root canal with calcium hydroxide using a lentulo spiral or a syringe with a special cannula. Seal the coronal cavity with zinc oxide-eugenol cement.
(5) In cases of acute periapical osteitis and swelling, treat the root canal with, e.g., 2% potassium iodine; eventually administer antibiotics for 7 days before filling with calcium hydroxide.
(6) Control radiographically at 3- to 6-month intervals. If radiographic signs of healing are not present, the root canal should be retreated and refilled with calcium hydroxide. Furthermore, when the level of calcium hydroxide in the root canal retracts to the cervical part of the canal, it should be refilled with calcium hydroxide.
(7) Permanent filling with gutta-percha is completed when follow-up examination shows periradicular healing, including arrested inflammatory root resorption, and an apical hard-tissue barrier which clinically is found to be continuous.
(8) Choose the thickest gutta-percha point that can easily fit to the apical barrier.
(9) Warm the tip of the gutta-percha point by passing it once through an alcohol flame; introduce it immediately into the root canal and press it steadily but not too hard against the apical barrier (Fig. 22.52).
(10) Verify the position with a control radiograph.
(11) Fill the root canal completely with additional gutta-percha points using lateral condensation.
(12) Follow-up: clinical and radiographic controls after 6 months, 1 year and annually for at least 4 years.

*Prognosis*: periapical healing and formation of an apical hard tissue barrier in 75–96%.

## *Mature permanent teeth*

(1) Isolate with a rubber dam and wash with a disinfectant.
(2) Establish access to the root canal.
(3) Remove necrotic pulp with a barbed broach and clean the canal mechanically with files and a copious flow of 0.5% sodium hypochlorite solution.
(4) After antibacterial treatment, e.g. with 2 % potassium iodide, fill the root canal with gutta-percha, using resin-chloroform or a sealer. If periapical healing is desired before filling with gutta-percha, or if inflammatory root resorption is present, the tooth should be treated initially with calcium hydroxide. Permanent filling with gutta-percha is carried out when follow-up examination shows periradicular healing and arrest of the inflammatory processes.
(5) Follow-up: clinical and radiographic controls after 6 months, 1 year and annually for at least 4 years.

*Prognosis*: periapical healing in 79–95%.

## Late external cervical root resorption

According to location and esthetic demands, one of the following treatment procedures can be chosen:

• Gingivectomy and removal of soft tissue from the resorption cavity followed by insertion of a dentin-bonded composite resin or glass ionomer cement.
• A gingival flap is raised, a dentin bonded composite placed in the resorption cavity, and the flap replaced (Fig. 22.67).
• The tooth is surgically or orthodontically extruded, thereafter the resorption defect is cleaned and repaired e.g. with dentin-bonded composite restoration.

*Prognosis*: not known.

## Internal resorption

Teeth with progressive internal root resorption are treated according to common endodontic principles. In case of a large resorption area, and in order to remove inflamed tissue in the lesion, the following procedure can be employed (Fig. 22.68).

(1) Clean the root canal mechanically, flush constantly with sodium hypochlorite and fill with calcium hydroxide.
(2) Flush the canal with sodium hypochlorite and re-fill with calcium hydroxide at 2- to 3-week intervals until all pulp tissue in the lesion has been dissolved, i.e. when calcium hydroxide is radiographically seen to fill the entire resorption cavity.
(3) Obturate the canal with gutta-percha and lateral condensation.

*Prognosis*: not known.

## Pulp canal obliteration with subsequent pulp necrosis

Endodontic treatment is performed in teeth in which a periapical radiolucency has developed.

(1) Isolate with a rubber dam and wash with a disinfectant.
(2) Establish access through the crown to the cervical part of the root.
(3) Search for the canal with the finest file.
(4) If the canal is not found, prepare the cavity a step deeper and continue the search.
(5) Clean the disclosed canal without unnecessary pressure, using the thinnest file until the apex is reached (Fig. 22.78). Do not use solutions capable of dissolving dentin.
(6) Enlarge the root canal mechanically.
(7) Fill the root canal with gutta-percha and a sealer.
(8) Follow-up: clinical and radiographic controls after 6 months, 1 year and annually for at least 4 years.

*Prognosis*: periapical healing in 80%.

## Crown malformation with pulp necrosis

• To prevent infection of the pulp through hypomineralized parts of the dentin, the tooth should be restored as soon as possible.
• Non-vital teeth are treated by conventional endodontic therapy.

## References

1. STEWART JK. The immediate response of odontoblasts to injury. *Odont T* 1965;**73**:417–23.
2. GARBEROGLIO R, BRÄNNSTRÖM M. Scanning electron microscopic investigation of human dentinal tubules. *Arch Oral Biol* 1976;**21**:355–62.
3. OLGART L, BRÄNNSTROM M, JOHNSSON G. Invasion of bacteria into dentinal tubules. Experiments in vivo and in vitro. *Acta Odontol Scand* 1974;**32**:61–70.
4. BRÄNNSTRÖM M. Observations on exposed dentine and corresponding pulp tissue. A preliminary study with replica and routine histology. *Odont Revy* 1952;**13**: 253–45.
5. DARLING AI. Response of pulpodentinal complex to injury. In: Gorlin RJ, Goldman H. eds. *Thoma's oral pathology*. 6th edn. St. Louis: CV Mosby Co, 1970:308–34.
6. MJÖR IA, TRONSTAD L. The healing of experimentally induced pulpitis. *Oral Surg Oral Med Oral Pathol* 1974;**38**:115–21.
7. BERGENHOLTZ G, REIT C. Pulp reactions on microbial provocation of calcium hydroxide treated dentin. *Scand J Dent Res* 1980;**88**:187–92.
8. KAKEHASHI S, STANLEY HR, FITZGERALD RJ. The effect of surgical exposures on dental pulps in germ-free and conventional laboratory rats. *Oral Surg Oral Med Oral Pathol* 1965;**20**:340–9.
9. SHEININ A, POHTO M, LUOSTARINEN V. Defense reactions of the pulp with special reference to circulation. An experimental study in rats. *Int Dent J* 1967;**17**:461–75.
10. LUOSTARINEN V, POHTO M, SHEININ A. Dynamics of repair in the pulp. *J Dent Res* 1966;**45**:519–25.

11. Cvek M. A clinical report on partial pulpotomy and capping with calcium hydroxide in permanent incisors with complicated crown fracture. *J Endod* 1978;**4**:232–7.

12. Smukler H, Tagger N. Vital root amputation. A clinical and histologic study. *J Periodontol* 1976;**47**:324–30.

13. Cvek M, Cleaton-Jones P, Austin J, Andreasen JO. Pulp reactions to exposure after experimental crown fractures or grinding in adult monkeys. *J Endod* 1982;**8**:391–7.

14. Heide S, Mjör IA. Pulp reactions to experimental exposures in young permanent monkey teeth. *Int Endod J* 1983;**16**:11–19.

15. Fusayama T, Maeda T. Effect of pulpectomy on dentin hardness. *J Dent Res* 1969;**48**:452–60.

16. Trabert KC, Caput AA, Abou-Rass M. Tooth fracture – a comparison of endodontic and restorative treatments. *J Endod* 1978;**4**:341–5.

17. Andreasen JO. Luxation of permanent teeth due to trauma. A clinical and radiographic follow-up of 189 injured teeth. *Scand Dent Res* 1970;**78**:273–86.

18. Eklund G, Stålhane I, Hedegård B. A study of traumatized permanent teeth in children aged 7–15. Part III. A multivariate analysis of post-traumatic complications of subluxated and luxated teeth. *Svensk Tandläk T* 1976;**69**:179–89.

19. Masterton JB. The healing of wounds of the dental pulp of man. A clinical and histological study. *Br Dent J* 1966;**120**:213–24.

20. Weiss M. Pulp capping in older patients. *NY State Dent J* 1966;**32**:451–7.

21. Haskell EW, Stanley HR, Chellemi J, Stringfellow H. Direct pulp capping treatment: a long-term follow-up. *J Am Dent Assoc* 1978;**97**:607–12.

22. Heyduck G, Wegner H. Klinische, röntgenologische and histologische Ergebnisse nach Vitalbehandlung der freigelegten Pulpa. *Stomat DDR* 1978;**28**:614–19.

23. Seltzer S, Bender IB. *The dental pulp*. 2nd edn. Philadelphia: JB Lippincott Co, 1975:356.

24. Bernick S, Adelman C. Effect of aging on the human pulp. *J Endod* 1975;**1**:88–94.

25. Stanley HR. Management of the aging patient and the aging pulp. *J Calif Dent Assoc* 1978;**57**:25–8.

26. Toto PD, Staffileno H, Weine FS, Das S. Age change effects on the pulp in periodontitis. *Ann Dent* 1977;**36**:13–20.

27. Krakow AA, Berk H, Grön P. Therapeutic induction of root formation in the exposed incompletely formed tooth with a vital pulp. *Oral Surg Oral Med Oral Pathol* 1977;**43**:755–65.

28. Berg C, Mårtensson K. Pulpabehandling av mjölktænder. En efterundersökning av pulpaamputationer och överkappningar. *Odont Revy* 1965;**6**:135–62.

29. Patterson SS. Pulp calcification due to operative procedures – pulpotomy. *Int Dent J* 1967;**17**:490–505.

30. Masterton JB. The healing of wounds of the dental pulp. An investigation of the nature of the scar tissue and of the phenomena leading to its formation. *Dent Pract* 1966;**16**:325–39.

31. Granath L-E, Hagman G. Experimental pulpotomy in human bicuspids with reference to cutting technique. *Acta Odontol Scand* 1971;**29**:155–63.

32. Zander HA. Reaction of the pulp to calcium hydroxide. *J Dent Res* 1939;**18**:373–9.

33. Glass RL, Zander HA. Pulp healing. *J Dent Res* 1949;**28**:97–107.

34. Mejare I, Hasselgren G, Hammarström LE. Effect of formaldehyde-containing drugs on human dental pulp evaluated by enzyme histochemical technique. *Scand J Dent Res* 1976;**84**:29–36.

35. Schröder U, Granath L-E. Early reaction of intact human teeth to calcium hydroxide following experimental pulpotomy and its significance to the development of hard-tissue barrier. *Odont Revy* 1971;**22**:379–96.

36. Schröder U. Reaction of human dental pulp to experimental pulpotomy and capping with calcium hydroxide. *Odont Revy* 1973;**24**:*(Suppl 25)*:1–97.

37. Stanley HR, Lundi T. Dycal therapy for pulp exposures. *Oral Surg Oral Med Oral Pathol* 1972;**34**:818–27.

38. Tronstad L, Mjör IA. Capping of the inflamed pulp. *Oral Surg Oral Med Oral Pathol* 1972;**34**:477–85.

39. Brännström M, Nyborg H, Strömberg T. Experiments with pulp capping. *Oral Surg Oral Med Oral Pathol* 1979;**48**:347–52.

40. Schröder U. Effect of extra-pulpal blood clot on healing following experimental pulpotomy and capping with calcium hydroxide. *Odont Revy* 1973;**24**:257–68.

41. Cabrini RI, Maisto OA, Manfredi EE. Internal resorption of dentine. Histopathologic control of eight cases after pulp amputation and capping with calcium hydroxide. *Oral Surg Oral Med Oral Pathol* 1957;**10**:90–6.

42. James VE, Englander HR, Massler M. Histologic response of amputated pulps to calcium compounds and antibiotics. *Oral Surg Oral Med Oral Pathol* 1957;**10**:975–86.

43. Masterton JB. Internal resorption of dentine. A complication arising from unhealed pulp wounds. *Br Dent J* 1965;**118**:241–9.

44. Schröder U, Granath L-E. On internal dentin resorption in deciduous molars treated by pulpotomy and capped with calcium hydroxide. *Odont Revy* 1971;**22**:179–88.

45. Malone AJ, Massler M. Fractured anterior teeth – diagnosis, treatment and prognosis. *Dent Dig* 1952;**58**:442–7.

46. Nygaard-Östby B. Uber die Gewebsveränderungen im apikalen Paradentium des Menschen and verschidenartigen Eingriffen in den Wurzelkanälen. *Det Norske Videnskaps Akademi Oslo*, 1939 no.4.

47. Kuttler Y. Analysis and comparison of root canal filling techniques. *Oral Surg Oral Med Oral Pathol* 1967;**48**:153–9.

48. Engström B, Spångberg L. Wound healing after partial pulpectomy. A histologic study performed on contralateral tooth pairs. *Odont T* 1967;**75**:5–18.

49. Holland R, de Mello MJ, Nery MJ, Bernabe PFE, de Souza V. Reaction of human periapical tissues to pulp

extirpation and immediate root canal filling with calcium hydroxide. *J Endod* 1977;**3**:63–7.

50. Nyborg H. Pulpaöverkappning och vitalamputation in permanenta tänder. In: Holst JJ, Nygaard Östby O, Osvald O. eds. Copenhagen: Nordisk Kinisk Odontologi, A/S Forlaget for Faglitteratur, Copenhagen, 1965 (Chapters 10–11):1–18.

51. Kozlowska I. Pokrycie bezposrednie miazgi preparatem krajowej produkcji. *Czas Stomat* 1960;**13**:375–88.

52. Ravn JJ. Follow-up study of permanent incisors with complicated crown fractures after acute trauma. *Scand J Dent Res* 1982;**90**:363–72.

53. Hallet GE, Porteous JR. Fractured incisors treated by vital pulpotomy. A report on 100 consecutive cases. *Br Dent J* 1963;**115**:279–87.

54. Strinberg L-Z. The dependence of the results of pulp therapy on certain factors. An analytic study based on radiographic and clinical follow-up examinations. *Acta Odont Scand* 1956;**14**: (Suppl 21).

55. Grossman LI, Sheppard LI, Pearson LA. Roentgenologic and clinical evaluation of endodontically treated teeth. *Oral Surg Oral Med Oral Pathol* 1964;**17**:368–74.

56. Adenubi JO, Rule DC. Success rate for root fillings in young patients. A retrospective analysis of treated cases. *Br Dent J* 1976;**141**:237–41.

57. Grahnén H, Hansson L. The prognosis of pulp and root canal therapy. A clinical and radiographic follow-up examination. *Odont Revy* 1961;**12**:146–65.

58. Andreasen JO, Hjörting-Hansen E. Intraalveolar root fractures: radiographic and histologic study of 50 cases. *J Oral Surg* 1967;**25**:414–26.

59. Lindahl B. Transverse intra-alveolar root fractures: Roentgen diagnosis and prognosis. *Odont Revy* 1963;**9**:10–24.

60. Andreasen JO. Relationship between surface and inflammatory root resorption and pathologic changes in the pulp after replantation of mature incisors in monkeys. *J Endod* 1981;**7**:194–301.

61. Michanowicz AE. Root fractures. A report of radiographic healing after endodontic treatment. *Oral Surg Oral Med Oral Pathol* 1963;**16**:1242–8.

62. Feldman G, Solomon G, Notaro PJ. Endodontic treatment of traumatized tooth. *Oral Surg Oral Med Oral Pathol* 1966;**21**:100–12.

63. Michanowicz AE, Michanowicz JP, Abou-Rass M. Cementogenic repair of root fractures. *J Am Dent Assoc* 1971;**82**:569–79.

64. Andreasen JO. Treatment of fractured and avulsed teeth. *ASDC J Dent Child* 1971;**38**:29–48.

65. Cvek M. Treatment of non-vital permanent incisors with calcium hydroxide. IV. Periodontal healing and closure of the root canal in the coronal fragment of teeth with intra-alveolar fracture and vital apical fragment. *Odont Revy* 1974;**25**:239–45.

66. Ravn JJ. En klinisk og radiologisk undersøgelse of 55 rodfrakturer i unge permanente incisiver. *Tandlægebladet* 1976;**80**:391–6.

67. Arwill T. Histopathologic studies of traumatized teeth. *Odont T* 1962;**70**:91–117.

68. Arwill T, Henschen B, Sundwall-Hagland I. The pulpal reaction in traumatized permanent incisors in children aged 9–18. *Odont T* 1967;**75**: 130–47.

69. Stanley HR, Weismann MI, Michanowicz AE, Bellizzi R. Ischemic infarction of the pulp: sequential degenerative changes of the pulp after traumatic injury. *J Endod* 1978;**4**:325–35.

70. Hasselgren G, Larsson A, Rundquist L. Pulpal status after autogenuous transplantation of fully developed maxillary canines. *Oral Surg Oral Med Oral Pathol* 1977;**44**:106–12.

71. Makkes PCH, Thoden van Velzen SK, van den Hooff A. Response of the living organism to dead and fixed dead, enclosed isologous tissue. *Oral Surg Oral Med Oral Pathol* 1978;**46**:131–44.

72. Grossman LI. Origin of micro-organisms in traumatized, pulpless, sound teeth. *J Dent Res* 1967;**46**:551–3.

73. Bergenholtz G. Micro-organisms from necrotic pulps of traumatized teeth. *Odont Revy* 1974;**25**:347–58.

74. Sundqvist G. *Bacteriological studies of necrotic dental pulps.* Umeå: Umeå University Odontological Dissertations, No 7, 1976:1–94.

75. Ravn JJ, Helbo M. Replantation of akcidentelt exartikulerede tinder. *Tandlægebladet* 1966;**70**: 805–15.

76. Frank AL. Therapy for the divergent pulpless formation. *J Am Dent Assoc* 1966;**72**:87–93.

77. Rule DC, Winter GB. Root growth and apical repair subsequent to pulpal necrosis in children. *Br Dent J* 1966;**120**:586–90.

78. Heithersay GS. Stimulation of root formation in incompletely developed pulpless teeth. *Oral Surg Oral Med Oral Pathol* 1970;**29**:620–30.

79. McDonald RE, Avery DR. *Dentistry for the child and adolescent.* 3rd edn. St. Louis: CV Mosby Co, 1978: 640.

80. Hotz R. Die Bedeutung, Beurteilung and Behandlung beim Trauma in Frontzahngebiet vom Standpunkt des Kieferorthopäden. *Dtsch Zahnärtzl Z* 1958;**13**:42–51.

81. Schröder U, Wennberg E, Granath L-E, Möller H. Traumatized primary incisors follow-up program based on frequency of periapical osteitis related to tooth color. *Swed Dent J* 1977;**1**:95–8.

82. Seltzer S, Bender IB, Zionz M. The dynamics of pulp inflammation: correlations between diagnostic data and actual histologic findings in the pulp. *Oral Surg Oral Med Oral Pathol* 1963;**16**:846–71.

83. Mumford JM. Pain reception threshold in stimulating human teeth and histologic condition of the pulp. *Br Dent J* 1967;**123**:427–33.

84. Stenberg S. Vitalitetsprövning med elektrisk ström av incisiver i olika genombrottsstadier. *Svensk Tandläkare Tidskrift* 1950;**43**:83–6.

85. Skieller V. The prognosis of young loosened teeth after mechanical injuries. *Acta Odont Scand* 1960;**18**:181–8.

86. Magnusson B, Holm A-K. Traumatized permanent teeth in children – a follow-up. I. Pulpal complications and root resorption. *Svensk Tandläkare Tidskrift* 1969;**62**:61–70.

87. Öhman A. Healing and sensitivity to pain in young replanted teeth. An experimental, clinical and histological study. *Odont T* 1965;**73**:165–228.

88. Jacobsen I, Kerekes K. Long-term prognosis of traumatized permanent anterior teeth showing calcifying processes in the pulp cavity. *Scand J Dent Res* 1977;**85**:588–98.

89. Rohner A. Calxyl als Wurzelfüllungsmaterial nach Pulpaextirpation. *Schweiz Monatschr Zahnheil* 1940;**50**:903–48.

90. Heithersay GS. Calcium hydroxide in the treatment of pulpless teeth with associated pathology. *J Br Endod Soc* 1962;**8**:74–93.

91. Martin DM, Crabb HSM. Calcium hydroxide in root canal therapy. A review. *Br Dent J* 1977;**142**:277–83.

92. Herforth A, Strassburg M. Zur Therapie der chronisch apikalen Paradontitis bei traumatisch beschädigten Frontzähnen mit nicht abgeschlossenen Wurzelwachstum. *Dtsch Zahnärtzl Z* 1977;**32**:453–9.

93. Cvek M. Treatment of non-vital permanent incisors with calcium hydroxide. I. Follow-up of periapical repair and apical closure of immature roots. *Odont Revy* 1972;**23**:27–44.

94. Kerekes K, Heide S, Jacobsen I. Follow-up examination of endodontic treatment in traumatized juvenile incisors. *J Endod* 1980;**6**:744–8.

95. Cvek M, Sundström B. Treatment of non-vital permanent incisors with calcium hydroxide. V. Histologic appearance of roentgenologically demonstrable apical closure of immature roots. *Odont Revy* 1974;**25**:379–92.

96. Heide S, Kerekes K. Endodontisk behandling av rotöpne permanente incisiver. En histologisk undersökelse over hårdvevsdannelse etter rotfylling med kalsiumhydroxid. *Norske Tandlägeforen Tid* 1977;**87**:426–30.

97. Holland R, de Souza V, Tagliavini RT, Milanezi LA. Healing processes of teeth with open apices: histologic study. *Bull Tokyo Dent Coll* 1971;**12**:333–8.

98. Dylewski JJ. Apical closure of non-vital teeth. *Oral Surg Oral Med Oral Pathol* 1971;**32**:82–9.

99. Steiner JC, van Hassel HJ. Experimental root apexification in primates. *Oral Surg Oral Med Oral Pathol* 1971;**31**:409–15.

100. Ham JW, Patterson SS, Mitchell DF. Induced apical closure of immature pulpless teeth in monkeys. *Oral Surg Oral Med Oral Pathol* 1972;**33**:438–49.

101. Holland R, de Souza V, de Campos Russo M. Healing processes after root canal therapy in immature human teeth. *Rev Fac Odont Aracatuba* 1973;**2**:269–79.

102. Binnie WH, Rowe AHR. A histological study of the periapical tissues of incompletely formed pulpless teeth filled with calcium hydroxide. *J Dent Res* 1973;**52**:1110–16.

103. Castagnola L. *Die Lebenderhaltung der Pulpa in der konservierenden Zahnheilkunde.* Munchen: Carl Hanser Verlag, 1953:1–127.

104. Matsumiya S, Kitamura K. Histopathological and histobacteriological studies of the relation between the condition of sterilisation of the interior of the root canal and the healing process of periapical tissues in experimentally infected root canal treatment. *Bull Tokyo Dent Coll* 1960;**1**:1–19.

105. Cvek M, Hollender L, Nord C-E. Treatment of non-vital permanent incisors with calcium hydroxide. VI. A clinical, microbiological and radiological evaluation of treatment on one sitting of teeth with mature and immature roots. *Odont Revy* 1976;**27**:93–108.

106. Vernieks AA, Masser LB. Calcium hydroxide induced healing of periapical lesions. A study of 78 non-vital teeth. *J Br Endod Soc* 1978;**11**:61–9.

107. Frank AL, Weine FS. Non-surgical therapy for the perforative defect of internal resorption. *J Am Dent Assoc* 1973;**87**:863–8.

108. Stewart GG. Calcium hydroxide-induced root healing. *J Am Dent Assoc* 1975;**90**:793–800.

109. Lambjerg-Hansen L, Levin A. Kofferdam. *Tandlægebladet* 1967;**81**:714–16.

110. Friend A. The treatment of immature teeth with non-vital pulps. *J Br Endod Soc* 1967;**1**:28–33.

111. Torneck CD, Smith JS, Grindahl P. Biologic effects of endodontic procedures on developing incisor teeth. III. Effect of debridement and disinfection procedures in treatment of experimentally induced pulp and periapical disease. *Oral Surg Oral Med Oral Pathol* 1973;**35**:532–40.

112. Torneck CD, Smith JS, Grindahl P. Biologic effects of endodontic procedures on developing incisors teeth. II. Effect of pulp injury and oral contamination. *Oral Surg Oral Med Oral Pathol* 1973;**35**:378–88.

113. Cvek M, Nord C-E, Hollender L. Antimicrobial effect of root canal debridement in teeth with immature root. *Odont Revy* 1976;**27**:1–10.

114. Spångberg L, Rutberg M, Rydinge E. Biologic effects of endodontic antimicrobial agents. *J Endod* 1979;**5**:166–75.

115. Holland R, Nery MJ, de Mello W, de Souza V, Bernabé PFE, Otoboni Filho JA. Root canal treatment with calcium hydroxide. I. Effect of overfilling and refilling. *Oral Surg Oral Med Oral Pathol* 1979;**47**:87–92.

116. Holland R, Nery MJ, de Mello W, de Souza V, Bernabé PFE, Otoboni Filho JA. Root canal treatment with calcium hydroxide. III. Effect of debris and pressure filling. *Oral Surg Oral Med Oral Pathol* 1979;**47**:185–8.

117. Torneck CD, Smith JS, Grindahl P. Biologic effects of endodontic procedures in developing incisor teeth. IV. Effect of parachlorophenol paste in the treatment of experimentally induced pulp and periapical disease. *Oral Surg Oral Med Oral Pathol* 1973;**35**:541–4.

118. Simpson TH, Natkin E. Guttapercha techniques for filling canals of young permanent teeth after induction of apical root formation. *J Br Endod Soc* 1972;**5**:35–9.

119. Andreasen JO, Hjörting-Hansen E. Replantation of teeth. II. Histological study of 22 replanted anterior teeth in humans. *Acta Odont Scand* 1966;**24**:287–306.

120. Cvek M. Treatment on non-vital permanent incisors with calcium hydroxide. II. Effect on external root resorption in luxated teeth compared with effect of root filling with gutta percha. *Odont Revy* 1973;**24**:343–54.

121. Lustman J, Ehrlich J. Deep external resorption: treatment by combined endodontic and surgical approach. A report of 2 cases. *Int Dent J* 1974;**2**:203–6.

122. Stålhane I. Permanenta tänder med reducerat pulpalumen som följd av olycksfallsskada. *Svensk Tandläkare Tidskrift* 1971;**64**:311–16.

123. Patterson SS, Mitchell DF. Calcific metamorphosis of the dental pulp. *Oral Surg Oral Med Oral Pathol* 1965;**20**:94–101.

124. Fischer C-H. Hard tissue formation of the pulp in relation to treatment of traumatic injuries. *Int Dent J* 1974;**24**:387–96.

125. Holcomb JB, Gregory WB Jr. Calcific metamorphosis of the pulp: its incidence and treatment. *Oral Surg Oral Med Oral Pathol* 1967;**24**:825–30.

126. Lundberg M, Cvek M. A light microscopy study of pulps from traumatized permanent incisors with reduced pulpal lumen. *Acta Odont Scand* 1980;**38**:89–94.

127. Cvek M, Granath L-E, Lundberg M. Failures and healing in endodontically treated non-vital anterior teeth with posttraumatically reduced pulpal lumen. *Acta Odont Scand* 1982;**40**:223–8.

128. Hasselgren G, Strömberg T. The use of iodine as a contrast medium in endodontic therapy. *Oral Surg Oral Med Oral Pathol* 1976;**41**:785–8.

129. Castaldi CR. Traumatic injury to unerupted incisors following a blow to the primary teeth. *J Can Dent Assoc* 1959;**25**:752–62.

130. Cutright DE. The reaction of permanent tooth buds to injury. *Oral Surg Oral Med Oral Pathol* 1971;**32**:832–9.

131. Andreasen JO, Sundström B, Ravn JJ. The effect of traumatic injuries to primary teeth on their permanent successors. I. A clinical and histologic study of 117 injured permanent teeth. *Acta Odont Scand* 1971;**79**:219–83.

132. van Gool AV. Injury to the permanent tooth germ after trauma to the deciduous predecessor. *Oral Surg Oral Med Oral Pathol* 1973;**35**:2–12.

133. Szpringer M. Pourazowe znieksztalcenie przednich zebów stalych i zwiazane z tym trudnosci leczmeze. *Czas Stomat* 1973;**26**:855–60.

134. Warfvinge J, Bergenholtz G. Healing capacity of human and monkey dental pulps following experimentally induced pulpitis. *Endod Dent Traumatol* 1986;**2**:256–62.

135. Bergenholtz G. Relationship between bacterial contamination of dentin and restorative success. In: Rowe NH. ed. *Proceedings of symposium: Dental pulp – reactions of restorative materials in presence or absence of infection.* Michigan: University of Michigan, School of Dentistry, 1982.

136. Setcos JC. Dentin bonding in perpective. *Am J Dent* 1988;**6**:*(Spec Issue)*:173–5.

137. Rees JS, Jacobsen PH, Koiiniotou-Kubia E. The current status of composite materials and adhesive systems. Part 4. Some clinically related research. *Rest Dent* 1990;**6**:4–8.

138. Hörsted-Bindslev P. Monkey pulp reactions to cavities treated with Gluma dentin and restored with a microfilled composite. *Scand J Dent Res* 1987;**95**:347–55.

139. Cox CG, Felton D, Bergenholtz G. Histopathological response of infected cavities treated with Gluma and Scotchbond dentine bonding agents. *Am J Dent* 1988;**6**:*(Spec Issue)*:189–94.

140. Andreasen JO. Periodontal healing after replantation of traumatically avulsed human teeth. Assessment by mobility testing and radiography. *Acta Odontol Scand* 1975;**33**:325–35.

141. Stanley HR, Bowen RL, Cobb EN. Pulp responses to a dentin and enamel adhesive bonding procedures. *Oper Dent* 1988;**13**:107–13.

142. Chohayeb AA, Bowen RL, Adrian J. Pulpal response to a dentin and enamel bonding system. *Dent Mater* 1988;**4**:144–6.

143. Franquin C, Brouillet JL. Biocompatibility of an enamel and dentin adhesive under different conditions of applications. *Quintessenz Int* 1988;**19**:813–26.

144. Felton D, Bergenholtz G, Cox C. Inhibition of bacterial growth under composite restorations following Gluma pretreatment. *J Dent Res* 1989;**68**:1–5.

145. Virgillito A, Holz J. Produits adhésifs dentinaires et de scellement soumis au contrôle biologique in vivo. *J Biol Buccale* 1989;**17**:209–24.

146. Bowen RL, Ropp NW, Eichmiller FC, Stanley HR. Clinical biocompatibility of an experimental dentine-enamel adhesive for composites. *Int Dent J* 1989;**39**:247–52.

147. Blosser RL, Rupp NW, Stanley HR, Bowen RL. Pulpal and micro-organisms response to two experimental dental bonding systems. *Dent Mat* 1989;**5**:140–4.

148. Lundin S-A, Norén JG, Warfvinge J. Marginal bacterial leakage and pulp reactions in Class II composite resin restorations in vivo. *Swed Dent J* 1990;**14**:185–92.

149. Grieve AR, Alani A, Saunders WP. The effects on the dental pulp of a composite resin and two dentin bonding agents and associated bacterial microleakage. *Int Endod J* 1991;**24**:108–18.

150. Elbaum R, Pignoli C, Brouillet J. A histologic study of the biocompatiliblity of a dentinal bonding system. *Quintessenz Int* 1991;**22**:901–10.

151. Warfvinge J, Rozell B, Hedström K-G. Effect of calcium hydroxide treated dentin on pulpal responses. *Int Endod J* 1987;**20**:183–93.

152. Pashley DH, Kaiathor S, Burham D. The effects of calcium hydroxide dentin permeability. *J Dent Res* 1986;**65**:417–20.

153. Mejare B, Mejare I, Edwardsson S. Acid etching and composite resin restorations. A culturing and histologic study on bacterial penetration. *Endod Dent Traumatol* 1987;**3**:1–5.

154. Andreasen FM, Noren JG, Andreasen JO, Englehardtsen S, Lindh-Strömberg U. Long-term survival of fragment bonding in the treatment of fractured crowns: a multicenter clinical study. *Quintess Int* 1995;**26**:669–81.

155. Robertson A, Andreasen FM, Andreasen JO, Noren JG. Long-term prognosis of crown fractured permanent incisors: the effect of stage of root development and associated luxation injury. *Int J Paediatr Dent* 2000;**10**:191–9.

156. Cvek M. Results after partial pulpotomy in crown fractured teeth 3–15 years after treatment. *Acta Stomatol Croat* 1993;**27**:167–73.

157. Cox CF, Bergenholtz G, Fitzgerald M, Heys DR, Avery JK, Baker JA. Capping of the dental pulp mechanically exposed to the oral microflora – a 5 week observation of wound healing in monkey. *J Oral Pathol* 1982;**11**:327–39

158. Hermann BW: *Biologische Wurzelbehandlung*. Frankfurt am Main: von Kramer Co, 1936:272.

159. Foreman PC, Barnes IE. A review of calcium hydroxide. *Int Endod J* 1990;**23**:83–97.

160. Cvek M, Granath L, Cleaton-Jones P, Austin J. Hard tissue barrier formation in pulpotomized monkey teeth capped with cyanoacrylate or calcium hydroxide for 10 and 60 minutes. *J Dent Res* 1987;**66**:1166–74.

161. Granath L. Pulp capping materials. In: Smith DC, Williams DF. eds. *Biocompatibility of dental materials*, Vol. II. Boca Raton, FL: CRC Press Inc., 1982:253–67.

162. Cox CF, Keall HJ, Ostro E, Bergenholtz G. Biocompatibility of surface-sealed dental materials against exposed pulps. *Prosthet Dent* 1987;**57**:1–8.

163. Heys DR, Fitzgerald RJ, Heys RJ, Chiego DJ. Healing of primate dental pulps capped with Teflon. *Oral Surg Oral Med Oral Pathol* 1990;**69**:227–37.

164. Gordon TM, Randly DM, Boyan BD. The effects of calcium hydroxide on bovine pulp tissue: Variations in pH and calcium concentration. *J Endod* 1985;**11**:156–60.

165. Tronstad L. Reaction of the exposed pulp to Dycal treatment. *Oral Surg Oral Med Oral Pathol* 1974;**34**:477–85.

166. Heys DR, Heys RJ, Cox CF, Avery JK. The response of four calcium hydroxides on monkey pulp. *J Oral Pathol* 1989;**9**:372–9.

167. Cox CF, Bergenholtz G, Heys DR, Syed SA, Fitzgerald M, Heys RJ. Pulp capping of dental pulp mechanically exposed to oral microflora: a 1–2 year observation of wound healing in the monkey. *J Oral Pathol* 1985;**14**:156–68.

168. Schröder U. Effects of calcium hydroxide-containing pulp capping agents on pulp cell migration, proliferation and differentiation. *J Dent Res* 1985;**64**:(*Spec issue*):541–8.

169. Seltzer S, Bender IB. *The dental pulp. Biologic considerations in dental procedures*. 3rd edn. Philadelphia: JB Lippincott Co, 1984:356.

170. Berkman D, Cucolo FA, Levin MP, Brunelle LJ. Pulpal response to isobutyl cyanoacrylate in human teeth. *J Am Dent Assoc* 1971;**83**:140–5.

171. Heys DR, Cox CF, Heys RJ, Avery JK. Histological considerations of direct pulp capping agents. *J Dent Res* 1981;**60**:1371–9.

172. Heller AL, Koenings JF, Brilliant JD, Melfi RC, Dribkell TD. Direct pulp capping of permanent teeth in primates using resorbable form of tricalcium phosphate ceramics. *J Endod* 1975;**1**:95–101.

173. Fuks A, Chosak A, Klein H, Eidelman E. Partial pulpotomy as a treatment alternative for exposed pulps in crown fractured permanent incisors. *Endod Dent Traumatol* 1987;**3**:100–2.

174. Cvek M, Lundberg M. Histological appearance of pulps after exposure by a crown fracture, partial pulpotomy and clinical diagnosis of healing. *J Endod* 1983;**9**:8–11.

175. Mesic-Par N, Pecina-Hrncevic A, Stipetic S. Clinical and histological examination of young permanent teeth after vital amputation of the pulp. *Acta Stomatol Croat* 1990;**24**:253–62.

176. Heide S, Kerekes K. Delayed direct pulp capping in permanent incisors of monkeys. *Int Endod J* 1987;**20**:65–74.

177. Pitt Ford TR, Roberts GJ. Immediate and delayed direct pulp capping with the use of a new visible light-cured calcium hydroxide preparation. *Oral Surg Oral Med Oral Pathol* 1991;**71**:388–42.

178. Bergenholtz G, Cox CF, Loeshe WJ, Syed SA. Bacterial leakage around dental restorations: its effect on the dental pulp. *J Oral Pathol* 1982;**11**:439–50.

179. Bergenholtz G. Bacterial leakage around dental restorations – impact on the pulp. In: Anusavice KJ. ed. *Quality Evaluation of Dental Restorations*, Lombard IL: Quintessence Publishing Co., 1989:243–54.

180. Pashley DH. Clinical considerations of microleakage. *J Endod* 1990;**16**:70–7.

181. Schröder U, Granath L-E. Scanning electron microscopy of hard tissue barrier following experimental pulpotomy of intact human teeth and capping with calcium hydroxide. *Odont Revy* 1974;**25**:57–67.

182. Ulmansky M, Sela J, Sela M. Scanning electron microscopy of calcium hydroxide induced bridges. *J Oral Pathol* 1972;**1**:244–8.

183. Goldberg F, Nassone EJ, Spielberg C. Evaluation of the dentinal bridge after pulpotomy and calcium hydroxide dressing. *J Endod* 1984;**10**:318–20.

184. Möller AJR. *Microbiologic examination of root canals and periapical tissues of human teeth* (Thesis). Gothenburg: Akademiförlaget, 1966:380.

185. Plant CG. The effect of polycarboxylate cement on the dental pulp. A study. *Br Dent J* 1970;**129**:424–6.

186. Prader F. *Diagnose and Therapie des infizierten Wurzelkanales*. Basel: Beno Schwabe Co., 1949:1–224.

187. Pereira JC, Stanley HR. Pulp capping: influence of the exposure site on pulp healing – histologic and radiographic study. *J Endod* 1981;**7**:213–23.

188. Fuks AB, Bielak S, Chosak A. Clinical and radiographic assessment of direct pulp capping and pulpotomy in young permanent teeth. *Pediatr Dent* 1982;**4**:240–4.

189. Gelbier MJ, Winter GB. Traumatized incisors treated by vital pulpotomy: a retrospective study. *Br Dent J* 1988;**164**:319–23.

190. Hörsted P, Söndergaard B, Thylstrup A, El Attar K, Fejerskov O. A retrospective study of direct pulp capping with calcium hydroxide. *Endod Dent Traumatol* 1985;**1**:29–34.

191. Delessert Y, Holz J, Baume L-J. Contrôle radiologique a court et à long terms du traitement radiculaire de la catégorie III de pulpopathies. *Schweiz Monatschr Zahnheil* 1980;**90**:585–607.

192. Jacobsen I, Kerekes K. Diagnosis and treatment of pulp necrosis in permanent anterior teeth with root fracture. *Scand J Dent Res* 1980;**88**:370–6.

193. Andreasen FM, Andreasen JO, Bayer T. Prognosis of root-fractured permanent incisors – prediction of healing modalities. *Endod Dent Traumatol* 1989;**5**:11–22.

194. ANDREASEN FM, ANDREASEN JO. Resorption and mineralization processes following root fracture of permanent incisors. *Endod Dent Traumatol* 1988;**4**:202–14.

195. CVEK M, CLEATON-JONES P, AUSTIN J, KLING M, LOWNIE J, FATTI P. Effect of topical application of doxycycline on pulp revascularization and periodontal healing in reimplanted monkey incisors. *Endod Dent Traumatol* 1990;**6**:1706.

196. ANDREASEN FM, VESTERGAARD-PEDERSEN B. Prognosis of luxated permanent teeth – the development of pulp necrosis. *Endod Dent Traumatol* 1985;**1**:207–20.

197. CIPRIANO TJ, WALTON RE. The ischemic infarct pulp of traumatized teeth: A light and electron microscopic study. *Endod Dent Traumatol* 1986;**2**:196–204.

198. TZIAFAS D. Pulpal reactions following experimental acute trauma of concussion type on immature dog teeth. *Endod Dent Traumatol* 1988;**4**:27–31.

199. OIKARINEN K, GUNDLACH KKH, PFEIFER G. Late complications of luxation injuries to teeth. *Endod Dent Traumatol* 1987;**3**:296–303.

200. ANDREASEN FM. A histological and bacteriological investigation of pulps extirpated following luxation injuries. *Endod Dent Traumatol* 1988;**4**:170–81.

201. CVEK M, CLEATON-JONES P, AUSTIN J, LOWNIE J, KLING M, FATTI P. Pulp revascularization in reimplanted monkey incisors – predictability and the effect of antibiotic systemic prophylaxis. *Endod Dent Traumatol* 1990;**6**:1567–9.

202. KOCH G, ULLBRO C. Klinisk funktionstid hos 55 exartikulerade och replanterade tänder. *Tandläkartidningen* 1982;**74**:18–24

203. KLING M, CVEK M, MEJARE I. Rate and predictability of pulp revascularization in therapeutically reimplanted permanent incisors. *Endod Dent Traumatol* 1986;**2**:83–9.

204. DELIVANIS PD, FAN VSC. The localization of blood-borne bacteria in instrumented and overinstrumented canals. *J Endod* 1984;**10**:521–4.

205. BARRET AP, READE PC. Revascularization of mouse tooth isographs and allographs using autoradiography and carbon perfusion. *Arch Oral Biol* 1981;**26**:541–5.

206. ANDREASEN FM. Transient apical breakdown and its relation to color and sensitivity changes after luxation injuries to teeth. *Endod Dent Traumatol* 1986;**2**:9–19.

207. JACOBSEN I. Criteria for diagnosis of pulp necrosis in traumatized permanent incisors. *Scand J Dent Res* 1980;**88**:306–12

208. ANDREASEN FM. Pulpal healing after luxation injuries and root fracture in the permanent dentition. *Endod Dent Traumatol* 1989;**5**:11–31.

209. FULLING H-J, ANDREASEN JO. Influence of maturation status and tooth type of permanent teeth upon electrometric and thermal pulp testing. *Scand J Dent Res* 1976;**84**:286–90.

210. FULLING H-J, ANDREASEN JO. Influence of splints and temporary crowns upon electric and thermal pulp-testing procedures. *Scand J Dent Res* 1976;**84**:291–6.

211. GAZELIUS B, OLGART L, EDWALL B. Restored vitality in luxated teeth assessed by laser Doppler flowmeter. *Endod Dent Traumatol* 1988;**4**:265–8.

212. OLGART L, GAZELIUS B, LINDH-STRÖMBERG U. Laser Doppler flowmetry in assessing vitality in luxated permanent teeth. *Int Endod J* 1988;**21**:300–6.

213. MÖLLER AJR, FABRICIUS L, DAHLÉN G, ÖHMAN AE, HEYDEN G. Influence on periapical tissues of indigenous oral bacteria and necrotic pulp tissue in monkeys. *Scand J Dent Res* 1981;**89**:475–84.

214. ANDREASEN JO. The effect of pulp extirpation or root canal treatment on periodontal healing after replantation of permanent incisors in monkeys. *J Endod* 1981;**7**:245–52.

215. NICHOLLS E. Endodontic treatment during root formation. *Int Dent J* 1981;**31**:49–59.

216. GHOSE LJ, BAGHDADY VS, HIKMAT BYM. Apexification of immature apices of pulpless permanent anterior teeth with calcium hydroxide. *J Endod* 1987;**13**:285–90.

217. MACKIE IC, BENTLEY EM, WORTHINGTON HV. The closure of open apices in non-vital immature incisor teeth. *Br Dent J* 1988;**165**:169–73.

218. MATES JA. Barrier formation time in non-vital teeth with open apices. *Int Endod J* 1988;**21**:313–19.

219. CHAWLA HS. Apical closure in a non-vital permanent tooth using one Ca(OH)$_2$ dressing. *ASDC J Dent Child* 1986;**53**:44–7.

220. KLEIER DJ, BARR ES. A study of endodontically apexified teeth. *Endod Dent Traumatol* 1991;**7**:112–7.

221. CVEK M. Prognosis of luxated non-vital maxillary incisors treated with calcium hydroxide and filled with guttapercha. *Endod Dent Traumatol* 1992;**8**:45–55.

222. HERFORTH A, SEICHTER U. Die apikale Hartsubstanzbarriere nach temporären Wurzelkanalfüllungen mit Kalziumhydroxid. *Dtsch Zahnärtzl Z* 1980;**35**:1053–7.

223. JAVELET J, TORABINEJAD M, BAKLAND L. Comparison of two pH levels for the induction of apical barriers in immature teeth of monkeys. *J Endod* 1985;**11**:375–8.

224. BYSTRÖM A, CLAESSON R, SUNDQVIST G. The antibacterial effect of camphorated paramonochlorophenol, camphorated phenol and calcium hydroxide in the treatment of infected root canals. *Endod Dent Traumatol* 1985;**1**:170–5.

225. SAFAVI KE, DOWDEN WE, INTROCASO JH, LANGELAND K. A comparison of antimicrobial effects of calcium hydroxide and iodine-potassium iodide. *J Endod* 1985;**11**:454–6.

226. ALLARD U, STRÖMBERG U, STRÖMBERG T. Endodontic treatment of experimentally induced apical periodontitis in dogs. *Endod Dent Traumatol* 1987;**3**:240–4.

227. SJÖGREN U, FIGDOR D, SPÅNGBERG L, SUNDQVIST G. The antibacterial effect of calcium hydroxide as a short-term intracanal dressing. *Int Endod J* 1991;**24**:119–25.

228. ÖRSTAVIK D, KEREKES K, MOLVEN O. Effects of extensive apical reaming and calcium hydroxide dressing on bacterial infection during treatment of apical periodontitis. *Int Endod J* 1991;**24**:1–7.

229. HAAPASALO M, ÖRSTAVIK D. *In vitro* infection and disinfection of dentinal tubules. *J Dent Res* 1987;**66**:1375–9.

230. SAFAVI KE, SPÅNGBERG LSW, LANGELAND K. Root canal dentinal tubule disinfection. *J Endod* 1990;**16**:207–10.

231. Hasselgren G, Olsson B, Cvek M. Effects of calcium hydroxide and sodium hypochlorite on the dissolution of necrotic porcine muscle tissue. *J Endod* 1988;**14**:125–7.

232. Andersen M, Lund J, Andreasen JO, Andreasen FM. In vitro solubility of human pulp tissue in calcium hydroxide and sodium hypochlorite. *Endod Dent Traumatol* 1992;**8**:104–8.

233. Metzler RS, Montgomery S. The effectiveness of ultrasonic and calcium hydroxide for the debridement of human mandibular molars. *J Endod* 1989;**15**:373–8.

234. Mitchell DF, Shankwalker GB. Osteogenetic potential of calcium hydroxide and other materials in soft tissue and bone wounds. *J Dent Res* 1958;**37**:1157–63.

235. Rasmussen P, Mjör IA. Calcium hydroxide as an ectopic bone inductor in rats. *Scand J Dent Res* 1971;**79**:24–30.

236. Rönning O, Koski AK. The fate of anorganic implants in the subcutaneous tissue in rat. *Plast Reconstr Surg* 1966;**37**:121–4.

237. Trope M, Tronstad L. Long-term calcium hydroxide treatment of a tooth with iatrogenic root perforation and lateral periodontitis. *Endod Dent Traumatol* 1985;**1**:35–8.

238. Pettersson K, Hasselgren G, Tronstad L. Endodontic treatment of experimental root perforations in dog teeth. *Endod Dent Traumatol* 1985;**1**:22–8.

239. Nordenwall K-J, Holm K. Management of cervical root perforation: report of a case. *ASDC J Dent Child* 1990;**57**:454–8.

240. Ohara PK, Torabinejad M. Apical closure of an immature root subsequent to apical curretage. *Endod Dent Traumatol* 1992;**8**:134–7.

241. Byström A, Sundqvist G. The antibacterial action of sodium hypochlorite and EDTA in 60 cases of endodontic therapy. *Int Endod*, 1985;**18**:35–40.

242. Byström A, Happonen R-P, Sjögren U, Sundqvist G. Healing of periapical lesions of pulpless teeth after endodontic treatment with controlled asepsis. *Endod Dent Traumatol* 1987;**3**:58–63.

243. Chong BS, Pitt Ford TR. The role of intracanal medication in root canal treatment. *Int Endod J* 1992;**25**:97–106.

244. Örstavik D. Endodontic materials. *Adv Dent Res* 1988;**2**:12–24.

245. Kerekes K, Tronstad L. Long-term results of endodontic treatment performed with a standardized technique. *J Endod* 1979;**5**:83–90.

246. Tronstad L, Andreasen JO, Hasselgren G, Kristerson L, Riis I. pH changes in dental tissues after root canal filling with calcium hydroxide. *J Endod* 1981;**7**:17–21.

247. Hammarström LE, Blomlöf LB, Feiglin B, Lindskog S. Effect of calcium hydroxide treatment on periodontal repair and root resorption. *Endod Dent Traumatol* 1986;**2**:1849.

248. Blomlöf L, Lindskog S, Hammarström L. Influence of pulpal treatments on cell and tissue reactions in the marginal periodontium. *J Periodontol* 1988;**59**:577–83.

249. Lengheden A, Blomlöf L, Lindskog S. Effect of immediate calcium hydroxide treatment and permanent root-filling on periodontal healing in contaminated replanted teeth. *Scand J Dent Res* 1991;**99**:139–46.

250. Lengheden A, Blomlöf L, Lindskog S. Effect of delayed calcium hydroxide treatment on periodontal healing in contaminated replanted teeth. *Scand J Dent Res* 1991;**99**:147–53.

251. Makkes PG, Thoden van Velzen SK. Cervical external root resorption. *J Dent Res* 1975;**3**:217–22.

252. Tronstad L. Pulp reactions in traumatized teeth. In: Guttman, JI, Harrison JW. eds. *Proceedings of the International Conference on Oral Trauma.* Chicago: American Association of Endodontists Endowment and Memorial Foundation, 1984:55–77.

253. Tronstad L. Root resorption – etiology, terminology and clinical manifestations. *Endod Dent Traumatol* 1988;**4**:241–52.

254. Rud J, Rud V, Munksgaard EC. Retrograd rodfyldning med plast og dentinbinder: Indikation og anvendelsesmuligheder. (Retrograde root filling with resin and a dentin bonding agent: indication and applications). *Tandlægebladet* 1989;**93**:223–9.

255. Frank AL, Bakland LK. Non-endodontic therapy for supraosseous extracanal invasive resorption. *J Endod* 1987;**13**:348–55.

256. Heithersay GS. Combined endodontic-orthodontic treatment of transverse root fractures in the region of the cervical alveolar crest. *Oral Surg Oral Med Oral Pathol* 1973;**36**:404–15.

257. Malmgren O, Malmgren B, Frykholm A. Rapid orthodontic extrusion of crown-root and cervical root fractured teeth. *Endod Dent Traumatol* 1991;**7**:49–54.

258. Tegsjö U, Valerius-Olsson H, Olgart K. Intra-alveolar transplantation of teeth with cervical root fractures. *Swed Dent J* 1978;**2**:73–82.

259. Kahnberg K-E. Intraalveolar transplantation of teeth with crown-root fractures. *J Oral Maxillofac Surg* 1985;**43**:38–42.

260. Malmgren B, Cvek M, Lundberg M, Frykholm A. Surgical treatment of ankylosed and infrapositioned reimplanted incisors in adolescents. *Scand J Dent Res* 1984;**92**:391–9.

261. Wedenberg C, Zetterqvist L. Internal resorption in human teeth – a histological, scanning electron microscopic and enzyme histochemical study. *J Endod* 1987;**13**:255–9.

262. Wedenberg C, Lindskog S. Experimental internal resorption in monkey teeth. *Endod Dent Traumatol* 1985;**1**:221–7.

263. Walton RE, Leonard LE. Cracked tooth: an etiology for 'idiopathic' internal resorption? *J Endod* 1986;**12**:167–9.

264. Smith JW. Calcific metamorphosis: a treatment dilemma. *Oral Surg Oral Med Oral Pathol* 1982;**54**:441–4.

265. Schindler WG, Gullickson DC. Rationale for the management of calcific metamorphosis secondary to traumatic injuries. *J Endod* 1988;**14**:408–12.

266. SELDEN HS. The role of a dental operating microscope in improved non-surgical treatment of 'calcified' canals. *Oral Surg Oral Med Oral Pathol* 1989;**68**:93–8.

267. FRANK AL. Bleaching of vital and non-vital teeth. In: Cohen S, Burns RC. eds. *Pathways of the pulp*. 2nd edn. St. Louis: C.V. Mosby Co 1980:568–75.

268. NUTTING EB, POE GS. A new combination for bleaching teeth. *J South Calif Dent Assoc* 1963;**31**:289–91.

269. GROSSMAN LI. *Endodontic practice*. 9th edn. Philadelphia: Lea & Febiger, 1978:440.

270. VAN DER BURGT T. *Tooth color and tooth discoloration. In vitro studies on tooth color and tooth discoloration related to endodontic procedures.* Thesis, Catholic University of Nijmegen, 1985.

271. STEWART GG. Bleaching discolored pulpless teeth. *J Am Dent Assoc* 1965;**70**:325–8.

272. LEMON RR. Bleaching and restoring endodontically treated teeth. *Current Opinion Dentistry* 1991;**1**: 754–9.

273. HARRINGTON GW, NATKIN E. External resorption associated with bleaching of pulpless teeth. *J Endod* 1979;**5**:344–8.

274. LADO AE, STANLEY HR, WEISMAN MI. Cervical resorption in bleached teeth. *Oral Surg Oral Med Oral Pathol* 1983;**55**:78–80.

275. MONTGOMERY S. External cervical resorption after bleaching a pulpless tooth. *Oral Surg Oral Med Oral Pathol* 1984;**57**:203–6.

276. CVEK M, LINDWALL A-M. External root resorption following bleaching of pulpless teeth with oxygen peroxide. *Endod Dent Traumatol* 1985;**1**:56–60.

277. FRIEDMAN S, ROTSTEIN I, LIBFELD H, STABHOLTZ A, HELING I. Incidence of external root resorption and esthetic results in 58 bleached pulpless teeth. *Endod Dent Traumatol* 1988;**4**:23–6.

278. FUSS Z, SZAJKIS S, TAGGER M. Tubular permeability to calcium hydroxide and to bleaching agents. *J Endod* 1989;**15**:362–4.

279. MADISON S, WALTON R. Cervical root resorption following bleaching of endodontically treated teeth. *J Endod* 1990;**16**:570–4.

280. ROTSTEIN I, FRIEDMAN S, MOR C, KATZNELSON J, SOMMER M, BAB I. Histological characterization of bleaching-induced external root resorption in dogs. *J Endod* 1991;**17**:436–41.

281. ROTSTEIN I, TOREK Y, LEVINSTEIN I. Effect of bleaching time and temperature on the radicular penetration of hydrogen peroxide. *Endod Dent Traumatol* 1991;**7**: 196–8.

282. ROTSTEIN I, TOREK Y, MISGAV R. Effect of cementum defects on radicular penetration of 30% $H_2O_2$ during intracoronal bleaching. *J Endod* 1991;**17**: 230–3.

283. SPASSER HF. A simple bleaching technique using sodium perborate. *NY State Dent J* 1961;**27**:332–4.

284. SARP OP. Blegning of rodfyldte, misfarvede taender. *Tandlaegebladet* 1978;**82**:73–7.

285. HOLMSTRUP G, PALM AM, LAMBJERG-HANSEN H. Bleaching of discoloured root-filled teeth. *Endod Dent Traumatol* 1988;**4**:197–201.

286. HO S, GOERIG A. An in vitro comparison of different bleaching agents in the discoloured tooth. *J Endod* 1989;**15**:106–11.

287. HOLMSTRUP G, PALM AM, LAMBJERG-HANSEN H. Blegning of misfarvede rodfyldte tænder. Resultater efter 3 og 5 års observationstid. *Tandlægebladet* 1989;**93**:445–9.

288. ROTSTEIN I, ZALKIND M, MOR C, TAREBAH A, FRIEDMAN S. *In vitro* efficacy of sodium perborate preparations used for intracoronal bleaching of discoloured non-vital teeth. *Endod Dent Traumatol* 1991;**7**:177–80.

289. SCHRÖDER U, HEIDE S, HÖSKULDSSON O, RÖLLING I. Endodontics. In: Koch G, Modeer TH, Poulsen S, Rasmussen P. eds. *Pedodontics – a clinical approach*. Copenhagen: Munksgaard 1991:185–210.

290. ROBERTSON A, ANDREASEN FM, BERGENHOTZ G, ANDREASEN JO, MUNKSGAARD EC. Pulp reactions to restoration of experimentally induced crown fractures. *J Dent* 1998;**26**:409–16.

291. COX CF, SUZUKI S. Re-evaluating pulp protection: calcium hydroxide liners vs. cohesive hybridization.(Review). *J Am Dent Assoc* 1994;**125**:823–31.

292. SWIFT EJ Jr, TROPE M. Treatment options for the exposed vital pulp. *Pract Periodont Aesthet Dent* 1999;**11**:735–9.

293. OLBURGH S, JACOBY T, KREJCI I. Crown fractures in the permanent dentition: pulpal and restorative considerations. *Dent Traumatol* 2002;**18**:103–115.

294. DE SOUZA COSTA CA, HEBLING J, HANKS CT. Current status of pulp capping with adhesive systems: a review. *Dent Mater* 2000;**16**:199–7.

295. FUKS A, GAVRA S, CHOSAK A. Long-term follow-up of traumatized incisors treated by partial pulpotomy. *Pediatric Dentistry* 1993;**15**:334–6.

296. BLANCO L, COHEN S. Treatment of crown fractures with exposed pulps. *J Calif Dent Assoc* 2002;**30**:419–25.

297. RAM D, HOLAN G. Partial pulpotomy in a primary incisor with pulp exposure: a case report. *Pediatric Dentistry* 1994;**16**:46–8.

298. CVEK M, ANDREASEN JO, BORUM MK. Healing of 208 intra-alveolar root fractures in patients aged 7–17 years. *Dent Traumatol* 2001;**17**:53–62.

299. ANDREASEN JO, ANDREASEN FM, MEJARE I, CVEK MI. Healing of 400 intra-alveolar root fractures. 1. Effect of pre-injury and injury factors such as sex, age, stage of root development, fracture type, location of fracture and severity of dislocation. *Dent Traumatol* 2004;**20**:192–202.

300. ANDREASEN JO, ANDREASEN FM, MEJARE I, CVEK M. Healing of 400 intra-alveolar fractures. 2. Effect of treatment factors, such as treatment delay, repositioning, splinting type and period and antibiotics. *Dent Traumatol* 2004;**20**:203–11.

301. CVEK M, MEJARE I, ANDREASEN JO. Healing and prognosis of teeth with intra-alveolar fractures involving the cervical part of the root. *Dent Traumatol* 2002;**18**:57–65.

302. CVEK K, MEJARE I, ANDREASEN JO. Conservative endodontic treatment of teeth fractured in the middle or

apical part of the root. *Dent Traumatol* 2004;**20**: 261–9.

303. YANPISET K, TROPE M. Pulp revascularization of replanted immature dog teeth after different treatment methods. *Dent Traumatol* 2000;**16**:211–7.

304. RITTER ALS, RITTER AV, SIGURDSSON A, TROPE M. Pulp revascularization of replanted immature dog teeth after treatment with minocycline and doxycycline assessed by laser Doppler flowmetry, radiography, and histology. *Dent Traumatol* 2004;**20**:75–84.

305. LOVE RM. Bacterial penetration of the root canal of intact incisor teeth after a simulated traumatic injury. *Endod Dent Traumataol* 1996;**12**:289–93.

306. YAMPISET K, VONGSAVAN N, SIGURDSSON A, TROPE M. Efficacy of laser Doppler flowmetry for the diagnosis of reimplanted immature dog teeth. *Dent Traumatol* 2001;**17**:63–70.

307. MACKIE IC, WORTHINGTON HV, HILL FJ. A follow-up study of incisor teeth which have been treated by apical closure and root filling. *Brit Dent J* 1993;**175**:99–101.

308. SCEEHY EC, ROBERTS GJ. Use of calcium hydroxide for apical barrier formation and healing in non-vital immature permanent teeth: a review. *Br Dent J* 1997;**183**:241–6.

309. MORFIS AS, SISKOS G. Apexification with the use of calcium hydroxide: a clinical study. *J Clin Pediatr Dent.* 1991;**16**:13–19.

310. MACKIE IC, HILL FJ, WORTHINGTON HV. Comparison of two calcium hydroxide pastes used for endodontic treatment of non-vital immature incisor teeth, *Endod Dent Traumatol* 1994;**10**:90–99.

311. CHAWLA HS. Apexification. Follow-up after 6–12 years. *J Ind Soc Pedodont Prev Dent* 1991;**8**:38–40.

312. GEORGOPOULOU M, KONTAKIOTIS E, NAKOU M. *In vitro* evaluation of the effectiveness of calcium hydroxide and paramonochlorophenol on anaerobic bacteria from the root canal. *Endod Dent Traumatol* 1993;**9**:249–53.

313. TURKUN M, GENGIZ T. The effects of sodium hypochlorite and calcium hydroxide on tissue dissolution and root canal cleanliness. *Int Endod J* 1997;**30**:135–42.

314. KEREZOUDDIS NP, VALAVANIS D, PROUNTZOS F. A method of adapting gutta-percha cones for obturation of open apex cases using heat. *Int Endod J* 1999;**32**:53–60.

315. ROS F. Fracture susceptibility of endodontically treated teeth. *J Endod* 1980;**6**:560–5.

316. HELFER AR, MELNICK S, SCHILDER H. Determination of the moisture content of vital and pulpless teeth. *Oral Surg Oral Med Oral Pathol* 1972;**34**:661–70.

317. ANREASEN JO, FARIK B, MUNKGSGAARD EC. Long-term calcium hydroxide as root canal dressing may increase risk of root fracture. *Dent Traumatol* 2002;**18**: 134–7.

318. SIM TPC, KNOWLES JC, NG Y-L, SHELTON J, GULABIVALA K. Effect of sodium hypochlorite on mechanical properties of dentin and tooth surface strain. *Int Dent J* 2001;**34**:120–32.

319. GRIGORATOS D, KNOWLES J, NG Y-L, GULABIVALA K. Effect of exposing dentine to sodium hypochlorite and

calcium hydroxide on its flexural and elastic modules. *Int Endod J* 2001;**34**:313–9.

320. RABIE G, TROPE M, TRONSTAD L. Strengthening of immature teeth during long-term endodontic therapy. *Endod Dent Traumatol* 1986;**2**:43–7.

321. RABIE G, TROPE M, GARCIA C, TRONSTAD L. Strengthening and restoration of immature teeth with an acid etch resin technique. *Endod Dent Traumatol* 1985;**1**:246–56.

322. RENE JR, NICHOLLS JI, HARRINGTON GW. Evaluation of fiber-composite laminate in the restoration of immature, nonvital maxillary central incisors. *J Endod* 2001;**27**:18–22.

323. HAMMARSTRÖM L, BLOMLÖF L, FEIGLIN B, ANDERSON L, LINDSKOG S. Replantation of teeth and antibiotic treatment. *Endod Dent Traumatol* 1986;**2**:51–7.

324. HAMMARSTRÖM L, PIERCE A, BLOMLÖF L, FEIGLIN B, LINDSKOG S. Tooth avulsion and replantation: a review. *Endod Dent Traumatol* 1986;**2**:1–9.

325. SAE-LIM V, WANG C-J, CHOI G-V, TROPE M. The effect of systemic tetracycline on resorption of dried replanted dog's teeth. *Endod Dent Traumatol* 1998;**14**:27.

326. SAE-LIM V, WANG C-J, TROPE M. Effect of systemic tetracycline and amoxicilline on inflammatory root resorption of replanted dog's teeth. *Endod Dent Traumatol* 1998;**14**:216–28.

327. DUMSHA T, HOVLAND EJ. Evaluation of long-term calcium hydroxide treatment in avulsed teeth – an *in vitro* study. *Int Endod J* 1995;**28**:7–11.

328. TROPE M. Short versus long-term CaOH$_2$ treatment of established inflammatory root resorption in replanted dog teeth. *Endod Dent Traumatol* 1995:**11**:121–9.

329. AMIR FA, GUTMANN JL, WITHERSPOON DE. Calcific metamorphosis: A challenge in endodonic diagnosis and treatment. *Quintessence Int* 2001;**32**:447–55.

330. HEITHERSAY GS, DAHLSTRÖM SW, MARIN PD. Incidence of invasive cervical resorption in bleached root-filled teeth. *Aust Dent J* 1994;**39**:82–7.

331. KLEIER DJ, BARR ES. A study of endodontically apexified teeth. *Endod Dent Traumatol* 1991;**7**:112–17.

332. CALISKAN MK, SEN BH. Endodontic treatment of teeth with apical periodontitis using calcium hydroxide: a long-term study. *Endod Dent Traumatol* 1996;**12**: 215–21.

333. FINUCANE D, KINIRONS MJ. Non-vital immature permanent incisors: factors that may influence treatment outcome. *Endod Dent Traumatol* 1999;**15**:273–7.

334. CHOSACK A, SELA J, CLEATON-JONES P. A histological and quantitative histomorphometric study of apexification of nonvital permanent incisors of vervet monkeys after repeated root filling with calcium hydroxide paste. *Endod Dent Traumatol* 1997;**13**: 211–17.

335. MANDEL E, BOURGUIGNON-ADELLE C. Endodontic retreatment: a rational approach to non-surgical root canal therapy of immature teeth. *Endod Dent Traumatol* 1996;**12**:246–53.

336. ANDREASEN JO, KRISTERSON L. The effect of extra-alveolar root filling with calcium hydroxide on periodontal healing after replantation of permanent incisors in monkeys. *J Endod* 1981;**7**:349–54.

337. ANDREASEN JO. A time-related study of periodontal healing and root resorption activity after replantation of mature permanent incisors in monkeys. *Swed Dent J* 1980;**4**:101–10.

338. GREGOIOU AP, JEANSONNE BG, MUSSELMAN RJ. Timing of calcium hydroxide therapy in the treatment of root resorption in replanted teeth in dogs. *Endod Dent Traumatol* 1994;**10**:268–75.

339. KINIRONS MJ, BOYD DH, GREGG TA. Inflammatory and replacement resorption in reimplanted permanent incisor teeth: a study of the characteristics of 84 teeth. *Endod Dent Traumatol* 1999;**15**:269–72.

# 23

# New Endodontic Procedures using Mineral Trioxide Aggregate (MTA) for Teeth with Traumatic Injuries

L. K. Bakland

## Introduction

The scope of endodontics includes vital pulp therapy in addition to managing teeth with pulp necrosis (1). So it should come as no surprise that endodontic specialists have been active in developing new procedures to preserve pulp vitality in developing teeth and to treat immature teeth with pulp necrosis. Techniques using a new material, mineral trioxide aggregate (ProRoot MTA®), will be described for teeth with traumatic pulp exposures (pulpotomy) and teeth with pulp necrosis and incompletely formed apexes (apexification). In addition, the use of MTA will be described for situations in which teeth with horizontal root factures require root canal therapy.

Until recent years, calcium hydroxide has been the gold standard for dental therapeutic materials; it has been used successfully for pulp capping (2), pulpotomies (3–5), apexifications (6–11), and for treating root fractured teeth that require endodontic therapy (12), as well as an antibacterial root canal medication (13, 14). It has both advantages and disadvantages.

The therapeutic advantages are well known and have been recognized since the material was first recommended in the 1930s (15, 16). It has antibacterial properties (13, 14) and it appears to stimulate hard tissue formation when applied to tissues with such potential, for instance pulp and periradicular tissues (3–11). While calcium hydroxide is a caustic material with a high alkaline pH (12.5), it appears to be very biocompatible and is not associated with untoward tissue reactions (17).

The disadvantages of the use of calcium hydroxide are procedure related. When it is used for pulp capping or pulpotomy, it is advisable to re-enter the capping site after hard tissue bridge formation to remove the combination of necrotic tissue and remnants of calcium hydroxide material so that bacterial microleakage can be prevented (3, 4) (Fig.

23.1). Recently, it has been recognized that calcium hydroxide has an effect on dentin that weakens dentin's resistance to fracture (18–21). As noted by Cvek (18), teeth in young children are more susceptible to cervical root fracture following calcium hydroxide treatment. This has been further elucidated by two research projects at Loma Linda (44, 82), in which the age of the animals from which teeth were harvested for testing with exposure to calcium hydroxide appeared to make a difference. Younger teeth were more likely to fracture than teeth from older animals, confirming the results of Andreasen et al. (19). For these reasons it has been desirable to develop dental materials without calcium hydroxide's disadvantages, but at the same time retaining its advantages. Mineral trioxide aggregate (MTA) is a material that appears to be a good alternative to calcium hydroxide.

Since its development in the early 1990s by Torabinejad and colleagues at Loma Linda University in California, USA, MTA has been tested and applied to numerous dental situations by researchers and clinicians worldwide.

When first developed, MTA was a gray powder, which has since been modified to a white color for esthetic reasons, without any apparent physical or therapeutic changes (22–25). This change has been made possible by the reduction of ferrite ($Fe_3O_3$) in the making of white MTA (22). MTA has a pH range of 10.2–12.5 that is time related during the first 3 hours of setting time, after which it remains constant. While MTA sets in about 3 hours, its compressive strength continues to increase over a period of 3 weeks (26).

Mineral trioxide aggregate consists of *calcium silicate* ($CaSiO_4$), *bismuth oxide* ($Bi_2O_3$), *calcium carbonate* ($CaCO_3$), *calcium sulfate* ($CaSO_4$), and *calcium aluminate* ($CaAl_2O_4$). MTA is mixed (3:1, MTA:$H_2O$) with water or other fluids such as saline, to form an amorphous structure of calcium crystals consisting of 33% calcium, 49% phosphate, 2% carbon, 3% chloride, and 6% silica (26). MTA is a hydrophilic material that sets in the presence of any moisture, including blood (27).

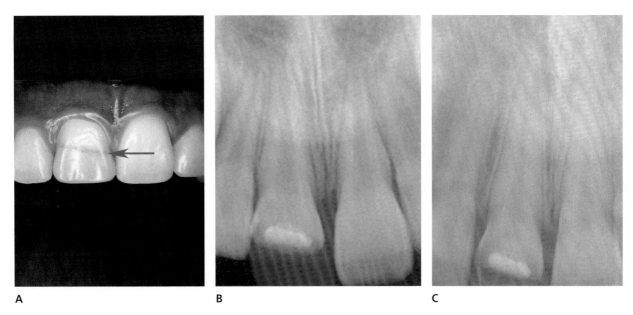

**Fig. 23.1** Secondary pulp necrosis after partial pulpotomy. A. Maxillary right central incisor as it appears seven years after receiving a calcium hydroxide partial pulpotomy. Note dark line (arrow) indicating microleakage between the tooth structure and the composite restoration. B. Radiographic appearance immediately following the pulpotomy seven years earlier, and C. radiograph taken at the same time as the photograph in A. The microleakage resulted in pulpitis requiring root canal therapy; the initial treatment, however, assured the tooth's continued development and root canal therapy could be done on a fully developed, mature tooth.

One of the major advantages of MTA is its demonstrated biocompatibility and non-mutagenicity. Numerous studies have shown that it is well tolerated by tissue cells both in the pulp and periradicular areas (28–35), and it appears to have a mechanism of action that encourages hard tissue deposition similar to that of calcium hydroxide (23).

Since bacterial microleakage is a major concern with any dental material, it is noteworthy that MTA has been shown to resist bacterial penetration quite favorably compared to other materials (36–38). Recently, Murray et al. (39) demonstrated that the pulp's reparative activity occurs more readily beneath capping materials that prevent bacterial microleakage, a feature favoring the use of MTA.

The reason for MTA's resistance to bacterial penetration is said to be related to its adaptation to adjacent dentin, a tight physical adaptation that includes penetration of MTA into dentinal tubules. The result is a low tendency to microleakage (26, 27, 29).

Mineral trioxide aggregate is a biological active material which induces hard tissue formation through mechanisms that are still being investigated (40). Koh et al. (33) noted that it stimulates interleukin formation and provides a substrate for osteoblasts, a finding also noted by Perez et al. (41), though the latter observed that osteoblasts did not survive as long on white MTA as on gray MTA. The bioactivity of MTA may be similar to that of calcium hydroxide; Friedland and Rosado (42, 43) described the results of exposing set MTA to water and found that calcium hydroxide is released from MTA (for at least up to 3 months), which can explain the stimulation of hard tissue formation against the material. Holland et al. (23) found that calcite crystals formed, similarly to that found with calcium hydroxide, when MTA comes in contact with water.

Another recognized advantage of MTA is its prevention of leakage of bacteria into a healing tissue wound, whether it is pulp or periradicular tissue (36–38). It is certainly true that the dental pulp's reparative activity can occur beneath capping materials in the absence of bacterial microleakage and that success is increased with materials that prevent bacterial leakage (39); the same can probably be said for apexification and repair of root fractures.

In spite of the similarity to calcium hydroxide (42, 43), MTA does not appear to have a detrimental effect on dentin (44), a problem noted with calcium hydroxide (18–21). This makes MTA especially well suited for treatment involving pulp necrosis in immature, developing teeth (e.g. teeth needing apexification and teeth with root fractures in which the coronal pulp tissue deteriorates and becomes infected).

The bioactive property of MTA has resulted in superior (when compared to calcium hydroxide and other materials) dentin bridges after pulp capping and pulpotomies (32, 40, 45–52) and apexifications (30, 31). The best explanation is probably that MTA provides an excellent protection against bacterial leakage (39) and possesses a biocompatible quality that allows tissue repair (28–35), along with providing stimulation for hard tissue deposition (23).

## Pulp capping and partial pulpotomy

Crown fractures in children and young teenagers in which the dental pulps are exposed can have severely detrimental effects on the long-term survival of such teeth if pulp necrosis results. The capacity for pulp cells to resist and repair injuries is fundamental to maintenance of the integrity and

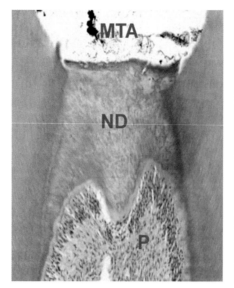

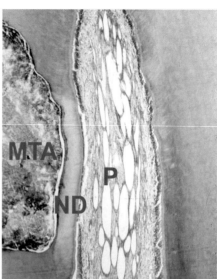

**A**                                                                **B**

**Fig. 23.2** Histologic response to partial pulpotomy and pulp capping. A. Partial pulpotomy on a dog's tooth shows healthy, normal appearing new dentin (MTA – position of MTA during treatment; ND – new dentin formed under MTA; P – pulp). B. Pulp capping on a monkey's tooth. Bridge formation at site of mechanical pulp exposure.

homeostasis of the dental organ (53). Incompletely developed teeth are more prone to cervical root fractures (18–21, 54) if they lose pulp vitality and require root canal therapy. Thus, every effort should be made to protect such exposed pulps to allow completion of root development, which means thickening of the root along with closing of the apical opening.

To date, the most commonly used procedure for pulp protection in teeth with traumatic pulp exposures has been the technique popularized by Cvek (3), often referred to as Cvek-pulpotomy (see Chapter 22). The technique relies on the use of calcium hydroxide as the active agent to promote hard tissue formation and perhaps secondarily to serve as an antibacterial agent at the site of the pulp wound. The technique has proven to be very successful and used worldwide (2–5). One drawback is that one needs to re-enter the site of calcium hydroxide placement after dentin bridge formation to remove remnants of necrotic tissue which can serve as nutrients for bacteria that may have gained access through microleakage between the restoration and the tooth structure (Fig. 23.1).

The new material, mineral trioxide aggregate (MTA), which has been described in the Introduction, offers many advantages as an agent for use in pulpotomies. It is biocompatible (28–35), provides excellent resistance to microleakage (36–38), allows opportunity for dentin bridging at the site of pulp exposure (32, 40, 45, 46, 48, 49) (Fig. 23.2), and appears to be associated with a very positive clinical outcome (47, 50, 51) (Fig. 23.3). And since MTA does not deteriorate over time, it is not necessary to re-enter the site of material placement at a later time to remove the material.

Since the development of white MTA, this version of the material is recommended for coronal aspects of teeth for cosmetic reasons. As noted, the difference in the two MTA types does not seem to result in any differences in quality or biocompatibility (22–25).

The action of MTA on exposed pulp tissue is similar to calcium hydroxide (40). A slight layer of necrotic pulp tissue superficial to the bridge, suggests a similar action (40). Initially a superficial zone of extracellular matrix forms, which is followed by hard tissue depositions, under which formative cells (odontoblast-like cells) produce reparative dentin as a

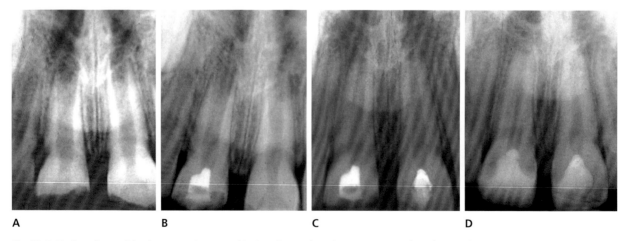

**A**                    **B**                    **C**                    **D**

**Fig. 23.3** Healing after partial pulpotomy. A. Two central incisors fractured in a boy age 8. B. First the right central incisor received an MTA pulpotomy, following which the left central incisor was also treated in the same manner. C. The teeth one year postoperatively. D. The MTA was changed from gray to white for cosmetic reasons after 3 years. Note continued root development.

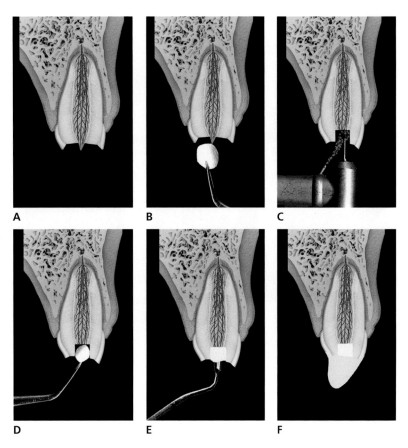

**Fig. 23.4** Recommended steps for MTA pulpotomies in teeth with reversible pulpitis. A. Administer local anesthetic and isolate the tooth with rubber dam. B. Disinfect the exposed dentin and pulp with either sodium hypochlorite or chlorhexidine. C. Remove pulp and surrounding dentin to a depth of 2 mm from the level of exposure, using a round diamond bur and water or saline spray. D. Place a saline-moistened cotton pellet onto the pulpal wound until bleeding has ceased, or nearly so. Slight hemorrhage does not affect placement of MTA. E. A mixture of MTA and saline or water can now be placed into the prepared cavity, against the pulpal wound and filling the entire cavity. F. After setting (4–6 hours) a restoration can be placed to restore the tooth or bond the fractured crown fragment. While setting the MTA serves as a temporary restoration. The patient should be instructed to avoid chewing or biting, because the material is initially quite soft.

sign that the pulp is back to normal function (49). The main difference between MTA and calcium hydroxide may be that MTA provides a good protective barrier against microleakage (36–38) and does not break down requiring replacement as is the case with calcium hydroxide (3, 4). If microleakage occurs in the case of calcium hydroxide, it allows bacteria to reach the dentin bridge which usually has numerous tunnel defects (55), a factor not of significance when MTA is used (49).

Finally, several studies have shown MTA to be superior to other alternative capping agents (e.g. resins) (51, 52). While there are promising possibilities with the use of resins for protecting the exposed pulp, the available evidence raises questions about their safety (56–59).

The technique for using MTA is in many ways similar to the partial pulpotomies in which calcium hydroxide is used. A major difference is that control of pulpal bleeding is less of a problem when MTA is used compared to calcium hydroxide. While calcium hydroxide should be placed on the exposed pulp tissue only after bleeding has completely stopped (and after washing away the blood clot), MTA can be placed on pulp tissue that may still be bleeding slightly, since MTA requires presence of fluid for the setting process, and blood has been shown to provide such a stimulus (27).

These are the recommended steps for MTA pulpotomies in teeth with reversible pulpitis (Fig. 23.4):

- See Fig. 23.4A,B. After anesthetizing the tooth, isolate it with a rubber dam and disinfect the operative site. Sodium hypochlorite or chlorhexidine are excellent agents for disinfection.

- See Fig. 23.4C–E. Using a round diamond (about the size of a #4 round bur) in the high speed handpiece and with a water coolant spray, gradually remove pulp tissue from the site of the exposure to a depth of about 2 mm into the pulp proper. Use a cotton pellet for a short time to reduce the initial brisk bleeding, after which MTA can be placed directly on the pulp wound. Mixed to manufacturer's recommendations (3 : 1, MTA : H$_2$O), the prepared MTA has the consistency of wet sand. Excess moisture can be soaked up from the material, using a cotton pellet. Before restoring the fractured tooth crown, it is necessary to wait about 4–6 hours for the MTA to cure. If an adequate thickness of MTA is present (at least 2 mm) it is not necessary to protect the MTA filling while it is curing, but the patient should refrain from using the tooth until the MTA has hardened. Exposure to saliva will provide needed moisture for the material to cure. If the tooth fracture is such that a temporary filling can be placed above the MTA material, one must place a moist cotton pellet between the MTA and the temporary filling.

- See Fig. 23.4F. After the MTA has cured, one can restore the tooth, either by using a bonded composite resin restoration or if it is available, bonding the fractured tooth fragment to the remaining tooth structure.

Teeth that have been treated with MTA pulpotomy may be monitored in several ways: development of a dentin bridge, continued root development, positive response to pulp testing, freedom from symptoms, and lack of radiographic abnormalities (60).

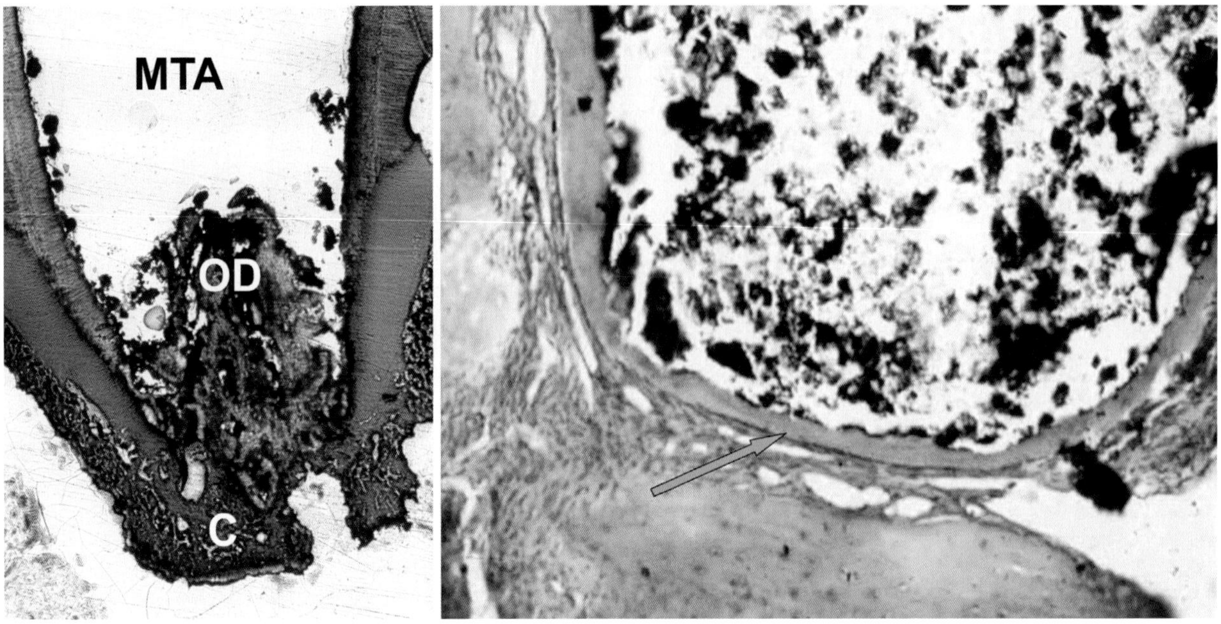

**Fig. 23.5** Apexification using MTA as a root-filling material. A. Apexification performed on a dog's tooth shows apical cementum (C) developing below the initial osteodentin (OD) which formed under MTA (MTA – space where MTA was placed). The stain is Masson's trichrome. (Courtesy of Dr. Shahrokh Shabahang, Loma Linda University, California, USA). B. An example of apical cementum (arrow) forming under MTA placed as retrofilling material. (Courtesy of Dr. Mahmoud Torabinejad, DMD, MSD, PhD, Loma Linda University, California, USA.)

## Apexification

When a child's tooth is traumatized, the pulp may not survive the injury. If that happens, the tooth ceases to develop, resulting in a tooth with thin, fragile root canal walls and an open apex. The necrotic pulps in such teeth frequently become infected, which promotes root resorption and periradicular disease. If left untreated, the end result is loss of the tooth (6, 60).

For many years, the recommended treatment for developing teeth with pulp necrosis has been apexification using calcium hydroxide (6, 8, 9). The technique has enjoyed good success and many teeth, otherwise doomed to extraction, have been saved. It has been recognized, however, that such treated teeth have a high rate of cervical root fracture during the years after treatment (18, 54, 60).

Recently, Andreasen et al. (19) demonstrated that immature sheep teeth filled with calcium hydroxide became increasingly less resistant to fracture when exposed to calcium hydroxide for long periods of time. In another recent study, when MTA was used to fill the root canals, the resistance to fracture was equal to controls, thus giving better results than roots treated for long periods of time with calcium hydroxide (44).

In addition to frequent cervical root fractures associated with the use of calcium hydroxide in immature teeth (7, 54), this technique for apexification has the disadvantage of increased treatment time, unpredictable results and delays in completing final restoration (61–63).

Alternatives to the use of calcium hydroxide for producing an apical barrier have been recommended (64, 65); it appears that MTA provides an excellent means of generating an apical plug above which either gutta-percha or resin can be placed (Fig. 23.5). Shabahang et al. (66) demonstrated that MTA promoted apical repair (Table 23.1), and

**Table 23.1** A comparison of the outcomes of three apexification materials and a control. SHABAHANG et al. (66), Masson's trichrome stain.

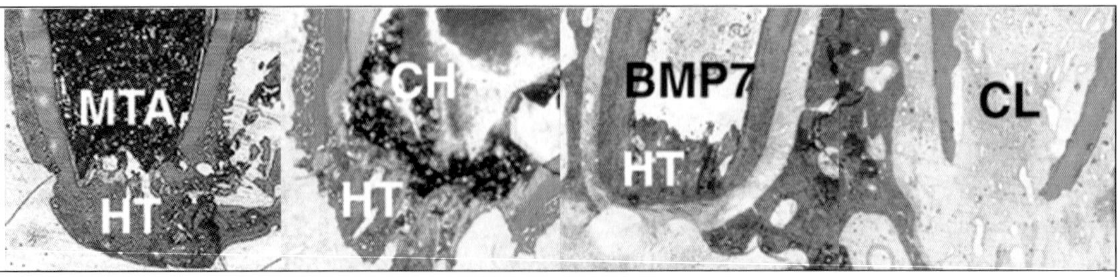

| | MTA | CH | BMP7 | CL |
|---|---|---|---|---|
| Successful | 13 | 5 | 5 | 0 |
| Failures | 1 | 8 | 8 | 11 |
| **Total** | **14** | **13** | **13** | **11** |

HT: hard tissue; MTA: mineral trioxide aggregate; CH: calcium hydroxide; BMP7: bone morphogenic protein; CL: collagen carrier (for BMP7).

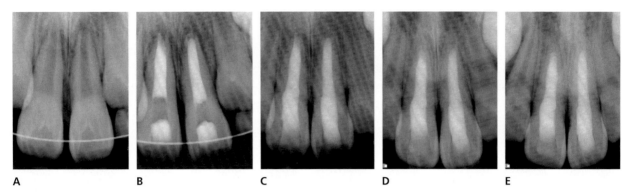

**Fig. 23.6**  A. Luxation injury to both maxillary central incisors resulted in pulp necrosis. The pulps were extirpated and calcium hydroxide placed in the canals. B. One month later, the canals were filled with MTA, covered with wet cotton pellets and a temporary restoration. A few days later, the coronal accesses were filled with composite resin. C. Six-month follow-up. D. Two-year follow-up. E. Three-year follow-up shows good periapical repair.

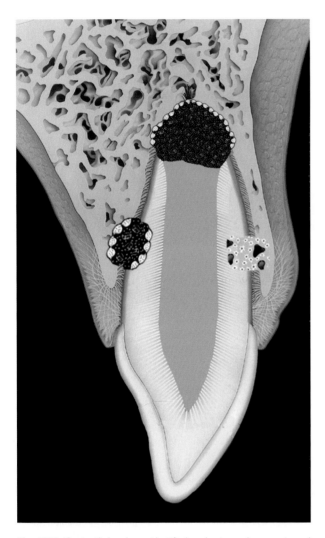

**Fig. 23.7**  The tooth has been identified as having pulp necrosis and external root resorption.

Since the introduction of MTA for use as an apical barrier, there have been several reports of successful outcomes (61, 68–72, 74) (Fig. 23.6). The recommended size of apical MTA plug is 4 mm (70, 73) and Lawley et al. (73) have suggested that ultrasonic placement is advisable, followed by a resin filling in the coronal section of the canal.

The recommended steps in the placement of an apical plug of MTA in root canals with open apices appear in Figs 23.7 and 23.8.

One of the problems in managing immature teeth with pulp necrosis is the frequent occurrence of cervical root fractures during and after apexification procedures (7, 54). Because of the thin, weak dentinal walls of the roots of developing teeth, it would be desirable to strengthen these roots to prevent accidental fracture. Several reports (77–81) have shown that the cervical area can be strengthened both before and after apexification procedures by bonding resin materials into the potentially fracture-prone areas. While long-term results are lacking, the initial observations are encouraging.

When apexification is done using MTA as an apical plug, the length of time during which the canal is exposed to calcium hydroxide is quite short – usually less than one month. Thus, there does not appear to be any advantage in placing a resin in the cervical area prior to apexification. Instead, the resin can be placed into the canal to a level well below the crest of alveolar bone *after* the MTA has cured (see Fig. 23.8I, J). A study by Hernandez et al. (81) showed that the new generation of dentin bonding systems appear to strengthen endodontically treated teeth to levels close to that of intact teeth. One can hope that the same holds true for immature teeth as well.

## Root fractures

Tittle et al. (67) also showed that MTA was an acceptable apical barrier that promoted apical healing. They pointed out that the induction of an apical hard tissue barrier was not necessary, since MTA itself used as an apical plug provides the necessary apical stop for root canal fillings (67).

Root fractures usually heal with either a hard tissue or a connective tissue union (or a combination of both) or by interposition of bone; a relatively small percentage of teeth with root fractures develop coronal canal infection leading to periradicular disease associated with the fracture site (76).

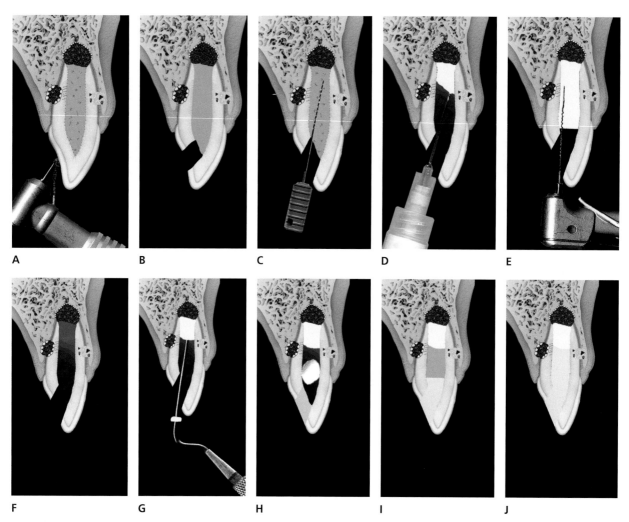

**Fig. 23.8** Apexification with MTA. A and B. The tooth is anesthetized (if needed) and isolated with a rubber dam and disinfected with sodium hypochlorite or chlorhexidine. Access is obtained to the root canal space in the usual manner. C. Carefully remove necrotic tissue to the level at which bleeding is first encountered (but not to exceed the length of the root canal). Instead of aggressively filing the thin root canal walls, it is preferable to gently brush the walls and use a liberal amount of irrigation with sodium hypochlorite. An effective 'brush' can be made by wrapping cotton around the shank of an endodontic file. D and E. Because the mechanical cleansing of the root canal is somewhat limited, and since removal of dentin from the already thin root canal walls will further weaken the tooth, disinfection must be obtained by the use of sodium hypochlorite and medication with calcium hydroxide. Keeping in mind that some formulations of calcium hydroxide can make the root canal dentin more brittle (21) it is important to limit the exposure to calcium hydroxide to one month or less (19). There is good evidence that the use of intracanal calcium hydroxide is very effective if left in place for up to two weeks (13). After placing the calcium hydroxide, a cotton pellet is placed over the calcium hydroxide, followed by a temporary restoration that will provide good protection for the period of time until the appointment for completing the treatment (maximum one month). F. At the next visit, again anesthetize (if needed), isolate with rubber dam, and re-enter the root canal. Gently remove the calcium hydroxide medication, flush the canal liberally and gently dry the canal, being careful not to stimulate bleeding from the level at which vital tissue is present. If bleeding inadvertently occurs, it can be stopped with the use of a cotton pellet coated with calcium hydroxide powder, following which the canal can again be dried with paper points. It is helpful to keep in mind that a totally dry canal is not required – MTA needs moisture to cure. With regards to any remnant of calcium hydroxide left on the root canal wall it does not affect the MTA seal (70). G. The placement of the mixed MTA material can be challenging for the dentist doing this for the first time. The consistency is similar to wet sand so handling can be difficult. But since it does not set immediately it can be removed by irrigation if needed. Positioning the material to the desired depth in the root canal starts with accurate determination of the desired apical level and preparing pluggers with the proper length marked with rubber stoppers. Place a small amount of the mixed MTA into the coronal chamber and use pluggers considerably smaller than the root canal diameter to carefully push the material toward apical level where vital tissue is present. An ultrasonic device can be used against the plugger to assist in compacting the MTA into the apical location. If the entire canal is empty because all the pulp tissue was necrotic, then the MTA should be placed to the apical opening of the root canal. H. Prior to placing the MTA in the root canal, a decision must be made about how much of the canal is to be filled with MTA. One can use a 'plug' of apical MTA (at least 4 mm) and fill the rest of the canal with gutta-percha (after the apical plug has cured), or fill the entire canal with MTA. In either approach, it is recommended to wait until the MTA has cured (a minimum of 4–6 hours) before completing the treatment. During the curing period, a moist cotton pellet is kept coronal to the MTA and the access opening is closed with a temporary filling. I and J. After the MTA has cured, the coronal access opening can be restored with a bonded composite resin. A tooth that has had an apexification procedure with MTA should be monitored radiographically and clinically. The desirable outcome is an asymptomatic tooth around which the alveolar supporting tissue is radiographically acceptable without evidence of resorption or periapical disease. Recent clinical reports show positive outcomes (68, 69, 71, 72, 74).

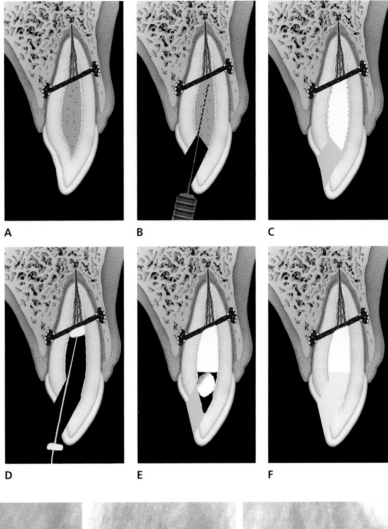

**Fig. 23.9** MTA used in the treatment of a root fracture with coronal pulp necrosis. A. The tooth that has been diagnosed as having pulpal/periradicular disease, usually evidenced by a circumradicular lesion associated with the fracture site, is anesthetized if needed and isolated with a rubber dam and disinfected with either sodium hypochlorite or chlorhexidine. B and C. A standard type coronal access to the root canal system is made. The necrotic tissue to the level of root fracture is removed; the canal is biomechanically prepared to that level and irrigated with sodium hypochlorite. Depending on the dentist's choice, the canal (to the fracture level only) can be filled with MTA immediately, or calcium hydroxide can be used as an interim medication between appointments. D, E and F. As with apexification cases, a decision must be made to either use a 'plug' of MTA at the fracture level of the coronal canal, or fill the entire coronal level with MTA. (See Apexification for suggestions for managing MTA.) In either case, it is recommended to let the MTA cure before either adding gutta-percha to the remainder of the coronal canal, followed by the access opening filling, or placing the access opening filling directly on top of the MTA if it was placed to the cervical level.

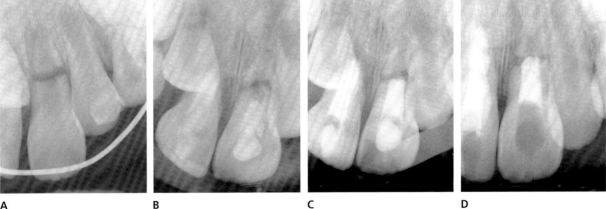

**Fig. 23.10** MTA used in root fracture treatment. A. A 9-year-old boy was in an accident in which the right central incisor was avulsed and the coronal segment of the root fractured left central incisor was also avulsed. Both teeth were replanted within a few minutes. B. Three weeks after replantation, calcium hydroxide was placed in the canals of both teeth. C. Two weeks later, MTA was placed in the canals, but only to the fracture line in the left incisor. D. Nine-month follow-up shows good repair.

The latter outcome is the only one requiring root canal treatment (or extraction).

When a tooth with root fracture develops pulpal and periradicular disease, root canal treatment has been recommended (77). Recently the various treatment procedures were compared based on a retrospective study of 98 teeth with root fractures (12). The best results were observed in situations in which only the coronal root canal segment was filled, following long term use of calcium hydroxide in

that segment to produce a hard tissue barrier at the canal opening at the fracture level. Considering the possible weakening effect on dentin from long term calcium hydroxide exposure, and the fact that calcium hydroxide treatment usually takes several months (3–24 months), it would be desirable to use a material that has no detrimental effect and can save time of treatment. MTA is such a material.

The recommended steps in using MTA for treating teeth with horizontal root fractures appear in Fig. 23.9. Monitoring the outcome of using MTA for root canal treatment of teeth with root fractures and pulp necrosis can be done radiographically and clinically (68). Desirable outcomes include radiographic evidence of healing if circumradicular disease was present at the level of fracture, and an asymptomatic, functioning tooth. At the present time, there is not enough information available to evaluate clinical outcomes of root canal treatments using MTA in teeth with horizontal root fractures. Individual case reports, however, are positive (68) (Fig. 23.10).

## Essentials

Mineral trioxide aggregate (MTA) may be used instead of calcium hydroxide in many endodontic procedures. MTA consists of a mixture of calcium silicate, bismuth oxide, calcium carbonate, calcium sulphate and calcium aluminate. Mixed with water it sets to an amorphous hard cement. MTA has the following properties which appear to be useful in its use as an endodontic material:

- It has during setting time a pH of 10.2–12.5, a characteristic which may be useful for hard tissue induction
- It requires a moist environment during setting, a characteristic useful in the apical area
- It creates a bacteria-tight seal
- It is biocompatible, implying that dentin and cementum may be formed on top of it

In dental traumatology MTA can be used in the following situations:

- Pulpotomy
- Apexification in luxated or replanted teeth
- Root fracture treatment

Long-term studies will demonstrate its potential for replacing calcium hydroxide in the endodontic procedures described.

## References

1. COMMISSION ON DENTAL ACCREDITATION. *Accreditation standards for advanced specialty education programs in endodontics.* American Dental Association, (Adopted December, 1983).
2. CVEK M. *Calcium hydroxide in treatment of traumatized teeth.* Knivsta, Sweden: Scania Dental, 1989.
3. CVEK M. A clinical report on partial pulpotomy and capping with calcium hydroxide in permanent incisors with complicated crown fracture. *J Endod* 1978;**4**:232–7.
4. CVEK M. Partial pulpotomy in crown fractured incisors: results 3 to 15 years after treatment. *Acta Stomatol Croat* 1993;**27**:167–73.
5. FUKS AB, CHOSACK A, KLEIN H, EIDELMAN E. Partial pulpotomy as a treatment alternative for exposed pulps in crown fractured permanent incisors. *Endod Dent Traumatol* 1987;**3**:100–2.
6. FRANK AL. Therapy for the divergent pulpless tooth by continued apical formation. *J Am Dent Assoc* 1966;**72**:87–93.
7. CVEK M. Treatment of non-vital permanent incisors with calcium hydroxide. Part I. Periodontal healing and apical closure of immature roots. *Odont Revy* 1972;**23**:27–44.
8. HEITHERSAY GS. Calcium hydroxide in the treatment of pulpless teeth with associated pathology. *J Br Endod Soc* 1975;**8**:74–93.
9. KEREKES K, HEIDE S, JACOBSEN I. Follow-up examination of endodontic treatment in traumatized juvenile incisors. *J Endod* 1980;**6**:744–8.
10. FEIGLIN B. Differences in apex formation during apexification with calcium hydroxide paste. *Endod Dent Traumatol* 1985;**1**:195–9.
11. SHEEHY EC, ROBERTS GJ. Use of calcium hydroxide for apical barrier formation and healing in non-vital immature permanent teeth: a review. *Br Dent J* 1997;**183**:241–6.
12. CVEK M, MEJÀRE I, ANDREASEN JO. Conservative endodontic treatment of teeth fractured in the middle or apical part of the root. *Dent Traumatol* 2004;**20**:261–9.
13. BYSTRÖM A, CLAESSON R, SUNDQVIST G. The antibacterial effect of camphorated paramonochlorophenol, camphorated phenol and calcium hydroxide in the treatment of infected root canals. *Endod Dent Traumatol* 1985;**1**:170–5.
14. SJÖGREN U, FIGDOR D, SPÅNGBERG L, SUNDQVIST G. The antimicrobial effect of calcium hydroxide as a short-term intracanal dressing. *Int Endod J* 1991;**24**:119–25.
15. HERMAN BW. *Biologische Wurzelbehandlung.* Frankfurt am Main: W Kramer & Co., 1936.
16. ZANDER FJ. Reaction of the pulp to calcium hydroxide. *J Dent Res* 1939;**6**:373–9.
17. SCHRÖDER U, GRANATH L-E. Early reaction of intact human teeth to calcium hydroxide following experimental pulpotomy and its significance to the development of hard tissue barrier. *Odont Revy* 1971;**22**:379–96.
18. CVEK M. Prognosis of luxated non-vital maxillary incisors treated with calcium hydroxide and filled with gutta percha. *Endod Dent Traumatol* 1992;**8**:45–55.
19. ANDREASEN JO, FARIK B, MUNKSGAARD EC. Long-term calcium hydroxide as a root canal dressing may increase risk of root fracture. *Dent Traumatol* 2002;**18**:134–7.
20. GRIGORATOS D, KNOWLES J, NG Y-L, GULABIVALA K. Effect of exposing dentine to sodium hypochlorite and calcium hydroxide on its flexural strength and elastic modulus. *Int Endod J* 2001;**34**:113–19.
21. YOLDAŞ O, DOGAN C, SEYDAOGLU G. The effect of two different calcium hydroxide combinations on root dentine microhardness. *Int Endod J* 2004;**37**:828–31.
22. PROROOT MTA, *Product Literature.* Tulsa, OK: Dentsply Tulsa Dental.
23. HOLLAND R, DE SOUZA V, NERY MJ, FARACO IM, Jr., BERNABÉ PFE, OTOBONI FILHO JA, DEZAN E Jr. Reaction of rat connective tissue to implanted dentin tubes filled with a white mineral trioxide aggregate. *Braz Dent J* 2002;**13**:23–6.
24. FERRIS DM, BAUMGARTNER JC. Perforation repair comparing two types of mineral trioxide aggregate. *J Endod* 2004;**30**:422–4.

25. Menezes R, Bramante CM, Letra A, Carvalho VG, Garcia RB. Histologic evaluation of pulpotomies in dog using two types of mineral trioxide aggregate and regular and white Portland cements as wound dressings. *Oral Surg Oral Med Oral Pathol Oral Radiol Endod* 2004;**98**:376–9.

26. Torabinejad M, Hong CU, McDonald F, Pitt Ford TR. Physical and chemical properties of a new root-end filling material. *J Endod* 1995;**21**:349–53.

27. Torabinejad M, Higa RK, McKendry DJ, Pitt Ford TR. Dye leakage of four root-end filling materials: Effects of blood contamination. *J Endod* 1994;**20**:159–63.

28. Torabinejad M, Hong CU, Pitt Ford TR, Kettering JD. Cytotoxicity of four root end filling materials. *J Endod* 1995;**21**:489–92.

29. Kettering JD, Torabinejad M. Investigation of mutagenicity of mineral trioxide aggregate and other commonly used root end filling materials. *J Endod* 1995;**21**:537–9.

30. Koh ET, Torabinejad M, Pitt Ford TR, Brady K, McDonald F. Mineral Trioxide Aggregate stimulates a biological response in human osteoblasts. *J Biomed Mater Res* 1997;**37**:432–9.

31. Torabinejad M, Pitt Ford TR, McKendry DJ, Abedi HR, Miller DA, Kariyawasam SP. Histologic assessment of mineral trioxide aggregate as a root-end filling material in monkeys. *J Endod* 1997;**23**:225–8.

32. Pitt Ford TR, Torabinejad M, Abedi HR, Bakland LK. Using mineral trioxide aggregate as a pulp-capping material. *J Am Dent Assoc* 1996;**127**:1491–4.

33. Koh ET, McDonald R, Pitt Ford TR, Torabinejad M. Cellular response to mineral trioxide aggregate. *J Endod* 1998;**24**:543–7.

34. Mitchell PJ, Pitt Ford TR, Torabinejad M, McDonald F. Osteoblast biocompatibility of mineral trioxide aggregate. *Biomaterials* 1999;**20**:167–73.

35. Keiser K, Johnson CC, Tipton DA. Cytotoxicity of mineral trioxide aggregate using human periodontal ligament fibroblasts. *J Endod* 2000;**26**:288–91.

36. Lee SJ, Monsef M, Torabinejad M. The sealing ability of a mineral trioxide aggregate for repair of lateral root perforations. *J Endod* 1993;**19**:541–4.

37. Torabinejad M, Rastegar AF, Kettering JD, Pitt Ford TR. Bacterial leakage of mineral trioxide aggregate as a root end filling material. *J Endod* 1995;**21**:109–21.

38. Bates CF, Carnes DL, Del Rio CE. Longitudinal sealing ability of mineral trioxide aggregate as a root-end filling material. *J Endod* 1996;**22**:575–8.

39. Murray PE, Hafez AA, Smith AJ, Windsor LJ, Cox CF. Histomorphometric analysis of odontoblast-like cell numbers and dentin bridge secretory activity following pulp exposure. *Int Endod J* 2003;**36**:106–16.

40. Faraco IM Jr, Holland R. Response of the pulp of dogs to capping with Mineral Trioxide Aggregate or a calcium hydroxide cement. *Dent Traumatol* 2001;**17**:163–6.

41. Perez AL, Spears R, Gutmann JL, Opperman LA. Osteoblasts and MG-63 osteosarcoma cells behave differently when in contact with ProRoot MTA and white MTA. *Int Endod J* 2003;**36**:564–70.

42. Friedland M, Rosado R. Mineral trioxide aggregate (MTA) solubility and porosity with different water-to-powder ratios. *J Endod* 2003;**29**:814–17.

43. Friedland M, Rosado R. MTA solubility: a long term study. *J Endod* 2005;**31**:376–9.

44. Ilapogu S, Bakland LK, Peterson J, Kim J. *The effect of NaOCL, Ca(OH)₂, MTA and MTAD on root dentin fracture resistance.* Master's thesis, Graduate School, Loma Linda University, 2004.

45. Abedi HR, Torabinejad M, Pitt Ford TR, Bakland LK. The use of mineral trioxide aggregate cement (MTA) as a direct pulp capping agent. *J Endod* 1996;**22**:199 (Abstract 44).

46. Myers K, Kaminski E, Lautenschlager E, Miller D. The effects of mineral trioxide aggregate on the pulp. *J Endod* 1996;**22**:198 (Abstract 39).

47. Junn DJ. *Quantitative assessment of dentin bridge formation following pulp-capping with Mineral Trioxide Aggregate.* Master's thesis, Graduate School, Loma Linda University, 2000.

48. Koh ET, Pitt Ford TR, Kariyawasam SP, Chen NN, Torabinejad M. Prophylactic treatment of dens evaginatus using Mineral Trioxide Aggregate. *J Endod* 2001;**27**:540–2.

49. Tziafas D, Pantelidou E, Alvanou A, Belibasakis G, Papadimitriou S. The dentinogenic effect of mineral trioxide aggregate (MTA) in short-term capping experiments. *Int Endod J* 2002;**35**:245–54.

50. Aeinenchi M, Eslami B, Ghanbariha M, Saffat AS. Mineral trioxide aggregate (MTA) and calcium hydroxide as pulp-capping agents in human teeth: a preliminary report. *Int Endod J* 2002;**36**:225–31.

51. Dominguez MS, Witherspoon DR, Gutmann JL, Opperman LA. Histological and scanning electron microscopy assessment of various vital pulp therapy materials. *J Endod* 2003;**29**:324–33.

52. Salako N, Joseph B, Ritwik P, Salonen J, John P, Junaid TA. Comparison of bioactive glass, mineral trioxide aggregate, ferric sulfate, and formocreosol as pulpotomy agents in rat molars. *Dent Traumatol* 2003;**19**:314–20.

53. Mitsiadis TA, Rahiotis C. Parallels between tooth development and repair: conserved molecular mechanisms following carious and dental injury. *J Dent Res* 2004;**83**:896–902.

54. Störmer K, Jacobsen I, Attramadal A. *How functional are root filled young permanent incisors? Nordisk Forening for Pedodonti.* Bergen, Norway: Aarsmöte, 1988.

55. Cox CF, Bergenholtz G, Heys DR, Syed SA, Fitzgerald M, Heys RJ. Pulp capping of dental pulp mechanically exposed to oral microflora: a 1–2 year observation of wound healing in monkeys. *J Oral Pathol* 1985;**14**:156–68.

56. Schuurs AHB, Gruythuysen RJM, Wesselink PR. Pulp capping with adhesive resin-based composite vs. calcium hydroxide: a review. *Endod Dent Traumatol* 2000;**16**:240–50.

57. Olsburgh S, Jacoby T, Krejci I. Crown fractures in the permanent dentition: pulpal and restorative considerations. *Dent Traumatol* 2002;**18**:103–15.

58. Costa CAS, Oliveira MF, Giro EMA, Hebling J. Biocompatibility of resin-based materials used as pulp-capping agents. *Int Endod J* 2003;**36**:831–9.

59. Hörsted-Bindslev P, Vilkinis V, Sidlauskas A. Direct capping of human pulps with dentin bonding system or calcium hydroxide cement. *Oral Surg Oral Med Oral Pathol Oral Radiol Endod* 2003;**96**:591–600.

60. Bakland LK, Andreasen JO. Dental traumatology: essential diagnosis and treatment planning. *Endodontic Topics* 2004;**7**:14–34.

61. Linsuwanont P. MTA apexification combined with conventional root canal retreatment. *Aust Endod J* 2003;**29**:45–9.

62. Finucane D, Kinirons MJ. Non-vital immature permanent incisors: factors that may influence treatment outcome. *Endod Dent Traumatol* 1999;**15**:273–7.

63. Kleier DJ, Barr ES. A study of endodontically apexified teeth. *Endod Dent Traumatol* 1991;**7**:112–17.

64. Coviello J, Brilliant JD. A preliminary clinical study on the use of tricalcium phosphate as an apical barrier. *J Endod* 1979;**5**:6–13.

65. Pitts DL, Jones JE, Oswald RJ. A histologic comparison of calcium hydroxide plugs and dentin plugs used for control of gutta-percha root canal filling material. *J Endod* 1984;**10**:283–93.

66. Shabahang S, Torabinejad M, Boyne PP, Abedi H, McMillan P. A comparative study of root-end induction using osteogenic protein-1, calcium hydroxide, and mineral trioxide aggregate in dogs. *J Endod* 1999;**25**:1–5.

67. Tittle KW, Farley J, Linkhardt T, Torabinejad M. Apical closure induction using bone growth factors and mineral trioxide aggregate. *J Endod* 1996;**22**:198 (Abstract 41).

68. Schwartz RS, Mauger M, Clement DJ, Walker WA. Mineral trioxide aggregate: a new material for endodontics. *J Am Dent Assoc* 1999;**130**:967–75.

69. Shabahang S, Torabinejad M. Treatment of teeth with open apices using mineral trioxide aggregate. *Pract Periodont Aesthet Dent* 2000;**12**:315–20.

70. Hachmeister DR, Schindler WG, Walker WA, Thomas DD. The sealing ability and retention characteristics of Mineral Trioxide Aggregate in a model of apexification. *J Endod* 2002;**28**:386–90.

71. Giuliani V, Baccetti T, Pace R, Pagavino G. The use of MTA in teeth with necrotic pulps and open apices. *Dent Traumatol* 2002;**18**:217–21.

72. Steinig TH, Regan JD, Gutmann JL. The use and predictable placement of mineral trioxide aggregate in one-visit apexification cases. *Aust Endod J* 2003;**29**: 34–42.

73. Lawley GR, Schindler WG, Walker WA, Kolodrubetz D. Evaluation of ultrasonically placed MTA and fracture resistance with intracanal composite resin in a model of apexification. *J Endod* 2004;**30**:167–72.

74. Maroto M, Barbería E, Planells P, Vera V. Treatment of a non-vital immature incisor with mineral trioxide aggregate (MTA). *Dent Traumatol* 2003;**19**:165–9.

75. Andreasen JO, Hjörting-Hansen E. Intraalveolar root fractures. Radiographic and histologic study of 50 cases. *J Oral Surg* 1967;**25**:414–26.

76. Cvek M. Treatment of non-vital permanent incisors with calcium hydroxide IV. Periodontal healing and closure of the root canal in the coronal fragment of teeth with intraalveolar fracture and vital apical fragment. *Odont Revy* 1974;**25**:239–46.

77. Trope M, Maltz DO, Tronstad L. Resistance to fracture of restored endodontically treated teeth. *Endod Dent Traumatol* 1985;**1**:108–11.

78. Rabie G, Trope M, Garcia C, Tronstad L. Strengthening and restoration of immature teeth with an acid-etch resin technique. *Endod Dent Traumatol* 1985;**1**:246–56.

79. Rabie G, Trope M, Tronstad L. Strengthening of immature teeth during long term endodontic therapy. *Endod Dent Traumatol* 1986;**2**:43–7.

80. Katebzadeh N, Dalton C, Trope M. Strengthening immature teeth during and after apexification. *J Endod* 1988;**24**:256–9.

81. Hernandez R, Bader S, Boston D, Trope M. Resistance to fracture of endodontically treated premolars restored with new generation dentin bonding systems. *Int Endod J* 1994;**27**:281–4.

82. Sturz K, Peterson J, Bakland LK. *The effect of different commercially available calcium hydroxide pastes on root dentin fracture resistance.* Master's thesis, Graduate School, Loma Linda University, 2006.

# 24

# Orthodontic Management of the Traumatized Dentition

O. Malmgren & B. Malmgren

Treatment planning for patients with traumatized teeth involves a detailed evaluation of both the prognosis for the injured teeth and treatment of an eventual malocclusion. A coordinated treatment plan, incorporating clinical and radiographic findings of healing and of complications must be established before orthodontic treatment is initiated. This plan should be based on a realistic evaluation of the prognosis for the injured teeth.

## Diagnosis and treatment planning

### Preventive orthodontics

Dental injuries in the mixed and permanent dentitions are most frequent in children from 8 to 9 years of age and most injuries involve the upper incisors. Boys are injured twice as often as girls. Patients with an increased overjet are at significantly greater risk of dental injury (1–22). One study has shown that an increase of the overjet from 0–3 mm to 3–6 mm doubles the extent of traumatic dental injuries. With an overjet exceeding 6 mm, the severity is tripled (20, 139). An additional trauma factor is insufficient lip closure, which often leaves the upper incisors unprotected (10–11, 14, 137–140). Many authors claim that this is the most important factor (141). Patients treated for dental injuries often sustain repeated trauma to the teeth (13), particularly if the first trauma occurs before the age of 11 years (142).

Considering the frequency of traumatic dental injuries in school-age children, it is apparent that the majority of children with increased maxillary overjet will have sustained a traumatic dental injury prior to school-leaving age (13, 20, 23–25). The treatment of increased maxillary overjet should therefore begin early, as a precaution against traumatic dental injuries (81–82, 143). If this is not possible, the child should be provided with a mouthguard during contact sports. Such a mouthguard can even be combined with a fixed orthodontic appliance (see Chapter 30).

### Primary dentition

Avulsion or extraction of primary incisors can lead to drifting of adjacent teeth as well as disturbances in eruption of the permanent successors (145). Early loss of primary teeth sometimes leads to delayed eruption of the permanent successors often in a more labial position (26–28). Conversely, loss of primary teeth at a later stage of development can lead to premature eruption of permanent teeth (27). However, these disturbances do not usually lead to loss of space and consequently do not require space maintenance or other orthodontic treatment (29).

### Mixed dentition

To minimize the risk of injuries in patients with proclined upper incisors, orthodontic treatment should be planned at the mixed dentition stage (144). Treatment of skeletal and dento-alveolar deviations, particularly in patients with Angle Class II, division 1 and 2 malocclusions, should be based on individual growth rate (30).

In the case of accidental loss of one or more incisors, it should be decided at the mixed dentition stage whether to partially or completely close the space or to maintain it. Rapid mesial tipping of the incisor and midline shift may jeopardize later careful treatment planning. This is particularly true during eruption of the upper canines. It is therefore important to use a space maintainer to avoid such side effects (Fig. 24.1).

In patients with skeletal deviations, extraoral forces can be used. But in some Class II division 1 cases with accidental loss of one or more permanent incisors, it may be better to leave the molars in their distoocclusion and close the space anteriorly. Mesial movement of lateral incisors to substitute a lost central incisor can however be complicated because of the anatomy and inclination of the lateral (see p. 691).

In patients with normal skeletal sagittal relations without crowding, it is usually better to postpone orthodontic therapy until the permanent dentition stage.

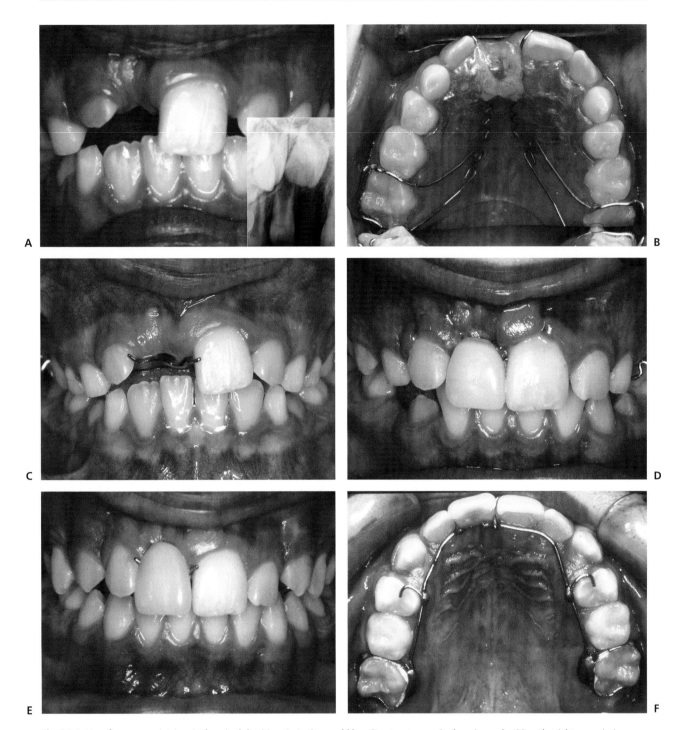

**Fig. 24.1** Use of a space maintainer in the mixed dentition. A. An 8-year-old boy. Due to a trauma in the primary dentition, the right upper incisor was malformed, and adjacent teeth were tilting towards the area of the impacted incisor. The radiograph shows the condition at 8 years of age. Due to the immature root development of the lateral incisor, surgery was postponed for 2 years. B. A removable plate with Adam's clasps and fingersprings was inserted for uprighting the tilted incisors. Due to large difference in incisor width and wide apical base conditions, space closure was not indicated. C and D. When the teeth had been up righted, a prosthetic tooth was fitted to the plate. E and F. After eruption of the first bicuspids, and during eruption of the canines, a lingual arch was soldered to molar bands. Occlusal stops on the first bicuspids and stops on both sides of a prosthetic tooth were used. When the upper canines were fully erupted, an acid-etch bridge was constructed.

## Permanent dentition

If trauma occurs in the permanent dentition, it must be determined whether any growth potential remains. Especially in cases with skeletal deviations, it is essential to coordinate the remaining growth potential with the proposed orthodontic treatment.

## Factors in treatment planning

A treatment plan that involves the various dental specialities (i.e. pedodontics, endodontics, oral surgery, orthodontics and general dentistry) must be based on a realistic evalua-

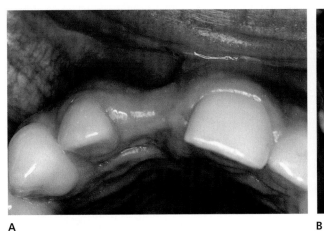 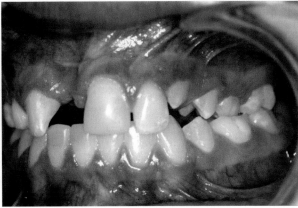

**Fig. 24.2** Reduced volume of the alveolar bone in buccal/palatinal direction after loss of a permanent tooth. A. An 18-year-old boy whose left upper incisor was extracted conventionally at the age of 12 years. B. A 10-year-old girl whose left upper incisor was avulsed two years earlier.

tion of orthodontic treatment possibilities and optimal treatment of the traumatized dentition. Before orthodontic treatment of a traumatized dentition is initiated, a number of factors should be evaluated. It must also be considered that orthodontic movement of teeth with less favorable prognosis might be justified to preserve the alveolar crest during growth of the jaws (146). Even an uncomplicated extraction of a tooth leads to loss of alveolar bone especially in the labio-lingual direction which makes insertion of future implants difficult (Fig. 24.2).

## Treatment sequence and timing

Sequence and timing of treatment is essential in all dentitions. Dental injuries to the primary teeth most often occur at 2 to 4 years of age. There is a close relationship between the apices of the primary incisors and the permanent successors. Thus a trauma to the primary dentition may cause disturbances in development and eruption of the permanent successors (Fig. 24.3).

In general, orthodontic treatment should be initiated in the mixed dentition. In cases of trauma at an early age, treatment can be shorter and performed with less complicated appliances if the age of the patient as well as the dental and skeletal development and maturity are considered (Fig. 24.4).

## Observation periods prior to orthodontic treatment

### Crown and crown-root fractures

Crown fractures and crown-root fractures without pulpal involvement have a good prognosis if properly treated. An observation period of about 3 months prior to initiation of treatment is sufficient.

A crown and crown-root fracture with pulpal involvement can be treated orthodontically after partial pulpectomy, once a hard tissue barrier has been established. As a

rule, such a barrier can be diagnosed radiographically 3 months after treatment.

### Root fractures

While an observation period of 2 years has been recommended before orthodontic movement of root-fractured teeth (31), clinical experience indicates that most complications (e.g. pulp necrosis) occur during the 1st year after the trauma (83–84, 147–148). Thus the observation period may be shortened if no complications occur.

### Luxated teeth

After luxation of teeth, a number of complications (e.g. pulp necrosis, root resorption and loss of marginal bone) may occur. Clinical experience indicates an observation period of at least 3 months after a mild injury (e.g. concussion and subluxation).

Pulp canal obliteration as a consequence of trauma indicates repair of the traumatized pulp. However, a repeated trauma or a heavy orthodontic force may cause further damage to the pulp.

After a moderate or severe luxation injury, endodontic treatment is most often needed. Then orthodontic movement should be postponed until there is radiographic evidence of healing. A follow-up period with clinical and radiographic controls of the endodontic treatment during 3 to 4 years has been advocated (Chapter 22). If orthodontic treatment is indicated, however, it is *not* reasonable to wait such a long time before start or continuing treatment in most cases. But it is advisable from clinical experience to delay start of the orthodontic movement until a permanent root filling has been performed.

## Endodontically-treated teeth

The risk of root resorption during movement of endodontically treated teeth has been debated for years. A slightly

### Fig. 24.3 Treatment sequence and timing
A 2-year-old boy with both central primary incisors intruded.

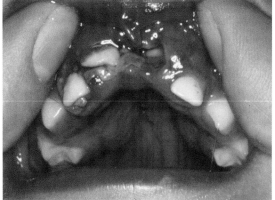
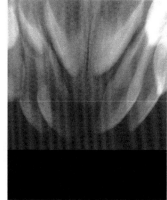

### Follow-up at 6 years of age
Both upper incisors and the right lateral are dilacerated and the right lower incisor is tipped distally.

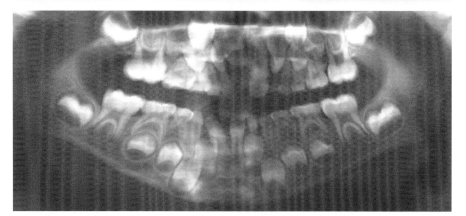

### Clinical appearance at 8 years of age
To avoid involvement of the pulp and ensure further root development, the hypomineralized crowns are restored. Note midline shift in the lower jaw.

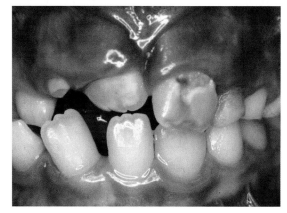
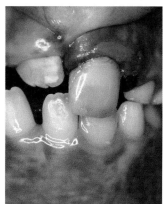

### Panoramic radiograph at 11 years of age
Due to a second traumatic injury the left upper incisor has been treated endodontically. Crowding in the right sides in both jaws is seen. Auto-transplantation of the second right upper premolar and the first right lower premolar is decided. Note difference in root development of the premolars.

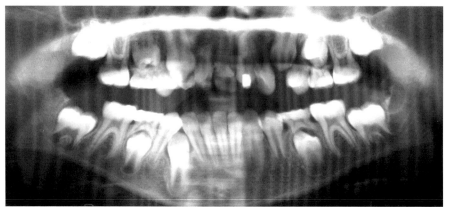

**Extraction of the right upper incisor**
Note crown dilaceration.

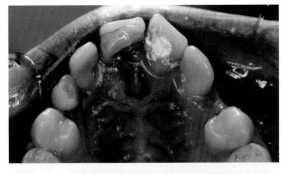
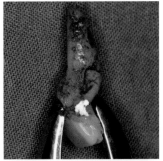

**Extraction of the right lower first premolar**

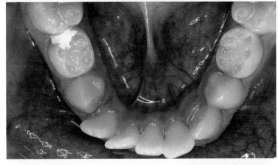
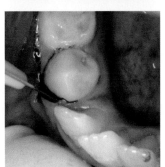

**Right lower first premolar transplanted into right central incisor position**
Radiograph two months after auto-transplantation. Note damage to the lateral.

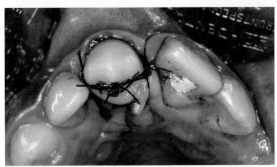
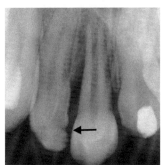

**Right upper second premolar transplanted into left central incisor position**
The first transplant restored with composite as well as the hypomineralized lateral. Radiograph 1 year after the first autotransplantation.

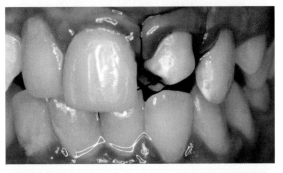
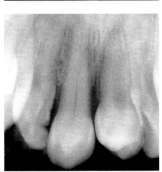

**Condition 3 years after first auto-transplantation**
No orthodontic treatment performed.

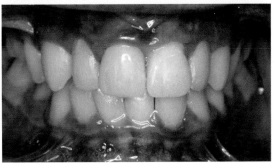
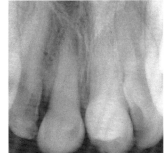

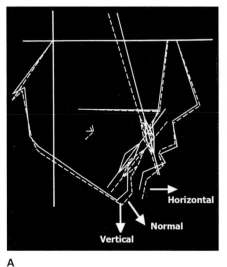
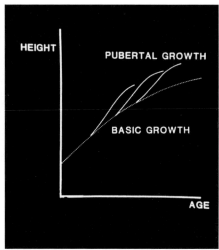

**Fig. 24.4** Skeletal development of the face as well as the skeletal maturation are important factors to consider. A. Annual profile radiographs can be used to evaluate the growth intensity and direction of the jaws. B. Annual standing height measurements can be used to evaluate the actual growth period of the patient; normal growth or pubertal growth spurt.

**A**

**B**

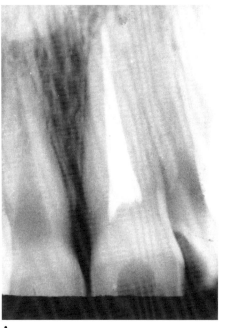
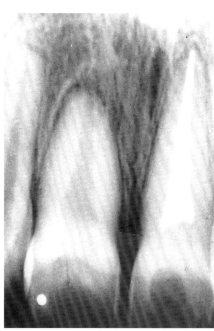

**Fig. 24.5** Response of a vital and a root filled tooth to orthodontic movement. The patient had a Class II div. 1 malocclusion and was treated with fixed appliances for 18 months. A. Condition before orthodontic treatment. Both central incisors sustained traumatic dental injury. As a result, the left central incisor was treated endodontically due to pulp necrosis. B. After orthodontic treatment, the left central incisor demonstrates slight apical root resorption and the right central incisor, with a vital pulp, severe root resorption. Both teeth were moved orthodontically in the same manner.

**A**

**B**

greater frequency of root resorption after orthodontic treatment has been reported in endodontically-treated compared to vital teeth by Wickwire et al. (32). Remington et al. (85) found that root-filled teeth sometimes resorb less than their vital antimeres (Fig. 24.5). Even though these differences were statistically significant they were minimal (0.7 mm) (85). Similar observations have been reported by Spurrier et al. (86). Mirabella and Artun (149) claim that endodontic treatment is a preventive factor. A few root-filled teeth, however, resorb for unknown reasons (Fig. 24.6). An experimental study by Hunter et al. (138) showed no difference in the frequency of root resorption after orthodontic movement when comparing vital and endodontically-treated teeth. In a comprehensive literature review, Hamilton and Gutman conclude that minimal resorptive/remodeling changes occur apically in teeth that are being moved orthodontically and that are well cleaned, shaped and three-dimensionally root canal obturated (Fig. 24.5) (150). These

conclusions coincide with the authors´ observation that root-filled teeth without signs of already existing root resorption can normally be moved without extensive root resorption (91).

## Pulp canal obliterated teeth

Pulp canal obliteration is a common sequel after luxation of immature teeth. It has been debated whether these teeth can be moved without losing pulp vitality or severe apical resorptions. This has been examined in a clinical study of 9 teeth by the author. No apical resorptions or radiolucency were seen (91). Obliteration is also always seen after auto-transplantation of immature teeth and even those teeth can be moved with only a limited risk of negative effects (see p. 689) (122). However it is essential to closely monitor obliterated teeth during orthodontic movement.

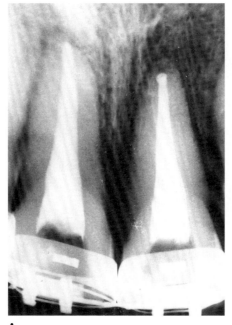 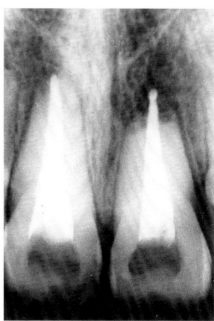

**Fig. 24.6** Different responses to orthodontic movement of 2 endodontically treated teeth. Both teeth were moved in the same manner. The patient had a Class II div. 1 malocclusion and was treated with fixed appliances for 19 months. A. Before orthodontic treatment. Both central incisors were traumatically injured and root filled. B. After orthodontic treatment, the right central incisor demonstrates slight root resorption, while the left central incisor demonstrates unusually extensive root resorption.

**A**                                         **B**

## Root surface resorption (external root resorption)

Damage to the periodontal ligament after a trauma can result in three types of external root resorption: surface resorption, inflammatory resorption and replacement resorption.

*Surface resorption (repair-related resorption)* implies a self-limiting resorption process, which is repaired with new cementum. Teeth with minor surface resorptions can be moved orthodontically with a prognosis similar to that of uninjured teeth.

*Inflammatory resorption (infection-related resorption)* implies a rapid resorption of both cementum and dentin with inflammation of adjacent periodontal tissue. This type of resorption is related to an infected and necrotic pulp and can usually be seen 3 to 6 weeks after injury. It is essential that proper endodontic treatment be initiated immediately. Arrest of the inflammatory resorption can be seen in about 96% of cases (87) (see Chapter 22, p. 635). Orthodontic treatment should be postponed until radiographic healing is seen and at least one year should elapse before orthodontic treatment is instituted. Teeth with evidence of root resorption appear to be more liable to further resorption during orthodontic movement (32–35, 88, 91) (Fig. 24.7). This does not necessarily contraindicate orthodontic treatment; but special care should be taken to avoid excessive pressure during movement (Fig. 24.8).

*Replacement resorption (ankylosis)* implies fusion of the alveolar bone and root substance and disappearance of the periodontal ligament space. This type of resorption is progressive, eventually involving the entire root. The rate of resorption varies with the degree of damage of the periodontal ligament and age and growth rate of the patient (168).

In children and adolescents, the ankylosed tooth prevents growth of the jaw segment. The ankylosed tooth may thus become infraoccluded, permitting the adjacent teeth to tilt towards the affected tooth. Ankylosed teeth do not respond to orthodontic movement (Fig. 24.9). This resorption entity can be recognized clinically during the first 2 months after injury and most often within 1 year after a severe trauma. The tooth becomes immobile and percussion produces a high tone compared with adjacent uninjured teeth. If the patient is in a period of rapid growth and the degree of infraocclusion is more than $1/4$ of the crown length, the tooth should be removed. A special extraction technique is then needed to avoid excessive loss of alveolar bone (90) (see page 700).

## General treatment principles

During orthodontic treatment, special care should be taken to avoid excessive pressure on traumatized teeth to reduce the risk of root surface resorption.

It is necessary to carefully study the anatomy of the roots before treatment (Fig. 24.10). An assessment of the radiographic outline of the apex provides useful information regarding the risk of root resorption during orthodontic treatment (88) (Fig. 24.11). Roots with pipette shaped, blunt or bent apices are more liable to root resorption than teeth with normal root forms (Figs 24.12 and 24.13). A root resorption index permits quantitative assessment of root conditions prior to treatment and can be used for evaluation of further resorption (88) (Fig. 24.14).

It has been shown that movement into labial or lingual cortical bone can initiate extensive root resorption; it is therefore important to establish the borders of the cortical bone, based on profile radiographs, prior to initiation of orthodontic therapy (37–38, 93) (Fig. 24.15). Particularly if

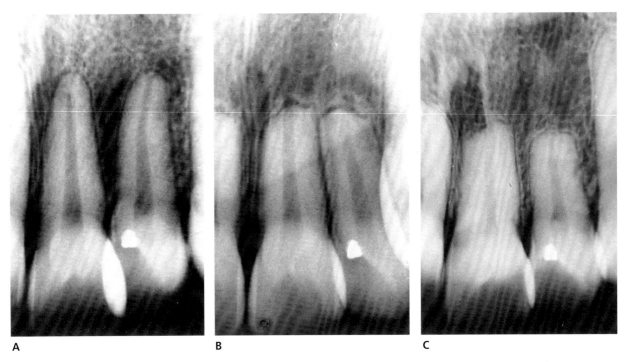

**A**          **B**          **C**

**Fig. 24.7** Vital teeth with signs of root resorption before orthodontic treatment. A. The lateral incisor shows an irregular root contour due to root resorption prior to initiation of orthodontic treatment. B. Conditions after orthodontic treatment with fixed appliances for 20 months. Extensive root resorption of the incisors has taken place. C. At a 10-year follow-up, slight rounding of the resorbed root surface can be seen. Otherwise, there has been no progression of the root resorption.

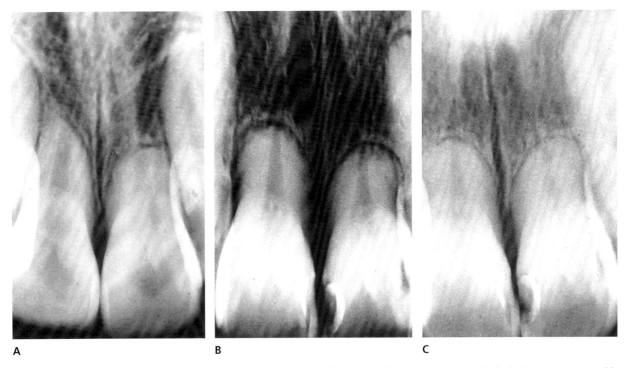

**A**          **B**          **C**

**Fig. 24.8** Patient with Class II div 1 malocclusion and severe root resorption of both central incisors due to trauma. Orthodontic treatment is possible if it is performed carefully. A. Condition before orthodontic treatment. Activator treatment was carried out for 2 years. B. Seven years later, slight rounding of the root surfaces is seen. Secondary crowding developed later, and 4 first premolars were extracted. Fixed appliances were then used for 18 months. C. Control after 20 years. There has been no progression of the resorptive process.

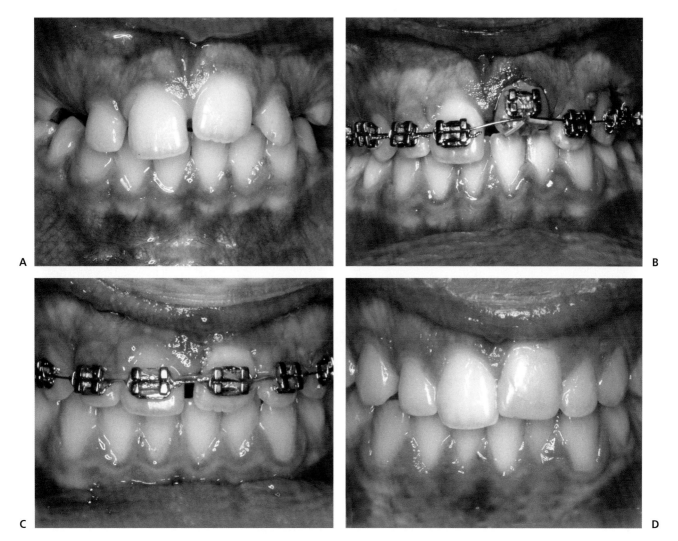

**Fig. 24.9** Treatment failure due to ankylosis. A. An 11-year-old girl with an ankylosed left upper incisor in infraposition. B. An orthodontic appliance with an extrusion force was applied. C. 6 months later, there is intrusion of all adjacent teeth. D. Relapse after treatment. Despite composite build-up, the outcome is a failure.

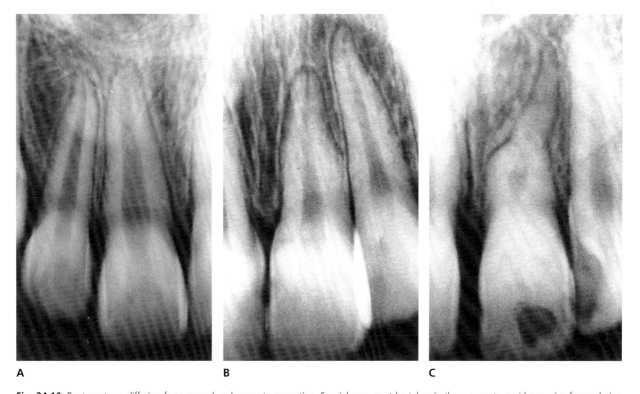

**Fig. 24.10** Root anatomy differing from normal and prone to resorption. Special care must be taken in these cases to avoid excessive forces during tooth movement. A. Incisors with slightly irregular apical root contour. B. Concavity along the distal surface of the root (surface resorption). C. Root malformation.

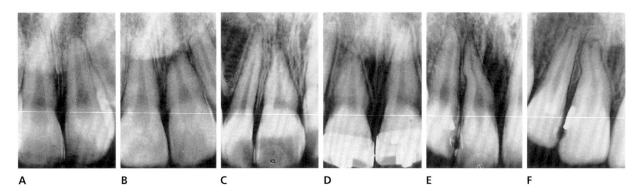

**Fig. 24.11** Root resorption developing during orthodontic treatment in teeth with abnormal root anatomy. A. Slightly irregular apical contour of a left central incisor. B. Marked root resorption after treatment. C. Right central incisor with a concavity along the distal root surface. D. Root resorption seen after treatment. E. Malformed root of a right central incisor. F. Marked root resorption is evident after treatment. All patients were treated with fixed appliances for 18–21 months.

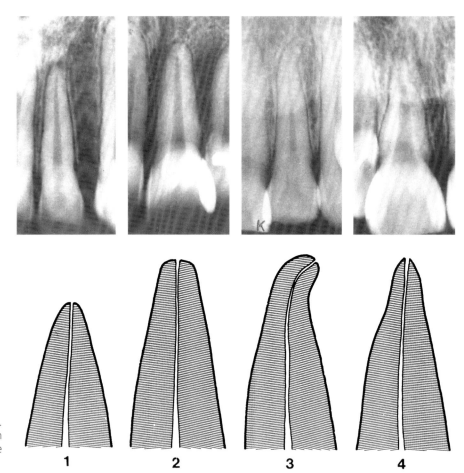

**Fig. 24.12** Deviating root forms. 1. Short root. 2. Blunt root. 3. Root with apical bend. 4. Root with apical pipette shape.

the alveolar crest is narrow, resorption can easily occur (Fig. 24.15B). During retraction of the maxillary incisors, it is necessary to avoid juxtaposition with the palatal or buccal cortical plates (Fig. 24.15C, D). In many situations, the incisors are protrusive and require palatal root torque during retraction. It is then advisable to perform this root movement in the roomier cancellous bone than in the compact cortical bone of the maxillary alveolus (Fig. 24.15E). It is therefore desirable to use a treatment approach that can intrude the anterior segment at the onset of orthodontic therapy (39).

There are some factors, which, alone or in combination, can contribute to the development of root resorption. The importance of forces has been discussed for years. Most authors consider only heavy forces to be responsible for root resorption (33–34, 40–41). Intensity and duration of forces are, however, also of great importance (94).

Continuous heavy forces could cause resorption (42). Prolonged tipping can also cause resorption of a tooth as well as resorption of the alveolar crest, especially in adult patients (42, 95). Thus, there is no single explanation

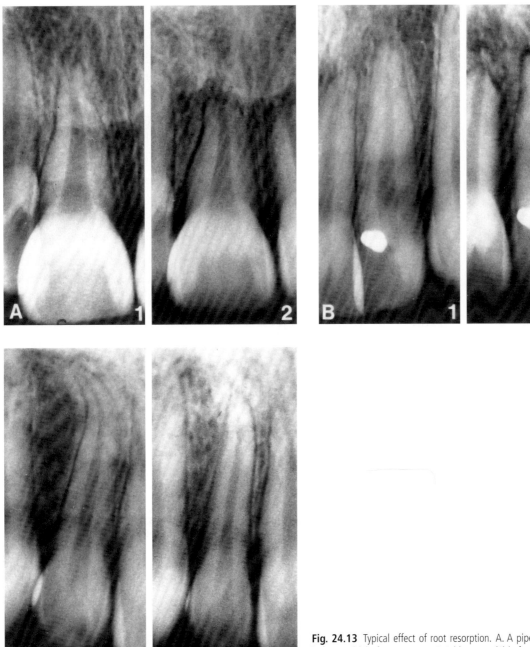

**Fig. 24.13** Typical effect of root resorption. A. A pipette-shaped root (1) before and (2) after treatment. B. A blunt root (1) before and (2) after treatment. C. A root with an apical bend (1) before and (2) after treatment.

as to why certain teeth resorb severely; but one factor often mentioned in the literature is a previous dental trauma.

In a study of root resorption after orthodontic treatment of traumatized teeth, 55 traumatized incisors were analyzed (91). All teeth had been examined at the time of injury by experienced pedodontists at the Eastman Institute in Stockholm according to standardized procedures. The types of injury were: crown fracture in 18 teeth and periodontal injury in 37 (i.e. concussion, subluxation or luxation). Signs of root resorption before and after treatment were registered with scores from 0 to 4 (Fig. 24.16).

After orthodontic treatment, 49% of the traumatized incisors showed an irregular root contour, 32% minor

resorption, 15% moderate root resorption and only 4% (2 teeth) showed severe resorption. The resorptions were more frequent in teeth with luxation injuries, but the difference was not significant (Fig. 24.16, top). The extent of root resorption was the same in the traumatized and in the contra lateral control uninjured teeth in the same individual.

The extent of root resorption in the traumatized teeth was also compared with that of uninjured incisors in a group of 55 consecutive patients treated with fixed appliances (edgewise and Begg technique) and extraction of 4 first bicuspids. No significant difference was found in the tendency towards root resorption of traumatized and uninjured teeth (Fig. 24.16). However, a few teeth that exhibited resorption

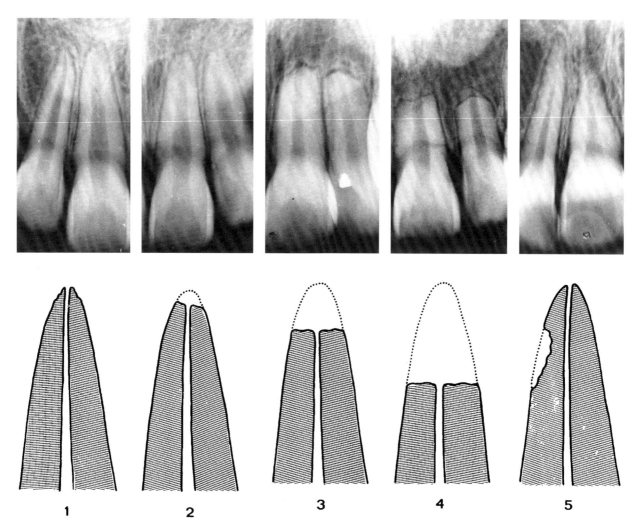

**Fig. 24.14** Root resorption index used for quantitative assessment of root resorption. Score description: 1. Irregular root contour; 2. Root resorption apically amounting to less than 2 mm of the original root length; 3. Root resorption apically amounting to from 2 mm to one-third of the original root length; 4. Root resorption exceeding one-third of the original root length; 5. Lateral root resorption.

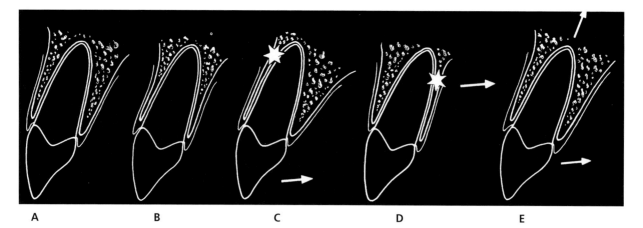

**Fig. 24.15** Schematic drawing illustrating the importance of examining the relation between the position of the root and cortical bone prior to ortho-dontic treatment. A. An alveolar crest with a wide cancellous bone area. B. An alveolar crest with a narrow cancellous bone area. C. Lingual tipping of the crown moves the root into juxtaposition with the buccal cortical plate, which can initiate root resorption. D. Lingual root torque during retraction can move the root into juxtaposition with the palatal cortical bone, which can initiate root resorption. E. Intrusion of an incisor into the roomier can-cellous part of the bone area is probably the best procedure.

**Fig. 24.16** Degree of root resorption after orthodontic treatment of 55 traumatized teeth. From MALMGREN et al. (91) 1982.

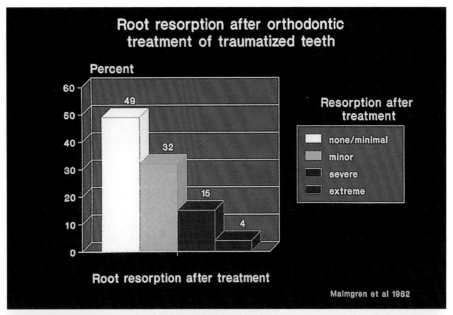

Root resorption in 264 incisors without trauma treated with edgewise technique.

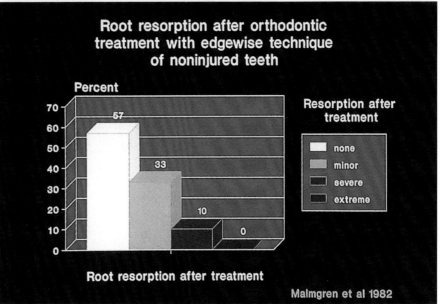

Root resorption in 176 incisors without trauma, treated with Begg technique.

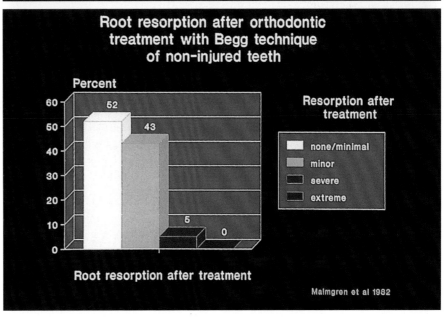

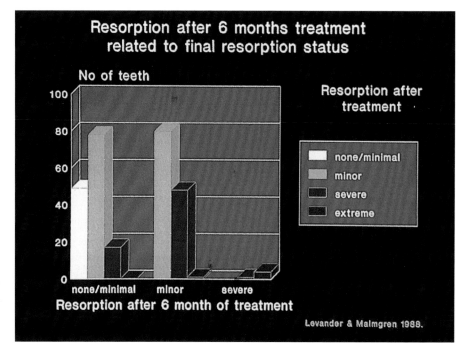

**Fig. 24.17** Frequency of root resorption after orthodontic treatment with fixed appliances in a study of 390 incisors. The radiographic examinations were performed before treatment, after 6 to 9 months and finally after completion of treatment. The index scores presented in Fig. 24.14 were used. From LEVANDER & MALMGREN (88) 1988.

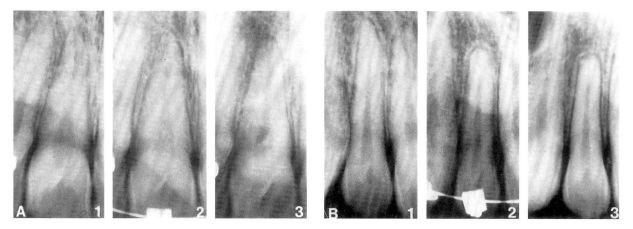

**Fig. 24.18** Root resorption after completion of treatment in relation to initial resorption status. A. (1) Status before treatment. (2) After 6 months there is no resorption. (3) At the end of treatment, minor resorption and blunting of the apex is seen. B. (1) Before treatment. (2) After 6 months, minor resorption is seen. (3) At the end of treatment, severe resorption is seen.

before orthodontic treatment were severely resorbed during treatment.

The risk of root resorption during orthodontic treatment with fixed appliances was studied in relation to initial resorption 6–9 months after start of treatment in 98 consecutive patients. The mean treatment time was 19 months. A total of 390 incisors were examined (Fig. 24.17). The same type of index as illustrated in Fig. 24.14 was used. The results are illustrated in Figs 24.17 and 24.18. Minor resorption was found in 33% of the teeth and severe resorption in 1%. No severe resorption after treatment was found in any teeth without resorption after initial treatment (i.e. 6–9 months). In teeth with an irregular root contour, 12% showed severe resorption at the end of treatment. In teeth with minor resorption after initial treatment, 38% showed severe resorption. Extreme resorption was registered in 4 of 5 teeth with severe resorption after initial treatment.

The conclusions are: if a severe resorption is found after

half a year of treatment with a fixed appliance, there is a high risk of extreme resorption at the end of treatment; minor resorption at that time indicates a moderate risk of severe resorption; irregular root contour indicates a limited risk of severe resorption at the end of treatment.

Therefore, regular radiographic controls are necessary in order to check if any root resorption occurs or increases during treatment. It is advisable to make the first control 6–9 months after the start of treatment. If signs of root resorption are seen, controls every 2 months are recommended. A pause in treatment for about 3 months can reduce the risk of further resorption (89) (Fig. 24.19). Marked root resorption diagnosed at this time should lead to re-evaluation of the treatment goal.

Thus, in trauma patients it is imperative to start treatment with light, preferably intermittent forces, avoid prolonged tipping, aim at a limited goal and in this way achieve a shorter treatment procedure.

**Fig. 24.19** Root resorption in relation to two orthodontic treatment regimens. Material of 62 upper incisors was studied. In all teeth, a minor apical root resorption was observed after the initial 6 to 9 months of treatment with a fixed appliance. In 20 patients (group I) treatment continued according to the original plan and 20 patients had a treatment pause of 2 to 3 months (group II). There was significantly less root resorption in patients treated with a pause than in those without. From LEVANDER et al. (89) 1994.

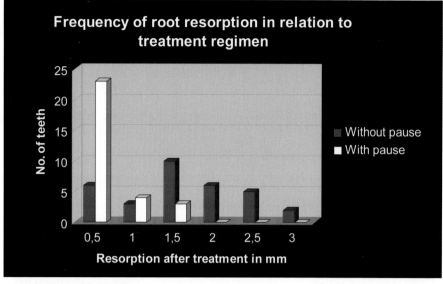

**Continuous treatment**
An upper lateral incisor before treatment; after 6 months when a minor resorption is seen; and at the end of treatment when the resorption is severe. Treatment was performed without pause.

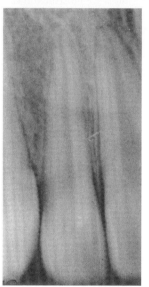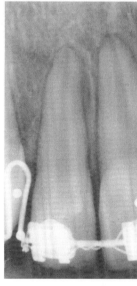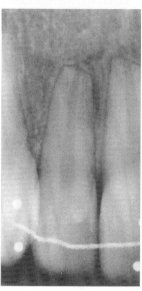

**Treatment with pause**
An upper incisor before treatment; after 6 months when a minor resorption is seen; and at the end of treatment, when no further resorption is observed.

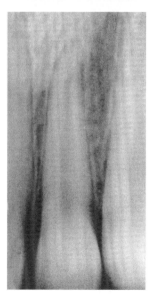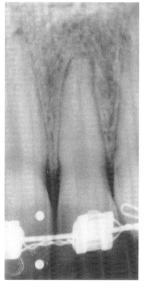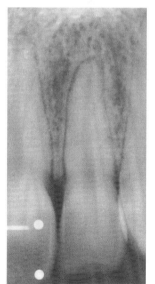

In the following, orthodontic treatment of various types of dental injuries will be discussed.

## Specific treatment principles for various trauma types

### Crown and crown-root fractures

It is essential that, even in teeth with slight injuries such as uncomplicated crown fractures, tests for sensibility and a radiographic examination are made before the start of orthodontic treatment. When in doubt as to the clinical condition of the pulp, a 3-month observation period with repeated sensibility tests is recommended before initiating orthodontic treatment.

A complicated crown fracture implies involvement of enamel, dentin and pulp. A complicated crown-root fracture also involves the root cement.

Capping of the pulp or partial pulpotomy on proper indications followed by a calcium hydroxide cover will in most cases preserve the vitality of the pulp (see Chapter 22, p. 600).

It is recommended that orthodontic movement of the injured immature teeth is postponed until root development is seen to resume. Clinical and radiographic controls should be carried out after 6 months, 1 year and 2 years.

### *Extrusion of crown-root and cervical root fractures*

To complete a crown restoration of a tooth with a crown-root or a cervical root fracture, it is often necessary to extrude the fractured root orthodontically (69–74, 97–103). Different types of fractures amenable to orthodontic extrusion are illustrated in Figs 24.20 and 24.21.

**Fig. 24.20 Rapid extrusion of a crown-root fractured central incisor**
A steel hook is cemented in the root canal. Traction with an elastic thread is applied axially.

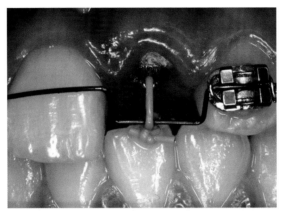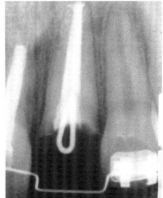

**Condition after 4 weeks**
The root is fully extruded and retained with a stainless steel ligature wire.

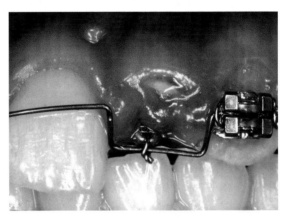

**Condition after raising a muco-periosteal flap**
No coronal shift of the bone margin is found. Note the rapid remodelling of bone surrounding the apex.

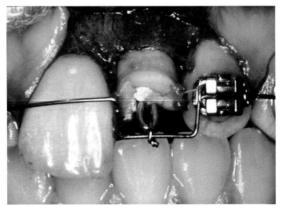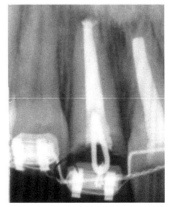

**Fig. 24.21 Orthodontic extrusion of teeth with crown-root fractures reaching below the marginal level**
Oblique crown-root fracture below the marginal bone buccally.

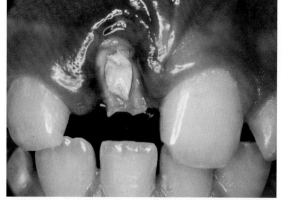 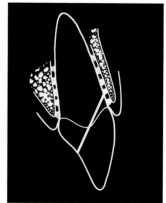

Oblique crown-root fracture below the marginal bone palatally.

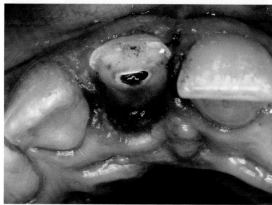 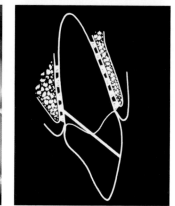

Crown-root fracture extending below marginal bone proximally.

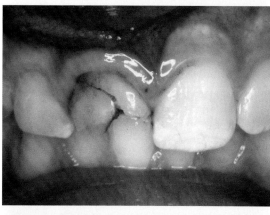 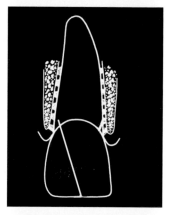

Transverse root fracture.

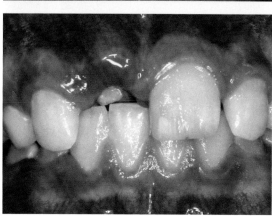 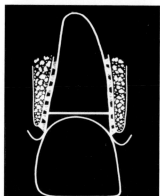

**Fig. 24.22 Orthodontic extrusion of a crown-root fractured central incisor**
The coronal fragment has been used as a temporary crown, cemented with a screw post in the root canal.

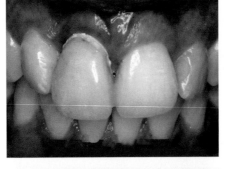
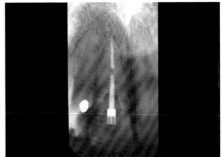

**Orthodontic appliance**
A heat-treated spring of Elgiloy® wire (0.016 × 0.016 inches) with a force of approximately 60 to 70 p is used for the extrusion.

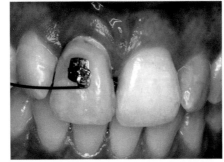
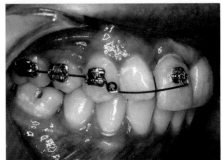

**Condition after 1 week**
The tooth has been extruded 1.5 mm. The crown is shortened to enable further extrusion.

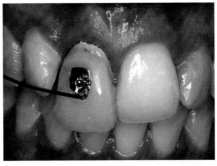
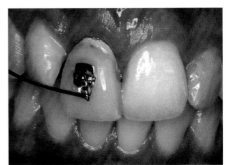

**Condition after 2 weeks**
The tooth has been extruded another 1.5 mm and the root is now available for preparation.

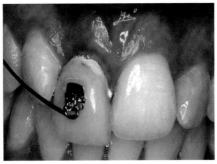
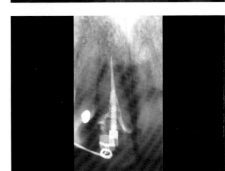

Orthodontic extrusion can be performed with a variety of orthodontic appliances. A rapid extrusion technique to save such teeth was introduced by Heithersay in 1973 (69) and further developed by Ingber in 1976 (71). Endodontic treatment of the root portion is usually performed before the orthodontic phase of treatment.

Orthodontic extrusion normally leads to a coronal shift of the marginal gingiva (40, 77) caused by growth of the attached gingiva and not by coronal displacement of the muco-gingival junction (Fig. 24.20). The increase of gingival tissue may partially mask the extent of root extrusion.

Rapid extrusion involves stretching and readjusting of the periodontal fibres, thereby avoiding marked bone remodelling by virtue of the rapid movement. It can thus be achieved without a coronal shift of marginal bone, thereby facilitating the coronal restoration, as there is no need to reshape bone.

Relapse may follow orthodontic extrusion, the prime reason being the stretched state of marginal periodontal fibres (72). To avoid relapse, fibrotomy should be performed before the retention period, which should last at least 3–4 weeks (101–102) (Fig. 24.22).

A non-vital tooth can be extruded, 3–5 mm during 3–4 weeks. Rapid movement is possible because stretching and readjusting the fibres accomplish bone remodelling. Rapid extrusion of teeth, in comparison to conventional orthodontic extrusion, may in rare cases elicit root resorption (103). However, both histological and clinical studies of extruded teeth indicate that root resorption after extrusion is very rare (69–75, 97–102).

**Fig. 24.22 (*cont.*)**
**Fibrotomy**
A fibrotomy extending below the level of marginal bone is performed prior to the retention period.

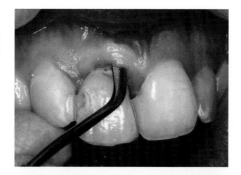

**Retention**
The extruded tooth is splinted to adjacent teeth.

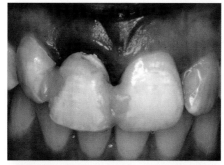

**Final restoration**
A post-retained crown is fabricated. Radiographically there is no sign of resorption after 2 years.

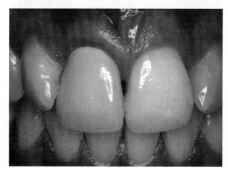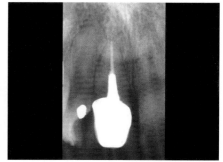

For a tooth with a complicated crown-root or cervical root fracture, two types of therapy are available, orthodontic or surgical extrusion (104–106, 164–165). In fractures below the marginal bone palatally surgical extrusion combined with rotation of the root 180°, less extrusion is needed favoring the bone support of the root (see Chapter 11). In teeth with thin root canal walls, i.e. teeth treated endodontically at an early stage of root formation, orthodontic extrusion seems to be less traumatic.

## Root fractures

Orthodontic management of root-fractured teeth depends on the type of healing and location of the fracture (31, 107–108). Radiographic and histological observations have shown different types of healing after root fracture: healing with calcified tissue and with interposition of connective tissue, sometimes combined with ingrowth of bone between fragments (107–109).

Healing with calcified tissue means that the fracture is healed with dentin and cementum. The bridging of the fracture may not be complete, but the fracture is consolidated. Tooth mobility is normal, as is response to pulpal sensibility testing. Orthodontic movement of a root-fractured tooth, which has healed with a hard tissue callus, can be per-

formed without breaking up the fracture site (Fig. 24.23).

Healing with interposition of connective tissue means that the fracture edges are covered with cementum and PDL. Orthodontic movement of a root-fractured tooth where the fragments are separated by connective tissue leads to further separation of the fragments (Fig. 24.24). A common finding after treatment is rounding of fracture edges. In planning orthodontic therapy, it must therefore be realized that a fractured root with interposition of connective tissue should be looked upon as a tooth with a short root. As a result, such a tooth must be evaluated with respect to the length of the coronal fragment. This means that teeth with fractures in the apical third of the root generally have enough periodontal support to allow orthodontic movement (Fig. 24.25A). Teeth with fractures located in the middle third of the root represent a hazard to tooth integrity because of the risk of further shortening of the very short coronal fragment (Fig. 24.25B). Orthodontic movement of such a tooth may result in a root with very little periodontal support. In cervical root fractures, the apical fragment can sometimes be extruded with a rapid extrusion technique or by surgical means (Fig. 24.25C).

Movement of root-fractured teeth with an adequate root filling may be performed with the same prognosis as when the coronal fragment is vital.

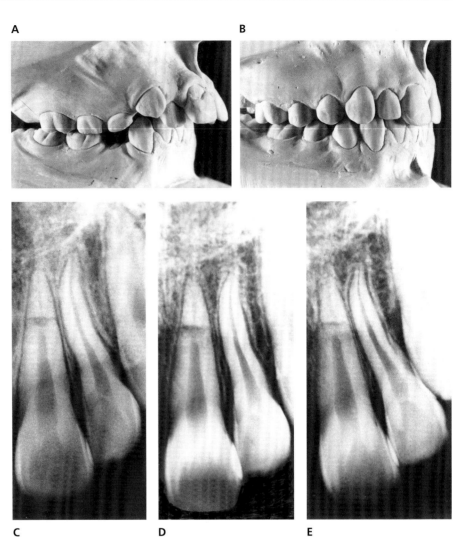

**A**                                          **B**

**Fig. 24.23** Orthodontic movement of a root fractured tooth healed by a hard tissue callus. A. Models of a Class II div. 1 malocclusion with deep bite before and B. after treatment. The patient was treated with extraoral traction and an activator for 2 years. C. The root fractured incisor before treatment. Note internal surface resorption at the level of the root fracture, which is typical for hard tissue healing. D. Immediately after active treatment. There is obliteration of only the apical part of the root canal, also an indication of continued hard tissue fracture healing. E. Condition 4 years after active treatment. Note that tooth movement was achieved without separating the fragments.

**C**                     **D**                     **E**

## Luxated teeth

It has not yet been clearly established whether luxated teeth are more liable to resorb during orthodontic treatment than non-injured teeth (68). In one study, luxated teeth were reported to develop more root resorption than their non-injured antimeres (43). However, in the evaluation of the results, the different types of luxation injuries were not taken into account. With respect to the occurrence of root resorption, it has been observed clinically that luxated teeth without root resorption can be moved with the same prognosis as non-injured teeth (91). Teeth with repaired surface resorption or repaired inflammatory resorption should be followed carefully during orthodontic treatment. A radiographic assessment of the outline of the roots prior to treatment gives information of some risk factors, such as an irregular root contour, concavities along the surface of the root, or root malformation (88). Regular radiographic controls are necessary in order to disclose early root resorption. An index provides a useful tool for quantitative assessment of root conditions during treatment (85, 88–89, 91).

Inflammatory and replacement resorption can be clearly related to traumatic injuries and have never been reported as a result of orthodontic treatment alone. Luxated teeth, which have developed inflammatory resorption, should be treated endodontically and observed for arrest of root resorption prior to initiation of orthodontic movement. Teeth with ankylosis (replacement resorption) do not respond to orthodontic treatment (Fig. 24.9).

## Avulsed teeth

### Primary teeth

Traumatic loss of a primary tooth is no indication for orthodontic treatment (29). A secondary effect of the traumatic episode might be malformation or impaction of the succedaneous tooth. The orthodontic implication of this will be discussed later in this chapter.

### Permanent teeth

After traumatic loss of permanent teeth, orthodontic treatment planning becomes relevant (46–54, 110–114). The main question is whether the space should be maintained for tooth replacement by autotransplantation, implant insertion or fixed bridgework. (An analysis of the long-term prognosis for these treatment procedures is given in Chapter 26.)

An unfavorable development of the width and height of the alveolar crest is often seen in growing individuals with missing

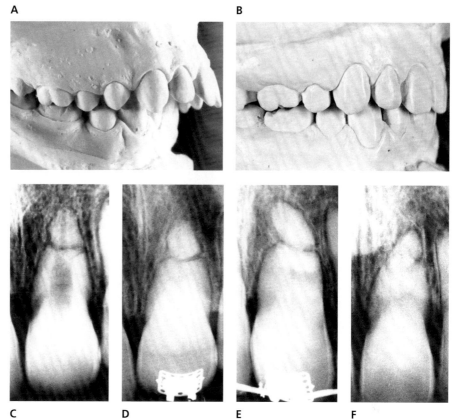

**Fig. 24.24** Orthodontic movement of a root-fractured tooth with healing by interposition of connective tissue. A. Models of a Class II div. 1 malocclusion with deep bite before and B. after treatment. The patient was treated with a fixed appliance for 19 months. C. The fractured incisor 3 years prior to treatment. Note initial obliteration of the apical and coronal aspects of the root canal. D. Condition at the start of orthodontic treatment. There is rounding of the fracture edges and obliteration of the entire root canal, and indications of interposition of connective tissue between root fragments. E. Four months after the start of orthodontic treatment. F. Condition 2 years after orthodontic treatment.

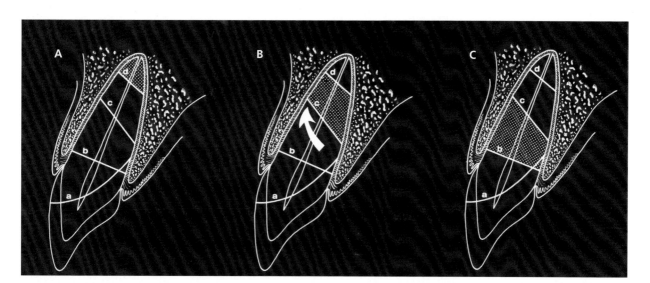

**Fig. 24.25** Evaluation of the prognosis for orthodontic treatment of root-fractured teeth healed with interposition of connective tissue. A. Root fractures apically of line d. The coronal part of the root is so long that movement of the root is possible without impairment of the prognosis. B. Root fractures between d and c. The coronal portion of the root is long enough to withstand careful orthodontic movement. Note the thin labial part of the root (arrow) which can easily resorb during orthodontic movement and which will lead to a significant shortening of the root length. C. Root fractures between c and b. The coronal part of the root is usually too short to assure enough periodontal support and orthodontic treatment is therefore contraindicated. If the fracture line is too close to b, extrusion of the apical fragment is an alternative.

maxillary incisors (Fig. 24.2). Severe traumatic injuries can also damage the alveolar ridge. Autotransplantation of premolars to replace missing incisors can contribute to favorable development of the alveolar bone (115–116).

Autotransplantation can be performed with both immature and mature teeth, but most reports conclude that auto-transplantation has the best prognosis if performed when the tooth germ has developed to three-fourths of its anticipated root length or to full length with a wide open apex (117–121) (see Chapter 27). At this stage of root development, vitality of the pulp can be maintained and root development continued (Fig. 24.26). Transplanted teeth can be

### Fig. 24.26 Combined orthodontic treatment and premolar auto-transplantation after anterior tooth loss

Three maxillary incisors have been avulsed in a 10-year-old girl. Note the extensive loss of alveolar bone buccally. Radiographic examination revealed that the mandibular second premolars were suitable as grafts.

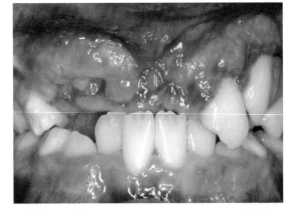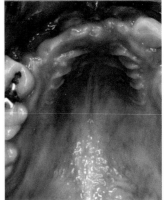

### Temporary restoration

A temporary plate with 2 incisors is used as a space maintainer. After 5 months the upper right cuspid has erupted in a mesial position. The cuspid was therefore moved distally with elastics to make room for the 2 transplants.

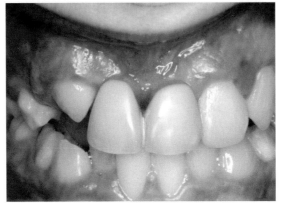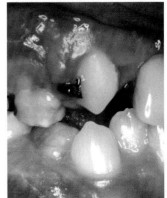

### Autotransplantation of premolars

Two years after the trauma, the roots of the premolars have developed to ³/₄ of anticipated root length. The premolars are then transplanted to the central incisor region. The teeth are aligned with a fixed appliance 6 months after transplantation.

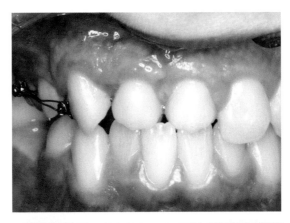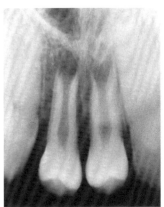

### Completion of treatment

At the end of treatment the premolars and the cuspid are recontoured with composite resin. The clinical and radiographic situation is shown 6 years after trauma and 4 years after transplantation.

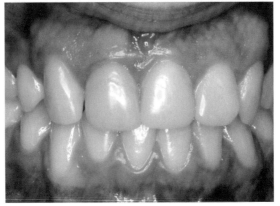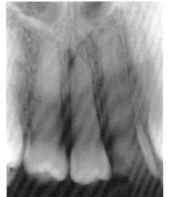

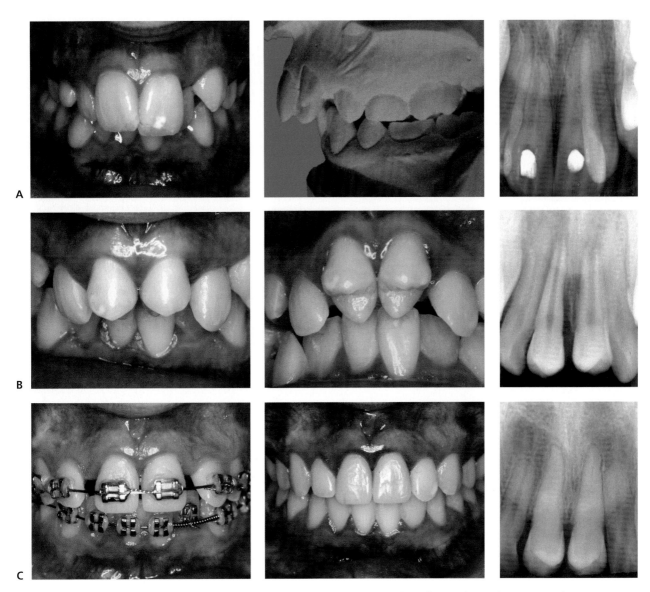

**Fig. 24.27** Orthodontic movement of autotransplanted teeth. A. A 12.5-year-old boy with bimaxillar crowding. Both upper incisors have poor prognosis due to ankylosis after a traumatic injury. B. Both maxillary second permanent premolars transplanted to incisor position. Note position of the lingual cusps. C. Orthodontic treatment and composite restoration, with radiograph 3 years after orthodontic treatment.

moved with only a minor loss of root length (122) (Fig. 24.27).

Osseointegrated implants have been used extensively during the last years to substitute missing anterior teeth. The implants are stationary in the jaws and do not erupt during the dental and alveolar development. It is therefore important to ensure that growth and development has ceased before the implant is placed. Periodic supervision of growth increments is essential for the result. The dental age must be fully erupted permanent teeth, and the skeletal maturation must be nearly completed, confirmed by a growth curve or a hand-wrist radiograph (Chapter 28).

### Space closure

Space closure is of prime importance in patients with maxillary arch length deficiency in Class I and II malocclusions. Treatment should start early or at least be planned in the mixed dentition. It is then possible by extraction or interproximal reduction of deciduous molars to guide molars, premolars and canines mesially. An intact dental arch can then be obtained with minor or no appliance therapy.

Space closure for a missing maxillary lateral incisor usually implies mesial positioning of the maxillary cuspid in the lateral incisor region. Periodontal status has been reported to be better in patients with closed lateral incisor spaces than in patients with prosthetic lateral incisors (55). Treatment of missing maxillary lateral incisors in patients with Class I malocclusion is schematically illustrated in Fig. 24.28A–F (114). The same principles can be applied in cases with loss of central incisors.

Mesial movement of a lateral with fixed appliance to replace a missing upper central incisor is complex. There is a risk of space reopening, increased load on the root to

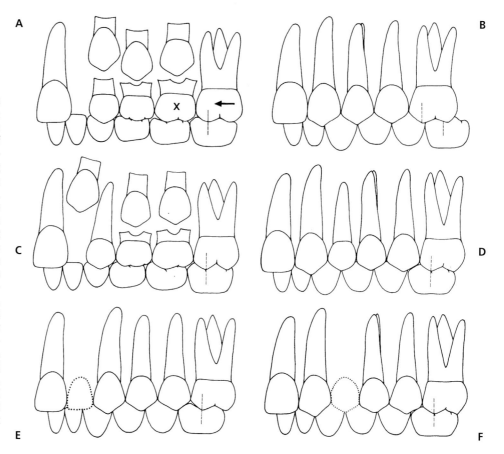

**Fig. 24.28** Treatment alternatives when a lateral incisor is avulsed in a Class I malocclusion arch length deficiency. A. Early extraction of the primary second molar facilitates mesial movement of the first permanent molar, arch length in the upper jaw is thereby reduced. B. The canine and premolars have moved mesially one tooth width and a Class II occlusion without spacing has been achieved. No arch length deficiency. C. The canine is positioned mesially. The root of the primary canine demonstrates no extensive resorption. D. The canine replaces the avulsed lateral incisor and the primary canine is used as a space maintainer as long as possible. E. A space maintainer is constructed while awaiting permanent therapy. F. The canine is used as a lateral incisor and a space is maintained between the canine and the first premolar.

support a larger crown and unfavorable fit of the prosthetic crown in the cervical area. Czochrowska et al. (151), however, found in a follow-up study of 20 consecutively treated patients that most patients (85%) were satisfied regarding the esthetic result, but only 50% of the professionals. Another study showed that unilateral space closure often resulted in a high degree of patient dissatisfaction (see Chapter 29). Crown form and inclination of the lateral incisors and canines must be favorable. The lateral must be properly uprighted both in mesial-distal and labio-lingual direction (Figs 24.29–24.31).

Crown form, dental arch symmetry and lip seal are important factors for an acceptable end result. Altering the crown forms with composite material in the mixed dentition and later on with porcelain veneers in the permanent dentition and grinding of canines, sometimes supplemented with gingivectomy to adjust differences in clinical crown height can contribute to an esthetically pleasing result (57–59, 152) (Fig. 24.32).

In cases where there is doubt about the functional or esthetic result of space closure after incisor loss, it is advisable to wait until growth of the jaws is finished (153). Meanwhile, the space can be maintained prosthetically (60, 61).

When treatment is planned, arch length and form, crown form and inclination of the anterior teeth should be studied carefully on casts and radiographs. Different alternatives of tooth position and compensatory extractions can be studied

on diagnostic set-up models. The set-up model also facilitates discussion with the patient, parents and colleagues (Fig. 24.33).

### Space maintenance

When space closure is contraindicated, a space maintainer can be constructed. This situation arises if more than one incisor is lost in the same arch. It is also true in patients with good alignment of teeth and normal occlusion, and in patients with spaces between teeth. If a tooth is lost in the upper jaw in a Class II division 2 or a Class III malocclusion, a space maintainer is often the treatment of choice.

For esthetic reasons, space maintainance is indicated if there is great discrepancy in crown form between central and lateral incisors. The crown form of cuspids sometimes also contraindicates space closure. Asymmetry of the upper incisors after space closure could be very obvious in patients with incomplete lip seal. A space maintainer followed by autotransplantation, a fixed bridge or an implant is then to be preferred.

A fixed space maintainer followed by bridgework is sometimes the only possible treatment in an uncooperative patient who does not want appliance therapy. Various space maintainers can be used. The easiest method is to use the traumatized tooth for as long as possible, even when the prognosis is poor. It is, however, important to control such a tooth. If it becomes ankylosed, it should be extracted

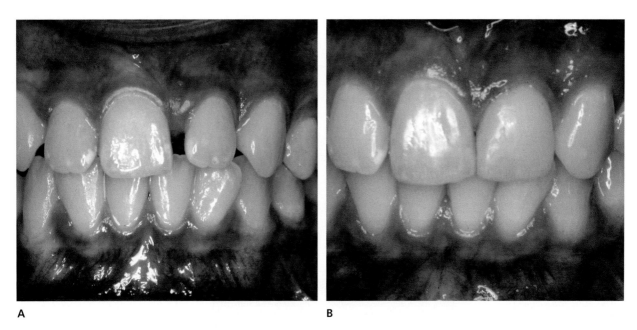

**Fig. 24.29** Closure of the space resulting from avulsion of a permanent left central incisor. A. The lateral incisor has moved mesially and has a fairly good position, which would have been better if the tooth had been uprighted. Note the mesial drift of the central incisor. A base plate or a lingual arch wire with a stop could have prevented this. B. The lateral incisor has been recontoured by selective grinding and the crown form reshaped with composite resin.

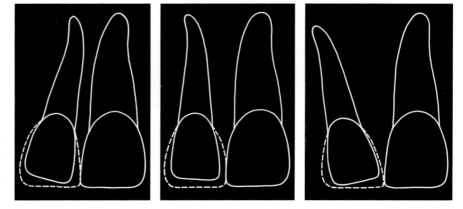

**Fig. 24.30** Schematic illustration of the need for mesio-distal up righting of a lateral incisor which has been moved mesially to replace a missing maxillary central incisor.

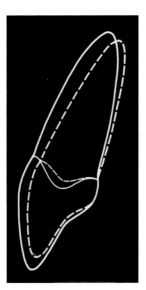

**Fig. 24.31** Schematic illustration of buccal root torque of a lateral incisor which is moved mesially to replace a missing maxillary central incisor. The solid line illustrates the inclination of a central incisor and the dotted line a lateral incisor.

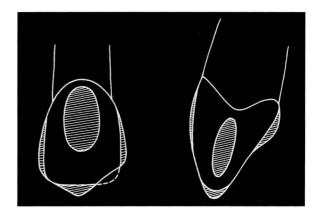

**Fig. 24.32** Reduction of a canine to simulate a lateral or central incisor. The shaded areas illustrate the spots of grinding. The dotted line indicates where a corner can be enhanced by composite resin build-up.

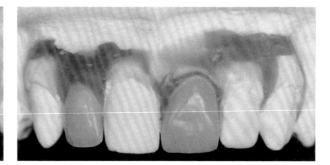

**Fig. 24.33** A model set-up for a patient with aplasia of the maxillary right lateral incisor and traumatic loss of left central incisor. Treatment planning involves mesial movement of the maxillary right central incisor, distal movement of left canine and alignment of the maxillary teeth. Acrylic teeth are used as space maintainers during treatment and retention (to be continued in Fig. 24.36) can be decided how space closure can be achieved. In cases with extreme crowding, however, it can be done at the time of initial treatment.

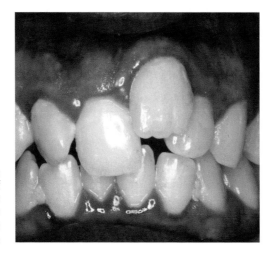

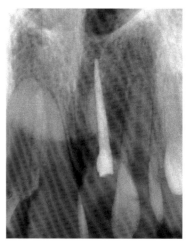

**Fig. 24.34** Severe infraocclusion of a central incisor with mesial tipping of adjacent teeth and a midline deviation in a 16-year-old boy. To avoid such complications, the ankylosed tooth should have been decoronated earlier.

before severe infraocclusion and tipping of adjacent teeth has occurred (Fig. 24.34).

The most common space maintainer is a removable appliance with a prosthetic tooth (Fig. 24.1D). An alternative is a lingual arch soldered to bands on the molars with a prosthetic tooth fixed to the arch. In the early mixed dentition it is often favorable to place the bands on the second primary molars to avoid interference with eruption of the first molars (Fig. 24.35). Later in the mixed dentition prior to eruption of the canines bands should be placed on the first permanent molars. Occlusal stops to prevent pressure on the alveolar ridge are important (Fig. 24.1E and F).

Various types of bonded appliances can also be used. An important factor is that the different appliances do not interfere with eruption of teeth and growth of jaws. In many cases, space maintainers can be combined with orthodontic appliances (Fig. 24.36). The crown of the extracted incisor can also be used as a pontic.

Autotransplantation of bicuspids to maintain the alveolar arch width and length in a growing child is illustrated in Fig. 24.27. The anatomy of the transplant is subsequently altered by a composite resin restoration. Both pre- and post surgical treatment planning is important, to make transplantation possible at an optimal stage of root development of the

bicuspids and to minimize the post surgical movement of the transplant (66, 67, 115, 117–121, 154).

Insertion of implants is important to consider but can only be used when growth of the jaws and alveolar crest is complete (see Chapter 28, p. 775).

If space maintenance is indicated, preprosthetic orthodontic therapy is often necessary. Malocclusions due to skeletal deviations (primarily open and deep bites, cross bites and Class II malocclusions) should be treated in the early permanent dentition. Remaining growth can thereby facilitate orthodontic therapy. After this treatment, semipermanent prosthetic therapy can be provided. In other malocclusions, treatment can be performed in close association with the definitive therapy. This facilitates both orthodontic and prosthetic treatment planning and shortens the retention period.

## Crown and root malformations

Malformations of permanent teeth due to traumatic injuries to primary predecessors often lead to impaction (28). If root development is reasonably advanced, combined surgical and orthodontic realignment is possible. Thus, teeth with crown or root dilacerations can be moved into a normal position

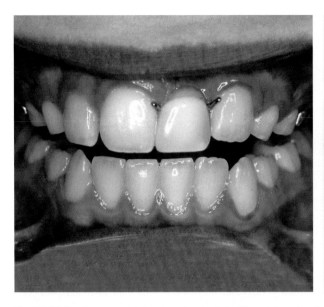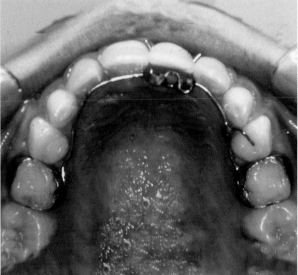

**Fig. 24.35** Fixed space maintainer in early mixed dentition. A lingual arch wire is soldered to bands on the primary second molars. Axial view; note the mesial and distal stops around the prosthetic tooth.

**Fig. 24.36 Combination of space maintainer and orthodontic appliance**
Acrylic teeth, right lateral and left central incisors, used as space maintainers during orthodontic treatment. Two acrylic teeth are replacing the missing incisors.

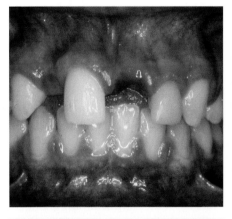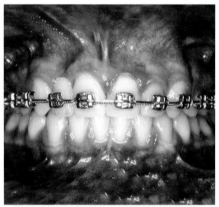

**Frontal and occlusal view of retainer**
After treatment the same teeth are used in the retainer. Note the occlusal stops on the retainer used to avoid excessive pressure on the alveolar ridge.

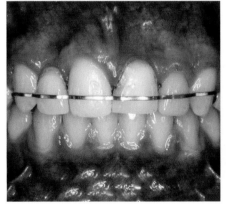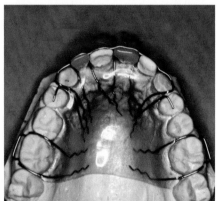

orthodontically. Treatment, however, should be postponed until the mixed dentition stage.

## Intruded teeth

Intrusion of a permanent tooth into the alveolar bone is a severe traumatic injury. The trauma can cause pulp necrosis, root resorption and ankylosis. The risks of pulpal damage and ankylosis are important considerations in treatment planning. Orthodontic movement of a tooth with small areas of replacement resorptions may be moved initially. Many years after treatment it will be obvious that ankylosis further developed and the tooth is infraoccluded.

Pulp canal obliteration as a consequence of intrusive luxation can be seen in immature teeth (127,171). Special care should be taken during orthodontic treatment of such teeth.

In experimental studies of intruded mature premolars in dogs, Turely et al. (166, 167) found that when an intrusive injury to the teeth was severe, orthodontic extrusion had little effect on repositioning of the teeth but resulted in undesirable effects on the anchorage teeth. When the injury was less severe the orthodontic forces could favorably reposition the affected teeth. A literature review by Chaushu et al. (155) concludes that treatment of intruded teeth is based largely on empirical experience rather than on scientific data.

### Immature teeth

Intruded immature teeth may be left to erupt spontaneously (128, 129, 169), or slightly loosened with finger pressure if the intrusion is not too severe. Orthodontic extrusion is indicated if the intrusion is severe or if the tooth has not begun erupting within 2–4 weeks. A plate with an extrusion spring is recommended for the extrusion in order to avoid pressure on neighbouring teeth (Figs 24.37 and 24.38). Intrusion always leads to pulpal damage. Sometimes the pulp may heal with subsequent obliteration of the pulpal lumen. Providing ankylosis does not develop, these teeth may have a good prognosis, as might teeth with pulp necrosis after adequate endodontic treatment.

### Mature teeth

Intrusion of mature teeth always leads to pulp necrosis. Prophylactic endodontic treatment is therefore recommended, as a necrotic and infected pulp can lead to rapidly progressive inflammatory root resorption. The critical period for the onset of external root resorption is 2 to 3 weeks. Therefore, in order to facilitate endodontic therapy, the intruded tooth must be at least partly repositioned within the first 3 weeks after injury. This can be accomplished either orthodontically or surgically (130–134, 169).

Before treatment, there are some factors that must be considered. If the intrusion is severe, there is a risk that orthodontic extrusion will have little effect. The tooth might be tightly locked in bone and orthodontic forces may not be able to overcome this mechanical barrier. This may cause ankylosis and make orthodontic extrusion impossible. To avoid this complication, the intruded incisor can be slightly luxated before orthodontic extrusion. Severe intrusion is often accompanied by fracture and displacement of the labial alveolar bone plate. Immediate surgical repositioning is then indicated, whereby the fractured labial bone plate is also repositioned.

As a clinical guideline, teeth with severe intrusive luxations can be surgically repositioned if the intrusion is accompanied by fracture of the alveolar walls. Teeth with less severe intrusion might be orthodontically extruded. If the tooth is firmly locked within bone, slight luxation facilitates the orthodontic therapy. If surgical repositioning of the intruded incisor is desired, optimal healing with respect to marginal bone support and periodontal ligament is achieved if the tooth is only repositioned partially. Repositioning can then be completed either by orthodontic traction or by spontaneous reeruption.

## Replanted teeth

In cases where an avulsed tooth has been replanted, it may later be necessary to move the replanted tooth. The problem then arises whether orthodontic movement of the replanted tooth is possible without a significant risk of root resorption. Preliminary clinical studies (43, 45) as well as an experimental study in monkeys (44) indicate that severe root resorption can be elicited after orthodontic movement. Most root resorptions after replantation are seen during the 1st year after injury (see Chapter 17). Thus, if no such complication is seen in this period, movement of the replanted tooth is possible. However, it must be considered that both replanted and intruded teeth may show progressive root resorption 5 or 10 years after trauma despite more optimistic evaluation earlier in the course of healing (see Chapters 17 and 31). Such teeth are often candidates for single implants after the growth period.

### Ankylosis

Replantation of avulsed teeth is frequently complicated by dentoalveolar ankylosis (156–158). The root of the reimplanted tooth is gradually resorbed and replaced by bone. Providing no other changes are seen, the ankylosed tooth can be retained until the crown breaks off, or is removed with forceps when most of the root substance has been replaced by bone. An ankylosed tooth does not follow development of the occlusion during growth. It must therefore be decided whether to extract the tooth or keep it as a space maintainer until complete resorption of the root has taken place. In young growing children and in adolescents particularly during growth spurts, the ankylosis is accompanied by increasing infraposition of the tooth, often with tilting of adjacent teeth (135, 159). The tooth shall therefore be removed before these changes become so advanced that a satisfactory orthodontic or prosthetic therapy becomes difficult (Fig. 24.34). A composite build up of the incisal edge can only be used temporarily to compensate for the infraocclusion (Fig. 24.39). If ankylosis is diagnosed later in adolescents when the alveolar growth is finished or almost finished, only a minor infraocclusion can be expected. Then a composite build up of the incisal edge is a more permanent option. Even in young adults, however a slight increase of the infraocclusion can be expected (158).

When alveolar growth is judged near completion, surgical block osteotomy and distraction osteogenesis to reposition the tooth at the proper vertical position in the arch has been suggested in a few case reports (160–162) (see Chapter 28, p. 781). The purpose with the method is to adjust the bone level in order to facilitate later prosthetic restoration (36). It must however be remembered that progression of replacement resorption will proceed.

### Fig. 24.37 Orthodontic extrusion of an intruded incisor

An 8-year-old boy suffered intrusion of an immature maxillary right incisor. Over a period of 2 months there has been no sign of reeruption.

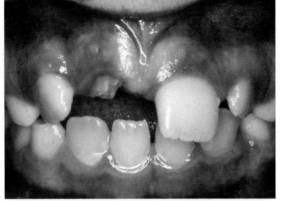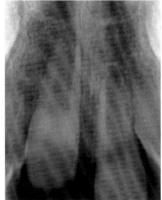

### Orthodontic appliance

A removable appliance with an extrusion spring acting on a bracket bonded to the injured tooth. A light force was used to avoid damage to the pulp.

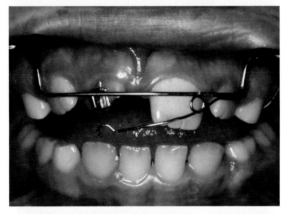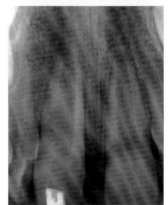

### Extrusion completed

The extrusion was complete within 2 months. Pulp necrosis and inflammatory resorption necessitated endodontic treatment.

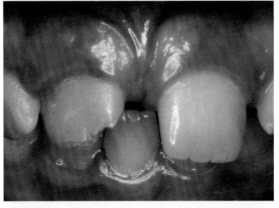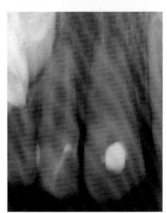

### Follow-up

The clinical and radiographic condition is shown 4 years after trauma.

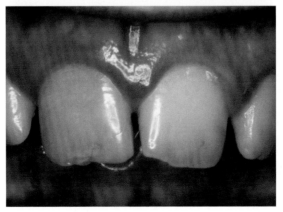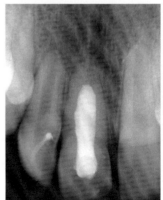

**Fig. 24.38 Loosening of two severely intruded central incisors with finger pressure combined with orthodontic extrusion**
Preinjury condition: this 8-year-old boy suffered intrusion of both central incisors 1 week after this photo was taken.

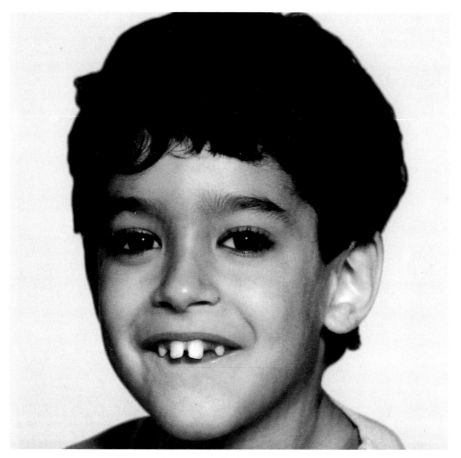

**Post injury condition**
The patient suffered intrusion of both central incisors.

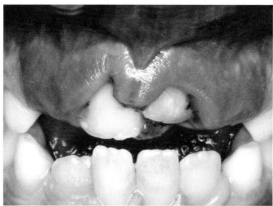
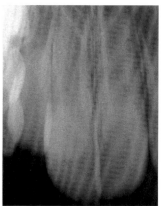

**Loosening of the incisors**
Both incisors were loosened with finger pressure. If this is not possible, forceps may be used. The radiograph is taken after orthodontic extrusion. Note inflammatory root resorption in the left incisor.

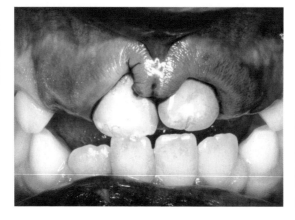
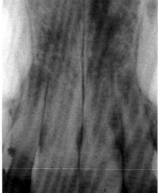

**Fig. 24.38 (*cont.*)**
**Status 2 months after injury**
There was no spontaneous reeruption. Orthodontic extrusion was therefore initiated. Endodontic treatment was performed in the left incisor due to pulp necrosis.

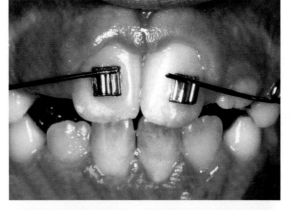 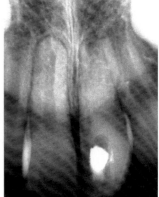

**Status after 1 and 4 years**
Clinical condition after 1 year and radiographic follow-up after 4 years. Note the partial pulp canal obliteration in the coronal part of the pulp chamber of the right incisor.

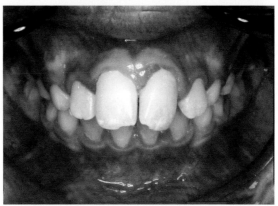 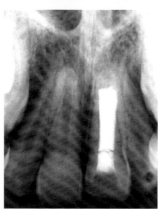

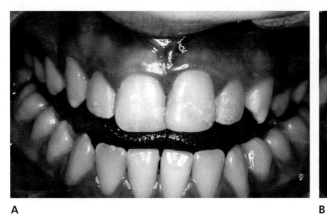 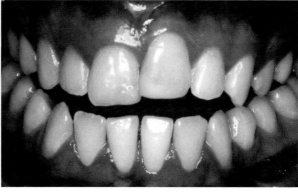

A                                         B

**Fig. 24.39** Incisal build-up of an ankylosed infrapositioned incisor. A. This is a 13-year-old girl. An incisal build-up was performed in the left upper ankylosed infrapositioned incisor. B. 3 years later the infraposition has increased and the esthetic effect is unsatisfactory. Observe that the level of infraposition is best evaluated at the gingival marginal.

Progression of the infraposition varies individually and is related to age, growth intensity (Figs 24.40 and 24.41) and growth direction of the jaws (Fig. 24.42). The risk of severe infraposition is particularly great if the ankylosis is diagnosed during eruption of teeth before and during the age interval, ten to twelve years due to the rapid alveolar growth during tooth eruption. In these cases the ankylosed tooth must be removed within 2 to 3 years after diagnosis. If ankylosis develops after this period the intensity and direction of growth of the alveolar bone and jaws varies and the tooth must be observed regularly. An individual

growth curve based on age in combination with body height measurements can aid in evaluation of the patient's growth status and annual cephalometric analysis is important for evaluation of the growth direction of the jaws (135, 157, 159). Study models are recommended for evaluation of the development of the infraocclusion. No active treatment is necessary as long as the adjacent teeth do not tilt and the extent of infraposition is minor and stable. In all other cases, the affected tooth must be removed and replaced by autotransplantation, orthodontic closure or fixed prosthetics.

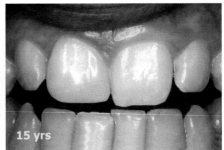

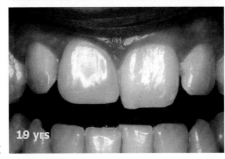

A  B

C

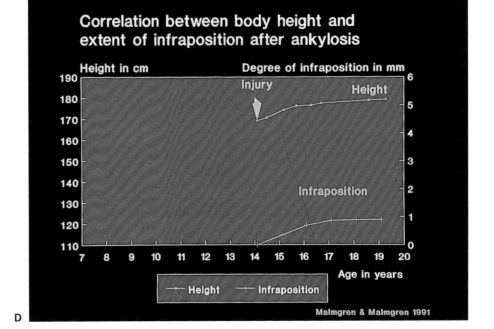

**Fig. 24.40** Relationship between general growth and infraposition of an ankylosed central incisor. A. The right central incisor was replanted in a boy at 14 years of age. B. Slight infraposition can be seen after 1 year. C. At 5-year control, there is a slight increase in infraposition. D. Annual body height measurements were registered for the patient and showed almost completed growth 2 years after the injury. The degree of infraposition was measured in mm.

D

### Extraction of ankylosed incisors (decoronation)

Extraction of an ankylosed incisor may involve vertical and horizontal loss of alveolar bone (Fig. 24.43). If infraposition is allowed to progress, even an uncomplicated extraction may lead to loss of large parts of the alveolar ridge (Fig. 24.44). To avoid such bone loss, a technique for extracting ankylosed teeth, called *decoronation*, has been developed (Fig. 24.45) (90, 163). The crown of the tooth is removed and the ankylosed root is left in the alveolus to be substituted by bone (Figs 24.46–24.48). In children, new marginal bone will then be formed coronal to the resorbing root. The height of the alveolar bone is thus improved vertically and preserved in the facio-lingual direction. The initial study using this method comprised 24 replanted maxillary incisors exhibit-

ing ankylosis and some degree of infraposition. The crown of the tooth was removed and the ankylosed root left in the alveolus to be substituted by bone (Figs 24.46–24.48). New marginal bone was formed coronal to the resorbing root in patients treated before or during pubertal periods of growth. A follow-up study of 77 decoronations was performed in 1999 (163). The age of the patients at the time of decoronation was 10 to 22 years (mean 14.8). The follow-up period varied from one to 14 years (mean 4.3). Radiographs were taken immediately before and after decoronation, after six months and then annually for up to 14 years. In 30 patients only normal alveolar bone was seen in the radiographs after 18 months, and in the remaining 47 patients remnants of the root were still present. The height of the alveolar bone was improved vertically in the patients treated before the age of

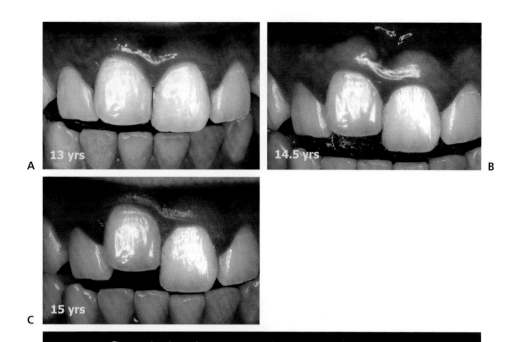

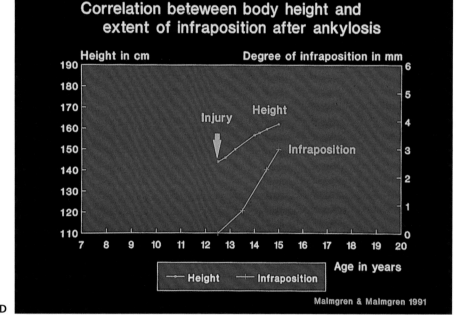

**Fig. 24.41** Relation between general growth and infraposition of an ankylosed central incisor. A. The right central incisor was replanted in a boy at 12 years of age. Slight infraposition can be seen after 1 year. B and C. At 2- and 2¹/₂-years after injury there is a marked increase in infraposition. D. There is a marked growth spurt in this patient which correlates with the marked infraposition.

13 years (Fig. 24.48), and the alveolar ridge was maintained in the facio-lingual direction in all patients. In conclusion, the conditions for subsequent orthodontic and prosthetic therapy were thereby improved. Moreover, the possibility of placing an implant was facilitated.

An ankylosed incisor can be extracted even if there is a risk of alveolar bone loss if it is going to be substituted by an autotransplanted tooth. It has been found that bone regeneration is induced from the intact periodontal ligament of the transplant and the transplant will be surrounded by new bone (see Chapter 27).

## Retention

Space closure or space maintenance during treatment determines the demands for retention.

Retention planning can be divided into three categories:

(1) No retention
(2) Limited retention
(3) Semi-permanent or permanent retention.

The need for retention in orthodontically treated patients with traumatic injuries depends on several factors. The following are the most important:

(1) Elimination of the cause of the malocclusion
(2) Proper occlusion
(3) Reorganization of bone and soft tissues around newly positioned teeth
(4) Correction of skeletal deviations during the growth period.

In cases where all of these objectives have been met, the need for retention is limited.

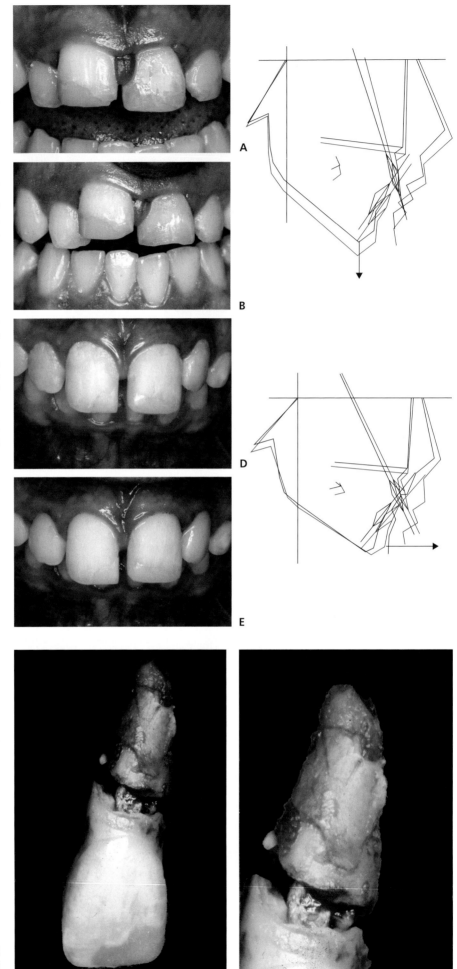

**Fig. 24.42 Relation between growth direction of the mandible and infraposition of ankylosed central incisors in a 14-year-old boy with a vertical growth direction of the mandible**
A. At the age of 14 years there was a minimal infraposition of the maxillary right incisor. The body height was 170 cm. B. At the age of 16 years the infraposition of the ankylosed incisor had increased markedly. Note incisal attrition of the maxillary left central incisor. The right lateral incisor has tilted mesially. The body height was 176 cm. C. Schematic illustration of the cephalometric changes of the face shows a vertical growth of the mandible.

**An 8-year-old boy with a horizontal growth direction of the mandible**
D. At the age of 8.2 years, 3 months after replantation, his body height was 129 cm. E. At the age of 9.6 years only a minimal infraposition can be seen. The body height was 137.5 cm. F. Schematic illustration of the cephalometric changes of the face shows a horizontal growth of the mandible.

**Fig. 24.43** Extraction of an ankylosed incisor where the bone plate was simultaneously removed.

**Fig. 24.44 Severe loss of alveolar bone after ankylosis of two incisors**
An 18-year-old boy with ankylosed incisors due to a trauma 10 years earlier. Infraposition was allowed to progress.

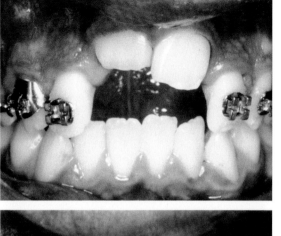
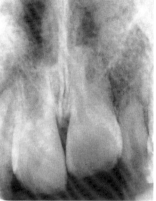

**Status after extraction**
An undesirable arrested development of the alveolar ridge is seen as a result of treatment neglect of the ankylosed teeth.

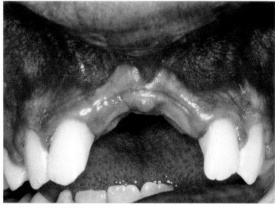
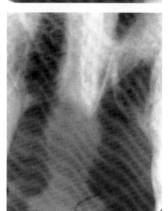

## Space closure

The need for retention is reduced if the roots of the teeth are parallel after treatment. Selective grinding and composite restorations can adjust tooth size discrepancies between the mesio-distal widths of the upper and lower teeth. This procedure might reduce the problem to one of limited retention, consisting of a removable or fixed appliance.

In cases where only a limited treatment goal can be achieved, semi permanent or permanent retention may be the only alternative. Semi permanent retention consists of a removable appliance, a lingual arch wire or a bonded appliance.

## Space maintenance

In cases where the space is maintained throughout treatment and the teeth are moved to positions best suited for a forthcoming bridge or implant, retention usually presents no problem. Permanent retention will then usually consist of a fixed prosthesis or a single standing implant.

## Prognosis

Very little is known today about the prognosis of orthodontic movement of traumatized teeth. A study, from the Eastman Institute in Stockholm, involving orthodontic treatment of 27 patients with 55 traumatized teeth and 60 non-traumatized teeth has been performed (91). Registration of the extent of root resorption before and after orthodontic movement showed a slight increase in the extent of root resorption in both traumatized and non-traumatized teeth, but with no significant difference between the two groups.

There is also a lack of information as to the risk of root resorption among the individual trauma entities. Empirical observations indicate that teeth with mild or moderate luxation injuries (i.e. concussion or subluxation) can be moved orthodontically with limited risk of root resorption if treatment is performed carefully. This means using light orthodontic forces, avoiding contact with cortical bone and ensuring a short period of treatment. After severe luxation (i.e. extrusion, lateral luxation, intrusion and after replantation), movement of a tooth is more hazardous. However, if no ankylosis has occurred 1 year after trauma, orthodontic therapy can be performed.

A recent study was performed of 15 patients orthodontically treated at Eastman Institute in Stockholm, Sweden, with complete records from a trauma episode. The study comprised 34 incisors with severely luxated teeth, follow-up after trauma, and during and after orthodontic treatment. One tooth was lost at the trauma episode and 6 teeth were extracted during follow-up after trauma.

**Fig. 24.45 Surgical treatment of an ankylosed and infrapositioned incisor**

Moderate infraposition of a right upper central incisor due to ankylosis in a 14-year-old boy.

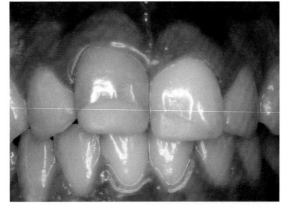 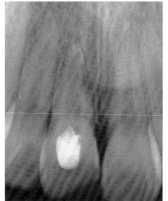

**Sectioning the crown from the root (decoronation)**

A mucoperiosteal flap is raised. The crown is removed with a diamond bur under a continuous flow of saline.

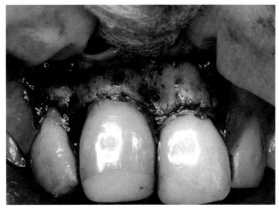 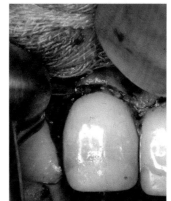

**Removing of the root filling**

The crown has been removed and the root filling removed with an endodontic file.

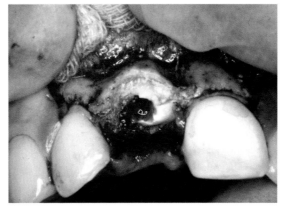 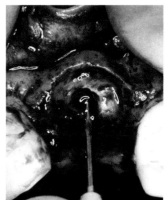

**Preparation of the root**

The coronal part of the root surface is reduced to a level of 2.0 mm below the marginal bone. The empty root canal is thoroughly rinsed with saline and thereafter allowed to fill with blood.

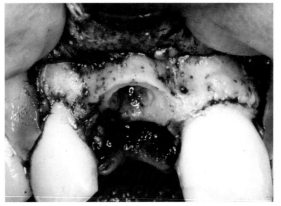 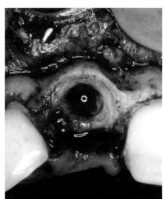

### Suturing the flap

The mucoperiosteal flap is pulled over the alveolus and sutured with single sutures. A blood clot is formed in the gap between the labial and palatal mucosa.

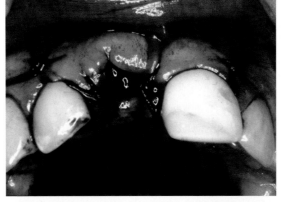 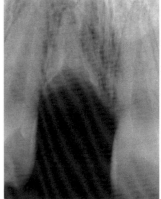

### Temporary restoration

The removed crown is shaped as a pontic with composite material and splinted to the adjacent teeth with acid-etch technique and an enamel composite bond.

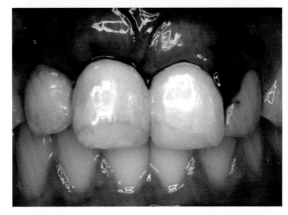 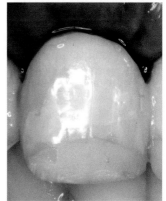

### Follow-up 1 year after treatment

A resin-retained bridge has been inserted. Note coronal growth of bone.

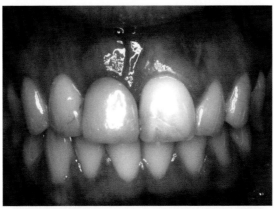 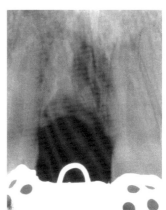

### 10 years after decoronation

The alveolar ridge has a favorable width and height for inserting an implant.

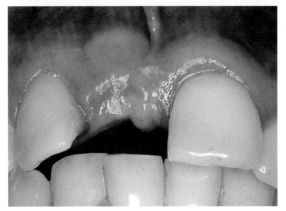 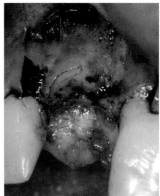

**Fig. 24.45 (*cont.*)**
**Insertion of implant**
A root remnant maintains in the alveolar ridge. It makes no obstacle for the insertion and integration of the implant.

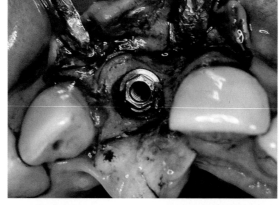
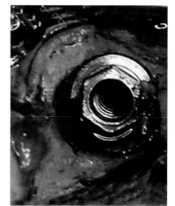

**Five-year follow-up after insertion of implant**

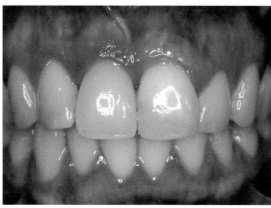
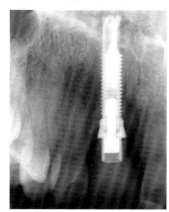

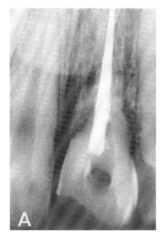
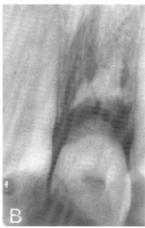
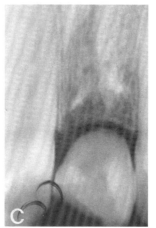
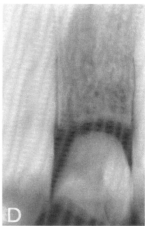

**Fig. 24.46** Decoronation of an ankylosed maxillary incisor in infraposition. There is continuous resorption of the ankylosed root and replacement with bone. Note shortened pontic and formation of new marginal bone coronal to the root remnants.

The conclusions from this study were that after a severe trauma, teeth with a poor prognosis should be extracted or looked upon as space maintainers prior to orthodontic treatment. Injured teeth properly treated and with a normal periodontal ligament might be moved with a normal risk of root resorption (169). Evaluation of the risk of root resorption after 6 months initial orthodontic treatment is important. If progressive resorption is seen at this stage a three months pause might reduce the risk of severe resorption at the end of treatment.

It is possible to move root-fractured teeth, if the fracture is healed with a hard tissue callus, with almost the same prognosis as a non-injured tooth. If the fragments are separated by connective tissue, further separation can be expected and the tooth should be evaluated according to the length of the coronal segment.

The prognosis after orthodontic extrusion of crown-root fractured teeth depends upon the technique used. Relapse after orthodontic extrusion can be minimized by a cervical fibrotomy.

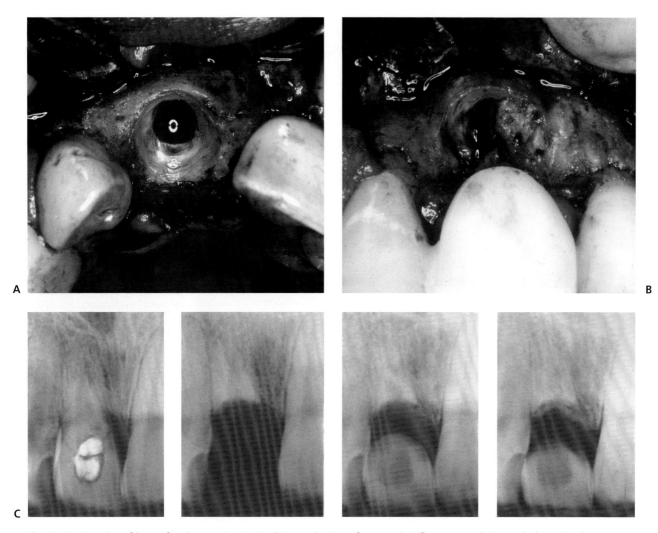

**Fig. 24.47** Formation of bone after decoronation. A. Condition at the time of surgery. B. A flap was raised 10 months later. New bone is seen replacing the resorbed root remnants. C. Radiographs immediately before and after surgery and at 6- and 18-month follow-ups. Note regeneration of coronal bone.

In treatment planning, it is essential to coordinate the prognosis for the traumatized tooth with the treatment of the malocclusion. Consequently, prognosis for the total treatment can be classified as follows:

- Good prognosis for the traumatized tooth; good prognosis for the malocclusion. The treatment procedure for the malocclusion does not differ from orthodontic treatment in patients without injured teeth.
- Good prognosis for the traumatized tooth; poor prognosis for the malocclusion. The orthodontic treatment is complicated, e.g. prolonged treatment time and severe anchorage problems. A limited goal must often be accepted in order not to overload the traumatized tooth.
- Poor prognosis for the traumatized tooth, good prognosis for the malocclusion. The traumatized tooth must often be extracted, but can otherwise serve as a space maintainer. The orthodontic treatment has a good prognosis and can provide optimal results. This is particularly true

if the malocclusion is caused by habits and the habits are stopped. Malocclusions combined with skeletal deviations have a better prognosis if they are treated during periods of active growth. The orthodontic treatment can in most cases provide optimal results with either space closure or space maintenance.

- Poor prognosis for the traumatized tooth; poor prognosis for the malocclusion. The traumatized tooth must often be extracted, but can serve as a space maintainer for some time. Prosthetic therapy, autotransplantation of a premolar or an implant to the trauma region can be indicated, depending upon the age of the patient. Orthodontic treatment in combination with orthognathic surgical correction is sometimes the treatment of choice.

The clinical sequelae to severe resorption are of major concern. In a study by Levander and Malmgren (170), increased mobility was found in incisors with a total root length of less than 9 mm. There was no difference between central and lateral incisors. Loss of root length moves the

**Fig. 24.48. Development of the alveolar ridge over 13 years after decoronation in a young girl**
(Left) At the age of 9 years, one year after replantation, the left central incisor is ankylosed and infrapositioned. Note build-up of the incisal edge. (Right) 3 years later, after orthodontic treatment, decoronation is performed. The removed crown is shaped as a pontic with composite and attached to the orthodontic appliance.

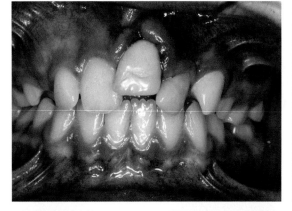
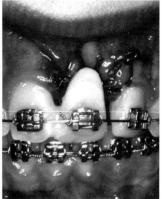

**Two years after decoronation**
Proliferation and down growth of the gingiva can be seen. A resin retained bridge has been inserted. Schematic illustration of the cephalometric changes of the face shows a vertical growth of the mandible.

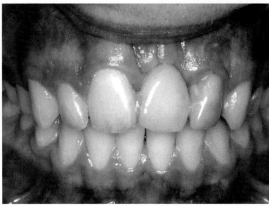
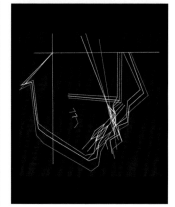

**At 21 years of age**
The situation at the time for insertion of an implant.

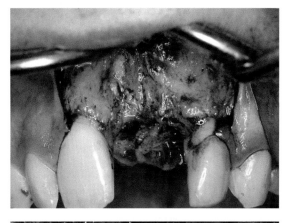
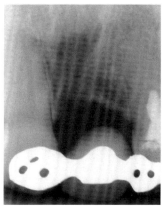

**Implant insertion**
The alveolar ridge has been maintained in buccopalatal direction and the implant could be inserted in perfect position.

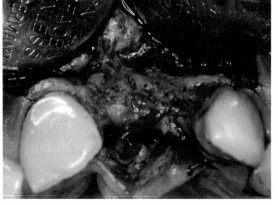
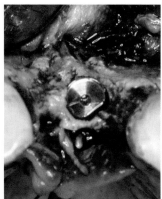

center of resistance coronally; thus the same amount of force will have a greater impact than on an intact root. The results of the study indicate enhanced risk of tooth mobility associated with a crown/root ratio greater than 1:1. Alveolar bone loss increases with age. This implies that the stability of incisors with resorption may decrease with time. The increased mobility of teeth with short roots should therefore be regarded as a long-term risk factor. Such teeth should be carefully monitored, particularly if the final root length is less than the crown height (<9 mm).

## Essentials

### Primary dentition

There is normally no need for interceptive orthodontic therapy.

### Mixed dentition

#### Risk factors

- Increased overjet and proclined upper incisors.
- Insufficient lip closure.

#### Prevention

- Children should be provided with a mouth guard to protect the teeth during sport activities.
- Early orthodontic treatment to minimize risk factors is indicated.
- Treatment shall be based on the individual growth intensity and direction of the jaws if the malocclusion is combined with skeletal deviations.

### Permanent dentition

#### Factors in treatment planning

- Evaluation of the remaining skeletal growth of the jaws and the remaining alveolar development of children and adolescents with severely traumatized teeth and malocclusions is important.
- Teeth with a poor long-term prognosis due to trauma can sometimes be part of the orthodontic therapy to avoid alveolar bone loss during development of the jaws.
- Ankylosed teeth should be decoronated or extracted before infraposition becomes so advanced that a satisfactory orthodontic or prosthetic therapy becomes difficult.

### Observation period after trauma prior to orthodontic treatment

- Mild injury (e.g. concussion, subluxation): 3 months
- Moderate or severe injury (e.g. extrusion, intrusion, lateral extrusion, replantation): 6 months
- Root-fractured teeth: 1 year

- In endodontically treated teeth, orthodontic treatment should be postponed until radiographic evidence of healing is seen.

### General treatment principles for orthodontic treatment of traumatized teeth

Orthodontic treatment represents an extra hazard to the periodontium and pulp.

#### Factors of importance

- The anatomy of the root
- Borders of cortical bone
- The use of light and short-acting orthodontic forces, possibly aimed at a limited goal

### Endodontically treated teeth

There is no evidence of a greater risk of root resorption of root filled teeth than vital teeth.

### Pulp canal obliteration

There is no evidence of a greater risk of root resorption of teeth with pulp canal obliteration than vital teeth.

### Root resorption subsequent to orthodontic treatment

Regular radiographic controls are necessary in order to check if any root resorption occurs or increases during treatment.

- The first control should be 6–9 months after initiation of treatment.
- Signs of root resorption indicate controls every 2 months.
- A suspension of treatment for about 3 months can reduce the risk of further resorption if signs of resorptions are seen.

### Specific treatment principles for orthodontic treatment of different types of trauma

#### Avulsion

##### A. Primary teeth
No immediate orthodontic treatment is indicated.

##### B. Permanent teeth
*Lateral incisor loss:*
- The space can be closed orthodontically.
- The space can be maintained for later prosthetic treatment. A space maintainer can be used in the interim.
- The space can be closed by an autotransplanted tooth.

*Central incisor loss:*
- Space closure seldom leads to optimal esthetic results.

- The space can be maintained for later prosthetic treatment. Space maintainers are important particularly during eruption of canines to avoid tooth migration and midline shifts.
- The space can be maintained by autotransplantation of premolars when their roots are developed to $3/4$ of full root length.

## Luxation

- Teeth with pulp necrosis and/or inflammatory root resorption should be treated endodontically prior to orthodontic treatment.
- Orthodontic movement of luxated teeth with initial signs of resorption should be carefully checked for further resorption. The first observation should be made after 6 months and thereafter at 3-month intervals.

## Crown-root fracture

- A non-vital tooth can be extruded over a period of 3–4 weeks.
- After a retention period of 4 weeks, the tooth can be restored.

## Root fracture

Orthodontic treatment possibilities are related to the type of healing and location of the fracture.
- Root-fractured teeth healed with *calcified tissue* can be moved without breaking the callus.
- Root-fractured teeth healed by *interposition of connective tissue* must be looked upon as teeth with short roots. Further shortening can be expected during orthodontic treatment.
- Teeth with fractures located in the apical third can normally be moved without impaired prognosis whereas teeth with fractures located in the middle third should be evaluated for adequate periodontal support.

## Crown or root malformation

- Impacted teeth with crown or root dilacerations can be moved into a normal position after surgical exposition if the damages are not too severe.
- Treatment shall be postponed until the mixed dentition stage.
- Crown and root malformed teeth can be used as space maintainers during growth and development of the jaws.

## Intruded teeth

### Immature teeth

- Intruded immature teeth may be left to erupt spontaneously if the intrusion is not too severe or slightly loosened with finger pressure.

- Orthodontic extrusion is indicated if the intrusion is severe or if the tooth has not begun erupting within two weeks.

### Mature teeth

- The critical period for onset of external root resorption is 2 to 3 weeks.
- Intruded teeth must be repositioned within the first 3 weeks after injury.
- Repositioning can be accomplished either orthodontically or surgically.
- If the tooth is tightly locked in bone it must be slightly luxated before orthodontic extrusion.

## Replanted teeth

### Normal periodontal ligament

Replanted teeth with a normal periodontal ligament can be moved orthodontically with the same prognosis as uninjured teeth.

### Ankylosis

There is no treatment known for dentoalveolar ankylosis *per se*, but an early overall treatment plan for the patient is of importance when the diagnosis has been established. An individual growth curve based on age in combination with body height measurements can aid in evaluation of the patients growth status and annual cephalometric analyses is important for evaluation of the growth direction of the jaws. Study models are recommended for evaluation of the development of the infraocclusion.

### Treatment options

#### Composite build-up of incisal level
If ankylosis is diagnosed late in adolescents when the alveolar growth is finished or almost finished, only a minor infraocclusion can be expected. Then a composite build up of the incisal edge is a more permanent option. Even in young adults, however a slight increase of the infraocclusion can be expected.

#### Extraction
Providing no adverse changes are seen, an ankylosed tooth can be retained until the crown breaks off, or is removed with forceps when most of the root substance has been replaced by bone.

#### Decoronation
Extraction of an ankylosed incisor may involve vertical and horizontal loss of alveolar bone. If infraposition is allowed to progress, even an uncomplicated extraction may lead to loss of large parts of the alveolar ridge. To avoid such bone loss, a technique for extracting ankylosed teeth, called decoronation, has been developed. The crown of the tooth is

removed and the ankylosed root is left in the alveolus to be substituted by bone. In children, new marginal bone will then be formed coronal to the resorbing root.

### Autotransplantation

An ankylosed incisor can be extracted even if there is a risk of alveolar bone loss if it is going to be substituted by an auto transplanted tooth. It has been found that bone regeneration is induced from the intact periodontal ligament of the transplant and the transplant will be surrounded by new bone.

### Dento-osseous osteotomy and distraction osteogenesis

When alveolar growth is judged near completion surgical block osteotomy, and distraction osteogenesis to reposition the tooth at the proper vertical position in the arch has been suggested.

### Surgical repositioning

For adult patients with ankylosed teeth in infraposition, dento-osseous osteotomy with immediate manual repositioning followed by orthodontic movement has been suggested. The purpose with the method is to adjust the bone level in order to facilitate later prosthetic restoration.

## Retention

Retention follows the same principles as for non-traumatized teeth.

## Prognosis

### A. Teeth with an intact periodontal ligament prior to orthodontic treatment

Movement can be performed with a prognosis, with respect to root resorption, comparable to that of non-traumatized teeth.

### B. Incisor roots shortened due to trauma or a combination of trauma and orthodontic movement

- If the final root length is less than the crown height (<9 mm), the teeth have a tendency to mobility.
- If the final root length is longer than the crown height (>9 mm) the tendency to mobility is minimal.

## References

1. SCHÜTZMANNSKY G. Unfallverletzungen an jugendlichen Zähnen. *Dtsch Stomat* 1963;**13**:919–27.
2. SCHÜTZMANNSKY G. Statistisches über Häufigkeit und Schweregrad von Unfalltraumen an der Corona Dentis im Frontzahn-bereich des kindlichen und jugendlichen Gebisses. *Z Gesamte Hyg* 1970;**16**:133–5.
3. GLUCKSMANN DD. Fractured permanent anterior teeth complicating orthodontic treatment. *J Am Dent Assoc* 1941;**28**:1941–3.
4. HARDWICK JL, NEWMAN PP. Some observations on the incidence and emergency treatment of fractured permanent anterior teeth of children. *J Dent Res* 1954;**33**:730.
5. LEWIS TE. Incidence of fractured anterior teeth as related to their protrusion. *Angle Orthod* 1959;**29**:128–31.
6. HALLET GEM. Problems of common interest to the paedodontist and orthodontist with special reference to traumatized incisor cases. *Eur J Orthod Soc Trans* 1953;**29**:266–77.
7. EICHENBAUM IW. A correlation of traumatized anterior teeth to occlusion. *J Dent Child* 1963;**30**:229–36.
8. BÜTTNER M. Die Häufigkeit von Zahnunfällen im Schulalter. *Zahnärztl Prax* 1968;**19**:286.
9. WALLENTIN I: Zahnfrakturen bei Kindern and Jugendlichen. *Zahnärztl Mitt* 1967;**57**:875–7.
10. McEWEN JD, McHUGH WD, HITCHIN AD. Fractured maxillary central incisors and incisal relationships. *J Dent Res* 1967;**46**:1290 (Abstract no. 87).
11. McEWEN JD, McHUGH WD. Predisposing factors associated with fractured incisor teeth. *Eur Orthod Soc Trans* 1969;**45**:343–51.
12. JOHNSON JE. Causes of accidental injuries to the teeth and jaws. *J Public Health Dent* 1975;**35**:123–31.
13. RAVN JJ. Dental injuries in Copenhagen school children school years 1967–1972. *Community Dent Oral Epidemiol* 1974;**2**:231–45.
14. O'MULLANE DM. Some factors predisposing to injuries of permanent incisors in schoolchildren. *Br Dent J* 1973;**134**:328–32.
15. BERZ H, BERZ A. Schneidezahnfrakturen and sagitale Schneidezahnstufe. *Dtsch Zahnärztl Z* 1971;**26**:941–4.
16. WÓJCIAK L, ZIÓLKIEWICS T, ANHOLCE H. Trauma to the anterior teeth in school-children in the city of Poznan with reference to masticatory anomalies. *Czas Stomat* 1974;**27**:1355–61
17. ANTOLIC I, BELIC D. Traumatic damages of teeth in the intercanine sector with respect to the occurrence with schoolchildren. *Zoboz Vestn* 1973;**28**:113–20.
18. PATKOWSKA-INDYKA E, PLONKA K. The effect of occlusal anomalies on fractures of anterior teeth. *Protet Stomatol* 1974;**24**:375–9.
19. DE MUNIZ BR, MUNIZ MA. Crown fractures in children. (Relationship with anterior occlusion.) *Rev Asoc Odont Argent* 1975;**63**:153–7.
20. JÄRVINEN S. Incisal overjet and traumatic injuries to upper permanent incisors. A retrospective study. *Acta Odontol Scand* 1978;**36**:359–62.
21. FERGUSON FS, RIPA LW. Incidence and type of traumatic injuries to the anterior teeth of preschool children. *I.A.D.R.* Abstract no. 401, 1979.
22. GAUBA ML. A correlation of fractured anterior teeth to their proclination. *J Indian Dent Assoc* 1967;**39**:105–12.
23. HELM S. Prevalence of malocclusion in relation to development of the dentition. *Acta Odontol Scand* 1970;**28**:Suppl. 58.
24. HELM S. Indikation af behov for ortodontisk behandling. En kritisk litteraturoversigt. *Tandlaegebladet.* 1980;**84**:175–85.

25. ANDREASEN JO, RAVN JJ. Epidemiology of traumatic dental injuries to primary and permanent teeth in a Danish population sample. *Int J Oral Surg* 1972;**1**:235–9.

26. ASH AS. Orthodontic significance of anomalies of tooth eruption. *Am J Orthod* 1957;**43**:559–76.

27. KORF SR. The eruption of permanent central incisors following premature loss of their antecedents. *ASDC J Dent Child* 1965;**32**:39–44.

28. ANDREASEN JO, SUNDSTRÖM B, RAVN JJ. The effect of traumatic injuries to primary teeth on their permanent successors. I. A clinical and histologic study of 117 injured permanent teeth. *Scand J Dent Res* 1971;**79**:219–83.

29. DRUSCH-NEUMANN D. Über die Lücken bei fehlenden Milchfront-Zähnen. *Fortschr Kieferorthop* 1969;**30**:82–8.

30. BJÖRK A. Käkarnas tillväxt och utveckling i relation till kraniet i dess helhet. In: Holst JJ, Nygaard Östby B, Osvald O. eds. *Nordisk Klinisk Odontologi*. Copenhagen: À/S Forlaget for Faglitteratur 1973, Chapter 1-I:1–44.

31. ZACHRISSON BU, JACOBSEN I. Response to orthodontic movement of anterior teeth with root fractures. *Eur Orthod Soc Trans* 1974;**50**:207–14.

32. WICKWIRE NA, McNEIL MH, NORTON LA, DUELL RC. The effects of tooth movement upon endodontically treated teeth. *Angle Orthod* 1974;**44**:235–42.

33. PHILLIPS JR. Apical root resorption under orthodontic therapy. *Angle Orthod* 1955;**25**:1–22.

34. DE SHIELDS RW. A study of root resorption in treated Class II Division I malocclusions. *Angle Orthod* 1969;**39**:231–45.

35. GOLDSON L, HENRIKSSON CO. Root resorption during Begg treatment: a longitudinal roentgenologic study. *Am J Orthod* 1975;**68**:55–66.

36. EPKER BN, PAULUS PJ. Surgical – orthodontic correction of adult malocclusions: single tooth dento-osseous osteotomies. *Am J Orthod* 1978;**74**:551–63.

37. TENHOEVE A, MULIE RM. The effect of antero-postero incisor repositioning on the palatal cortex as studied with laminagraphy. *J Clin Orthod* 1976;**10**:804–22.

38. MULIE RM, TENHOEVE A. The limitations of tooth movement within the symphysis studied with laminagraphy and standardized occlusal films. *J Clin Orthod* 1976;**10**:882–99.

39. EDWARDS JG. A study of the anterior portion of the palate as it relates to orthodontic therapy. *Am J Orthod* 1976;**69**:249–73.

40. REITAN K. Initial tissue behavior during apical root resorption. *Angle Orthod* 1974;**44**:68–82.

41. MASSLER M, MALONE AJ. Root resorption in human permanent teeth. A roentgenographic study. *Am J Orthod* 1954;**40**:619–33.

42. REITAN K. Biomechanical principles and reactions. In: Graber TM, Swain BF. eds. *Current orthodontic concepts and techniques*. Philadelphia: W. B. Saunders Company, 1975. Vol I:111–29.

43. HINES FB Jr. A radiographic evaluation of the response of previously avulsed teeth and partially avulsed teeth to orthodontic movement. *Am J Orthod* 1979;**75**:1–19.

44. GORDON NS. Effects of orthodontic force upon replanted teeth: a histologic study. *Am J Orthod* 1972;**62**:544.

45. GRAUPNER JG. The effects of orthodontic force on replanted teeth: a radiographic survey. *Am J Orthod* 1972;**62**:544–5.

46. ANTOLIC I. Functional treatment of traumatic teeth in children and youth. *Zobozdravstveni vestnik* 1973;**28**:121–7.

47. WOJTOWICZ N. Orthodontic-prosthetic management in cases of absent permanent incisors in children. *Czas Stomat* 1971;**24**:1067–73.

48. RAVN JJ. En redegörelse for behandlingen efter eksartikulation of permanente incisiver i en skolebarnspopulation. Tandlaegebladet. 1977;**81**:563–9.

49. SELMER-OLSEN R. Hvordan skal vi bedst mulig hjelpe barn som har slått ut en eller flere av sine permanente fortenner i overkjeven? *Norske Tandlaegeforen Tid* 1975;**45**:41–50.

50. VAN DER LINDEN FPGM. De orthodontische behandeling van een geval met agenesie van een premolaar en verlies door trauma van een central incisief in dezelfde vobenkaakhelft. *Ned T Tandheelk* 1972;**79**:436–43.

51. DORENBOS J. Algemeen tandheelkundige en orthodontische aspecten bij traumata van fronttanden. *Ned T Tandheelk* 1972;**79**:398–405.

52. DROSCHL H. Kieferorthopädisch-prophylaktische Massnahmnen beim Frontzahntrauma. *Öst Z Stomat* 1974;**71**:459–64.

53. PHILIPPE J. Remplacement d'une incisive centrale et orthodontie. *Actual Odontostomatol* 1972;**99**:389–93.

54. BRÜCKL H, BIRKE P. Zur kieferorthopädischen Behandlung des traumatischen Frontzahnverlustes. *Fortschr Kieferorthop* 1964;**25**:289–94.

55. NORDQUIST GG, McNEIL RW. Orthodontic vs. restorative treatment of the congenitally absent lateral incisor – long term periodontal and occlusal evaluation. *J Periodontol* 1975;**46**:139–43.

56. RAMFJORD SP, ASH MM Jr. *Occlusion*. Philadelphia: W. B. Saunders Company, 1966:333.

57. ZACHRISSON BU, MJÖR IA. Remodelling of teeth by grinding. *Am J Orthod* 1975;**68**:545–53.

58. ZACHRISSON BU. Improving orthodontic results in cases with maxillary incisors missing. *Am J Orthod* 1978;**73**:274–89.

59. MONEFELDT I, ZACHRISSON B. Adjustment of clinical crown height by gingivectomy following orthodontic space closure. *Angle Orthod* 1977;**47**:256–64.

60. HALLONSTEN A-L, KOCH G, LUDVIGSSON N, OLGART K, PAULANDER J. Acid-etch technique in temporary bridgework using composite pontics in the juvenile dentition. *Swed Dent J* 1979;**3**:213–19.

61. RAKOW B, LIGHT EI. Enamel-bonded immediate tooth replacement. *Am J Orthod* 1978;**74**:430–4.

62. DIXON DA. Autogenous transplantation of tooth germs into the upper incisor region. *Br Dent J* 1971;**131**:260–5.

63. KRISTERSON L. Unusual case of tooth transplantation: report of case. *J Oral Surg* 1970;**28**:841–4.

64. SLAGSVOLD O, BJERCKE B. Applicability of autotransplantation in cases of missing upper anterior teeth. *Am J Orthod* 1978;**74**:410–21.

65. SLAGSVOLD O. Autotransplantation of premolars in cases of missing anterior teeth. *Eur Orthod Soc Trans* 1970;**46**:473–85.

66. ANDREASEN JO. *Atlas of replantation and transplantation of teeth*. Fribourg: Mediglobe, 1992.

67. KUGELBERG R, TEGSJÖ U, MALMGREN O. Autotransplantation of 45 teeth to the upper incisor region. *Swed Dent J* 1994;**18**:165–72.

68. RÖNNERMAN A. Orthodontic movement of traumatized upper central incisors. Report of two cases. *Swed Dent J* 1973;**66**:527–34.

69. HEITHERSAY GS. Combined endodontic-orthodontic treatment of transverse root fractures in the region of the alveolar crest. *Oral Surg Oral Med Oral Pathol* 1973;**36**:404–15.

70. WOLFSON EM, SEIDEN L. Combined endodontic-orthodontic treatment of subgingivally fractured teeth. *J Canad Dent Assoc* 1975;**11**:621–4.

71. INGBER JS. Forced eruption: Part II. A method of treating nonrestoreable teeth – periodontal and restorative considerations. *J Periodontol* 1976;**47**:203–16.

72. PERSSON M, SERNEKE D. Ortodontisk framdragning av tand med cervikal rotfraktur för att möjliggöra kronersättning. *Tandläkartidningen* 1977;**69**:1263–9.

73. DELIVANIS P, DELIVANIS H, KUFTINEC MM. Endodontic-orthodontic management of fractured anterior teeth. *J Am Dent Assoc* 1978;**97**:483–5.

74. SIMON JHS, KELLY WH, GORDON DG, ERICKSEN GW. Extrusion of endodontically treated teeth. *J Am Dent Assoc* 1978;**97**:17–23.

75. BESSERMANN M. Ny behandlingsmetode of krone-rodfrakturer. *Tandlaegebladet* 1978;**82**:441–4.

76. BESSERMANN M. Personal communication.

77. OPPENHEIM A. Artificial elongation of teeth. *Am J Orthod Oral Surg* 1940;**26**:931–40.

78. RIEDEL RA. Retention. In Graber TM, Swain BF. eds. *Current orthodontic concepts and techniques*. Philadelphia: W. B. Saunders Company, 1975. Vol I:1095–37.

79. DAVILA JM, GWINNET AJ. Clinical and microscopic evaluation of a bridge using the acid-etch resin technique. *ASDC Dent J Child* 1978;**45**:228–32.

80. JORDAN RE, SUZUKI M, SILLS PS, GRATTON DR, GWINNET AJ. Temporary fixed partial dentures fabricated by means of the acid-etch resin technique: a report of 86 cases followed for up to three years. *J Am Dent Assoc* 1978;**96**:994–1001.

81. MACKIE IC, WARREN VN. Avulsion of immature incisor teeth. *Dent Update* 1988:406–8.

82. MOHLIN B. Early reduction of large overjet. Proceedings of the Second International Conference on Dental Trauma. Folksam IADT, 1991:88–95.

83. ANDREASEN FM, ANDREASEN JO, BAYER T. Prognosis of root-fractured permanent incisors – prediction of healing modalities. *Endod Dent Traumatol* 1989;**5**:11–22.

84. ANDREASEN FM, VESTERGAARD-PEDERSEN B. Prognosis of luxated permanent teeth – the development of pulpal necrosis. *Endod Dent Traumatol* 1985;**1**:202–20.

85. REMINGTON DN, JOONDEPH DR, ARTÜN J, RIEDEL RA, CHAPKO MK. Long term evaluation of root resorption occurring during orthodontic treatment. *Am J Orthod Dentofacial Orthop* 1989;**98**:43–6.

86. SPURRIER SW, HALL SH, JOONDEPH DR, SHAPIRO PA, RIEDEL RA. A comparison of apical root resorption during orthodontic treatment in endodontically treated and vital teeth. *Am J Orthod Dentofacial Orthop* 1990;**97**:130–4.

87. CVEK M. Treatment of non-vital permanent incisors with calcium hydroxide. An effect on external root resorption in luxated teeth compared with effect of root filling with guttapercha. A follow-up. *Odont Revy* 1973;**24**:343–54.

88. LEVANDER E, MALMGREN O. Evaluation of the risk of root resorption during orthodontic treatment. *Eur J Orthod* 1988;**10**:30–8.

89. LEVANDER E, MALMGREN O, ELIASSON S. Evaluation of root resorption in relation to two orthodontic treatment regimes. A clinical experimental study. *Eur J Orthod* 1994;**16**:223–8.

90. MALMGREN B, CVEK M, LUNDBERG M, FRYKHOLM A. Surgical treatment of ankylosed and infrapositioned reimplanted incisors in adolescents. *Scand J Dent Res* 1984;**92**:391–9.

91. MALMGREN O, GOLDSON L, HILL C, ORWIN A, PETRINI L, LUNDBERG M. Root resorption after orthodontic treatment of traumatized teeth. *Am J Orthod Dentofacial Orthop* 1982;**82**:487–91.

92. LINGE L, LINGE BO. Patient characteristics and treatment variables associated with apical root resorption during orthodontic treatment. *Am J Orthod Dentofacial Orthop* 1991;**99**:35–43.

93. WEHRBEIN H, BAUER W, SCHNEIDER B, DIETRICH P. Experimentelle körperliche Zahnbewegung durch den knöchernen Nasenboden-eine Pilotstudie. *Fortschr Kieferorthop* 1990;**51**:271–6.

94. GÖS G, RAKOSI T. Die apikale Wurzelresorption unter kieferorthopädischer Behandlung. *Fortschr Kieferorthop* 1989;**50**:196–206.

95. HIRSCHFELDER U. Nachuntersuchung zur Reaktion des marginalen and apikalen Parodontiums unter kontinuerlicher Kraftapplikation. *Fortschr Kieferorthop* 1990;**51**:82–9.

96. STÅLHANE I, HEDEGARD B. Traumatized permanent teeth in children aged 7–15 years. Part II. *Swed Dent J* 1975;**68**:157–9.

97. BENENATI FW, SIMON JHS. Orthodontic root extrusion: its rationale and uses. *Gen Dent* 1986;**34**:285–9.

98. WEISSMAN J. Orthodontic extrusion of endodontically treated anterior teeth. *Can Dent Assoc J* 1983;**11**:21–4.

99. GHAREVI N. Extrusions-Therapiemöglichkeiten bei tieffrakturierten Zähnen. *Konservierende Zahnheilkunde* 1986;**4**:67–81.

100. KING NM, SO L. A laboratory fabricated fixed appliance for extruding anterior teeth with subgingival fractures. *Pediatr Dentistry* 1988;**10**:108–10.

101. PONTORIERO R, CELENZA F, RICCI G, CARNEVALE G. Rapid extrusion with fiber resection: a combined orthodontic–periodontic treatment modality. *Int J Period Rest Dent* 1987;**5**:31–43.

102. MALMGREN O, MALMGREN B, FRYKHOLM A. Rapid orthodontic extrusion of crown root and cervical root fractured teeth. *Endod Dent Traumatol* 1991;**7**:49–54.

103. ÅRTUN J, AAMDAL HMA. A Severe root resorption of fractured maxillary lateral incisor following endodontic treatment and orthodontic extrusion. *Endod Dent Traumatol* 1987;**3**:263–7.

104. Tegsjö U, Valerius-Olsson H, Frykholm A, Olgart K. Clinical evaluation of intra-alveolar transplantation of teeth with cervical root fractures. *Swed Dent J* 1987;**11**:235–50.

105. Kahnberg K-E. Intra-alveolar transplantation of teeth with crown-root fractures. *J Oral Maxillofac Surg* 1985;**43**:38–42

106. Kahnberg K-E. Surgical extrusion of root-fractured teeth – a follow-up study of two surgical methods. *Endod Dent Traumatol* 1988;**4**:85–9.

107. Andreasen FM, Andreasen JO, Bayer T. Prognosis of root-fractured permanent incisors – prediction of healing modalities. *Endod Dent Traumatol* 1989;**5**: 11–22.

108. Andreasen FM. Pulpal healing after luxation injuries and root fracture in the permanent dentition. *Endod Dent Traumatol* 1989;**5**:111–31.

109. Zachrisson BU, Jacobsen I. Long term prognosis of 66 permanent anterior teeth with root fracture. *Scand J Dent Res* 1975;**83**:345–54.

110. Schopf P. Frontzahntrauma/Frontzahnverlust – epidemiologische and kieferorthopädische Aspekte. *Fortschr Kieferorthop* 1989;**50**:564–98.

111. Joho JP. Das Zahntrauma aus kieferothopädischer Sicht. *Schweiz Monatsch Zahnheilk* 1974;**84**:934–46.

112. Kraft J, Hertrich J, Spitzer WJ, Hickel R, Mussig D. Das Frontzahntrauma bei Kindern and Jugendlichen. *ZWR* 1986;**95**:915–21.

113. Newsome PRH, Cook MS. Modifying upper lateral incisors to mimic missing central incisors: New ways to overcome old problems? *Restorative Dentistry* 1987;**13**:91–9.

114. Schröder U, Granath L. A new interceptive treatment of cases with missing maxillary lateral incisors. *Swed Dent J* 1981;**5**:155–8.

115. Kristerson L, Lagerström L. Autotransplantation of teeth in cases with agenesis or traumatic loss of maxillary incisors. *Eur J Orthod* 1991;**13**:486–92.

116. Bowden DEJ, Patel HA. Autotransplantation of premolar teeth to replace missing maxillary central incisors. *Br J Orthod* 1990;**17**:21–8.

117. Kristerson L. Autotransplantation of human premolars. A clinical and radiographic study of 100 teeth. *J Oral Surg* 1985;**14**:200–13.

118. Andreasen JO, Paulsen HU, Yu Z, Ahlquist R, Bayer T, Schwartz O. A long-term study of 370 autotransplanted premolars. Part I. Surgical procedures and standardized techniques for monitoring healing. *Eur J Orthod* 1990;**12**:3–13.

119. Andreasen JO, Paulsen HU, Yu Z, Bayer T, Schwartz O. A long-term study of 370 autotransplanted premolars. Part II. Tooth survival and pulp healing subsequent to transplantation. *Eur J Orthod* 1990;**12**:14–24.

120. Andreasen JO, Paulsen HU, Yu Z, Schwarz O. A longterm study of 370 autotransplanted premolars. Part III. Periodontal healing subsequent to transplantation. *Eur J Orthod* 1990;**12**:25–37.

121. Andreasen JO, Paulsen HU, Bayer T. A long-term study of 370 autotransplanted premolars. Part IV. Root development subsequent to transplantation. *Eur J Orthod* 1990;**12**:38–50.

122. Lagerström L, Kristerson L. Influence of orthodontic treatment on root development of autotransplanted premolars. *Am J Orthod Dentofacial Orthop* 1986;**89**:146–50.

123. Årtun J, Zachrisson U. New technique for semipermanent replacement of missing incisors. *Am J Orthod Dentofacial Orthop* 1984;**85**:367–75.

124. Adell R, Eriksson B, Lekholm U, Brånemark P-I, Jemt T. A long term follow-up study of osseointegrated implants in treatment of totally edentulous jaw. *Int J Oral Maxillofac Implants* 1990;**5**:347–59.

125. Jemt T, Lekholm U, Gröndahl K. A three year follow-up study of early single implant restorations ad modum Brånemark. *Int J Period Restor Dent* 1990;**5**:341–9.

126. Ödman J, Gröndahl K, Lekholm U, Thilander B. The effect of osseointegrated implants on the dento-alveolar development. A clinical and radiographic study in growing pigs. *Eur J Orthod* 1991;**13**:279–86.

127. Andreasen FM, Yu Z, Thomsen BL, Andersen PK. Occurrence of pulp canal obliteration after luxation injuries in the permanent dentition. *Endod Dent Traumatol* 1987;**3**:103–15.

128. Bruszt P. Secondary eruption of teeth intruded into the maxilla by blow. *Oral Surg Oral Med Oral Pathol* 1958;**11**:146–9.

129. Ravn JJ. Intrusion af permanente incisiver. *Tandlaegebladet* 1975;**79**:643–6.

130. Turley PK, Joiner MW, Hellström S. The effect of orthodontic extrusion on traumatically intruded teeth. *Am J Orthod Dentofacial Orthop* 1984;**85**:47–56.

131. Vinckier F, Lambrechts W, DeClerck D. Intrusion de l'incisive définitive. *Rev Belge Med Dent* 1989;**44**:99–106.

132. Jacobsen I. Clinical follow-up study of permanent incisors with intrusive luxation after acute trauma. *J Dent Res* 1983;**62**: Abstract No 37.

133. Perez B, Becker A, Chosak A. The repositioning of a traumatically intruded mature rooted permanent incisor with removable orthodontic appliance. *J Pedod* 1982;**6**:343–54.

134. Shapira J, Regev L, Liebfeld H. Re-eruption of completely intruded immature permanent incisors. *Endod Dent Traumatol* 1986;**2**:113–16.

135. Malmgren B, Malmgren O. Rate of infraposition of reimplanted ankylosed incisors related to age and growth in children and adolescents. *Dent Traumatol* 2002;**18**:28–36.

136. Albers DD. Ankylosis of teeth in the developing dentition. *Quintessence Int* 1986;**17**:303–8.

137. Ghose LJ, Baghdady VS, Enke H. Relation of traumatized permanent anterior teeth to occlusion and lip condition. *Community Dent Oral Epidemol* 1980;**8**:381–4.

138. Hunter ML, Hunter B, Kingdon A, Addy M, Dummer PMH, Shaw WC. Traumatic injury to maxillary incisor teeth in a group of South Wales school children. *Endod Dent Traumatol* 1990;**6**:260–4.

139. Forsberg CM, Tedestam G. Etiological and predisposing factors related to traumatic injuries to permanent teeth. *Swed Dent J* 1993;**17**:183–90.

140. Otuyemi OD. Traumatic anterior dental injuries related to incisor overjet and lip competence in 12-year-old Nigerian children. *Int J Paediatr Dent* 1994;**4**:81–5.

141. Soriano EP, Caldas AF Jr, Goes PS. Risk factors related to traumatic dental injuries in Brazilian schoolchildren. *Dent Traumatol* 2004;**20**:246–50.

142. Glendor U. On dental trauma in children and adolescents. Incidence, risk, treatment, time and costs. *Swed Dent J Suppl* 2000;**140**:1–52.

143. Bauss O, Rohling J, Schwestka-Polly R. Prevalence of traumatic injuries to the permanent incisors in candidates for orthodontic treatment. *Dent Traumatol* 2004;**20**:61–6.

144. Koroluk LD, Tulloch JF, Phillips C. Incisor trauma and early treatment for Class II Division 1 malocclusion. *Am J Orthod Dentofacial Orthop* 2003;**123**:117–25; discussion 125–6.

145. Brin I, Ben-Bassat Y, Zilberman Y, Fuks A. Effect of trauma to the primary incisors on the alignment of their permanent successors in Israelis. *Community Dent Oral Epidemiol* 1988;**16**:104–8.

146. Schwartz-Arad D, Levin L, Ashkenazi M. Treatment options of untreatable traumatized anterior maxillary teeth for future use of dental implantation. *Implant Dent* 2004;**13**:120–8.

147. Cvek M, Andreasen JO, Borum MK. Healing of 208 intra-alveolar root fractures in patients aged 7–17 years. *Dent Traumatol* 2001;**17**:53–62.

148. Cvek M, Mejare I, Andreasen JO. Healing and prognosis of teeth with intra-alveolar fractures involving the cervical part of the root. *Dent Traumatol* 2002;**18**:57–65.

149. Mirabella AD, Artun J. Risk factors for apical root resorption of maxillary anterior teeth in adult orthodontic patients. *Am J Orthod Dentofacial Orthop* 1995;**108**:48–55.

150. Hamilton RS, Gutmann JL. Endodontic-orthodontic relationships: a review of integrated treatment planning challenges. *Int Endod J* 1999; **32**:343–60.

151. Czochrowska EM, Skaare AB, Stenvik A, Zachrisson BU. Outcome of orthodontic space closure with a missing maxillary central incisor. *Am J Orthod Dentofacial Orthop* 2003;**123**:597–603.

152. Robertsson S, Mohlin B. The congenitally missing upper lateral incisor. A retrospective study of orthodontic space closure versus restorative treatment. *Eur J Orthod* 2000;**22**:697–710.

153. Antosz, M. Space closure for a missing central incisor. *Am J Orthod Dentofacial Orthop* 2003;**124**:18A; author reply 18A–19A.

154. Czochrowska EM, Stenvik A, Zachrisson BU. The esthetic outcome of autotransplanted premolars replacing maxillary incisors. *Dent Traumatol* 2002;**18**:237–45.

155. Chaushu S, Shapira J, Heling I, Becker A. Emergency orthodontic treatment after the traumatic intrusive luxation of maxillary incisors. *Am J Orthod Dentofacial Orthop* 2004;**126**:162–72.

156. Malmgren B, Malmgren O. Studies concerning the problem and management of replacement resorption in

the developing dentition – infraposition of reimplanted ankylosed incisors related to growth in children and adolescents. IX World Congress on Dental Trauma. Eilat, Israel. 1998.

157. Andersson L, Malmgren B. The problem of dentoalveolar ankylosis and subsequent replacement resorption in the growing patient. *Aust Endod J* 1999;**25**:57–61.

158. Kawanami M, Andreasen JO, Borum MK, Schou S, Hjörting-Hansen E, Kato H. Infraposition of ankylosed permanent maxillary incisors after replantation related to age and sex. *Endod Dent Traumatol* 1999;**15**:50–6.

159. Steiner DR. Timing of extraction of ankylosed teeth to maximize ridge development. *J Endod* 1997;**23**: 242–5.

160. Isaacson RJ, Strauss RA, Bridges-Poquis A, Peluso AR, Lindauer SJ. Moving an ankylosed central incisor using orthodontics, surgery and distraction osteogenesis. *Angle Orthod* 2001;**71**:411–18.

161. Kofod T, Wurtz V, Melsen B. Treatment of an ankylosed central incisor by single tooth dento-osseous osteotomy and a simple distraction device. *Am J Orthod Dentofacial Orthop* 2005;**127**:72–80.

162. Medeiros PJ, Bezerra AR, Treatment of an ankylosed central incisor by single-tooth dento-osseous osteotomy. *Am J Orthod Dentofacial Orthop* 1997;**112**:496–501.

163. Malmgren B. Decoronation: How, why, and when? *J Cal Dent Assoc* 2000;**28**:846–54.

164. Kahnberg KE. Intra-alveolar transplantation. I. A 10-year follow-up of a method for surgical extrusion of root fractured teeth. *Swed Dent J* 1996;**20**:165–72.

165. Warfvinge J, Kahnberg KE. Intraalveolar transplantation of teeth. IV. Endodontic considerations. *Swed Dent J* 1989;**13**:229–33.

166. Turley PK, Joiner MW, Hellstrom S. The effect of orthodontic extrusion on traumatically intruded teeth. *Am J Orthod* 1984;**85**:47–56.

167. Turley PK, Crawford LB, Carrington KW. Traumatically intruded teeth. *Angle Orthod* 1987;**57**:234–44.

168. Andersson L, Bodin I, Sorensen S. Progression of root resorption following replantation of human teeth after extended extraoral storage. *Endod Dent Traumatol* 1989;**5**:38–47.

169. Morin AC, Levander E, Malmgrem O. The risk of root resorption during orthodontic movement of severely traumatized incisors. In preparation.

170. Levander E, Malmgrem O. Long-term follow-up of maxillary incisors with severe apical root resorption. *Eur J Orthod* 2000;**22**:85–92.

171. Andreasen JO, Bakland LK, Andreasen FM, Traumatic injuries of permanent teeth. Part 3. A clinical study of the effect of treatment variables such as treatment delay, method of repositioning, type of splint, length of splinting and antibiotics on 140 teeth. *Dent Traumatol* 2006;**;22**:99–111.

# 25
# Restoration of Traumatized Teeth with Resin Composites

U. Pallesen & J. W. V. van Dijken

The primary choice for initial restoration of a crown-fractured front tooth has for a long time been resin composite material. The restoration can in most cases be performed immediately after injury if there is no sign of periodontal injury and the tooth responds to a sensibility test. The method's adhesive character is conservative to tooth-structure and with minimal risk of pulpal complication. In addition it offers an esthetic solution to the patient immediately after an injury, which may bring a little joy in a sad situation.

The resin composite build-up is often changed or repaired a couple of times, before the tooth is restored with a porcelain or porcelain fused to metal crown, at a time when the pulp is out of danger for a more invasive preparation. In some cases an endodontic treatment is still necessary. After crown therapy a gingival inflammation may occur due to the usual sub-gingival preparations. After some years *in situ*, the crowns may present an esthetic problem due to exposure of un-esthetic crown-margins. The invasive permanent crown restorations are therefore often not successful on a long-term scale. On the other hand a conservative direct restoration of an extensively fractured incisor crown with composite may be an exceedingly demanding procedure, involving esthetic acceptability, function and biological aspects and require significant skills, which may influence durability.

When are we ready to consider the non-invasive resin composite crown build-up as a permanent restoration? Has its durability improved? Do today's materials and techniques result in a better prognosis? Where are the problems? In this chapter these matters will be discussed with focus on factors in clinical procedures, which can influence the longevity of the restoration.

## Long-term prognosis of composite restorations

Traumatic injuries to anterior teeth in children and adolescents are a common problem. About 50% of children are exposed to dental trauma before the age of 15 and the majority of these injuries result in crown fractures which imply a great need for composite restoration (1) (Fig. 25.1). Unfortunately very few follow-up studies have been published on the long term fate of these restorations (1). One of the earliest studies of Class IV restorations was a 5-year follow-up of children with crown fractured permanent incisors reported by Ulvestad in 1978 (2). Three conventional resin composites were used following enamel etching. Among the 253 composite restorations, fracture of the composites was observed in 9–14% and fracture of enamel in 2–3%. A high frequency of marginal discoloration was reported (17–19%), but no case of secondary caries. Abrasion was seen in 52–79%. Robertson et al. in 1997 (3) evaluated crown fractures restored with resin composite materials, which were carried out during a 15-year period. In this study all restorations had been replaced at least once and 19% of the restorations had been replaced 10 times or more; in fact the majority of the restorations had been in service for only 2–4 years. In a retrospective cohort study published by Borssén and Holm in 2000 (4), 44% of the 16-year-old patients, where crown fractures were restored with composite, had the composite revised one or more times.

Only one longitudinally clinical study has been published by Spinas in 2004, where modern resin composites were used to restore traumatically injured teeth (5) (Fig 25.2.). Here 70 restorations were followed during 7 years with modified USPHS criteria. A total-etch technique and third or fourth generation bonding systems were used. The number of necessary restoration replacements increased and reached 100% after 7 years. The main reasons for replacement were: loss of the restoration; loss of marginal integrity; discoloration caused by the loss of pulp vitality. At the end of the study 48% of the replaced restorations had been replaced at least one more time.

Because only few publications on longevity of crown build-ups are available, the long-term prognosis may also be based on the experience of caries lesions in anterior teeth restored with Class IV restorations. The class of anterior cavity preparation substantially affects the resin composite

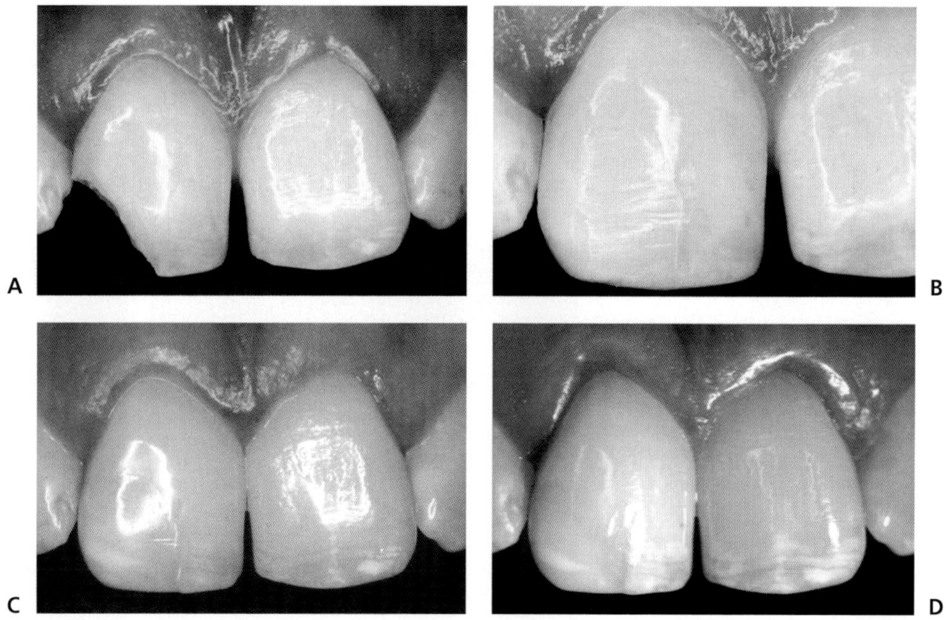

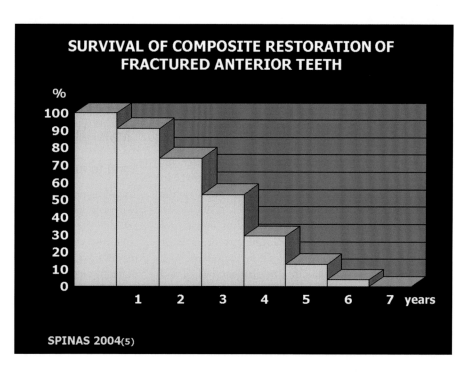

**Fig. 25.1** Initial result and durability of a composite crown build-up. A. The fractured incisor before restoration. B. The restored tooth at baseline. Morphology and white spots of the synergist tooth has been immitated. Horizontal lines in the surface structure mask the preparation line. C. Acceptable result after 5 years. D. Acceptable result after 10 years with no re-treatment between baseline and 10 years.

**Fig. 25.2** Long-term survival of composite restorations of trauma fractured teeth. From SPINAS (5) 2004.

survival (6–8). Unfortunately, most anterior resin studies do not distinguish between cavity classes and therefore limited clinical evidence has been published concerning the longevity of the more difficult Class IV resin composite restoration. Tyas in 1990 (9) restored 102 Class IV cavities with microfilled and hybrid composite materials. A cumulative failure rate of 26% was observed after 3 years. The 2 microfilled resin composite materials showed the highest failure rates (40% and 42%) compared to the hybrid materials (5% and 9%). Smales in 1991 (10) reported the survival of a conventional anterior resin composite with a low viscosity enamel bonding resin. The median survival time for Class III restorations was 9.8 years and for Class IV 4.1 years.

He attributed the losses to increased wear and occlusal stresses. Smales & Hawthorne in 1996 (11) examined in a retrospective study the survival and cost-effectiveness of restorations in various classes of cavity preparation in permanent teeth placed before 1980. For Class III resin composite restorations 72% survived for 10 years and for Class IV 48% survived 15 years. Browning & Dennison in 1996 (12) investigated the modes by which Class IV restorations failed. The main reason for replacement of Class IV was secondary caries (19%), marginal discoloration (11%) fracture of tooth (10%) and fracture of composite (47%) and 50% had failed by 5 years. The high failure rate of Class IV restorations was also shown by Miller et al. in 1997 (13),

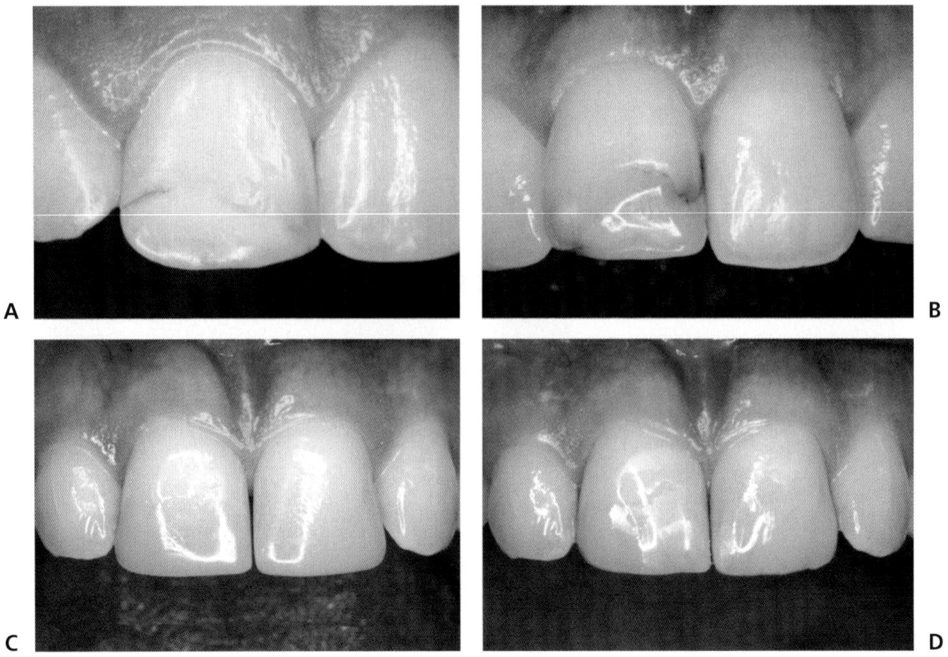

**Fig. 25.3** Common causes of failures of composite crown build-ups of fractured teeth. A. Marginal discoloration, lack of color-match and insufficient morphology. B. Marginal leakage leading to secondary caries. C. Incorrect morphology of restorations in both central incisors is the reason for an unacceptable esthetic result. D. After shaping the old restorations in C to a better morphology replacement could be postponed.

however based on very few restorations. Recently Burke et al. in 1999 (14) examined Class IV resin composite restorations and the mean longevity was 3.9 years.

Adhesive techniques and materials may influence longevity. Recent results from a 12-year still ongoing study of 464 anterior restorations of various modern anterior restorative materials showed a mean survival age (range) for the 30 Class IV restorations of 9.8 (7–12) years, where 22 of the 30 Class IV restorations were still in place (73.3%) at the last evaluation (15).

In conclusion, findings of the few studies on longevity of direct crown build-ups of fractured teeth have lead to the concept that these composites should be considered as a *semi-permanent restoration* with a median survival of 4–5 years. However, a few studies of modern composites have shown a potential for an improved longevity in the case of Class IV restorations.

The most frequent reasons for failures appear to be marginal leakage, bulk discoloration and fractures of the composite (Fig. 25.3), which presents the profession with a great challenge. Probably many of the old studies used non-optimal dentin bonding systems. Modern hybrid composites contain ultrafine inorganic filler particles with a mean diameter below 1 micron. They provide superior abrasion resistance and mechanical properties when compared with conventional or microfilled composites. Also the esthetic properties of new materials have been improved. However, resin composites should not be considered as a single product but as part of a complete system. The modern resin composite includes an enamel/dentin etchant, an enamel/dentin adhesive system, a resin composite and a light curing device. It is reasonable to believe that improvement in the retention and esthetics of Class IV restorations can be achieved with improvements in preparation and

bonding techniques as well as in filling, finishing and polishing procedures.

## Material considerations

### Bond to enamel

Traditional mechanical methods of retaining dental restorative materials required in most cases removal of sound tissue. These techniques have now been replaced largely with adhesive techniques. Buonocore's pioneering work, noticing the industrial use of phosphoric acid to improve adhesion of paints on cars, led to major changes in operative dentistry. Large preparations and extension for prevention have been gradually replaced by minimally invasive techniques. The basic mechanism of bonding to enamel for resin based materials is a micromechanical bond. It is essentially a replacement of minerals by resin monomers that after setting becomes interlocked in the irregularities and porosities created by conditioning. Adhesive restorations are tooth substance saving, and prevent microleakage along the cavity walls, which may improve the longevity of the restoration. The strength and durability of the adhesive bond depends on several factors: the physicochemical properties of the adhesive and adherent adhesive technique applied, polymerization stresses developed during curing and the continuous stress in the oral environment.

Adhesive dentistry started with the first commercial systems in the mid-1960s, followed in the early 1970s with the introduction of the acid-etch technique in the clinic. Since then there has been a continuous development and improvement in bonding agents. Effective bonding to enamel was achieved early and was proven to be durable and

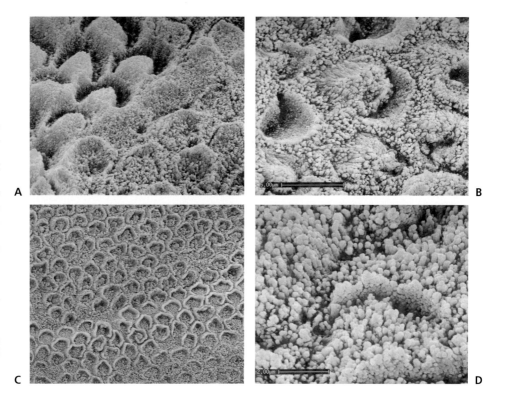

**Fig. 25.4** Unprepared (non-ground) buccal surface of a pre-molar acid etched with 37% phosphoric acid for 15 s. Different etch patterns can be observed. A. Two etch patterns with different degrees of demineralization between rod and interrod enamel. Original magnification 3600×. B. Etch pattern with high dissolution between rod and inter-rod enamel. Observe increase of surface area. Original magnification 7200×. C. Etch pattern with highest demineralization in the rod enamel. Original magnification 1200×. D. Higher magnification of C showing the various degrees of peripheral dissolution of the apatite crystals. Original magnification 12000×.

reliable in the clinic. Enamel etching transforms the smooth enamel surface into an irregular surface with a surface energy twice of that of unetched enamel (about 72 dynes/cm). An unfilled, low viscosity resin wets the high-energy surface and is drawn into the micro porosities by capillary attraction. Acid etching removes about 10 μm from the surface and creates irregularities from 5–50 μm deep. Different enamel-etching patterns can be observed after etching (Fig. 25.4). Generally, a 32–40% phosphoric acid etching time of 15 seconds for instrumented enamel, and rinsing times of 10–20 seconds are recommended to achieve the most receptive enamel surface for bonding.

## Bond to dentin

Adhesion to dentin was more difficult to obtain. Only recently developed dentin adhesive systems have produced bond strength approaching that of enamel bonding and have achieved higher levels of clinical success. The early selective enamel-etching was replaced in the 1990s by the total-etch technique with simultaneous conditioning and priming of the enamel and dentin. Chronological, dentin bonding systems have been classified in generations. In the first and second generations, enamel was acid etched separately, while the dentin adhesive mechanism to dentin involved an ionic interaction to the positively charged calcium-ions. Modest bond strength and high clinical failure rates were observed. In the early to mid-1990s many dentin adhesives in the third and fourth generations were based on the dentin etching technique. Most of these 3-step adhesive systems required a first step of dentin conditioning to decalcify the intertubular and peritubular dentin. In the second

step a primer with amphiphilic monomers, displaces the dentinal liquid and infiltrates the collagen network of the demineralized dentin. The third step with adhesive monomers enhances the bond with the hydrophobic resin composite. The production of a high micromechanical bond to the tooth tissue is ensured by formation of the so-called hybrid layer. The degree of monomer penetration is enhanced by water chasing solvents in the primer step and the collagen fibrils have to be coated optimally by the primer monomers to obtain a high bond. The multiple-step procedure is technique sensitive and the clinical success may depend on the handling of the system (16). Developments in adhesive dentistry are the simplification of the multi-step systems, to reduce their technique sensitivity during clinical handling, in the fifth and six generation systems. Several simplified, one-bottle and self-etching primer systems have recently been introduced to decrease the technique sensitivity and allergic potential of the 3-step systems. In the one-bottle or two-step systems, primer and adhesive are combined in one step. Commonly this step was applied twice, but in recently marketed systems a single application is recommended. In the self-etching primer systems, unsaturated, potentially polymerizable organic acids or acidic monomers are incorporated, and etching and priming of the dentin occur simultaneously. They are based on infiltration and modification of the smear layer by acidic monomers or by dissolving of the smear layer and demineralizing of the underlying outer layer of the dentin followed by infiltrating the smear layer covered dentin with acidic monomers of the primer (17). In one type of self etching primer system, an adhesive is applied on top, while in other systems, the 'all-in-one' systems, all 3 steps are applied simultaneously.

## Glass ionomer bond

Parallel to the progress made with resin-based adhesives, glass ionomer cement technology has been modified and improved. Glass ionomer-based materials have a chemical bond to tooth tissues based on their specific chemical formula. Developments during the 1990s combined glass ionomer and resin composite in new adhesive materials with mixed characteristics. Improved modifications, the resin-modified glass ionomer cements (RMGIC) were introduced in 1988. Addition of light-curing resin components led to a higher resistance to early moisture contact and desiccation, and higher mechanical characteristics. RMGIC were used first as bases or restoratives, and in1995, a modern RMGIC was developed as dentin-enamel adhesive. After pretreatment of the cavity with a weak polyalkenoic acid, self adhesion of the adhesive is obtained by both a micromechanical interlocking by a submicron hybrid layer (0.5–1 µm) and a chemical bond through ionic bonds between the carboxyl groups of the glass ionomer and calcium of hydroxyapatite that remains around the collagen. Kemp-Scholte and Davidsson (18) showed that a material with enhanced flow and reduced elastic modulus may function as a stress-absorbing layer and improve marginal sealing. Resin composites have a higher Young's modulus of elasticity which results in a relative high remaining contraction stress compared to poly-acid modified resin composites (PMRC) and RMGIC.

## Resin materials

Historically, restoring of fractured anterior teeth has evolved from the use of stainless steel crowns to the current procedures of bonded esthetic resin based materials. The commercial introduction of resin composites in the late 1960s led to their widespread use in the restoration of Class IV cavities. Retention of the resin restorations relied for the most part on the effectiveness of the bonding systems utilized. Preparation techniques recommended have varied over time such as butt joint margins, feathered edge margins, bevels, threaded pin and retention slot preparations, long bevels and chamfer preparation. Retentive pins improve the retention of Class IV restorations only to a small extent (10%), and have risks such as perforation of the pulp chamber, inflammatory responses of the pulp, dentin cracks, perforation of the root surface, and increase in fracture susceptibility (19, 20). Semi-permanent restoration of an incisor with a composite resin material, following acid etching of the enamel became a frequently used method during the 1970s (2). Resin composites used at that time in anterior build-ups lacked color stability, polishability and physical properties. These limitations could not compete with the esthetics of the laboratory produced porcelain or porcelain-fused-to-metal crowns. Patients demand superior esthetics for anterior restorations. They have to simulate the natural tooth in color, texture and translucency. The materials must have adequate strength, good wear characteristics, good marginal adaptation and sealing, color stability, insolubility and biocompatibility. Resin composites are currently the direct restorative materials that best fulfil these requirements.

A resin composite contains four components: a polymer matrix, filler particles, a silan coupling agent and an initiator system. Newer formulations of resin composites with improved particle size distribution have imparted additional strength and polishability, allowing the materials to be used in rather high stress bearing areas. Varying degrees of opacity are available required for the different areas of the tooth. Undesirable characteristics of resin composites are their volumetric shrinkage and coefficient of thermal expansion. Shrinkage stresses during the post-gel phase may cause crack and marginal gap formation between the resin composite and the walls of the preparation with the weakest bonds. Gap formation may result in postoperative sensitivity, marginal leakage, marginal discoloration and secondary caries. The size of stress formation on the bonding surface depends partly on the configuration of the cavity. The higher the number of bonded surfaces in the cavity, the higher the stress formation on the bonded margins. Occlusal Class I cavities show the highest configuration-factor (21), while the Class IV cavity with more unbounded surfaces has a more favourable configuration.

The majority of currently used resin composites are hybrid resin composites. Hybrid resin composites are a combination of conventional and microfiller technology. They contain a blend of submicron (0.04 µm) and small particles (1–4 µm), allowing a high level of filler loading resulting in improved physical properties. They are often the materials of choice for the whole restoration, but may also be used as only the bulk/dentin part of Class III and IV restorations. Microfilled resin composites contain submicron inorganic fillers. They are not as strong as the hybrid composites but can be used as the enamel part, veneering of anterior restorations due to their high polishability and translucency. Glass ionomer restorative materials are not commonly used in anterior restorations when esthetics is a major consideration. They are indicated in cavities with deep cervical located margins or high caries risk patients. Recently, so called nanofiller resin composite materials have been introduced. These materials contain fillers in the size of microfillers (4–40 nm) claiming a high polishability and high abrasion resistance.

## Curing of materials

Autocured resin composites were the first resin composite materials used for treatment of anterior cavities. A major drawback was their bulk discoloration over time. Light cured resin composites became therefore increasingly popular since their introduction in the mid-1970s, making dental restorations more conservative and esthetic. The degree of polymerization in cross-linked resin based systems plays a potentially significant role in determining the ultimate physical and mechanical properties of the material. Inadequate polymerization results in inferior biological and physico-mechanical properties, such as poor resistance to wear, increased rates of water absorption and poor color stability (22–25). The degree of cure is affected by the power density of the curing unit, the exposure time, the resin shade, and the filler size (26). As light passes through the bulk of the restoration, its intensity decreases greatly, thus decreasing the curing efficacy and limiting the depth of cure (27). Power density is fundamental for an adequate depth of cure.

The use of high intensity light sources to improve composite properties has recently been introduced. High intensity lights provide higher values of the degree of conversion and superior mechanical and physical properties but produce on the other hand also higher contraction strain rates during the polymerization of resin composites (28). The most widely used curing units today are quartz tungsten halogen (QTH) units. Their bulb is filled with iodine or bromine gas and contains a tungsten filament. When connected to an electric current the tungsten filament glows and produces a very powerful light (29). White light is produced, which is then filtered to the range of blue light (400–500 nm). However, only part of the emitted spectrum of light is effective for activating the photoinitiators. A QTH curing unit should deliver a power density of 350–400 mW/cm$^2$ to adequately cure. Heat generation is a major disadvantage of QTH units and increases with increasing radiation time (25, 30, 31). Other drawbacks are limited lifetime of the bulb and degradation of the reflector and filter over time. It has been reported that 2 mm increment of resin composite should be placed combined with a 40–60 second light cure (32, 33). However, newer curing units are more powerful and may offer higher depth of cure or reduced exposure time. Other QTH curing units feature so-called soft-start programs, e.g. two-step curing and pulse-delay curing, according to which an initial exposure at relatively low power density is followed by exposure at higher power density. The aim is to improve marginal adaptation by prolonging the phase during which the resin composite may flow and thus compensate for polymerization shrinkage and stress (28, 34–36).

To overcome some of the problems inherent to QTH units, light emitting diode (LED) technology has been introduced in operative dentistry (37). In these devices junctions of doped gallium nitride semiconductors (p-n junctions) are subject to an electric current and generate blue light. LED's curing units have a narrower wavelength spectrum compared to QTH curing units and require no filters. In contrast to QTH units, 100% of the light emitted by blue LEDs lies within the spectrum that can be used to cure most resin composites (450–490 nm), i.e. resin composites initiated by camphoroquinone (31). LED curing units have significant advantages compared with the QTH curing units. The diodes have a life-time of more than 10,000 hours compared with the 40–100 hrs effective lifetime of QTH bulbs, and there is no degrading of bulb, reflector or filter over time which results in reduction of curing effectiveness. They produce little heat and no fan is needed. Whereas the first LED units were characterized by relatively low power density, more recently marketed LED units display higher power density and/or wider wavelength spectrum resulting in curing efficiency comparable to halogen lights regardless of curing modes (38, 39).

## Clinical implications

The need for a high level of esthetics is obvious when an anterior fractured tooth is restored. This, together with already mentioned problems of too early replacements of Class IV composite restoration, presents the profession with a great challenge. Quality of restoration at baseline highly influences longevity. The right choice of material, bonding system and curing method has already been mentioned as important matters, but also other aspects in the clinical procedure as preparation techniques, shade selection, filling and finish/polish techniques must be optimized. The better longevity, the closer to the goal, where this non invasive restoration technique can be considered as a permanent restoration (Fig. 25.1A–D).

## Critical points in the restorative procedure

### Preparation techniques

In order to prevent loss of the restoration, marginal chipping and marginal discoloration, preparation technique should be carefully considered. Also the esthetic appearance is influenced by the preparation technique. Most often a bevel or a chamfer preparation is applied. Either should be 1–1$^1$/$_2$ mm width, go half way through the enamel, and surround the periphery of the fracture line. A bevel compared to a chamfer preparation is conservative concerning removal of tooth substance and gives a more gradient color change from the tooth-structure to the restoring material. On the other hand, the fragile margins of the restoring material frequently deteriorate over the years and may lead to marginal chipping and discoloration. A chamfer is more invasive and provides more bulk to the restoring material at the margins, but may fail to blend in with tooth color at the fracture line. To overcome this, the stair-step or wave preparation technique has been recommended, in which the preparation follows the anatomical contour of the human incisors (Fig. 25.5). Another mentioned advantage of the chamfer compared to the bevel is the increased enamel surface area providing a better bond to tooth surface (20). Both preparation types will provide sufficient retention for even large crown-build-ups.

### Shade selection

In contrast to old composite resin materials, the new generations have shown acceptable color stability and smoother surface characteristics. Shade selection plays an important role for the esthetic outcome of an anterior restoration and requires knowledge of colors and careful analysis of the

## Fig. 25.5 Anatomical layering technique for restoration of an incisor with incisal translucency

A. The crown-fractured incisor. B. A 1–1¹/₂ mm wide wave-shaped bevel preparation has been made using a flame shaped diamond bur, here visualized by a pencil line.

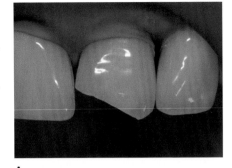

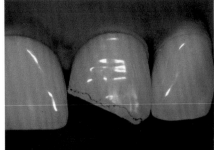

**A**

**B**

### Silicone mould mock-up

C. An impression of the old crown build-up or of an indirect wax-up/direct composite mock-up provides a mould for the lingual and incisal areas. Control of the layering technique is hereby made easier. D. After bonding procedures the palatinal part is built up with a thin layer of enamel material (transparent). The silicone mould is used to form the palatinal surface in the right place.

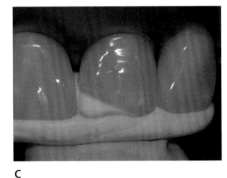

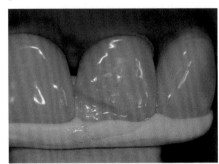

**C**

**D**

### Build-up of the palatal surface

E. The first enamel layer in place. Color of the enamel has been selected before treatment by using a shade guide in the incisal area of the synergist tooth. F. A matrix fixed by a wedge helps to control form in the mesial area.

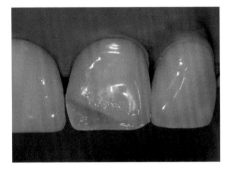

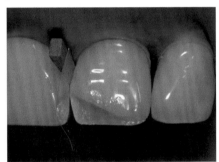

**E**

**F**

### Build-up of the mesial surface

G. The mesial enamel is built up with enamel material. H. The first layer of dentin material (opaque) is placed. The color of this layer should have the same hue but a higher chroma than the second dentin layer. Here an A3 has been used.

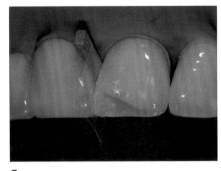

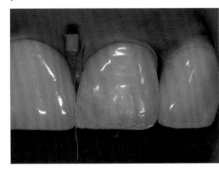

**G**

**H**

### Build-up of the facial dentin surface

I. The second dentin layer should conform with the facial surface and leave space for the enamel layer. The mammelons are shaped, and for masking purpose the bevel may be partly covered. Selection of color for this second/last dentin layer has been done in the gingival area of an upper canine, where the enamel is thin and the dentin saturated. Here an A1 has been used. J. To imitate translucency incisally in the mesial and distal areas and below/between the mammelons a translucent blue material is added here (arrows).

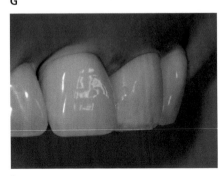

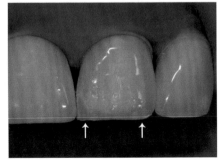

**I**

**J**

## Building up the incisal edge

K. The incisal halo effect is made by amber/yellow colored material closest to the incisal edge (arrow). L. Finally the whole facial surface is covered with a thin layer of enamel-material. The facial morphology should only be slightly overextended, in order to facilitate finishing.

## Finishing the restoration

M. Incisal aspect before finish. The silicone mould has helped placing the incisal edge in the right position. N. Final result after polish. Diamonds burs and abrasive disks have been used for shaping the morphology and fine disks and rubber polishers for the polish. The finial gloss is obtained by polishing paste. Notice the important reflexes placed as in the neighboring teeth. The halo and the mesial and distal translucencies are visible in the incisal area.

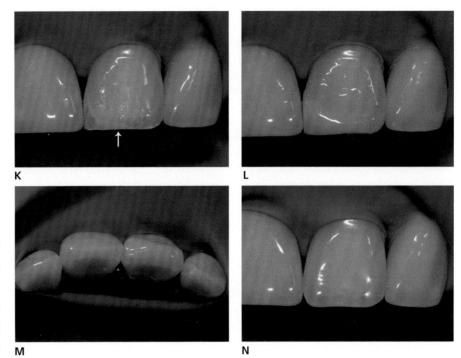

K          L

M          N

remaining tooth-structure and of the adjacent teeth. The same color-layering technique as used by the dental technician for indirect esthetic restorations may be applied. Resin composites with different hues, chroma and values have been used for a long time, but properties as high/low translucencies, opalescence and fluorescence – known from ceramic materials – have lately been added. It would go too far in this chapter, to include information of shade selection at a high level, and only a few definitions and recommendations will be mentioned (40, 41).

*Hue* is the basic shade of the tooth and can be assigned to the dentin. Hue is often referred to as the A, B, C or D in the Vita shade-guide.

*Chroma* is a further refinement of the hue that defines the quality of color, strong or weak, or saturation/intensity of the color. Chroma is often referred to as the 1, 2, 3 or 4 in the Vita shade-guide. Hue and chroma may be evaluated in the cervical area of a canine, where the enamel is thin and the dentin thick. The hue is usually uniform in a person's teeth, whereas the chroma may vary from tooth to tooth.

*Value* is the degree of brightness or darkness in the tooth, or the amount of white reflected from the tooth. Value is assigned to the enamel, and although the enamel itself is colorless, it projects the underlying color in the dentin. Value is evaluated at the incisal third of the tooth.

*Translucency* in a tooth expresses how much light is able to pass through the tooth-substance. Part of the light is absorbed, part is diffused and part is transmitted.

*Opalescence* is the enamel's capacity to distinguish wavelength in the light. The short wavelengths are reflected (appear blue) and the long wavelengths pass through the enamel and appear orange.

*Fluorescence* in natural teeth will reflect blue light, when exposed to incident UV light. A material without fluorescence will look dark e.g. in a nightclub.

*Identifying characteristics of tooth color* is of significant importance, when decision of shades for a crown-build up is made (42–44). Natural tooth architecture affects color by the different layers, by its composition and by the quality of dentin and enamel. Dentin is more opaque than enamel, and enamel translucency is high. At the incisal edge and in the periphery of a crown the enamel is thick and without underlying dentin, which makes these areas translucent (appearing gray or blue). In the cervical area enamel is thin and supported by dentin, which makes the area more opaque (appearing yellow/brown). Wear of the enamel in the incisal area will remove the translucent area (the mammelons will disappear) and in general a worn tooth will appear more saturated (higher chroma) and more opaque. Formation of tertiary dentin will also lead to a higher saturation of the dentin. Different kinds of mineralization disturbances in enamel may give special characteristics to the tooth. Each tooth has its own characteristics to be mimicked in the crown build-up.

Decision of colors and form should always be performed before isolation with rubberdam or cotton rolls, when the tooth is still moistened with saliva and in its natural surroundings. Commercial shade guides do not usually show the real tones and are only of limited assistance. It can be recommended to make a diagnostic mock-up before acid etching, where the different selected colors and translucencies are applied in the right thickness and place, and with the natural background (often the dark oral cavity). Evaluating colors of the wet mock-up after light curing will also give an impression of the color change from before and after curing.

## Anatomical layering technique

Natural upper incisors often have palatal ridges in the proximal areas – like a shovel form – and if this is reproduced in the restoration, fracture resistance may be improved. Also other information of form, colors, translucencies and special characteristics obtained from the remaining tooth-structure and from the adjacent teeth should be reproduced. The so-called anatomical layering technique may be preferred to control the different elements (Fig. 25.5A–N) (45–47). By this method the restoration is built up with 2–3 layers of dentin material (opaque) of the same hue, but with different chroma (highest saturation of the first lingual layer) and a facial layer of enamel material (translucent). The preparation line may be masked by partly covering the preparation with the last dentin layer, but without extending it to the prepared margin. Special effects in the restoration like mottled enamel, white or yellow spots, halo effect, mammelons can be added by tints between the last dentin and the enamel layer, or by using special enamel material containing the characteristics. If high translucency is needed in the incisal and approximal areas – typically for young people – these areas may be built up of only enamel materials. Each composite system has its own color-system with different intensities of hue, chroma, value, translucency etc. influencing the layering thickness and the characterization of the restoration.

Different insertion techniques can be used to obtain the correct morphology and to control the layering technique (46):

- An impression of an of an old crown build-up to be replaced or of an indirect wax-up/direct composite mock-up can provide an excellent matrix for the lingual, proximal and incisal areas. Control of the layering technique is hereby made possible (Fig. 25.5C, D).
- A finger-hold matrix band or a fingertip protected by tape may also give support for the first lingual layer. In both cases the exact position of the lingual surface may be difficult to control. The uncured resin material should due to its allergic potential never be touched by fingers. Monomers from resin materials also penetrate gloves within a short time (48–51).
- A crown matrix (Odus Pella® Crown or CoForm Angulus®) may also provide possibilities for the layering technique (Fig. 25.6A–L). The facial part of the matrix can be filled with enamel-material followed by 1–2 dentin colors. This method, however, makes control of the layers more difficult.

## Finish and polish

An optimal finish and polish of the restoration improves fracture resistance, prevents periodontal problems and improves esthetics. If morphology of the restoration is not in accordance with tooth anatomy during placement, finish and polish may be time-consuming. Time spent on the modelling procedure before light curing will richly be gained during finish.

### Occlusion/articulation control

As already mentioned clinical studies have shown fracture to be one of the main reasons for early failure of class IV restorations. This may be caused by insufficient adjustment of occlusion and articulation. Although nowadays hybrid materials have improved mechanical properties, inadvertently left supra-contacts during eccentric movements may lead to cohesive fracture of the composite material. Therefore, care should be taken to provide light group contact in centric, protrusive, and protrusive lateral positions if contact is necessary.

### Finishing in general

Diamonds, carbide burs, stones, disks, strips, knives etc. may all be used to remove excess material and shaping to correct morphology. The transition line between tooth and resin material can be masked by letting structures in the natural tooth surface such as curves, grooves or crests cross the preparation and continue in the surface of the restoration. It may be difficult to distinguish between composite material and tooth structure, and care should be taken not to remove sound tooth structure. Overheating is another option that harms the pulp and deteriorates composite material creating visible white lines along the margins. Therefore, water-cooling should be applied in all finishing procedures.

Surface polish can be made by fine polishing disks or rubber polishers, but care should be taken not to sacrifice morphology of the finished surface. Finally a highly reflective surface gloss may be obtained using abrasive polishing paste applied with a brush of fine diamond bur. In teeth of young people natural surface texture reflects light in many different directions, which makes them look shiny and lively (Fig. 25.7A). In older people wear or erosion has often removed surface structure and the reflection of light will be from only one or two reflexes (Fig. 25.7B). A composite crown build-up should have the same surface texture as the adjacent natural teeth. Texture of a restoration can be made with a sharp edged stone after polish, but before the final polishing paste. Creating surface texture when needed will often give the final touch to an esthetic direct crown build-up.

## Indications

The initial treatment of a fractured front tooth will most often be a composite crown build-up. Concerning the final treatment the pros and cons for the direct composite restoration, the porcelain full/partial crown or the porcelain-fused-to-metal crown should be discussed in every case. Age of the patient, size of the fracture, bite function/occlusion, para-functions, esthetic need, economy and not least the skills of the dentist – and the technician – should be included in the decision.

A disadvantage with composite crown build-ups is the lack of information on durability. However, durability of Class IV restorations with newer materials and bonding systems have improved – as already mentioned – and

**Fig. 25.6 Restoring technique using a crown matrix**
A. A fractured central incisor. B. Preparation of a facial bevel with a flame shaped diamond.

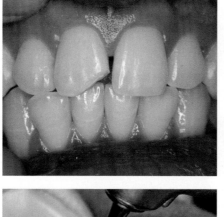

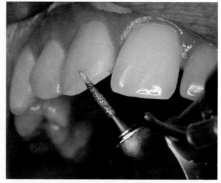

**Palatal chamfer**
C. Preparation of a palatal chamfer using a round stone or a rounded conic diamond. D. If sufficient enamel in the gingival area is left, a bevel can be made using a metal polishing strip.

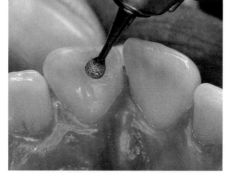

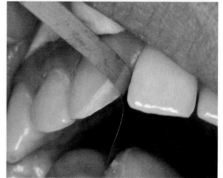

**Final preparation and shade selection**
E. The final preparation. F. Shade selection for the enamel is made in the incisal area of the neighboring tooth, whereas dentin color can be selected in the gingival area of the canine.

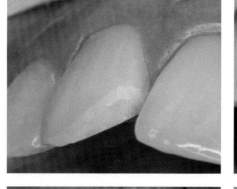

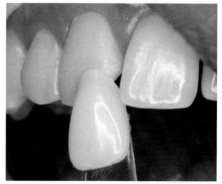

**Adjustment of a matrix**
G. A corner matrix is adjusted to cover only 1–2 mm outside the preparation. The right wedge is selected. H. After acid etching and bonding the dentin part of the restoration is built up by hand using dentin material (opaque) followed by light-curing.

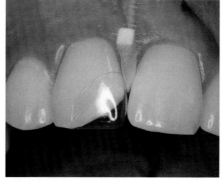

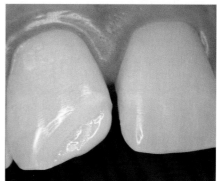

although longevity of ceramic restorations still is better, the biological consequences by the invasive treatment and the high initial cost for the patient should be included in the treatment decision.

Full coverage should be avoided in the young adolescent or the early adult dentition in order to prevent a negative pulp response of the combined irritants of trauma, extensive preparation, temporization and cementation. Young anterior teeth may not have reached the state of full erup-

tion, and the gingival response to placement of a crown margin beneath the free gingival crest is often less than positive (52). Fracture resistance with modern resin and bonding materials is acceptable, and in case of occurrence of a fracture, it is easily and reliably repaired (53). Chipping at the margins and marginal discoloration appearing over time may be removed by finishing the margins. Therefore, composite resin crown build-ups will often be able to cover the demand for esthetics, biological acceptability and resist-

**Fig. 25.6 (*cont.*)**
**Application of enamel composite**
I. For restoration of the enamel part the corner matrix is used. Only the facial and palatal part of the matrix is filled with enamel-material (translucent). This can be done before the bonding procedure starts, as long as the filled matrix is kept protected from light. After placement surplus of material is removed before light curing. J. After light-curing and removal of matrix and wedge.

**Finished restoration**
K. The restoration is polished to mimic the synergist tooth by morphology, surface structure and reflexes. L. The lingual aspect of the final restoration.

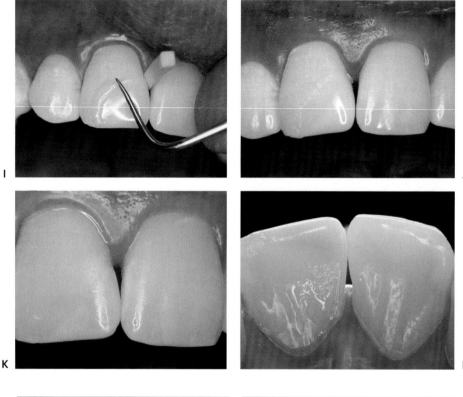

**Fig. 25.7** Surface structure is important. A composite crown build up should have the same surface texture as the adjacent natural teeth. A. In teeth of young people natural surface texture reflects light in many different directions, which makes them look shiny and lively. B. In older people wear or erosion has often removed surface structure and the reflection of light will be from only one or two reflexes.

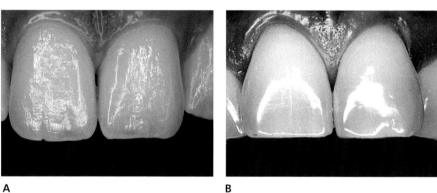

ance to abrasive wear, where the size of the fracture is small to medium, and should be first choice of permanent treatment in such cases both in young and older patients (54). For larger crown fractures the choice of treatment may more often be a ceramic restoration, which also depends on both the skills of the dentist and the economic resources of the patient. If in any doubt the least invasive treatment should always be preferred. If it does not meet the expectation of the patient or the dentist, the non-invasive treatment may always be changed to a more invasive treatment later in life, whereas the opposite is not possible.

## Essentials

### Indications

Resin composites offer a conservative restoration of crown-fractured teeth with a minimal risk of pulpal and periodontal complications in both children and adults.

Restoration can be performed immediately after injury if there is no associated periodontal or supporting bone injury.

Hybrid composites and amphiphilic bonding systems are especially useful.

### Durability

Class IV resin restorations have a shorter longevity than Class III, and also a shorter longevity than full ceramic and porcelain fused to metal crowns.

### Biology and economy

A composite build-up of a fractured tooth is more conservative to the hard tooth-structures, the pulp and the surrounding soft tissue than a crown.

Considering that the composite build up may need replacement 2–3 times to equal the durability of a crown, the economical consequences for the patients over time may be the same for both treatments.

## Treatment

(1) Shade selection and preparation of matrix system.

(2) Select resin composites for layering technique.

(3) Prepare a 1–1¹/₂ mm wide chamfer or bevel around the fracture. To mask the transition line between tooth and resin material the facial part may be shaped like a stair-step or a wave.

(4) A pulp protective agent should be applied only on localizations in the dentin with very close distance to the pulp.

(5) Enamel and dentin bonding.

(6) Insert the composite material in opaque (dentin) and translucent (enamel) layers of max. 2 mm. Characterization resin material may be added below the last enamel layer or may be part of the enamel layer, depending on the resin system.

(7) Each layer is formed to right morphology and polymerized for at least 20 sec each.

(8) Remove matrix and major excess of material.

(9) Trim cavity margins and finish to correct morphology with diamonds, burs or discs. Polish with rubber polisher, abrasive discs and paste.

(10) Surface texture can be made using a sharp stone or a diamond bur before final polish.

## Survival of composites

Survival of crown build-ups are dependent on:

- Size of restoration
- Skill of the dentist
- Bruxism/clenching
- Oral hygiene
- Material properties
- Enamel and dentin bonding systems

Composite restorations should be considered semipermanent restorations with an expected average of 3–4 years lifetime.

## References

1. Andreasen JO, Andreasen FM. Dental traumatology: quo vadis. *Endod Dent Traumatol* 1990;**6**:78–80.
2. Ulvestad H. A 5-year evaluation of semipermanent composite resin crowns. *Scand J Dent Res* 1978;**86**:163–8.
3. Robertson A, Robertson S, Norén JG. A retrospective evaluation of traumatized permanent teeth. *Int J Pediatric Dent* 1997;**7**:217–26.
4. Borssén E, Holm A-K. Treatment of traumatic dental injuries in a cohort of 16-year-olds in northern Sweden. *Endod Traumatol* 2000;**16**:276–81.
5. Spinas E. Longevity of composite restorations of traumatically injured teeth. *Am J Dent* 2004;**17**:407–11.
6. Mjör IA. Placement and replacement of restorations. *Operative Dent* 1981;**6**:49–54.
7. Dijken van JWV. A clinical evaluation of anterior conventional, microfiller, and hybrid composite resin fillings. *Acta Odontol Scand* 1986;**44**:357–67.
8. Allander L, Birkhed D, Bratthall D. Quality evaluation of anterior restorations in private practice. *Swed Dent J* 1989;**13**:141–50.
9. Tyas MJ. Correlation between fracture properties and clinical performance of composite resins in Class IV cavities. *Austr Dent J* 1990;**35**:46–9.
10. Smales RJ. Effects of enamel-bonding, type of restoration, patient age and operator on the longevity of an anterior composite resin. *Am J Dent* 1991;**4**:130–3.
11. Smales RJ, Hawthorne WS. Long-term survival and cost-effectiveness of five dental restorative materials used in various classes of cavity preparations. *Int Dent J* 1996;**46**:126–30.
12. Browning WD, Dennison JB. A survey of failure modes in composite resin restorations. *Operative Dent* 1996;**21**:160–6.
13. Miller BJ, Robinson PB, Inglis AT. Clinical evaluation of an anterior hybrid composite resin over 8 years. *Brit Dent J* 1997;**182**:26–30.
14. Burke FJT, Cheung SW, Mjör IA, Wilson NHF. Restoration longevity and analysis of reasons for the placement and replacement of restorations provided by vocational dental practitioners and their trainers in the United Kingdom. *Quintessence Int* 1999;**30**:234–42.
15. Dijken van JWV, Pallesen U. Long-term survival of Class IV restorations restored with new anterior restorative materials. In preparation.
16. Sano H, Kanemura N, Burrow MF, et al. Effect of operator variability on dentin adhesion: students vs dentists. *Dent Mat* 1998;**17**:51–8.
17. Van Meerbeek B, Inoue S, Perdigao J, et al. Enamel and dentin adhesion. In: Summitt JB, Robbins JW, Schwartz RS. eds. *Fundamentals of operative dentistry, a contemporary approach.* Singapore: Quintessence Publishing Co., 2001:178–235.
18. Kemp-Scholte CM, Davidsson CL. Complete marginal seal of Class V resin composite restorations effected by increased flexibility. *J Dent Res* 1990;**69**:1240–3.
19. Felton SA. Pulpal response to threaded pin and retentive slot techniques. *J Prosth Dent* 1991;**66**:597–602.
20. Eid H. Retention of composite resin restorations in class IV preparations. *J Clin Pediat Dent* 2002;**26**:251–6.
21. Feilzer AJ, de Gee AJ, Davidson CL. Setting stress in composite resin in relation to configuration of the restoration. *J Dent Res* 1987;**66**:1636–9.
22. Venhoven BA, de Gee AJ, Davidsson CL. Polymerization contraction and conversion of light-curing bisGMA-based methacrylate resins. *Biomaterials* 1993;**14**:871–5.
23. Pearson GJ, Longman CM. Water sorption and solubility of resin-based materials following adequate polymerization by a visible-light curing system. *J Oral Rehab* 1989;**16**:57–61.
24. Caughman WF, Caughman GB, Shiflett RA, Rueggeberg F, Schuster GS. Correlation of cytotoxicity, filler loading and curing time of dental composites. *Biomaterials* 1991;**12**:737–40.
25. Davidsson CL, Feilzer AJ. Polymerization shrinkage and polymerization shrinkage stress in polymer-based restoratives. *J Dent* 1997;**25**:435–40.

26. RUEGGENBERG FA, CAUGHMAN WF, CURTIS JW, DAVIS HC. Factors affecting cure at depths within light-activated resin composites. *Am J Dent* 1993;**6**:91–5.

27. RUYTER IE, ÖYSAED H. Conversion in different depth of ultraviolet and visible light activated composite materials. *Acta Odont Scand* 1982;**40**:179–92.

28. UNO S, ASMUSSEN E. Marginal adaptation of a restorative resin polymerized at reduced rate. *Scand J Dent Res* 1991;**99**:440–4.

29. MEYER GR, ERNST C-P, WILLERSHAUSEN B. Decrease in power output of new light-emitting diode (LED) curing devices with increasing distance to filling surface. *J Adhes Dent* 2002;**4**:197–204.

30. SHORTALL AC, HARRINGTON E. Temperature rise during polymerization of light-activated resin composites. *J Oral Rehab* 1998;**25**:908–13.

31. TARLE Z, MENIGA A, KNEZEVIC A, ŠUTALO J, RISTIC M, PICHLER G. Composite conversion and temperature rise using a conventional, plasma arc, and an experimental blue LED curing unit. *J Oral Rehab* 2002;**29**:662–7.

32. CAUGHMAN WF, RUEGGEBERG FA. Shedding new light on composite polymerization. *Operative Dent* 2002;**27**:636–8.

33. RUEGGEBERG FA, CAUGHMAN WF, Curtis JW Jr. Effect of light intensity and exposure duration on cure of resin composite. *Operative Dent* 1994;**19**:26–32.

34. RUEGGEBERG FA, CAUGHMAN WF, CHAN DN. Novel approach to measure composite conversion kinetics during exposure with stepped or continuous light-curing. *J Esthetic Dent* 1999;**11**:197–205.

35. ASMUSSEN E, PEUTZFELDT A. Influence of pulse-delay curing on softening of polymer structures. *J Dent Res* 2001;**80**:1570–3.

36. UNTERBRINK GL, MUESSNER R. Influence of light intensity on two restorative systems. *J Dent* 1995;**23**:183–9.

37. KNEZEVIC A, TARLE Z, MENIGA A, SUTALO J, PICHLER G, RISTIC M. Degree of conversion and temperature rise during polymerization of composite resin samples with blue diodes. *J Oral Rehab* 2001;**28**:586–91.

38. SOH MS, YAP AUJ, YU T, SHEN ZX. Analysis of the degree of conversion of LED and halogen lights using micro-raman spectroscopy. *Operative Dent* 2004;**29**:571–7.

39. LINDBERG A, NAZANIN E, VAN DIJKEN JWV. A FT-Raman spectroscopy analysis of the degree of conversion of a universal hybrid resin composite cured with light-emitting diode curing units. *Biomaterials.* Submitted for publication.

40. ZYMAN P, JONAS P. Shade selection. Rational protocol selection. *Réalités Cliniques* 2003;**4**:379–91.

41. FELIPPE LA, MONTEIRO S, CALDEIRA DE ANDRADA CA, DIXON DI, CERQUEIRA A, RITTER AV. Clinical strategies for successs in proximoincisal composite restorations. Part I: Understanding color and composite selection. *J Esthet Restor Dent* 2004;**16**:336–47.

42. WINTHER R. Visualizing the natural dentition. *J Esthet Dent* 1993;**5**:103–17.

43. MILLER LL. Shade matching. *J Esthet Dent* 1993;**5**:143–53.

44. VANINI L. Light and color in anterior composite restorations. *Pract Periodont Esthet Dent* 1996;**8**:673–82.

45. DIETSCHI D. Layering concepts in anterior composite restorations. *J Adhes Dent* 2001;**3**:71–80.

46. DIETSCHI D. Freehand composite restorations: a key to anterior esthetics. *Pract Periodont Esthet Dent* 1995;**7**:15–25.

47. MAGNE P, HOLZ J. Stratification of composite restorations: systematic and durable replication of natural esthetics. *Pract Periodont Esthet Dent* 1996;**8**:61–8.

48. MUNKSGAARD EC. Permeability of protective gloves to (di)methacrylates in resinous dental materials. *Scand J Dent Res* 1992;**100**:189–92.

49. MUNKSGAARD EC. Permeability of protective gloves by HEMA and TEGDMA in the presence of solvents. *Acta Odontol Scand* 2000;**58**:57–62.

50. LÖNROTH E-C, WELLENDORF H, RUYTER IE. Permeability of different types of medical protective gloves to acrylic monomers. *Eur J Oral Sci* 2003;**111**:440–6.

51. ANDREASSON H, BOMAN A, JOHNSSON S, KARLSSON S, BARREGAARD L. On permeability of methyl methacrylate, 2-hydroxyethyl methacrylate and triethyleneglycol methacrylate through protective gloves in dentistry. *Eur J Oral Sci* 2003;**111**:529–35.

52. DELLO RUSSO NM. Replacement of crown margins in patients with altered passive eruption. *Int J Periodont Restor Dent* 1984;**4**:58–65.

53. CHAN RC, BOYER DB. Repair of conventional and microfilled composite resins. *J Prosthet Dent* 1983;**50**:345–50.

54. JORDAN RE, SUZUKI M, GWINNETT AJ. Conservative application of acid etch resin techniques. *Dent Clin North Am* 1981;**25**:307–36.

# 26

# Resin-related Bridges and Conventional Bridges in the Anterior Region

N. H. J. Creugers & C. M. Kreulen

Resin-retained bridges can be used both as transitional (interim) and long-term treatment in the traumatized dentition. Compared to the conventional fixed prostheses and the implant-retained (single) tooth replacement, there are some advantages, which make this treatment especially useful following dental trauma. Advantages of resin-bonded bridges compared to conventional bridges include: minimal tooth preparation, i.e. reversible procedures and no pulpal involvement; as well as short working time, thereby implying lower costs. The ultra-conservative approach makes the resin-bonded bridge a standard treatment option in the case of uncertain prognosis, which is often the case in dental trauma. A disadvantage associated with resin-bonded bridges may be the anticipated limited length of clinical service.

## Treatment planning

In the treatment of missing anterior teeth, the following factors must be considered (1):

• Age of the patient
• General condition of the dentition
• Occlusion
• Location and width of the edentulous space
• Quality of the teeth adjacent to the edentulous space
• Amount and quality of alveolar bone.

There are several treatment options, such as orthodontic closure (see Chapter 24), autotransplantation of teeth (see Chapter 27) and implants (see Chapter 28). The main advantages and disadvantages of these treatments are discussed in Chapter 29 which concentrates on esthetics and function.

Indications for resin-bonded bridges include almost all situations where interim or transitional treatment is desired.

The classical indication for a resin-bonded bridge is replacement of a single tooth with 2 intact abutment teeth (Fig. 26.1), and improvement of the bonding capacities of

luting cements and quality of composites have enlarged this indication substantially.

In general there are no absolute contraindications for resin-bonded bridges. Nonetheless, in specific situations, such as moderate or severe trauma to dentitions, there may be complications that influence the prognosis and quality of service negatively. These complications may be present displacement of the abutment teeth with crown or root fractures, pulpal involvement of the abutment teeth and atrophy of alveolar bone. A non-favorable position of an abutment tooth, for instance, can make an esthetic solution impossible.

The treatment sequence and timing for resin-bonded bridges depends on the presence or absence of complicating factors mentioned above. In many cases an observation period of several months is necessary before treatment can be initiated. If a resin-bonded bridge is to serve as a long-term therapy the complicating factors should be eliminated. Because of the reversible character of the system, early application of the resin-bonded bridge may be appropriate in some situations, and the resin-bonded bridge can serve as an interim or transitional restoration during evaluation or treatment of the complicating factors (Fig. 26.2). This treatment strategy is gaining more and more attention in contemporary prosthodontics and is called 'the dynamic treatment approach'. In this approach, which is very useful in the treatment of traumatized dentitions, the goals of treatment are less oriented towards the traditional aim of long-lasting restorations than to solve functional problems by applying customized solutions to current situations. For a better understanding of the goals and tools used in this approach, and its use in the treatment of dental trauma, this concept is described in the next section.

## The 'dynamic treatment' concept

The ultimate goal of restorative dental care is to maintain a healthy and functional dentition for life (2). The traditional

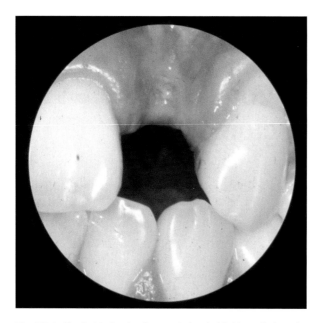

**Fig. 26.1** Classical indication for a resin-bonded bridge, which is the replacement of a single tooth and the presence of sound adjacent abutment teeth.

follow-up periods may be necessary before key questions concerning the prognosis of individual or multiple teeth can be answered. In the mean time, basic function and acceptable esthetics must be provided to the patient. In this respect, the transitional restoration is becoming increasingly important, as long as an appropriate life span is provided.

The impact of this treatment concept is becoming even clearer when comparing it to the traditional concepts. In the traditional treatment plan, the key factor is the diagnosis. Textbooks then provide standard guidelines for indications following the diagnosis, emphasizing mainly morphological reconstruction of what is impaired. These guidelines are extremely static and will lead to uniform treatments. The problem-solving concept on the other hand allows individual variation and is an excellent basis for a dynamic treatment approach.

It is difficult to give a definition for the term 'dynamic treatment approach'. Nevertheless it is possible to give a number of characteristics to help understanding. One characteristic is that the approach is 'moderate' in the sense of 'acting with restraint' or 'careful'. The dynamic treatment approach is problem-oriented, meaning that where there is no problem, solutions are not required. The approach is flexible at different levels. It offers flexibility during the different treatment phases, but also in the longer run. At certain stages, especially when uncertainties are involved, an evaluation period is built in. Furthermore there is interaction with the adaptive capacity of the patient in both active and passive ways. A big difference between the dynamic treatment approach and the traditional treatment approach is that where the traditional approach is aimed at longevity of restorative work, the dynamic approach is based on generations of restorative work, which offer the patient optimal service at different stages of his life at relative low costs and with minimal invasive techniques. The restorative materials used for this purpose are challenged, as they have to offer maximum flexibility during the different treatment phases, should provide adequate protection to the tooth and surrounding tissues, must be economically acceptable, and have to keep subsequent treatment options open. Key issues in this approach are: functionality rather than longevity, repair rather than renewal, and limited treatment goals rather than maximal result, all of them aiming to maintain a healthy and functional dentition for life.

concept and sequence of restorative care is to eliminate pathological factors, to reconstruct the dentition and to maintain this situation as long as possible. To avoid a repair cycle, the durability of restorations plays an important role. However, depending on specific situations, a relatively high price has to be paid to achieve this, both in economic as well as in biological terms. There are many circumstances in which such an investment is not justified, and where the treatment should primarily aim at functional goals rather than at durability demands. Examples may be found in the field of pediatric, geriatric and social dentistry and also in the treatment of dentitions after traumatic injuries. Not only in these fields, the traditional morphological concept is declining in favor of more problem-oriented concepts. For instance, contemporary prosthodontic treatment strategies show a trend to postpone 'final' treatments until interim or transitional treatment phases are completed, and – if possible – avoid 'definitive' prosthetic reconstructions. During interim phases, causes for decay and breakdown have to be eliminated and conditions can be improved. Substantial

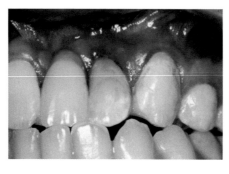

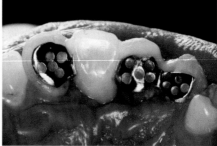

**Fig. 26.2** Rochette bridge in a patient where the left central incisor was lost and the left lateral incisor was replanted after avulsion; the prognosis of the lateral incisor is uncertain. Courtesy of Dr. F. J. M. ROETERS.

## Direct resin-bonded bridges

Although clinical studies have indicated that indirect resin-bonded bridges are more durable than direct ones, there is still a need for directly applied resin-bonded bridges, especially in cases where the device is meant as an interim solution (3). The direct technique provides a restoration at relatively low cost and with good esthetics and oral comfort. The direct-pontic systems that have been described in the literature include: the *acrylic tooth pontic*, the *all-composite pontic*, and the *natural tooth pontic*. In general the pontic is retained by resin composite material that acts as an adhesive paste at the approximal areas of the teeth. The reported survivals for these systems from a number of clinical studies vary from 30% up to 100% after 4 years (4–10). The greatest advantage of the direct resin-bonded bridge is that it is a very cost-effective technique with minimal biological damage. If required, alternative tooth replacement techniques are still open in a later stage.

The main disadvantage of the direct-pontic technique is the inherent lack of strength against tensile and torqueing forces of the resin composite fixation material. Especially at the connector areas direct resin-bridges tend to fail. To strengthen the relatively weak connector areas metal wire and mesh 'reinforcements' have been employed. Because of the weak adhesion to the resinuous material they showed a questionable value in this respect. Recently developed fiber systems (FRCs: fiber-reinforced composites) are capable of increasing the fracture resistance of direct-pontic systems substantially, bypassing the need for bulky connector areas (11). This is especially the case if the fibers are combined with all-composite pontics (Fig. 26.3). Generally fiber materials combine a high tensile strength with sufficient adhesion to resin composites. The materials science and properties of glass-fibers are well described in the (dental) literature (12–15). Since a detailed presentation of this knowledge is beyond the scope of this book, only some principles of their reinforcing effect are presented. The mechanical properties of FRCs are influenced by:

- Adhesion of fibers to the pontic material. The best adhesion can be expected in combination with all-composite pontics.
- Fiber orientation. A direction parallel to the tensile stress of unidirectional fibers provides highest strength and enables the fibers to absorb or intercept the majority of tensile forces.
- Fiber placement. Fibers are most effective when placed in the zone where tensile stress is expected.
- Fiber quantity. More fibers provide better reinforcement than fewer.

## Indirect resin-bonded bridges

There are two major types of indirect resin-bonded bridges: the cast metal resin bonded bridge and the fiber-reinforced resin-bonded bridge. The cast metal resin-bonded bridge consists of a pontic and a cast metal framework. The resin based bridge is constructed of a fiber-polymer frame that is veneered with composite material.

The success of both restoration types is directly related to the quality of the bond at the resin-tooth interface and to the physical and chemical properties of the luting cement. Moreover, the adhesive strength at the resin-metal interface is directly of importance to the clinical performance of the metal based resin bonded bridge, while for the resin based bridge the strength of the fiber frame and the bond strength to the veneering composite is critical (delamination). The bond strength of composite cements that can be achieved at the resin-tooth interface is in the order of 20–25 MPa. For the resin-metal interface bond strengths may vary from less than 10 MPa to over 40 MPa (16–20), depending on differences in surface treatments of the metal, the type of metal alloy, and the luting cement used. Analogously, the inherent characteristics of different fiber systems do not allow being conclusive as to strength compared to the metal resin-bonded bridge.

The strength of the system is significantly affected by the design of the framework and abutment tooth preparation. The design has to be such that the framework, whether metal or fibers, absorbs forces that are applied to the pontic during function. For this purpose, many suggestions have been made as to their design (20–24). The preparation design principles are based on the provision of a certain minimal volume of construction material and on the creation of shear resistance forms. These principles have consequences for abutment tooth modifications and for the outline form of the retention wings. If a truly adhesive restoration is desired, there is the dilemma that resistance against tensile and oblique forces must be sufficiently provided by tooth preparation, while from a minimal intervention approach only minimal tooth preparation is preferred.

## Cast metal resin-bonded bridges

The following factors must be taken into consideration in planning a cast resin-bonded bridge (Fig. 26.4):

- the design of the retention wings
- tooth preparation
- the number of abutment teeth.

The *retention wings* should cover a maximal surface of the enamel while not compromising esthetics. Incisal translucency of the abutment teeth must also be taken into consideration. Proximal wrap around is preferable when esthetics do permit. Plaque-retentive areas must be avoided, implying marginal placement at least 1 mm from the gingival margin. The patient's occlusion must also be considered in the design of the retention wings in order to avoid premature contacts or excessive loading during excursions. Occlusion on the retention wings is preferable to occlusion on the abutment tooth enamel as occlusal forces load the retention wing in the direction of the tooth, while occlusion

### Fig. 26.3 Direct all-composite fiber-reinforced pontic system

A 15-year-old girl with a traumatized central incisor which had to be extracted due to external resorption.

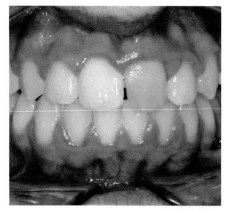

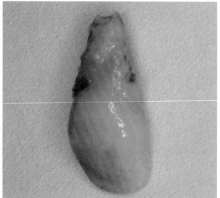

### Application of glass fiber Periostick®

Immediately after extraction, a rubber-dam was placed. After etching the tooth, the central and lateral incisors and two pieces of the glass fiber Periostick® were bonded to the palatal surface of these teeth.

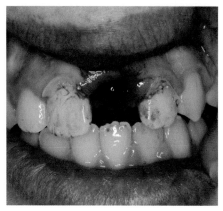

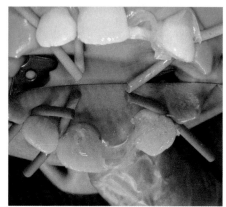

### Application of pontic

A precured round piece of composite was pushed in the extraction alveolus and bonded to the Periostick®. Then the pontic was built up with a highly filled hybrid composite resin in combination with an anterior hybrid composite resin. Finally the patient was instructed how to clean the pontic area.

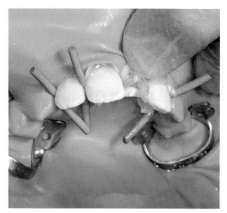

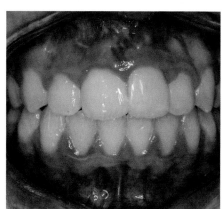

### Control of pontic bridge

Six weeks later the patient came for a final examination and minor adjustments of the bridge. The extraction alveolus was well healed and there is a good shape of the interdental papilla as a result of the way the pontic was made. Occlusal view after six weeks shows a retention wire on the palatal surfaces that was applied by her orthodontist. Courtesy of Dr. F. J. M. ROETERS and Dr. M. SIERS.

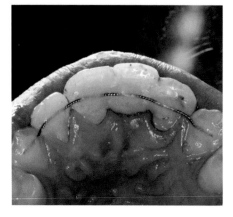

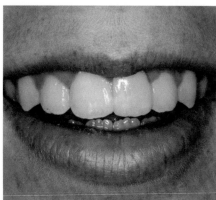

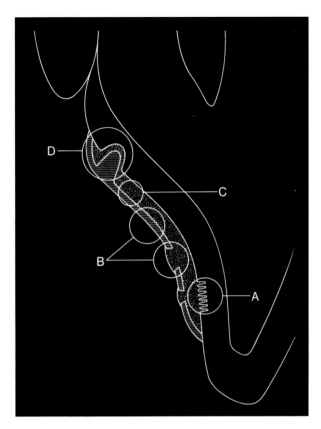

**Fig. 26.4** Schematic representation of the weak points in cast metal resin-bonded bridges. A. The interface between resin cement and the tooth enamel. B. The resin-cement/metal interface. C. Physical and chemical properties of the composite resin-cement. D. The design of the bridge.

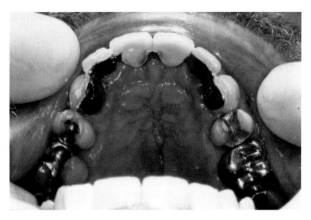

**Fig. 26.6** Palatal view of a 6-unit resin-bonded bridge. More than 2 abutment teeth were used as the lateral incisors demonstrated increased mobility.

on the tooth itself forces the tooth away from the resin-bonded bridge (25).

With respect to *tooth preparation* there are divergent opinions. Some authors recommend extensive preparation while others advocate a more conservative design. Tooth preparation should always be included in the design of the bridge in cases of insufficient interocclusal space and increased mobility of the abutment teeth. Tooth preparation is also indicated in cases where more than 2 abutment teeth are involved in the construction or when there is an unclear seat or an unclear path of insertion (Fig. 26.5).

Finally, preparation of grooves may be indicated, to increase shear resistance. A useful anatomical guide for

enamel reduction during preparation for resin-bonded bridges has been published by Ferrari et al. (26). The choice of the optimal *number of abutment teeth* depends on the situation. Usually 2 abutment teeth are sufficient for 3- or 4-unit bridges. If 3 or more teeth are to be replaced, or in cases where the abutment teeth have increased mobility, more abutment teeth can be used for retaining the bridge (Fig. 26.6).

Orthodontic pre-treatment may be another indication for the use of extra abutment teeth and tooth preparation. Fig. 26.7 presents a patient with missing cuspids and lateral incisors, who is orthodontically pre-treated. A central diastema was closed with a simple orthodontic method. To prevent any relapse, the bridge was cast as a single unit crossing the midline.

## Fiber-reinforced resin-bonded bridges

Initially developed in the aerospace industry, fiber-reinforced constructions have been used for diverse applications in daily life for several decades. In many instances the material replaces metal, leading to light constructions that can bear heavy loads. In dentistry the optimal combination of clinically applied resin composite materials with specific

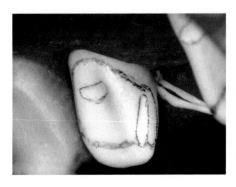

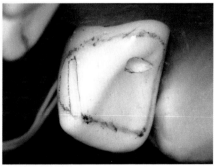

**Fig. 26.5** Model set-up demonstrating the preparation form for a resin-bonded bridge in the anterior region.

fiber materials is as yet being studied. So far adequate materials have been introduced to the market and the application of fiber-reinforced composite (FRC) constructions is expanding.

Principally the indication of the indirectly fabricated fiber-reinforced resin-bonded bridge does not differ from the cast metal type (Fig. 26.8). The greatest advantage of FRCs is their esthetic appearance, which makes constructions possible that are not realistic using metals. Moreover, once the bridge has been placed adaptations with directly applied composite materials, in order to change form or treat parts of the tooth that are not involved in the bridge, are possible due to the use of comparable resin composite materials in the bridge (27).

The actual lines to use fiber material are not different from the use described for direct resin-bonded bridges. Like the cast metal resin-bonded bridge, which is made in an indirect restorative technique, the operator should bear in mind comparable clinical guidelines making the FRC resin-bonded bridge, being:

- The design of the retention wing
- Tooth preparation
- The number of abutment teeth.

The idea to cover most of the palatal surface of an abutment tooth is valid, just as the instructions to consider the gingival margin and the location of occlusal contacts. However, enclosure of abutment teeth is not difficult to achieve, since buccal outlines of palatal retainers are no problem from an esthetic point of view.

Tooth preparation is subject to dicussion. Least invasive concepts recommend to grind tooth material only to create sufficient volume of the construction interocclusally and to secure a clear path of insertion approximally, while refraining from providing resistance pits (palatal) or grooves

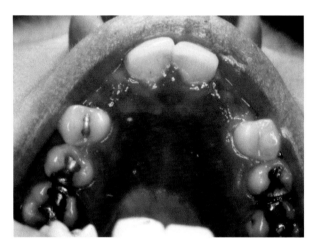 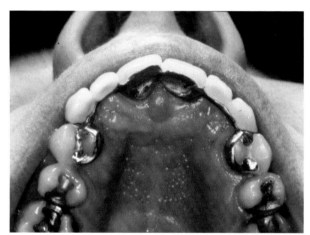

**Fig. 26.7** Example of a six-unit resin-bonded bridge after orthodontic pre-treatment. Before (left) and after (right) placement of the restoration.

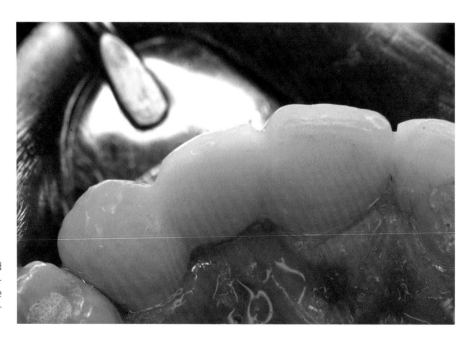

**Fig. 26.8** Indirect fiber-reinforced resin-bonded bridge replacing an unesthetic cast metal Rochette bridge that has been in function for approximately 10 years.

(approximal). Others refer to the analogy with the cast metal resin-bonded bridge, for which the construction itself is not the weak link of the restorative provision, but merely the luting resin composite material. To cope with shear stress due to occlusal forces, resistance forms in the tooth surfaces are then recommended additionally.

The number of abutment teeth that are required is expected to be in line with the choices that have to be made with cast metal resin-bonded bridges. Due to the limited long-term clinical experience with FRC bridges it is not known whether constructions with more than 2 adjacent pontics can reliably be made.

Finally, FRC resin-bonded bridges can be repaired during their lifecycle, since resin composite is an adjustable material. This too is an advantage of FRC constructions over metal-ceramic constructions. It is an appealing characteristic in view of the dynamic treatment approach.

## Conventional bridges

The retention and resistance form of conventional bridges is mainly based on the preparation and subsequent restoration of the abutment teeth. In most cases the bridge is retained by crowns; in some situations (mostly posterior) inlay restorations provide the retention of the bridge. Conventional bridges are durable restorations and may provide satisfactory function (including esthetics) for a long period. The materials conventional bridges are made of are usually durable and they have high resistance to fatigue and deterioration. As a result conventional bridges show almost no ageing effects: they are very stable in their performance. This latter characteristic – which is a very useful one in many cases – is, however, a serious drawback for the use of conventional bridges in trauma cases. A traumatic injury is always followed by a period of healing and adaptation in which the affected tissues and structures may change during periods of months or years. This process may include the pulp (delayed necrosis), the surrounding soft tissues (loss of attachment) and the bone (continuous bone atrophy). As a result an initially perfectly well-adapted conventional bridge may easily become inconvenient and eventually a threat to its surroundings. On top of this intrinsic risk, the clinical procedures making a conventional bridge increase the risk of complications substantially. This is especially the case in young patients where the pulp is large and the clinical crowns are relatively short. In these cases the trauma from tooth preparation might exceed the trauma from the injury. The biological price is not in balance with the expected benefits, therefore a conventional bridge is not a treatment option in these cases and the making of it should be avoided until all trauma related complications are under control. It is beyond the scope of this book to present the many details about materials, designs and clinical procedures of conventional bridges that can be applied; these can be found in the many excellent prosthodontic textbooks that are available.

## Prognosis of resin-bonded bridges and comparison with alternative prosthodontic treatments

Clinical data on the efficacy of resin-bonded bridges include data from both retrospective clinical studies and from prospective trials. The durability data reported in the literature are not especially representative for the resin-bonded bridges in the case of trauma. It is reported that resin-bonded bridges in young patients with trauma tend to fail more frequently than in 'average' patients (28, 29). In one study (30–32) the reasons for anterior tooth loss of the 'average' patient was described in detail: about a quarter of the cases resulted from trauma, about 40% were related to dental diseases, and in 33% of the cases there was no real tooth loss, but bridge constructions were related to aplasia or spacing (5%). Although it is not proven that the 'average patient' in the described study is representative, it may be expected that the populations of other studies do not differ substantially regarding anterior tooth loss.

The reported survivals in clinical studies vary widely, and the conclusions are sometimes conflicting. The heterogeneity of the results indicates that interpretation of only one study may significantly mislead clinicians. Powerful tools to deal with different outcomes of different studies are the systematic review and the meta-analysis. These methods are increasingly being used in different fields of dentistry. Regarding the hierarchy of strength of evidence in medical (33, 34) and dental (35) clinical studies, it is stated that the strongest evidence can be found from at least one published systematic review of multiple, well-designed randomized controlled trials (RCT). However, it then appears that only a few randomized controlled trials on tooth replacement are available. Moreover reviews on this topic are unsuitable to be used as evidence for relative risks or benefits of therapies, as they are not based on randomized controlled trials only (36). If uncontrolled studies are included, these kinds of research questions cannot be answered adequately, since it is well known that studies without a control group are prone to bias and generally show too positive effects of treatments. Although outcomes of these reviews provide no strong evidence that efficacies of therapies differ, systematic reviews including non-RCTs can provide useful information for the clinician and evidence for prognosis of treatments (37).

With respect to tooth replacement, five systematic reviews have been published so far (38–42). Overall survivals of resin-bonded bridges, conventional fixed bridges and crowns on single tooth implants of 3 systematic reviews are shown in Fig. 26.9 (38, 39, 42). Although relative risks cannot be inferred and direct comparison is not allowed, they are shown in one figure for practical reasons. The outcomes from two other systematic reviews (40, 41) are not shown in the diagram, although the results are almost similar to those depicted in the graph. The overall survival of resin-bonded bridges appears to be 74% after 4 years. Unfortunately, the included studies did not allow calculating an overall survival

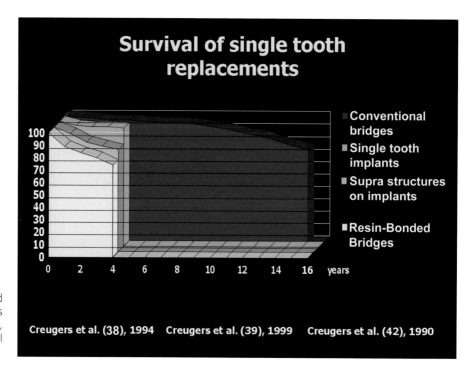

**Fig. 26.9** Survival curves adapted from 3 different systematic reviews on respectively resin-bonded bridges, single tooth implants and conventional bridges.

for periods over 4 years at the time the study was performed. One single RCT showed a survival up to 58% after 10 years follow-up for anterior resin-bonded bridges (43). The same is true for implant survival; here also the included studies allow no calculation of overall survival beyond 4 years follow-up. The predicted overall survival for single implants was 97% after 4 years, but the study showed uncomplicated crown maintenance of 83% (42). From a durability point of view, the conventional fixed bridge still reflects the gold standard with a predicted survival of 74 ± 2% after 15 years (39). This predicted outcome has been confirmed later by another systematic review (41).

Unfortunately survival data on FRC resin-bonded bridges are scarce at the time of publication of this book. One observational study (44) reported a survival probability of 75% for glass-fiber reinforced resin-bonded bridges at 5 years. Another study, including 61 anterior and 26 posterior FRC resin-bonded bridges, reported 88% survival after 2 years (45).

## Factors influencing the survival of resin-bonded bridges

Mobility of the abutment teeth has been found to be a significant risk factor for failure (46). Excessive occlusal loading due to premature contacts on the abutment teeth or the pontic has also been recognized as an important cause of failure in several studies (46–48). Anterior resin-bonded bridges show better prognosis than posterior resin-bonded bridges. Besides the risk factors adapted from longitudinal clinical studies, it is worth mentioning a few limitations brought up by clinicians, such as bruxism and parafunctional habits, deep-bite occlusion and long-span bridges.

One of the main advantages of resin-bonded bridges is the possibility of rebonding in case of loosening. For cast metal resin-bonded bridges the survival of these restorations increases up to 77% after 10 years if they are once rebonded (43). However, rebounded bridges are susceptible to new failure. Hence the failure rate has been found higher than the failure rate of originally bonded bridges (46, 47, 49). The risk of failure after rebonding is estimated to be about twice the risk of failure after original bonding (31). Before rebonding the causes of loss of retention must be investigated carefully.

FRC bridges can fail in a dramatic way as they can break due to high impacts. Generally, broken FRC bridges must be replaced by new ones.

In conclusion, resin-bonded bridges have been evaluated extensively over the past 25 years. The value of resin-bonded bridges is their cost-effectiveness and the possibility of providing the patient with a minimal invasive treatment that leaves all future treatments open. Cast metal resin-bonded bridges show reasonably high survival rates. The indirect FRC resin-bonded bridge is a relatively new development. This type of bridge has enlarged the indication of resin-bonded bridges to situations where high esthetic demands must be encountered. Although no long-term data are available yet, the experiences so far are encouraging.

## Essentials

### Indications

• Individuals with intact or almost intact abutment teeth and an intact alveolar process. In case of spacing between teeth, cast metal bridges are contraindicated for esthetic reasons; direct or indirect resin composite techniques are advocated.

- Interim solution in cases of waiting for diagnosis of eventual complications.

## Treatment planning

- Depends on the age of the patient and presence or absence of complicating factors.
- A direct resin-bonded bridge can serve very well as a transitional provision and can be made immediately after the loss of a tooth. Depending on the skills of the operator a direct resin-bonded bridge may be effective in the long run.
- An indirect resin-bonded bridge can serve as a long-term solution.

## Clinical procedure

### All-composite tooth pontic

- If required, grinding of the palatal surface of the abutment teeth to create interocclusal space
- Cleaning and isolation of the abutment teeth
- Etching of the enamel and application of bonding agent
- Preferably application of a fiber reinforcement from one abutment tooth to the other, or alternatively a stainless steel mesh
- Building up of the pontic in layers, and covering the palatal surface of the abutment teeth
- Finishing the restoration

### Acrylic denture tooth or natural tooth pontic

- Molding, fitting and aligning of the pontic tooth into a proper position
- Fabrication of a silicone matrix for orienting the pontic in the desired position
- Retentive preparation of the proximal surfaces of the pontic
- If required, grinding of a horizontal palatal groove in the pontic and creating interocclusal space at the abutment teeth (for the benefit of fiber integration)
- Etching of the enamel and application of bonding agent
- If required, application of a fiber reinforcement
- Application of resin composite in the preparations and on the proximal palatal surfaces of the abutment teeth
- Finishing of the restoration

### Cast metal resin-bonded bridge

#### First session
- Cleaning of the abutment teeth
- Preparation of abutment teeth
- Selection of shade and color taking
- Impression taking

#### Second session
- Cleaning of the abutment teeth
- Checking of the fit, color and occlusion

- Application of rubber dam
- Cleaning of the bridge
- Etching, bonding and cementation
- Check of the occlusion and removal of the excess cement

#### Third session
- Re-check of the occlusion and finishing
- Oral hygiene instruction

### Indirect fiber-reinforced resin-bonded bridge

#### First session
- Same procedure as for cast resin-bonded bridges

#### Second session
- Cleaning of the abutment teeth
- Checking of the fit, color and occlusion
- Application of rubber dam
- Preparing the adhesive (internal) surface of the bridge for bonding
- Etching, bonding and cementation
- Check of the occlusion and removal of the excess cement

#### Third session
- See cast resin-bonded bridges

## Follow-up

- Checking of retention and verifying proper function
- Application of normal prosthodontic maintenance program

## Prognosis

- 4-years cast metal resin-bonded bridge survival: 74%
- Direct and indirect fiber-reinforced resin composite bridge survival: presently unknown

## Risk factors

- Mobility of abutment teeth
- Excessive occlusal loading
- Posterior location (versus anterior)
- Diastema >2 teeth

## References

1. KÄYSER AF, CREUGERS NHJ, PLASMANS PJJM, POSTEMA N, SNOEK PA. Kroon – en brugwerk. Uitgangspunten bij de diagnostiek van het gemutileerde gebit en de behandeling ervan met vaste voorzieningen. Houten: Bohn Stafleu van Loghum, 1995.
2. SHEIHAM A. Public health aspects of periodontal diseases in Europe. J Clin Periodontol 1991;**18**:362–9.
3. HOWE DF, DENEHY GE. Anterior fixed partial dentures utilizing the acid–etch technique and a cast metal framework. J Prosthet Dent 1977;**37**:28–31.

4. Hallonsten A–L, Koch G, Ludvigsson N, et al. Acid–etch technique in temporary bridgework using composite pontics in the juvenile dentition. *Swed Dent J* 1979;**3**:213–19.

5. Ibsen RL. Fixed prosthetics with a natural crown pontic using an adhesive composite. *J Cal Dent Assoc* 1973;**41**:100–2.

6. Ibsen RL. One-appointment technic using an adhesive composite. *Dent Survey* 1973;**49**:30–2.

7. Jenkins CBG. Etch retained anterior pontics, a 4-year study. *Br Dent J* 1978;**144**:206–8.

8. Jordan RE, Suzuki M, Sillis PS, et al. Temporary fixed partial dentures fabricated by means of the acid-etched resin technique: a report of 86 cases followed for up to three years. *J Am Dent Assoc* 1978;**96**:994–1001.

9. van Hoeve JP. Directly etched bridges. Experiences in 33 patients. *Ned Tijdschr Tandheelkd* 1996;**103**:208–9.

10. de Kloet HJ, van Pelt AW. The all composite adhesive dental bridge. *Ned Tijdschr Tandheelkd* 1996;**103**:477–9.

11. Vallittu PK. Prosthodontic treatment with a glass fiber-reinforced resin-bonded fixed partial denture: a clinical report. *J Prosthet Dent* 1999;**82**:132–5.

12. Dyer SR, Lassila LV, Jokinen M, Vallittu PK. Effect of fiber position and orientation on fracture load of fiber–reinforced composite. *Dent Mater* 2004;**20**:947–55.

13. Lassila LV, Vallittu PK. The effect of fiber position and polymerization condition on the flexural properties of fiber–reinforced composite. *J Contemp Dent Pract* 2004;**5**:14–26.

14. Murphy J. *Reinforced plastics handbook.* 2nd edn. Oxford: Elsevier Science, 1998.

15. Nohrstrom TJ, Vallittu PK, Yli-Urpo A. The effect of placement and quantity of glass fibers on the fracture resistance of interim fixed partial dentures. *Int J Prosthodont* 2000;**13**:72–8.

16. Hill GL, Zidan O, Marin O. Bond strength of etched base metals: effects of errors in surface area estimation. *J Prosthet Dent* 1986;**56**:41–6.

17. Creugers NHJ, Welle PR, Vrijhoef MMA. Four bonding systems for resin-retained cast metal protheses. *Dent Mater* 1988;**3**:85–8.

18. Wirz J, Besimo C, Schmidli F. Verbundfestigkeit von Metallgerüst und Haftvermittler in der Adhäsivbrückentechnik. *Schweiz Monatsschr Zahnmed* 1989;**99**:24–39.

19. Zardiackas LD, Caldwell DJ, Caughman WF, et al. Tensile fatigue of resin cements to etched metal and enamel. *Dent Mater* 1988;**4**:163–8.

20. Aquillino SA, Diaz–Arnold AM, Piotrowski TJ. Tensile fatigue limits of prosthodontic adhesives. *J Dent Res* 1991;**70**:208–10.

21. Lividitis GJ. Resin bonded cast restorations: clinical study. *Int J Periodont Rest Dent* 1981;**1**:70–9.

22. Simonsen R, Thompson VP, Barrack G. *Etched cast restorations: clinical and laboratory techniques.* Chicago: Quintessence, 1983.

23. Lividitis GJ. Cast metal resin–bonded retainers for posterior teeth. *J Am Dent Assoc* 1980;**101**:926–9.

24. Marinello CP, Lüthy H, Kerschbaum TH, et al. Die Flächen- und Umfangbestimmung bei Adhäsivhalteelementen: eine Möglichkeit der Langzeitprognose. *Schweiz Monatsschr Zahnmed* 1990;**100**:291–9.

25. Creugers NHJ, Snoek PA, Van't Hof MA, Käyser AF. Clinical performance of resin–bonded bridges: a 5-years prospective study. Part II: The influence of patient-dependent variables. *J Oral Rehabil* 1989;**16**:521–7.

26. Ferrari M, Gagidiaco MC, Bertelli E. Anatomic guide for reduction of enamel for acid–etched retainers. *J Prosthet Dent* 1987;**58**:521–7.

27. Vallittu PK. Prosthodontic treatment with a glass fiber-reinforced resin-bonded fixed partial denture: a clinical report. *J Prosthet Dent* 1999;**82**:132–5.

28. Bergendal B, Hallonsten AL, Koch G, et al. Composite retained onlay bridges. *Swed Dent J* 1983; **7**:217–25.

29. Edwards GD, Mitchell L, Welbury RR. An evaluation of resin-bonded bridges in adolescent patients. *J Ped Dent* 1989;**5**:107–14.

30. Creugers NHJ. *Clinical performance of adhesive bridges.* Thesis, Nijmegen, the Netherlands, 1987.

31. Creugers NHJ, Käyser AF, Van't Hof MA. A seven-and-a-half-year survival study on resin-bonded bridges. *J Dent Res* 1992;**71**:1822–5.

32. Creugers NHJ, de Kanter RJAM, Van't Hof MA. Long-term survival data from a clinical trial on resin-bonded bridges. *J Dent* 1997;**25**:239–42.

33. US Department of Health and Human Services, Public Health Service, Agency for Health Care Policy and Research (AHCPR). *Acute pain management: operative or medical procedures and trauma.* Rockville, MD: AHCPR, 1992.

34. Guyatt GH, Sackett DL, Sinclair JC, Hayward R, Cook DJ, Cook RJ. Users' guides to the medical literature. IX. A method for grading health care recommendations. *J Am Med Assoc* 1995;**274**:1800–4.

35. Richards D, Lawrence A. Evidence based dentistry. *Br Dent J* 1995;**179**:270–3.

36. Creugers NHJ, Kreulen CM. Systematic review of 10 years of systematic reviews in prosthodontics. *Int J Prosthodont* 2003;**16**:123–7.

37. Black N. Why we need observational studies to evaluate the effectiveness of health care. *Br Med J* 1996;**312**:1215–8.

38. Creugers NHJ, Van't Hof MA. An analysis of clinical studies on resin-bonded bridges. *J Dent Res* 1990;**70**:146–9.

39. Creugers NHJ, Käyser AF, Van't Hof MA. A meta-analysis of durability data on conventional fixed bridges. *Community Dent Oral Epidemiol* 1994;**22**:448–52.

40. Lindh T, Gunne J, Tillberg A, Molin M. A meta-analysis of implants in partial edentulism. *Clin Oral Implants Res* 1998;**9**:80–90.

41. Scurria MS, Bader JD, Shugars DA. Meta-analysis of fixed partial denture survival: Prostheses and abutments. *J Prosthet Dent* 1998;**79**:459–64.

42. Creugers NHJ, Kreulen CM, Snoek PA, de Kanter RJAM. A systematic review of single-tooth restorations supported by implants. *J Dent* 2000;**28**:209–17.

43. Creugers NHJ, de Kanter RJAM, Van't Hof MA. Long-term survival data from a clinical trial on resin-bonded bridges. *J Dent* 1997;**25**:239–42.

44. VALLITTU PK. Survival rates of resin-bonded, glass fiber-reinforced composite fixed partial dentures with a mean follow-up of 42 months: a pilot study. *J Prosthet Dent* 2004;**91**:241–6.

45. KREULEN CM, CREUGERS NHJ. Clinical performance of three-unit fiber reinforced composite fixed partial dentures. *Int J Prosthodont*. In press.

46. PASZYNA CN, MAU J, KERSCHBAUM TH. Riskofactoren dreigliederiger Adhäsivbrücken. *Dtsch Zahnärtzl Z* 1989;**44**:328–31.

47. CREUGERS NHJ, SNOEK PA, VAN'T HOF MA, KÄYSER AF. Clinical performance of resin-bonded bridges: a 5-years prospective study. Part III: Failure characteristics and survival after rebonding. *J Oral Rehabil* 1990;**17**:179–86.

48. CLYDE CS, BOYD T. The etched cast metal resin-bonded (Maryland) bridge: a clinical review. *J Dent* 1988;**16**:22–6.

49. MARINELLO CP, KERSCHBAUM TH, PFEIFFER P, et al. Success rate experience after rebonding and renewal of resin-bonded fixed partial dentures. *J Prosthet Dent* 1990;**63**:8–11.

# 27
# Autotransplantation of Teeth to the Anterior Region

J. O. Andreasen, L. Andersson & M. Tsukiboshi

Autotransplantation of teeth is today a well documented treatment method and is well suited for treatment of anterior tooth loss (1–12, 17–20, 32–37). Due to the unique osteogenic capacity of the graft, this procedure offers a treatment alternative, where both the lost tooth and the atrophied alveolar process can be replaced (Fig. 27.1). Studies have demonstrated good long-term survival of these transplants, thus providing a realistic treatment alternative for tooth replacement in young individuals (see Appendix 4, p. 882).

Furthermore this treatment procedure has its optimum of success in early childhood, a period where implants are definitively contraindicated (see Chapter 28).

The key to successful tooth transplantation has been shown clinically and experimentally to be proper selection of grafts with adequate root development as well as the design of surgical techniques for atraumatic graft removal and graft insertion. These techniques are described in detail in published textbooks on tooth replantation and transplantation (21, 38) and survey articles (35, 39).

## Treatment planning

When a tooth has been lost after trauma there are many factors that have to be taken into consideration when a long-term treatment plan is made. A multidisciplinary approach is recommended with many specialists involved. When anterior tooth loss occurs before completion of skeletal growth a panoramic radiograph should be taken, in which potential grafts, such as canines, premolars and in some cases diminutive third molars, can be identified. When donor teeth are available, the cost–benefit of autotransplantation should be weighted against other treatment solutions, such as orthodontic space closure (see Chapter 24), fixed prosthetics (see Chapter 26) and implants (see Chapter 28). As optimal prognosis depends upon teeth with incomplete root formation, the patient group best suited for this procedure is from

10 to 13 years old. At this age, alveolar growth is not yet complete, thereby contraindicating implants and fixed prosthetics (except for resin-retained bridges). An important question is whether to close the space of the lost tooth or keep the space open for replacement with a transplant. In some patients it may be preferable to close the space by orthodontic space closure. The choice between autotransplantation and orthodontic space closure depends upon an orthodontic analysis of growth and occlusion (see Chapters 24 and Chapter 29).

## Autotransplants versus implants

Most traumatic tooth losses occur in young, growing patients. Implants are contraindicated in growing patients because they interfere with the growth of the alveolar process resulting in an infraocclusion (see Chapter 28). Implant treatment must therefore often be postponed until

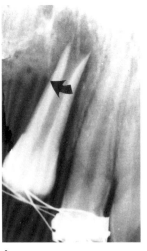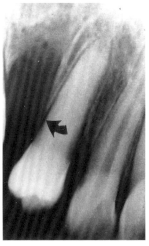

A                                    B

**Fig. 27.1** Alveolar bone induction by a premolar transplant to the canine region. A. Due to a severe trauma considerable bone has been lost in the region (arrow). B. The autotransplanted premolar has induced formation of alveolar bone distal to the transplant (arrow). From KRISTERSON (10) 1985.

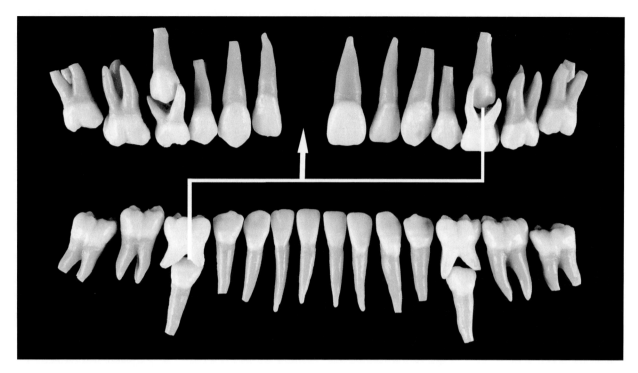

**Fig. 27.2** Central incisor loss, possible donor teeth. Except for mandibular first premolars, all premolars can serve as donor teeth. In rare cases, diminutive maxillary third molars can also be used.

growth is finished. During this waiting period there is a risk of atrophy of the alveolar crest: when it is time for implant installation this cannot be done without bone grafting prior to implant treatment to achieve an esthetically optimal situation.

Autotransplantation of teeth to the region of tooth loss is a method that can be applied regardless of whether the patient has finished growth or not. In most cases, autotransplantation is a permanent choice, but can also be applied temporarily in young patients to preserve the alveolar bone volume until growth is finished. The ultimate goal of autotransplants in growing individuals is the potential of not only maintaining bone but also creating a new alveolar bone by periodontal ligament induction and the eruption process (Fig. 27.1).

Implant treatment can be a good choice for replacing a lost tooth in adult patients, who have finished growth. The completion of growth must be confirmed by height measurement or a hand-wrist radiograph before implant treatment can start.

A comparison between autotransplant and implant reveals almost identical long-term prognosis (see Chapter 29) and good esthetics can be achieved with both methods.

There is, however, a significant difference in the cost efficiency (see Chapter 34) as autotransplantation does not carry the high cost of implant treatment. This is an especially important consideration for those individuals throughout the world who cannot afford implant treatment.

## Graft selection

The primary goals in graft selection are to ensure optimal periodontal healing and pulp survival, which in turn ensures optimal root development after transplantation. In the selection of donor teeth, crown and root anatomy should be considered.

With respect to coronal anatomy, reduction of tooth structure should generally be limited to enamel. Dentin exposure should be limited due to the risk of exposure of soft tissue inclusions which are found in post-transplantation dentin and which can imply a risk of subsequent pulp necrosis (see later). However, in cases with compatible root anatomy but less than optimal crown anatomy, crown anatomy following transplantation can be modified significantly by the use of porcelain crowns or veneers following interceptive endodontic treatment (see the section on restoration of transplanted teeth).

Concerning root anatomy, the graft should fit the recipient site loosely, avoiding contact with adjacent bone and providing at least 1 mm to the adjacent roots. Many potential grafts will exceed the existing labio-palatal dimension, especially if atrophy of the alveolar process has taken place. However, special surgical techniques, such as intentional fracture of the labial bone plate or a composite tooth-labial bone plate graft can solve this problem (see p. 744). An important aspect is the dimension at the cervical aspect of the graft. This must be in reasonable harmony with its antimere. Such harmony can often be obtained if the graft is rotated 45° or 90°. Moreover, if possible the donor tooth should be harvested from the opposite side of the arch to the recipient site.

With these limitations in mind, the following grafts (in order of preference) appear to be suitable for the *maxillary central incisor* region: second mandibular premolars, canines, first mandibular premolars, second maxillary premolars and diminutive third molars (Figs 27.2–27.4). Maxillary first premolars should generally not be used because

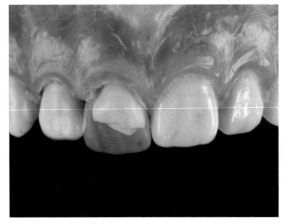

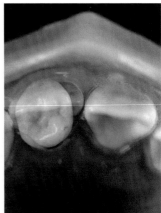

**Fig. 27.3** Central incisor region, transplantation of a mandibular second premolar. The double exposure illustrates where crown substance should be added or reduced.

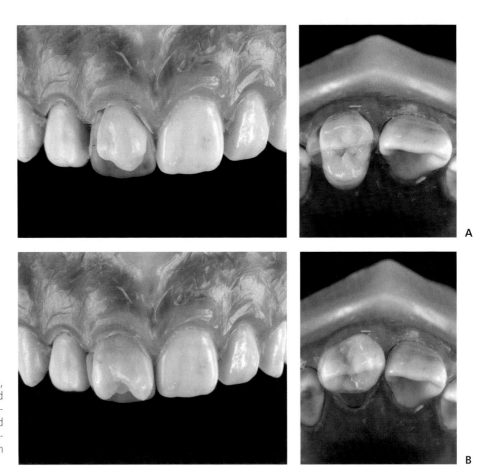

**Fig. 27.4** Central incisor region, transplantation of a maxillary second premolar. The double exposure illustrates where crown substance should be added or reduced when the transplant is positioned without (A) or with (B) rotation.

A

B

of their bifid roots, which present surgical obstacles to atraumatic graft removal.

In the *lateral incisor* region, the mandibular first premolar is, because of its size, the only good candidate for transplantation (Figs 27.5 and 27.6). In the *canine* region, all premolars, except the maxillary first, can be used (Figs 27.7 and 27.8). In general, grafts should be selected with three-quarter to full root formation with a wide open apex. At this stage of development, the graft is easy to remove and both

periodontal and pulpal healing are very predictable (see p. 758).

## Analysis of the recipient site

A radiographic examination is necessary to analyze the vertical bone level and space available between adjacent teeth. As a rule, the crown of the potential graft should fit into the space available mesiodistally above bone level. Furthermore,

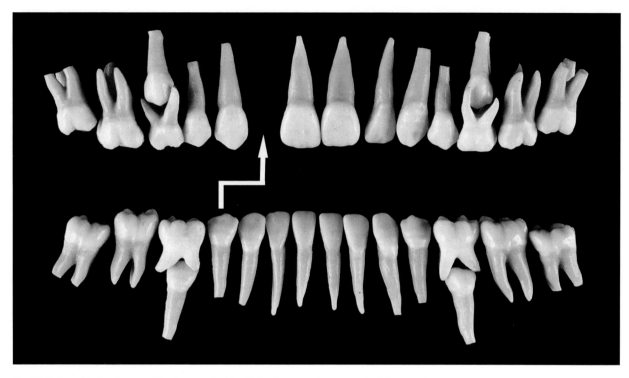

**Fig. 27.5** Lateral incisor loss, possible donor teeth. Mandibular first premolars are optimal donor teeth.

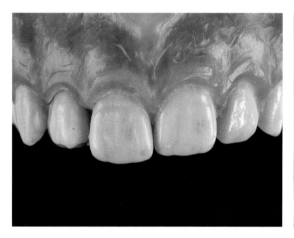
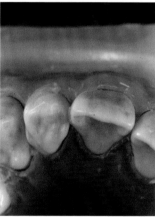

**Fig. 27.6** Lateral incisor region, transplantation of a mandibular first premolar. The double exposure illustrates where crown substance should be added or reduced.

dimensions of the root of the graft should ensure 1 mm of bone between itself and the roots of adjacent teeth.

The labio-palatal dimension of the alveolar process can be estimated by inspection clinically. In case of doubt as to whether a potential graft can fit into the recipient site, an open surgical procedure should be chosen (see p. 747).

## Surgical procedure

In this context only certain principles of graft removal and recipient site preparation will be presented. Readers interested in details about the surgical procedures are referred to recently published textbooks on this subject (21, 38).

## Preparation of the recipient site

Based on the radiographic and clinical examination, and depending on the fit of the graft in the existing alveolar process, a *closed* (without raising a flap) or *open* (with flap exposing the buccal alveolar bone area) procedure is selected. As a rule, the recipient site is prepared prior to graft removal in order to shorten the extra-alveolar period for the graft. Before the surgical procedure, antibiotic coverage is achieved (e.g. phenoxymethylpenicillin 2 g) 1 hour before surgery and maintained for a period of 4 days (at doses of 1 g twice daily). (The doses mentioned are for a normallly weighted 70 kg man and should be reduced accordingly for persons with a lower body weight such as children and adolescents.)

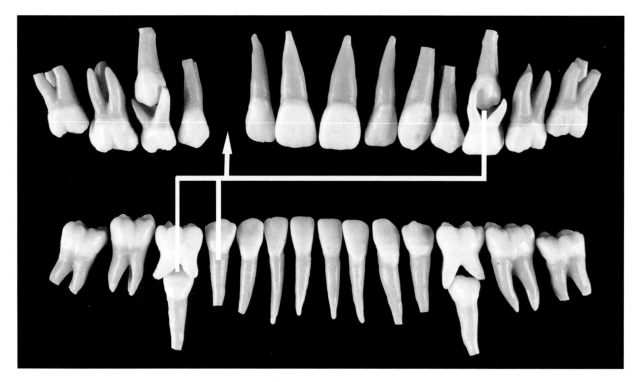

**Fig. 27.7** Canine loss, possible donor teeth. Mandibular premolars are optimal donor teeth.

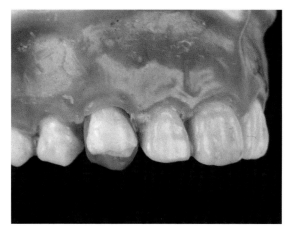
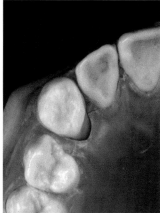

**Fig. 27.8** Canine region, transplantation of a mandibular first or second premolar. The double exposure illustrates where crown substance should be added or reduced.

If a tooth is present at the recipient site, it is extracted and the socket enlarged so that the future graft will be surrounded by a 1–2 mm coagulum (Fig. 27.9). This will optimize periodontal and pulpal healing (13). The socket preparation should be performed atraumatically using a bur with internal saline cooling (15). Thereafter the entrance to the socket is covered with a gauze sponge while awaiting the graft.

### Open procedure

A trapezoid incision is made in the attached labial gingival mucosa. The affected tooth is extracted (Fig. 27.10) and an osteotomy cut is made with a thin bur at the site of the future alveolus. The labial bone plate is then removed with a chisel and stored in saline. Thereafter the socket is prepared with

a bur with internal saline cooling. Finally, the socket is covered with a gauze sponge in order to prevent saliva contamination during graft removal.

### Graft removal and insertion

The donor tooth is removed atraumatically, usually implying a flap procedure and removal of marginal bone labially in the case of mandibular premolars or palatally in the case of maxillary premolars. The graft is placed in a semi-erupted position in the new socket and stabilized with a suture cervically.

In an open procedure, the dissected labial bone plate is cut lengthwise with a heavy scissors into 2–3 pieces. These grafts are placed so that they cover the labial part of the root

**Fig. 27.9 Autotransplantation of a premolar to the central incisor region using a closed procedure**
The treatment plan is to transplant a maxillary second premolar to the central incisor region. The incisor is to be removed due to root resorption subsequent to replantation.

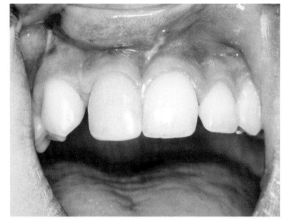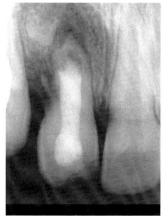

### Extracting the incisor
The incisor is extracted. Note the extensive root resorption.

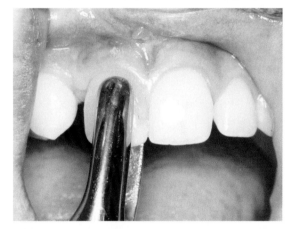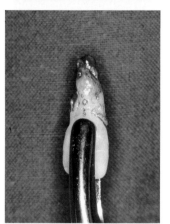

### Preparing the socket
The socket is enlarged with a surgical bur with internal saline cooling. The socket is expanded palatally. The socket is then rinsed with saline.

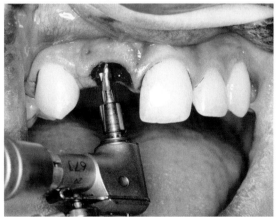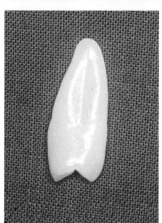

### Testing the size of the socket
Using a porcelain replica of a premolar, the size of the socket is tested. Thereafter the socket is washed with saline.

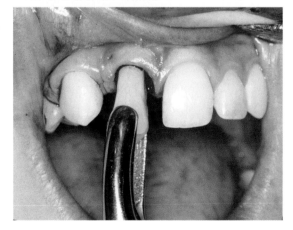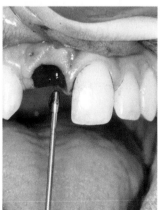

**Fig. 27.9 (cont.)**
**Removing the maxillary second premolar**
After making a gingival incision and incising the cervical part of the PDL, the tooth is extracted using gentle luxation movements.

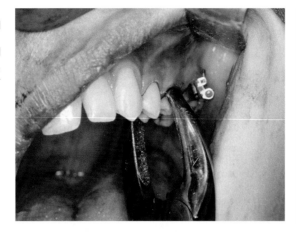
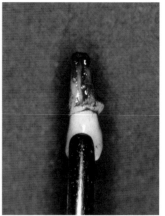

**Repositioning the graft**
The graft is placed in a 45° rotated position in order to achieve sufficient cervical width.

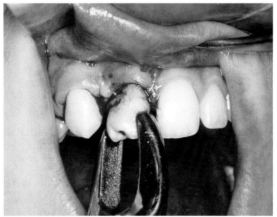
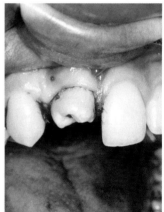

**Splinting the graft**
The tooth is splinted with an 0.2 mm stainless steel wire placed around the necks of the adjacent teeth. The position for the wire is ensured by etching the labial enamel of the adjacent teeth and incorporating the wire in composite.

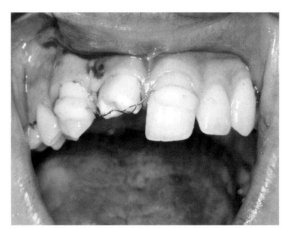
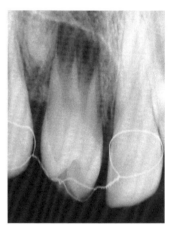

with cortical bone facing the root. Thereafter the labial flap is elongated using periosteal incisions and then sutured tightly around the neck of the transplant. As experimental studies have shown that rigid splinting is detrimental to both pulpal and periodontal healing, this procedure should be avoided (13, 40). To prevent vertical displacement during healing, a suture is placed over the occlusal surface of the graft. Alternatively, a figure-of-eight stainless steel wire (diameter 0.2 mm) inserted between adjacent teeth may serve the same purpose. The stabilizing sutures or wires can be removed after 1 week.

## Follow-up period

Clinical and radiographic controls should be made 4 and 8 weeks after grafting, where healing complications, such as pulp necrosis or external root resorption (i.e. inflammatory or replacement resorption) can be diagnosed (13). After 4 months, the graft can be restored (see later). Further clinical and radiographic controls should be performed at the following intervals: 6 months, 1 year, 2 years and 5 years after grafting in order to assess pulpal and periodontal healing (Fig. 27.11).

**Fig. 27.10 Autotransplantation of a premolar to the central incisor region using an open procedure**

The treatment plan is to transplant a right maxillary premolar to the central incisor region where there is marked vertical and horizontal bone atrophy.

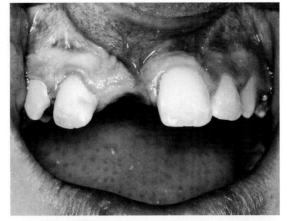 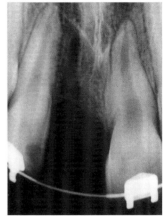

**Flap procedure and socket preparation**

A trapezoidal incision is made and the atrophied alveolar ridge exposed. Osteotomy cuts through the labial bone plates and subsequent removal of bone plate with a chisel will expose the future socket. The socket is prepared with a bur with internal saline cooling.

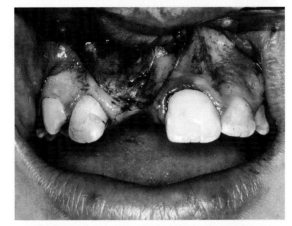 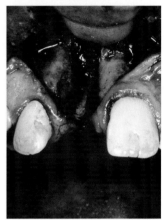

**Transplanting the premolar**

The premolar is seated in the socket and fixed in its new position with a suture placed cervically. Thereafter, the labial bone plate is cut lengthwise in 2-mm wide strips with heavy scissors and placed over the transplant, with the concave cortical surface against the periodontal ligament (arrow).

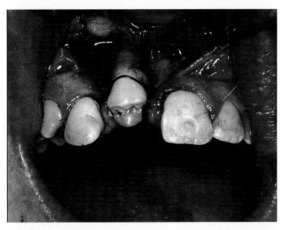 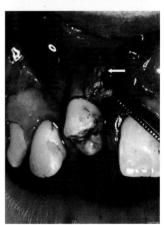

**Flap repositioning and splinting**

The flap is lengthened via periosteal incisions at its base and then sutured. A thin (0.2 mm) stainless steel wire anchored between the right lateral incisor and the left central incisor stabilizes the tooth during initial healing.

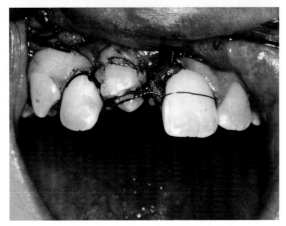 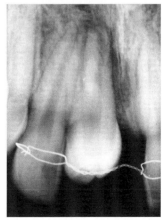

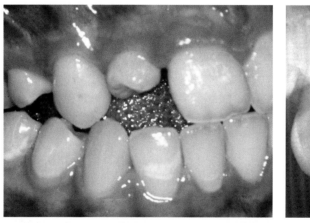

**Fig. 27.11** Tooth survival of auto-transplanted teeth used in the treatment of anterior tooth loss. A life table analysis of two clinical studies representing 50 and 130 transplants to the anterior region. From KRISTERSON & LAGERSTRÖM (20) 1991 and ANDREASEN et al. (22) 2005.

**Fig. 27.12 Long-term survival of a grafted premolar**
A maxillary second premolar transplanted to the lateral incisor region.

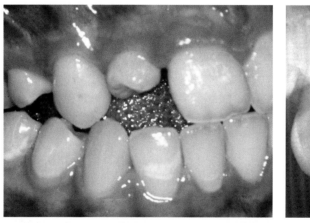
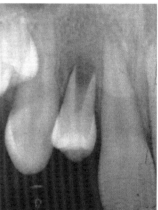

**10-year control**
Stable periodontal and pulpal healing is evident 10 years after transplantation.

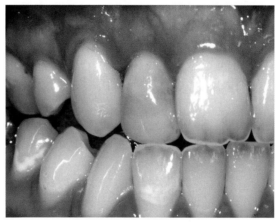
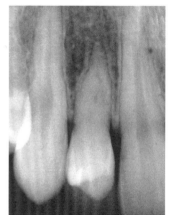

## Pulpal healing

Three to 6 months after transplantation, pulpal healing can be diagnosed clinically by a positive sensibility response as well as radiographically by pulp canal obliteration (Fig. 27.12), which is a sign of reinnervation and revascularization of the traumatized pulp (14). Pulp necrosis due to infection can usually be diagnosed after 4 to 8 weeks. Treatment of pulp necrosis is outlined in Chapter 22. Secondary pulp necrosis may occur following pulp canal

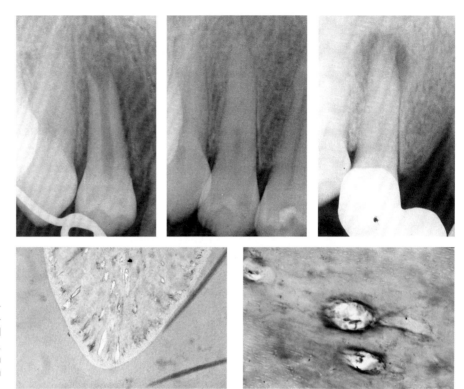

**Fig. 27.13** Pulpal complications subsequent to crown preparation. The histologic slides show extreme canal obliteration with vascular inclusions. One year after crown preparation, a periapical radiolucency is seen. From KRISTERSON (10) 1985.

obliteration and is suspected to be related to a new trauma or dentin exposure during crown preparation (10).

## Periodontal healing

The earliest radiographic signs of healing (i.e. reformation of the periodontal ligament space) can be seen after 4 weeks and are usually manifest after 8 weeks. Inflammatory and replacement resorption are usually evident after 4–8 weeks. These complications were found with a frequency of 7% in the authors' material (22). The treatment of both resorption types follows the principles outlined for avulsed and replanted teeth (see Chapter 17, p. 470).

## Root development

When transplanting teeth with an open apex a continuing root development is seen (Fig. 27.12).

## Orthodontic treatment of transplanted teeth

In many trauma cases, where autotransplantation to the anterior region has been performed, it is often necessary to reduce a maxillary overjet orthodontically.

Clinical studies indicate that orthodontic treatment is possible 3–6 months after autotransplantation without a significant risk of progressive resorption (15, 20, 22).

## Restoration of transplanted teeth

The general principles for restoration of transplanted teeth should imply a minimum interference with the health of the pulp and the gingiva. In a tooth transplanted with an incompletely formed root, revascularization of the pulp normally occurs, but as a rule with pulp canal obliteration to follow. Pulp canal obliteration can usually be diagnosed 3–6 months after transplantation. This newly formed dentin differs from normal dentin by virtue of its cellular content and many vascular inclusions (21). Thus, any exposure of dentin, as during crown preparation or caries, may permit progressive bacterial invasion. As an adequate secondary dentin response in the pulp is not possible due to the constricted root canal, an infected pulp necrosis may occur (Fig. 27.13). For this reason, it is suggested that restorative procedures are performed prior to total canal obliteration, i.e. 3–9 months after transplantation.

Before restoration, the contour of the gingival margin should also be considered. If a gingivectomy is to be performed, coronal regrowth of approximately 1 mm in the anterior region should be expected (24).

Safe restoration of transplanted teeth implies the following considerations:

(1) Pulpal status should be determined prior to restoration, i.e. a positive sensibility response should be elicited.
(2) The restoration should be made so that no or only a minimum of dentin is exposed. At least no post-transplantation dentin must be exposed.
(3) The restorative procedure used should prevent or limit microleakage, which leads to bacterial invasion, hyper-

sensibility and discoloration of the restoration. The use of the new dentin-bonding agents may help to eliminate these problems related to bacteria invasion following tooth reduction.

If the tooth has been endodontically treated, the first two considerations can usually be ignored.

The restorative procedures are presently confined to two types: *composite resin restoration* or *ceramic laminate veneers*, both employed after adequate enamel reduction.

## Composite restoration

These restorations can be performed very soon after transplantation. After necessary enamel reduction, the crowns are built up according to the principles described for the use of composite resin in the treatment of crown fractures. Figs 27.14–27.16 demonstrate examples of final treatment results of autotransplantation in the treatment of anterior tooth loss.

An important aspect in the restoration of the traumatized dentition is the restoration of symmetry in the dental arch. A decisive factor is the cervical dimension of the graft, which can be adjusted during the surgical phase of treatment by graft rotation at the recipient site. However, in the case of anterior asymmetry, either due to deviation of graft dimension with its antimere, or where adjacent teeth have migrated into the site of tooth loss or infraocclusion in the case of protracted ankylosis, and where for various reasons orthodontic realignment is not possible, the problem arises as to how to re-establish lost symmetry.

Slight reduction of the proximal surface of the adjacent incisor may compensate for some space loss. There should be maximal length of the restored transplanted tooth to enhance the illusion of symmetry. The facial surface should be flattened, with maximum separation between mamelons, and acute proximal angles to allude to a broader tooth. Finally, the mesial and distal corners of the incisal edge should be squared (21).

Another situation can arise when the mesiodistal dimension of the transplant is greater than its antimere, as when a maxillary premolar has been transplanted and rotated 90°. In this situation, the opposite optical effect can be used to achieve optimal symmetry (21). The transplant should be restored to maximum length, with the facial surface as well as the mesial and distal corners rounded and minimal distance between mamelons. This technique will deflect light and suggest smaller dimensions. Moreover, the size of the contralateral can also be enhanced to improve symmetry (21).

Finally, in teeth with diminutive cervical dimensions, cervical build-up in ceramic, similar to that done in the case of single tooth implants can provide another solution to anterior asymmetry (25). In case of replacement of lateral incisors very minimal composite restoration is necessary (Fig. 27.17).

## Ceramic laminate veneers

The conservative preparation necessary for veneer restoration makes this treatment procedure suitable for restoring the esthetics to the anterior region following premolar autotransplantation while preserving pulpal vitality following post-transplantation canal obliteration (25) (Fig. 27.18). Although the crown height in younger individuals is very likely to undergo changes, the gingival margin of ceramic veneers cemented with a composite luting agent is esthetically acceptable despite its eventual visibility. Patient satisfaction with these restorations, including the prospect of revision at a later date due to maxillary skeletal growth, is more than adequate.

Special problems arise with respect to preparation of premolars for anterior restorations. Often orthodontic adjustment of the transplant is necessary prior to definitive restoration. In such cases, the period of retention must be complete before preparation for veneers. Otherwise, there is a risk of tooth migration. Alternatively, a retention wire should be applied palatally to assure transplant orientation even after restoration.

Other problems that also present in these cases concern the proximal extension of the preparation to ensure adequate ceramic bulk to withstand occlusal loading during function, as well as the extent of reduction of the palatal cusp to ensure occlusal stability. It is still a matter of debate whether a bulky palatal cusp invites lingual pressure that could force the transplant facially or whether occlusion in the central fossa stabilizes the tooth. Esthetic demands might well dictate cusp reduction. Whatever decision is made with regard to tooth preparation, caution must be exercised if dentin is exposed during tissue reduction. In such cases, it is advisable that the exposed dentin be treated with a dentin-bonding agent and a thin layer of composite resin immediately after preparation and prior to impression taking in order to seal dentinal tubules until veneer cementation.

The following procedures have been suggested for detecting exposed dentin: search under magnification or with an explorer where dentin feels and looks smooth compared to a roughened, prepared enamel, or by a 5-second etch where enamel looks frosty and dentin dull. Provisional restoration would seem appropriate in such situations; also in the case of palatal-occlusal reduction (i.e. a reverse 3/4 crown) in order to maintain interdental and intermaxillary relationships. When provisional restorations are indicated, they can be retained either as a resin splint by spot-etching the prepared and adjacent teeth or as a provisional veneer with a eugenol-free luting agent (27–29).

In unpublished clinical material, porcelain veneers were used to restore autotransplanted premolars. The conservative approach which was necessary in order to avoid exposure of post-transplantation dentin often demanded an unfortunate compromise in porcelain construction. It is, therefore, suggested that if crown anatomy demands such compromises, the graft be endodontically treated when adequate root development is achieved.

**Fig. 27.14 Maxillary central incisor replacement using autotransplantation**
Right central incisor replaced with a left mandibular second premolar. The tooth has been restored with composite.

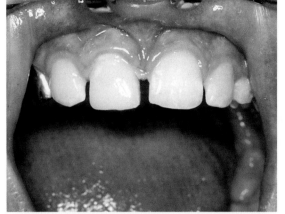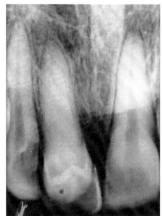

**Right central incisor replacement**
The incisor was replaced with a left mandibular second premolar. The tooth has been restored with composite.

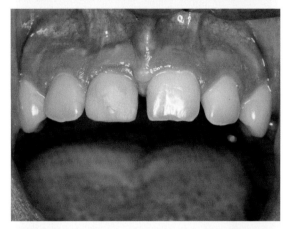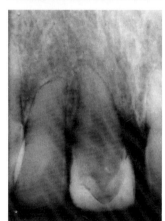

**Right central incisor replacement**
The incisor was replaced with a right maxillary second premolar. The tooth has been restored with composite.

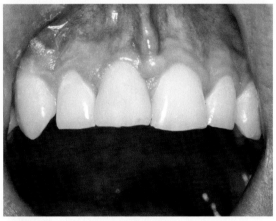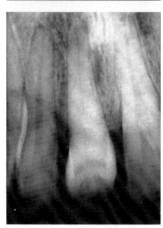

**Left central incisor replacement**
The incisor was replaced with a left maxillary third molar. The tooth has been restored with composite.

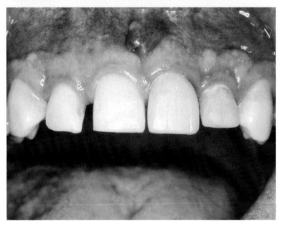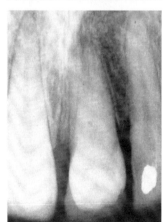

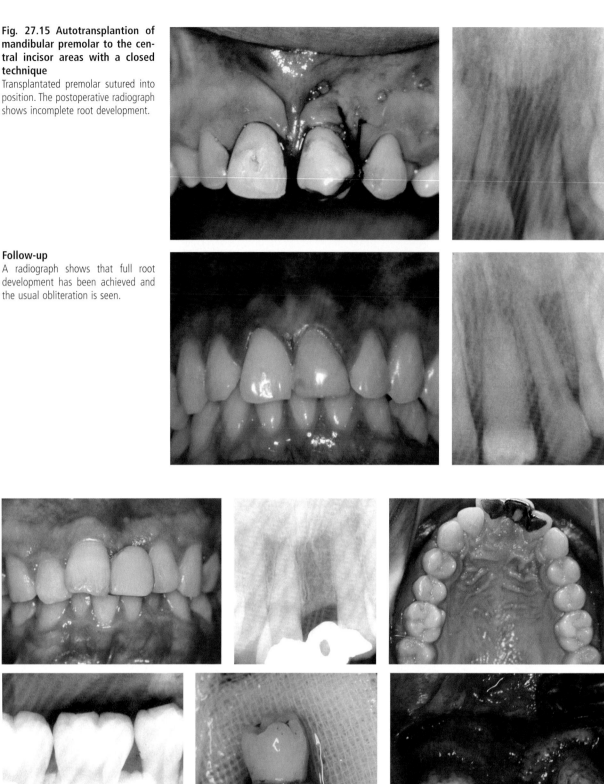

**Fig. 27.15 Autotransplantion of mandibular premolar to the central incisor areas with a closed technique**
Transplantated premolar sutured into position. The postoperative radiograph shows incomplete root development.

**Follow-up**
A radiograph shows that full root development has been achieved and the usual obliteration is seen.

A

B

**Fig. 27.16** Autotransplantation of a supernumerary premolar to the anterior region. A. Frontal view of a 21-year-old man at first examination. His chief complaint was the replacement of an anterior bridge with an implant. The left central incisor was avulsed due to a traumatic injury and replaced by a Maryland bridge. B. A supernumerary tooth was found between the right second premolar and the first molar. The extracted donor tooth shows a root form optimal for transplantation. When the flap was raised, it was realized that the alveolar ridge was too thin to accommodate the donor tooth.

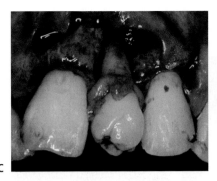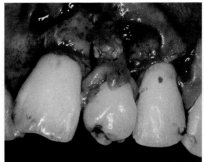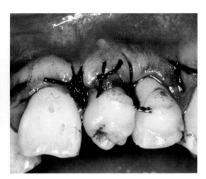

C

**Fig. 27.16** C. The buccal bone plate was removed first and stored extra-orally in saline during socket preparation and replaced upon the transplant. The flap was sutured tightly around the transplant, and the transplant was splinted to adjacent tooth with wire and resin. A root canal treatment of transplants was started two weeks after surgery and finished with gutta-percha three months later.

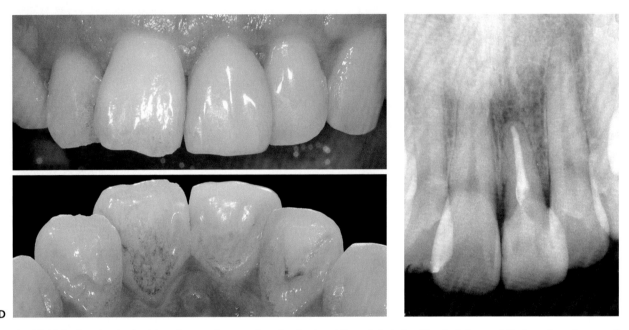

D

**Fig. 27.16** D. Buccal and palatal view six years after transplantation. Tooth mobility and gingival probing depth is normal. On the radiograph a normal PDL space is found around the root and no sign of progressive root resorption.

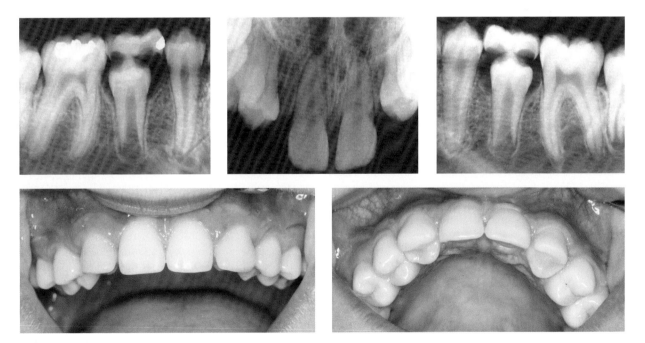

**Fig. 27.17** Maxillary lateral incisors replaced by mandibular second premolar transplants. This patient suffered lateral incisor and canine aplasia. Orthodontic evaluation showed that mandibular second premolar transplantation to the lateral incisor position, together with anterior orthodontic movement of the distally placed teeth was indicated in order to compensate for the missing teeth. The two mandibular premolars are at an optimal stage of root development, with three-quarters of the anticipated root length. The clinical condition is shown 5 years after transplantation and after completion of orthodontic treatment.

**Fig. 27.18 Autotransplanted pre-molars restored with a porcelain laminate veneer**
Two restored central incisors were replaced with 2 second maxillary pre-molars. The transplants were later restored with porcelain.

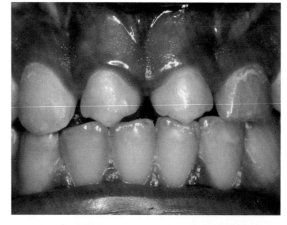
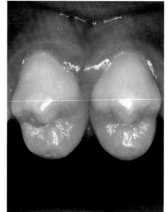

**Final result**
The transplants, after grinding were restored with porcelain laminates.

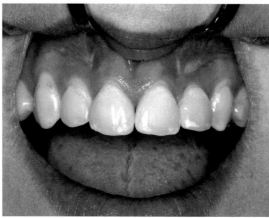
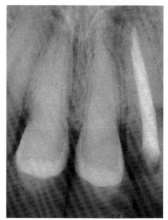

## Combined orthodontic closure and autotransplantation

In some cases it might be an advantage in the case of loss of two incisors to close one of the sites and autotransplant the second (Fig. 27.19).

## Autotransplantation of teeth with completed root formation

Recently a technique for autotransplantation of teeth with completed root formation has been used in the initial or late treatment of acute dental trauma (30, 31) (Fig. 27.20).

In this technique, the socket is prepared atraumatically with surgical burs to a size which is slightly larger than the donor tooth. The graft tooth is luxated and extracted after incision of the periodontal ligament with a thin scalpel blade and immediately transferred to the new socket and placed slightly out of occlusion. The graft is splinted for 8 weeks with a flexible wire splint and an acid-etch/composite technique.

After 3 to 4 weeks, endodontic treatment can be performed using an interim dressing of calcium hydroxide followed by a gutta-percha root filling (see Chapter 22).

In cases of acute trauma, this technique can also be used to place the tooth in a site of less injury (Fig. 27.21).

In a recent study, the gingival and periodontal condition of transplanted premolars to the anterior region by Czochrowska et al. was compared to adjacent natural incisors (41, 42). Identical gingival and periodontal conditions were found, a finding which is rare with regard to implants. Furthermore, the esthetic outcome of autotransplanted premolars was analyzed. In a study of 22 transplants, a satisfactory or acceptable esthetic outcome was found in 86% of the cases (41, 42).

## Prognosis

In several studies a success rate (i.e. without progressive root resorption) of 87–93% was found for transplants and a tooth survival rate of 90–98% (Table 27.1) (13–16, 20, 41–47). With respect to pulpal and periodontal healing, it should be, however, mentioned that 10–20% of cases may show complications at a later date, such as primary or secondary pulp necrosis as well as external (cervical) root resorption, which may require additional treatment.

In long-term studies of autotransplanted teeth with immature root development, where data allow *life table analysis* of the prognosis, there appears to be almost identical survival: *5-year survival* ranges of 98–99%; and *10-year survival* of 87–95% and 80% (20–23). The longest study of autotransplanted premolars showed 90% survival after 39 years, a record that neither prosthetics nor implantology can surpass (43) (Fig. 27.22). This survival rate thus appears to be equal to alternative treatment approaches, such as implants and for certain fixed prosthetic appliances (see Chapters 26 and 28).

**Fig. 27.19 Maxillary lateral and central incisor replacement with combined orthodontic space closure and premolar transplantation**

Two incisors have been avulsed in a 9-year-old girl. The treatment plan is to orthodontically move the canine into the lateral incisor position, the first premolar into the canine position, and finally to transplant the mandibular second premolar into the central incisor position.

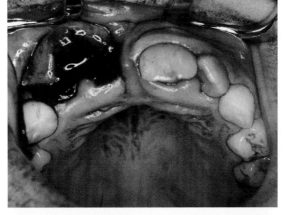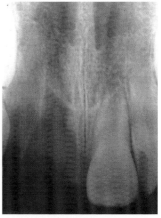

**Restoration of the anterior segment**

The premolar has been moved into the canine position, rotated 45° and the oral cusp reduced. The canine has been moved into the lateral incisor position and its cusp and proximal surfaces reduced. The transplanted premolar has been restored with composite. From ANDREASEN et al. (12) 1989.

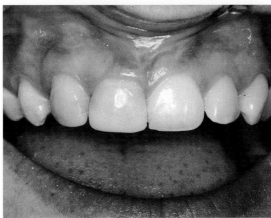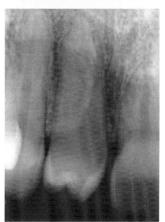

**Fig. 27.20 Autotransplantation of two premolars with complete root formation to the central incisor region**

This 14-year-old girl had lost her two central incisors due to progressive root resorption subsequent to replantation after avulsion. In conjunction with orthodontic reduction of a maxillary overjet, two second mandibular premolars were extracted and transplanted to cental incisor region.

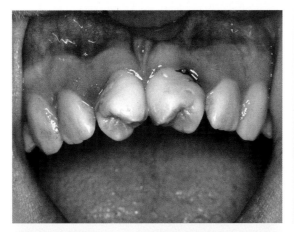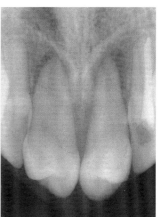

**10-year follow-up**

The clinical and radiographic condition is shown 10 years after transplantation. The transplanted teeth have been treated endodontically and later restored with post-retained crowns.

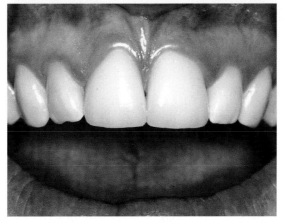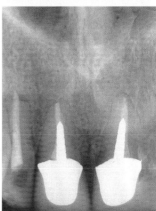

### Fig. 27.21 Autotransplantation of an intruded central incisor with completed root formation

Radiographic and clinical condition at the time of injury in a 32-year-old woman. There is extrusion of the right maxillary lateral incisor with associated gingival laceration. The right central and left lateral incisors have been avulsed and the left central incisor intruded with severe crushing of the associated alveolar process.

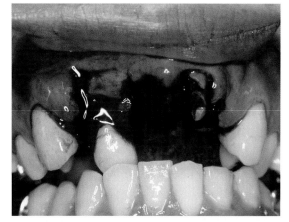 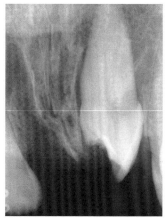

### Treatment plan

Treatment includes autotransplantation of the left central incisor to a site with least bony injury in order to avoid later bone loss (i.e. the right central incisor socket) and repositioning of the extruded right lateral incisor.

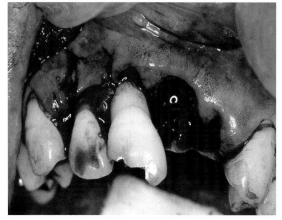 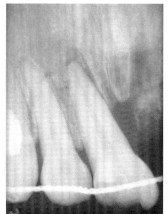

### Clinical and radiographic condition after treatment

The teeth are repositioned and the gingiva sutured. The teeth are splinted with flexible wire and an acid-etch/composite resin technique for 3 months. The root canals were initially treated with a calcium hydroxide dressing for 3 months prior to final root filling with gutta percha and sealer.

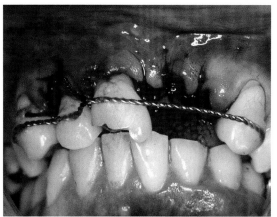 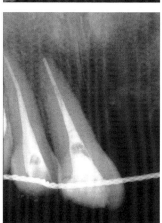

### Follow-up

The clinical condition is shown 4 years after completed prosthetic treatment. Radiographic condition 6 years after completed treatment shows slight apical surface resorption of the transplanted central incisor.

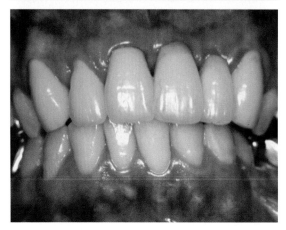 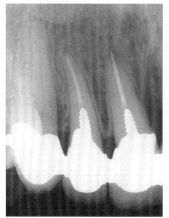

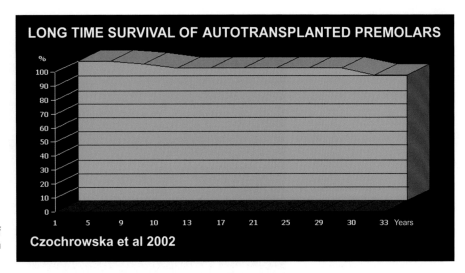

**Fig. 27.22** Long-term prognosis of autotransplanted premolars. From CZOCHROWSKA et al. (43) 2002.

With respect to the restorative procedures presently available, little is known of long-term success when applied to autotransplanted teeth.

In conclusion, autotransplantation of premolars (and sometimes diminutive molars) when indicated due to problems of crowding offers a unique treatment possibility of restoring the bone, gingiva and the tooth in a trauma region. Such a treatment solution should therefore be considered in all cases of early loss of anterior teeth and when found indicated performed with due regards to the prognosis related factor.

## Predictors for healing

The strongest predictor for optimal healing appears to be the *stage of root development* and *apical diameter* at the time of grafting (14–16, 38, 39) (Fig. 27.23). This factor appears to influence both pulp and periodontal healing and to a less degree also graft survival (Figs 27.24 and 27.25).

A very significant factor appears to be the *experience of the oral surgeon*: individuals who had performed more that 25 autotransplants had a significantly higher success rate (48, 49).

Another parameter shown to influence graft survival was a structured *follow-up regimen* to monitor periodontal and pulpal complications. Thus, it was found to be able to increase the survival rate of autotransplants in 30% (48, 49).

Finally, the type of graft is of importance, with maxillary first premolars haring significantly less healing potential (14, 15).

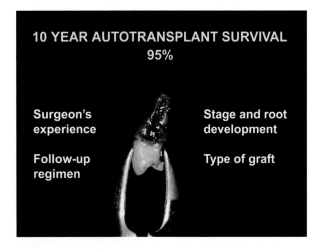

**Fig. 27.23** Predictors for successful autotransplantation of premolar.

**Table 27.1** Success rate of transplanted premolars to the anterior region.

|  | No. of teeth | Success rate (%) | Survival rate (%) |
|---|---|---|---|
| Andreasen et al. (13–16) 1990 | 33 | 88 | 98 |
| Kristerson & Lagerström (20) 1991 | 23 | 87 | 96 |
| Kugelberg et al. (44) 1994 | 31 | 87 | 90 |
| Czochrowska et al. (41, 42) 2000 | 45 | 93 | 93 |

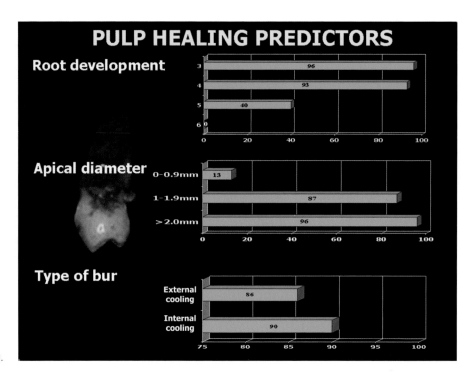

**Fig. 27.24** Predictors for pulp healing.

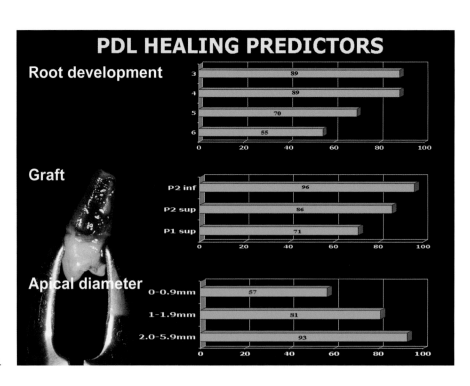

**Fig. 27.25** Predictors for PDL healing.

## Essentials

### Indications

- All cases where an early loss of permanent incisors could be anticipated – in that case a panoramic radiograph should be taken in order to detect possible tooth grafts.
- The advantage of tooth autotransplantation in comparison to alternative treatment procedures is the establishment of a functional tooth unit, which allows tooth eruption and development of the alveolar process.

### Graft selection

*Central maxillary incisor region*
- All premolars except maxillary first premolars, sometimes canines or maxillary third molars of small size

*Lateral maxillary incisor region*
- Only mandibular first premolars

*Canine region*
- All premolars except maxillary first premolars

### Stage of graft removal

- $^3/_4$ or full root development with wide open apex is optimal; however, full root development with subsequent endodontic therapy is also an option.

### Surgical procedures

- Atraumatic surgery and experience is the key to success.
- Closed procedure in cases with adequate bone support (Fig. 27.9).
- Open procedure in cases with composite bone-tooth grafting (Fig. 27.10).
- Atraumatic graft removal and graft insertion is essential for successful long-term results.

### Orthodontic treatment

- If orthodontic treatment is necessary, it can be performed when revascularization of the pulp has been completed, i.e. after 4 months.

### Prosthetic restoration

- Autotransplanted teeth can be restored by a composite technique after 3 months with a porcelain laminate technique.
- Minimal or no dentin exposure during crown preparation is essential. Eventual prophylactic endodontic intervention at the time of adequate root development to ensure optimal preparation for porcelain construction.

### Prognosis

- 5-year graft survival: 98–99%
- 10-year graft survival: 87–95%

## References

1. SLAGSVOLD O. Autotransplantation of premolars in cases of missing anterior teeth. *Trans Eur Orthod Soc* 1970;**66**:473–85.
2. KRISTERSON L. Unusual case of tooth transplantation: Report of case. *J Oral Surg* 1970;**28**:841–4.
3. DIXON DA. Autogenous transplantation of tooth germs into the upper incisor region. *Br Dent J* 1971;**131**: 260–5.
4. KVAM E, BJERCKE B. Dentes confuse – en kasusrapport og et behandlingsalternativ. *Nor Tandlaegeforen Tid* 1976;**86**:305–8.
5. SLAGSVOLD O, BJERCKE B. Applicability of autotransplantation in cases of missing upper anterior teeth. *Am J Orthod* 1978;**74**:410–21.
6. BRADY J. Transplantation of a premolar to replace a central incisor with advanced resorption. *J Dent* 1978;**6**:259–60.
7. BJERCKE B. Autotransplantasjon av tenner på börn. In: Hjörting-Hansen E. ed. *Odontologi*. Copenhagen: Munksgaard, 1979:1–25.
8. SHULMAN LB. Impacted and unerupted teeth: donors for transplant tooth replacement. *Dent Clin North Am* 1979;**23**:369–83.
9. KRAGH MADSEN I. Autotransplantation i privat praksis. *Tandlaegebladet* 1984;**88**:373–4.
10. KRISTERSON L. Autotransplantation of human premolars. A clinical and radiographic study of 100 teeth. *Int J Oral Surg* 1985;**14**:200–13.
11. DERMAUT L, DE-PAUW G. L'autogreffe de dents: une dimension supplémentaire dans la practique dentaire. *Rev Belge Med Dent* 1989;**44**:85–98.
12. ANDREASEN JO, PAULSEN HU, FJELLVANG H, BARFOD K. Autotransplantation af praemolarer til behandling af tandtab i overkaebefronten. *Tandlaegebladet* 1989;**93**:435–40.
13. ANDREASEN JO, PAULSEN HU, YU Z, AHLQUIST R, BAYER T, SCHWARTZ O. A long-term study of 370 autotransplanted premolars. Part I. Surgical procedures and standardized techniques for monitoring healing. *Eur J Orthod* 1990;**12**:3–13.
14. ANDREASEN JO, PAULSEN HU, YU Z, BAYER T, SCHWARTZ O. A long-term study of 370 autotransplanted premolars. Part II. Tooth survival and pulp healing subsequent to transplantation. *Eur J Orthod* 1990;**12**:14–24.
15. ANDREASEN JO, PAULSEN HU, YU Z, SCHWARTZ O. A long-term study of 370 auto transplanted premolars. Part III. Periodontal healing subsequent to transplantation. *Eur J Orthod* 1990;**12**:25–37.
16. ANDREASEN JO, PAULSEN HU, YU Z, BAYER T. A long-term study of 370 autotransplanted premolars. Part IV. Root development subsequent to transplantation. *Eur J Orthod* 1990;**12**:38–50.

17. PAULSEN HU, ANDREASEN JO, SCHWARTZ O. Behandling of tab i fronten med autotransplantation of praemolarer. *Tandlaegernes Tidsskrift* 1990;**5**:70–5.

18. BOWDEN DEJ, PATEL HA. Autotransplantation of premolar teeth to replace missing maxillary central incisors. *Br J Orthod* 1990;**17**:21–8.

19. OIKARINEN K. Replacing resorbed maxillary central incisors with mandibular premolars. *Endod Dent Traumatol* 1990;**6**:43–6.

20. KRISTERSON L, LAGERSTRÖM L. Autotransplantation of teeth in cases with agenesis or traumatic loss of maxillary incisors. *Eur J Orthod* 1991;**13**:486–92.

21. ANDREASEN JO. *Atlas of replantation and transplantation of teeth.* Fribourg: Mediglobe, 1991.

22. ANDREASEN JO, ANDREASEN FM. Autotransplantation of premolars, canines and third molars to the anterior region. 2007. In preparation.

23. LAGERSTRÖM L, KRISTERSON L. Influence of orthodontic treatment on root development of autotransplantated premolars. *Am J Orthodont* 1986;**89**:146–9.

24. MONEFELDT I, ZACHRISSON BU. Adjustment of clinical crown height by gingivectomy following orthodontic space closure. *Angle Orthod* 1977;**47**:256–64.

25. ANDREASEN JO, DAUGAARD J, ANDREASEN FM. Autotransplantation of teeth to the anterior region. II. Restorative procedures. 2007. In preparation.

26. GOLDSTEIN RE. *Esthetics in dentistry.* Philadelphia: JB Lippincott Company, 1976.

27. BROOKS L. The porcelain bonded to tooth restoration. *J Pedod* 1987;**11**:269–80.

28. WILIS P. Temporization of porcelain laminate veneers. *Compendium of Continuing Education in Dentistry* 1987;**IX**:352–8.

29. GARBER DA, GOLDSTEIN RE, FEINMAN RA. *Porcelain laminate veneers.* Chicago: Quintessence Publishing, 1988:136.

30. TSUKIBOSHI M. Autogenous tooth transplantation-reevaluation. *Int J Periodontol Rest Dent.* 1993;**13**:126–49.

31. TSUKIBOSHI M. The efficacy of autogenous tooth transplantation. Abstract, AAP 79th Annual Meeting. Chicago, 1993.

32. NIELSEN IL. Autotransplante de un bicúspide como sustitución de in insisivo perdido. *Rev Esp Ortod* 2000;**30**:341–50.

33. SCHATZ JP, JOHO JP. Autotransplantations and loss of anterior teeth by trauma. *Endod Dent Traumatol* 1993;**9**:36–9.

34. KALWITZKI M, NEY T, GÖZ G. Transplantation of a lower bicuspid after traumatic loss of three upper incisors. *J Orofac Orthop* 2003;**64**:57–66.

35. STENVIK A, ZACHRISSON BU. Orthodontic closure and transplantation in the treatment of missing anterior teeth. An overview. *Endod Dent Traumatol* 1993;**9**:45–52.

36. STENVIK A, ZACHRISSON BU. A difficult agenesis case made easier by autotransplantation: deep overbite with one incisor and two second premolars missing in the mandible. *World J Orthod* 2001;**2**:45–50.

37. WATERHOUSE PJ, HOBSON RS, MEECHAN JG. Autotransplantation as a treatment option after loss of a maxillary permanent incisor tooth. A case report. *Int J Paediatr Dent* 1999;**9**:43–7.

38. TSUKIBOSHI M. *Autotransplantation of teeth.* Illinois: Quintessence Publishing, 2001:192.

39. TSUKIBOSHI M. Autotransplantation of teeth: requirements for predictable success. *Dent Traumatol* 2002;**18**:159–80.

40. BAUSS O, SCHILKE R, FENSKE C, ENGELKE W, KILIARIDIS S. Autotransplantation of immature third molars: influence of different splinting methods and fixation. *Int J Oral Maxillofac Surg* 2004;**33**:558–63.

41. CZOCHROWSKA EM, STENVIK A, ZACHRISSON BU. The esthetic outcome of autotransplanted premolars replacing maxillary incisors. *Dent Traumatol* 2002;**18**:237–45.

42. CZOCHROWSKA EM, STENVIK A, ALBUM B, ZACHRISSON BU. Autotransplantation of premolars to replace maxillary incisors: a comparison with natural incisors. *Am J Orthod Dentofacial Orthop* 2000;**118**:592–600.

43. CZOCHROWSKA EM, STENVIK A, BJERCKE B, ZACHRISSON BU. Outcome of tooth transplantation: survival and success rates 17–41 years post-treatment. *Am J Orthod Dentofacial Orthop* 2002;**121**:110–9.

44. KUGELBERG R, TEGSJÖ U, MALMGREN O. Autotransplantation of 45 teeth to the upper incisor region in adolescents. *Swed Dent J* 1994;**18**:165–72.

45. LUNDBERG T, ISAKSSON S. A clinical follow-up study of 278 autostransplanted teeth. *Br J Oral Maxillofac Surg* 1996;**34**:181–5.

46. SCHATZ JP, JOHO P. Long-term clinical and radiographic evaluation of autotransplanted teeth. *Int J Oral Maxillofac Surg* 1992;**21**:271–5.

47. ANDERSSON L, KVINT S, TEGSJÖ U. Transplantation av tänder. *Tandläkartidningen* 1996;**88**:873–81.

48. SCHWARTZ O, BERGMANN P, KLAUSEN B. Autotranplantation of human teeth. A life-table analysis of prognostic factors. *Int J Oral Surg* 1985;**14**:245–58.

49. SCHWARTZ O, BERGMANN P, KLAUSEN B. Resorption of autotransplanted human teeth: a retrospective study of 291 transplantations over a period of 25 years. *Int Endod J* 1985;**18**:119–31.

# 28
# Implants in the Anterior Region

J. O. Andreasen, J. Ödman, C. Hämmerle, D. Buser, T. von Arx, J. Jensen,
S. E. Nörholt & O. Schwartz

*J.O. Andreasen*

## Indications for implants in trauma patients

One of the largest achievements in dental history has been the development of implants as a reliable replacement for failing or missing teeth (Fig. 28.1). This evolution has been going on for more than three decades and has gradually evolved into a simplified and usually reliable treatment procedure. There are now reports on the long-term results in trauma patients of using this treatment entity (1).

With regard to the use of implants in trauma cases a series of questions occurs:

- What is the indication for using implants?
- Should implants be preferred to other tooth replacement procedures? (e.g. prosthodontics, autotransplantation of teeth or orthodontic closure)
- At what age can implant treatment be used? (A critical question as early adulthood is the most common time for dental traumas to occur.)
- At what time after an injury and/or an extraction can implant treatment be performed?

- Which technique should be used to optimize long-term esthetic and functional results?
- What are the long-term effects of implant treatment in regard to function and esthetics?
- Can failures be predicted?

These items will be discussed, but only aspects of implantology that are related to treatment of tooth loss after acute dental trauma will be presented. For a complete description of dental implantology the reader is referred to recent textbooks devoted to this topic. The evaluation of treatment options after tooth loss based on cost, economy and use in growing individuals in shown in Appendix 4, page 882.

## Treatment with implants in a trauma situation – when to give up?

Dental traumas may present such a variety of healing complications that it is sometimes difficult to decide when to give up and rely on other treatment solutions. As it appears from Fig. 28.2 the yellow and red trauma types represent potential tooth loss candidates; however, in relation to frequency, they represent a relatively small proportion of all traumas (see Chapter 34).

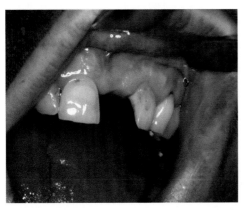
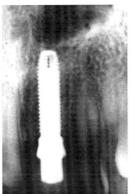
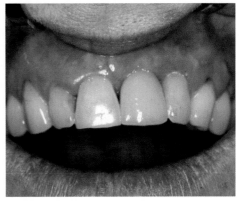

**Fig. 28.1** Treatment of a central incisor loss with an implant supported restoration. Prosthetics performed by Dr. B. Holm, Copenhagen.

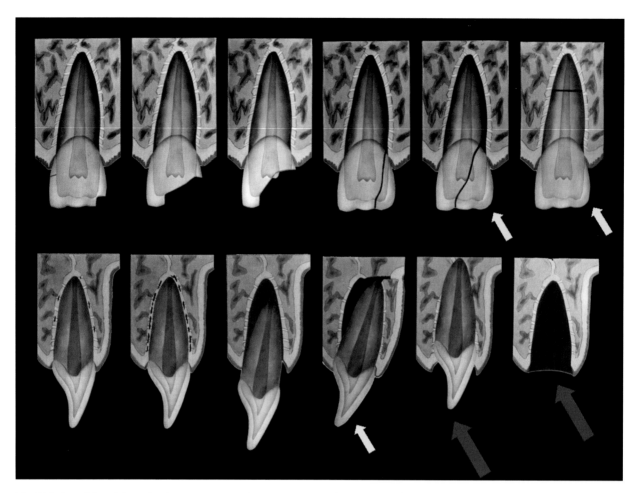

**Fig. 28.2** Potential tooth loss related to trauma type. Various trauma types in the permanent dentition, with yellow arrows indicating a certain risk of tooth loss and red arrows indicating frequent tooth loss.

## Avulsion without replantation

In these cases an immediate demand for tooth replacement arises. A decisive factor appears to be the age as installation of an implant demands completed alveolar growth (see p. 763).

## Avulsion and subsequent replantation

In case of replantation usually a number of complications arise, normally related to fast or protracted root resorption (see Chapter 17, p. 470). In case of fast root resorption (e.g. in children), a treatment solution has to be made very soon due to the fast infraposition of the tooth; in these cases decoronation is often the treatment of choice (see Chapter 24, p. 703). In case of protracted resorption (e.g. in adults) the tooth can be kept as space maintainer for a prolonged time.

## Intrusion

After replantation of an avulsed tooth, this is the most severe injury and usually implies severe periodontal and pulpal complications (see Chapter 16, p. 439). A common treatment procedure for implanted teeth such as orthodontic repositioning require many patient appointments (an average of nineteen) which makes the treatment expensive. When the chance of a successful healing outcome is consid-

ered, there is often a discrepancy between the effort used to solve an intruded permanent tooth in an adolescent and the chance of good long-term survival (see Chapter 16, p. 441). In these cases an analysis of the cost of repositioning plus surveillance of healing should also incorporate an analysis of alternative treatment, which may imply installation of an implant.

## Crown-root fractures

A certain number of crown-root fractures will not be suitable for restoration (see Chapter 11). In these cases implant installation may be the immediate option, considering the age of the patient (see p. 763).

## Root fractures

In the past healed root fractures with hard tissue interposition were not accepted as permanent healing and were therefore extracted and replaced by implants or fixed prosthodontics. With the present knowledge of root fracture healing, such an approach cannot be considered acceptable today, except in a few cases of cervical fracture where a hard tissue union has not occurred and permanent splinting is not indicated (see Chapter 12, p. 358). Cervical fractures related to endodontic treatment of immature teeth usually represent an indication (see Chapter 22, p. 631).

## Treatment planning

When anterior tooth loss has occurred or is anticipated (e.g. due to progressive root resorption) the most important factors to consider with respect to treatment planning are: *age of the patient, anticipated vertical growth* of the alveolar process, *space* available between crowns and roots of neighboring teeth, *occlusal relations,* and *condition of the alveolar process.* These factors usually determine the treatment of choice, whether orthodontic space closure, resin-retained or conventional fixed prosthetics, autotransplantation, or implantation. To aid in the choice between the treatment possibilities, study models, intraoral and panoramic radiographs, and sometimes CT scans are necessary.

*J. Ödman*

## Timing of implant insertion in relation to jaw growth

The vertical and horizontal growth of the alveolar process is strongly related to tooth eruption (2–4). Furthermore, tooth eruption is first of all related to genetic and hormonal factors which imply that tooth eruption stages can vary extensively in individuals with the same chronologic age. Erupting teeth, besides moving in occlusal direction, also perform a lateral movement in the mesio-distal and bucco-oral directions due to bone remodeling processes in the jaws (5).

In the 1980s there was intense discussion as to whether implants could be used in young individuals to replace missing teeth without interfering with growth of the jaw. The main question was at what chronologic age implants could be installed. To obtain an answer to this problem, a series of experimental and clinical studies were initiated and performed at the University of Gothenburg, Sweden (7–11). Subsequent to this, a consensus conference was held in Jonköping, Sweden, in 1990 to find answers to these problems (12).

The experimental study was carried out in young pigs with developing permanent premolars and showed that inserted implants behaved like ankylosed teeth, being integrated with bone. Accordingly, the implants did not erupt together with adjacent teeth and caused local arrest of the vertical alveolar growth process in the implant areas. The osseointegrated implants stayed in their original position and did not participate in the mesio-distal or buccal-oral growth (7–11).

In view of the results of this experimental study, placement of implants in growing regions or in the neighbourhood of developing or erupting teeth was found to be inappropriate in children and young adolescents (8). However, clinical trials were necessary to verify if implants were suitable to replace missing teeth in older adolescents.

Consequently a group of 15 adolescents (ages 13 to 19

years) with missing teeth were selected (9). All patients had the same dental stage and fully erupted permanent teeth (third molars excluded). There was, however, a difference in age, skeletal development and amount of remaining growth. Body height was recorded and skeletal maturation assessed from radiographs: this varied between MP3-FG and R-J, i.e. skeletal stages ranging from pubertal spurt termination to practically completed growth (13).

A total of 27 fixtures were placed, 19 in the upper jaw and 8 in the lower jaw, and the patients were followed during a 10-year period with photographs, study casts, periapical radiographs, lateral cephalograms, hand-wrist radiographs and body height measurements (11).

During the first three years the increase in body height of the patients varied between 0 and 18 cm and the infraocclusion of the implants in the incisor region varied between 0 and 1.6 mm (9) and in the canine and premolar regions from 0 to 0.6 mm. The most noticeable infra-occlusion took place in individuals with the largest increase in body height. Based on this study it could be concluded that even when all permanent teeth (except for third molars) are fully erupted it is important to check that skeletal maturation is completed before placing implants (9).

During the next six years of the follow-up no increase in body height took place. However, occlusal changes were detected. The infraocclusion of the implants in the upper incisor region increased from 0.6 mm to 1.0 mm during the six years and the range of the whole 10 year period was 0.1–2.2 mm (11) (Fig. 28.3A–D). This problem of continuing infraposition has later been supported by a study from Switzerland reported by Bernard et al. 2004 (13), where infrapositions ranged from 0.1–1.9 mm.

An explanation for this late infraposition is most likely the phenomenon of slight continuous eruption which takes place in the dentition even in adults. These events have been analyzed in long-term studies of normal patients and have revealed an annual vertical eruption of 0.07–0.1 mm of incisors in adults aged 20–40 years (14–18) (Fig. 28.4). Late condylar growth can possibly add to the infraposition problem.

Whereas bone level next to the implants appears to be stable, continuing proximal bone loss has been found to take place among neighboring teeth. Thus in a study of maxillary lateral incisor implants a bone loss of 2.2 and 4.3 mm was found in the canine and central incisor region, respectively (11) (Fig. 28.5). This continuing bone loss is naturally of concern and further studies should be performed to reveal whether this effect eventually plateaus.

The above mentioned clinical and experimental findings call for treatment guidelines concerning installation of implants in young adults. In general installations of implants should be postponed until major alveolar growth has terminated (Fig. 28.4). This event can be evaluated by using one or more of the following growth estimators (12, 17):

- Terminated growth in height (being stable for at least two years).
- Repeated cephalographs demonstrating arrest of alveolar growth.

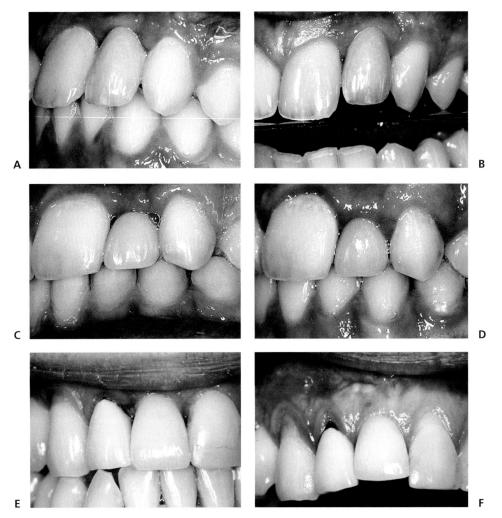

**Fig. 28.3** Infrapositions of implants over time. A–D. Two male patients, with implants in the same region and close in age, illustrating the importance of ceased craniofacial growth for the outcome of implant treatment. After THILANDER et al. 1994 (9). A. The patient had a fixture inserted in the upper left lateral region at the age of 14 years 10 months. The crown was placed when he was 15 years 5 months. The skeletal stage at the insertion of the osseointegrated implant was MP3-FG (according to HÄGG & TARANGER (17) 1980). Superimposition of the cephalograms from the crown placement and the three-year follow-up demonstrated large growth changes. In the same period the increase in body height was 18 cm. B. At the three-year follow-up there was a very evident infraocclusion of 1.6 mm and an apical shift of the gingival margin. The infraocclusion of the fixture crown increased during the next 7 years. C. Shows a patient with no change in vertical position of the implant crown during the three-year follow-up. The patient had a fixture inserted in the upper left lateral region at the age of 16 years and 4 months. The crown was placed when he was 16 years 11 months. D. There is no change in vertical position of the fixture crown 3 years later. During the 3 years and 7 months since fixture insertion the patient had an increase in body height of 0.5 cm, while superimposition of the cephalograms from the crown placement and the three-year follow-up demonstrated no craniofacial growth change during this time. During the following 7 years there was no evident change of the vertical position of the fixture crown. E and F. Adult patient with infraocclusion of the implant crowns. E. A 25-year-old female treated with single implant in the right central incisor region. F. The situation 9 years later at the age of 34 years. Note right central incisor in infraposition and with gingival recession. From JEMT et al. (19) 2005.

• Wrist radiographs with radius epiphysis line being closed or almost closed.

In spite of these precautions progressive infraposition of implants in the anterior region may occur with an annual risk of approximately 0.1 mm infraposition. This may, over the years, lead to esthetic problems due to an uneven incisal line (19) (Fig. 28.3E–F).

This problem is especially of concern in unilateral placed implants and especially in the central incisor region where comparison between the incisal line is so obvious. The implication of this is that young patients requiring anterior implants should be informed about the risk of infraposition.

*C. Hämmerle*

## Timing of implant placement following tooth extraction

When a tooth is scheduled for extraction and the treatment plan foresees replacement of the tooth by an endosseous implant, the clinician has to make a decision with respect to the best time for placing the implant following removal of the tooth. Implant replacement has previously been advocated either *immediately* following tooth extraction and thus during the same surgical intervention, or following certain time frames allowing for healing to proceed. These

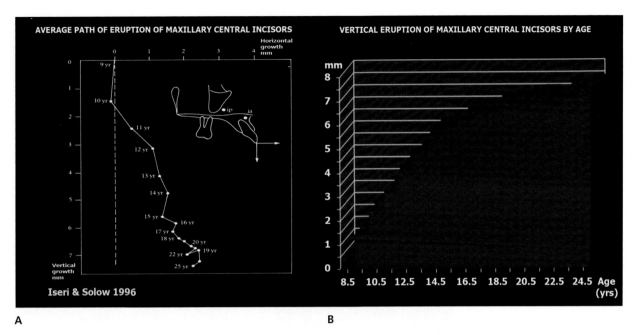

**Fig. 28.4** Estimate of expected infraposition for anterior dental implants inserted in children and young adults. A. Based on data from a longitudinal growth study of 14 girls from 8–25 years, the expected residual vertical and horizontal component of continued eruption of the upper central incisors can be estimated in relation to age for girls. This measure is also an estimate of the amount of infraposition to be expected in the adult for a dental implant inserted at the age in question. The graph is constructed according to the subject's age, and the expected infraposition can be determined from the vertical scale. Somewhat larger values can be expected for boys. B. Graphic illustration of vertical eruption (i.e. expected infraposition) related to age. Modified from ISERI & SOLOW (16) 1996.

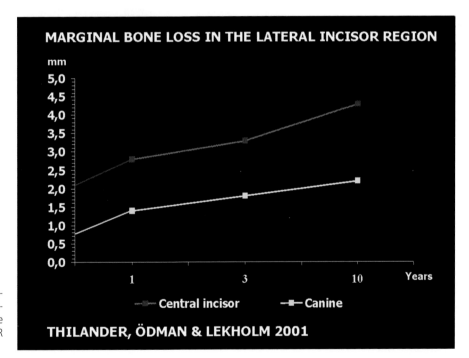

**Fig. 28.5** Marginal bone loss on adjacent teeth subsequent to implant insertion in adolescent patients in the lateral incisor region. After THILANDER et al. (11) 2001.

time frames include waiting for *soft tissue healing* over the extraction socket, waiting for *substantial bone fill* to occur within the socket, or waiting for *complete bone fill* triggered by the tooth extraction, to be completed (Fig. 28.6) (20, 21). All four of these approaches are associated with certain advantages and disadvantages (Table 28.1).

Important clinical problems are the lack of bone to place an implant in a congruent bony bed and the relative lack of soft tissues for primary wound closure. In a well designed

controlled clinical trial it has recently been demonstrated that when implants are placed into extraction sockets, where the distance from the implant surface to the surrounding bone walls is less that 2 mm, spontaneous bone fill of the gap and osseointegration of the previously exposed implant surface will predictably occur (22). Furthermore, evidence from series of case reports indicates that gaps larger than 2 mm may also spontaneously heal with bone at implants placed immediately into extraction sockets (23, 24).

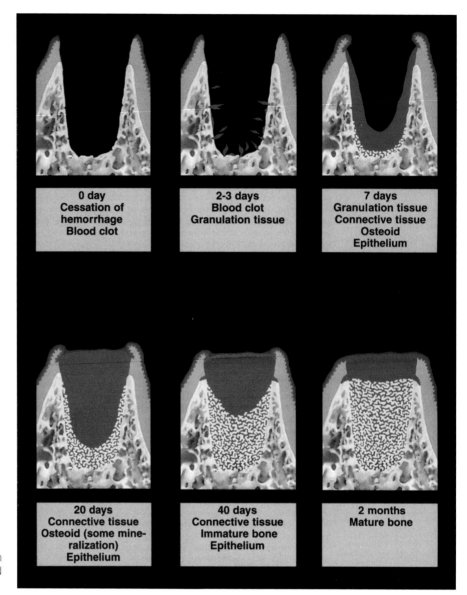

**Fig. 28.6** Healing stages after tooth extraction in man. From ANDREASEN et al. (20) 1994.

**Table 28.1** Treatment options for implant replacement into extraction sockets.

| Approach | Advantages | Disadvantages |
|---|---|---|
| Immediate implant placement following tooth extraction | • Reduced number of surgical procedures<br>• Reduced overall treatment time<br>• Optimal availability of existing bone | • Site morphology may complicate optimal placement and anchorage<br>• This tissue biotype may compromise optimal outcome<br>• Potential lack of keratinized mucosa for flap adaption<br>• Adjunctive surgical procedures may be required<br>• Technique-sensitive procedure |
| Complete soft tissue coverage of the socket (4 to 8 weeks) | • Increased soft tissue area and volume facilitated soft tissue flap management<br>• Allows resolution of local pathology to be assessed | • Site morphology may complicate optimal placement and anchorage<br>• Increased treatment time<br>• Varying amounts of resorption of the socket walls<br>• Adjunctive surgical procedures may be required<br>• Technique-sensitive procedure |
| Substantial clinical and/or radiographic bone fill of the socket (12 to 16 weeks) | • Substantial bone fill of the socket facilitates implant placement<br>• Mature soft tissue facilitates flap management | • Increased treatment time<br>• Adjunctive surgical procedures may be required<br>• Varying amount of resorption of the socket walls |
| Healed site (>16 weeks) | • Clinically healed ridge<br>• Mature soft tissue facilitates flap management | • Increased treatment time.<br>• Adjunctive surgical procedures may be required<br>• Large variations in available bone volume |

Clinical studies in humans have demonstrated that bone remodeling initiated by extraction of the tooth leads to morphological changes of the ridge (25–27). These changes are characterized by internal bone fill of the socket and external resorption of the socket walls. It has recently been demonstrated that in situations where implants are placed immediately into the extraction socket, such alterations also occur (24). As a result of internal bone formation, the exposed implant surface was covered by bone at the time of re-entry surgery 4 months following implant placement. However, the external dimension of the socket was diminished by an average of 56% from the buccal direction and 30% from the lingual direction (25).

The above described data suggest that immediate placement of implants into extraction sockets will lead to bone anchorage of the implants. This bone integration takes place in the absence of specific therapeutic steps aimed at improving spontaneous soft and hard tissue healing. In contrast, the loss of ridge volume, in particular from the buccal aspect, prevents this clinical approach from being used in esthetically demanding situations. Loss of soft and hard tissue often compromises optimal esthetic results (28). In such situations adjunctive measures are necessary to prevent bone resorption and, if necessary, to augment the bone and soft tissue to the desired volume.

Two basic strategies aimed at improving hard and soft tissue volumes have been advocated for the replacement of teeth by implants in esthetic sites. The first one calls for implant placement immediately following tooth extraction. Protocols following this treatment take advantage of the maximum availability of existing bone contours. Maintenance of these bone contours is achieved by placing barrier membranes with or without membrane supporting materials. Insufficient soft tissue for primary coverage of the implant, or for tension-free adaptation of the flap towards the neck of the implant, is a significant clinical problem of this approach. Techniques have been described utilizing pedicle grafts, free grafts or stretching of the buccal mucosa towards the palatal flap margin to obtain gap closure. Whereas bone augmentation is highly successful, complication-free healing of soft tissue is less reliable. In addition, the optimal technique for obtaining the desired level of soft tissue healing has not been determined in experimental or clinical studies (Table 28.1).

The second strategy calls for a waiting time of several weeks, which allows complete healing of the soft tissue over the extraction socket. Subsequently, implants are placed and the missing bone volume is regenerated by use of guided bone regeneration. By using this approach the increased amount of soft tissue facilitates flap closure and thus improves the predictability of complication-free integration of the implant. This approach is often preferred in sites where esthetics are highly important, where successful treatment outcome is more important than increased treatment time and an additional surgical intervention (Table 28.1).

Although, good clinical results have been presented using both strategies, studies comparing the two are presently lacking.

*D. Buser and T. von Arx*

## Biologic and surgical aspects for implant therapy after loss of traumatized teeth

### The patient's expectations

Initiation of therapy starts with an understanding of the patient's desires. In most cases, the patient's primary demand is an esthetic tooth replacement offering a nice smile. Furthermore, the patient usually expects a life long treatment result with a minimum of maintenance. Finally, patients are usually concerned by the cost of the treatment.

For the clinician, the reestablishment of esthetics and function requires knowledge of all treatment options. Conventional fixed partial dentures and implant-supported restorations should be objectively evaluated for their potential to provide long-term function and stability (see Chapter 26). Today, implant-supported restorations often represent the best solution since intact tooth structure and supporting tissues of neighboring teeth can be preserved (67) (see also Chapter 26).

### The challenges for the clinician

Tooth replacement in the anterior maxilla is challenging, since poor judgement during preoperative analysis, the selection of an inappropriate treatment approach, or the inappropriate execution of clinical procedures can lead to esthetic short-comings, esthetic failures, or even esthetic disasters. Esthetic complications with implant-borne restorations are either iatrogenic or anatomic in nature (29). Iatrogenic causes include implant placement in a malposition, the selection of an oversized implant, such as wide-platform implants, or the selection of an inappropriate treatment approach overstressing the biologic healing capacity of the oral tissues. Anatomic causes include bone deficiencies in the horizontal or vertical direction, combined bone and soft tissue defects, or implant sites with multiple missing teeth leading to the placement of adjacent implants.

These considerable challenges make implantology in the anterior region one of the most demanding procedures in implantology (29, 221).

To successfully meet the challenges of esthetic implant dentistry in daily practice, a team approach is advantageous and highly recommended. The team includes an *implant surgeon*, a *restorative dentist*, and a *dental technician* who preferably all have advanced knowledge and clinical experience. A successful implant surgeon working in the esthetic arena has a good biologic understanding of tissue response to implant placement, a thorough surgical education and the skills to perform precise and low-trauma surgical procedures, and a large patient pool providing sufficient surgical experience of esthetic implant placement.

### Biologic aspects in esthetic implant sites

It is important for the clinician to understand that ridge anatomy includes the soft tissues and the supporting bone

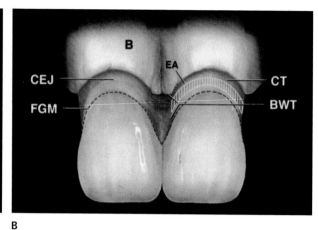

**A**    **B**

**Fig. 28.7** PDL conditions in a natural and healthy dentition. A. Illustration demonstrates the relationship between the free gingival margin (FGM), bone crest (BC) scalloping, and the cementum-enamel junction (CEJ) in a healthy dentition. A 5-mm distance is present from the interproximal bone crest to the contact point. Note the supracrestal connective tissue (CT) the junctional epithelium (JE) and the gingival sulcus. B. Illustration demonstrates the supracrestal position of the biologic width (BWT) and epithelium on healthy teeth. From ELIAN et al. (43) 2003.

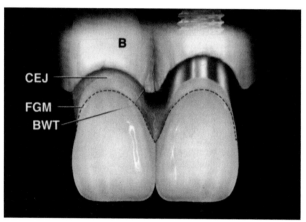
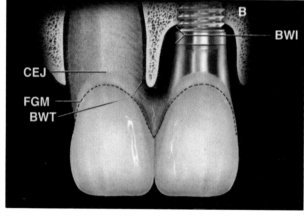

**A**    **B**

**Fig. 28.8** Placement of one implant next to a natural tooth. A. Implant placement adjacent to healthy dentition does not affect the interdental papilla due to the supracrestal position of the biologic width (BWT). B. Removal of buccal bone to visualize the interproximal bone level midway between buccal and palatal corticals. Note position of biologic width around implant (BWI) in comparison to the tooth (BWT). From ELIAN et al. (43) 2003.

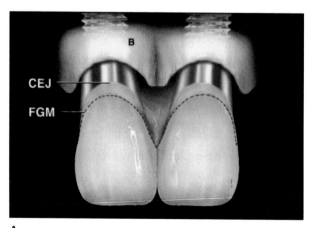
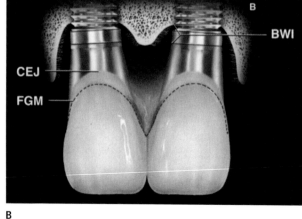

**A**    **B**

**Fig. 28.9** Placement of two adjacent implants. A. The placement of two adjacent implants results in the loss of the supracrestal biologic width. This means the soft tissue papilla will be higher. B. Buccal cortical plate removal to visualize the interproximal bone level midway between the buccal and palatal corticals. Note the position of the biologic width around the implant in relation to the contact point. From ELIAN et al. (43) 2003.

in all dimensions, and that the soft tissue contours around implants are heavily influenced by bone anatomy. In recent years, numerous studies revealed that the concept of the *biologic width*, once described for natural teeth by Gargiulo et al. (30) (Fig. 28.7), is also valid for osseointegrated implants, since soft tissues also demonstrate relatively constant dimensions around implants (31, 32, 43) (Figs 28.8 and 28.9). These studies have demonstrated a thickness of the peri-implant soft tissues of approximately 3 mm on the facial aspect, and of approximately 4.5 to 5.0 mm at interproximal areas. The size of this soft tissue cuff dictates the position of the bone level. In addition, there are differences in soft tissue thickness among different gingival biotypes (68). A thin biotype with a highly scalloped gingival architecture has a reduced soft tissue thickness when compared with a thick biotype featuring a blunted contour of papillae (34).

Keeping these relatively constant dimensions of peri-implant soft tissues in mind, the underlying bone structure plays the key role in the establishment of esthetic soft tissue contours in the anterior maxilla. Two anatomic structures are of importance: the bone height of the alveolar crest at interproximal areas, and the height and thickness of the facial bone wall. The interproximal crest height plays a role in the presence or absence of peri-implant papillae. Today, it is well accepted that a distance of more than 5 mm from the alveolar crest to the contact point reduces the probability of intact papillae not only at teeth, but also at implants (35, 36). It has also been shown that the height of peri-implant papillae in single-tooth gaps is *independent* of the proximal bone level next to the implant, but depends upon the interproximal bone height at adjacent teeth (68). Clinical situations with reduced vertical bone on adjacent teeth are challenging, since there are currently no surgical techniques available to predictably regain lost crest height.

Having a facial bone wall of sufficient height and thickness is important for the long-term stability of a harmonious gingival margin on the facial aspect without changes in tissue height. Patients with traumatic tooth loss frequently present with a bone wall that is missing or is insufficient in height and/or thickness. Thus, various surgical techniques have been proposed in the past 15 years to correct such bone defects at the facial aspect of potential implant sites. The best documented technique is *guided bone regeneration* (GBR) using barrier membranes, which can be carried out using a simultaneous or a staged approach (37, 38). Clinical studies and experience demonstrate that horizontal bone augmentation can be predictably obtained with the GBR technique (82), whereas vertical bone augmentation is much more difficult to obtain (39).

## Ideal implant position in esthetic sites

Placement of implants in the correct three-dimensional position is the key to the outcome of esthetic treatment, regardless of the implant system used (29, 46, 47). The rela-tionship between the position of the implant and the proposed restoration should be based upon the position of the implant shoulder. The implant shoulder position can be viewed in three dimensions: *oro-facial*, *mesio-distal* and *corono-apical*.

In the *oro-facial* direction, an implant shoulder placed too far facially will result in the risk of soft tissue recession, since the thickness of the facial bone wall is clearly reduced by the malpositioned implant. In addition, potential prosthetic complications could result in restoration–implant axis problems, making the implant difficult to restore. Implants positioned too far palatally can result in emergence problems, as seen with ridge–lap restorations.

Improper *mesio-distal* positioning of implants can have a substantial effect on the generation of interproximal papillary support in addition to the osseous crest on the adjacent natural tooth. Placing the implant too close to the adjacent tooth can cause resorption of the interproximal aveolar crest to the level of that on the implant. With this loss of the interproximal crest height comes a reduction in papillary height. The loss of crest height at adjacent teeth is caused by bone saucerization, routinely found around osseointegrated implants. This saucerization has a horizontal and vertical component (Fig. 28.10). Radiographs demonstrate that the horizontal component of proximal bone saucerization measures about 1.0 to 1.5 mm from the implant surface (40). This minimal distance needs to be respected at implant placement to prevent vertical bone loss on adjacent teeth. Too close a position results in loss of proximal bone (40, 42) and thereby the height of the interdental papilla (33).

The vertical component of saucerization amounts to approximately 2 mm at interproximal areas, measured from the implant shoulder. This radiographic observation routinely seen in patients (40, 41, 44) has been confirmed by an experimental study (45).

With regard to the *corono-apical* position of the implant shoulder, the same study (45) demonstrated that the position of the implant/abutment interface, often called the microgap, has an important influence on the hard and soft tissue reactions around osseointegrated implants. The further apically the microgap is located, the more bone resorption is observed. Clinically, if an implant is inserted with an excessive countersinking procedure, an unnecessary amount of bone loss will occur. Since this resorption will take place circumferentially (Fig. 28.10), it will affect not only the proximal bone structure, but also the height of the facial bone wall, and can lead to undesired soft tissue recession (29). This phenomenon is also important in sites with two adjacent implants since the inter-implant bone will be resorbed, leading to a shortened interimplant papilla (Fig. 28.10).

Esthetic failures can also be caused by improper implant selection, mainly due to the use of oversized implants. The use of 'tooth analogous' implant diameters based solely upon the mesio-distal dimension of the tooth to be replaced should be avoided. With such wide-platform or wide-neck implants, the implant shoulder could be placed too close to adjacent teeth and too far facially, leading to the complications mentioned above.

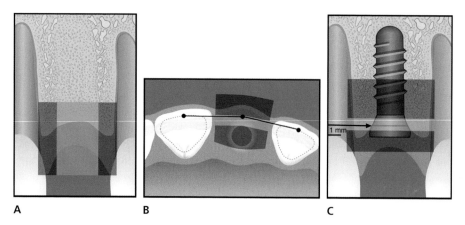

**Fig. 28.10** Comfort and risk zones in implant insertion. A. Correct implant position in the mesiodistal dimension. The implant shoulder should be positioned within the comfort zone, avoiding the danger zones, which are located close to adjacent root surfaces. The danger zone is about 1.0–1.5 mm wide. B. Correct implant position in the orofacial dimension. The implant shoulder is positioned about 1 mm palatal to the point of emergence at adjacent teeth. The danger zone is clearly entered when the implant is placed too far facially; this can cause resorption of the facial bone wall with subsequent recession. C. Correct implant position in the apicocoronal dimension. The implant shoulder is positioned about 1 mm apical to the CEJ of the contralateral tooth in patients without gingival recession. The danger zone is entered when the implant is placed too far apically using excessive countersinking, or too far coronally, which results in implant shoulder exposure at the mucosa. From BUSER et al. (29) 2004.

## The concept of comfort and danger zones

When planning for an ideal three-dimensional implant position, a distinction is made between '**comfort**' and '**danger**' zones in each dimension (mesio-distal, oro-facial, and corono-apical) (29) (Fig. 28.10). Selection and placement of the dental implant should be based on the planned restoration in these zones (29, 43, 46, 47). If the implant shoulder is positioned within the danger zones, one of the above mentioned complications could occur, potentially resulting in esthetic shortcomings.

Respecting the comfort zones in three dimensions results in an implant shoulder located in an ideal position, allowing for an esthetic implant restoration with stable, long-term peri-implant tissue support.

### Mesio-distal dimension

In the mesio-distal dimension, the *danger zones* are located next to adjacent teeth. It is recommended that the implant shoulder and the adjacent root surface be at least 1–1.5 mm apart (Fig. 28.10). The critical distance between two implants has been found to be 3 mm. Too close a position results in loss of intraproximal bone from saucerization around the implant shoulders (41–43) and thereby the height of the interdental papilla (33, 36).

### Oro-facial dimension

With regard to the oro-facial dimension, the *facial danger zone* is located anywhere facially to the imaginary line highlighted from the point of emergence of the adjacent teeth and/or planned restoration (Fig. 28.10). The *palatal danger zone* starts about 2 mm from this point of emergence, and leads to an increased risk of a ridge-lap restoration. Place-

ment of the implant oro-facially in the comfort zone, which is located anywhere in between these areas, will allow for a restoration with a proper emergence profile to maintain the harmonious scalloping of the gingival margins.

### Coronal-apical positions

Tooth loss will, as a rule, result in not only loss of the oro-facial dimension but also the vertical height. This phenomenon becomes excessive if tooth loss occurs early or is followed by gradual infraposition of an ankylosed tooth (18, 48, 49). In these cases the installation of implants will result in a significant esthetic problem due to gingival asymmetry.

Another disturbing phenomenon is that the position of the gingiva will be below the interdental crest, and this may lead to subsequent loss of interdental bone (42). Furthermore, if implants are placed too deep the saucerization will interfere with labial bone, leading to retraction of the papilla (29).

The corono-apical positioning of the implant shoulder follows the philosophy 'as shallow as possible, as deep as necessary', being a compromise between esthetic and biologic principles. The position of the implant shoulder should be approximately 2 mm apical to the mid-facial gingival margin of the planned restoration (78). This can be accomplished through the use of surgical templates highlighting the gingival margin of the planned restoration. In patients without vertical tissue deficiencies, the use of periodontal probes leveled on the adjacent cemento-enamel junction (CEJ) in single-tooth gaps has proven to be a valid alternative. Implant placement within the *apical danger zone* (located anywhere 3 mm or greater apically from the proposed gingival margin) can result in undesired facial bone resorption and subsequent gingival recession. The *coronal danger zone* is invaded with a supragingival shoulder position leading to a visible metal margin and poor emergence profile (Fig. 28.10).

## To create and maintain a normal appearing gingiva

Soft tissue appearance is related to the level, color and texture of the gingiva. The interdental papilla will be described separately.

### Gingival level and appearance

#### Labial and oral

Repeated surgical incisions in the implant area (e.g. to insert bone transplant and/or membranes) may create scar tissue. If repeated surgical intervention has to be made incisions should be made along previous incision lines.

In case that a choice can be made between vertical bone augmentation and vertical bone distraction it should be considered that the latter preserves the gingival texture (see p. 783).

The location of the gingival margin labially is primarily determined by the depth and installation of the implant. According to the abutment plateau the level of the labial and palatal gingiva will be approximately 2.5 mm coronally (Fig. 28.8). This means a 5–7 mm-deep interproximal position of the implant shoulder due to the gingival scallop. Such a deep position may prevent satisfactory cementation and call for screw retention of the restoration (47).

In follow-up studies it has been found that retraction of the gingival margin takes place, and the extent of this has been found normally to be in the range of 0.6–1 mm; however, predictors for this retraction have not yet been identified (50–52). Such a retraction may have serious consequences by exposing crown margins, abutments and fixtures.

### Interdental papilla

The creation or maintenance of an interdental papilla has been a serious challenge in implantology (43). A normal tooth has gingival collagen fibers inserted in cementum which support and maintain the interdental papilla, but the circumferential collagen fibers around an implant do not have the same capacity.

In several studies it has been found that creation of an interdental papilla with adequate fill out of the interdental space is related to a number of factors:

- The original soft tissue level at the implant site
- The proximal bone level at the implant site
- The presence of a natural tooth or another implant in the region
- Position of the contact point to neighboring teeth
- Surgical techniques (see later)
- Time after implant installation
- Whether or not a customized temporary restoration is used.

Since Tarnow's classical studies on the relation between the position of the interdental septa in natural teeth and the position of the interdental papilla (35) a similar relation has been found in regard to implants next to natural teeth (36, 43, 53). Thus when the distance from the interproximal contact point to the top of the bone crest was 3–4 mm, the chance of a gingival papilla filling the interdental space was found to be 100%, whereas the chance was reduced to 50–60% when the distance was 6 mm (36, 53).

The strong relation between an adjacent neighboring tooth with normal periodontal conditions implies that the natural tooth is the essential host for the papilla and will determine the position of the papilla (68). This principle can be used to create a more favorable position of the interdental papilla next to an implant by orthodontic extrusion of neighboring teeth whereby the interdental bone height is increased (54, 55).

A different problem arises if two implants are placed next to each other (Fig. 28.9). In this case the height of the papilla will be approximately 3 mm above bone level (43, 53, 56), a situation that usually implies that a 1–2 mm reduced gingival papilla will be found between the two implants (43, 53, 56).

Another factor that determines the presence of a papilla is the distance of the cervical level between implant to adjacent teeth or implant-to-implant. The chance of a 100% papilla fill is found when this distance is less than 2.5 mm (53).

The volume and position of the interdental papilla has been found to increase over time (50, 57–59). Furthermore, customized intermediate restorations that are slightly oversized may induce growth of the interdental papilla (58). However, it appears that the inherent spontaneous growth of the papilla over a two-year period of time will give the same result (58, 59).

### Gingival pocket depth

This feature appears to be quite stable over the years, thus in a 1–9 year follow-up study no significant deepening took place (59, 62).

## To create and maintain a normal appearing alveolar process

In almost all trauma cases alveolar bone has been lost and needs to be recreated. A variety of methods are available today, with varying success rates (see p. 773).

### Proximal bone

The maintenance of proximal alveolar bone is of interest as loss of this bone may endanger an adjacent natural tooth. In a 10-year study in young adolescents a loss ranging from 0.5–1.5 mm took place (63). Such an amount may be of concern if this rate of bone loss continues. In adults, however, the bone loss appeared to be more confounded and leveled out after some years (64, 68, 187). A new concept, scalloped parabolic implant design, could possibly lead to less proximal bone loss (65, 66).

**Fig. 28.11 Preoperative radiographic evaluation, angulated exposure**
The space needed cervically amounts to the cervical diameter of the abutment plus adequate space to adjacent teeth, i.e. 1–1.5 mm mesially and distally. The length of the implant cannot be accurately determined radiographically due to the oblique projection in the maxillary anterior region.

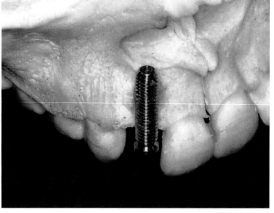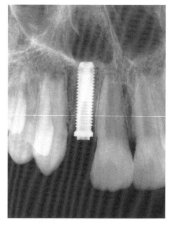

**Preoperative radiographic evaluation, horizontal exposure**
It appears that the actual distance between the crest of marginal bone and the nasal floor is approximately 1 mm shorter than the radiographic distance shown with angulated exposure.

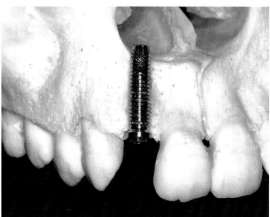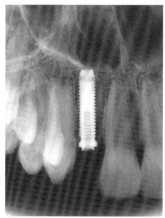

## Labio-lingual bone

This has been very little researched due to limitations in the standard of radiographic procedures. However, the development of Micro CT scan (see Chapter 9, p. 270) provides a new method to measure this parameter. From clinical experience, it has been noted that atrophy of labial bone often takes place and, in some cases, leads to gingival retraction.

*J.O. Andreasen*

## Preoperative evaluation

### Prosthetic aspects

The prosthetic aspects of implant selection for restoring lost anterior teeth depend upon various situations. These include:

- *The condition of the adjacent teeth.* Thus, if the adjacent teeth are crowned or have large restorations, a conventional bridge could be considered.
- *Occlusal relationships and/or habits.* Patients with deep overbite and/or severe parafunctional habits may present contraindications.
- *Interdental space relationships.* The minimum space required between adjacent teeth is 6–7 mm for implant placement, as well as to permit adequate crown form and size (see later).
- *Cuspid guidance.* In restoring a cuspid, one should be aware of the occlusion. A cuspid-protected occlusion on an implant should be avoided due to the great forces a cuspid can exert.
- *Esthetic limits of an implant-borne crown, due to lack of bone or alignment of the fixture.* These problems have become less significant as the latest implant techniques use surgical reconstruction of the alveolar process (see later).

The restorative dentist should guide the surgeon in placing the implant in the correct horizontal and axial orientation. This can be done in several ways, either indirectly by the use of surgical stents or directly by the restorative dentist being present during fixture insertion. A good general rule is that the axis of the implant should ideally be placed identically to the long axis of the tooth to be replaced.

There are several different types of surgical stent that can be used. All are aimed at aiding the orientation of the labial surface of the future restoration.

### Surgical aspects

Vertical and horizontal alveolar bone atrophy is a common problem following anterior tooth loss. This can be extreme following early tooth loss or in cases where the labial bone plate has been lost due to tooth avulsion. In order to evaluate osseous condition at the proposed implant site, periapical orthoradial radiographs should be taken (Fig. 28.11). With respect to the recipient site, there should be a distance of 1–1.5 mm between the potential position of the implant and adjacent teeth. This distance is especially important in the cervical region where the width of the cervical part of

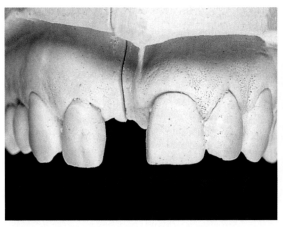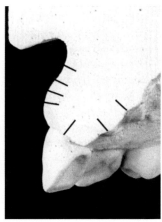

**Fig. 28.12** Estimating the bony dimensions of a reduced alveolar process. An impression is taken and the model sectioned at the potential implant site. After administration of a local anesthetic, the mucosa is penetrated with a periodontal probe. These measurements are then transferred to the sectioned plaster model. In this way the sagittal extension of the alveolar process is accurately determined.

the fixture and the abutment should be considered (Fig. 28.11). If the distance appears critical, orthodontic expansion should be considered or a smaller implant size chosen.

To estimate the extent of labial bone atrophy, several methods have been advocated, such as sagittal CT scanning and direct probing under local anesthesia, using a measuring instrument which penetrates the gingival and alveolar mucosa (Fig. 28.12). These techniques can determine whether or not there is sufficient horizontal bone support for the implant. CT scanning is useful to determine in three-dimensions the amount of bone (and its quality) and should definitely be used in cases where more than one tooth is being replaced. If very precise assessment of alveolar atrophy is required, a plaster model is cast and sectioned at the implant site. The soft tissue depth is then marked after direct probing through the mucosa (Fig. 28.12). It is not unusual for a soft tissue thickness of 5–6 mm to be present, so care should be taken not to overestimate existing bone volume.

The surgical procedure is entirely determined by the status of the alveolar process. In the following text, different treatment solutions will be presented according to the condition of the alveolar bone.

## Standard insertion in single gaps with good bone volume

In this situation, the tooth to be replaced may be either present or recently extracted. In both cases traumatic tooth removal is of the utmost importance with respect to the maintenance of an intact labial bone plate. Special instruments have been designed to facilitate tooth removal by severing cervical periodontal ligament fibers (70).

To install the fixture, a trapezoidal flap is raised which avoids the marginal gingiva of adjacent teeth, as this appears to result in less proximal bone loss (215). Implant placement without flap elevation (often called 'flapless surgery') is considered experimental since no proper scientific documentation is available yet. The implant site is then prepared according to the implant system used (Fig. 28.13). The axis of the implant should ideally follow the axis of the tooth to be replaced and be directed at the proposed incisal edge. The

ideal position and alignment of the implant is one in which the fixture resembles that of the natural tooth. If a compromise is necessary, the axis of the implant can be deviated to some extent in most implant systems.

In some cases a large incisal canal may prevent optimal placement of the implant. In these cases it has been shown that elimination of the canal content and replacement with an autogenous bone graft (see later) can solve this problem (71).

The cervical level of the implant is important in ensuring an optimal esthetic suprastructure. Thus, in the central incisor region, this level should be 2 mm apical to the mid-facial gingival margin of the planned restoration (78). In the lateral direction a distance of 1–1.5 mm is desirable (see p. 769). After implant insertion, the flap is repositioned and sutured.

Although the value of antibiotics has not been definitively shown it seems advisable to administer penicillin for 2–4 days following fixture installation (212). The peri- and postoperative use of 0.12 chlorhexidine rinse is also recommended (213).

*D. Buser and T. van Arx*

## Surgical procedure in single tooth gaps with doubtful bone volume

Today, the majority of implants in the anterior maxilla are placed in combination with an augmentation in areas with local bone deficiencies (Fig. 28.14). Thus, an open flap procedure is necessary to allow for bone augmentation. In daily practice, facial line-angle relieving incisions are most often necessary to allow sufficient access to the surgical site. In patients requiring bone augmentation, this flap design allows for tension-free wound closure with the release of the periosteum and coronal mobilization of the flap.

Following degranulation of the surgical site, the implant is placed in the correct three-dimensional position as described on p. 769. Primary stability of the implant is a prerequisite for successful osseointegration. If a local defect is present, a simultaneous GBR procedure is performed as long as a bone defect with a two-wall morphology is present. For implant sites with a one-wall defect, a staged approach using

### Fig. 28.13 Use of an implant to treat anterior tooth loss

A 24-year-old man has suffered anterior tooth loss due to trauma. The alveolar process was intact.

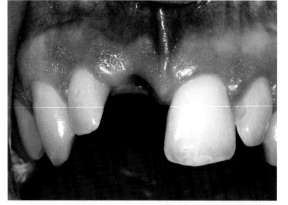
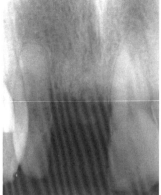

### Raising a flap

A trapezoidal labial flap is raised which respects the interdental papillae. The flap is extended palatally so that sutures are not placed directly over the implant.

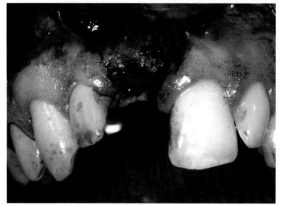
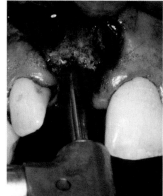

### Insertion of the implant

The level of the implant before insertion of the healing cap should be 3 mm below the labial gingival margin of the homologous tooth.

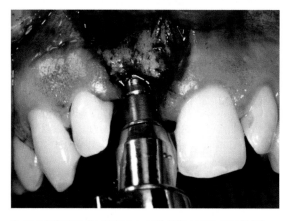
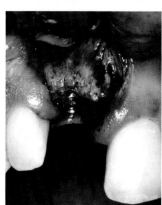

### Completed restoration

After a healing period of 6 months and installation of an abutment a porcelain crown is fabricated.

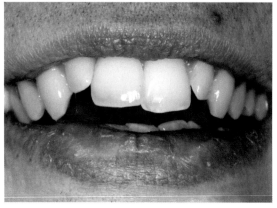
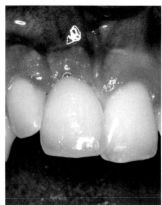

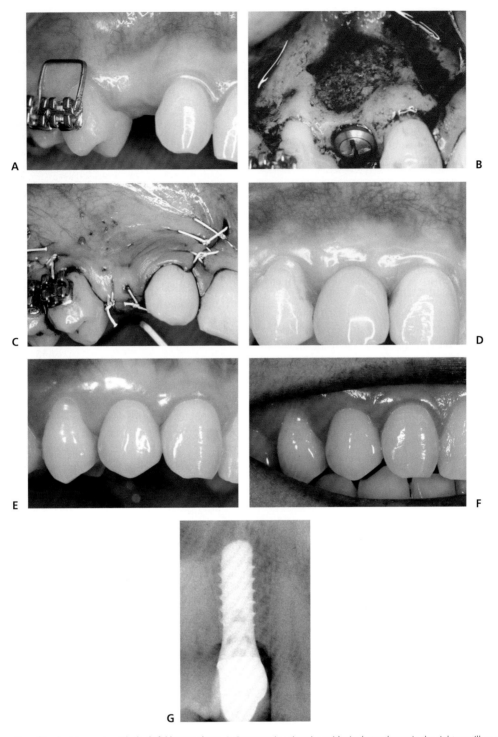

**Fig. 28.14** Insertion of implant in a case with doubtful bone volume. A. Preoperative situation with single tooth gap in the right maxillary canine region. B. Intrasurgical status following placement of a standard implant in a correct 3-dimensional position and an intact facial bone wall in crestal area. A small apical fenestration defect was augmented with locally harvested autogenous bone grafts. C. Submerged implant healing was chosen for 3 months at that time. D. The implant was first restored with a provisional acrylic crown to condition the peri-implant soft tissues. E, F. Clinical status 12 years following implant placement demonstrates absolute stability of the gingival margin at the implant crown and a nice convexity in the alveolar crest. A good esthetic result is achieved, an important feature considering the high line. G. The periapical radiograph at 12 years following implant placement confirms stable bone crest levels around the implant.

primary bone augmentation without implant placement is recommended (see p. 773). The implant is precisely inserted avoiding the danger zones as previously described. The bone augmentation procedure is performed using autogenous bone grafts usually combined with a bone substitute with a low substitution rate such as deproteinized bovine bone mineral. The augmentation material is covered with a

barrier membrane preferably made of collagen to avoid a second surgical procedure for membrane removal. Finally, tension-free primary flap closure is performed using a submerged implant during the healing period.

This method requires the site to be reopened to gain access to the integrated implant to initiate prosthetic therapy. The healing period prior to reopening varies from 6 to 12 weeks depending on the extent of the peri-implant bone defect present at implant placement. The reopening is made with a punch technique using a 12b blade. Subsequently, prosthetic therapy includes most often a provisional single crown to condition the peri-implant soft tissues followed by the final ceramo-metal or full ceramic crown.

## Horizontal augmentation

### Introduction

One important prerequisite of implant treatment is sufficient bone volume at the recipient site to allow correct three-dimensional positioning of the implant and primary implant stability. The time has gone when implantation was controlled by bone structure. Prosthetic- and/or esthetic-driven implant placement often require enhancement of remaining bone structures. As a consequence, planning of implant therapy always includes a thorough investigation of the bone quality and quantity of the recipient site. Additionally, adjacent anatomical structures such as the nasal and maxillary sinus cavities, the mandibular canal, and the mental foramen must be taken into account during treatment planning. If the clinical and standard radiographic (periapical and panoramic radiographs) examination reveals compromised bone volume, further clinical (bone mapping) and or radiographic evaluations (cross-sectional images) are recommended for preoperative site analysis.

Depending on the extent and morphometry of the bone deficiency, on the number of implants to be placed, on soft tissue characteristics and esthetic demands, the sequence and type of bone surgery will be determined. If alveolar ridge atrophy mainly involves a lateral component, horizontal augmentation of the residual ridge is the objective of bone surgery.

### Horizontal augmentation techniques

In the last two decades, a number of horizontal augmentation techniques have been described, including:

- Use of bone grafts
- Use of barrier membranes with autografts and/or bone substitutes
- Use of titanium mesh with autografts
- Bone splitting

With respect to time sequence, ridge augmentation is either performed simultaneously with implant placement, or as a preparatory step in a staged procedure before implant placement.

### Onlay and veneer grafts

Autogenous block grafts are applied for lateral ridge augmentation as an onlay or veneer graft (72, 73). Block grafts should be fixed to the residual bone using fixation screws gliding through the bone block and engaging the lingual or palatal bone wall. This results in optimal stability and absence of micro-movements that allows for fast integration of the bone blocks (74, 75). However, considerable surface resorption of so-called non-protected bone blocks has been reported (76). This bone loss must be taken into account and overcorrection is recommended when using this technique before subsequent implant placement (77).

### Guided bone regeneration (GBR)

The use of barrier membranes has become widely accepted in periodontology and implant dentistry. Although in the past clinicians have advocated the use of barrier membranes for space secluding, it is now recognized that membranes collapse into the defect resulting in limited success of the treatment (78). Therefore, it is now unequivocally recommended that a block or particulate material be used for membrane support (79–84).

Early clinical and experimental studies on GBR reported the use of a non-resorbable expanded polytetrafluoroethylene (ePTFE) membrane, but nowadays resorbable collagen or polyester (polylactide, polyglycolide) membranes have become widely accepted (85–87). Although ePTFE membranes show excellent biocompatible properties they have an increased risk of wound dehiscence with possible site infection and/or reduced volume of bone healing (88–91, 123). Additionally, the hydrophobic ePTFE-material has poor handling and adaptation properties and requires fixation to the underlying bone. Another disadvantage is the necessity of a second flap procedure for membrane removal. To improve their mechanical stability, ePTFE-membranes were reinforced with titanium but this did not help to reduce their significant drawbacks.

In contrast, resorbable barrier membranes made of collagen or polyesters are hydrophilic compared to ePTFE making membrane management easier and faster. Furthermore, no additional flap surgery is required for membrane removal. However, resorbable membranes show an increased tendency to collapse (92–94). For polyester membranes, inflammatory tissue responses have also been reported following membrane degradation (83, 94, 95, 122).

Several clinical and experimental studies have proven that bone regenerated with the GBR technique reacts to implant placement like pristine bone, and this bone is load-bearing over the evaluated periods (81, 96–98).

### Use of titanium mesh

Titanium mesh has been used for ridge augmentation procedures because of its enhanced mechanical properties (99–101). However, titanium mesh has no barrier effect and neighboring soft tissues grow through it. Therefore, some authors have combined titanium mesh with barrier membranes (102). Because the mesh is rigid it must be perfectly adapted to the bone contour and must be secured with small fixation screws to prevent mucosal perforations (103). A second surgical procedure is also necessary for mesh removal. Since handling and application of a titanium mesh is a rather technique-sensitive procedure, it has not gained wide acceptance. However, recent clinical studies have pointed to the benefit of using a titanium mesh for vertical alveolar ridge augmentation (104, 105).

## Bone splitting

The crest of an edentulous ridge is expanded by splitting the two cortical plates. This technique is most often combined with immediate implant placement which reduces treatment time (106–109). Since no blockgrafts are used the need for a second surgical site is eliminated.

## GBR technique: simultaneous approach (Fig. 28.15)

Provided the clinical and radiographic site analyses have shown that a simultaneous approach is feasible, the patient is scheduled for implant placement with concomitant ridge augmentation. Following local anesthesia a crestal incision (in esthetic sites, the incision is moved to the palatal aspect of the crest) is made with intrasulcular incisons on facial and lingual aspects of the adjacent teeth. Two vestibular divergent release incisons are placed at the line angle of adjacent teeth. Full mucoperiosteal flaps are raised on the facial and lingual aspects and are retracted with retraction sutures. All remaining soft tissues are thoroughly cleaned off and the crest is slightly scalloped with a large round bur.

The implant bed is prepared according to the implant surgery protocol. Correct three-dimensional implant placement is essential for prosthetic (and esthetic) tooth restoration (78, 110). In esthetic sites, the implant shoulder should be placed 1–2 mm below the cemento-enamel junction (CEJ) of the adjacent teeth with respect to vertical implant position. In the horizontal direction, the implant shoulder should be located slightly inside the CEJ of the adjacent teeth. Both measures are important to ensure an optimal emergence profile of the implant restoration. An appropriate closure screw is placed on top of the implant.

The bone adjacent to the area to be augmented is perforated with a small round bur for bone marrow penetration. The exposed implant surface is covered with bone chips harvested from nearby cortical bone surfaces using bone scrapers or bone chisels. A layer of *anorganic bovine bone mineral* (ABBM) particles which have been soaked in blood is applied above the autogenous bone particles for recontouring and protection of the augmentation area. A collagen membrane is trimmed to the appropriate size and is placed to fully cover the augmentation material. The membrane is soaked in blood for tight adaptation but it is not secured with screws or tacks. A second membrane is positioned to form a double layer to enhance barrier function.

Following a periosteal release incision, the flap is repositioned in a coronal direction and primary wound closure is accomplished with single interrupted sutures. No tension should be exerted on the wound margins. In non-esthetic sites or in fenestration-type defects, transgingival or semi-submerged implant healing is possible. Any removable provisional prosthesis must be adapted to avoid pressure to the augmented tissues. Sutures are removed within 7–10 days.

For the same period, chemical plaque control is instituted with chlorhexidine-digluconate 0.1–0.2%. Perioperative, short-term antibiotic prophylaxis is recommended for up to 3 days post-closure.

After a healing period of 8–12 weeks the submerged implant is uncovered with a punch incision, and a transgingival healing cap is placed for peri-implant soft tissue healing. The provisional or definitive restoration is fabricated within 1–3 weeks.

## GBR technique: staged approach (Fig. 28.16)

In sites with severe bone deficiencies, where implant placement and implant stability are compromised, a staged approach should be chosen. A thorough clinical and radiographic examination (including cross-sectional imaging) is mandatory to analyze both the augmentation and possible harvest sites. Since staged horizontal augmentation requires larger volumes of bone grafts, donor sites for bone blocks must be evaluated before surgery. Potential intraoral donor sites for block grafts include the retromolar area and the symphysis (111–114).

This surgical technique often involves a second surgical site with prolonged surgical time. Therefore, patients are normally given a sedative premedication, but surgeries are still performed under local anesthesia. The site to be augmented is prepared with similar incisions as those utilized in the simultaneous procedure. Full mucoperiosteal flaps are raised again on both aspects of the deficient alveolar ridge. The bony surfaces are cleaned with a large round bur in counter clockwise rotation. The cortex is perforated with a small drill for early blood supply from the bone marrow. It has been shown that this procedure enhances fusion and integration of the block grafts (115). The dimensions of the defect are measured with a calliper or probe and a corresponding block graft is harvested in the retromolar area or in the symphysis. The block graft is adapted to the recipient site for horizontal augmentation, and it is fixated with one or two fixation screws (diameter 1.5 mm) to the residual bone wall. The screws should glide in the block graft and only engage the host bone (lag screw principle).

Following block graft fixation, any sharp corners or edges are smoothed. Voids around the block graft are filled with additional bone chips. ABBM particles that have been soaked in blood are placed in a thin layer over the block graft to prevent surface resorption. In order to avoid displacement of the particles, a collagen membrane is adapted to cover the entire augmentation site. A second layer of collagen membrane is positioned to enhance barrier function and membrane stability. Membranes are not secured *per se* with screws or tacks, but soaking with blood or saline is recommended for membrane adaptation. Following a periosteal release incision ensuring full flap mobilization, the flap is coronally repositioned and the incision is reapproximated with single interrupted sutures.

In distal extension situations, the patient should refrain from wearing a provisional prosthesis, whereas for esthetics,

### Fig. 28.15 GBR technique: simultaneous approach

Maxillary left central incisor shows external root resorption (replacement resorption) following crown fracture and avulsion at the age of 14 years. The ankylotic left incisor presents with a gingival step of 2 mm and an incisal step of 1 mm. It was decided to remove the incisor and to keep the right central incisor.

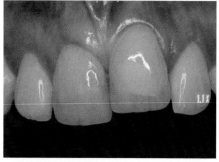
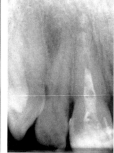
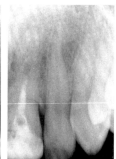

### Placing a gingival graft

Following removal of the incisor, a free gingival connective tissue graft from the palate was placed to optimize the width of the keratinized tissues. There is only a slight concavity on the facial aspect of the alveolar crest.

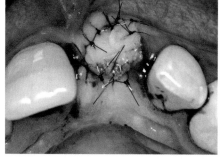
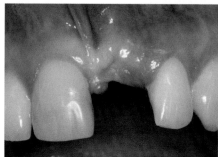

### Mucoperiosteal flaps

Full mucoperiosteal flaps are raised on facial and palatal aspects. The bone height is good. The occlusal view clearly shows the horizontal bone deficiency.

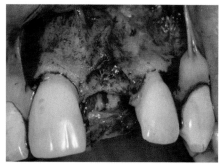
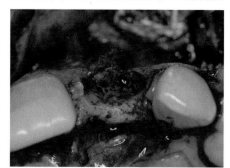

### Placing the implant

An ITI implant is placed with the implant shoulder slightly below the CEJ of the adjacent teeth. The bony deficiency on the facial aspect of the implant is visible.

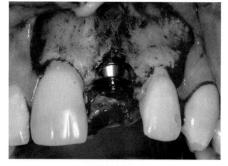
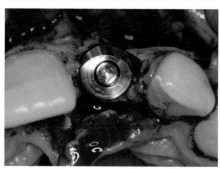

### Placing bon chips and ABBM particles

Bone chips harvested from the nearby cortical bone surfaces are used to cover the exposed implant surface. The site is also augmented with ABBM particles.

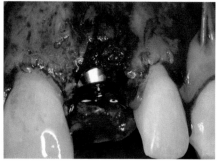
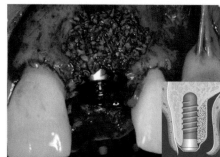

**Placing a collagen membrane**
The occlusal view demonstrates that the facial contour has been over-corrected. A collagen membrane is adapted to fully cover the implant and augmentation site.

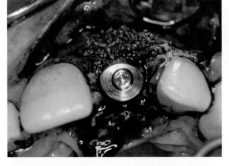 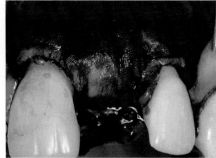

**Flap repositioning**
Following periosteal release, the flap is repositioned in a coronal direction and primary wound closure is accomplished with multiple interrupted sutures. Eight weeks later, the implant is uncovered and a larger healing cap is placed.

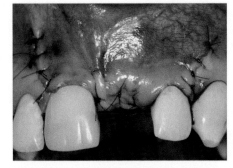 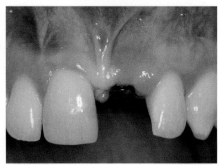

**Final restoration**
The final clinical view shows good esthetics and harmonious gingival contours. The radiograph demonstrates optimal crown-implant position with healthy peri-implant bone structures. Endodontic revision has been performed on the right central incisor. (Prosthetic work by Dr H. Müller, Neuenkirch/Switzerland.)

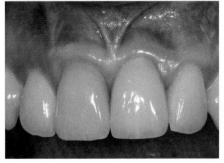 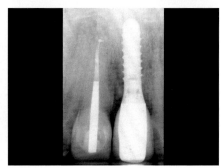

the prosthesis must be carefully adapted to avoid pressure by the pontic or flange onto the augmentation site. Sutures are removed after 10–14 days, and patients are instructed to rinse with chlorhexidine-digluconate 0.1–0.2% twice daily. Perioperative antibiotic coverage should be given for 6 days after the procedure.

After a healing period of 5–6 months the augmentation site is reentered using a similar incision and flap technique. The bone block fixation screws are located and removed. Implant placement is now performed according to the standard implant surgical protocol.

## Rationale for the described techniques

Both presented simultaneous and staged augmentation techniques use three distinctive surgical steps, and materials respectively: placement of autogenous bone, application of ABBM particles, and use of a collagen membrane.

Autogenous bone is considered as the gold standard for ridge augmentation in implant dentistry. However, non-protected bone grafts can undergo severe surface resorption with a compromised treatment outcome (76–77). Experimental and clinical studies have shown, that membrane pro-

tection of grafted bone ensures volume stability and graft integration (90, 116–117). In particular in the aesthetic zone, contour preservation is of highest importance to warrant the aesthetic outcome following implant placement.

With the emergence of non-resorbable barrier membranes which are liable to degradation or resorption within weeks (92, 118–119), the protection of grafted bone is only assured for a limited period. Thereafter, the bone grafts may undergo surface resorption comparable to non-protected grafts. One option to circumvent this problem is to cover the bone graft with a slow or non-resorbable material, such as hydroxyapatite. Anorganic bovine bone mineral has been shown to fulfil these criteria. Once inserted in host tissue, this bone substitute is not resorbed following bony integration (84, 91, 120–121). When located at the periphery of bone defects, ABBM particles are embedded in fibrous tissue with very slow resorption if at all (91, 99). Therefore, the rationale of covering bone grafts with ABBM particles in augmentation sites is twofold: 1) to maintain the contour of the augmented site, and 2) to protect the bone grafts from surface resorption.

The use of a collagen membrane in a double layer technique assures that the applied filler particles are not dislodged until they have become encapsulated with fibrous connective tissue.

### Fig. 28.16 GBR technique: staged approach

This 40-year old female patient presents with a single tooth gap. The occlusal view depicts a marked depression of the facial bone contour.

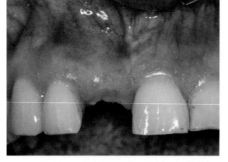
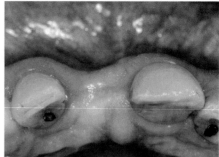

### Alveolar bone condition

The bone height of the alveolar ridge is intact. The bone width along two thirds of the bone height is noticeably reduced.

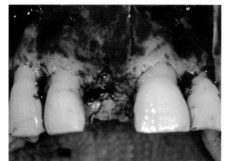
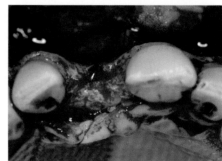

### Harvesting a bone graft

A rectangular block graft is harvested from the symphysis. The block graft is fixed in a vertical position using two lag screws.

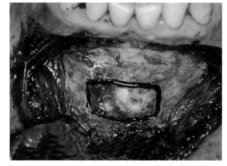
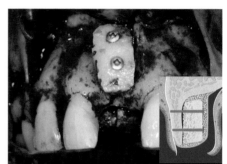

### Application of bone graft and anorganic particles

Subsequently, the blockgraft is covered with anorganic bone particles (Bio-Oss®). The occlusal view demonstrates overcorrection of the facial contour at the augmentation site.

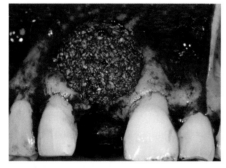
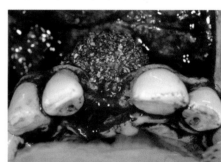

### Application of collagen membrane

A collagen membrane is placed to prevent dislodgement of the graft particles. Primary and tension-free wound closure is accomplished following periosteal release and flap repositioning.

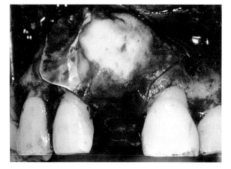
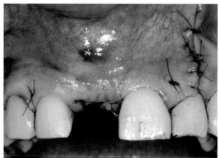

**Condition after 5 months**
Five months after ridge augmentation, healthy soft tissues are present. The occlusal view now shows a convexity of the facial aspect in the region.

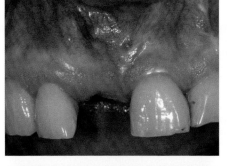
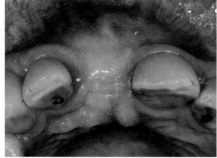

**Re-entry**
The bone block shows good integration into the host tissues. The occlusal view clearly demonstrates that the head of the fixation screw rests on the block graft indicating that no surface resorption has occurred.

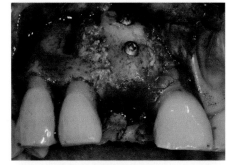
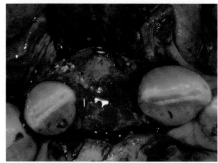

**Placing the implant**
The implant is placed with its shoulder slightly inside the CEJ of the adjacent teeth. Ideal maintenance of the facial bone contour is obvious. In a vertical direction the implant shoulder is positioned slightly below the CEJ of the adjacent teeth.

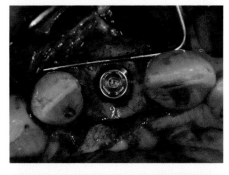
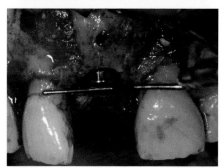

**Final restoration**
Facial view of the final restoration taken 18 months following implant placement; a provisional crown was in situ for 14 months. The periapical radiograph shows ideal implant bone levels. (Prosthetic work by Dr F. Piatti, Rüfenacht/Switzerland.)

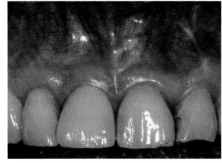
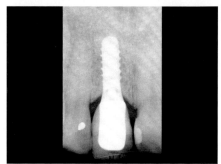

*J. Jensen*

## Vertical augmentation by bone transplantation

Traumatic tooth loss usually leads to alveolar resorption of the alveolar ridge in sagittal and vertical dimension. Augmentation of both hard and soft tissues before implant therapy is, therefore, an essential part of the reconstructive procedures (see p. 769).

At the present time, transplantation of autogenous bone is the golden standard against which all techniques of osseous reconstruction of the maxillofacial skeleton must be judged. Bone grafting studies have shown that autogenous bone produces successful and predictable results (124). However, bone grafts resorb and may cause failures of implant treatment. Free bone grafts act mostly as scaffolds and are thus more osteoconductive than osteoinductive even though osteogenic activity may have remained in the spongious part of graft (125). The other disadvantage of autogenous grafts is the need for a second surgical site and its associated morbidity (126). Autogenous grafts can be taken from the maxillofacial region such as anterior or posterior mandible, maxillary tuberosity and zygoma or from distant sites such as iliac crest, tibia and calvarium.

It has been shown that bone grafts taken from the jaws resorb more slowly than other grafts (127–129). It seems to be due to the fact that jaw bone has a relatively greater frac-

**Table 28.2** Advantages and disadvantages of intraoral donor sites.

| Parameters | Symphysis | Ramus/coronoid process | Tuberosity |
|---|---|---|---|
| Access | good | fairly | fairly |
| Cosmetic concern | high | low | low |
| Graft shape | block | thinner | thinner |
| Morphology | cortico-cancellous | cortical | cortico-cancellous |
| Graft size | 4–8 cc | 3–10 cc | <2 cc |
| Graft resorption | minimal | minimal | more |
| Pain/edema | moderate | minimal | minimal |
| Sensitivity changes | temporary | uncommon | uncommon |
| Dehiscense | occasional | uncommon | uncommon |

tion of cortical bone. This supports the hypothesis that architectural differences of bone grafts determine long-term volume maintenance (130). Advantages and disadvantages of intraoral donor sites are listed in Table 28.2.

## One- or two-stage bone grafting and implant installation?

Resorption of autogenous onlay bone grafts used for augmentation of severely atrophied alveolar ridges has been a frequent problem in preprosthetic surgery, with resorption rates up to 100% within the first 3 years being reported (131). Therefore, when implants have been placed into onlay grafts, the loss of marginal bone height is one of the most important variables to be monitored. Resorption of onlay grafts that have been used with primary or secondary implant placement (one- or two-stage surgery), has been found to be considerably lower than with onlay grafts alone (132). This has been attributed to a functionally stimulating effect of the implants (133). The loss of marginal bone height around these implants has been shown to range between 1.5 and 5 mm during the first 3 years when performed as a one-stage procedure (134–136).

In the last 10 years results from clinical studies indicate that two-stage bone grafting and implant installation is superior to one-stage procedures (137–143).

Increased maturation of the grafted bone before implant installation when using a two-stage technique may result in an improved apposition of bone onto the implant surface compared with the one-stage technique (138, 143). Furthermore, using the two-stage technique may reduce the continuous amount of crestal bone graft resorption around implants (138, 140, 143, 144). It also seems to be of importance that staged surgery permits implant placement that optimizes prosthodontic alignment without the need to consider graft fixation or bone remodeling (140, 143). Possibly the only draw-back of the two-stage procedure compared with the one-stage procedure is the prolonged period of treatment. The possible advantages and disadvantages of one- versus two-stage procedures are listed in Table 28.3.

## Surgical technique

All bone grafting procedures are performed through a vestibular incision. Following submucosal infiltration of a local anesthetic in the anterior labial vestibule and palatal mucosa adjacent to the atrophied region, a standard, full-thickness, vestibular mucoperiosteal flap is raised. The vestibular incision commences approximately 10 mm superior to the mucogingival junction and is extended horizontally to the distal aspect of the teeth adjacent to the atrophied region. A periosteal elevator is used to reflect the flap towards the alveolar crest. Necessary mobility of the soft tissues is obtained by undermining the attached gingiva around the necks of the teeth adjacent to the edentulous region (Fig. 28.17).

Cortico-cancellous bone block grafts corresponding to the size of the maxillary alveolar defect are obtained from either the mandibular retromolar or symphyseal region. The bone graft consists of the buccal cortex and adjacent cancellous bone. Before harvesting, the cortical bone is drilled and countersunk to allow placement of an osteosynthesis screw for later fixation of the graft to the residual ridge. Osteotomes are used to free the grafts, and curved chisels are used to harvest additional cancellous bone. Bone forceps or an acrylic bur are used to contour the bone graft to fit the maxillary defect and it is fixed either as an onlay or a saddle graft with a titanium osteosynthesis screw (Fig. 28.17). Additional cancellous bone is used to fill any voids. Prior to suturing the wound, releasing incisions are made in the periosteum of the flap to achieve a tension-free closure. The incisions are closed with 5-0 Vicryl interrupted and mattress sutures. Provisional removable partial dentures are adjusted to avoid contact with the area. Prophylactic antibiotic treatment (usually penicillin) is initiated at the time of surgery and continued for 5–7 days postoperatively.

**Table 28.3** Possible advantages and disadvantages of one-stage and two-stage bone graft and implant reconstruction techniques. ↑ = increased risk; ↓ = decreased risk.

| | One-stage | Two-stage |
|---|---|---|
| Risk of wound dehiscence | ↑ | ↓ |
| Risk of implant failure | ↑ | ↓ |
| Difficulty of surgery | ↑ | ↓ |
| Amount of marginal bone resorption | ↑ | ↓ |
| Improved alignment of implants | ↓ | ↑ |
| Increased period of treatment | ↓ | ↑ |

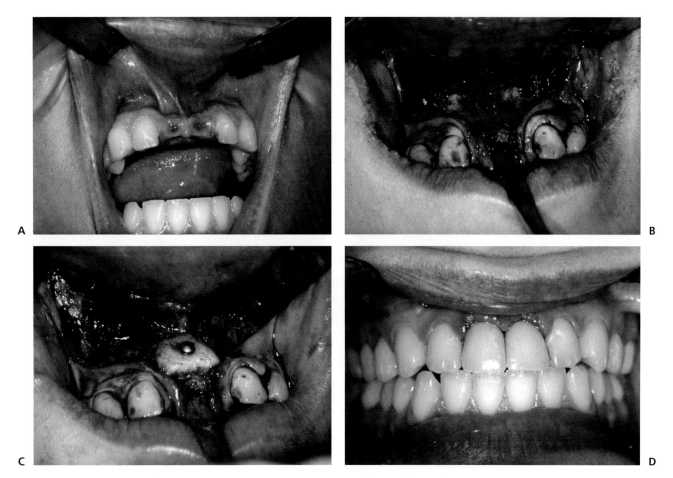

**Fig. 28.17** Reconstruction of alveolar process after loss of 2 central incisors. A. A dentoalveolar trauma to the central incisal region has resulted in alveolar atrophy in both vertical and sagittal dimensions. B. Surgical exposure of the alveolar bone ridge through a vestibular incision followed by mobilization of the surrounding soft tissue. C. Bone graft adapted and fixed by an osteosynthesis-screw to the residual ridge as a saddle graft. D. Final prosthetics.

Four months later, the osteosynthesis screws are removed under local anesthesia using a standard crestal incision and the implant is installed in the grafted region. After a healing period of 4 months prosthetics can be performed (Fig. 28.17).

In Fig. 28.18 reconstruction of a total maxillary segment with a bone graft is shown (129).

*S.E. Nörholt and O. Schwartz*

## Vertical augmentation by alveolar distraction osteogenesis

Reconstruction of the traumatized atrophic alveolus by use of bone grafting techniques is sometimes compromised by bone resorption, wound dehiscence or by the amount and structure of the soft tissues, which can result in lack of attached gingiva. Bone augmentation by gradual distraction of the hard and soft tissues is a method that aims at reducing these problems.

The principles of ossseodistraction were first applied in orthopedic surgery by Ilizarov 1975 (145) and were applied

in maxillofacial surgery by McCarthy et al. 1992 (146) for mandibular lengthening, and later used for alveolar process reconstruction (147–164).

When a traumatic injury in the maxillofacial region leads to loss of teeth and alveolar bone, the use of distraction osteogenesis may be indicated to treat a severe deficiency of the alveolar bone. In such cases reconstruction by other techniques is often unpredictable, and especially in the anterior maxilla where esthetic demands are highest optimal position and volume of hard and soft tissues is essential.

The indications for alveolar distraction osteogenesis after traumatic injuries are mainly in the anterior maxilla and mandible. The timing of the treatment should allow for implant installation shortly after consolidation of the reconstructed bone; that is to say, growth of the jaw must be complete.

The aim of alveolar distraction osteogenesis is to reconstruct bone and soft tissue (in particular attached gingiva) in order to make it possible to install dental implants in an optimal esthetic position. Therefore, preoperative planning including radiographs (and in some cases CT scans), dental casts, prosthetic considerations and a diagnostic wax-up is necessary to estimate the size and vector of distraction needed.

**Fig. 28.18 Loss of several teeth and alveolar ridge reconstructed by mental bone grafts and implants**
This 18-year-old man suffered avulsion of most of the right pre-maxilla including first premolar, canine, second and first incisors in a traffic accident. Only the bony floor of the nasal cavity remains.

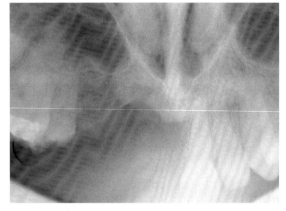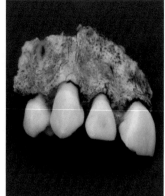

**Immediate treatment and later reconstruction**
Due to an associated jaw fracture an intermaxillary splint was applied. The alveolar ridge was reconstructed using bone harvested from the mental region fixed to residual bone by 4 implants. At the time of abutment implantation, a vestobuloplasty with a palatal mucosal graft was performed to improve lip contour and width of attached gingiva.

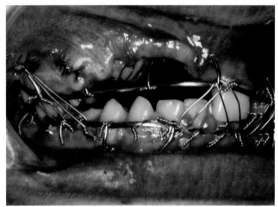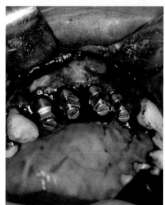

**Follow-up 4 years after surgery**
The implants have been restored with porcelain crowns. Note the very limited resorption of the bone graft. From JENSEN & SINDET-PEDERSEN (129) 1991.

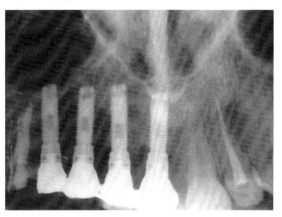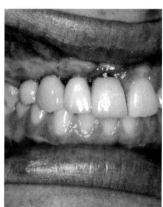

The alveolar defect must be assessed according to the vertical and transversal deficiency. In cases with a very thin alveolar ridge, bone grafting may be needed before or after distraction.

When the initial planning has been done the choice of distraction device can be made. There are presently numerous commercial devices for alveolar distraction on the market and many custom-made devices have been described. The choice includes extraosseous or intraosseos; unidirectional or adjustable, titanium or resorbable materials. Some of the most commonly used devices have been described in detail in a comprehensive textbook on this topic published by Jensen 2002 (154).

Only a limited number of long-term follow-up studies on alveolar distraction have been published in the literature and, as it can be seen from Table 28.4, the number of treatments included is often limited. Implant survival rate was high (90–100%) but esthetic results were not always optimal. This probably reflects the fact that many of the treatments reported were early cases and the technology and surgical techniques were still under development at that time.

There is, however, no doubt that distraction osteogenesis will continue to be a method of choice for bone reconstruction. With the correct patient profile and indications it provides superior esthetic results, in large part due to the fact that keratinized mucosa is transposed to a coronal position, which helps to optimize esthetic appearance.

## Surgical technique

Treatment of localized defects can be done under local anesthetic, but larger defects should be treated using general

**Table 28.4** Results of vertical alveolar distraction.

| Authors | No. of patients | Type of device | Observation period (months) | Vertical bony gain (mm) | Esthetic result | Device failures | Implant survival | |
|---|---|---|---|---|---|---|---|---|
| Chin & Toth (148) 1996 | 5 | Intraosseous (LEAD®) | ? | 9.6 | ? | no | ? | |
| Hidding et al. (149) 1999 | 5 | ExtraosseousMartin® | 12 | 13.6 (6–15) | ? | no | 100% | |
| Gaggl et al. (151) 2004 | 35 | Intraosseous | 12 | ? | acceptable | 2/35 | 60/62 | (97%) |
| Rachmiel et al. (164) 2001 | 14 | Intraosseous (LEAD®) | 16 | 10.3 (8–13) | ? | ? | 21/22 | (95%) |
| Raghoebar et al. (162) 2002 | 10 | IntraosseousMartin® | (6–20) 11.2 | 6.8 (6–8) | acceptable | no | 9/10 | (90%) |
| Jensen OT et al. (153) 2002 | 28 | Intraosseous (3i) Orthodontic | 54 | 6.5 | acceptable | 6/28 | 76/84 | (90%) |
| Chiapasco et al. (160, 161) 2004 | 37 | Extraosseous | 34 | 9.9 (4–15) | acceptable | ? | 130/138 (94%) | |

? not documented.

anesthetic. Prophylactic antibiotics are administered during and 5–7 days after surgery.

The technique can be used in adult patients to move an ankylosed infrapositioned incisor into an occlusal position (167, 168) (Fig. 28.19). It is also valuable when a whole alveolar segment is moved in an occlusal direction (Fig. 28.20).

For the placement of an extraosseous distraction device (commercial or custom made) a high vestibular incision is made and the buccal side of the alveolus is exposed. Periosteum on the top and lingual aspect of the alveolus is left attached to bone. The distraction device is placed into the correct position and the level of osteotomy is marked. The device is removed and an osteotomy of the transport segment is made with thin burs, saw and osteotomes. Free mobility of the transport segment is secured and the distraction device is repositioned and activated 3–5 mm to ensure it functions. Before wound closure the device is deactivated.

A temporary prosthesis is used when possible; in some cases a prosthesis is used to support the distraction rod to ensure the distraction is being done in the correct direction. Following a resting period of 5–7 days the patient is instructed to activate the distraction device 0.5–1.0 mm per day. The patient is followed closely to ensure problem-free distraction and for inspection of the wound. The distraction is complete when the desired level has been obtained (including 3–4 mm over-correction to compensate for any relapse). After this the device is left passive for 2 months.

Implant installation can usually be done when the distraction device is removed and, if there has been an over-correction, contouring of the bone may be needed. Overcorrection represents an opportunity to make a scalloped bone edge which is important for supporting interdental papillas (see p. 771).

*J.O. Andreasen*

## Long-term results

In the past a number of long-term studies of the survival of single standing implants have been published. However, few of those contain adequate information to be considered reliable for a meta-analysis (165–166) (see also Chapters 26 and 31). Thus, in the latest review of single standing implants only four studies qualified for such an analysis. Fig. 28.21 illustrates the survival analysis of 459 single standing implants and covers observations periods of up to 4 years. It shows 97% implant survival after 4 years and 83% survival of implant supported crowns, a figure which compares well with fixed prostodontics (see Chapter 26).

Unfortunately, it is not possible from such an analysis to differentiate between healing rates for implants inserted for trauma-related reasons and those inserted due to other causes, such as tooth aplasia, apical or marginal periodontitis. One cannot assume that these very different situations would have identical prognoses.

## Causes and predictors of failure

Although a multitude of studies have examined the overall healing and survival rates of implants, few investigations have analyzed the cause of failures (169, 170, 172). In a definitive study by Exposito and coworkers (169, 170), it was found that most failures occur during graft insertion, i.e. before abutment stage, and such cases can be considered *iatrogenic* or *host-related* (Fig. 28.22). The next most likely period for implant loss is within the first and second years, where *overload* and *host-related* factors possibly play a role (169–170). From three to five years and beyond, there are rather fewer implant losses and those that do occur are likely related to *overload* and /or *peri-implantitis* (Fig. 28.22).

Perusal through the literature reveals that several preoperative and operative factors have been identified that are significantly related to an increased risk of failure (Fig. 28.23). A short description of these factors will be given, with special consideration of how they relate to dental trauma patients.

### Sex and age
At least for younger ages there is no significant relation between these two factors and implant survival (176).

### Fig. 28.19 Treatment of an ankylosed permanent incisor and alveolar bone with alveolar distraction

Condition 4 years after trauma. Ankylosis of right central incisor with severe vertical infraocclusion and horizontal malposition.

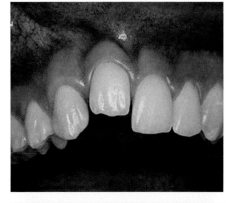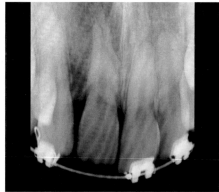

### Surgical procedure
The transport segment is mobilized.

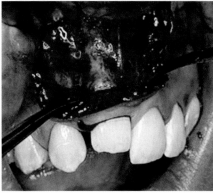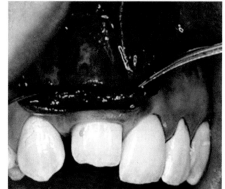

### Distraction device
An extraosseous anchored device (Martin® Track 1) is formed and applied. The vector of distraction is adjusted.

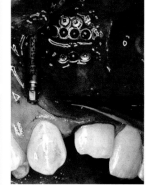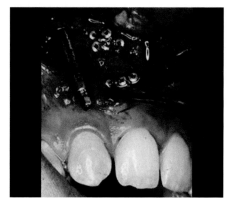

### The use of a screwdriver 3 times a day for distraction
0.3 mm for each turn of the screwdriver, leading to 0.9 mm distraction per day for 8 days.

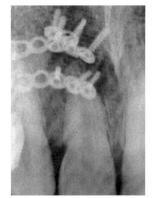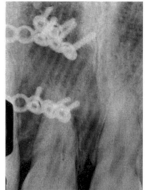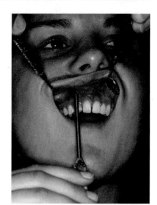

### Final treatment result
Replacement resorption will, within several years, lead to replacement of the root with bone, ideally formed for replacement by an implant without bone grafting when the crown is eventually lost. In the meantime, the ankylosed tooth has been esthetically and functionally satisfactory for years.

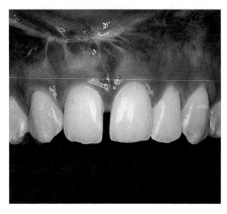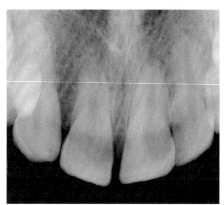

**Fig. 28.20 Treatment of loss of 4 anterior teeth and alveolar bone with alveolar distraction and implants**
Condition after trauma. Severe vertical and horisontal deficiency. Surgical procedure. The transport segment is mobilized.

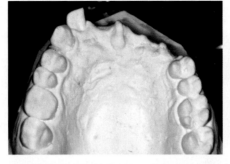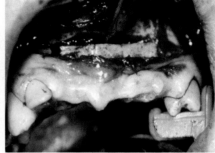

**Distraction device**
An orthodontically anchored custum made device has been applied. The vector of distraction is adjustable. The right image shows the condition after distraction. The clinical appearance compared to the atrophy seen on a plaster model.

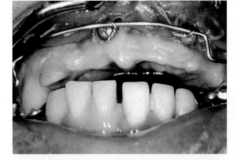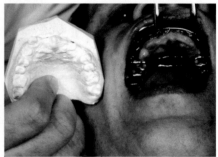

**Installation of implants and final prosthetic treatment**
Note the optimal bone volume as well as keratinized gingiva next to the implant.

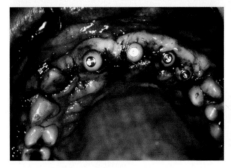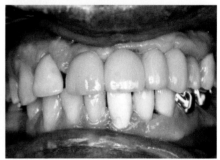

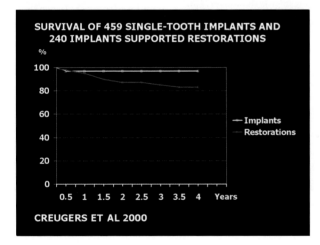

**Fig. 28.21** Survival of 459 single tooth implants and 240 implant-supported single-tooth restorations based on a meta-analysis. From CREUGERS et al. (166) 2000.

### Anatomical region

In a recent literature survey it was found that the latest studies do not show any significant difference in implant survival in the maxilla compared to the mandible, or posterior compared to anterior regions (174).

### Smoking

In several studies it has been demonstrated that smoking increases the chance of implant failure. A recent and large study showed a 3% reduction in the healing rate in smokers (175) (Fig. 28.23).

### General health

Only a few studies have examined this factor. No significant relationship has been found with regard to ASA-status 1 and 2 (176) (Fig. 28.23).

### Diabetes

Several studies have shown that type II diabetes (NIDDM) has only a very small influence upon implant survival (177) (Fig. 28.23). Presently no data exist for type I diabetes (IDDM).

### Wound healing capacity

In several studies a clustering effect of implant failures has been noticed (178, 179). The effect of that could be related to an IL-1-positive genotype (180) (Fig. 28.23). This factor possibly works synergistically with smoking (181, 182).

### Bone volume and quality

In earlier studies it was found that these two factors have a very significant influence upon implant survival (183, 184,

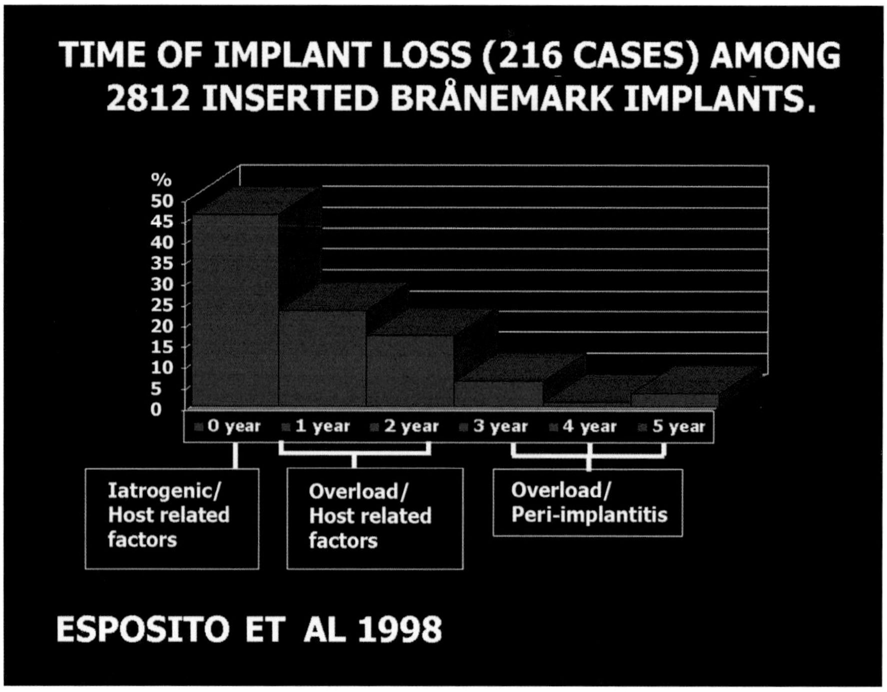

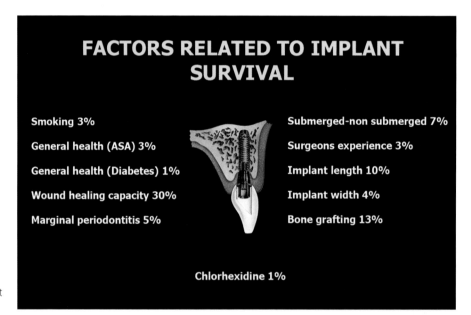

**Fig. 28.22** Time relation to implant failure. From ESPOSITO et al. 1998 (169, 170).

**Fig. 28.23** Factors related to implant survival.

187), but it is remarkable that more recent studies do not show a significant difference in graft survival which could be related to bone volume and quality (179, 185, 186). This may possibly be related to the optimized surface texture of most modern implants (188) or better treatment indications.

### Influence of existing marginal periodontitis

In traumatic injury of young individuals marginal peri-odontitis is rare. The latest research shows that preexisting chronic marginal periodontitis only has a very limited effect on long-term survival of the implant (189, 190). Whereas survival of implants does not appear to be affected, a higher risk of peri-implantitis has been found (223) (Fig. 28.23).

### Surgeon experience

In several studies this factor has been found to be of only moderate importance (191) (Fig. 28.23).

### Submerged and non-submerged

This factor has been examined in a number of studies. In a recent meta-analysis it was found that non-submerged implants had a significant higher failure rate (192) (Fig. 28.23).

### Immediate or delayed implant insertion

In a recent meta-analysis it was found that immediate or delayed insertion had no influence upon implant survival (193).

### Immediate or delayed loading

In a few randomized studies on the mandible no significant influence was found between immediate (2–3 days) or delayed loading (3–8 months) (194). The amount of loading has been found to influence implant survival both experimentally (195–197) and clinically (198). In a recent study of implants placed in the anterior region with and without immediate loading the same healing rate was found (199). However, the mean bone level change at prosthetic seating was significantly higher in loaded versus non-loaded implants (200). Furthermore, where implants were placed immediately into the extraction socket with immediately loading a 20% risk of implant was found (201).

### Implant dimensions

In several studies it has been found that the length of an implant is important. An implant length of more than 10 mm has been found to result in fewer implant losses than shorter implants (179, 202, 214) (Fig. 28.23).

The diameter of the implant has also been found to have some influence upon implant survival (204). In the lateral maxillary incisor region and in the mandibular incisor region a small diameter implant is often required. In a recent study a narrow diameter implant (3 mm) was compared with a 3.75 mm implant. A slightly higher failure rate was found for the narrower diameter implant (205) (Fig. 28.23).

### Types of implants

In a recent review by Cochran no significant difference in healing was found between six different implant systems (206) (Fig. 28.23).

### Implant surface

The relationship between surface characteristics of implants (rough or smooth) and implant success is still unclear. In one meta-analysis study rough surface implants were found to give significantly better success rates than smooth implants (206). However, the validity of this study has been questioned (207, 219, 220).

A recent Cochrane review came to the conclusion that insufficient data exists at present to relate implant survival to surface characteristics of the implant. However, implants with smooth surfaces showed a 20% reduction in the risk of being affected by peri-implantitis over a 3-year period (210).

### Implants placed in transplanted bone

In a recent survey of implant success in autotransplantated bone it was found that if the implant was installed at the time of bone transplantation this resulted in approximately a 25% reduction in implant survival (211). However, if the implant was inserted after healing of the bone transplant no increase in implant loss was seen compared with transplantation to a normal bone site (211) (Fig. 28.23).

### Antibiotics

There is no reliable scientific evidence to recommend or discourage the use of prophylactic antibiotics to prevent complications and failures of dental implants (212) (Fig. 28.23).

### Chlorhexidine digluconate rinses

In one study the use 0.12% chlorhexidine rinse perioperatively was found to significantly reduce the number of infection complications (213) (Fig. 28.23).

## In conclusion

There are presently very few contraindications for the use of implants. Risk predictors appear to be *smoking* and at least temporary cessation of smoking should be attempted. *Previous implant loss* is also a warning sign about potential healing problems. A recently introduced interleukin test may be of importance to identify patients with such a problem. However, this has not yet been verified in larger patient studies. *Proper length and diameter* of the implants should be selected.

## Patient satisfaction

In several studies it has been found that 95% or more patients are very satisfied with the treatment result (1, 216–218).

## Essentials

### Indications

- Lost teeth
- Teeth with progressive resorption
- Teeth with non-restorable crown-root fractures
- Teeth with non-healed cervical root fractures

### Timing of implant insertion in relation to jaw growth

Await termination of alveolar growth monitored by:
- Terminated growth in height
- Repeated cephalographs
- Wrist radiographs

## Timing of implant insertion in relation to tooth loss or extraction

- Immediate
- Delayed (soft tissue coverage, partial bone fill, full bone fill)

## Planning of implant insertion

A clinical and radiographic intra-oral and panoramic examination and/or CT scan should reveal the hard and soft tissue topography in all three dimensions.

## Surgical procedures

### No bone atrophy

Standard insertion ensuring correct mesio-distal, oro-facial and apico-coronal positioning.

### Horizontal atrophy

- Bone grafts
- Barrier membranes with autografts and/or bone substitutes
- Titanium mesh with autografts
- Bone splitting

### Vertical atrophy

- Bone grafts with or without barrier membrane
- Alveolar distraction

### Long-term prognosis (Fig. 28.21)

- Four year survival of implant: 97%
- Four year survival of implant supported crowns: 83%

### Predictors of healing or failures (Fig. 28.23)

- Smoking
- Diabetes
- Wound healing capacity
- Pre-existing marginal periodontitis
- Surgeon experience
- Immediate or delayed loading
- Implant dimensions
- Implants placed in transplanted bone
- Chlorhexidine rinse

## References

1. ANDERSSON L, EMAMI-KRISTIANSEN Z, HÖGSTRÖM J. Single tooth implant treatment in the anterior region of the maxilla for treatment of tooth loss after trauma: a retrospective clinical and interview study. *Dent Traumatol* 2003;**19**:126–31.

2. BRODIE AG. The growth of the alveolar bone and eruption of teeth. *Oral Surg Oral Med Oral Pathol* 1948;**1**:342–5.

3. MOOREES CF. *The dentition of the growing child.* Cambridge, Massachusetts: Harvard University Press, 1959.

4. LINDEN FPGM, VAN DER DUTERLOO HS. *Development of the human dentition.* New York: Harper & Row Publisher Inc, 1976.

5. ENLOW DH. *Handbook of facial growth*, 2nd ed. Philadelphia: WB Saunders Company, 1982.

6. ÖDMAN J, GRÖNDAHL K, LEKHOLM U, THILANDER B. The effect of osseointegrated implants on dento-alveolar development. A clinical and radiographic study in growing pigs. *Eur J Orthodont* 1991;**13**:279–86.

7. THILANDER B, ÖDMAN J, GRÖNDAHL K, LEKHOLM U. Aspects of osseointegrated implants inserted in growing jaws. A biometric and radiographic study in the young pig. *Eur J Orthodont* 1992;**14**:99–109.

8. SENNERBY L, ÖDMAN J, LEKHOLM U, THILANDER B. Tissue reactions towards titanium implants inserted in growing jaws. *Clin Oral Implant Res* 1993;**4**:65–75.

9. THILANDER B, ÖDMAN J, GRÖNDAHL K, FRIBERG B. Osseointegrated implants in adolescents. An alternative in replacing missing teeth? *Eur J Orthodont* 1994;**16**:84–95.

10. THILANDER B, ÖDMAN J, JEMT T. Single implants in the upper incisor region and their relationship to the adjacent teeth. An 8-year follow-up study. *Clin Oral Implant Res* 1999;**10**:346–55.

11. THILANDER B, ÖDMAN J, LEKHOLM U. Orthodontic aspects of the use of oral implants in adolescents: a 10-year follow-up study. *Eur J Orthodont* 2001;**23**:715–31.

12. KOCH G, BERGENDAL T, KVINT S, JOHANSSON U. *Consensus conference on oral implants in young patients.* Jönköping, Sweden: Gothia A, 1996.

13. BERNARD JP, SCHATZ JP, CHRISTOU P, BELSER U, KILIARIDIS S. Long-term vertical changes of the anterior maxillary teeth adjacent to single implants in young and mature adults. A retrospective study. *J Clin Periodontol* 2004;**11**:1024–8.

14. TALLGREN A, SOLOW B. Age differences in adult dentoalveolar heights. *Eur J Orthodont* 1991;**13**:149–56.

15. FORSBERG C-M, ELIASSON S, WESTERGREN H. Face height and tooth eruption in adults. A 20-year follow-up investigation. *Eur J Orthodont* 1991;**13**:249–54.

16. ISERI H, SOLOW B. Continued eruption of maxillary incisors and first molars in girls from from 9 to 25 years, studied by the implant method. *Eur J Orthodont* 1996;**18**:245–56.

17. HÄGG U, TARANGER J. Skeletal stages of the hand and wrist as indicators of the pubertal growth spurt. *Acta Odontol Scand* 1980;**38**:187–200.

18. KAVANAMI M, ANDREASEN JO, BORUM MK, SCHOU S, HJØRTING-HANSEN E, KATO H. Infraposition of anklosed permanent maxillary incisors after replantation related to age and sex. *Endod Dent Traumatol* 1999;**15**:50–6.

19. JEMT T. Measurements of tooth movements in relation to single implant restorations: a case report. *Clin Implant Dent Relat Res* 2005;**1**:200–8.

20. ANDREASEN JO, SINDET-PETERSEN S. Wound healing after surgery. In: Andreasen JO, Kölsen Pedersen A,

Laskin D, eds. *Textbook and color atlas of tooth impaction.* Copenhagen: Munksgaard, 1994.

21. HÄMMERLE CHF, CHEN ST, WILSON TG. Consensus statements and recommended clinical procedures–group 1. *Int J Oral Maxillofac Impl* 2004;**19**(Suppl):26–8.

22. PAOLANTONIO M, DOLCI M, SCARANO A, D'ARCHICIO D, DI PLACIDO G, TUMINI V, PIATTELLI A. Immediate implantation in fresh extraction sockets. A controlled clinical and histological study in man. *Oral Surg Oral Med Oral Pathol* 2001;**72**:1560–71.

23. WILSON TG Jr, SCHENK R, BUSER D, COCHRAN D. Implants placed in immediate extraction sites: a report of histologic and histometric analysis of human biopsies. *Oral Surg Oral Med Oral Pathol* 1998;**13**:333–41.

24. BOTTICELLI DT, BERGLUND H, LINDHE J. Hard-tissue alterations following immediate implant placement in extraction sites. *J Clin Periodontol* 2004;**31**:820–8.

25. SCHROPP L, WENZEL A, KONTOPOULOS L, et al. Bone healing and soft tissue contour changes following single-tooth extraction: a clinical and radiographic 12-month prospective study. *Int J Periodont Restor Dent* 2003;**23**:313–23.

26. SCHROPP L, KOSTOPOULOS L, WENZEL A. Bone healing following immediate versus delayed placement of titanium implants into extraction sockets: a prospective clinical study. *Int J Oral Maxillofac Implants* 2003;**18**:189–99.

27. AMLER MH, JOHNSON PL, SALMAN I. Histological and histochemical investigations of human alveolar socket healing in undisturbed extraction wounds. *Oral Surg Oral Med Oral Pathol* 1960;**61**:32–44.

28. GRUNDER U. Stability of the mucosal topography around single-tooth implants and adjacent teeth: 1-year results. *Int J Periodont Restor Dent* 2000;**20**:11–17.

29. BUSER D, MARTIN W, BELSER C. Optimizing esthetics for implant restorations in the anterior maxilla: anatomic and surgical considerations. *Int J Oral Maxillofac Implants* 2004;**19**(Suppl):43–61.

30. GARGIULO AW, WENTZ FM, ORBAN B. Dimensions and relations of the dentogingival junction in humans. *J Periodontol* 1961;**32**:261–7.

31. BERGHLUND T, LINDHE J. Dimension of the peri-implant mucosa. Biological width revisited. *J Clin Periodontol* 1996;**23**:971–3.

32. COCHRAN DL, HERMANN JS, SCHENK RK, HIGGINBOTTOM FL, BUSER D. Biologic width around titanium implants. A histometric analysis of the implanto-gingival junction around unloaded and loaded nonsubmerged implants in the canine mandible. *J Periodontol* 1997;**68**:186–98.

33. TARNOW DP, CHO SC, WALLANCE SS. The effect of interimplant distance on the height of inter-implant bone crest. *J Periodontal* 2000;**71**:546–9.

34. KOIS JC. Predictable single tooth peri-implant esthetics: five diagnostic keys. *Compend Contin Educ Dent* 2001;**22**:19–206.

35. TARNOW DP, MAGNER AW, FLETCHER P. The effect of the distance from the contact point to the crest of bone on the presence or absence of the interproximal dental papilla. *J Periodontol* 1992;**63**:995–6.

36. CHOQUET V, HERMANS M, ADRIAENSSENS P, DAELEMANS P, TARNOW DP, MALEVEZ C. Clinical and radiographic

evaluation of the papilla level adjacent to single-tooth dental implants. A retrospective study in the maxillary anterior region. *J Periodontol* 2001;**2**:1364–71.

37. NYMAN S, LANG NP, BUSER D, BRÄGGER U. Bone regeneration adjacent to titanium dental implants using guided tissue regeneration: a report of two cases. *Int J Oral Maxillofac Implants* 1990;**5**:9–14.

38. BUSER D, DAHLIN C, SCHENK RK (eds). *Guided bone regeneration in implant dentistry.* Chicago: Quintessence, 1994.

39. SIMION M, BALDONI M, ZAFFE D. Jawbone enlargement using immediate implant placement associated with a split-crest technique and guided tissue regeneration. *Int J Periodontics Restor Dent* 1992;**12**:462–73.

40. ESPOSITO M, EKKESTUBE A, GRÖNDAHL K. Radiological evaluation of marginal bone loss at tooth surfaces facing single Brånemark implants. *Clin Oral Implants Res* 1993;**4**:151–7.

41. THILANDER B, ÖDMAN J, LEKHOLM U. Orthodontic aspects of the use of oral implants in adolescents: a 10-year follow-up study. *Eur J Orthod* 2001;**23**:715–31.

42. THILANDER B, ÖDMAN J, JEMT T. Single implants in the upper incisor region and their relationship to the adjacent teeth. An 8-year follow-up study. *Clin Oral Implants Res* 1999;**10**:346–55.

43. ELIAN N, JALBOUT ZN, CHO SC, FROUM S, TARNOW DP. Realities and limitations in the management of the interdental papilla between implants. Three case reports. *Pract Proceed Aesthet Dent* 2003;**15**:737–44.

44. JEMT T, LEKHOLM, U, GRÖNDAHL K. A 3-year follow-up study of early single implant restorations and modern Brånemark. *Int J Periodont Res Dent* 1990;**5**:341–9.

45. HERMANN JS, COCHRAN DL, NUMMIKOSKI PV, BUSER D. Crestal bone changes around titanium implants. A radiographic evaluation of unloaded non submerged and submerged implants in the canine mandible. *J Periodontol* 1997;**68**:1117–30.

46. HIGGINBOTTOM FL, WILSON TG Jr. Three-dimensional templates for placement of root-form dental implants: a technical note. *Int J Oral Maxillofac Implants* 1996;**11**:787–93.

47. HIGGINBOTTOM F, BELSER U, JONES JD, KEITH S. Prosthetic management of implants in the esthetic zone. *Int J Oral Maxillofac Implants* 2004;**19**:62–72.

48. ROSSI E, ANDREASEN JO. Maxillary bone growth and implants positioning in a young patient: a case report. *Int J Periodontics Restorative Dent* 2003;**23**:113–19.

49. MALMGREN B, CVEK M, LUNDBERG M, FRYKHOLM A. Surgical treatment of ankylosed and infrapositioned reimplanted incisors in adolescents. *Scand J Dent Res* 1984;**92**:391–9.

50. GRUNDER U. Stability of the mucosal topography around single-tooth implants and adjacent teeth: 1-year results. *Int J Periodont Rest Dent* 2000;**20**:11–17.

51. OATES TW, WEST J, JONES J, KAISER D, COCHRAN DL. Long-term changes in soft tissue height on the facial surface of dental implants. *Implant Dent* 2002;**11**:272–9.

52. SMALL PN, TARNOW DP. Gingival recession around implants: a 1-year longitudinal prospective study. *Int J Oral Maxillofac Implants* 2000;**15**:265–71.

53. CASTALDO JF, CURY PR, SENDYK WR. Effect of the vertical and horizontal distances between adjacent

implants and between a tooth and an implant on the incidence of interproximal papilla. *J Periodontol* 2004;**75**:1242–6.

54. Salama H, Salama M. The role of orthodontic extrusive remodelling in the enhancement of soft and hard tissue profile prior to implant placement: a systemic approach to the management of extraction site defects. *Int J Periodont Restor Dent* 1993;**13**:312–34.

55. Goldberg PV, Higginbottom FL, Wilson TG. Periodontal considerations in restorative and implant therapy. *Periodontol 2000* 2000;**25**:100–9.

56. Tarnow D, Elian N, Fletcher P, Froum S, Magner A, Cho SC, Salama M, Salama H, Garber DA. Vertical distance from the crest of bone to the height on the interproximal papilla between adjacent implants. *J Periodontol* 2003;**74**:1785–8.

57. Jemt T. Regeneration of gingival papillae after single-implant treatment. *Int J Periodont Restor Dent* 1997;**17**:326–33.

58. Jemt T. Restoring the gingival contour by means of provisional resin crowns after single-implant treatment. *Int J Periodont Restor Dent* 1999;**19**:20–9.

59. Priest G. Predictability of soft tissue form around single-tooth implant restorations. *Int J Periodont Restor Dent* 2003;**23**:19–27.

60. Chang M, Wennström JL, Ödman P, Andersson B. Implant-supported single-tooth replacements compared to contralateral natural teeth. Crown and soft tissue dimensions. *Clin Oral Implants Res* 1999;**10**:185–94.

61. Chang M, Ödman P, Wennström JL, Andersson B. Esthetic outcome of implant-supported single-tooth replacements assessed by the patient and by prosthodontists. *Int J Prosthodont* 1999;**12**:335–41.

62. Giannopoulou C, Bernard JP, Buser D, Carrel A, Belser UC. Effect of intracrevicular restoration margins on peri-implant health: clinical, biochemical and microbiologic findings around esthetic implants up to 9 years. *Int J Oral Maxillofac Implants* 2003;**18**:173–81.

63. Thilander B, Ödman J, Jemt T. Single implants in the upper incisor region and their relationship to the adjacent teeth. An 8-year follow-up study. *Clin Oral Implants Res* 1999;**10**:346–55.

64. Palmer RM, Palmer PJ, Smith BJ. A 5-year prospective study of Astra single tooth implants. *Clin Oral Implants Res* 2000;**11**:179–82.

65. Holt RL, Rosenberg MM, Zinser PJ, Ganeles J. A concept for a biologically derived, parabolic implant design. *Int J Periodont Restor Dent* 2002;**5**:64–73.

66. Wohrle PS. Nobel Perfect esthetic scalloped implant: rationale for a new design. *Clin Implant Dent Relat Res* 2003;**5**:64–73.

67. Belser UC, Bernhard JP, Buser D. Implant placement in the esthetic zone. In: Lindhe J, Karring T, Lang NP (eds). *Clinical periodontology and implant dentistry*, 4th edition. Oxford: Blackwell Munksgaard, 2003.

68. Kan JY, Rungcharassaeng K, Umezu K, Kois JC. Dimensions of peri-implant mucosa: an evaluation of maxillary anterior single implants in humans. *J Periodontol* 2003;**4**:557–62.

69. Buser D, Brägger U, Lang NP, Nyman S. Regeneration and enlargement of jaw bone using guided tissue regeneration. *Clin Oral Implants Res* 1990;**1**:22–32.

70. Quale AA. A traumatic removal of teeth and root fragments in dental implantology. *Int J Oral Maxillofac Implants* 1990;**5**:293–6.

71. Rosenquist JB, Nyström E. Occlusion of the incisal canal with bone chips. A procedure to facilitate insertion of implants in the anterior maxilla. *Int J Oral Maxillofac Surg* 1992;**21**:210–11.

72. Bedrossian E, Tawfilis A, Alijanian A. Veneer grafting: a technique for augmentation of the resorbed alveolus prior to implant placement. A clinical report. *Int J Oral Maxillofac Implants* 2000;**15**:853–8.

73. Sethi A, Kaus T. Ridge augmentation using mandibular block bone grafts: preliminary results of an ongoing prospective study. *Int J Oral Maxillofac Implants* 2001;**16**:378–88.

74. Phillips JH, Rahn BA. Fixation effects on membranous and endochondral onlay bone-graft resorption. *Plast Reconstr Surg* 1988;**82**:872–7.

75. Raghoebar GM, Batenburg RHK, Vissink A, Reintsema H. Augmentation of localized defects of the anterior maxillary ridge with autogenous bone before insertion of implants. *J Oral Maxillofac Surg* 1996;**54**:1180–5.

76. Widmark G, Andersson B, Ivanoff CJ. Mandibular bone graft in the anterior maxilla for single-tooth implants. Presentation of a surgical method. *Int J Oral Maxillofac Surg* 1997;**26**:106–9.

77. Chiapasco M, Abati S, Romeo E, Vogel G. Clinical outcome of autogenous bone blocks or guided bone regeneration with e-PTFE membranes for the reconstruction of narrow edentulous ridges. *Clin Oral Implants Res* 1999;**10**:278–88.

78. Buser D, von Arx T. Surgical procedures in partially edentulous patients with ITI implants. *Clin Oral Implants Res* 2000;**11**(Suppl 1):83–100.

79. Buser D, Dula K, Belser U, Hirt HP, Berthold H. Localized ridge augmentation using guided bone regeneration. I. Surgical procedure in the maxilla. *Int J Periodont Restor Dent* 1993;**13**:29–45.

80. Buser D, Dula K, Belser U, Hirt HP, Berthold H. Localized ridge augmentation using guided bone regeneration. II. Surgical procedure in the mandible. *Int J Periodont Restor Dent* 1995;**15**:10–29.

81. Buser D, Ruskin J, Higginbottom F, Hardwick WR, Dahlin C, Schenk RK. Osseointegration of titanium implants in bone regenerated in membrane-protected defects. A histologic study in the canine mandible. *Int J Oral Maxillofac Implants* 1995;**10**:652–66.

82. Buser D, Dula K, Hirt HP, Schenk RK. Lateral ridge augmentation using autografts and barrier membranes: a clinical study with 40 partially edentulous patients. *J Oral Maxillofac Surg* 1996;**54**:420–32.

83. Hürzeler MB, Quinones CR, Hutmacher D, Schüpbach P. Guided bone regeneration around dental implants in the atrophic alveolar ridge using a bioresorbable barrier. An experimental study in the monkey. *Clin Oral Implants Res* 1997;**8**:323–31.

84. Hockers T, Abensur D, Valentini P, Legrand R, Hämmerle CHF. The combined use of bioresorbable membranes and xenografts or autografts in the treatment of bone defects around implants. A study in beagle dogs. *Clin Oral Implants Res* 1999;**10**:487–98.

85. VERT M, LI SM, SPENLEHAUER G, GUERIN P. Bioresorbability and biocompatibility of aliphatic polyesters. *J Mat Science Mat Med* 1992;**3**:432–46.

86. BUNYARATAVEJ P, WANG HL. Collagen membranes: a review. *J Periodontol* 2001;**72**:215–29.

87. PATINO MG, NEIDERS ME, ANDREANA S, NOBLE B, COHEN RE. Collagen as an implantable material in medicine and dentistry. *J Oral Implantol* 2002;**28**:220–5.

88. BECKER W, DAHLIN C, BECKER BE, LEKHOLM U, VAN STEENBERGHE D, HIGUCHI K, KULTJE C. The use of e-PTFE barrier membranes for bone promotion around titanium implants placed into extraction sockets: a prospective multicenter study. *Int J Oral Maxillofac Implants* 1994;**9**:31–40.

89. GHER ME, QUINTERO G, ASSAD D, MONACO E, RICHARDSON AC. Bone grafting and guided bone regeneration for immediate dental implants in humans. *J Periodontol* 1994;**65**:881–91.

90. ANTOUN H, SITBON JM, MARTINEZ H, MISSIKA P. A prospective randomized study comparing two techniques of bone augmentation: onlay graft alone or associated with a membrane. *Clin Oral Implants Res* 2001;**12**:632–9.

91. ZITZMANN NU, NAEF R, SCHÄRER P. Resorbable versus nonresorbable membranes in combination with Bio-Oss for guided bone regeneration. *Int J Oral Maxillofac Implants* 1997;**12**:844–52.

92. ZELLIN G, GRITLI-LINDE A, LINDE A. Healing of mandibular defects with different biodegradable and non-biodegradable membranes: an experimental study in rats. *Biomaterials* 1995;**16**:601–9.

93. KOHAL RJ, WIRSCHING C, BÄCHLE M. Geführte Knochenregeneration um dentale Implantate mit einer bioresorbierbaren Membran. Eine tierexperimentelle Pilot-Untersuchung. *Schweiz Monatsschr Zahnmed* 2001;**111**:1397–405.

94. VON ARX T, COCHRAN DL, SCHENK RK, BUSER D. Evaluation of a prototype trilayer membrane (PTLM) for lateral ridge augmentation: an experimental study in the canine mandible. *Int J Oral Maxillofac Surg* 2002;**31**:190–9.

95. SCHLIEPHAKE H, DARD M, PLANCK H, HIERLEMANN H, JAKOB A. Guided bone regeneration around endosseous implants using a resorbable membrane vs a PTFE membrane. *Clin Oral Implants Res* 2000;**11**:230–41.

96. BUSER D, DULA K, LANG NP, NYMAN S. Long-term stability of osseointegrated implants in bone regenerated with the membrane technique. Five-year results of a prospective study with 12 implants. *Clin Oral Implants Res* 1996;**7**:175–83.

97. NEVINS M, MELLONIG JT, CLEM DS, REISER GM, BUSER D. Implants in regenerated bone: long-term survival. *Int J Periodont Restor Dent* 1998;**18**:35–45.

98. BUSER D, INGIMARSSON S, DULA K, LUSSI A, HIRT HP, BELSER UC. Long-term stability of osseointegrated implants in augmented bone: a 5-year prospective study in partially edentulous patients. *Int J Periodont Restor Dent* 2002;**22**:108–17.

99. VON ARX T, HARDT N, WALLKAMM B. The TIME technique: a new method for localized alveolar ridge augmentation prior to placement of dental implants. *Int J Oral Maxillofac Implants* 1996;**11**:387–94.

100. VON ARX T, KURT B. Implant placement and simultaneous ridge augmentation using autogenous bone and a microtitanium mesh: a prospective clinical study with 20 implants. *Clin Oral Implants Res* 1999;**10**:24–33.

101. MAIORANA C, SANTORO F, RABAGLIATI M, SALINA S. Evaluation of the use of iliac cancellous bone and anorganic bovine bone in the reconstruction of the atrophic maxilla with titanium mesh: a clinical and histologic investigation. *Int J Oral Maxillofac Implants* 2001;**16**:427–32.

102. ASSENZA B, PIATTELLI M, SCARANO A, IEZZI G, PETRONE G, PIATTELLI A. Localized ridge augmentation using titanium micromesh. *J Oral Implantol* 2001;**27**:287–92.

103. EISIG SB, HO V, KRAUT R, LALOR P. Alveolar ridge augmentation using titanium micromesh: an experimental study in dogs. *J Oral Maxillofac Surg* 2003;**61**:347–53.

104. ARTZI Z, DAYAN D, ALPERN Y, NEMCOVSKY CE. Vertical ridge augmentation using xenogenic material supported by a configured titanium mesh: clinicohistopathologic and histochemical study. *Int J Oral Maxillofac Implants* 2003;**18**:440–6.

105. ROCCUZZO M, RAMIERI G, SPADA MC, BIANCHI SD, BERRONE S. Vertical alveolar ridge augmentation by means of a titanium mesh and autogenous bone grafts. *Clin Oral Implants Res* 2004;**15**:73–81.

106. ENGELKE WG, DIEDERICHS CG, JACOBS HG, DECKWER I. Alveolar reconstruction with splitting osteotomy and microfixation of implants. *Int J Oral Maxillofac Implants* 1997;**2**:310–18.

107. SETHI A, KAUS T. Maxillary ridge expansion with simultaneous implant placement: Five-year results of an ongoing clinical study. *Int J Oral Maxillofac Implants* 2000;**15**:491–9.

108. COATOAM GW, MARIOTTI A. The segmental ridge-split procedure. *J Periodontol* 2003;**74**:757–70.

109. OIKARINEN KS, SANDOR GK, KAINULAINEN VT, SALONEN-KEMPPI M. Augmentation of the narrow traumatized anterior alveolar ridge to facilitate dental implant placement. *Dent Traumatol* 2003;**19**:19–29.

110. BUSER D, MARTIN W, BELSER UC. Optimizing esthetics for implant restorations in the anterior maxilla: anatomic and surgical considerations. *Int J Oral Maxillofac Implants* 2004;**19**(Suppl):43–61.

111. MISCH CM. Comparison of intraoral donor sites for onlay grafting prior to implant placement. *Int J Oral Maxillofac Implants* 1997;**12**:767–76.

112. NKENKE E, SCHULTZE-MOSGAU S, RADESPIEL-TRÖGER M, KLOSS F, NEUKAM FW. Morbidity of harvesting of chin grafts: a prospective study. *Clin Oral Implants Res* 2001;**12**:495–502.

113. NKENKE E, RADESPIEL-TRÖGER M, WILTFANG J, SCHULTZ-MOSGAU S, WINKLER G, NEUKAM FW. Morbidity of harvesting of retromolar bone grafts: a prospective study. *Clin Oral Implants Res* 2002;**13**:514–21.

114. CLAVERO J, LUNDGREN S. Ramus or chin grafts for maxillary sinus inlay and local onlay augmentation: comparison of donor site morbidity and complications. *Clin Implants Dent Rel Res* 2003;**5**:154–60.

115. De Carvalho PSP, Vasconcellos LW, Pi J. Influence of bed preparation on the incorporation of autogenous bone grafts: a study in dogs. *Int J Oral Maxillofac Implants* 2000;**15**:565–70.

116. Von Arx T, Cochran DL, Hermann J, Schenk RK, Buser D. Lateral ridge augmentation using different bone fillers and barrier membrane application. A histologic and morphometric pilot study in the canine mandible. *Clin Oral Implants Res* 2001;**12**:260–9.

117. Araujo MG, Sonohara M, Hayacibara R, Cardaropoli G, Lindhe J. Lateral ridge augmentation by the use of grafts comprised of autologous bone or a biomaterial. An experiment in the dog. *J Clin Periodontol* 2002;**29**:1122–31.

118. Zhao S, Pinholt EM, Madsen JE, Donath K. Histological evaluation of different biodegradable and non-biodegradable membranes implanted subcutaneously in rats. *J Cranio Maxillofac Surg* 2000;**28**:116–22.

119. Owens KW, Yukna RA. Collagen membrane resorption in dogs: a comparative study. *Implant Dent* 2001;**10**:49–56.

120. Jensen SS, Aaboe M, Pinholt EM, Hjørting-Hansen E, Melsen F, Ruyter IE. Tissue reaction and material characteristics of four bone substitutes. *Int J Oral Maxillofac Implants* 1996;**11**:55–66.

121. Skoglund A, Hising P, Young C. A clinical and histologic examination in humans of the osseous response to implanted natural bone mineral. *Int J Oral Maxillofac Implants* 1997;**12**:194–9.

122. Hürzeler MB, Kohal RJ, Naghshbandi J, Mota LF, Conradt J, Hutmacher D, Caffesse RG. Evaluation of a new bioresorbable barrier to facilitate guided bone regeneration around exposed implant threads. An experimental study in the monkey. *Int J Oral Maxillofac Surg* 1998;**27**:315–20.

123. Zitzmann NU, Schärer P, Marinello CP, Schüpbach P, Berglundh T. Alveolar ridge augmentation with Bio-Oss: a histologic study in humans. *Int J Periodont Restor Dent* 2001;**21**:288–95.

124. Marx RE. Clinical application of bone biology to mandibular reconstruction. *Clin Plast Surg* 1994;**21**:377–92.

125. Burchard T. The biology of bone graft repair. *Clin Orthop Rel Res* 1983;**174**:28–42.

126. Caminiti MF, Sandor GKB, Carmichael RP. Quantification of bone harvested from the iliac crest using a power-driven trephine. *J Oral Maxillofac Surg* 1999;**57**:801–6.

127. Smith JD, Abrahamson M. Membraneous vs. endochondral bone autografts. *Arch Otolaryngol* 1974;**99**:203–5.

128. Zins JE, Whitaker LA. Membranous versus endochondral bone: implications for craniofacial reconstruction. *Plast Reconstr Surg* 1983;**72**:778–85.

129. Jensen J, Sindet-Pedersen S. Autogenous mandibular bone grafts and osseointegrated implants for reconstruction of severely resorbed maxilla: a preliminary report. *J Oral Maxillofac Surg* 1991;**49**:1277–87.

130. Chen NT, Glowacki J, Bucky LP, Hong HZ, Kim WK, Yaremchuk MJ. The roles of revascularization and resorption on endurance of craniofacial onlay bone grafts in the rabbit. *Plast Reconstr Surg* 1994;**93**:714–22.

131. Koberg W. Spätergebnisse nach Augmentationsplastiken. *Dtsch Z Zahnärztl Implantol* 1985;**1**:239–47.

132. Listrom RD, Symington JS. Osseointegrated dental implants in conjunction with bone grafts. *Int J Oral Maxillofac Surg* 1988;**17**:116–18.

133. Kent JN, Block MS. Simultaneous maxillary sinus floor bone grafting and placement of hydroxyapatite coated implants. *J Oral Maxillofac Surg* 1989;**47**:238–42.

134. Åstrand P, Nord PG, Brånemark P-I. Titanium implants and onlay bone graft to the atrophic edentulous maxilla: a 3-year longitudinal study. *Int J Oral Maxillofac Surg* 1996;**25**:25–9.

135. Adell R, Lekholm U, Gröndahl K, Brånemark P-I, Lindström J, Jacobsson M. Reconstruction of severely resorbed edentulous maxillae using osseointegrated fixtures in immediate autogenous bone grafts. *Int J Oral Maxillofac Implants* 1990;**5**:233–46.

136. Jensen J, Sindet-Pedersen S, Enemark H. Reconstruction of residual alveolar cleft defects with one-stage mandibular bone grafts and osseointegrated implants. *J Oral Maxillofac Surg* 1998;**56**:460–6.

137. Tolman DE. Reconstructive procedures with endosseous implants in grafted bone: a review of the literature. *Int J Oral Maxillofac Implants* 1995;**10**:275–94.

138. Misch CM, Misch CE. The repair of localized severe ridge defects for implant placement using mandibular bone grafts. *Implant Dent* 1995;**4**:261–7.

139. Widmark G, Andersson B, Ivanoff C. Mandibular bone graft in the anterior maxilla for single-tooth implants. Presentation of a surgical method. *Int J Oral Maxillofac Surg* 1997;**26**:106–9.

140. Jensen J. *Reconstruction of residual cleft defects with mandibular onlay bone grafts and osseointegrated implants.* Thesis, Faculty of Health Sciences, University of Aarhus, 1998.

141. Raghoebar GM, Batenburg RHK, Vissink A, Reintsema H. Augmentation of localized defects of the anterior maxillary ridge with autogenous bone before insertion of implants. *J Oral Maxillofac Surg* 1996;**54**:1180–5.

142. Cordaro L, Amade DS, Cordaro M. Clinical results of alveolar ridge augmentation with mandibular bone grafts in partially edentulous patients prior to implant placement. *Clin Oral Implants Res* 2002;**13**:103–11.

143. Lundgren S, Rasmusson L, Sjöström M, Sennerby L. Simultaneous or delayed placement of titanium implants in free autogenous iliac bone grafts. Histological analysis of bone-titanium interface in 10 consecutive patients. *Int J Oral Maxillofac Surg* 1999;**28**:31–7.

144. Raghoebar GM, Schoen P, Meijer HJ, Stellingsma K, Vissink A. Early loading of endosseous implants in the augmented maxilla: a 1-year prospective study. *Clin Oral Implants Res* 2003;**14**:697–702.

145. Ilizarov GA. Basic principles of transosseous compression and distraction osteosynthesis. *Orthop Traumatol Protez* 1971;**32**:7–15.

146. McCarthy JG, Schreiber J, Karp N, et al. Lengthening the human mandible by gradual distraction. *Plast Reconstr Surg* 1992;**89**:1–10.

147. HOFFMEISTER B, MARCKS CH, WOLFF KP. The floating bone concept in intraoral distraction. *J Craniomaxillofac Surg* 1998;**26**:76–81.

148. CHIN M, TOTH B. Distraction osteogenesis in maxillofacial surgery using internal devices: review of five cases. *J Oral Maxillofac Surg* 1996;**54**:45–53.

149. HIDDING J, LAZAR F, ZOLLER JE. Initial outcome of vertical distraction osteogenesis of the atrophic alveolar ridge. *Mund Kiefer Geschtschir* 1999;**3**(Suppl 1):79–83.

150. GAGGL A, SCHULTES G, KÄRCHER H. Vertical alveolar ridge distraction with prosthetic treatable distractors: a clinical investigation. *Int J Maxillofac Implants* 2000;**15**:701–10.

151. GAGGL A, OFNER C, RAINER H, CHIARI FM. Distraction implants in vertical ridge distraction. In: Balaji SM, ed. *Craniofacial distraction osteogenesis.* 2004.

152. GAGGL A, RAINER H, CHIARI FM. Horizontal distraction of the anterior maxilla in combination with bilateral sinuslift operation: preliminary report. *Int J Oral Maxillofac Surg* 2005;**34**:37–44.

153. JENSEN OT, COCKRELL R, KUHIKE L, REED C. Anterior maxillary alveolar distraction osteogenesis: a prospective 5-year clinical study. *Int J Oral Maxillofac Implants* 2002;**17**:52–68.

154. JENSEN OT. *Alveolar distraction osteogenesis* 2002.

155. APARICIO C, JENSEN OT. Alveolar distraction to gain width. In: Jensen OT (ed). *Alveolar distraction osteogenesis.* 2002.

156. TAKAHASHI T. Widening of the alveolar ridge. In: Balaji SM, ed. *Craniofacial distraction osteogenesis.* 2004.

157. STUCKI-MCCORMICK S, MOSES JJ. Vector and stabilization during alveolar lengthening by distraction osteogenesis. In: Jensen OT (ed). *Alveolar distraction osteogenesis.* 2002.

158. KOFOD T, WURTZ V, MELSEN B. Treatment of ankylosed central incisor by single tooth dento-osseous osteotomy and simple distraction device. *Am J Orthod Dentofac Orthop* 2005;**127**:72–80.

159. EWERS R, FOCK N, MILLESI-SCHOBEL G, ENISLIDIS G. Pedicled sandwich plasty: a variation on alveolar distraction for vertical augmentation of the atropic mandible. *Br J Maxillofac Surg* 2004;**42**:445–7.

160. CHIAPASCO M, CONSOLO U, BIANCHI A, RONCHI P. Alveolar distraction osteogenesis for the correction of vertically deficient edentulous ridges: a multicenter prospective study on humans. *Int J Oral Maxillofac Implants* 2004;**19**:299–407.

161. CHIAPASCO M, ROMEO E, CASENTINI P, RIMONDINI L. Alveolar distraction osteogenesis vs. vertical guided bone regeneration for the correction of vertically deficient edentulous ridges: a 1–3 year prospective study in humans. *Clin Oral Implants Res* 2004;**15**:82–95.

162. RAGHOEBAR GM, LIEM RS, VISSINK A. Vertical distraction of the severely resorbed edentulous mandible. A clinical, histological and electron microscopic study of 10 treated cases. *Clin Oral Implants Res* 2002;**13**:558–65.

163. ROBIONY M, CORRADO T, STUCKI-MCCORMICK SU, ZERMAN N, COSTA F, POLITI M. The floating alveolar device: a bi-directional distraction system for distraction osteogenesis of the alveolar process. *J Oral Maxillofac Surg* 2004;**62**:136–42.

164. RACHMIEL A, SROUJI S, PELED M. Alveolar ridge augmentation by distraction osteogenesis. *Int J Oral Maxillofac Surg* 2001;**30**:510–17.

165. LINDH T, GUNNE J, TILLBERG A, MOLIN M. A meta-analysis of implants in partial edentulism. *Clin Oral Implants Res* 1998;**9**:80–90.

166. CREUGERS NHJ, KREULEN CM, SNOEK PA, DE KANTER RJAM. A systematic review of single-tooth restorations supported by implants. *Dent Jour* 2000;**28**:209–17.

167. KOFOD T, WÜRTZ V, MELSEN B. Treatment of an ankylosed central incisor by single tooth dento-osseous osteotomy and a simple distraction device. *Am J Orthod Dentofac Orthoped* 2005;**127**:72–80.

168. ISAACSON RJ, STRAUSS RA, BRIDGES-POQUIS A, PELUSO AR, LINDAUER SJ. Moving an ankylosed central incisor using orthodontics, surgery and distraction osteogenesis. *Angle Orthod* 2001;**71**:411–18.

169. ESPOSITO M, HIRSCH JM, LEKHOLM U, THOMSEN P. Biological factors contributing to failures of osseointegrated oral implants. *J Oral Sci* 1998;**106**:527–51.

170. ESPOSITO M, HIRSCH JM, LEKHOLM U, THOMSEN P. Biological factors contributing to failures of osseointegrated oral implants. II. Etiopathogenesis. *J Oral Sci* 1998;**106**:721–64.

171. BERGLUNDH T, PERSSON L, KLINGE B. A systematic review of the incidence of biological and technical complications in implant dentistry reported in prospective longitudinal studies of at least 5 years. *J Periodont* 2002;**29**:197–212.

172. SNAUWAERT K, DUYCK J, VAN STEENBERGHE D, QUIRYNEN M, NAERT I. Time dependent failure rate and marginal bone loss of implant supported prostheses: a 15-year follow-up. *Clin Oral Invest* 2000;**4**:13–20.

173. DUYCK J, NAERT I. Failure of oral implants: aetiology, symptoms and influencing factors. *Clin Oral Invest* 1998;**2**:102–14.

174. BELSER UC, SCHMID B, HIGGINBOTTOM F, BUSER D. Outcome analysis of implant restorations located in the anterior maxilla: review of the recent literature. *Int J Oral Maxillofac Implants* 2004;**19**(Suppl):30–42.

175. LAMBERT PM, MORRIS HF, OCHI S. The influence of smoking on 3-year clinical success of osseointegrated dental implants. *Ann Periodontol* 2005;**5**:79–89.

176. ORENSTEIN IH, PETRAZZUOLO V, MORRIS H, OCHI S. Variables affecting survival of single tooth hydroxyapatite-coated implants in anterior maxillae at 3 years. *Ann Periodontol* 2000;**5**:68–78.

177. MORRIS HF, OCHI S, WINKLER S. Implant survival in patients with type 2 diabetes: placement to 36 months. *Ann Periodontol* 2000;**5**:157–65.

178. WEYANT RJ, BURT BA. An assessment of survival rates and within-patient clustering of failures for endosseous oral implants. *J Dent Res* 1993;**72**:2–8.

179. VAN STEENBERGHE D, BOLENDER C, HENRY P, HIGUCHI K, LINDÉN U. The applicability of osseointegrated oral implants in the rehabilitation of partial edentulism: a prospective multicenter study on 558 fixtures. *Int J Oral Maxillofac Implants* 1990;**5**:272–81.

180. SHIMPUKU H, NOSAKA Y, KAWAMURA T, TACHI Y, SHINOHARA M, OHURA K. Genetic polymorphisms of the interleukin-1 gene and early marginal bone loss

around endosseous dental implants. *Clin Oral Implants Res* 2003;**14**:423–9.

181. FELOUTZIS A, LANG NP, TONETTI MS, et al. IL-1 gene polymorphism and smoking as risk factors for peri-implant bone loss in a well-maintained population. *Clin Oral Implants Res* 2003;**14**:10–17.

182. GRUICA B, WANG HY, LANG NP, BUSER D. Impact of IL-1 genotype and smoking status on the prognosis of osseointegrated implants. *Clin Oral Implants Res* 2004;**15**:393–400.

183. JAFFIN RA, BERMAN C. The excessive loss of Brånemark fixtures in type IV bone: a 5-year analysis. *J Periodontol* 1991;**62**:2–4.

184. HUTTON JE, HEATH MR, CHAI JY, HARNETT J, JEMT T, JOHNS RB, et al. Factors related to success and failure rates at 3-year follow-up in a multicenter study of overdentures supported by Brånemark implants. *Int J Oral Maxillofac Implants* 1995;**10**:33–42.

185. TRUHLAR R, MORRIS HF, OCHI S. Implant surface coating and bone quality-related survival outcomes through 36 months post-placement of root form endosseous dental implants. *Ann Periodontol* 2000;**5**:109–18.

186. STACH RM, KOHLES SS. A meta-analysis examining the clinical survivability of machine-surfaced and osseotite implants in poor-quality bone. *Implant Dent* 2003;**12**:87–96.

187. FRIBERG B, JEMT T, LEKHOLM U. Early failures in 4641 Brånemark implants. *Int J Oral Maxillofac Implants* 1991;**6**:142–6.

188. KHANG W, FELDMAN S, HAWLEY CE, GUNSOLLEY J. A multicenter study comparing dual acid-etched and machined-surfaced implants in various bone qualities. *J Periodontol* 2001;**72**:1384–90.

189. KAROUSSIS IK, SALVI GE, HEITZ-MAYFIELD LJA, BRÄGGER U, HÄMMERLE CHF, LANG NP. Long-term implant prognosis in patients with and without a history of chronic periodontitis: a 10-year prospective cohort study of the ITI® Dental Implant System. *Clin Oral Implants Res* 2003;**14**:329–39.

190. HARDT CRE, GRÖNDAHL K, LEKHOLM U, WENNSTRÖM JL. Outcome of implant therapy in relation to experienced loss of periodontal bone support. A retrospective 5-year study. *Clin Oral Implants Res* 2002;**13**:488–94.

191. LAMBERT PM, MORRIS HF, OCHI S. Positive effect of surgical experience with implants on second-stage implant survival. *J Oral Maxillofac Surg* 1997;**55**: 12–18.

192. BOION LT, PENAUD J, MILLER N. A meta-analytic, quantitative assessment of osseointegration establishment and evolution of submerged and non-submerged endosseous titanium oral implants. *Clin Oral Implants Res* 2001;**12**:579–88.

193. ESPOSITO M, HIRSCH JM, LEKHOLM U, THOMSEN P. Biological factors contributing to failures of osseointegrated oral implants. II Etiopathogenesis. *Eur J Oral Sci* 1998;**106**:721–64.

194. ESPOSITO M, WORTHINGTON HV, COULTHARD P. *Interventions for replacing missing teeth: different times for loading dental implants.* The Cochrane Library Issue 1, 2004. Chichester: John Wiley & Sons, Ltd.

195. ISIDOR F. *Occlusal loading in implant dentistry.* Proceedings of the 3rd European Workshop on Periodontology and Implant Dentistry, 1999.

196. ISIDOR F. Loss of osseointegration caused by occlusal load of oral implants. A clinical and radiographic study in monkeys. *Clinical Oral Implants Res* 1996;**7**:143–52.

197. ISIDOR F. Histological evaluation of peri-implant bone at implants subjected to occlusal overload or plaque accumulation. *Clinical Oral Implants Res* 1997;**8**:1–9.

198. RANGERT B, ENG M, KROGH PHJ, LANGER B, ROEKEL NV. Bending overload and implant fracture: a retrospective clinical analysis. *Int J Oral Maxillofac Implants* 1995;**10**:326–34.

199. LORENZONI M, PERTL C, ZHANG K, WIMMER G, WEGSCHEIDER WA. Immediate loading of single-tooth implants in the anterior maxilla. Preliminary results after one year. *Clin Oral Implants Res* 2003;**14**:180–7.

200. LORENZONI M, PERTL C, ZHANG K, WEGSCHEIDER WA. In-patient comparison of immediately loaded and non-loaded implants within 6 months. *Clin Oral Implants Res* 2003;**14**:273–9.

201. CHAUSHU G, CHAUSHU S, TZOHAR A, DAYAN D. Immediate loading of single-tooth implants: immediate versus non-immediate implantation. A clinical report. *Int J Oral Maxillofac Implants* 2001;**16**:267–72.

202. LEKHOLM U. The Brånemark implant technique: a standardized procedure under continuous development. In: Laney WR, Tolman DE, eds. *Tissue integration in oral, orthopedic and maxillofacial reconstruction.* Chicago: Quintessence, 1990.

203. VAN STEENBERGHE D, JACOBS R, DESNYDER M, MAFFAEI G, QUIRYNEN M. The relative impact of local and endogenous patient-related factors on implant failure up to the abutment stage. *Clin Oral Implants Res* 2002;**13**:617–22.

204. WINKLER S, MORRIS H, OCHI S. Implant survival to 36 months as related to length and diameter. *Ann Periodontal* 2000;**5**:22–31.

205. ANDERSEN E, SAXEGAARD E, KNUTSEN BM, HAANAES HR. A prospective clinical study evaluating the safety and effectiveness of narrow-diameter threaded implants in the anterior region of the maxilla. *Int J Oral Maxillofac Implants* 2001;**16**:217–24.

206. COCHRAN DL. A comparison of endosseous dental implant surfaces. *J Periodontol* 1999;**70**:1523–39.

207. ALBREKTSSON T, SENNERBY L. Letters to the editor. *J Periodontol* 2000;**71**:1054–6.

208. WENNSTRÖM JL, EKESTUBBE A, GRÖNDAHL K, KARLSSON S, LINDE J. Oral rehabilitation with implant-supported fixed partial dentures in periodontitis-susceptible subjects. A 5-year prospective study. *J Clin Periodontol* 2004;**31**:713–24.

209. JUNGNER M, LUNDQUIST P, LUNDGREN S. Oxidized titanium implants (Nobel Biocare® TiUnite™) compared with turned titanium implants (Nobel Biocare® Mark III™) with respect to implant failure in a group of consecutive patients treated with early functional loading and two-stage protocol. *Clin Oral Implants Res* 2005;**16**:308–12.

210. ESPOSITO M, COULTHARD P, THOMSEN P, WORTHINGTON HV. The role of implant surface modifications, shape and material on the success of osseointegrated dental

implants. A Cochrane systematic review. *Eur J Prosthodont Restor Dent* 2005;**13**:15–31.

211. LEKHOLM U, WANNFORS K, ISAKSSON S, ADIELSSON B. Oral implants in combination with bone grafts. A 3-year retrospective multicenter study using the Brånemark implant system. *Int J Oral Maxillofac Surg* 1999;**28**:181–7.

212. ESPOSITO M, COULTHARD P, OLIVER R, THOMSEN P, WORTHINGTON HV. *Antibiotics to prevent complications following dental implant treatment (Cochrane Review).* The Cochrane Library, Issue 1, 2004. Chichester: John Wiley & Sons, Ltd.

213. LAMBERT PM, MORRIS HF, OCHI S. The influence of 0.12% chlorhexidine digluconate rinses on the incidence of infectious complications and implant success. *J Oral Maxillofac Surg* 1997;**55**:25–30.

214. FRIBERG B, JEMT T, LEKHOLM U. Early failure in 4641 conceedutively placed Brånemark dental implants: a study from stage 1 surgery of the connection of completed protheses. *Int J Oral Maxillofac Implants* 1991;**6**:142–6.

215. GOMEZ-ROMAN G. Influence of flap design on peri-implant interproximal crestal bone loss around single-tooth implants. *Int J Oral Maxillofac Implants* 2001;**16**:61–7.

216. DE BRUYN H, LINDEN U, COLLAERT B, BJORN AL. Quality of fixed restorative treatment on Brånemark implants. A 3-year follow-up study in private dental practices. *Clin Oral Implants Res* 2002;**13**:359–64.

217. VERMYLEN K, COLLAERT B, LINDEN U, BJORN AL, DE BRUYN H. Patient satisfaction and quality of single-tooth restorations. *Clin Oral Implants Res* 2003;**14**:119–24.

218. LEVI A, PSOTER WJ, AGAR JR, REISINE ST, TAYLOR TD. Patient self-reported satisfaction with maxillary anterior dental implant treatment. *Int J Oral Maxillofac Implants* 2003;**18**:113–20.

219. WEST W, LANGER L, KARABIN S, GRBIC V, BUDASOFF D, GOTTEGEN R, et al. Letter to the editor. *J Periodontol* 2000:**71**;1051–3.

220. BECKER W, BAHAT O, ISRAELSON H. Letter to the editor. *J Periodontol* 2000:**71**;1053–4.

221. BELSER UC, BERNHARD JP, BUSER D. Implant-supported restorations in the anterior region: prosthetic considerations. *Pract Periodontics Aesthet Dent* 1996;**8**:875–83.

222. HERMANN JS, BUSER D, SCHENK RK, COCHRAN DK. Crestal bone changes around titanium implants. A histometric evaluation of unloaded nonsubmerged and submerged implants in the canine mandible. *J Periodontol* 2000;**71**:1412–24.

223. SCHOU S, HOLMSTRUP P, WORTHINGTON HV, ESPOSITO M. Outcome of implant therapy in patients with previous tooth loss due to periodontitis: a systematic review. *Clin Oral Implants Res* 2006;**17**(Suppl. 1):104–23.

# 29

# Esthetic Considerations in Restoring the Traumatized Dentition: a Biologic Approach

B. U. Zachrisson & S. Toreskog

One of the most challenging problems in dental traumatology is the choice of treatment for replacement of one or more maxillary incisors that have been lost as a result of traumatic injuries. The task is to restore optimal function and esthetics; the latter effect especially is seldom reached today.

In order to produce an optimal treatment result, it is frequently necessary to utilize the combined efforts of a multidisciplinary team of experts, representing orthodontics, prosthodontics, periodontics, oral surgery and dental technology. By using the skills of such a team, the beauty and function of the natural dentition can sometimes be recreated, a fact that can have a significant psychological impact upon a previous trauma victim (see Chapter 6).

The problem of recreating esthetics and function varies significantly according to the *age* of the patient, the trauma *location*, and the *extent* of the traumatic injury. These three factors will be considered in this chapter. Furthermore, a minimally invasive porcelain laminate veneer and onlay technique will be presented, with the main emphasis on restoring teeth after crown fractures.

## Replacement of a missing maxillary central incisor

Several options are available for the treatment of accidentally lost maxillary central incisors in children and adults. This is the most challenging treatment situation in dental traumatology. In the maxillary anterior region there is a maximum demand for an esthetically satisfactory solution that mimics the contralateral non-injured incisor. Any flaws in the appearance of the replacement can easily be seen by a comparison of the anatomy and color of the two adjacent teeth.

The situation generally calls for cooperation among orthodontist, restorative dentist, endodontist and oral surgeon. The armamentarium used by these specialists may include the following techniques:

- Individualized orthodontic extrusion and intrusion to create optimal alveolar bone and gingival contours (1)
- Localized simple minor surgeries (2)

- Use of ultra-thin porcelain veneers and new hybrid resins for build-ups on mesially repositioned teeth or transplanted premolars (1)
- Vital bleaching of selected teeth (e.g. for canines that have been moved mesially to the position of the lateral incisors)
- Incisal edge contouring
- Reshaping of mesially repositioned canines by grinding (3–5)
- Mesio-distal stripping to solve problems with crowding, interdental gingival recession ('black triangles'), and tooth size discrepancies between the maxillary and mandibular dentition (1, 6).

Basically, there are 4 ways of replacing lost central incisors:

- Orthodontic space closure
- Premolar autotransplantation
- Placement of a single-tooth implant
- Conventional or cantilever bridge-work.

Each of these options will be briefly discussed below.

## Orthodontic space closure treatment

The movement of the entire lateral segment mesially with the lateral incisor replacing the missing central incisor is indicated when there is a concomitant malocclusion that has to be corrected by orthodontic means. The result of orthodontic space closure is rarely ideal, but the use of several techniques adopted from esthetic dentistry, coupled with careful orthodontic treatment, may provide an outcome that approximates that of a natural dentition (Fig. 29.1) (6–8). This is a biologic approach with good long-term prognosis (7).

The primary concern in order to obtain a satisfactory esthetic result with space closure is a good alignment of the long axis of the lateral incisor (8), and to secure an adequate width along the gingival margin of the replacement porcelain laminate veneer bonded onto the lateral incisor (Fig. 29.1) (7). It is also emphasized that the canine, now placed in the lateral incisor location, and the first premolar in the canine position, normally need correction of their anatomy and axial inclination (torque), and frequently adjustment of

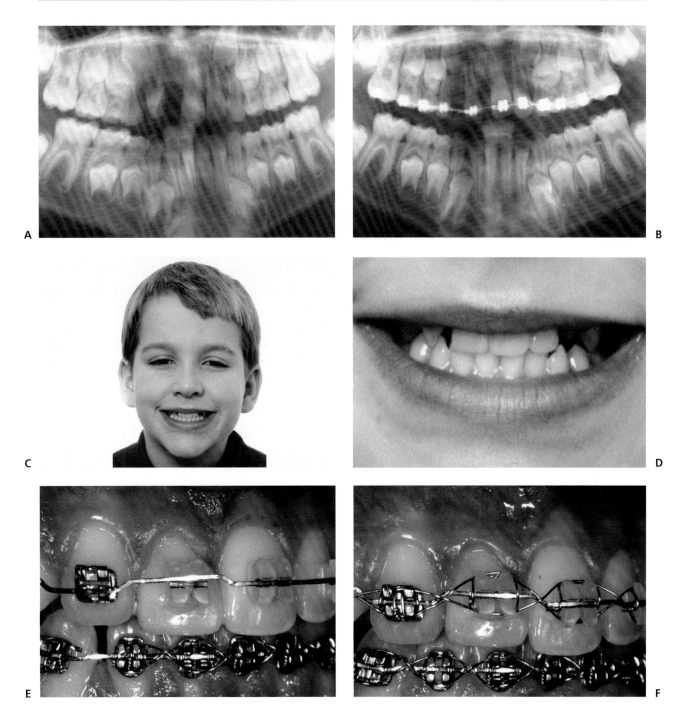

**Fig. 29.1** Orthodontic space closure combined with minimally invasive esthetic dentistry to replace maxillary right central incisor after traumatic accident in 8-year-old boy. Radiographic and clinical appearance is given in A–D. The lateral incisor was moved mesially to the midline with push-coil. Marginal gingival leveling was made by intrusion of lateral incisor, extrusion of the canine, and intrusion of the first premolar, respectively (E–H). The lateral incisor was restored to central incisor shape by a porcelain laminate veneer (I, J). The canine was restored to lateral incisor morphology by grinding and a hybrid composite 'corner' mesially. The first premolar was intruded orthodontically and built-up incisally with hybrid composite (J). Note naturally looking dentition with good occlusal interdigitation and good axial inclinations of all teeth after treatment (K, L). (*continues overleaf*)

the color. By extruding the canine during the orthodontic treatment, the gingival margin is moved in an incisal direction, and the incisal portion can be ground with diamond burs to lateral incisor shape (4, 5). Sometimes a composite resin mesial 'corner' is useful to obtain better lateral incisor morphology. The first premolar should be intruded to move the gingival margin in an apical direction, and be built up incisally with a hybrid composite resin (1) (Fig. 29.1).

Color differences between canines and incisors may vary. The canines are usually more yellowish and/or darker than the incisors, accentuating the contrast between the maxillary central incisors and the 'new' lateral incisors (1). The color difference can be handled by in-office or at-home vital bleaching of single teeth (see below).

The crown torque difference between canines and lateral incisors, and the marked individual variation in crown torque of maxillary canines, must be taken into account and

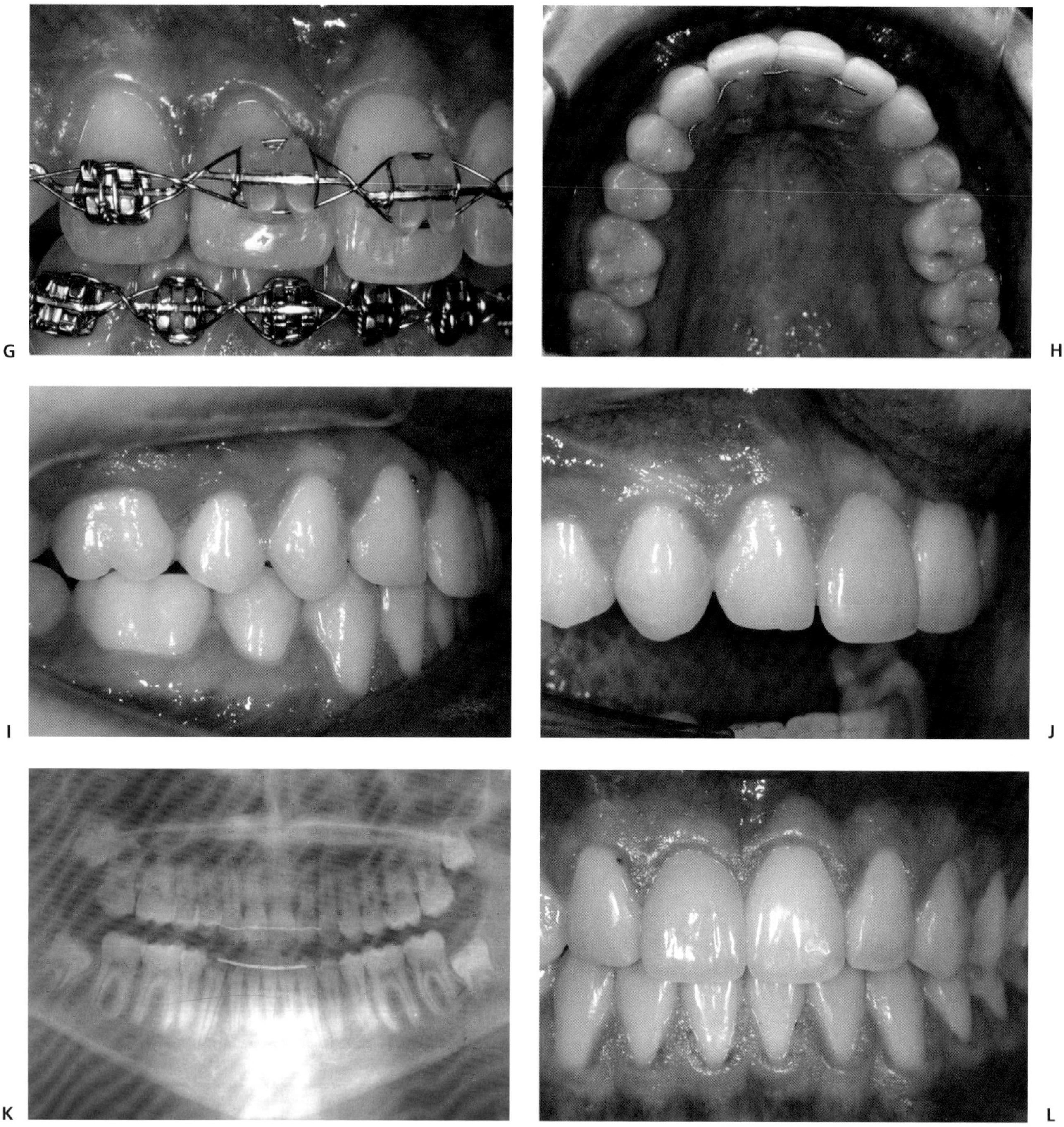

**Fig. 29.1** (*cont.*)

corrected. In a follow-up study 10 years after orthodontic treatment of space closure cases where the canines had been moved mesially to replace the lateral incisors, the most common mistake was inadequate crown torque of the mesially relocated canines (5). The lateral incisors normally have labial crown inclination, whereas the canines most often have a lingual crown inclination. If the crown torque of a canine that has been moved mesially is not corrected, the 'new' lateral incisor will not look natural (5, 6).

There is usually a marked tendency for spaces to reopen in the maxillary anterior region after orthodontic space closure and conventional retention with removable plates or splints. For this reason, the retention of space closure cases

must not be taken lightly. We recommend long-term (10 years or more) or even permanent retention with lingually bonded multistranded wire retainers over 6 teeth, combined with a removable plate to be used continuously for the first 6 months and then at night (1).

## Keys to esthetically optimal treatment

### Set-ups

A diagnostic set-up on plaster models can identify the tooth-size problems and the amount of crown reshaping that will be needed. It is also advisable to make a pictorial set-up with the patient smiling and/or speaking (1). This will allow the clinician to focus on the crucial aspects of the tooth display – the relationship between teeth, gingiva and lips – and make it age- and sex-related (9–11). The 'visual set-up' procedure is helpful in planning any intrusion and extrusion of different teeth that is needed to obtain normal relationships for the marginal gingival contours. The central incisors and the 'new' canine (i.e. first premolar) should have the gingival margins at the same level, with the 'lateral incisor' (canine) at a more incisal level (Fig. 29.1), to provide a natural exposure of the gingiva on smiling. This usually implies that the canines have to be extruded and the first premolars be intruded during the orthodontic treatment (Fig. 29.1A, B, D). Because the canines are thicker buccolingually than the lateral incisors, their extrusion should be coupled with moving them labially, increasing their lingual root torque, and grinding their incisal and lingual surfaces.

## Cosmetic contouring of canines to simulate lateral incisors

As demonstrated in 1970 by Tuverson (3), it is possible to recontour a canine to almost an ideal lateral incisor shape by grinding with diamond instruments. Iatrogenic effects of grinding, such as increased sensitivity to hot and cold, and other pulp and dentin reactions, can be prevented with careful attention to adequate cooling (4) with abundant water and air spray, and preparation of smooth and self-cleansing surfaces (4, 5). When this technique is used, no harmful pulp or dentin reactions have been observed, even with extensive grinding and incisal dentin exposure. Gross recontouring can be done in one session at the start of orthodontic treatment, with the fine tuning delayed until the end of treatment, if necessary. Since the labial enamel of canines may be thin in the gingival parts, it may be safer to avoid flattening of the labial surfaces of canines and accept a somewhat more rounded labial shape than what is seen on natural lateral incisors. The mesiodistal dimension can also be reduced, particularly on the the distal surface, which may be too convex compared to a lateral incisor. The mesial margins can be corrected with composite resin 'corners' (1). Mesial and incisal build-ups are relatively easy to make with one of the new hybrid resin restorative materials. They will effectively conceal the difference in morphology between first premolars, canines, and lateral incisors (Fig. 29.1).

With the use of esthetic porcelain laminate veneers, it is possible to recontour mesially relocated premolars and canines into, respectively, 'normal' canine and lateral incisor shapes (Figs 29.1 and 29.2). Porcelain veneers on the first premolars and canines are more expensive than grinding and resin build-ups, but compare favorably with the cost of restorations on single-tooth implants or conventional composite restorations with their short life-span (see Chapter 25).

## Surgical crown lengthening

When orthodontic space closure is performed in young patients, the marginal gingiva around the mesially moved canine may sometimes become hyperplastic, which can significantly reduce its crown length. A simple localized gingivectomy to the bottom of the clinical pocket will increase the crown length. The same procedure can be used on the first premolar moved into the canine position. As shown in humans, nearly 50% of the excised tissue will regenerate and become indistinguishable from normal gingiva (2). This means, for example, that if the labial probing pocket depth on the canine is 4 mm, a permanent gain of 2 mm in crown length can be anticipated. Electrosurgery and diode soft tissue laser can be used, but are no more effective than using a scalpel. Even if the excision is extended into the alveolar mucosa, the coronal part of the regenerated gingiva will still become keratinized (12). Careful oral hygiene procedures, using single-tufted brushes, are required for 2 months after the gingivectomy so that the regenerated gingiva will appear entirely normal (2).

If a greater crown length increase than 50% of the probing depth is wanted, a surgical flap must be raised, and bone recontouring should be made to about 3 mm away from the desired future gingival margin (13).

## Whitening (vital bleaching of the translocated canine)

The problem of a relocated canine being more yellowish than the intact lateral incisor can be solved reasonably easy and predictably with either at-home or in-office vital bleaching procedures (14–16) (see Chapter 33). It is generally agreed in esthetic dentistry that yellow discolorations are the easiest to improve. Nocturnal use of 10% hydrogen peroxide gel in a tray is a convenient way of bleaching teeth (14). If only one canine is to be whitened, the bleaching gel is injected only into the canine reservoir. In-office bleaching with stronger gel concentrations may sometimes be preferable for single teeth (15). Recent evidence indicates that the clinical use of light and/or heat during in-office bleaching does not make teeth lighter than with bleach alone, once the teeth have rehydrated for 2 to 5 days following treatment (16).

## Conclusion

Orthodontic space closure with the lateral incisor replacing the missing central incisor, and mesial movement of the entire lateral segment, may be a good option for treatment of patients who have traumatically lost a maxillary central incisor. This treatment alternative is particularly indicated when there is a concomitant malocclusion that has to be corrected by orthodontic means. The use of several techniques adopted from esthetic dentistry, together with careful orthodontic treatment, may provide an outcome that approximates the looks of a natural dentition (Fig. 29.1G–K). This biologic approach has a good long-term prognosis, when bonded lingual retainers are used to maintain the treatment outcome.

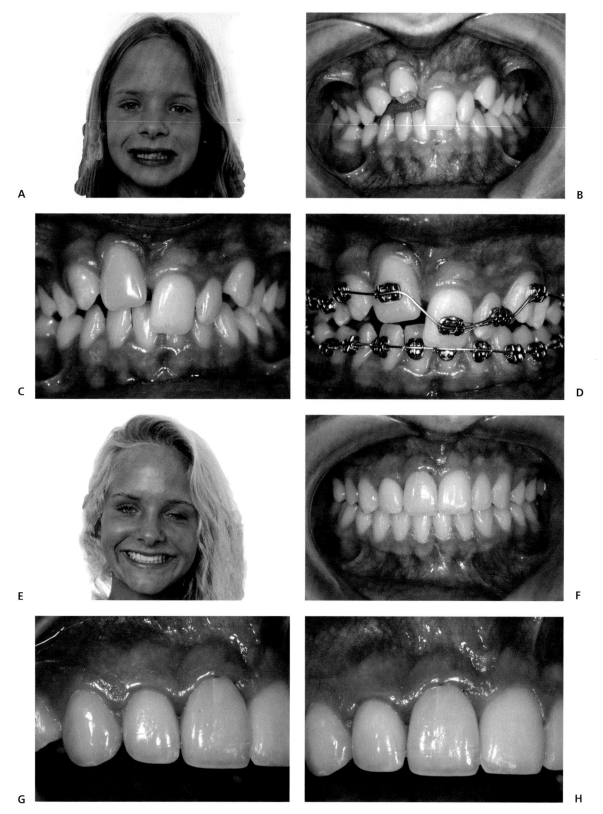

**Fig. 29.2** Autotransplantation of mandibular right second premolar to region in maxilla where both the right lateral and central incisors were lost in traumatic injury (A, B). The premolar crown was restored initially with composite resin (C). Orthodontic treatment was performed to close all spaces, upright the teeth, and level the gingival margins (D). Clinical result after orthodontic treatment and three porcelain laminate veneers shows an almost natural dentition (E–H). Note the change in axial inclinations of the canines and premolars (compare C and F) to broaden the smile. During treatment, the canine to replace the lateral incisor was extruded, and the first premolar to replace the canine was intruded, in order to level the gingival margins before the ultrathin porcelain veneers were made.

## Autotransplantation of premolars

Over 40 years ago, Slagsvold and Bjercke (17) developed a method of transplanting teeth with partly formed roots. After transplantation, root growth continues, and the teeth maintain their capacity for functional adaptation, and endodontic treatment is usually not necessary. Since then, a series of investigations have supported these findings (see Chapter 27). With regard to graft selection, mandibular premolars appear to be optimal for transplantation to the maxillary incisor region (Figs 29.2 and 29.3) (see Chapter 27). The optimal time for autotransplantation of premolars to the maxillary anterior region is when the root development has reached two-thirds to three-quarters of the final root length. The prognosis for complete periodontal healing at this stage of root development is better than 90% (17, 18). Patients suited for autotransplantation of premolars to the maxillary anterior region are about 9 to 12 years of age, which corresponds with the period when most serious traumatic injuries occur in children. It is remarkable that tooth transplants have inherent potential for bone induction (6, 17) and reestablishment of a normal alveolar process (Figs 29.2 and 29.3).

### Long-term survival and success rates

The long term outcome of tooth transplantation, including gingival and periodontal conditions, was examined in a recent study from the University of Oslo (19). Patient's attitudes about treatment and outcome was also evaluated. The follow-up period for 33 transplanted premolars ranged from 17 to 41 years, with a mean of 26.4 years. Both the survival (teeth still present at the examination) and success (teeth fulfilling defined success criteria) rates were high – 90% and 79%, respectively. The patients generally responded favorably regarding their perception of the treatment. The study showed that autotransplantation of teeth with partly formed roots compares favorably in a long-term perspective with other treatment modalities for substituting missing teeth.

### Orthodontic and restorative treatment for autotransplanted premolars

Because the root of an autotransplanted premolar continues to develop and a normal periodontal ligament is established, such teeth can be moved orthodontically like any other tooth that has erupted into occlusion (20–22). It is generally recommended to wait for an observation period of 3–4 months before orthodontic treatment is started. Premolar crowns can be reshaped to resemble incisor morphology (Figs 29.2 and 29.3). A direct composite resin build-up can be performed and later replaced with a porcelain laminate veneer (PLV) (Fig. 29.2). There are some drawbacks with the composite resin build-ups because it is difficult to establish normal incisor width along the gingival margin, and the build-ups tend to get a triangular crown form (Fig. 29.2C, D). Furthermore, some composite resins tend to discolor

with time. Both problems can be solved by using thin PLVs instead (Fig. 29.2E–H). The 2 main reasons to avoid cemented crowns in children and adolescents – that the large pulp chambers limit preparation and that the gingival retraction over time could lead to unesthetic root display – are not valid for PLVs. The reflection of light will not be stopped by an enamel-bonded PLV, and any later root exposure will display a normal color and no darkening of the gingiva (Fig. 29.3M, N).

In a recent study, 45 premolars autotransplanted to the maxillary incisor region in 40 adolescent patients were evaluated, after restoration, with a mean observation period of 4 years (20). Mean age at surgery was 11 years. Clinical criteria assessed tooth mobility, plaque and gingival conditions, probing pocket depths, and reaction to percussion. The interproximal gingival papilla fill was assessed according to an index. Pathosis, pulp obliteration, root length, and crown-root ratios were studied on standardized radiographs. The result showed that the clinical variables for transplants did not differ from those of the natural incisors, except for some increased mobility and more plaque in a few transplanted premolars (20, 21). The interproximal gingival papilla adjacent to all transplanted teeth were normal or slightly hyperplastic, and no interdental gingival recesssion (black triangles) were seen.

### Esthetic outcome and patient satisfaction

A comprehensive study comparing the esthetics of 22 autotransplanted premolars reshaped to incisor morphology with their natural, intact, contralateral incisor was made (21). Features considered important for esthetics (color, soft tissue appearance, tooth morphology and position) were compared. Most of the transplanted teeth matched the contralateral incisor, and most patients were satisfied with the appearance of the transplant. The distribution in set categories assessed professionally and by the patient was not significantly different. However, the color and the gingival width of the transplanted tooth were scored as different from the natural incisor when the restorations were made with composite resin. Thus, the findings demonstrated that interdisciplinary treatment planning is important for successful esthetic results and that porcelain laminate veneers rather than composite build-ups should be used for restoration of the crowns (Figs 29.2 and 29.3).

### Conclusion

Premolar autotransplantation represents an attractive, and maybe the best, solution to difficult treatment planning problems when a maxillary incisor is traumatically lost in young patients (Fig. 29.2). The transplanted tooth represents a normal root with normal periodontal membrane, and it can be moved orthodontically like any other natural tooth. The 'abnormal' crown should be restored with a porcelain veneer. Transplantation represents a biologic approach in which the transplanted tooth germ retains the potential to induce alveolar bone growth.

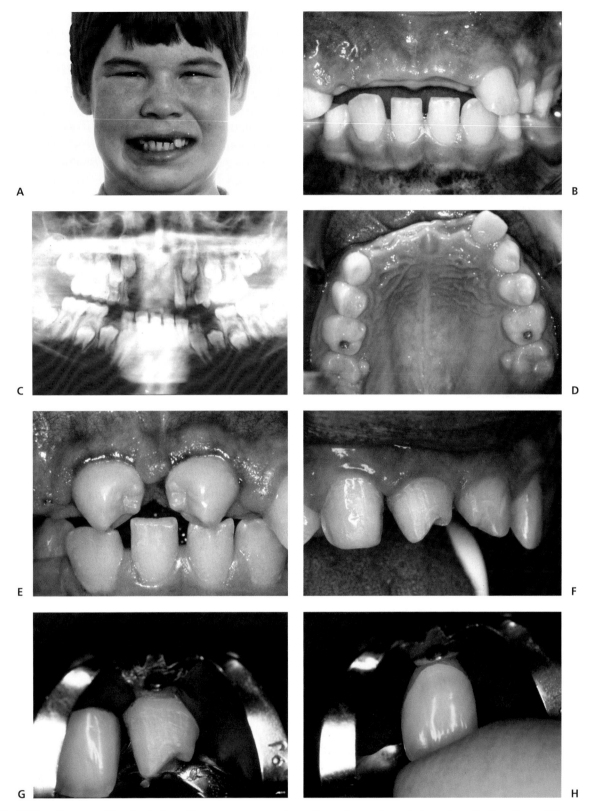

**Fig. 29.3** Replacement of three lost incisors with two autotransplanted premolars and space closure in the canine region in a 10-year-old boy due to trauma. Note the loss of horizontal bone in the trauma region (B–D). E–H. Premolar transplantation and restoration. Two mandibular premolars were transplanted to the central incisor region and later restored with porcelain laminate veneer crowns. The canine was orthodontically moved into the lateral incisor region and restored in the same way.

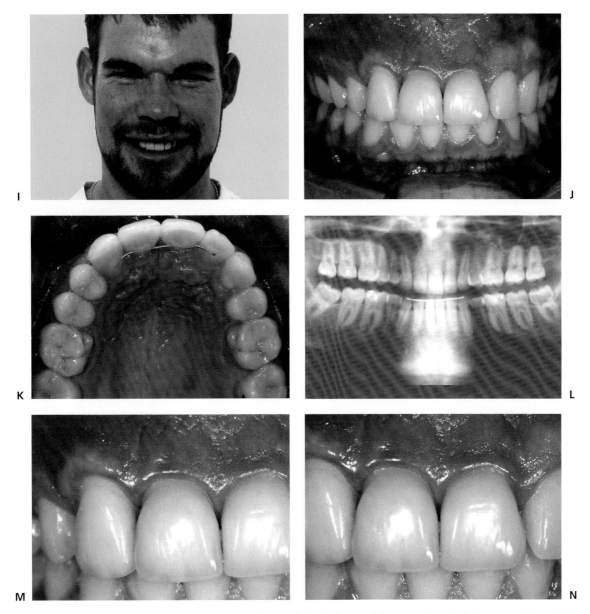

**Fig. 29.3** (*cont.*) I–L. Clinical result after 12 years. Note optimal shape of alveolar bone and dental arch form (J, K) (compare with the clinical situation before restoration, B, D). M, N. Clinical result after 14 years. The gingival recessions that occurred show a natural appearance, since the thin veneers reflect light like intact teeth. There is no darkening effect along the exposed root surfaces.

## Single-tooth implants

Within the last 2 decades, the use of osseointegrated implants to replace missing incisors has become a common treatment solution for patients 20 years of age and older (see Chapter 28). Experience gained to date with single-tooth implants is favorable, with survival rates of about 90% after 10 years in multicenter studies. However, filling an anterior space with an implant-supported porcelain crown is a major challenge from both the esthetic and functional aspects (Chapter 28, p. 767). Clinical success depends not only on persisting osseointegration but also on harmonious integration of the crown in the dental arch (Fig. 29.4).

Recent studies indicate that the esthetic result for single implants in the maxillary anterior region is sometimes suboptimal (23–26). There are several potential esthetic

problems associated with the long-term use of implant-supported crowns.

## Age changes in tooth position

An implant is, by definition, ankylosed and cannot change position, in contrast to the neighboring natural teeth. Occlusion over time is a result of developmental and adaptive processes in which facial growth, dynamic interrelationships between aging facial structures, dental eruption, function, tooth wear and orthodontic relapse can contribute (23). These processes show much individual variation throughout life (23, 26–28). Even small tooth movements after implant placement can cause esthetic problems (25, 26, 28). Complications like tooth-implant contact displacements after completed orthodontic treatment can also occur, for example as a consequence of unwanted tipping of neigh-

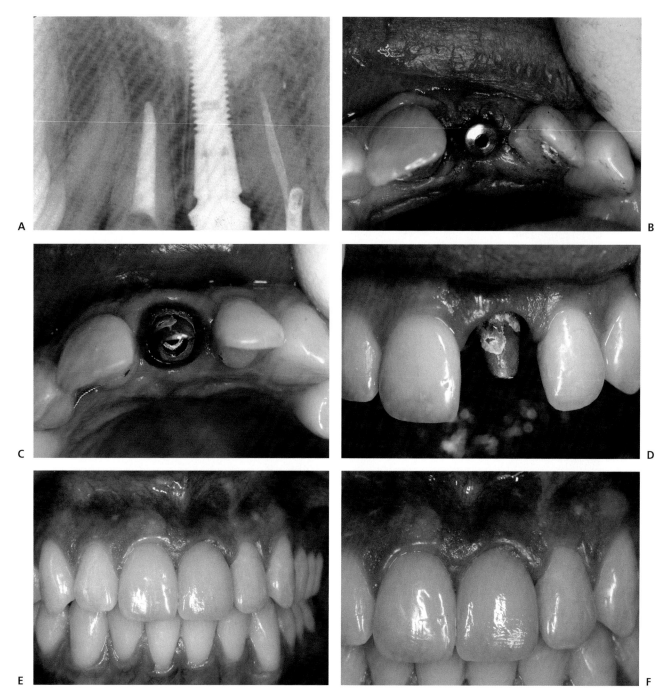

**Fig. 29.4** Implant-supported porcelain crown used to replace a central incisor. A 24-year-old female patient has, due to trauma, lost a left maxillary central incisor. A, B. Condition immediately after implant insertion. C, D. Sculpting the gingiva. By the use of a temporary crown the labial and interdental gingivae have been optimally reshaped. E, F. A good esthetic result has been achieved; however, there is a slight reduction in the height of the distal papilla.

boring teeth after retention (23). A recent study from the University of Geneva documented clinical infraocclusion of implant-borne restorations not only in a group of young adults (15–21 years) but also in most of the patients in a group of mature adults between 40 and 55 years of age (26).

## Gingival recession and dark margins along porcelain crowns

An implant-supported crown placed in a young adult should be expected to have a long life. During this time, which might span 60 or more years, the marginal and interdental gingival

tissue surrounding the implant crown is unlikely to remain unchanged. Gingival recession might occur due to overzealous toothbrushing or to periodontal disease in adult and elderly patients. Gingival recession may result in a darkening effect along the exposed implant crown.

## Lack of gingival papilla fill, probing depths, and bleeding

The difficulties in obtaining natural marginal gingival contours around implant-supported porcelain crowns is partly a result of the relationship between implants and the bone and gingiva surrounding them. The reduction in osseous scallop from facial to interproximal areas and lack of difference in gingival heights above bone from facial to interproximal, compared with those of natural teeth, may lead to a flat gingival form (29). In 2 studies comparing the soft tissue characteristics of implant-supported single-tooth crowns and their contralateral natural teeth in the esthetic zone of the maxilla (24, 30), it was demonstrated that most implant crowns displayed some lack of interdental papilla fill, particularly on the distal papilla (Fig. 29.4). Such 'dark triangles' between teeth are rarely, if ever, observed with orthodontic space closure treatment (7) or after premolar autotransplantation (20–22, 31). In addition, implant crowns have more mucositis/gingivitis, increased probing depths, and more bleeding on probing (24) than natural teeth.

## Buccal alveolar bone loss and gingival discoloration

In an award-winning 10-year follow-up study by Thilander et al. (23) of implant-supported crowns replacing maxillary incisors, some patients showed progressive loss of marginal bone support at the buccal aspects of the implant. The ongoing buccal bone resorption resulted in discolored soft tissue, gingival retraction, or a denuded implant due to vigorous toothbrushing. The buccal bone plate in the incisor region is often very thin. Sometimes resorption can occur even when the implant had sufficient alveolar bone support at time of placement (32).

## Conclusion

The single-tooth implant may be a useful treatment option in adults when a maxillary central incisor has been accidentally lost. Implants should normally not be placed until the skeletal growth is completed. Careful procedures, including gingival sculpting with the provisional crown are needed to obtain adequate soft tissue thickness interdentally and labially (Fig. 29.4E, F). Independent recent studies indicate that the clinical long-term result for single implants replacing maxillary incisors is sometimes esthetically suboptimal. Extended long-term evaluations are needed.

## Fixed prosthetics

Although this treatment appears to have reasonably good long-term success (36), it has several shortcomings related to the common alveolar process atrophy in the trauma region. Furthermore, conventional abutment preparation may compromise the long-term esthetics (see Chapter 26). Fixed prosthetics appears today not to be an attractive treatment option in young patients.

## Replacement of a missing maxillary lateral incisor

The cause for absence of the maxillary lateral incisor may be traumatic loss of the tooth or congenital agenesis. This is a relatively frequent problem. Basically, there are four ways of replacing missing lateral incisors, namely *orthodontic space closure*, insertion of a *single implant* (directly, or after orthodontic space opening), *autotransplantation* of a developing premolar, or restoration with conventional or cantilever resin-bonded *bridge-work*. The longevity of these treatment solutions are described in Chapter 26. In the following, esthetic advantages or shortcomings will be described for these treatments.

## Orthodontic closure

When a maxillary canine is moved mesially to substitute for a missing lateral incisor, and the first premolar is used in place of the canine, the same esthetic problems occur as those discussed above for replacement of a missing central incisor. When careful orthodontic treatment procedures are combined with clinical techniques adapted from esthetic dentistry, the outcome with space closure can be very satisfying, and almost indistinguishable from a natural dentition (1, 3). Long-term periodontal and occlusal studies on congenitally missing lateral incisors have shown that space closure with premolar substitution for canines may lead to an acceptable functional relationship, with modified group function on the working side (33, 34).

In a recent study, the long-term result (mean 7 years after treatment) of prosthetic replacement of maxillary lateral incisors were compared with orthodontic space closure (34). The space closure patients were more satisfied with the treatment results than the prosthesis patients; there was no difference between the 2 groups in prevalence of signs and symptoms of temporomandibular joint (TMJ) dysfunction; and patients with prosthetic replacement had impaired periodontal health with accumulation of plaque and gingivitis. It was concluded that orthodontic space closure produced results that were well accepted by patients, did not impair TMJ function, and encouraged periodontal health in comparison with prosthetic replacement (34).

## Implants

Although this treatment solution is at present a popular option, it represents a considerable challenge from an esthetic point of view, particularly in the long-term perspective. An implant-supported crown placed in a young adult should have an expected life span of 60 or more years. It is difficult for dental technicians to make an implant-supported crown with optimal shade and translucency that blends perfectly with the neighboring teeth. In our experience, the color of a canine that has been moved mesially and vital-bleached (and/or restored with a thin translucent porcelain laminate veneer) frequently comes closer to that of adjacent teeth than the color of porcelain crowns on implants. Even in adults, the esthetic outcome of implant-supported crowns in the maxillary anterior region may sometimes lead to esthetic results that are less optimal than desired (23–26).

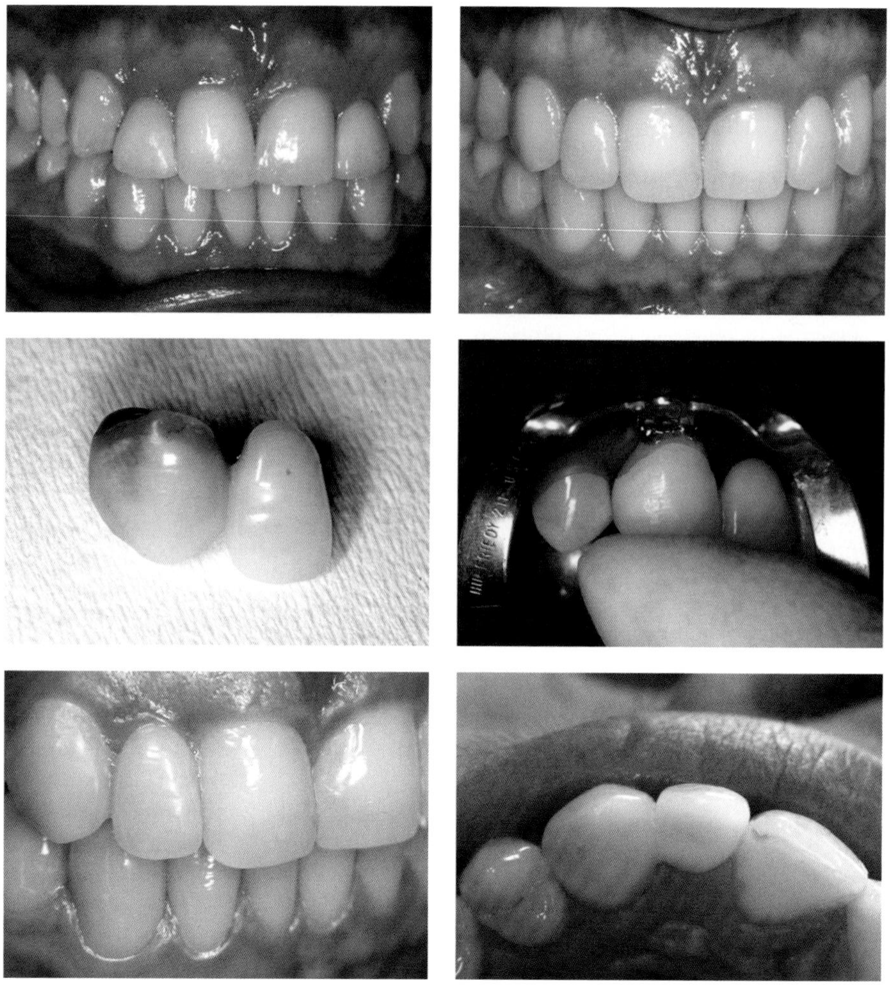

**Fig. 29.5** Cantilever fiber reinforced composite bridge. Patient with two existing unesthetic 3-unit Maryland bridges replacing congenitally missing upper laterals (A) and our substitute at 5 year follow up; two 2-unit cantilevered fiber reinforced (Stick Tech) bonded composite bridges (B). The shallow cervical preparation is illustrated by the translucency of the composite (C) as the blue cleaning acid is kept on the inside of the crown. The rubber dam placement exposes the bridge site plus the contact points of the adjacent teeth (D). Note also the cervical fit of the retainer on the prepared cuspid. The close up of the just bonded/cemented bridge shows the temporarily irritated gingiva (E) in comparison to the excellent gingival conditions, palatally as well as buccally, at the five year follow up (F).

## Autotransplants

Whereas premolar autotransplantation may represent the best treatment option for a lost maxillary central incisor in a young patient, it does not represent a common treatment choice for replacement of a missing lateral incisor. One of the reasons is that most premolars would normally be too wide mesiodistally, an exception being the mandibular first premolars. When selected, therefore, the transplantation generally is associated with some form of orthodontic treatment.

## Resin-bonded cantilever prosthetics

Since most maxillary lateral incisors are small teeth that take less load than the central incisors in occlusion and function, the use of recently introduced forms of fiber-reinforced resin-bonded cantilever prosthetics (35) represents an interesting esthetic treatment alternative for replacement of missing lateral incisors. Our clinical experience with this technique in the esthetic zone over the past few years is promising. Most commonly, we have used the canine as the abutment tooth, with a cantilever lateral incisor (Fig. 29.5). Since there are presently no translucent ceramic materials with adequate strength, we currently use a fiber-reinforced (Stick Tech®) indirect laboratory composite resin (Sinfony®,

3M ESPE Company) for the 2-unit bridge. Further clinical studies are needed to evaluate if such cantilever bridges can be used as a more permanent replacement for missing lateral incisors, compared with single tooth implants.

## Replacement of a canine

Because of the anatomy of the canines (massive crown and a long root), this tooth is rarely lost due to trauma (see Chapter 8). As for lost central and lateral incisors, the same 4 treatment solutions exist. In the following the esthetic considerations will be described for canine loss.

### Orthodontic closure

In these cases, a first premolar is moved mesially to replace the missing canine. Because of the shorter clinical crown length of the first premolar in comparison with the canine to be replaced (Fig. 29.3M), it is advisable to intrude the premolar and build it up incisally with hybrid composite resin (Fig. 29.1J) or a porcelain laminate veneer after treatment (Fig. 29.2E–H). For further details, see Zachrisson (37).

### Autotransplants

Mandibular premolars are very good candidates for transportation to replace maxillary canines, and due to their anatomy need little crown alteration. Necessary changes can be performed with either hybrid composite or porcelain laminates. Concerning the esthetic advantage of using transplants see p. 803.

### Implants

The esthetic problem using implants in the canine region is the same as for lateral incisors. However, the atrophy of the labial bone with related bluish gingival discoloration due to the implant is possibly even more marked in the canine location, due to the thin gingiva and the frequent gingival recessions often related to mechanical trauma (vigorous tooth brushing).

### Fixed prosthetics

The use of fixed prosthodontics to replace missing canines presents not only esthetic problems due to the common alveolar bone atrophy in the region (see Chapter 28), but also functional problems related to the canine location which imply a significant stress upon the tooth during articulation.

## Replacement after loss of multiple maxillary anterior teeth

Multiple losses of anterior teeth represent a significant increase in the number of esthetic problems. This is primarily due to the associated alveolar bone loss which may require both horizontal and vertical bone augmentation (see Chapter 28). Fortunately, in children the autotransplantation of developing premolars may induce alveolar bone growth and thus make it possible to restore the dental arch form using a combination of autotransplantation and orthodontic space closure after severe accidents with loss of several maxillary incisors. Fig. 29.4 shows such a case where 3 lost anterior teeth (2 central incisors and 1 lateral incisor) were reduced to two by orthodontic treatment, and where the 2 missing central incisors were replaced with autotransplanted mandibular premolars that received bonded porcelain veneer crowns. At a follow-up 14 years after treatment, satisfactory esthetic results are apparent. Despite considerable retraction of the marginal gingiva, there is no shadowing effect, and the exposed roots have a light and normal color.

In adults, a significant esthetic problem will occur when 2 implants are placed next to each other. In these instances, it is generally not possible to create a satisfactory gingival papilla between the two implants (29, 32), and an esthetic compromise has to be accepted (see Chapter 28, p. 771). One treatment principle to reduce this problem may be to combine orthodontic space closure and a surgical solution (e.g. implants).

## Restoring fractured teeth

Replacement of the tooth structure lost due to trauma provides both a practical and an ethical problem. How much more tooth substance can justifiably be removed in order to optimally restore the anatomy of the injured tooth? By tradition, it has been accepted in dentistry that removal of large amounts of healthy tissue is acceptable to restore an injured tooth esthetically and functionally. The main reason for this acceptance has been that the strength of various types of available restorations until recently have depended on the strength of the restoration as such. Consequently, it was necessary to design the remaining tooth substance in such a way that it favored the strength of the restoration rather than the strength of the tooth.

The conventional jacket crown preparation is a typical example, where the concept is to optimize the strength and survival of the porcelain crown without giving consideration to the biological drawbacks. Consequently, even after a minor injury, a fractured tooth would end up with a subgingivally located, circumferentially prepared 1.2 mm shoulder and a jacket crown as the permanent restoration. Still, even with these maximally invasive preparations, the fracture rate of the jacket crowns remained high (36).

In the late 1950s, the metal-ceramic concept was introduced and allowed fabrication of a crown that was both strong and esthetic. The metal-ceramic crown replaced the jacket crown as the permanent restoration for fractured incisors. However, the invasiveness of the preparation was not reduced. Therefore, the introduction of acrylic materials and, later, composite resins that could be bonded to enamel was welcome, since they made removal of healthy tooth substance obsolete. Acid etching of enamel became the retentive tool for tooth colored restorative materials, allowing a truly minimally invasive restorative technique. However, the composite build-ups did not represent a permanent restoration (see Chapter 25). The initial composite resin materials were weak, prone to wear, and they discolored extensively with time.

In 1983, Calamia and Simonsen (38) produced the idea of bonding thin pieces of porcelain to the labial part of a tooth – thus the porcelain laminate veneer concept was invented. By etching enamel with phosphoric acid and the inside of the porcelain veneer with hydrofluoric acid gel, it became possible to get enough micromechanical retention for a diluted composite material to bond to both sides, thus producing a strong veneered tooth. Later, the diluted composite resin was replaced with light cured composite cements (39, 40). This idea was effective, since only minimal reduction of tooth substance was necessary, and the preparation could thus be kept in enamel. Intact enamel provides the most reliable

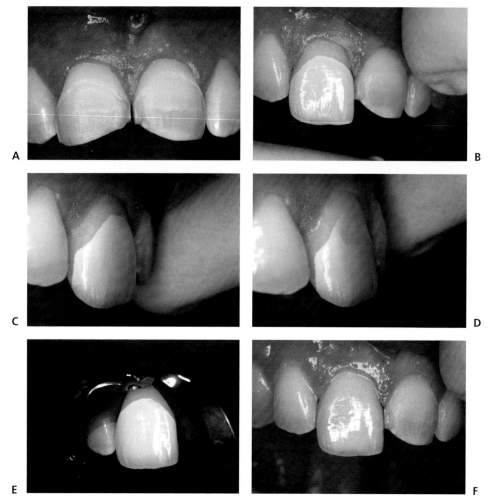

**Fig. 29.6** Supragingival laminate veneer preparations on centrals after fracture of both incisal edges (A). The apparent opacity of the veneer during try-in (B) is proven wrong as one drop of water enters in between the tooth and the veneer making the cervical part locally blend with the color of the tooth (C). This blending of the porcelain and the tooth is further illustrated by the frontal pictures (D, E) as compared to the picture of the just bonded/cemented veneer (F). It is naturally important to use a translucent composite cement for this to occur. Note that veneers are bonded/cemented one by one and the rubber dam applied so that immediate contact points are exposed for perfect seating of the veneer (E).

substrate for etched porcelain veneer restorations (41, 42). The porcelain cervically was very thin, so the supragingivally placed finishing line became virtually invisible.

Today, the original concept has been altered in accordance with knowledge obtained during past years (39, 40), and the *Toreskog/Myrin concept* to be described below represents ultrathin porcelain laminate veneers/crowns based upon a minimally invasive procedure, in which proper bonding to existing enamel is a basis (Figs 29.6 and 29.7) (40). Unfortunately, in some areas of the world the preparations for bonded veneers/crowns are much too extensive, and are carried far into dentin (41–44). This will produce problems with retention of the restoration and potential pulp problems. Leading experts in the USA claim that preserving existing enamel as much as possible is a worthy goal (41–44), and therefore, it is wise to always consider orthodontic treatment prior to tooth preparation in cosmetic dentistry (43). Even minor movement and derotation of anterior teeth can have a profound impact on enamel preservation, and the longevity of the porcelain veneer restorations (43). It is not acceptable treatment to casually prepare teeth in malocclusion for traditional crown restorations, and refer to them as 'veneer restorations', with no regard whatsoever for enamel preservation (41–44).

## The Toreskog/Myrin concept

### Don't cut through enamel just out of habit

By staying in enamel we will secure a long-term predictable bond to etched enamel. Even though dentine bonding works and should be used as soon as any part of the dentine is exposed, dentine bonding is still more technique sensitive and not as predictable in a long-term perspective. Furthermore, by staying in enamel we minimize the risk of pulp irritation during the entire procedure.

### Place cervical finishing line supragingivally

This will increase the chance to stay in enamel which has been shown to be of a positive long-term advantage. There are contraindications for the supragingival preparation, e.g. when caries or existing fillings are subgingivally placed. Furthermore, whenever changes of the cervical anatomy are planned or when the background color is very dark and should be brightened, the gingival finishing line has to be in the gingival area or sometimes even placed subgingivally, e.g. when a lateral has been placed in the central's position and should be restored to look like a central.

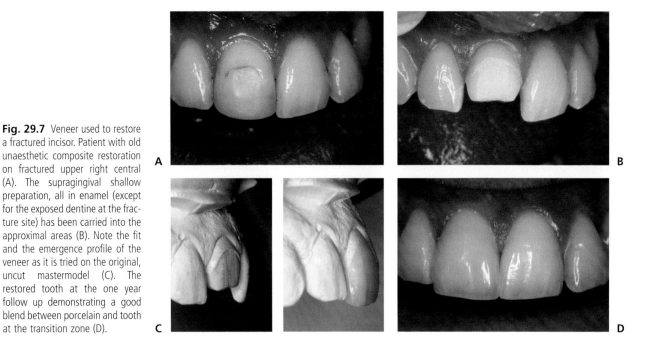

**Fig. 29.7** Veneer used to restore a fractured incisor. Patient with old unaesthetic composite restoration on fractured upper right central (A). The supragingival shallow preparation, all in enamel (except for the exposed dentine at the fracture site) has been carried into the approximal areas (B). Note the fit and the emergence profile of the veneer as it is tried on the original, uncut mastermodel (C). The restored tooth at the one year follow up demonstrating a good blend between porcelain and tooth at the transition zone (D).

## Make a very shallow cervical preparation (0.2–0.4 mm in depth)

This will again decrease the risk of exposing dentine during preparation and thus increase the positive prognosis of the veneer/crown. It also gives the best possibility of having an invisible finishing line that does not have to be hidden subgingivally.

The invisibility of the cervical margin comes from the fact that fairly translucent porcelain and translucent cement is used in this area letting the background color of the tooth shine through. As soon as the porcelain becomes thicker it is impossible to use as much translucency since the porcelain then will appear gray.

## Let the preparation be carried past existing proximal fillings

The quality of the bond to existing old composite fillings is not as good as that to enamel and dentine and the long-term survival of the veneer/crown will be endangered when the finishing line is in a filling or when too much of the prepared tooth constitutes the prepared bonding surface.

## Let porcelain cover the incisal edge

This is important for two reasons: to optimize the strength of the incisal part of the crown and to secure a definite seating of the restoration during the cementation procedure. Normally the incisal edge should be shortened 1–1.5 mm during the preparation. However, if the teeth are going to be lengthened, which is a very common situation, no reduction of the incisal edge has to be done.

## Use rubber dam for maximum control and expose one preparation at a time plus the immediate contact point(s). Cement one restoration at a time

The bonding and cementation procedure is technique sensitive and all efforts should be taken to optimize the circumstances during bonding. If a less than optimal bond is achieved the risk of fracture of the brittle restoration is critical.

## Use the all-etch technique with 35% phosphoric acid, dentin bonding and a translucent cement

It is virtually impossible to see if dentine is exposed so all surfaces have to be etched and subsequently dentine bonding has to be used all the time and on all surfaces.

## Essentials

Tooth loss requires a combination of esthetics and function. Methodology depends upon age, location and extent of traumatic injury.

## Replacement of a central incisor

- Orthodontic space closure.
- Premolar transplantation.
- Implant.
- Correctional or cantilever bridge work.

## Replacement of a lateral incisor

- Orthodontic closure.
- Premolar transplantation.
- Implant.
- Resin bonded cantilever prosthetics.

## Replacement of a canine

- Orthodontic closure.
- Autotransplants.
- Implants.
- Fixed prosthetics.

## Replacement after loss of multiple anterior teeth

- Combination of orthodontic closure and autotransplants.

## Restoring fractured teeth

- Porcelain laminate veneers using Toreskog/Myrin concept of preparation.
- Don't cut through enamel.
- Place cervical finishing line supragingivally.
- Make a very shallow cervical preparation.
- Let the preparation be carried past existing proximal fillings.
- Let porcelain cover the incisal edge.
- Use rubber dam, expose on preparation at a time plus the immediate contact point(s).
- Cement one restoration at a time.
- Use all-etch technique with 35% phosphoric acid, dentin bonding and a translucent cement.

## References

1. Rosa M, Zachrisson BU. Integrating esthetic dentistry and space closure in patients with missing maxillary lateral incisors. *J Clin Orthod* 2001;**35**:221–34.
2. Monefeldt I, Zachrisson BU. Adjustment of clinical crown height by gingivectomy following orthodontic space closure. *Angle Orthod* 1977;**47**:256–64.
3. Tuverson DL. Orthodontic treatment using canines in place of missing maxillary lateral incisors. *Am J Orthod* 1970;**58**:109–27.
4. Zachrisson BU, Mjör IA. Remodeling of teeth by grinding. *Am J Orthod* 1975;**68**:545–53.
5. Thordarson A, Zachrisson BU, Mjör IA. Remodeling of canines to the shape of lateral incisors by grinding. A long-term clinical and radiographic evaluation. *Am J Orthod* 1991;**100**:123–32.
6. Stenvik A, Zachrisson BU. Orthodontic closure and transplantation in the treatment of missing anterior teeth. An overview. *Endod Dent Traumatol* 1993;**9**:45–52.
7. Czochrowska EM, Skaare AB, Stenvik A, Zachrisson BU. Outcome of orthodontic space closure with a missing maxillary central incisor. *Am J Orthod Dentofac Orthop* 2003;**123**:597–603.

8. Zachrisson BU. Improving orthodontic results in cases with maxillary incisors missing. *Am J Orthod* 1978;**73**:274–89.
9. Tjan AHL, Miller GD, The JPG. Some esthetic factors in a smile. *J Prosthet Dent* 1984;**51**:24–8.
10. Dong JK, Jin TH, Cho HW, Oh SC. The esthetics of the smile: a review of some recent studies. *Int J Prosthodont* 1999;**12**:9–19.
11. Zachrisson BU. Esthetic factors involved in anterior tooth display and the smile: vertical dimension. *J Clin Orthod* 1998;**32**:432–45.
12. Wennström JL. Regeneration of gingiva following surgical excision. A clinical study. *J Clin Periodontol* 1983;**10**:287–97.
13. Bragger U, Lauchenauer D, Lang NP. Surgical lenghtening of the clinical crown. *J Clin Periodontol* 1992;**19**:58–63.
14. Cibirka RM, Myers M, Downey MC, Nelson SK, Browning WD, Hawkins IK, Dickinson GL. Clinical study of tooth shade lightening from dentist-supervised patient-applied treatment with two 10% carbamide peroxide gels. *J Esthet Dent* 1999;**11**:325–31.
15. Clark DM, Hintz J. Case report: In-office tooth whitening procedure with 35% carbamide peroxide evaluated by the Minolta cr-321 chroma meter. *J Esthet Dent* 1998;**10**:37–42.
16. CRA Newsletter Status Report. Why resin curing lights do not increase tooth lightening. *CRA Newsletter* 2000;**24**(8).
17. Slagsvold O, Bjercke B. Applicability of autotransplantation in cases with missing upper anterior teeth. *Am J Orthod* 1978;**74**:410–21.
18. Kristerson L. Autotransplantation of human premolars. A clinical and radiographic study of 100 teeth. *Int J Oral Surg* 1985;**14**:200–13.
19. Czochrowska EM, Stenvik A, Bjercke B, Zachrisson BU. Outcome of tooth transplantation. Survival and success rates 17 to 41 years posttreatment. *Am J Orthod Dentofac Orthop* 2002;**121**:110–19.
20. Czochrowska EM, Stenvik A, Album B, Zachrisson BU. Autotransplantation of premolars to replace maxillary incisors. A comparison with natural incisors. *Am J Orthod Dentofac Orthop* 2000;**118**:592–600.
21. Czochrowska EM, Stenvik A, Zachrisson BU. The esthetic outcome of autotransplanted premolars replacing maxillary incisors. *Dent Traumatol* 2002;**18**:237–45.
22. Zachrisson BU, Stenvik A, Haanæs HR. Management of missing maxillary anterior teeth with emphasis on autotransplantation. *Am J Orthod Dentofac Orthop* 2004;**126**:284–8.
23. Thilander B, Ödman J, Lekholm U. Orthodontic aspects of the use of oral implants in adolescents: a 10-year follow-up study. *Eur J Orthod* 2001;**23**:715–31.
24. Chang M, Wennström JL, Ödman J, Andersson B. Implant supported single-tooth replacement compared to contralateral natural teeth. Crown and soft tissue dimensions. *Clin Oral Impl Res* 1999;**10**:185–94.
25. Weisgold AS, Arnoux JP, Lu J. Single-tooth anterior implant: a word of caution. Part II. *J Esthet Dent* 1997;**9**:225–33.
26. Bernard JP, Schatz JP, Christou P, Belser U, Kiliaridis S. Long-term vertical changes of the anterior

maxillary teeth adjacent to single implants in young and mature adults. A retrospective study. *J Clin Periodontol* 2004;**31**:1024–8.

27. ISERI H, SOLOW B. Continued eruption of maxillary incisors and first molars in girls from 9 to 25 years studied by the implant method. *Eur J Orthod* 1996;**18**:245–56.

28. OESTERLEE LJ, CRONIN RJ Jr. Adult growth, aging, and the single-tooth implant. *Int J Oral Maxillofac Implants* 2000;**15**:252–60.

29. SPEAR FM. Restorative considerations in combined orthodontic-implant therapy. In: Higuchi KW. ed. *Orthodontic applications of osseointegrated implants.* Carol Stream, IL: Quintessence Publishing, 2000:121–32.

30. WEICHBRODT DJ, STENVIK A, HAANÆS HR. An intra-individual evaluation of implant-supported single tooth replacement for missing maxillary incisors (abstract). 18th Congress of the Nordic Association of Orthodontists, Loen, Norway, September 4–7, 2003.

31. ZACHRISSON BU, STENVIK A. Letter to the editor: single implants – optimal therapy for missing lateral incisors? *Am J Orthod Dentofac Orthop* 2004;**126**:13A–15A.

32. WENNSTRÖM JL. Personal communication, 2004.

33. NORDQUIST GG, MCNEILL RW. Orthodontic vs. restorative treatment of the congenitally absent lateral incisor – long term periodontal and occlusal evaluation. *J Periodont* 1975;**46**:139–43.

34. ROBERTSSON S, MOHLIN B. The congenitally missing upper lateral incisor. A retrospective study of orthodontic space closure versus restorative treatment. *Eur J Orthod* 2000;**22**:697–710.

35. KANGASNIEMI I, VALLITTU P, MEIERS J, DYER SR, ROSENTRITT M. Consensus statement on fiber-reinforced polymers: current status, future directions, and how they can be used to enhance dental care. *Int J Prosthodont* 2003;**16**:209.

36. VALDERHAUG J. A 15-year clinical evaluation of fixed prosthodontics. *Acta Odontol Scand* 1991;**49**: 35–40.

37. ZACHRISSON BU. First premolars substituting for maxillary canines – esthetic, periodontal and functional considerations. *World J Orthod* 2004;**5**:358–64.

38. CALAMIA JR, SIMONSEN RJ. Effect of coupling agents on bonding strength of etched porcelain. *J Dent Res* 1983;**63**:179.

39. TORESKOG S, REHNBERG P. *Protecting tissue with esthetic dental treatment – a visionary handbook.* Stockholm: Rehnberg Forlag, 1996.

40. TORESKOG S, MYRIN C. A minimal invasive and esthetic bonded porcelain technique – the concept and the vision. In: *Nordic Dentistry 2003, Year Book.* Copenhagen: Quintessence Publishing.

41. HEYMANN H. Is tooth structure not sacred anymore? (Editorial) *J Esthet Restor Dent* 2001;**13**:283.

42. FRIEDMAN MJ. Porcelain veneer restorations: a clinician's opinion about a disturbing trend. *J Esthet Restor Dent* 2001;**13**:318–27.

43. FRIEDMAN MJ. Novel porcelain laminate preparation approach driven by a diagnostic mock-up (commentary). *J Esthet Restor Dent* 2004;**16**:17–18.

44. CHRISTENSEN G. I have had enough! *J Esthet Restor Dent* 2004;**16**:83–6.

# 30

# Prevention of Dental and Oral Injuries

## A. Sigurdsson

## Introduction

Traumatic dental and maxillo-facial injuries are very common and appear worldwide to affect approximately 20–30% of permanent dentition and with often serious psychological, economic, functional and esthetic consequences for the individual (see Chapters 8 and 9). With such a high frequency of injuries prevention becomes a primary goal. Such an approach must take its origin in an identification of common causes for these injuries and whether such causes can be avoided or if preventive measures can be used to reduce the impact of such injuries (Fig. 30.1).

A number of epidemiological studies of traumatic injuries have examined the etiology of injury (see Chapter 8). However, only a few have offered such a detailed analysis that possible preventive measures can be related to the cause of injuries (1–3). In Fig. 30.1 a detailed analysis is shown for etiology of traumatic dental injuries. The various causes of injuries are related according to the possibility of using preventive measures to reduce the consequences of such injuries. It also appears from Fig. 30.1 that sports injuries for those older than 7 years of age represent about 20% of the trauma population (red columns) and it could be speculated that this is the most obvious activity where preventive measures would be possible and effective in reducing the rate of oral trauma. Traffic accidents appear to be the next frequent cause (blue columns) and also call for preventive measures to prevent or reduce the consequences of these usually severe impacts.

A significant number of oral and dental injuries result from participation in contact sports such as American football, basketball, rugby, soccer, boxing, wrestling or 'stick sports' (Fig. 30.2). However, there is a growing indication that oral and dental injuries occur as much if not more often during children's play or leisure activities (1, 2) (see Chapter 8). For example, in a study by Skaare and Jacobsen from Norway, in 2003 (2) nearly half (48%) of the 1275 injured individuals that were reported on in the study were injured at school. Sports and traffic accidents were less common in

their sample and organized sports accidents represented only 8% of the total number of injuries, the same as the number of individuals that were injured by violence. As importantly, the authors concluded that probably only one-third of the injuries were preventable.

Precisely the same results were reported by Andreasen in 2001 from a sample of 3655 dental casualty insurance claims from a major Danish insurance company (3). In this, 7% of the dental trauma claims were due to organized sports, while 93% were from various, unpreventable causes. In both studies, the authors felt that it is neither easy to prevent dental injuries nor to make guidelines on prevention. Based on this it should be clear that promoting mouthguards and facial masks is not the only preventive measure that needs to be taken.

The best prevention of dental and oral injuries is probably education; both how to avoid injuries as well as how to manage them at the site of the injury when they occur. This education should be targeted equally at children, teenagers and those who are around them when they are at risk of injuring themselves, e.g. parents, school officials and youth leaders. It should be the aim of every dentist to discuss risk factors that could lead to dental or oral injury during routine dental visits. (See also Chapter 35.) It is important to remember that this education should be aimed at both sexes equally. Even though some of the older epidemiological data indicated that boys were more prone to sustain oral and dental injury, with increased participation of girls in the more traditionally male sports, e.g. basketball and soccer, as well as in leisure activities, e.g. roller-blading and skate-boarding, that gap seems to be narrowing, at least in some areas (4).

Special emphasis should placed be on those who are at high risk, such as those with severe maxillary overjet, as it has been shown that the odds of dental trauma are significantly linearly related to the severity of the overjet (5, 6). It has even been suggested that a preventive orthodontic treatment should be initiated for these individuals and completed before the age of 11, i.e. in the early to middle mixed dentition in an attempt to reduce their risk of trauma (7).

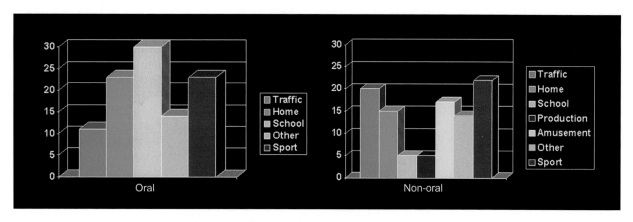

**Fig. 30.1** Injury environment for oral and non-oral injuries at various ages. An epidemiological study on injuries during one year in a Swedish county. From PETERSON et al. (1) 1997.

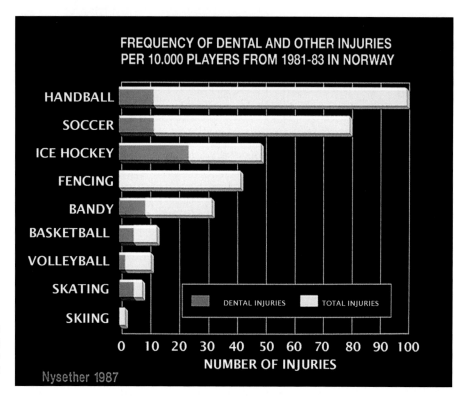

**Fig. 30.2** Dental injuries related to various sports, based on insurance records, which are precise documentation of dental and other injuries in Norway. From NYSETHER (85) 1987.

Another group that should receive special counseling are those who have already sustained an oral injury, for those seem to be much more likely to sustain another injury than those who have not (8, 9). It is of interest that the risk of sustaining multiple injuries has been reported as 8.4 times higher when the first trauma episode occurred at 9 years of age, compared with those occurring at age 12 (9). Therefore, young children should receive special attention. Their activities, games and sporting involvement should be carefully assessed; and any risk behavior should be discussed with them as well as with their parents or those who care for them. A typical example is the recent popularity of basketball hoops that can be lowered from standard height, so that 10- to 12-year-olds can 'slamdunk' or place the ball in the net by jumping up and hanging on the net ring that holds the net after letting go of the ball. Because their arms are short at that age, their maxillary incisors are often at the level with the basket net. This scenario has now been reported to

result in an increase in severe dental trauma, where multiple teeth are frequently avulsed (10).

All children should also be made aware of correct first aid when an injury does occur. Things like replanting avulsed teeth immediately if at all possible or alternatively storing them in milk, looking for all fragments of a broken tooth crown before running home or after help, should be discussed with them in clear, simple language. Posters like the one that the International Association of Dental Traumatology (IADT) and others have sponsored (Fig. 30.3) are likely to gain the attention of young individuals; and if widely displayed they should also reinforce their knowledge. (See also Chapter 35.)

Not only should young ones be educated about dental trauma but also those who care for them, especially those who are responsible for their safety during school and organized activities. A simple instruction sheet, like that in Table 30.1, is in many cases more than sufficient to ensure

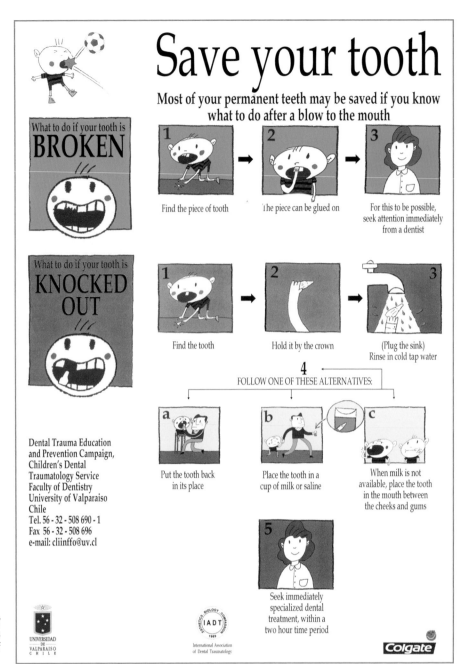

**Fig. 30.3** Poster co-sponsored by several national dental organizations and the International Association of Dental Traumatology.

**Table 30.1** Suggested review chart for athletic trainers or those who are responsible for children and teenagers in play.

| Term | Type of injury | Immediate treatment | Refer to a dentist |
|------|----------------|---------------------|--------------------|
| Uncomplicated crown fracture | Portion of the tooth broken, no bleeding from the fracture | None | Within 48 hours, especially if the patient has difficulty due to cold sensitivity |
| Complicated crown fracture | Portion of the tooth broken and bleeding from the fracture | None, do not place any medication on the bleeding pulp, stop the bleeding with sterile cotton gauge | As soon as logistically possible – could wait 48 hours, if the patient can tolerate cold and eat |
| Root fracture | Tooth might appear in normal position but bleeding from the gum around the tooth. The crown of the tooth might be pushed back or loose | None | As soon as possible |
| Concussion and subluxation | Tooth still in its normal place and firm or slightly loose | None | Within 48 hours, for evaluation only |
| Luxation | Tooth very loose and/or has moved from its normal position | Only move the tooth back to normal place if easy to move | As soon as possible, especially if it is not possible to reposition the tooth to its normal position |
| Avulsion | Tooth completely out of the mouth | Replace the tooth in its hole, if not possible then store the tooth in milk or saline | Immediately; it is extremely important for prognosis of the tooth to be treated immediately |

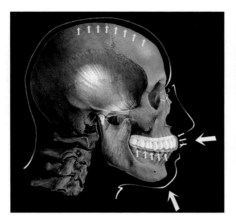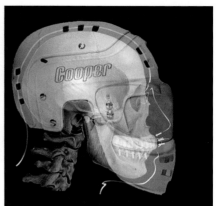

**Fig. 30.4** Mechanisms of mouthguard and facemask protection. The protection varies depending on the energy and direction of the impact. The full facemask protects the face and teeth from direct hits and the mouthguard protects the teeth from frontal impacts by distributing the forces over a greater area and from an impact on the base of the mandible by the cushioning effect between the maxilla and mandible.

that those who are injured receive proper emergency care at the site of the injury. When educating non-dentally trained persons it is important to remember to avoid complicated language. Table 30.1 shows a suggested communication form that is based on the recommendations of the IADT. Its language is clear; and it explains simply what to do and not to do immediately, as well as how urgent dental consultation is.

## Means to prevent dental maxillofacial injuries

The nature of a trauma implies acute delivery energy released upon soft and hard tissues and resulting in laceration, contusion or ablation of tissue. A protective device to reduce the consequences of such traumas can be devices which prevent the impact from getting in contact with the oral region or a cushioning device which absorbs and/or distributes the impact forces (mouthguards) (Fig. 30.4). Finally, restraining devices such as safety belts may absorb a significant part of the energy from the impact and thereby reduce the chance of the impact becoming delivered to the oral and maxillofacial region.

Not appearing in Fig. 30.1 is traumatic dental injuries occurring during oral endoscope and orotracheal intubations. By using preventive measures these injuries can be significantly reduced and these procedures will be described (see p. 829).

In the following a description will be given of possible ways to prevent dental and maxillofacial injuries in relation to various sports and traffic activities.

## Appliances to prevent dental injuries

During sports and other activities, where there is a risk of falling or being hit by an object, wearing a faceguard and/or mouthguard still seems to be the only way to prevent or at least significantly reduce the seriousness of dental injuries.

It has been reported that prior to the mandate of wearing face- and mouthguards in US high school football, facial and oral injuries constituted up to 50% of all reported football injuries (11, 12). Subsequent to that mandate a significant decrease was noted in reported injuries, down to a small percentage (11, 13).

Another common mechanism of oral injury is traffic accidents. Wearing seatbelts in a car, and when riding a motorcycle using a helmet with a chin arch, is in many places mandatory. The most commonly used bicycling helmets do provide very good protection against head injuries as shown in Victoria, Australia, when one year after mandatory helmet protection was introduced there was a 48% reduction of reported head injuries for bicyclists (14). Unfortunately these same helmets do not offer mouth or dental protection.

### Faceguards

Faceguards are usually a prefabricated cage of metal or composite that is attached to a helmet or a head strap (Fig. 30.5). Recently guards made out of clear polycarbonate plastic have become available, either as prefabricated or custom made. It would appear that these faceguards provide good protection to the face and the teeth, but are not applicable to all activities; and in many cases do not protect the teeth if the individual is hit under the chin.

Very few large-scale studies have been conducted on the actual benefits of wearing faceguards in games or practice; but it is clear that the introduction of mandatory helmet and facial protection has been effective in virtually eliminating ocular, facial and dental injuries in juvenile hockey (15). However, an unforeseen problem has been reported for the same groups of youths: while the number of head injuries has been reduced, an increase in catastrophic spinal injuries has been noted. It has been speculated that players get a false sense of security when donning the equipment, leading them to take excessive and unwarranted risks due to the protection they are supposedly afforded (15).

One of the few intervention studies on the effectiveness of faceguards was performed by Danis et al. (16) on a group of youth league baseball teams in the USA. Approximately

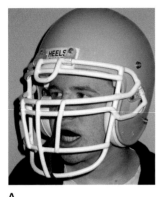 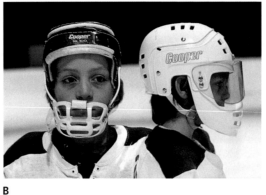 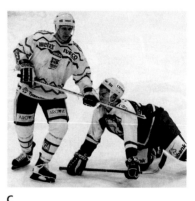

A  B  C

**Fig. 30.5** A. A typical cage-like face mask as worn by American football players. It provides good protection to the face and mouth but even with this extended type there is minimal protection from a blow under the chin. (Note the athlete is not wearing the mandatory chinstrap.) B. Full face masks are used in the junior level of ice hockey and they have been found effective in protecting the player from orofacial injuries. C. With a face mask, an injury like this could easily be avoided.

one-half of the teams were supplied with guard helmets (intervention); all others used this protection at their discretion (comparison). They found that the intervention teams reported a significant reduction in the incidence of oculofacial injuries compared to comparison team respondents ($p = 0.04$).

Half facemasks have been popular in hockey, as it has been speculated that a full face shield may increase the risk of concussions and neck injuries, offsetting the benefits of protection from dental, facial and ocular injuries. In a recent study, it was found that the use of full face shields is associated with a significantly reduced risk of sustaining facial and dental injuries without an increase in the risk of neck injuries, concussions or other injuries (17).

With the emergence of many new fiber-composites, custom fabricated faceguards will become more available and affordable. Studies confirming their benefits must be conducted.

## Mouthguards

Mouthguards have existed for well over a century. According to Reed (18) they were originally designed and fabricated in the late 19th century by a London dentist, Woolf Krause. They were initially made from gutta-percha and their main purpose was to protect boxers from lip lacerations and other soft tissue injuries. Philip Krause, son of W. Krause, a dentist as well as an amateur boxer, further developed the 'gum shield' to something that approaches what is known today. He used vella rubber rather than the relatively hard gutta-percha to create his mouthguards (18, 19).

The use of mouthguards in contact sports has been reported in the past to reduce the occurrence of dental injuries to over 90% (20–23). Since rules regarding the use of headgear and mouthguards in high school football were established in the 1960s, facial and dental injuries sustained on the field have dropped by approximately 48% (13).

Few studies have specifically investigated, prospectively or in real time, whether athletes who wear mouthguards sustain significantly fewer dental injuries than those who do not (24, 25). The first study to do so involved a sample population of 272 high school rugby players. The athletes received a pre-season clinical examination by a team of dentists and completed a questionnaire. Mouthguards were fitted one week later and the players were instructed in their use. At the end of the season, a follow-up questionnaire was completed. There was a significant difference in the number of tooth fractures between mouthguard wearers and non-mouthguard wearers (24). The second study, which evaluated US male college basketball players (age 18–22), collected 'real time' data (25). Trainers reported information about their teams on a weekly basis using an interactive website. The results of this study are likely to be significant, as it captured 70 936 athlete exposures (an athletic exposure is a one athlete participating in a game or practice, whether it was one play, one quarter, one half or the entire game). The study found that mouthguard users had significantly lower rates of dental injuries and dentist referrals than non-users. However, there was no significant difference between mouthguard users and non-users in the rate of soft tissue injuries. Of note, this study reported significantly more oral/dental injuries than that reported by the NCAA for the same season (25) (Table 30.2).

Not all studies have demonstrated a beneficial effect of mouthguards. In a cross-sectional study, a sample of 321 university rugby players participating on 555 player occasions was examined (26). The results of that study indicated no statistically significant association between oral, dental and lip injuries sustained during rugby playing with the use or non-use of mouthguards. This study, like most mouthguard studies, irrespective of whether they demonstrated a beneficial effect or not, is relatively small and therefore it is likely that it did not have enough statistical power. More large-scale studies are therefore needed.

## Function of mouthguards

The four main suggested functions of a mouthguard are (27):

**Table 30.2** Injury rate difference between mouthguard wearers and non-wearers for male college basketball players in a large real-time study including dental injuries. From LABELLA et al. (25) 2002.

| Injury rate per 100 players | Brain concussion | Mouth injuries | Dental injuries (fract/lux/avuls) | Dental referrals |
|---|---|---|---|---|
| Mouthguard | 6.2% | 13.0% | 0.6% | 1.6% |
| No mouthguard | 6.1% | 14.2% | 2.0% | 5.8% |
| | NS | NS | $P < 0.03$ | $P < 0.02$ |

(fract/lux/avuls) = fractures, luxations, avulsions.

(1) Preventing tooth injuries by absorbing and deflecting blows to the teeth

(2) Shielding the lips, tongue and gingival tissues from laceration

(3) Preventing opposing teeth from coming into violent contact

(4) Providing the mandible with resilient support, which absorbs an impact that might fracture the unsupported angle or condyle of the mandible.

Various materials and methods have been used to achieve these basic functions, as many test protocols and devices tried to investigate them and confirm the effectiveness. The main problem with testing these suggested functions are that there is no *in vivo* model ethically possible and *in vitro* models are at best crude approximations. To further complicate matters, large prospective cohort studies are very difficult to conduct, and to some degree are unethical as well, because of the need for crossover or control groups. One very interesting attempt to circumvent some of these problems was a study by Johnston and Messer (28), where they used mandibular sheep segments with incisors at four developmental stages. Customised pressure formed mouthguards were made for each mandibular segment and then trauma was inflicted with a servohydraulic materials testing machine. Injuries were examined clinically, radiographically and by dissection. The magnitude of lateral luxation measurements of individual teeth was reduced significantly by mouthguard protection in both deciduous and permanent dentitions. Fourteen- to 24-fold greater forces were required to cause an injury in the sheep mandibular dentition covered with a custom made mouthguard compared with dentition without mouthguard coverage. Of interest was their finding that the mouthguard tended to increase the mobility of the teeth it encompassed and, in some instances, promoted dentoalveolar injury of adjacent teeth.

Other studies have used the upper central incisors in a dry human skull that were excited by an electrodynamic shaker (29), or a simulated maxilla, constructed of polymethylmethacrylate, containing replaceable resin teeth where a steel ram was dropped on the maxillary incisor region. Changes in voltage, which were induced by a strain gauge at the back of the upper left incisor, were the measure of protection (30), or measuring the cushioning effect of the material directly, as by deflection caused by impact forces induced by a pendulum ram impact testing machine (31). The main concern with all these approaches it that it is not clear if they translate into true protection of the dentition and alveolus in humans.

In recent studies from a Japanese group an attempt was made to investigate real objects (steel balls, baseball, softball, ice hockey puck, cricket ball, wooden baseball bat) that could hit mouthguard and teeth during an athletic event rather than just a steel drop-ball that has been frequently used in studies on mouthguards (32). Their studies indicated that transmitted forces were less when a standard single layer mouthguard was used compared to no mouthguard, but as importantly they demonstrated that the effect was significantly influenced by the object type that hit the teeth. The steel ball showed the biggest (62.1%) absorption ability while the wooden ball showed the second biggest (38.3%). Other objects, baseball, field hockey ball and hockey puck, showed 0.6–6.0% absorbency. These results show that it is important to test the effectiveness of mouthguards on specific types of sports equipment rather than using some standard experimental equipment that might not give a realistic outcome. This group also investigated different sensors in a follow-up paper (33) and found that the sensor plays an important role in the measurement values reported for absorbency of mouthguard materials; they concluded that a standard sensor should be used for all experiments. It is therefore clear that further studies are warranted in standardizing this kind of test so that effectiveness of mouthguards can be compared with confidence.

How the mouthguard is able to achieve these suggested protective functions is not quite clear. Many studies have placed an emphasis on investigating the energy absorption of different materials with the idea in mind that the higher the absorption, the better protection the mouthguard provides. It has been shown that the physical and mechanical properties vary with their chemical composition and this itself varies with different brands of the same material (see later in this chapter). The resilience of PVAc-PE materials appears to vary inversely with the magnitude of the impact energy at which they are tested. A number of factors may be responsible for this variation including the degree of crosslinking between polymer chains, the proportion of plasticizer present and the volume of filler particles. It has been suggested that laminated thermoplastic mouthguards are dimensionally more stable in use (34). Again the clinical significance of these variations has not been determined; but it has been suggested that high energy absorption does not necessarily indicate that the material will give maximum protection, since some of the absorbed energy may be transmitted directly to the underlying dental structures (35). Research elucidating if this is the case is very much needed.

A fifth suggested function of the mouthguard has been that it prevents neck and cerebral brain injuries. Through the years there has been a great deal of discussion in the literature that the mouthguard prevents cerebral concussion in athletes (36–38). However, most of these papers have only been case reports or opinions, not based on controlled scientific studies. The two papers usually cited as a foundation of this presumed effect were written by Stenger et al. in 1964 (39) and Hickey et al. in 1967 (40).

The first article reported on only five football players who had a history of head and/or neck injuries. Three players gave a history of 'being concussion prone' and one had previous neck injuries. The fifth athlete experienced definite pain with crepitation on the left side when the temporomandibular joint was palpitated and cervical pain extending halfway down his shoulder. Each athlete wore a custom-fitted mouthguard when playing football in conjunction with daily intermaxillary acrylic splint therapy. Each player's symptoms were either eliminated or diminished. The author concluded that the custom-fitted mouthguard provided protection and relief for patients.

The second paper was a report on an *in vitro* study, where series of impact blows were applied to a single cadaver using an intracranial pressure transducer to measure pressure changes associated with the blows. The authors of that study concluded that 'there was a decided reduction in the amplitude of the intracranial pressure wave when the mouth protector was in place. Bone deformation was also decreased moderately when the mouth protectors were in place (40). However, the correlation between those factors and cerebral concussion is not at all clear (41). Recently, with more careful scrutiny of scientific evidence in the literature, this claim of protectiveness of the mouthguard has been called into question (19).

Two recent and very large studies using interactive websites to collect weekly information on the incidence of cerebral brain concussion in athletes have failed to show any benefits (25, 42) (Tables 30.2 and 30.3). In the former, a comparison was made between those who wore a mouthguard and those who did not in US college men's basketball. Almost 71 000 athletic exposures were reported; there was no significant difference in the rate of brain concussion between the groups (25). The second study compared 'boil

and bite' versus custom made mouthguards worn by American college football players (42). Over 500 000 athletic exposures were recorded; again, there was no significant difference in trauma risk between the two groups (25, 42). It is important to note that these two studies did not assess the mechanism of injury, for example blow under the chin versus fall to the ground. However and unfortunately, these two studies do not indicate that wearing a mouthguard helps reduce cerebral brain concussion in any significant way.

## Types of mouthguard

Mouthguards can be divided in to three basic types based on how they are manufactured and used:

- Stock – prefabricated
- Mouth formed
- Custom made.

Some of these basic types have now several sub-groups, especially the custom made ones.

*Stock* mouthguards may be made either from rubber or one of the plastic materials (Fig. 30.6). They are generally available in two or three sizes, and are supposed to have a

**Table 30.3** Athletic exposures and brain concussions reported by 87 USA NCAA Division I college football teams for the 2001 season. From LaBELLA et al. (25) 2002.

| | Total athletic exposures (contact practices and games; additional 168 800 exposures in non-contact practices excluded) | Brain concussions |
|---|---|---|
| Custom mouthguard | 141 165 | 166 (0.1%) |
| Boil-and-bite mouthguard | 196 332 | 199 (0.1%) |
| | | NS |

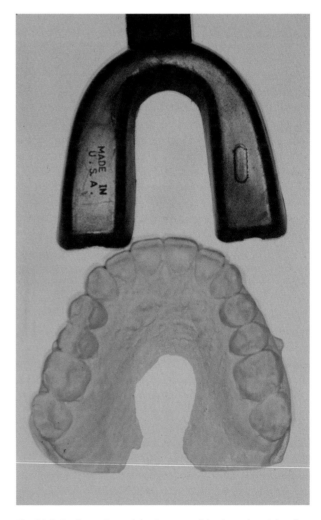

**Fig. 30.6** Stock mouthguard that is too small for the arch and therefore will not stay easily in place as it is not comfortable.

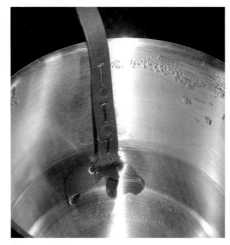 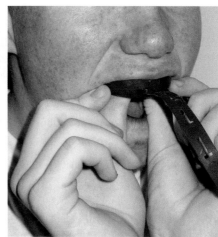

**Fig. 30.7** Boil-and-bite being formed in the mouth. A. The stock mouthguard is heated in boiling water for a few minutes and then inserted in to the mouth with care. B. The index fingers should be used to adapt the mouthguard as well as possible to the facial sides of the molars and the thumbs at the same time press on the palatal side.

**A**  **B**

universal fit, sometimes aided by flanges in the molar area. Modification is limited to trimming the margins to relieve the frenula. The loose fit means that the wearer must occlude to prevent the guard from being displaced. The main advantage of this type of mouthguard is that they are inexpensive and may be purchased by the public in sports shops. Also, because they do not require any preparation, a replacement is readily available at any time. Most reports agree (43, 44) that these types of mouthguard provide the least protection of all available types due to their poor fit, though admittedly there is no conclusive scientific data confirming this opinion. However, it is unquestioned that these mouthguards are uncomfortable for the wearers: they tend to obstruct speech and breathing because the wearer must keep them in place by either clenching or supporting with the tongue (45) and therefore are less likely to be worn, and when needed could be blown out of the mouth prior to impact with the ground or other obstacles.

There are two types of *mouth-formed mouthguards*. The first consists of a hard and fairly rigid outer shell that provides a smooth, durable surface and a soft, resilient lining that is adapted to the teeth (Fig. 30.7). The outer shell of vinyl chloride may be lined with a layer of self-curing methyl-methacrylate or silicone rubber. The outer shell is fitted and trimmed, if necessary, around the sulci and frenal attachments. It is filled with the soft lining and seated in the mouth. Care must be taken to ensure that it is centrally placed. The lining is allowed to polymerize for 3–5 minutes. Excess material is trimmed with a sharp knife and the margins smoothed with dental stones. This type of mouthguard tends to be bulky and the margins of the outer shell may be sharp unless protected by an adequate thickness of the lining material. The most commonly used type of mouth-formed protector is constructed from a preformed thermoplastic shell of PVAc-PE copolymer or PVC (43) that is softened in warm water and then molded in the mouth by the user (Fig. 30.7). These mouthguards have several distinct advantages over the stock mouthguard. If carefully adapted, they give a closer fit and are more easily retained than stock protectors. Care must be taken during the molding process

so that the mouthguard fits accurately. The temperature necessary to allow adequate adaptation to the teeth is fairly high, so additional care must be taken to prevent burning the gingiva. Similar to the stock mouthguard, this type of mouthguard is relatively inexpensive, readily available to the general public and can be formed into a decent appliance with some care.

*Custom mouthguards* are individually made in a laboratory, on plaster of Paris models poured from impressions of the player's mouth. Many studies have shown that these mouthguards are more acceptable and comfortable to athletes than the other types (46, 47) There is no evidence, however, that custom made protectors are more effective in preventing injuries.

Historically, three groups of materials were used to fabricate custom made mouth protectors: *molded velum rubber* (46), *latex rubber* (48) and *resilient acrylic resins*. Currently by far the most common material used for custom made mouthguards is ethylene vinyl acetate (EVA) copolymers. Previously polyvinylchloride, soft acrylic resins and polyurethane were also used; but the superiority of the EVA copolymers has practically eliminated the others. Its popularity is mainly due to its elastomeric softness and flexibility so that it can be relatively easily processed. Also, the material has good clarity and gloss, barrier properties, low-temperature toughness, stress-crack resistance and little or no odor (43, 49). Many prefabricated plates of EVA are now commercially available; but it is important to know that the percentage of vinyl acetate (often indicated as a percentage) can vary between manufactures and therefore show differences in properties. The more vinyl acetate is copolymerised (higher % marking), the more flexible, stretchable, softer and tougher is the material (49). This property will also lower the softening temperature, allowing manipulation of the material within a comfortable temperature. The most common material for mouthguards contains 28% vinyl acetate. It should be remembered that the actual performance of a mouthguard is just as dependent upon the design, thickness and manner of impact on the mouth as the base material used (49).

The EVA mouthguard material can now be bought in varying color, thickness and hardness. There has been some discussion about whether there should be different stiffness or hardness suggested for different sports. Thus, while the low-stiffness guards absorb shock during hard-object collisions (e.g. baseballs), they may not protect the tooth-bone during soft-object collisions (e.g. boxing gloves) (50). To date, clinical studies are lacking to substantiate such recommendations.

In 1985 Chaconas et al. (34) described a laminated thermoplastic mouthguard that showed significantly less dimensional change than other materials tested (i.e. poly vinyl acetate-ethylene) copolymer clear thermoplastic and polyurethane). This was the start of several different subcategories within custom fabricated mouthguards.

A few years ago, layered EVA stock plates were introduced (Fig. 30.8). The idea was to further strengthen the mouthguard without losing its protective capacity. When a stock plate of EVA is fabricated, it is drawn out in one direction so that the polymer chains are more or less parallel, like the grain in wood. This can theoretically make a difference in properties whether the 'grains' are running facio-palatally or mesio-distally on the crown of the tooth. To eliminate this and increase the stiffness without adding bulk, manufacturers have started to market 2- or 3-layered stock EVA, where the layers have been added perpendicular to each other. Some manufactures have even added a low percentage EVA plate between layers, which is designed to further stiffen the mouthguard palatally behind the anterior incisors (Figs 30.9 and 30.10). There is not much, if any, scientific proof that

this can increase the protectiveness of the mouthguard and again is a question of whether a too stiff mouthguard could not cause other damage to the tooth or alveolus. Some disturbing findings were reported in a recent study (51). It was found that a hard insert resulted in reduced energy absorption when compared with a control sheet of the same material and approximate thickness but without the hard inserts (51). The same research group has, however, shown improved impact characteristics of the EVA mouthguard material with regulated air inclusions (52). But as yet, there is no clinical data available to support this, and durability of air-included mouthguards is unknown.

Another version of this layered concept is the fusion of two plates of different stiffness. It is important to know that these only seem to improve the mouthguard when the softer material is next to the teeth. A study, using a finite element model, by Kim and Mathieu (35) showed that a soft outer layer covering a hard core had no significant difference from

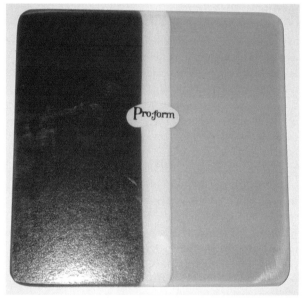

**Fig. 30.9** Mouthguard made of prefabricated double layered stock plate with a further added low percentage EVA plate between layers that is designed to stiffen the mouthguard on the palatal site of the anterior incisors. When making a mouthguard with these plates care must be taken to align the insert with the center and on the palatal site of the teeth.

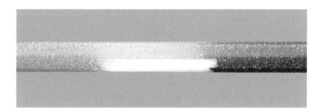

**Fig. 30.8** Prefabricated double layered mouthguard stock plate. Both layers are of the same vinyl acetate percentage but the top layer is clear and the bottom composed of three different colors, for esthetic reasons, all fused into one mass.

**Fig. 30.10** A. When making a boil and bite mouthguard, it is important to select a stock that fits the arch that it is going to be adapted to. B. If too small it is likely that the molar arch will not be properly covered and the retention and fit will be greatly reduced (B).

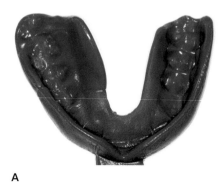

**A**

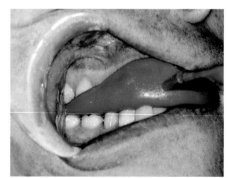

**B**

**Table 30.4** Athletic exposures and dental injuries reported by 87 USA NCAA Division I college football teams for the 2001 season. From WISNIEWSKY et al. (54) 2007.

| | Total athletic exposures (contact practices and games; additional 168 800 exposures in non-contact practices excluded) | Dental injuries (tooth fractures, luxations and avulsions) |
|---|---|---|
| Custom mouthguard | 141 165 | 13 (0.1%) |
| Boil-and-bite mouthguard | 196 332 | 21 (0.1%) NS |

a monolayer in stress distribution and impact force. However, a soft core was found to have a significant effect on stress distribution. This effect could be increased by controlling ratios of modulus and volume fractions of the core and outer layer.

The main question regarding these various types of mouthguard is whether there is any actual protective difference between them. Very few studies have investigated the efficacy of the different types in preventing dental injuries with large enough samples to have significant statistical power.

In one study on 98 professional rugby players, custom made mouthguards did not significantly reduce the amount of dental injuries sustained as compared to mouth-formed mouthguards (53). At a follow-up clinical examination, there was no damage to teeth when either custom made or boil-and-bite mouthguards were worn.

Stokes et al. compared mouth-formed and custom made mouthguards (46). They showed that although there were no dental injuries in either group, the users preferred laboratory-formed mouthguards because of comfort.

In a very large study on college football players, where their trainers reported every week for the entire season using an interactive website the number of players, mouthguard use and dental and oral injuries, there was no apparent difference between boil-and-bite or custom made mouthguards (54). The sample consisted of 87 (76%) out of a possible 114 Division I teams, with a total of 506 297 athletic exposures recorded (Table 30.4). Most of those teams had a mixed use of custom and boil-and-bite mouthguards and thereby there was a possibility that the benefits of one particular mouthguard would be obscured by these teams. Therefore the data was further analyzed where a subselection of fourteen teams was selected. Seven of these used exclusively custom made mouthguards and the other seven exclusively boil-and-bite. The results were the same: no statistically significant benefits of type of one mouthguard over another (54). It is important to emphasise that in this study there was no attempt to inspect the quality of the mouthguard used or the comfort of one type over the other.

Wear and tear will affect all mouthguards; it has been suggested that they should be replaced regularly, not only due to lack of fit, but also because of reduction in protective properties. Recently it has been shown in a simulated aging study on different types of custom made mouthguards, that

aging induced various dimensional changes. Most of the dimensional change for all mouthguards occurred at the central incisor region. Pressure-laminated mouthguard specimens showed the lowest range of changes at the central incisor region, suggesting potentially improved fit, comfort and protection (55).

## Fabrication of custom mouthguards

Organizations, such as the Federation Dentaire International (FDI) have created and published recommended criteria on the construction of an effective mouthguard (56). Most of these recommendations state the same criteria:

(1) The mouthguard should be made of a resilient material, which can be easily washed, cleaned and readily disinfected.
(2) It should have adequate retention to remain in position during sporting activity, and allow for a normal occlusal relationship to give maximum protection.
(3) It should absorb and disperse the energy of a shock by:
   - Covering the maxillary dental arch
   - Excluding interferences
   - Reproducing the occlusal relationship
   - Allowing mouth breathing
   - Protecting the soft tissues.

Furthermore, the FDI also recommends that mouthguards be made by dentists from an impression of the athlete's teeth.

### Mouth-formed mouthguards

Regardless of type, the key for functionality is selection of a stock that fits the arch. If too small, it is likely that the molars will not be properly covered, thereby reducing retention and fit (Fig. 30.10). Once the proper size is found and fitted, the mouthguard should be made strictly following the manufacture's guidelines or recommendations.

#### Common pitfalls in making mouth-formed mouthguards

- *Size*: Care must be taken to select the appropriate size that fits over the teeth in the dental arch. The mouthguard must cover at least one molar tooth on each side.
- *Adaptation to the teeth and surrounding tissue*: Care must be taken for optimal adaptation to the teeth and gums.
- *Trimming of the mouthguard*: After forming the mouthguard it should be carefully trimmed so that unnecessary excess is removed, without compromising the retention or strength.

### Custom mouthguards

The best way to construct a custom mouthguard is to take alginate impressions of both arches together with a wax bite

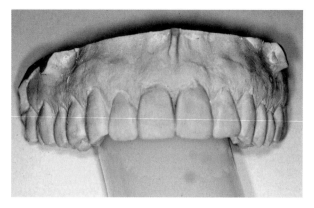
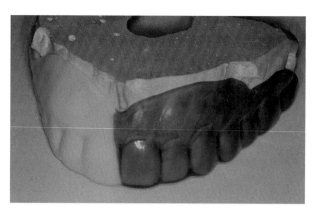

**Fig. 30.11** It is important to gain a good impression of the alveolus above all the teeth, even to the point that the vestibule is over-extended. The cast should reflect this with as much impression of the alveolar structure above the teeth as possible, especially in the anterior region. This will allow good adaptation of the mouthguard material to the soft tissue area and which in turn will ensure better retention as well as comfort.

**Fig. 30.12** The cast should be trimmed so that the vestibule is almost removed. This will ensure that there will be a good adaptation of the mouthguard material to the cast when it is sucked over the cast.

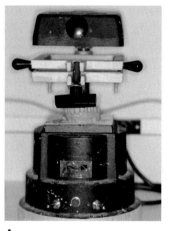
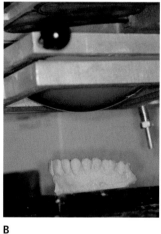
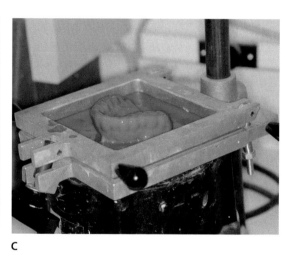

A                                       B                                       C

**Fig. 30.13** A. A traditional vacuum suction machine used to make custom made mouthguards. At top there is a heating element; the stock plate is sandwiched in a jig right underneath the element. The cast is placed on a perforated plate and care must be taken that it is as much in the center as possible. When the stock plate heats up it will start to droop, so care must be taken not to overheat it because that will result in too thin mouthguard. Most commonly used EVA materials should droop about 2–2.5 cm (3/4–1 inch) before being sucked down on the cast. C. The plate needs to completely cool down on the cast before it is removed from the cast.

taken with the patient's mandible in a physiological rest position. However, when time and cost is a major issue, impression of the maxilla can be considered sufficient. It is very important to get a good impression of the alveolus over all teeth, even to the point that the vestibule is overextended (Fig. 30.11). This will allow good adaptation of the mouthguard material to the soft tissue area and will in turn ensure better retention and comfort.

In a crossover study of different mouthguard extensions, McClelland et al. (57) found that comfort of wear was likely to be increased if the mouthguard was extended labially to within 2 mm of the vestibular fold, adjusted to allow even occlusal contact, rounded at the buccal peripheries, and tapered at the palatal edges. To further ensure good adaptation of the mouthguard material to the cast, the cast should be carefully trimmed so the vestibule is almost removed (Fig. 30.12). It has also been shown that residual moisture in the working cast is the most critical factor in determining the fit of the mouthguard made by vacuum-forming machines. The best fit was achieved when the working cast was thoroughly dried and its surface temperature was elevated (58).

There are two basic methods of fabricating a custom mouthguard: the first is with the more traditional vacuum suction machine (Fig. 30.13) that basically draws the EVA stock plate over the plaster cast. It is possible to use either the single layer or prefabricated multilayered EVA in these machines; but it is very difficult to create a multi-laminated mouthguard from separate plates using this technique, as adaptation of layers will always be poor. There is a high risk

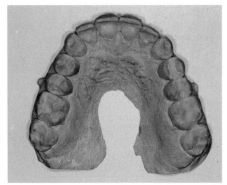
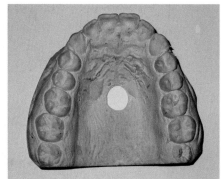

**Fig. 30.14** To improve the suction and thereby the adaptation drilling a hole in the palatal area of the cast in necessary. Alternatively trim the cast such that some of the palatal structure is removed. This is however only possible for individuals with a high palatal vault, because otherwise there is a danger of removing too much of the alveolar process.

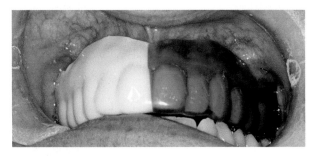

**Fig. 30.15** The mouthguard should extend as far up in the vestibule as tolerated by the patient, with appropriate clearance of the buccal and labial frenum.

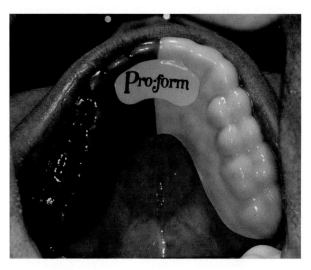

**Fig. 30.16** The mouthguard should extend as far back on the palate as reasonable to increase both anterior strength and retention, and it should distally cover up to the second molar at least if at all possible.

of the mouthguard coming apart during use and its benefit lost.

There are several critical steps that must be followed when this type of mouthguard is made. Each must be carefully followed, otherwise the benefits of the mouthguard could be severely compromised. First, to improve the suction and thereby adaptation, a hole is drilled in the palatal area of the cast (Fig. 30.14) to ensure good suction in the palatal region. Second, the EVA plate is heated to adapt well to the cast and cool in place. If the formed mouthguard is removed while still warm, there is great risk of deformation, which will result in poor adaptation to the teeth and surrounding tissue and thereby poor retention. The third step is the one that is most often overlooked, that is, proper trimming of the mouthguard after it has cooled completely.

As stated before, the mouthguard should extend as far into the vestibule as tolerated by the patient, with appropriate clearance of the buccal and labial frena. It should extend as far back on the palate as reasonable to increase anterior strength and retention (57) (Fig. 30.15). Distally, the mouthguard should cover at least up to the second molar (59) (Fig. 30.16). The mouthguard could be trimmed with a specially heated knife on the cast or removed from the cast and scissors used (Fig. 30.17). It is advisable to replace the mouthguard on the cast after trimming is complete and flame the edges with a torch. Smooth the flamed edges with wet fingers or a small spatula. Alternatively the edge can be smoothed with a small rag-wheel in a hand trimmer (Fig. 30.18). To further improve the athlete's comfort, it is possible to gently heat the occlusal surface and then have the athlete bite

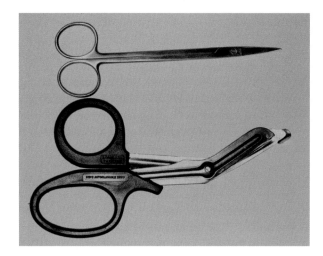

**Fig. 30.17** The mouthguard can be trimmed with a specially heated knife on the cast or removed from the cast. Heavy duty as well as fine curved scissors can be used.

together with the guard in place. This is done to even the occlusal contact between sides. Alternatively, this can be done on an articulator, if casts of both arches and bite registration are made.

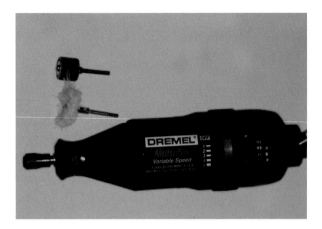

Fig. 30.18 The edges of the mouthguard can be smoothed with a small rag-wheel or sanding wheel in a simple hand trimmer that can even be taken to the field house.

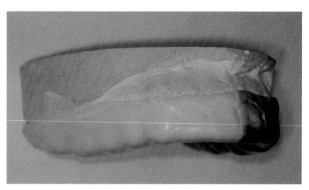

Fig. 30.20 An example of a poorly made mouthguard. First, the cast is not properly trimmed so that there is a lip in the vestibule area, preventing a good adaptation in that area. Second, the mouthguard is too thin as is evident from the color of the cast showing well through the blue EVA; the extensions into the vestibule are too short in the anterior area and the edges are not smooth.

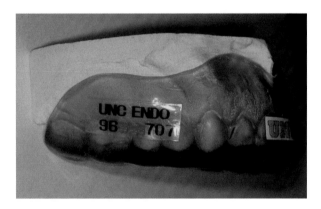

Fig. 30.19 An interesting possibility using the multilayered technique is the possibility to sandwich in names, numbers or logos.

The second method is with positive pressure machines, such as **Drufomat®**, **Erkopress-2004®** or **Biostar®**. In these machines, the stock plate is pressed, after being heated, onto the cast with pressure from above the plate rather than being drawn down onto the cast with negative pressure from below. This will ensure very close adaptation of the material to the cast and it is relatively easy to add multiple layers, as the positive pressure will always ensure that the new layer adapts to the existing one. It is much easier to control the thickness of the mouthguard using this technique and the stiffness of the mouthguard can quickly build up with multiple layers without losing much adaptability to the teeth. However, there must be some resilience in the mouthguard, so care must be taken not to make too stiff an appliance. An interesting possibility with this technique is the possibility of sandwiching names, numbers or logos between layers (Fig. 30.19). This will not only make it easier to know whose mouthguard is whose, but also might encourage the athlete to wear one if the team logo was clearly visible.

Once the mouthguard is made, it should be inspected for quality. The main issue, especially with the vacuum technique is thickness. There has been some effort made to find the most ideal thickness of a mouthguard to ensure comfort as well as yield optimal protection. Consensus seems to be that the thicker the mouthguard is, the more protection it affords. However, it would appear that if thickness exceeds more than 4 mm, performance is only improved marginally and is much less comfortable for the wearer (47, 60).

### Common pitfalls in fabricating custom made mouthguards (Fig. 30.20)

- *Extension above the teeth*: The more of the gums that are covered above the teeth, the greater the retention as well as increased strength of the mouthguard. Overextension is uncomfortable and could lead to injury in the vestibule. The mouthguard should be trimmed so that the frenum is free.
- *Extension over the molar area*: The mouthguard should cover at least one molar tooth on each side. Some extension over the gums in the molar region is recommended for retention.
- *Extension in the palatal area*: The mouthguard needs to cover some of the tissue above and behind the anterior teeth. This will both increase retention and strength of the mouthguard.
- *Rough edges*: Rough edges decrease comfort and could cause additional injuries. Smooth them with a flame, sandpaper or rag-wheel.
- *Too thin or too thick*: Too thin a mouthguard will not be strong enough to provide protection; too thick might be uncomfortable to wear.

## Special considerations for mouthguards

For patients undergoing orthodontic treatment involving fixed appliances, the brackets and arch wires may be covered with boxing wax before impressions are taken. The mouthguard may be made of a less elastic material to protect the teeth, but care should be taken not to increase the thickness

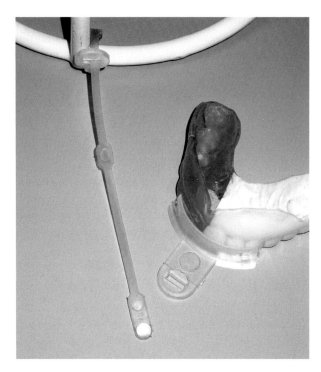

**Fig. 30.21** The connection between a facemask and the mouthguard should have self-releasing mechanisms so that if the helmet and/or the facemask comes off the athlete, there will not be a forceful pull on the mouthguard that could damage the teeth or the dental arch.

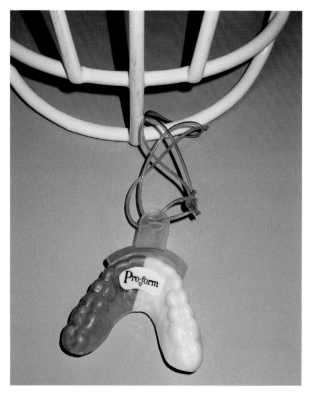

**Fig. 30.22** The mouthguard should never be tied to the facemask or other appliances that could come loose.

so that lips or other soft tissues are put under tension. It is not clear whether mouthguards that are specifically sold to athletes who wear orthodontic appliances appear to offer any protection. Adapting a boil-and-bit mouthguard might be more beneficial if cost or convenience is an issue. This also applies for children in mixed dentition. If a custom mouthguard is made for these children, it must be remade with new impressions at least every 6 months, thus making cost a strong factor. A well-made mouth-formed guard might be as effective.

In those sports where the athletes are wearing a helmet and some kind of facemask, the mouthguard is frequently attached to the mask for convenience. The issue has been raised there should be an automatic release mechanism, so that if the helmet and/or the facemask comes off the athlete, there will not be a forceful pull on the mouthguard and thereby the teeth or the dental arch (Figs 30.21, 30.22).

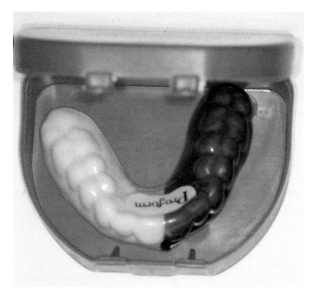

**Fig. 30.23** Everyone who receives a custom made mouthguard needs to be provided with an appropriate storage box that will allow ventilation and they should be taught how to regularly clean the mouthguard by brushing it with toothbrush and tooth paste.

## Care of mouthguards

When fitted, instructions should be given for the care of the mouthguard (Figs 30.23, 30.24). It has been reported in the past that only half of athletes clean their mouthguards after use. Eight percent even lend them to other athletes (61). Bacteriological studies have led to the recommendation that mouthguards should (a) be washed with soap and water immediately after use; (b) be dried thoroughly and stored in a perforated box; and (c) be rinsed in mouthwash or mild antiseptic (e.g. 0.2% chlorhexidine) immediately before use.

The mouthguard should be inspected regularly to check its fit, especially in children who are still growing. During use it may become distorted or torn by chewing. Athletes should be warned that chewing the mouthguard will shorten its life and could potentially diminish its protection.

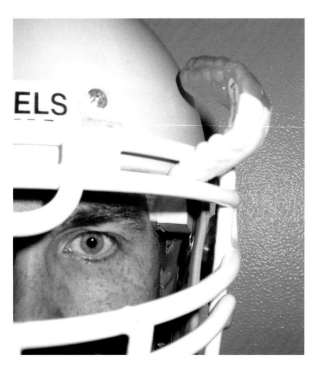

**Fig. 30.24** Athletes should also be taught proper care of the mouthguard during play, such as not chewing on it or placing it somewhere where it can easily be lost.

## Use of mouthguards and other protective appliances in various sports activities

Oral and dental injuries have been reported to be a relatively large portion of all injuries reported for certain sports (2, 62). Nysether found for example that approximately 20% of all reported injuries among Norwegian soccer players were dental injuries (62). In every fifth case the expenses for necessary dental treatment exceeded the maximum compensation from the insurance company. The best protection available for the oral and dental area should be a priority for everyone involved in sports activities, not only for the benefit of the participants but also to reduce the potential cost and liability of the organization.

### American football

As stated previously in this chapter the introduction of facemasks and proper helmets virtually eliminated oral and dental injuries (11–13). For dental protection the choice of mouthguard for American football does not appear to matter: boil-and-bite mouthguards appeared to provide as good protection as the custom made ones (54). However the comfort of the custom made is unquestioned especially for those who have to communicate frequently during the game.

### Baseball

The best protection for baseball players is a faceguard or a cage attached to the batting helmet. An intervention study

in juvenile baseball found that wearing a faceguard resulted in significantly less oculofacial injuries than not wearing one (16). For other players on the field it is possible that they would benefit from wearing a custom made mouthguard but as of yet no published study has investigated this.

### Basketball

Mouthguards have been shown to significantly reduce dental injuries and referral to dental offices for male players (25). For this sport there is no question that a custom made mouthguard is the only choice because both stock and boil-and-bite require the wearer to clench their jaws to keep it in place. The air flow is not affected by a custom made mouthguard but can be with a stock type (63).

### Boxing

Mouthguards were initially created for boxers to protect their soft tissue (18) but it soon became apparent that they protected the teeth much more than the lips and ginigiva (18, 19). There has been mandatory wear of a mouthguard in boxing at almost all levels for a long time and it is of note that despite repeated blows to the chin and face dental injuries appear to be relatively infrequent, most likely due to the mouthguards. It has been reported that none of 250 participants in an amateur boxing championship who were evaluated after the game had any visible dental trauma (64). All kinds of mouthguards have been suggested for boxers, both stock and custom made maxillary, as well as various forms of 'bimaxillar' that covers both arches. However once again no comprehensive study has been done to show that one type is more beneficial than other.

### Field and ice hockey

Hockey has been traditionally considered to be very dangerous for the oral and dental structures. A report from Helsinki, Finland found that of 106 patients with sports-related dental traumas, 39% of cases happened in ice hockey or skating. Many amateur and college level sports organizations have by now mandated faceguards as well as mouthguards for their players. Those actions have virtually eliminated lower facial injures (15), but only in the case of full facial guards because it has been shown that the so-called half mask that only covers the upper half of the face does not protect the jaws or oral cavity (17). The additional benefit of wearing a mouthguard to a full face mask in hockey is not clear and needs to be further investigated.

### Horseback riding

Facial injuries have been reported to be common among those who ride horses (65). However, the use of custom made mouthguards is not promoted by those in the equestrian industry. Use of helmets with face protectors have become more common, especially for the younger generation of riders but data is lacking about the effectiveness of those.

## Rugby

Several papers have reported on the protection, or lack thereof, of mouthguards (23, 26) in rugby. Once again a large intervention study is needed to clearly demonstrate how much a mouthguard does protect rugby players. Custom made mouthguards are probably the best for these players, primarily for comfort.

## Soccer

Soccer is without a doubt the most common sports activity in the world. The incidence of oral injuries has been reported surprisingly high, for example 28–32% in high school soccer players in a 2-year observation (66, 67). Yet in many areas there has been a very little discussion about need for dental protection. The risk seems to be especially high for goalkeepers and forwards, as well as for inexperienced teams (62). A custom mouthguard should be considered for those who are at risk.

## Team handball

Team handball is another aggressive contact sport where oral and dental protection does not seem to have gained much interest although there seems to be a high rate of injuries for participants (68). Effort should be made to make players aware of the risk as well as to investigate whether a custom mouthguard does offer protection.

## Cost–benefit of impact protecting devices

An unanswered question at present is how the cost of protecting individuals from injuries relates to the cost of treating actual injuries in a non-protected situation. This question becomes substantial in many sports activities where traumas are not that frequent (see Fig. 30.2). Before such a question can be answered for individual sports disciplines the following questions should be answered:

- What is the incidence of traumatic dental and maxillofacial injuries in that particular sport activity?
- Is there a typical trauma pattern in the particular sport?
- How effective are different protective devices?
- What are the costs of these devices?
- What is the cost of treating a typical traumatic injuries related to that particular sport activity?
- Can the protective device possibly cause a shift in injury pattern, like protecting the crown but causing instead alveolar or root fractures?

As stated previously very few studies have been conducted in a scientific manner and on a large scale on the actual effectiveness of all the above mentioned protective devices.

This was strongly highlighted in 2002 when a Task Force on Community Preventive Services (formed by the USA Government Agency: Centers for Disease Control and Prevention in Atlanta, GA) did systematic reviews of all papers that reported on effectiveness, applicability, other positive and negative effects, economic evaluations and barriers to use of selected population-based interventions intended to prevent or control sports-related craniofacial injuries (69). The report stated that there was not a single study that was sufficient to meet minimum requirements of the Task Force for inclusion in the report on the issue. The Task Force concluded: 'According to *Community Guide* rules of evidence, evidence is insufficient to determine the effectiveness of population-based interventions to encourage use of helmets, facemasks, and mouthguards in contact sports in increasing equipment use or reducing injury-related morbidity or mortality' (69).

There is no question that we need in the very near future multiple large epidemiological studies on sports injuries and their prevention, to confirm the clinical impression of effectiveness of protective devices. Detailed analysis of cost effectiveness should also be carried out for every sporting activity once that data is collected. This would be a good foundation for rational accident prevention in sports.

## Other applications for the use of mouthguards

### Protection of the dental tissues during general anesthesia

Oral endoscopy and orotracheal intubation may result in fracture or displacement of teeth (70–72). Damage may be inflicted by using the incisal edges of the anterior teeth as a fulcrum when inserting a laryngoscope, retractors or endoscopes. The fracture of prosthetic crowns has also been reported and injuries to the teeth are one of the most frequent complications during the delivery of general anesthesia (73). However, it is not at all clear how frequent this kind of trauma is, for it is likely that in many cases the damage is not discovered until months if not years later because the tooth or teeth only sustained mild luxation during the trauma rather than crown fracture or frank avulsion.

It has been suggested that patients who present with discolored and/or symptomatic anterior teeth for which there are no obvious etiologic factors should be carefully questioned regarding their past surgical history. If the patient denies a history of trauma yet relates a recent (2–5 years) history of general anesthesia, a differential diagnosis including trauma secondary to endotracheal intubation should be considered (74).

There are a number of injures to teeth during general anaesthesia. The most frequent of all anesthesia-related medicolegal claims was for dental injuries: up to one-third of all medicolegal claims against anesthetists (75). Concern for dental injuries of this type has increased due to an awareness of the medicolegal responsibility of the surgeon or anesthetist for iatrogenic injury (73). A number of methods have been recommended to prevent injuries in these circumstances; but there is little evidence of their success. Custom made mouthguards have not been considered cost-effective. This might be in part because anesthesiologists fear that the mouthguard could get in the way during intubation. However, a recent study showed that when comparing 80 patients, where half had a mouthguard and the other not, there was only on average 7 seconds difference between the two groups (76). When one considers the possible cost of legal action due to dental trauma, even as infrequent as they may be, the case for a dental protection of some sort during intubation becomes even stronger. At least in cases where there is a great risk of complications due to restorations, limited mouth opening etc., this approach might be advisable (77, 78).

## Prevention of oral injury from traffic accidents

As it appears from Fig. 30.1 traffic accidents are the cause of a significant amount of oral injuries. In that regard, some preventive measures can be made.

### Bicycle injuries

These injuries are very common in some countries, due to the popularity of bicycles. In addition, a relatively new extreme sport where a rider does tricks, jumps over obstacles and slides on rails etc. on BMX bikes has raised concerns by many dentists who treat dental injuries about the potential for serious injuries and the apparent lack of protectors for the lower portion of the face. No study has of yet has been completed on this subgroup of bicyclists but there is every indication that they do suffer as frequent and serious oral injuries as extreme skateboarders and rollerblades.

Bicycle riders are extremely exposed to head injury during accidents (14). In most of these injuries the impact direction is either direct and frontal or tangential to the face resulting in a combination of dental and soft tissue wounds when the face hits or slides along the ground (Fig. 30.25). The use of bicycle helmets has been common in professional bicycle sport and is now becoming popular among both children and adults. In some countries laws have been passed to require at least all children and even everyone riding a bicycle to wear an appropriate helmet. The bicycle helmet is primarily designed to prevent brain injuries and has been shown to reduce the risk of these injuries by 48% (14) but it offers no protection against injuries to the lower part to the face, including dental injuries (79–81).

### Motorcycle injuries

These traffic injuries are the most dangerous of all traffic accidents. In most countries the mandatory use of helmets has been legislated for. This preventive measure has been found to reduce the mortality rate significantly and also the

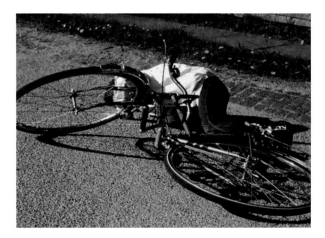

**Fig. 30.25** Head and facial injuries are frequent in bicycle accidents. In most of these injuries the impact direction is either direct and frontal or tangential to the face resulting in a combination of dental and soft tissue wounds when the face hits or slides along the ground.

frequency of oral and maxillofacial injuries (82, 83). Motorcycle helmets with chin-bars are likely to provide the best protection for the lower half of the face.

### Motor vehicle injuries

Head injuries are common in car accidents and vary significantly according to the person's position in the car. The driver is usually affected by direct impact with the steering wheel and/or the windscreen whereas the front seat passenger suffers from injuries related to a collision with the front seat panel and/or the windscreen. The back seat passenger usually faces collision with the front seat. In all of these instances a frontal impact is the result with a combination of soft tissue and dental and/or maxillofacial injuries.

Since the introduction of safety belts and later airbags a significant reduction in not only the mortality after automobile injuries has been noted but also a reduction in the severity of oral and maxillofacial injuries (Fig. 30.26) (84).

## Essentials

The majority of dental and oral injuries appear unexpectedly and during daily life activities which make their prevention difficult if not impossible. The best approach is education, both on how to avoid injuries as well as how to manage them when they occur.

At present preventive measures can be indicated in the following situations:

- Contact sports
- Certain traffic activities (bicycle, motorcycle, motor vehicle)
- Oral endoscopy and orotracheal intubation in cases with extensive restorations or a weakened periodontium.

Altogether, 7–25% of dental injuries appear to have a nature where preventive measures have a chance of reducing or preventing those from occurring.

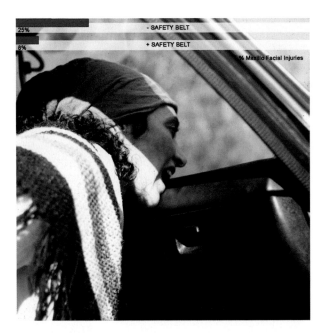

**Fig. 30.26** The introduction of safety belts and later airbags has significantly reduced not only mortality after automobile injuries but also the severity of oral and maxillofacial injuries.

## Preventive devices

- Helmets may prevent skull fractures and to a certain degree brain concussion but not dental injury if they are without faceguard or chin bar.
- Faceguards may prevent facial and oral injuries.
- Mouthguards may prevent or reduce the severity of oral traumas.

## Design of mouthguards

An ideal mouth guard should ideally have the following functions:

- Preventing or reducing injuries by absorbing or deflecting frontal and axial impacts
- Shielding the oral soft tissue
- Providing the mandible with resilient support during forceful occlusion that may prevent crown root fractures of premolars and molars, jaw fractures and brain concussion.

## Types of mouthguard

- Stock – prefabricated
- Mouth formed
- Custom made

Among these the custom made has the optimum comfort for the wearer and according to some the best trauma preventive capacity.

## Use of mouthguards and other preventive measures in sport

### American football

Helmets and face masks significantly reduce the chance of oral injury.

### Basketball

Mouthguards significantly reduce the frequency of oral injuries for males.

### Boxing

Mouthguards reduce the chance of dental injuries.

### Field and ice hockey

Face masks and/or mouth guards significantly reduce facial and oral injuries.

### Horseback riding

There is a high frequency of facial injuries. There is no report on the effect of preventive measures.

### Rugby

Mixed protection effects of mouthguards have been reported.

### Soccer

Possibly goal keepers and forwards may need mouth guard protection. Unfortunately no studies have verified this.

### Team handball

This sporting activity is attended by a number of injuries. There are no data of oral protective measures.

## Use of preventive measures in traffic

### Bicycle injuries

The use of helmets appears to reduce the frequency and severity of facial injuries.

### Motorcycle injuries

Helmets appear to reduce the frequency and severity of head injuries.

### Car injuries

Safety belts reduce the frequency, severity and mortality of facial injuries.

## Use of preventive measures in endoscopy and orotracheal intubation

Mouthguards are indicated in cases of maxillary anterior restoration (crowns, bridges and implants) or reduced periodontal support. The effectiveness of this procedure has not yet been documented.

## References

1. PETERSON EE, ANDERSSON L, SÖRENSEN S. Traumatic oral vs non-oral injuries. An epidemiological study during one year in a Swedish county. *Swed Dent J* 1997;**21**:55–68.
2. SKAARE AB, JACOBSEN I. Etiological factors related to dental injuries in Norwegians aged 7–18 years. *Dent Traumatol* 2003;**19**:304–8.
3. ANDREASEN FM. The price of a blue tooth – the cost of dental trauma. Presented at the World Congress on Sports Dentistry and Dental Traumatology. Boston, USA. June 20–24, 2001.
4. GUTMANN JK, GUTMANN MS. Cause, incidence, and prevention of trauma to teeth. *Dent Clin North Am* 1995;**39**:1–13.
5. EICHENBAUM I. A correlation of traumatised anterior teeth to occlusion. *ASDC J Dent Child* 1963;**30**:229–36.
6. SHULMAN JD, PETERSON J. The association between incisor trauma and occlusal characteristics in individuals 8–50 years of age. *Dent Traumatol* 2004;**20**:67–74.
7. BAUSS A, RÖHLING J, SCHWETKA-POLLY R. Prevalence of traumatic injuries to the permanent incisors in candidates for orthodontic treatment. *Dent Traumatol* 2004;**20**: 61–6.
8. GLENDOR U. On dental trauma in children and adolescents. Incidence, risk, treatment, time and costs. *Swed Dent J* Suppl 2000;**140**:1–52.
9. GLENDOR UB, KOUCHEKI B, HALLING A. Risk evaluation and type of treatment of multiple dental trauma episodes to permanent teeth. *Endod Dent Traumatol* 2000; **165**:205–10.
10. KUMAMOTO DP, WINTER J, NOVICKAS D, MESA KL. Tooth avulsions resulting from basketball net entanglement. *J Am Dent Assoc* 1997;**128**:1273–5.
11. HEINTZ WD. Mouth protectors: a progress report. Bureau of Dental Health Education. *J Am Dent Assoc* 1968;**77**:632–6.
12. BUREAU OF DENTAL HEALTH EDUCATION. Mouth protectors: 11 years later. *J Am Dent Assoc* 1973; **86**:1365–7.
13. GABON MA, WRIGHT JT. Mouth protectors and oral trauma: study of adolescent football players. *J Am Dent Assoc* 1986;**112**:663–5.
14. VULCAN AP, CAMERON MH, WATSON WL. Mandatory bicycle helmet use, experience in Victoria, Australia. *World J Surg* 1992;**16**:389–97.
15. MURRAY TM, LIVINGSTON A. Hockey helmets, face masks, and injurious behavior. *Pediatrics* 1995;**95**:419–21.
16. DANIS RP, HU K, BELL M. Acceptability of baseball faceguards and reduction of oculofacial injury in receptive youth league players. *Inj Prev* 2000;**6**:232–4.
17. BENSON BW, MOHTADI NG, ROSE MS, MEEUWISSE WH. Head and neck injuries among ice hockey players wearing full face shields vs half face shields. *J Am Med Assoc* 1999;**282**:2328–32.
18. REED RV. Origin and early history of the dental mouthpiece. *Br Dent J* 1994;**176**:478–80.
19. McCRORY P. Do mouthguards prevent concussion? *Br J Sports Med* 2001;**35**:81–2.
20. DAVIES RM, BRADLEY D, HALE RW, LARID WR, TOMAS PD. The prevalence of dental injuries in rugby players and their attitude to mouthguards. *Br J Sports Med* 1977;**11**:72–4.
21. HUGHSTON JC. Prevention of dental injuries in sports. *Am J Sports Med* 1980;**8**:61–2.
22. DE WET FA. The prevention of orofacial sports injuries in the adolescent. *Int Dent J* 1981;**31**:313–19.
23. CHAPMAN PJ, NASSER BP. Prevalence of orofacial injuries and use of mouthguards in high school Rugby Union. *Aust Dent J* 1996;**41**:252–5.
24. MORTON JG, BURTON JF. An evaluation of the effectiveness of mouthguards in high-school rugby players. *N Z Dent J* 1979;**75**:151–3.
25. LaBELLA CR, SMITH BW, SIGURDSSON A. Effect of mouthguards on dental injuries and concussions in college basketball. *Med Sci Sports Exerc* 2002;**34**:41–4.
26. BLIGNAUT JB, CARSTENS IL, LOMBARD CJ. Injuries sustained in rugby by wearers and non-wearers of mouthguards. *Br J Sports Med* 1987;**21**:5–7.
27. STEVENS OO. In: Andreasen JO. ed. *Traumatic injuries to the teeth*. Copenhagen: Munskgaard, 1981:442.
28. JOHNSTON T, MESSER LB. An *in vitro* study of the efficacy of mouthguard protection for dentoalveolar injuries in deciduous and mixed dentitions. *Endod Dent Traumatol* 1996;**12**:277–85.
29. MORIKAWA MH, TANIGUCHI H, OHYAMA T. Evaluation of athletic mouthguard through vibration test on maxillary teeth of human dry skull. *J Med Dent Sci* 1998;**45**:9–18.
30. BEMELMANNS P, PFEIFFER P. Shock absorption capacities of mouthguards in different types and thicknesses. *Int J Sports Med* 2001;**22**:149–53.
31. HOFFMANN J, ALFTER G, RUDOLPH NK, GOZ G. Experimental comparative study of various mouthguards. *Endod Dent Traumatol* 1999;**15**:157–63.
32. TAKEDA T, ISHIGAMI K, SHINTARO K, NAKAJIMA K, SHIMADA A, REGNER CW. The influence of impact object characteristics on impact force and force absorption by mouthguard material. *Dent Traumatol* 2004;**20**: 12–20.
33. TAKEDA T, ISHIGAMI K, JUN H, NAKAMIMA K, SHIMADA A, OGAWA T. The influence of the sensor type on the measured impact absorption of mouthguard material. *Dent Traumatol* 2004;**20**:29–35.
34. CHACONAS SJ, CAPUTO AA, BAKKE NK. A comparison of athletic mouthguard materials. *Am J Sports Med* 1985;**13**:193–7.
35. KIM HS, MATHIEU K. Application of laminates to mouthguards: finite element analysis. *J Mater Sci Mater Med* 1998;**9**:457–62.
36. CHAPMAN PJ. The bimaxillary mouthguard: a preliminary report of use in contact sports. *Aust Dent J* 1986;**31**:200–6.
37. CHAPMAN PJ. Mouthguard protection in sports. *Aust Dent J* 1996;**41**:212.

38. BIASCA NS, WIRTH S, TEGNER Y. The avoidability of head and neck injuries in ice hockey: an historical review. *Br J Sports Med* 2002;**36**:410–27.

39. STENGER JM, LAWSON E, WRIGHT JM, RICKETTS J. Mouthguards: protection against shock to head, neck and teeth. *J Am Dent Assoc* 1964;**69**:273–81.

40. HICKEY JC, MORRIS AL, CARLSON LD, SEWARD TE. The relation of mouth protectors to cranial pressure and deformation. *J Am Dent Assoc* 1967;**74**:735–40.

41. OMMAYA A. Head injury mechanisms and the concept of preventative management: a review and critical synthesis. *J Neurotrauma* 1995;**12**:527–46.

42. WISNIEWSKI JF, GUSKIEWICA K, TROPE M, SIGURDSSON A. Incidence of cerebral concussions associated with type of mouthguard used in college football. *Dent Traumatol* 2004;**20**:143–9.

43. GOING RE, LOEHMAN RE, CHAN MS. Mouthguard materials: their physical and mechanical properties. *J Am Dent Assoc* 1974;**89**:132–8.

44. CHALMERS DJ. Mouthguards. Protection for the mouth in rugby union. *Sports Med* 1998;**25**:339–49.

45. WALKER J, JAKOBSEN J, BROWN S. Attitudes concerning mouthguard use in 7- to 8-year-old children. *ASDC J Dent Child* 6 2002;**9**:207–11, 126.

46. STOKES AN, CROFT GC, GEE D. Comparison of laboratory and intraorally formed mouth protectors. *Endod Dent Traumatol* 1987;**3**:255–8.

47. CHAPMAN PJ. Mouthguard protection in sports injury. *Aust Dent J* 1995;**40**:136.

48. NICHOLAS NK. Mouth protection in contact sports. *N Z Dent J* 1969;**65**:14–24.

49. PARK JB, SHAULL KL, OVERTON B, DONLY KL. Improving mouth guards. *J Prosthet Dent* 1994;**72**: 373–80.

50. CUMMINS NK, SPEARS IR. The effect of mouthguard design on stresses in the tooth-bone complex. *Med Sci Sports Exerc* 2002;**34**:942–7.

51. WESTERMAN BP, STRINGFELLOW PM, ECCLESTON JA. The effect on energy absorption of hard inserts in laminated EVA mouthguards. *Aust Dent J* 2000;**45**:21–3.

52. WESTERMAN BP, STRINGFELLOW PM, ECCLESTON JA. Beneficial effects of air inclusions on the performance of ethylene vinyl acetate EVA mouthguard material. *Br J Sports Med* 2002;**36**:51–3.

53. UPSON N. Mouthguards, an evaluation of two types for Rugby players. *Br J Sports Med* 1985;**19**:89–92.

54. WISNIEWSKI JF, GUSKIEWICZ K, TROPE M, SIGURDSSON A. The incidence of dental trauma associated with type of mouthguard used in college football. *Dent Traumatol* 2007. In press.

55. WAKED EJ, LEE TK, CAPUTO AA. Effects of aging on the dimensional stability of custom made mouthguards. *Quintessence Int* 2002;**33**:700–5.

56. FEDERATION DENTAIRE INTERNATIONAL. Commission on dental products. Working Party No. 7. 1990.

57. MCCLELLAND C, KINIRONS M, GEARY L. A preliminary study of patient comfort associated with customised mouthguards. *Br J Sports Med* 1999;**33**: 186–9.

58. YONEHATA Y, MAEDA Y, MACHI H, SAKAGUCHI RL. The influence of working cast residual moisture and temperature on the fit of vacuum-forming athletic mouth guards. *J Prosthet Dent* 2003;**89**:23–7.

59. YAMANAKA T, UENO T, OKI M, TANIGUCHI H, OHYAMA T. Study on the effects of shortening the distal end of a mouthguard using modal analysis. *J Med Dent Sci* 2002;**49**:129–33.

60. WESTERMAN B, STRINGFELLOW PM, ECCLESTON JA. EVA mouthguards: how thick should they be? *Dent Traumatol* 2002;**18**:24–7.

61. NACHMAN BMS, SMITH JF, RICHARDSON FS. Football players opinions of mouthguards. *J Am Dent Assoc* 1965;**70**:62–9.

62. NYSETHER S. Dental injuries among Norwegian soccer players. *Comm Dent Oral Epidemiol* 1987;**15**:141–3.

63. AMIS T, DI SOMMA E, BACHA F, WHEATLEY J. Influence of intra-oral maxillary sports mouthguards on the airflow dynamics of oral breathing. *Med Sci Sports Exerc* 2000;**32**:284–90.

64. DE CARDENAS SO. Mouth protectors during the 1st World Amateur Boxing Championship. *Rev Cubana Estomatol* 1975;**12**:49–66.

65. DOUGLAS BL. Oral protection for equestrians. *CDS Rev* 1995;**88**:28–30.

66. YAMADA T, SAWAKI Y, TOMIDA S, TOHNAI I, UEDA M. Oral injury and mouthguard usage by athletes in Japan. *Endod Dent Traumatol* 1998;**14**:84–7.

67. KVITTEM B, HARDIE NA, ROETTGER M, CONRY J. Incidence of orofacial injuries in high school sports. *J Public Health Dent* 1998;**58**:288–93.

68. LANG B, POHL Y, FILIPPI A. Knowledge and prevention of dental trauma in team handball in Switzerland and Germany. *Dent Traumatol* 2002;**18**:329–34.

69. TRUMAN BI, GOOCH BF, SULEMANA I, GIFT HC, HOROWITZ AM, EVANS CA, GRIFFIN SO, CARANDE-KULIS VG. Reviews of evidence on interventions to prevent dental caries, oral and pharyngeal cancers, and sports-related craniofacial injuries. *Am J Prev Med* 2002;**23** (Suppl 1):21–53.

70. BAMFORTH BJ. Complications during endotracheal anaesthesia. *Anesth Analges* 1963;**42**:727–32.

71. WRIGHT RB, MANFIELD FFV. Damage to the teeth during the administration of general anaesthesia. Anesth Analges 1974;**53**:405–8.

72. MCCARTHY G, CARLSON O. A dental splint for use during peroral endoscopy. *Acta Otolaryngol* 1977;**84**: 450–2.

73. LOCKHART PB, FELDBAU EV, BABEL RA. Dental complications during and after tracheal intubation. *J Am Dent Assoc* 1986;**112**:480–3.

74. SIMON JH, LIES J. Silent trauma. *Endod Dent Traumatol* 1999;**15**:145–8.

75. CHADWICK RG, LINDSAY SM. Dental injuries during general anaesthesia: can the dentist help the anaesthetist? *Dent Update* 1998;**25**:76–8.

76. BROSNAN C, RADFORD P. The effect of a toothguard on the difficulty of intubation. *Anaesthesia* 1997;**52**: 1011–14.

77. CHADWICK RG, LINDSAY M. Dental injuries during general anaesthesia. *Br Dent J* 1996;**180**:255–8.

78. SKEIE A, SCHWARTZ O. Traumatic injuries of the teeth in connection with general anaesthesia and the effect of use of mouthguards. *Endod Dent Traumatol* 1999;**15**:33–6.

79. ACTON CH, NIXON JW, CLARK RC. Bicycle riding and oral/maxillofacial trauma in young children. *Med J Aust* 1996;**165**:249–51.

80. LINN S, SMITH D, SHEPS S. Epidemiology of bicycle injury, head injury and helmet use among children in British Colombia: a five year descriptive study. Canadian hospitals injury reporting and prevention program (CHIRPP). *Inj Prev* 1998;**4**:122–5.

81. THOMPSON DC, NUNN MF, THOMPSON RS, RIVARA FP. Effectiveness of bicycle safety helmets in preventing facial injury. *J Amer Med Ass* 1997;**276**:1774–5.

82. KELLY P, SANSON T, STRANGE G, ORSAY E. A prospective study of the impact of helmet usage on motorcycle trauma. *Ann Emerg Med* 1991;**20**:852–6.

83. BACHULIS BL, SANSTER W, GORRELL GW, et al. Patterns of injury in helmet and nonhelmet motorcyclists. *Am J Surg* 1988;**155**:708–11.

84. REATH DB, KIRBY J, LYNCH M, MAULL KI. Patterns of maxillofacial injuries in restrained and unrestrained motor vehicle crash victims. *J Trauma* 1989;**29**:806–9.

85. NYSETHER S. Traumatic dental injuries among Norwegian athletes. *Nor Tannlaegeforen Tid* 1987;**97**:512–14.

# 31

# Prognosis of Traumatic Dental Injuries: Statistical Considerations

P. K. Andersen, F. M. Andreasen & J. O. Andreasen

## Identifying prognosis related factors

### Univariate and stratified analysis

In most dental trauma studies, a univariate analysis is performed where healing outcomes are compared against various pre-injury and injury factors (e.g. age, root development, severity of trauma) and treatment factors (e.g. type of splinting, antibiotics, treatment delay). A minimum observation time should be used (usually one year) in order for a given complication to become manifest. A *univariate analysis* is then performed using Chi square or other tests. This will normally reveal a series of significant relations among which a number are due to associations between related parameters (e.g. age and root development). To reveal these associations a *stratified analysis* should be performed where for instance root development (mature and immature) is subdivided for given age groups. In this way a certain number of associations can be revealed and redundant factors can be excluded from having a significant influence on healing outcome.

## Expressing prognosis quantitatively

In the dental literature, the most frequently used method for expressing prognosis is as proportion survival, where n treatments are followed for time intervals of varying lengths and x/n ×100% of these procedures develop a given complication x. Prognosis is then related to an average or median interval (1, 2).

When analyzing the occurrence of events, such as pulp necrosis (PN), pulp canal obliteration (PCO) and root resorption (RR) after dental trauma, *time* becomes very important. First, from a clinical point of view, where the time after injury at which complications are likely to occur, and the order in which different complications can be anticipated, play an important role for clinical decision making.

As healing complications usually appear with some time variation, the length of observation period of patients followed is decisive (Fig. 31.1). If, for example, the observation period for an overwhelming majority of patients in a trauma study is so long that most complications will have appeared (period C), conventional frequency calculations will provide a reliable picture of the likelihood of a given event. However, if prognosis is calculated from a material with a very short observation period (period A), an unrealistically optimistic picture of complication events will be presented. In period B, a varied picture of the appearance of complications will be seen due to variation in length of observation periods and their relation to the chance of detecting a given complication (1).

It can be seen from Figs 31.2–31.4 that pulp necrosis, pulp canal obliteration and root resorption after luxation or avulsion with subsequent replantation of permanent teeth appear with relatively large variations in time (3–8). Thus, expression of prognosis for these complications will show great variation from one investigation to another, making comparison of results difficult, if not impossible. However, using the method of meta-analysis (see later), it is possible to summarize the results from similar investigations in a quantitative manner.

Also, from a statistical point of view, the time factor is important because teeth are observed at varying time intervals due to staggered entry and a fixed closing date, implying different probabilities of experiencing a given complication within the period of observation. This fact must be taken into account in statistical analyses of clinical data on dental trauma. This problem can be overcome by focusing on events during a time interval of fixed length and expressing prognosis as proportion survival as explained above; but such a procedure may involve a serious loss of information.

An informative expression of prognosis is achieved by means of *life table*, or *actuarial statistics*, by which variation in prognosis with variation in observation period can be described. Such an analysis permits full utilization of all 'survival' information accumulated up to the closing date of the

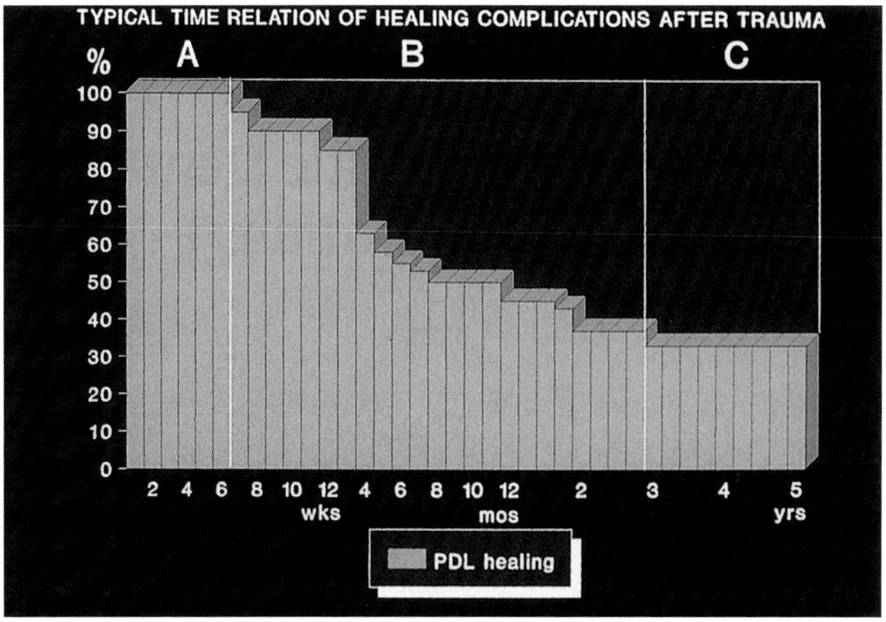

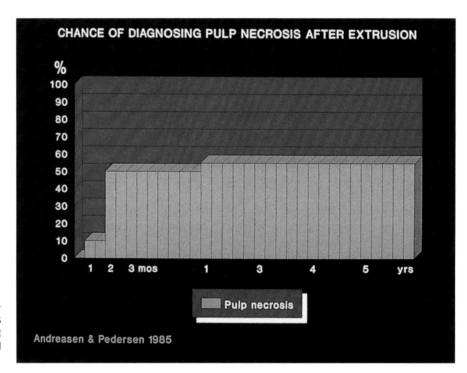

**Fig. 31.1** Typical time relation between occurrence of healing complications after dental trauma. From ANDREASEN (1) 1987.

**Fig. 31.2** Observation time and probability of diagnosis of pulp necrosis after extrusion of mature permanent teeth. From ANDREASEN & PEDERSEN (3) 1985.

study, including information from patients with partial follow-ups (i.e. patients not followed through to the occurrence of a given complication or terminal event). This form of analysis is well known and widely applied in studies of life expectancy with cancer (9–12). It has also been applied to long-term dental investigations, such as the longevity of dental filling materials (13–16), pulp capping procedures (17), tooth transplantation (18, 19), endodontic procedures (25–27, 29) and long-term prognosis of various dental trauma entities (3–8, 20, 21, 35–37). Non-technical text books on survival analysis are also available (12, 22–24).

A crucial difference in survival data from, e.g., cancer trials and data on occurrence of complications after dental trauma results from the non-fatal nature of the latter complications. Typically, the occurrence of a dental complication must be diagnosed in a clinical investigation, and this means that only at some predetermined observation periods can it be seen whether a given complication has arisen since the previous follow-up examination; but the precise time of occurrence in the time interval cannot be determined. Thus, the relevant statistical analysis of occurrences of complications is an analysis of *grouped survival data* (3).

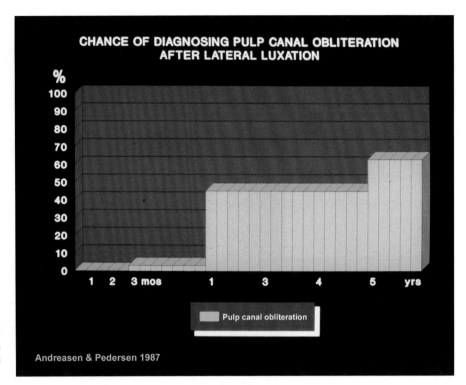

**Fig. 31.3** Observation time and probability of pulp canal obliteration subsequent to lateral or extrusive luxation of mature permanent teeth. From ANDREASEN et al. (5) 1987.

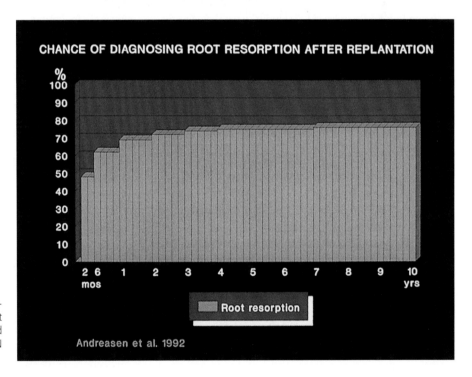

**Fig. 31.4** Observation time and probability of diagnosis of external root resorption after replantation of avulsed permanent teeth. From ANDREASEN et al. (7) 1995.

A calculation illustrating the principles of life-table analysis is presented in the following example of patients suffering dental trauma (e.g. replantation of avulsed teeth) (Fig. 31.5). Each patient will represent one of the following three outcomes:

• *Failed* – if the replanted tooth has developed one of the complications under study.
• *Withdrawn* – if the tooth (patient) is lost from the trial for any reason other than healing complications from the injury. For example, if a patient stopped attending recall examinations and was lost to follow-up, or if a tooth was lost due to causes unrelated to the initial trauma, e.g. a new acute injury.
• *Censored* – if the tooth is still in function at the end of the investigation and does not show the complications being studied.

The following example will show the principles of the calculations behind a tooth survival analysis: Ten patients with a total of 10 replanted incisors participate in a prospective investigation. There are no teeth showing failure at the end

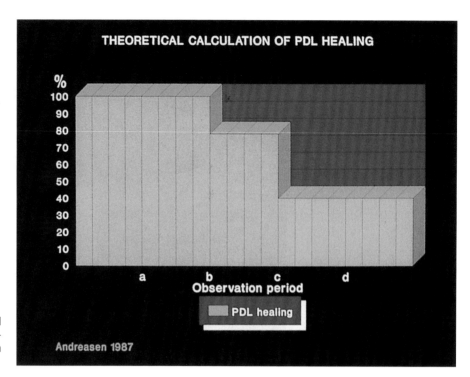

**Fig. 31.5** Calculation of periodontal ligament survival in a theoretical clinical dental trauma study. From ANDREASEN (1) 1987.

of the first observation period (a). Tooth survival at the end of the first interval is therefore 100%. At the end of the next interval (b), failure is seen in 2 teeth. Tooth survival is now:

$$(10 - 2) / 10 \times 100\% = 80\%$$

In the third observation period (c), there are now only 8 teeth at risk. Of these 8 teeth, 4 fail; that is, 4/8 of 80% have survived, yielding 40% survival. No complications are registered in the fourth interval (d), but 2 patients have such short observation periods that they are withdrawn from the study. There are now only 2 teeth left. Tooth survival is therefore 2/2 of 40% = 40%. It can be seen from Fig. 31.5 that the risk for a given complication can now be calculated for a given observation period (3).

Life table statistics are sensitive to a number of factors, such as definitions of failed, withdrawn and censored patients, as well as recall procedures and sample size. The significance of these factors will therefore be discussed.

## Importance of definition of failures

*Failures* can be defined according to the type of dental trauma analyzed, such as loss of tooth, root resorption, development of pulp necrosis, pulp canal obliteration or loss of marginal bone support. Each of these conditions (apart from tooth loss) represents unique diagnostic difficulties. Thus, *pulp necrosis* is dependent upon a number of diagnostic procedures, where none is conclusive (see Chapter 13, p. 378). *Pulp canal obliteration, root resorption* and *loss of marginal bone support* are primarily dependent upon radiographic examination procedures (see Chapter 13). This implies that a variation in technique could influence the sensibility of the analysis. Concerning *tooth loss*, it should be established whether the tooth in question was otherwise

intact and in function, and that the extraction was *not* related to the previous trauma (e.g. a traffic accident, extraction for orthodontic or prosthetic purposes). Otherwise serious bias might arise.

## Importance of censored patients

The definition of a censored event (i.e. tooth survival or tooth presence without pathology), like failures, is entirely dependent upon the established criteria for pathology. Furthermore, it is important that the majority of censored data represent adequate observation periods for the complication to have had a chance to appear. Otherwise problems may arise regarding the reliability of the survival analysis.

## Importance of withdrawn patients

The usual reason for withdrawal of patients from continuing examination appears to be one of the following:

- The patient cannot be traced (moved without a forwarding address, emigration, death).
- The patient has received a recall notice and chosen not to respond.
- The tooth in question is lost.
- The tooth in question has survived and the patient does not feel the need for a follow-up examination.
- The patient ignores the recall notice for other reasons (e.g. inconvenience or lack of interest).

If the reasons for no-show at a scheduled follow-up are centered around the first two reasons for withdrawal, the analysis may be seriously jeopardized. The relevance of no-shows has only been studied in a few dental investigations (25–27). Thus, it was shown in a long-term study of healing after surgical endodontics that patients not initially responding to recall notices, when later examined after extensive recall efforts demonstrated the same healing pattern as the rest of the material (27). This illustrates that, at least in the cited study, the no-shows were usually related to inconvenience for the patient of the scheduled examination. Also the situation where patients feeling well tend to withdraw may cause bias since the patients remaining in the study are no longer representative for the treated patient population (so-called 'dependent censoring').

## Importance of the length of the investigation period

This is a crucial factor and should be related to the mean or median observation period for the occurrence of the event under investigation. Thus, root resorption requires extended observation periods for the material before any meaningful survival statistics can be established (7, 8).

## Importance of sample size

The sample size becomes very important especially when the pathological event under investigation occurs infrequently.

## Effect of recall schedule

As mentioned above, it can usually only be established at some prescheduled follow-up examinations whether a given complication has arisen since the previous examination, whereas the precise time of occurrence within that period cannot be determined. The recall schedule is therefore important. Short time intervals between successive follow-up examinations are recommended when the rate of failure is high, whereas longer time intervals may be chosen when few failures are likely to occur.

## Comparing life tables

### The logrank test for comparison of life tables

Life table estimates for the survival probability in two groups, e.g. two randomized treatment groups, may be compared at a single point in time, t, using the variance estimate based on Greenwood's formula (12). It would be more efficient, however, to compare survival of the two groups on the entire survival functions and not only on their value at a single point in time. This may be done using the *logrank test statistic* for the case of continuously observed i.e. *non-grouped survival data* (9, 10). For *grouped survival data*, a similar test has been developed (12).

### Further treatment comparisons, multiple regression analysis

In almost all clinical investigations, the identification of clinical factors which have an effect on the occurrence of healing

**Table 31.1** Effect of antibiotics upon fracture healing.

|  | Infected cases | Healed cases | n |
|---|---|---|---|
| Antibiotics (intervention) | 10 (a) | 90 (b) | 100 (e) |
| Control | 20 (c) | 80 (d) | 100 (f) |

complications after trauma has been achieved using univariate statistical analysis, where it is assumed that all teeth in the group for which the estimate is calculated have the same survival probability. In this type of analysis, each potential causative factor is considered individually, usually with the result that numerous clinical factors can be identified that are significantly related to the given healing complication. In many cases, however, the groups are heterogeneous and the relationships found may have little biological relevance, as they may be due to associations between registered clinical parameters. As an example, assume that the stage of root development is the only clinical parameter related to a given complication, and a given type of treatment (e.g. repositioning and splinting) is chosen according to stage of root development. In such a case, in a univariate analysis, there may be a significant relationship between treatment procedure and complication due to this association.

In order to identify and eliminate such associations, various multiple regression analyses have been developed whereby the effect of several factors is studied simultaneously.

In the case of continuously observed data, the *Cox regression model* is frequently used (12, 22–24, 30). It is also possible to use such a model for grouped survival data when, e.g. treatment comparisons are to be made in the presence of other prognostic factors (3, 31). An alternative model which is frequently used is the *logistic regression model* for grouped survival data (30). This model leads to effects of prognostic factors being quantified as *odds ratios* (Table 31.1). Using such multiple regression models, associations can be disclosed and/or eliminated and this has been shown to significantly reduce the number of predictors for healing complications after dental traumas (3, 6–8, 32).

### Odds ratio (OR) and risk ratio (RR)

OR represents the risk for an experimental group compared to that of the control group. RR is defined as the ratio of risk in the intervention group to the risk in the control group. Risk is the ratio of people with an event in a group to the total in the group.

In the following example, the action of OR and RR is shown for a constructed example in a trauma situation (Table 31.1).

$$OR = \frac{a/b}{c/d} = \frac{10/90}{20/80} = 0.44$$

$$RR = \frac{a/e}{c/f} = \frac{10/100}{20/100} = 0.50$$

An OR or RR of 1 indicates no difference between comparison groups. For undesirable outcome, an OR that is <1 indicates that the intervention was effective in reducing the risk of outcome. Likewise figures above indicate increased risk in the intervention group.

## The use of predictors and confidence limits

From a regression model it is possible to estimate the probability that a given complication will arise during a given interval for a patient having a tooth with the given characteristics. Confidence limits for such a predictor may also be estimated. It is important to note that, due to the association between prognostic factors, such individual predictions *must* be based on a multiple regression model and cannot be obtained from a series of single-factor analyses.

## Comparing tooth survival or healing results from various studies

In the evaluation of the effect of various treatment modalities, the usual approach is to report the individual findings from clinical studies, the so-called narrative review (33). Such an analysis usually results in a range of treatment effects from which it is difficult to summarize the effect of a given treatment. To overcome this difficulty, *meta-analysis* can be used. This method uses statistical techniques to summarize estimates from a series of studies with common underlying characteristics (34) and thus allows estimation of the magnitude of a treatment effect. The principle is that when the effect of the same treatment has been estimated in a number of similar studies (together with confidence limits), a quantitative overview can be obtained as a weighted average of the individual estimates using as weights the precision of the individual estimates.

## Essentials

### Expressing prognosis quantitatively

- Percent calculation (i.e. disregarding relationship to observation period)
- Life table statistics (i.e. incorporating relationship to observation period)

### Factors of importance for life table analysis

- Definition of healing and non-healing
- Censored patients
- Withdrawn patients
- Length of period under consideration
- Sample size
- Recall schedule

### Comparing life tables

- Log rank test for treatment comparisons

## Multiple regression analysis
## Odds and risk ratio
## Predictors and confidence intervals
## Comparing healing results

- Meta-analysis

## References

1. ANDREASEN FM. Prognoser ved tandskader i det permanente tandsæt. *Odontologi '87.* Copenhagen: Munksgaards Forlag, 1987:149–64.
2. DAMES JA. Dental restoration longevity: a critique of the life table method of analysis. *Community Dent Oral Epidemiol* 1987;**15**:202–4.
3. ANDREASEN FM, PEDERSEN BV. Prognosis of luxated permanent teeth – the development of pulp necrosis. *Endod Dent Traumatol* 1985;**1**:207–20.
4. ANDREASEN F, YU Z, THOMSEN BL. The relationship between pulpal dimensions and the development of pulp necrosis after luxation injuries in the permanent dentition. *Endod Dent Traumatol* 1986;**2**:90–8.
5. ANDREASEN FM, YU Z, THOMSEN BL, ANDERSEN PK. The occurrence of pulp canal obliteration after luxation injuries in the permanent dentition. *Endod Dent Traumatol* 1987;**3**:103–15.
6. ANDREASEN JO, BORUM M, JACOBSEN HL, ANDREASEN FM. Replantation of 400 avulsed permanent incisors. II. Factors related to root growth after replantation. *Endod Dent Traumatol* 1995;**11**:59–68.
7. ANDREASEN JO, BORUM M, JACOBSEN HL, ANDREASEN FM. Replantation of 400 avulsed permanent incisors. IV. Factors related to periodontal ligament healing. *Endod Dent Traumatol* 1995;**11**:76–89.
8. ANDREASEN JO, BORUM MK, ANDREASEN FM. Progression of root resorption after replantation of 400 avulsed human incisors. In: Davidovitch Z. ed. *The biological mechanisms of tooth eruption, resorption and replacement by implants.* Boston: Harvard Society for the Advancement of Orthodontics, 1994:577–82.
9. PETO R, PIKE MC, ARMITAGE P, et al. Design and analysis of randomized clinical trials requiring prolonged observation of each patient. II. Analysis and examples. *Br J Cancer* 1977;**35**:1–39.
10. PETO R, PIKE MC, ARMITAGE P, et al. Design and analysis of randomized clinical trials requiring prolonged observation of each patient. I. Introduction and design. *Br J Cancer* 1976;**34**:585–612.
11. LEE ET. *Statistical methods for survival data analysis.* Belmont, California: Lifetime Learning Publications, 1980.
12. ANDERSEN PK, VÆTH M. *Statistisk analyse af overlevelsesdata ved lægevidenskabelige undersøgelser.* Copenhagen: FADL's Forlag, 1984.
13. THYLSTRUP A, RÖLLING I. The life table method in clinical dental research. *Commun Dent Oral Epidemiol* 1975;**3**:5–10.
14. WALLS AWG, WALLWORK MA, HOLLAND IS, MURRAY JJ. The longevity of occlusal amalgam restorations in first

permanent molars of child patients. *Br Dent J* 1985;**158**:133–6.

15. SMALES RJ. Effects of enamel-bonding, type of restoration, patient age and operator on the longevity of an anterior composite resin. *Am J Dent* 1991;**4**: 130–3.

16. SMALES RJ, WEBSTER DA, LEPPARD PI. Survival predictions of four types of dental restorative materials. *J Dent* 1991;**19**:278–82.

17. HÖRSTED P, SÖNDERGAARD B, THYLSTRUP A, EL ATTAR K, FEJERSKOV O. A retrospective study of direct pulp capping with calcium hydroxide compounds. *Endod Dent Traumatol* 1985;**1**:29–34.

18. SCHWARZ O, BERGMANN P, KLAUSEN B. Autotransplantation of human teeth. A life-table analysis of prognostic factors. *Int J Oral Surg* 1985;**14**:245–58.

19. ANDREASEN JO, PAULSEN HU, YU Z, BAYER T, SCHWARTZ O. A long-term study of 370 autotransplanted premolars. Part II. Tooth survival and pulp healing subsequent to transplantation. *Eur J Orthod* 1990;**12**:14–24.

20. ANDREASEN FM, ANDREASEN JO, BAYER T. Prognosis of root fractured permanent incisors – prediction of healing modalities. *Endod Dent Traumatol* 1989;**5**:11–22.

21. MITCHELL L, WALLS AWG. Survival analysis in practice. *Dental Update* 1990;April:125–8.

22. COLLETT D. *Modelling survival data in medical research.* London: Chapman and Hall, 1994.

23. PARMAR MKB, MACHIN D. *Survival analysis. A practical approach.* London: John Wiley and Sons, 1995.

24. MARUBINI E, VALSECCHI MG. *Analysing survival data from clinical trials and observational studies.* London: John Wiley and Sons, 1995.

25. STRINDBERG LZ. The dependence of the results of pulp therapy on certain factors. An analytic study based on radiographic and clinical follow-up examinations. *Acta Odontol Scand* 1956;**14**(Suppl):21.

26. MÜHLEMANN HR. Zur statistischen Beurteilung von Wurzelbehandlungserfolgen. *Schweiz Monatschr Zahnheilk* 1965;**75**:1135–42.

27. RUD J, ANDREASEN JO, MÖLLER JENSEN JE. A follow-up study of 1000 cases treated by endodontic surgery. *Int J Oral Surg* 1972;**1**:215–28.

28. FAZIO RC, BOFFA J. A study of 'broken appointment' patients in children's hospital dental clinic. *J Dent Res* 1977;**56**:1071–6.

29. APT H, DYRNA G, NITZSCHE W, VOLKER J. Mathematisch-statistische Aussagekraft klinisch-röntgenologischer Nachuntersuchungen von Wurzelbehandlungen. *Zahn Mund Kieferheilk* 1975;**63**:819–22.

30. COX DR. Regression models and life tables. *J Royal Stat Soc* 1972;**34**:187–220.

31. PRENTICE RL, GLOECKLER LA. Regression analysis of grouped survival data with applicaton to breast cancer data. *Biometrics* 1978;**34**:57–67.

32. ANDREASEN FM. Pulpal healing after luxation injuries and root fracture in the permanent dentition. *Endod Dent Traumatol* 1989;**5**:111–31.

33. EARLY BREAST CANCER TRIALISTS' COLLABORATIVE GROUP. Effects of adjuvant tamoxifen and of cytotoxic therapy on mortality in early breast cancer: an overview of 61 randomized trials among 28 896 women. *New Engl J Med* 1988;**319**:1681–92.

34. COHEN PA. Meta-analysis: application to clinical dentistry and dental education. *J Dent Education* 1992;**56**:172–5.

35. ANDREASEN JO, BAKLAND L, ANDREASEN FM. Traumatic intrusion of permanent teeth. Part 2. A clinical study of the effect of preinjury and injury factors, such as sex, age, stage of root development, tooth location, and extent of injury including number of intruded teeth on 140 intruded permanent teeth. *Dent Traumatol* 2006;**22**:90–98.

36. BARRETT E, HUMPHREY JA, KENNY D. An analysis of outcomes following intrusion of permanent maxillary incisors in children. *Int J Paediatric Dent* 1999;**9**:14–22.

37. HUMPHREY JM, KENNY DJ, BARRETT EJ. Clinical outcomes for permanent incisor luxation in a pediatric population. I. Intrusions. *Dent Traumatol* 2003;**19**:266–73.

38. WEIGER R, AXMANN-KRCMAR D, LÖST C. Prognosis of conventional root canal treatment reconsidered. *Endod Dent Traumatol* 1998;**14**:1–9.

# 32
# Splinting of Traumatized Teeth

K. S. Oikarinen

Until the 1970s, splinting of traumatized teeth was primarily accomplished using methods employed in the treatment of jaw fractures, with cap splints, arch bars and wires (1–3). This was not only because of a lack of knowledge of the healing mechanisms of injured teeth, but also because of lack of appropriate splinting materials. Since the discovery of adhesive techniques in the late 1960s, a wide range of splinting devices has been developed (4, 5). However, the most important discovery in recent decades has been that splinting in general can have an adverse effect on healing processes in the periodontium and pulp after trauma. Thus, non-physiologic fixation of displaced teeth can induce periodontal and pulpal healing problems; and long-term splinting may not only prolong the wound healing process in the periodontal ligament (6), but may also lead to preservation of an otherwise transient ankylosis (7–10). Arrest of revascularization of the pulpal has also been observed in animal experiments (9). In autotransplantation of teeth, both ankylosis and increased risk for pulp necrosis have been observed more frequently in rigidly splinted than in flexibly splinted autotransplanted molars in humans (11). In the following, the effect of various splinting devices on the healing of dental tissues after injury will be discussed.

## Influence of splinting on dental tissues

### Influence upon gingiva

It has been shown that gingival damage caused by arch bars fastened with steel wires is reversible if the periodontium was healthy before splinting (12–19). Wire-loop splints (used in intermaxillary splinting) have been found to lead to gingival changes which are, however, reversible after wire removal (20). The presence of wires placed in contact with the gingiva may lead to invasion of bacteria through rupture or tears in the epithelial attachment.

## Influence upon periodontal healing

An early experimental study in 1974 by Andreasen (7), and supported by later clinical (11, 21) and experimental (8–10, 22) studies, demonstrated that optimal periodontal healing (i.e. with minimal ankylosis) after extraction and replantation of teeth in animals was obtained in a non-splinted situation compared to rigid splinting. It is assumed that slight mobility in the initial healing period activates resorption of initially formed ankylosis sites. Only a single experimental study did not support these findings (23).

## Influence upon pulp healing

In a monkey model of extracted and replanted teeth, it was shown that splinting could decrease pulp revascularization and increase the extent of pulp necrosis and inflammatory root resorption compared to non-splinting (9). In humans, splinting of autotransplanted teeth for only one week (with a suture splint, see later) has been found to improve pulpal healing as compared to rigid splinting for four weeks (21).

## Enamel changes after splinting

The staining of labial enamel after acid etching could present a problem, especially if filled composite resin has been used, where there is no clear distinction between enamel and the splinting material. However, experimental studies have shown that treatment of enamel with methods simulating various phases of splinting does not cause permanent staining; and discoloration can be removed with careful polishing (24).

## Requirements for an acceptable splint

The splint should preferably have slightly vertical and horizontal flexibility in order to support healing (see above). In

**Table 32.1** Comparison of different types of splints. Various properties are assessed on a three-point system. Plus (+) illustrates that the property is strongly related, plus-minus (±) that the property is slightly related and minus (−) that the property is not related to the splint concerned.

| Type of splint | Accuracy of reposition | Easily discolored | Flexibility | Rigidity | Easily fractured | Easy to construct | Suitability after dental trauma |
|---|---|---|---|---|---|---|---|
| Suture splint | + | | + | − | + | + | ± |
| Arch bar splint | − | − | − | + | − | − | − |
| Arch bar splint with acrylic | − | − | − | + | − | − | − |
| Flexible wire-composite | + | ± | + | − | − | + | + |
| Rigid wire-composite | + | ± | − | + | − | + | ± |
| Composite splint | + | ± | − | + | + | + | ± |
| Protemp®, Luxatemp® | + | ± | + | − | ± | + | + |
| TTS splint | ± | ± | + | ± | − | ± | + |
| Orthodontic splint | ± | ± | ± | ± | − | ± | ± |

the following, the rigidity of splints will be described as: *flexible* i.e. more mobility than a non-injured tooth, *semi-rigid*: equal to normal tooth mobility, and *rigid*: less than normal tooth mobility. An optimal splint should fulfil most or all of the following requirements:

- Direct intraoral application
- Easy to construct with materials available in dental practice
- Does not increase periodontal injuries or promote caries
- Does not irritate oral soft tissues
- Passive; does not exert any orthodontic force on teeth
- Versatile in achieving rigid, semi-rigid or flexible splint
- Easy to remove and causes minimal or no permanent damage to the dentition
- Allows pulp testing and endodontic treatment
- Hygienic and esthetic.

## Splinting methods

Since the discovery of the acid etch technique of enamel by Buonocore in 1955 (4), this procedure has had a major influence on splinting devices (5). Since the 1970s, several splinting methods have been introduced which allow slight horizontal and vertical movement, many of which utilize the acid etch technique, various types of wires or orthodontic appliances (25–29). Thus composite and similar materials can be attached firmly to the enamel surface. The area needed for acid etching can be limited to a small surface of the crown (3).

## Testing the mechanical properties of various splinting types

An experimental *acrylic model* jaw-tooth was designed to simulate the clinical mobility of teeth and the influence of various splinting devices. The lateral and vertical flexibility of two *arch bar splints* (Schuchardt and Erich arch bars), which are frequently used in the immobilization of jaw fractures, and a *wire-composite splint* were examined (30). The tests showed that a 0.3 mm thick wire-composite splint had

a flexibility which closely resembled that of a control situation, while arch bar splints with and without acrylic coverage virtually prevented vertical movement (30).

In a second study, using a *sheep jaw model*, a variety of different splinting materials were tested for their flexibility and grouped into rigid, semi-rigid and flexible (31). In this study, light cured composite resin splints, Fermit® (Vivadent, Germany) and Triad® gel composite splint (light cured gel form acrylic, Dentsply, USA) yielded a *non-flexible* splint. *Semi-rigid* splinting was achieved by Kevlar®, Fiber-splint®, Protemp II® (multiple functional methylacrylic esters, Espe, Germany) and flexible wire-composite splint. The latter splint types provided adequate lateral support for a loose injured tooth and also allowed slight vertical flexibility.

In order to establish optimal splinting stability, the foremost requirement is to define to what extent a loose tooth or tooth-bone segment should be immobilized in order to ensure optimal healing. Unfortunately, no such analysis exists. However, experience from vertical distraction osteogenesis indicates that limited mobility can advance osteogenesis (see Chapter 28, p. 781).

Properties of various suitable splinting materials are compared in Table 32.1. The most versatile splints are resin splints (Protemp®, Luxatemp®), wire-composite and TTS splints (titanium trauma splint), all of which fulfil the demands of modern dental splinting.

In the following, the various types of splints will be described.

### Suture splint

The simplest type of splint is a suture placed over the incisal edge from the palatal/lingual gingiva to the buccal gingiva. This fixation can be used, for example, in preventing repositioned incisors from extruding, but will only be effective for a short period of time (32–34). After autotransplantation of premolars, the suture is placed over the occlusal surface of the transplant (see Chapter 27). Suture splints have been found to improve the prognosis of autotransplanted teeth compared to rigid splints (11).

### Arch bar splint

Several decades ago, rigid splinting of luxated teeth was considered necessary, and the types of splints used were either

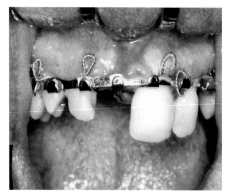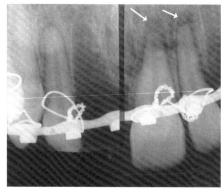

**Fig. 32.1** Displacement of an originally subluxated left central and lateral incisors by an Erich's arch bar (see arrows).

arch bars or cap splints. These splints caused considerable damage to the injured teeth, due to inaccurate repositioning, which could press the loose tooth against the socket wall (Fig. 32.1). Furthermore, there was risk of bacterial invasion into the periodontal wound due to the close proximity of the splints and wires to the gingival margin (35).

## Orthodontic appliances

Orthodontic ligature wire bonded with composite or attached to brackets has been advocated (36). However, orthodontic bracket wires and composite may cause irritation of oral mucosa, impairment of oral hygiene and discomfort, especially at the start of the splinting period (37). Furthermore, demands for a passive splinting (i.e. with the tooth in a neutral position) are endangered if brackets are united by rectangular orthodontic wires. It is therefore recommended that malleable steel wire is used (38).

## Composite resin

A splint composed entirely of composite resin is esthetic and easy to construct, but has been found to fracture in the interdental area, as the material is fragile. The splint is rigid and thereby violates the demands for splinting in most cases. Moreover, due to color match and bonding strength to etched enamel, it is difficult to remove without damaging underlying tooth structure. If a splint of this material must be used, it is advisable to splint the luxated tooth to only one adjacent tooth (39).

## Wire-composite splint

Wire-composite splinting was introduced in 1987 (40) and has since been reviewed (3) and tested both *in vitro* (12, 24, 30) and *in vivo* (39). One of the major benefits is that the splint is constructed of materials that are routinely available in dental offices. Detailed illustration of construction of a flexible wire-composite splint is illustrated in Fig. 32.2. Wire-composite splinting is easily modified into a rigid splint by changing the dimension of the wire or by adding composite along the labial wire up to the interdental space (Fig. 32.2). Examples of the use of wire-composite are shown in Figs 32.3 and 32.4. However, there is the same

problem concerning risk of potential damage to underlying enamel as with a composite splint.

In a recent comparative study of various types of splints in volunteers, a wire-composite splint proved to be well accepted, did not cause major damage to the oral mucosa and allowed the volunteer to maintain good oral hygiene (37).

In several studies the use of fiber glass instead of wires has been described and is frequently in use (27, 37, 42–44). Fiber glass ribbon is soaked in composite resin and no filler material is used. Flexibility can be varied with the numbers of layers and extension of the splint (27).

## Resin splint (e.g. Protemp® and Luxatemp®)

Protemp® and Luxatemp® are multi-phase resin materials used in temporary prosthetic restorations and for lining prefabricated crowns. Protemp® is chemically cured; whereas Luxatemp® is dual cured (i.e. chemical and light cured). It is possible to apply the material in stages, an advantage with multiple displaced and repositioned teeth (Fig. 32.5). These materials do not exert forces on teeth during application and are esthetically and hygienically acceptable. Furthermore, they have been shown to allow semi-rigid splinting (31).

In a case of missing teeth or in a mixed dentition, where neighboring teeth are not fully erupted, it is necessary to span the edentulous area. In these cases, reinforcement is necessary. This can be accomplished with metal bars, orthodontic wires, nylon lines, glass fibers, or synthetic fibers or tapes which are presently on the market (e.g. Kevlar®, Dupont Corp., Fiber-splint®, Polydent Corp., Mezzovico, Switzerland) and which can fuse with resin. If these are not available, even paperclips can be straightened out for the purpose. The material allows some flexibility and the splint is applied directly to etched crown surfaces.

## Prefabricated metal splinting materials

Commercially available dental splints have recently been introduced. Prefabricated splints made of titanium have been reported by von Arx and co-authors (37, 44, 45). The prefabricated titanium trauma splint (TTS) is only 0.2 mm thick and can easily be bent with fingers and adapted to the dental arch. Because of the rhomboid design of the splint, it

**Fig 32.2 Application of a wire composite splint**

(Left) Instruments needed. (Right) Loop of a 0.4 mm diameter soft round steel wire is twisted around the injured and neighboring teeth. Dental tooth picks both keep the labial part of the wire to the mid-portion of the crown and at the same time decrease papillary bleeding. It is important to ensure that the dental tooth picks keep the injured tooth in a neutral position and do not displace the loosened teeth. They should not be used to stabilize the luxated tooth.

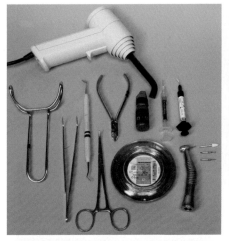
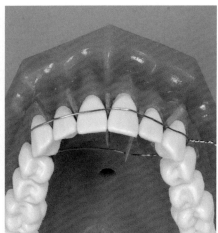

**Etching enamel and application of composite**

Only a small area on the mid-portion of the crown is etched. A small amount of resin is applied on the surface. Flowing light-cured composite is applied with a syringe. Composite is applied first on non-injured teeth. The luxated tooth is finally included in the splint. The position of the tooth is ensured with finger pressure.

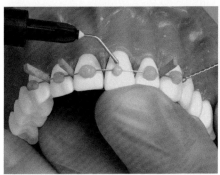
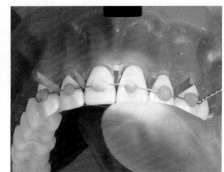

**Composite application and polymerization**

Flexibility of the splint is achieved by leaving some free wire interdentally. Wire is cut with a diamond bur at both distal ends.

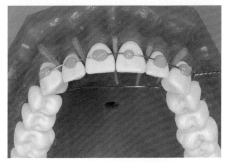
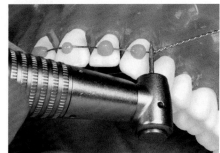

**Finished splint**

(Left) The splint is complete after the palatal part is removed and sharp edges of composite polished. (Right) Final splint from frontal view (upper view). The splint can be altered from a flexible into a rigid one by adding composite on the wire and also in the interdental areas as is done here in the right-hand-sided teeth (lower view).

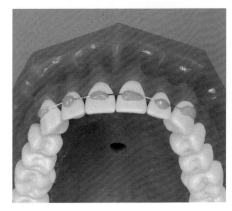
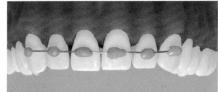
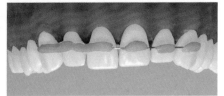

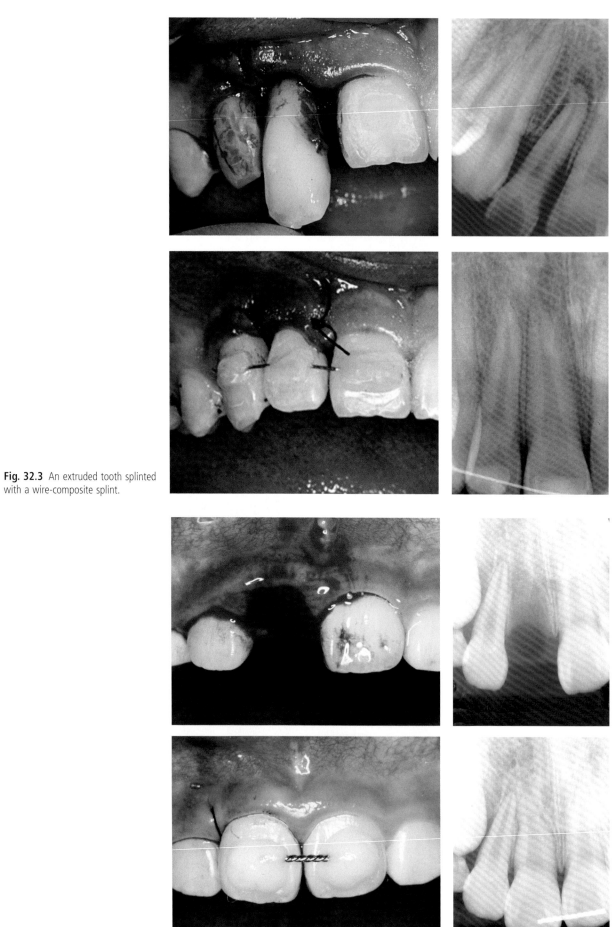

**Fig. 32.3** An extruded tooth splinted with a wire-composite splint.

**Fig. 32.4** An avulsed tooth splinted with a wire-composite splint.

**Fig. 32.5 Application of a Luxatemp®
splint**
(Left) Instruments needed. (Right) Extruded
central incisors repositioned with finger pressure.

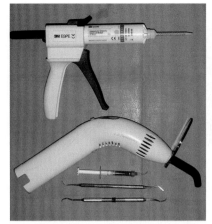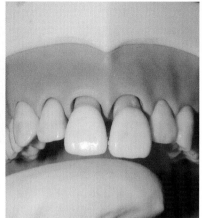

**Etching of enamel**
The now repositioned incisors are etched
incisally.

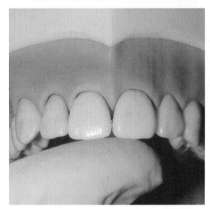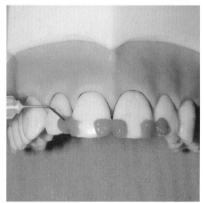

**Rinsing and application of Luxatemp®**
The acid etch gel is rinsed away with saline or
water and air dried, then Luxatemp® is applied
to the laterals and the centrals.

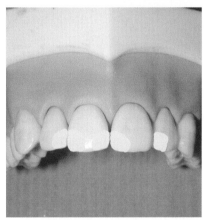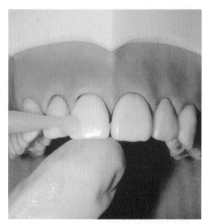

**Curing the splint**
The resin is immediately cured with UV light.
During this procedure the tooth is kept *in situ*
with finger pressure. This process is continued
until the four incisors are united with the resin
splint.

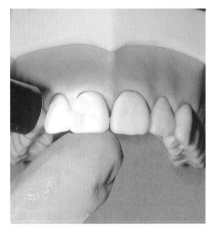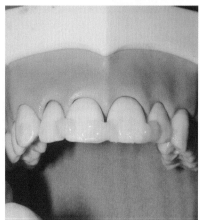

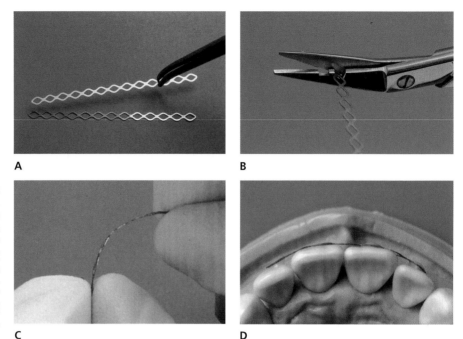

**Fig. 32.6** Construction of a Titanium Trauma Splint (TTS) (Mediartis AG, Switzerland). This is available in two lengths of 51 and 100 mm (A). The TTS is cut to the desired length with a pair of scissors (B). Since the TTS is only 0.2 mm thick, it can be easily bent with the fingers (C). A well adapted TTS is characterized by only small amounts of composite placed into the rhomboid openings (D). (Courtesy of Dr. von Arx, Berne, Switzerland).

can also be adapted in length. TTS is bonded to enamel with a light cured composite resin and removed by 'peeling' it off the tooth surface. The splints have been found to be well tolerated and cause only slight patient discomfort (45) (Fig. 32.6).

## Removable splint

Recently a new type of splint has been described where a removable splint made of polycarboxylate and polyacrylic was made after impression taking.

These splints were used in cases where initial reposition and splinting was not considered optimal, resulting in occlusal trauma (45). The indications for this splint appear questionable.

## Recommendations for splinting type and duration

Length and rigidity of splinting is primarily determined by the trauma scenario. In the following, various types of injuries will be described as well as their need for fixation and fixation period (see Table 32.2).

## Extrusion

Extrusive luxation implies rupture of the periodontal ligament fibers. It has been shown that the periodontal ligament achieves approximately 70% of its original strength 2–3 weeks after injury (6). Thus, extrusion represents a simple healing scenario and only 2 weeks of splinting is needed to allow healing of the PDL as well as to keep Hertwig's epithelial root sheath in immature teeth in position

adjacent to vital apical tissues to ensure continued root development (see Chapters 2 and 15). A semi-rigid splint is recommended.

## Lateral luxation

Traumatic dislocation in a lateral direction often causes damage to the PDL and bone. Hence the splinting time must be longer than for extrusively luxated teeth in which the alveolar socket is intact. In these cases a semi-rigid splint should be used for 4 weeks. Before removal of a splint a radiograph should be taken. If there are radiographic signs of periodontal breakdown, additional splinting time is necessary (usually 3–4 weeks) (see also Chapter 15).

## Intrusion

Intrusive luxation causes serious damage to the alveolar socket. If the tooth is surgically repositioned, the splinting time must be long enough to support the tooth during remodelling of the bony socket, a process which normally takes 6–8 weeks (see also Chapter 16). To prevent permanent ankylosis a semi-rigid splint should be used.

## Avulsion

The duration of splinting is dependent upon the extent and nature of additional damage to the socket (fracture). Replantation into an intact alveolar socket requires a splinting period of no longer than 7–10 days to prevent ankylosis (see Chapter 17). In cases with incomplete eruption a suture placed over the incisal edge can provide adequate support for an avulsed replanted tooth (34).

**Table 32.2** Fixation periods after various dental injuries. In multiple injuries, the length and rigidity is chosen according to the injury which requires the longest or the most rigid fixation.

| Type of injury | Extrusive luxation | Lateral luxation | Intrusive luxation | Avulsion | Root fracture in the cervical third | Root fracture in the middle or apical third | Alveolar fracture |
|---|---|---|---|---|---|---|---|
| Fixation period | 2 weeks* | 4 weeks* | 6–8 weeks | 1–2 weeks | 4 months | 4 weeks | 4 weeks |
| Type of fixation | Flexible | Flexible | Flexible | Flexible | Rigid | Flexible | Flexible |

\* Fixation period following lateral luxation starts at 4 weeks, but might be increased, depending upon healing of marginal bone. (See Chapter 15.)

## Autotransplantation

Autotransplantation can be considered a well-controlled avulsion, but differs in the initial instability due to the expanded socket. In autotransplanted teeth, healing usually takes place without ankylosis and with complete pulp revascularization. A suture placed across the occlusal surface is usually sufficient and has been found to lead to significantly better pulp and periodontal healing than a rigid splint (11, 21).

## Root fracture

Root fractures can be located in the apical, middle or cervical third of the root. Displacement of the coronal fragment can be classified as concussion, subluxation, extrusion and lateral luxation (see Chapter 12). Root fractures in the apical third of the root and without coronal fragment displacement do not normally require any splint.

In the past, root fractured teeth have been stabilized by a variety of splints, such as cap splints, orthodontic appliances, bonded metal wires, composites and fiber-glass splints.

Previous recommendations of rigid, long-term splinting for all root fractures have been questioned in recent studies (41, 46, 50). It has been shown that splinted and non-splinted teeth did not differ in outcome of treatment, i.e. whether the healing takes place by hard tissue union, interposition of connective tissue and/or bone or no healing (see Chapter 12). The type of splinting – cap splint or wire-composite splint – does not influence outcome either in transverse or in oblique cervical root fractures (41). Based on controversial results in recent studies, it has been recommended to splint root fractures located at mid-root for 4 weeks (47). In cervical root fractures, a longer splinting time might be indicated. However, a recent study could not demonstrate an effect in healing pattern (41).

## Alveolar bone fractures

The principles of treatment of alveolar fractures are related to the treatment of both jaw fractures and tooth luxations. After proper repositioning, splinting is assumed to support both PDL and bone healing. Fixation should be semi-rigid or rigid and the splinting period 4–6 weeks.

## Splinting in primary dentition

In most cases, splinting of luxated primary teeth is not possible due to lack of patient cooperation. In the case of alveolar or mandibular fractures, a resin or a cap splint is indicated. The cap splint should be cemented only on non-traumatized teeth, leaving the injured teeth free within the splint in order not to damage them when the splint is removed (48, 49).

## General comments

Gingival fibers heal within one week, which is enough to provide some stability. Where ankylosis may be a problem (avulsions), a short fixation period may in some cases prevent permanent ankylosis (see Chapter 17).

In cases where ankylosis is not a significant risk, a fixation period of 2–3 weeks is indicated. During the splinting period, it is essential that good oral hygiene be maintained. Careful toothbrushing and rinsing with chlorhexidine are recommended. When there is an associated injury to the bone, an additional 1–2 weeks is indicated. If remodeling of the socket takes place (e.g. following crushing injuries, as after intrusions and lateral luxation), 6–8 weeks of splinting may be required. Concerning length of the splint (number of adjacent teeth), mobility tests have shown that there is no need to extend the splint to more than one non-injured adjacent tooth to the injured tooth (39).

## Essentials

Splinting may negatively influence:

- Gingival healing
- Periodontal healing
- Pulp healing

## Splinting properties

- *Flexible* and *semi-rigid*: optimal for pulp and periodontal healing
- *Rigid*: to be used in cervical root fractures and replantation of teeth after PDL removal and fluoride treatment.

## Splinting types

a. Suture splint
b. Arch bar
c. Orthodontic appliances
d. Composite
e. Wire-composite
f. Resin
g. Metal(TTS)splint

Splint types e, f and g appear to be the most versatile in dental traumatology.

## Splinting periods

- Extrusive luxation: 2 weeks
- Lateral luxation: 4 weeks
- Intrusive luxation: 6–8 weeks
- Avulsion: 1–2 weeks
- Root fracture; middle or apical third: 4 weeks
- Root fracture; cervical third: 3 months
- Alveolar fracture: 4 weeks

## References

1. ANDREASEN JO. *Traumatic injuries of the teeth*. 2nd edn. Copenhagen: Munksgaard, 1981:168–9.
2. OIKARINEN K, GUNDLACH KKH, PFEIFER G. Late complications of luxation injuries to teeth. *Endod Dent Traumatol* 1987;**3**:296–302.
3. OIKARINEN K. Tooth splinting: a review of the literature and consideration of the versatility of a wire-composite splint. *Endod Dent Traumatol* 1990;**6**:237–50.
4. BUONOCORE MG. Simple mehod of increasing the adhesion of acrylic filling materials to enamel surface. *J Dent Res* 1955;**34**:849–51.
5. ANDREASEN JO. Buonocore memorial lecture. Adhesive dentistry applied to the treatment of traumatic dental injuries. *Oper Dent* 2001;**26**:328–35.
6. MANDEL U, VIDIK A. Effect of splinting on the mechanical and histological properties of the healing periodontal ligament in the vervet monkey (*Cercopithecus aethiops*). *Arch Oral Biol* 1989;**34**:209–17.
7. ANDREASEN JO. The effect of splinting upon periodontal healing after replantation of permanent incisors in monkeys. *Acta Odontol Scand* 1974;**33**:313–23.
8. NASJLETI CE, CASTELLI WA, CAFFESSE RG. The effects of different splinting times on replantation of teeth in monkeys. *Oral Surg Oral Med Oral Pathol* 1982;**53**:557–66.
9. KRISTERSON L, ANDREASEN JO. The effect of splinting upon periodontal and pulpal healing after autotransplantation of mature and immature permanent incisors in monkeys. *Int J Oral Surg* 1983;**12**:239–49.
10. ANDERSSON L, LINDSKOG S, BLOMLÖF L, HEDSTRÖM K-G, HAMMERSTRÖM L. Effect of masticatory stimulation on dentoalveolar ankylosis after experimental tooth replantation. *Endod Dent Traumatol* 1985;**1**: 13–16.
11. BAUSS O, SCHILKE R, FENSKE C, ENGELKE W, KILIARIDIS S. Autotransplantation of immature third molars: influence of different splinting methods and fixation periods. *Dent Traumatol*. 2002;**18**:322–8.
12. OIKARINEN KS, NIEMINEN TM. Influence of arch bar splinting on periodontium and mobility of fixed teeth. *Acta Odontol Scand* 1994;**52**:203–8.
13. ROED-PETERSEN B, MORTENSEN H. Periodontal status after fixation with Sauer's and Schuchardt's arch bars in jaw fractures. *Int J Oral Surg* 1972;**1**:43–7.
14. ROED-PETERSEN B, MORTENSEN H. Arch bar fixation of fractures in dentulous jaws: a comparative study of Sauer's and Erich's bar. *Danish Med Bull* 1973;**20**:164–8.
15. BIENENGRÄBER V, SONNENBURG I, WILKEN J. Klinische und tierexperimentelle Untersuchungen über den Einfluss von Drahtschienenverbänden auf das marginale Parodontium. *Dtsch Stomatol* 1973;**23**:84–6.
16. NGASSAPA DN, FREIHOFER H-PM, MALTHA JC. The reaction of the peridontium to different types of splints. (I). Clinical aspects. *Int J Oral Maxillofac Surg* 1986;**15**:240–9.
17. NGASSAPA DN, MALTHA JC, FREIHOFER H-PM. The reaction of the peridontium to different types of splints. (II). Histological aspects. *Int J Oral Maxillofac Surg* 1986;**15**:250–8.
18. HÄRLE F, KREKELER G. Die Reaktion des Parodontiums auf die Drahtligaturenschiene (Stout-Obwegeser). *Dtsch Zahnärztl Z* 1977;**32**:814–16.
19. FRÖHLICH M, GÄBLER K. Der Einfluss von Kieferbruchshienenverbänden auf das Parodont. *Stomatol DDR* 1981;**31**:238.
20. LELLO JL, LELLO GE. The effect of interdental continuous loop wire splinting and intermaxillary fixation on the marginal gingiva. *Int J Oral Maxillofac Surg* 1988;**17**:249–52.
21. ANDREASEN JO, PAULSEN HU, YU Z, BAYER T, SCHWARTZ O. A long-term study of 370 autotransplanted premolars. Part II. Tooth survival and pulp healing subsequent to transplantation. *Eur J Orthod* 1990;**12**:14–24.
22. WESSELINK PR, BEERTSEN W. Repair processes in the periodontium following dento-alveolar ankylosis: the effect of masticatory function. *J Clin Periodontol* 1994;**21**:472–8.
23. BERUDE JA, HICKS ML, SAUBER JJ, LI S-H. Resorption after physiological and rigid splinting of replanted permanent incisors in monkeys. *J Endod* 1988;**14**:592–600.
24. OIKARINEN K, NIEMINEN T. Influence of acid-etched splinting methods on discoloration of dental enamel in four media: an in vitro study. *Scand J Dent Res* 1994;**102**:313–18.
25. HEIMAN GR, BIVEN GM, KAHN H, SMULSON MH. Temporary splinting using an adhesive system. *Oral Surg Oral Med Oral Pathol* 1971;**31**:819–22.
26. NEAVERTH EJ, GEORIG AC. Technique and rationale for splinting. *J Am Dent Assoc* 1980;**100**:56–63.
27. ANDERSSON L, FRISKOPP J, BLOMLOF L. Fiber-glass splinting of traumatized teeth. *ASDC J Dent Child* 1983;**50**:21–4.
28. CROLL TP. Bonded composite resin/ligature wire splint for stabilization of traumatically displaced teeth. *Quintessence Int* 1991;**22**:17–21.

29. Dawoodbhoy I, Valiathan A, Lalani ZS, Cariappa KM. Splinting of avulsed central incisors with orthodontic wires: a case report. *Endod Dent Traumatol* 1994;**10**:149–52.

30. Oikarinen K. Comparison of the flexibility of various splinting methods for tooth fixation. *Int J Oral Maxillofac Surg* 1988;**17**:125–7.

31. Oikarinen K, Andreasen JO, Andreasen FM. Rigidity of various fixation methods used as dental splints. *Endod Dent Traumatol* 1992;**8**:113–19.

32. Artisuk A, Gargiulo AV Jr. Incisal edge splint – a case report. *Periodontal Case Rep* 1982;**4**:3–4.

33. Baar EH, Yarshansky OH, ben Yehuda A. Intracoronal incisal splint. *J Prosthet Dent* 1993;**70**:491–2.

34. Gupta S, Sharma A, Dang N. Suture splint: an alternative for luxation injuries of teeth in pediatric patients – a case report. *J Clin Pediatr Dent* 1997;**22**:19–21.

35. Ngassapa DN, Freihofer HP, Maltha JC. The reaction of the periodontium to different types of splints. (I). Clinical aspects. *Int J Oral Maxillofac Surg* 1986;**15**:240–9.

36. Croll TP, Helpin ML. Use of self-etching adhesive system and compomer for splinting traumatized incisors. *Pediatr Dent* 2002;**24**:53–6.

37. Filippi A, Von Arx T, Lussi A. Comfort and discomfort of dental trauma splints – a comparison of a new device (TTS) with three commonly used splinting techniques. *Dent Traumatol* 2002;**18**:275–80.

38. Prevost J, Louis JP, Vadot J, Granjon Y. A study of forces originating from orthodontic appliances for splinting of teeth. *Endod Dent Traumatol* 1994;**10**:179–84.

39. Ebeleseder KA, Glockner K, Pertl C, Stadtler P. Splints made of wire and composite: an investigation of lateral tooth mobility *in vivo*. *Endod Dent Traumatol* 1995;**11**:288–93.

40. Oikarinen K. Functional fixation for traumatically luxated teeth. *Endod Dent Traumatol* 1987;**3**:224–8.

41. Cvek M, Mejare I, Andreasen JO. Healing and prognosis of teeth with intra-alveolar fractures involving the cervical part of the root. *Dent Traumatol* 2002;**18**:57–65.

42. Strobl H, Haas M, Norer B, Gerhard S, Emshoff R. Evaluation of pulpal blood flow after tooth splinting of luxated permanent maxillary incisors. *Dent Traumatol* 2004;**20**:36–41.

43. Emshoff R, Emshoff I, Moschen I, Strobl H. Diagnostic characteristics of pulpal blood flow levels associated with adverse outcomes of luxated permanent maxillary incisors. *Dent Traumatol* 2004;**20**:270–5.

44. von Arx T, Filippi A, Lussi A. Comparison of a new dental trauma splint device (TTS) with three commonly used splinting techniques. *Dent Traumatol* 2001;**17**:266–74.

45. von Arx T, Filippi A, Buser D. Splinting of traumatized teeth with a new device: TTS (Titanium Trauma Splint). *Dent Traumatol* 2001;**17**:180–4.

46. Cvek M, Andreasen JO, Borum MK. Healing of 208 intra-alveolar root fractures in patients aged 7–17 years. *Dent Traumatol* 2001;**17**:53–62.

47. Andreasen JO, Oikarinen K. Dentale og orale skader. *Tandlægebladet* 2004;**108**:12–22.

48. Brown CL, Mackie IC. Splinting of traumatized teeth in children. *Dent Update* 2003;**30**:78–82.

49. Qin M, Ge LH, Bai RH. Use of a removable splint in the treatment of subluxated, luxated and root fractured anterior permanent teeth in children. *Dent Traumatol* 2002;**18**:81–5.

50. Andreasen JO, Andreasen FM, Mejare I, Cvek M. Healing of 400 intra-alveolar fractures. 2. Effect of treatment factors, such as treatment delay, repositioning, splinting type and period, and antibiotics. *Dent Traumatol* 2004;**10**:203–11.

# 33
# Bleaching of the Discolored Traumatized Tooth

## J. E. Dahl & U. Pallesen

This chapter focuses on the treatment of discolored traumatized teeth, most of them being non-vital and subsequently, endodontically treated. Tooth bleaching based upon hydrogen peroxide as the active agent, applied directly or produced in a chemical reaction from sodium perborate or carbamide peroxide, must be regarded as the treatment of choice, alone or preceding a prosthetic restoration. More than 90% immediate success has been reported for intracoronal bleaching of non-vital teeth, but in a period of 1–8 years after treatment, 10–40% of the initially successfully treated teeth needed retreatment (see p. 855).

## Etiology of discoloration

Discoloration of the traumatized tooth is a consequence of pulpal response to the trauma (1). The dark staining of non-vital teeth is caused by deposition of blood degradation products or necrotic pulp tissue in the dentinal tubules (2, 3). Formation of tertiary dentin may be an effect of pulp inflammation, and the dentin sclerosis affects the light-transmitting properties of the tooth resulting in a gradual darkening of the tooth. Trauma to the primary dentition may also damage the developing tooth that erupts discolored due to disturbances of matrix deposition and mineralization (4). These types of discoloration are termed intrinsic (1) and may be exaggerated by extrinsic discoloration from aging, coffee, tea, red wine, carrots, oranges and tobacco (1, 5).

## Medicaments

### Historical overview

The first publication on bleaching of discolored, pulpless teeth appeared in 1864 (6) and, since then, medicaments such as *chloride, sodium hypochlorite, sodium perborate* and *hydrogen peroxide*, have been used, alone, in combination,

and with and without heat activation (7). In the walking bleach technique that was introduced in 1961, the bleaching was performed between the visits (8). A mixture of sodium perborate and water was placed in the pulp chamber that was sealed off between the visits. The method was later modified replacing the water with 30–35% hydrogen peroxide to improve the whitening effect (9). The use of carbamide peroxide for bleaching teeth was first published in 1989 (10) and was based on an observation made in the late 1960s by an orthodontist who had prescribed an antiseptic containing 10% carbamide peroxide to be used in a tray for the treatment of gingivitis and found tooth lightening as an additional effect of the treatment (11).

## Today's medicaments and their mode of action

Tooth bleaching today is based upon hydrogen peroxide as the active agent. Hydrogen peroxide may be applied directly, or produced in a chemical reaction from sodium perborate (12) or carbamide peroxide (13). Hydrogen peroxide is a strong oxidizing agent through the formation of free radicals (14), reactive oxygen molecules, and hydrogen peroxide anions (15). These reactive molecules attack the long chained, dark colored chromophore molecules and split them into smaller, less colored and more diffusible molecules. Carbamide peroxide also yields urea (13) that theoretically can be further decomposed to carbon dioxide and ammonia. It is, however, unclear how much ammonia will be formed during tooth bleaching using carbamide peroxide. The high pH of ammonia facilitates the bleaching procedure (16). This can be explained by the fact that in a basic solution, lower activation energy is required for the formation of free radicals from hydrogen peroxide, and the reaction rate is higher resulting in an improved yield compared to an acidic environment (15). The outcome of the bleaching procedure depends mainly on the concentration of the bleaching agent, the ability of the agent to reach the chromophore molecules, and the duration and number of times the agent is in contact with chromophore molecules.

## Toxicity of bleaching agents

In animal experiments, exposure of the gingiva to 1% hydrogen peroxide for 6–48 hours resulted in epithelial damage and acute inflammation in the subepithelial connective tissue (17). Long-term application of 3% or 30% hydrogen peroxide in the hamster cheek pouch twice weekly resulted in inflammatory changes (18). In clinical trials using 10% carbamide peroxide in custom made trays, 25–40% reported gingival irritation during the treatment (19, 20).

A single dose of carbamide peroxide in rats induced a concentration dependent toxic reaction, including respiratory depression, reduced weight gain and water consumption, changes in estrous cycle, and, at necropsy, histological abnormalities of the stomach as ulceration, necrotic mucosa and disrupted gastric glands (21–23). Long term administration of hydrogen peroxide has resulted in deleterious localized effects on the gastric mucosa, decreased food consumption, reduced weight-gain, and blood chemistry changes in rats (24), and the formation of small duodenal mucosal hyperplasias in catalase deficient mice that seemed to be reversible during a 6-week recovery period (25). Catalase is a scavenger of reactive oxygen species, and long-term exposure to hydrogen peroxide reduced the plasma catalase levels significantly in rats (26). These results (25, 26) indicate that the toxicity of hydrogen peroxide is mediated through the formation of oxygen radicals.

Several studies of DMBA carcinogenesis in mice skin and hamster cheek pouch indicate that hydrogen peroxide may act as a tumour-promoter (18, 27). In an evaluation of the genotoxic potential of hydrogen peroxide in oral health products, it was concluded that oral health products containing or releasing hydrogen peroxide up to 3.6% hydrogen peroxide were unlikely to enhance the cancer risk in individuals except those that have an increased risk of oral cancer due to tobacco use, alcohol misuse or genetic predisposition (28). This is in line with statements from the International Agency for Research on Cancer that found limited evidence in experimental animals and inadequate evidence in humans for the carcinogenicity of hydrogen peroxide (29). The chemicals used for tooth bleaching have a toxic potential, and accidental ingestion may occur (30). However, based upon the amount of the chemicals used for the treatment of single tooth or few teeth that is the most likely situation in a trauma case, this treatment seems to represent little risk to the patient.

## Effects of bleaching agents on restorations

This has been reviewed recently (31) and it was unclear if the reported changes in surface structure caused by bleaching agents were of any clinical significance. The bond strength between enamel and resin based fillings was reduced in the first 24 hours after bleaching (32). This was explained by the presence of hydrogen peroxide residuals in the enamel that inhibit the polymerization of resin-based materials and thus reduce the bond strength. The length of time in which these radicals inhibit the polymerization is a

matter of controversy. Lag time from 24 hours (32, 33) up to 1–3 weeks (34, 35) has been suggested to obtain the best bond strength.

## Intracoronal bleaching

### Methods

Intracoronal bleaching is a conservative alternative to more invasive esthetic treatment of non-vital discolored teeth (Fig. 33.1). Several aspects of the methods have been reviewed recently (3, 30, 36). Careful examination of the

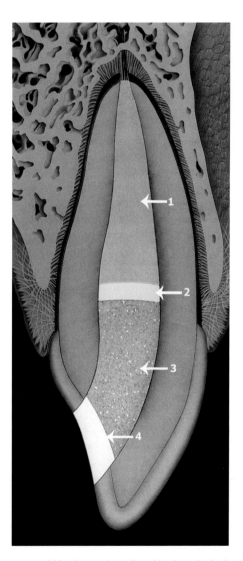

**Fig. 33.1** Internal bleaching – the walking bleach method. Sketch of a tooth where internal bleaching is being carried out. Arrows at root-filling material (gutta-percha) (1), coronal seal of the root-channel (e.g. IRM® or Cavit®) or glass ionomer cement (2), bleaching agent (sodium perborate suspended in water) (3), and temporary seal (e.g. IRM®-cement or Cavit®) (4). If the root is discolored it is necessary to remove 2–3 mm of the root filling material from the cervical part of the root canal. The depth can be estimated by measuring the distance between the incisal edge of the tooth to a level about 2–3 mm below the buccal gingival margin. The method is further described in Table 33.1.

teeth is necessary, as the method requires root canal that is properly obturated to prevent the bleaching agent from reaching the periapical tissues (37). In addition, it is suggested to remove any residual caries and restorations from the pulp chamber and to have a healthy periodontal tissue (37). Both hydrogen peroxide and sodium perborate have been used, and various heat sources have been applied to speed up the reaction and improve the bleaching effect (7). A combination of sodium perborate and water (8, 38) or hydrogen peroxide (9) has been employed in the 'walking bleach' (Fig. 33.1) technique. As an alternative, carbamide peroxide has been evaluated (39, 40). The medicament is placed into the pulp chamber, sealed, and left for 3–7 days; thereafter it is replaced regularly until acceptable lightening is achieved. If the tooth has not responded satisfactorily after 2–3 treatments, the 'walking bleach' technique can be supplemented with an in office bleaching procedure (37). The treatment may continue until an acceptable result is obtained. A modification of the method that reduces the number of in-office appointments has been suggested (41, 42). Access to the pulp cavity is gained, and the root filling is sealed off with a glass ionomer filling. The patient places the bleaching agent, usually 10% carbamide peroxide, intracoronally with regular intervals and covers the lingual aspect of the tooth with a plastic splint. By this method the pulp chamber is left unsealed during the weeks of treatment. If the seal of the root-filling is insufficient the periapical tissue may be contaminated leading to endodontic treatment failure. Bleaching agent left due to insufficient rinse of the sticky gel could be ingested, and intracoronal dentin is subjected to discoloration from pigments in food or beverage. The saved chair-side time using this bleaching method does not compensate for the adverse biological consequences.

## Efficacy

The efficacy of the different medicaments used for internal tooth bleaching has been evaluated *in vitro* on artificially stained teeth. The outcome of the 'walking bleach' method, the thermo-catalytic method, and a combination of the two methods using sodium perborate in 35% hydrogen peroxide and 35% hydrogen peroxide was compared and no difference was observed between the methods and medicaments (43). The results for sodium perborate in 30% hydrogen peroxide were superior to those of sodium perborate in water (93% versus 53% of the artificially stained and bleached teeth recovered their initial shade) (44, 45). Other studies found no difference in the bleaching efficacy using sodium perborate mixed with 30% hydrogen peroxide, sodium perborate mixed with 3% hydrogen peroxide, or sodium perborate mixed with water (46–48). Increased lightening of the teeth was observed with longer bleaching time. The immediate results after intracoronal bleaching with 10% carbamide peroxide was better than sodium perborate in 30% hydrogen peroxide, but the final outcome after 3 treatments over 14 days was in favor of sodium perborate in 30% hydrogen peroxide (39). Both 35% carbamide peroxide gel and 35% hydrogen peroxide gel

lightened artificially stained teeth to the same extent after 7 days with a somewhat better result for 35% carbamide peroxide gel after 14 days (40). In the same study, sodium perborate-treated teeth lightened significantly less. The cited *in vitro* studies showed that sodium perborate in water, sodium perborate in 30% hydrogen peroxide, and 10–35% carbamide peroxide all were efficient in the bleaching nonvital teeth. This conclusion is based on results from bleaching artificially stained teeth and that the clinical situation may give a different outcome.

## Esthetic results

The evaluation of the esthetic outcome of a bleaching treatment is subjective, and the patient may have a different opinion than the dental surgeon (49). In addition, different terms and definitions of the outcome have been applied, which make comparisons between studies difficult (38, 49, 50). Immediate treatment success has usually been defined as no or slight deviation in color between the treated teeth and the neighboring teeth (Figs 33.2–33.4). More than 90% immediate success rates have been reported using the thermo-catalytic method (7) or the conventional 'walking bleach' procedure (38). To evaluate the long-term esthetic results of internal bleaching, a determination of treatment failure rate may be useful. Failure was, however, not defined in the different long-term studies (38, 49–51), but the intuitive definition is teeth that need to be retreated. The need for retreatment increased with the observation time, 10% after 1–2 years (50), 20–25% after 3–5 years (38, 51) and 40% in teeth observed up to 8 years (50) (Fig. 33.4). In a more recent study the failure rate was reported to be 7% after 5 years, but the majority of cases in this study were defined as ideal for bleaching (no other filling than the palatal endodontic opening) (50). In a study of tetracycline-stained teeth that were endodontically treated, internally bleached and followed for 3–15 years, 4 out of 20 patients needed re-treatment (52). At present, there is no good predictor for the long-term outcome of internal bleaching, but for the recommendation that teeth with many fillings are not suitable for the procedure (7, 49).

## Adverse effects

A review of published case reports on cervical root resorption has revealed 28 such cases following internal bleaching (3, 30) (Figs 33.5 and 33.6). A majority of these cases involved teeth with a history of trauma, and trauma has been regarded as a risk factor for development of cervical root resorption after internal bleaching (53). The occurrence of cervical root resorption has also been evaluated in clinical studies. Fifty-eight bleached pulpless teeth (30% $H_2O_2$ and heating) were followed for 1–8 years, and 4 cases (7%) of external root resorption were observed (50). A study of 204 teeth treated with a combination of thermo-catalytic and 'walking bleach' techniques with an observation time of 1–19 years revealed 4 teeth with cervical resorption and all these had a history of trauma (54). Another 95 teeth

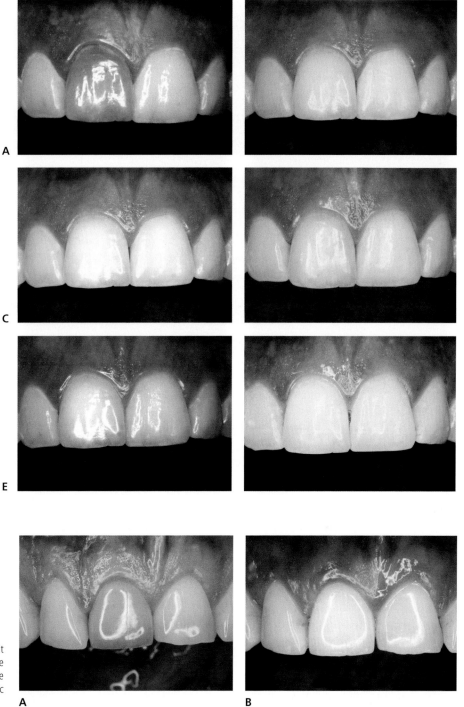

**Fig. 33.2** Long time result of internal bleaching. A. Central incisor in a 21-year-old woman had been endodontically treated 6 years earlier due to trauma. A discoloration was visible immediately after the endodontic treatment, which subsequently became more intense. B. Result after 3 weeks of internal bleaching with sodium perborate suspended in water and a weekly change of bleaching agent. C. 5 yrs after bleaching. A slight discoloration is visible, and no re-treatment was necessary. D. Condition after 8 years. E. 10 years after bleaching. Recurrence of the discoloration is visible and the patient was re-treated. F. 10 years after initial bleaching the tooth was re-bleached for 2 weeks to a satisfying color.

**Fig. 33.3** Internal bleaching. Result of bleaching with sodium perborate and water. A. Conditions before bleaching. B. A successful aesthetic result after 3 weeks of bleaching.

examined three years after treatment, using the walking bleach technique (sodium perborate in water), revealed no cervical resorption (38). In a four-year follow-up of 250 teeth with severe tetracycline discoloration using sodium perborate in oxygen-water as the bleaching agent, no evidence of external resorption was found (55). An analogous study comprising 112 teeth bleached with a paste of sodium perborate in 30% hydrogen peroxide and observed for 3–15 years, reported no external root resorption (52).

High concentration of hydrogen peroxide in combination with heating seems to promote cervical root resorption (50, 54), in line with observations made in animal experiments (56–58). The underlying mechanism for this effect is unclear, but it has been suggested that the bleaching agent reaches the periodontal tissue through the dentinal tubules and initiates an inflammatory reaction (59). It has also been speculated that the peroxides by diffusing through the dentinal tubules denature the dentin, and once denatured, the dentin becomes an immunologically different tissue and is attacked as a foreign body by the periodontal tissue (60). Frequently, the resorption was diagnosed several years after the bleaching (50, 60). *In vitro* studies using extracted teeth

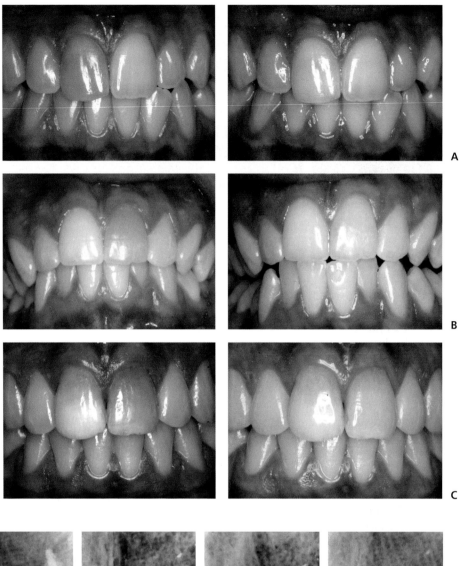

**Fig. 33.4** Examples of different aesthetic results after internal bleaching with sodium perborate. Conditions before and 3 years after bleaching. A. Good aesthetic result. B. Acceptable aesthetic result. C. Unacceptable aesthetic result.

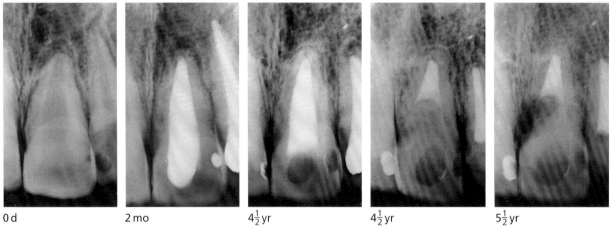

0 d          2 mo          $4\frac{1}{2}$ yr          $4\frac{1}{2}$ yr          $5\frac{1}{2}$ yr

**Fig. 33.5** Inflammatory root resorption after internal bleaching. Central incisor was bleached with 30% hydrogen peroxide and a light beam from a heat producing lamp. The tooth had previously suffered a luxation injury with subsequent pulp necrosis and root filling. Extensive cervical inflammatory root resorption is seen 1 year after bleaching. From CVEK & LINDVALL (59) 1985.

showed that hydrogen peroxide placed in the pulp chamber penetrated the dentin (61). Heat and cervical defects of the cementum increased the penetration (62–64). Hydrogen peroxide also increased the permeability of dentin (65), which may enhance the effects of hydrogen peroxide by repeated exposures. Most cases of cervical resorption of internally bleached teeth are associated with trauma to the tooth. It seems also that the use of thermo-catalytic bleaching procedure may constitute risk factor for the development of cervical resorption.

Tooth crown fracture has also been observed after internal bleaching (66) most probably due to extensive removal

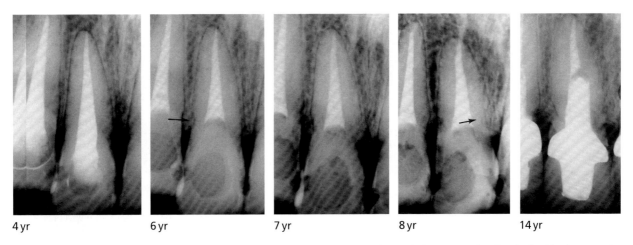

4 yr          6 yr          7 yr          8 yr          14 yr

**Fig. 33.6** Ankylosis after bleaching. A discolored central incisor crown was bleached with 30% hydrogen peroxide. After the first bleaching a cavity with arrested resorption was seen cervically (arrow). After the second series of bleaching 2 years after, a slowly progressing root resorption associated with ankylosis developed in the cervical part of root. From CVEK & LINDVALL (59) 1985.

of the intra-coronal dentin. In addition, internal bleaching with 30% hydrogen peroxide has been found to reduce the micro-hardness of dentin and enamel (67), especially when the thermocatalytic method was applied (68), and to weaken the mechanical properties of the dentin (69).

## External tooth bleaching

External tooth bleaching may be performed as the only treatment of the discolored traumatized tooth or complementary to internal tooth bleaching. The different approaches for tooth whitening relevant for such treatment are: (a) dentist administered bleaching – using high concentration of hydrogen peroxide (35–50%) or carbamide peroxide (35–40%) often supplemented with a heat source, and (b) dentist supervised bleaching – by means of a bleaching tray loaded with high concentration of carbamide peroxide (35–40%) that is placed in the patient's mouth for 30 minutes to 2 hours while the patient is in the dental office (70). The efficacy for treating discolored traumatized teeth has not been evaluated for these methods. Care must be taken to secure bleaching only of the traumatized teeth to prevent persisting color mismatch to the other teeth. Recently, a combination of irradiation and tooth bleaching agent has been introduced to improve the efficacy of in-office bleaching (71, 72). The immediate results of this method could favor the additional use of light/heat activation; however, the difference to teeth treated with bleaching agents without light/heat activation was insignificant after 6 months (73).

## Clinical recommendations

Based on the literature, bleaching of discolored traumatized teeth must be regarded as a safe and predictable biological treatment in most cases. Unquestionable contraindications

for bleaching the endodontically treated tooth are unhealthy periodontal tissue, insufficient root filling or a heavily restored tooth. Although the bleaching procedure may need to be repeated over the years, retreatment will also be necessary for more invasive and expensive treatments such as laminates or full-crowns after some years of service. Therefore, bleaching should be the initial treatment in both young and old patients, when a discolored, endodontically treated tooth needs esthetic improvement. Bleaching may be performed alone or as a supplement to composite or ceramic restoration of the injured tooth.

When discoloration is caused by degradation of necrotic material in the pulp chamber, internal bleaching should always be the treatment of choice. External bleaching only cannot be recommended, as this method gives the bleaching agent less favorable access to the discolored dentin. An example of a recommended protocol for internal bleaching – the 'walking bleach' method – where focus is put on proven efficacy and minimizing side effects, is shown in Table 33.1 and Fig. 33.1. If this method does not lead to a satisfactory result for the patient, it may be supplemented with in-office bleaching, both internally and externally. A recommended protocol for in-office bleaching as a supplement to walking bleach method is shown in Table 33.2.

In teeth with obliterated pulp chambers, the discoloration is not caused by pigments from blood degradation products, but as result of the light transmitting properties of thick dentin, known from yellow canines, and a successful and long-lasting effect of bleaching cannot be expected. Chromophore molecules may, however, be present in the superficial layers of the enamel. External in-office bleaching may thus give a minor effect provided the neighboring teeth are not bleached. To obtain this, the adjacent teeth have to be protected by rubber dam during the bleaching. The procedure in Table 33.2 may be used, omitting the internal placement of the bleaching agent. Long-lasting esthetic treatment of obliterated teeth is seldom possible to obtain without invasive treatment such as thick porcelain veneer or full crown.

**Table 33.1** Recommended protocol for internal bleaching – the walking bleach method – with focus on proven efficacy and minimizing side effects.

| Steps | Comments |
|---|---|
| Radiographic control | To secure healthy periodontium and complete root filling. |
| Opening | To all areas of the pulp chamber and pulp horns. Discolored dentin should not be removed. The superficial layers of old approximal restorations can be left in place, but must be non-leaking, and replacement due to lack of color match may be necessary after bleach. |
| Coronal seal of root filling | The entrance to the root channel is normally sealed off with a thin and tight layer of temporary cement (IRM®, Cavit®) or glass ionomer cement. If the root is discolored and needs bleaching, it is necessary to remove 2–3 mm of the coronal gutta-percha in the channel. |
| Preparation of the pulp chamber | The smear layer is removed by phosphoric acid-etch for 10 seconds, followed by water spray and dehydration with air and ethanol. |
| Bleaching agent | The pulp chamber is filled with a thick mix of sodium perborate and water, excess water is soaked by cotton pellets, and the mix is condensed by e.g. an amalgam condense. |
| Temporary seal | A 2 mm layer of Cavit® or IRM® cement (thick consistence) is pressed into undercuts and towards the clean cavosurface margin. |
| Bleaching time | The bleaching agent is changed weekly 2–4 times, until the tooth is slightly lighter than the adjacent teeth. |
| Restoration of the cavity | The cavity is filled with a dual cured white shaded resin material bonded to the tooth structure. The white color may lighten the tooth further and makes it possible to distinguish between dentin and resin material if re-treatment becomes necessary. The enamel part of the cavity is filled with a tooth colored light-cured resin material. It is recommended to have the final restoration placed 1–3 weeks after completion of the bleaching. |

**Table 33.2** A short protocol for in-office bleaching as a supplement to walking bleach of the discolored endodontically treated tooth, with focus on minimizing side effects and proven efficacy. Indication for this treatment is teeth where discoloration remains after 3–4 weeks of walking bleach procedure according to Table 33.1.

| Steps | Comments |
|---|---|
| Protection of the patient | Gingival tissue and adjacent teeth are covered with a well fitting rubber dam, and the patient is told to report pain from the gums during bleaching. The patient's eyes are shielded with safety glasses. |
| Pre treatment | The pulp chamber and tooth surface is cleaned and dried with air and ethanol. No acid etch is used. |
| Bleaching agent | 25–40% hydrogen peroxide or 35–40% carbamide peroxide gel is applied to the tooth internally and externally. Heating or light device is not recommended. |
| Bleaching time | Bleaching agent is changed every 10–15 min. The procedure is continued 1–1$\frac{1}{2}$ hour and may be repeated after 1–2 weeks. |
| Restoration of the cavity | See Table 33.1. |

The use of high percentages of hydrogen peroxide in bleaching procedures may impair the mechanical properties of dentin.

## Prognosis

The need for retreatment increases with observation time:

- 1–2 years: 10%
- 3–5 years: 20–25%
- 6–8 years: 40%

## Essentials

### Indications

Bleaching of discolored endodontically treated teeth can be regarded as a safe and predictable biological treatment in most cases.

### Efficacy

Internal bleaching has up to 90% immediate success.

### Precautions

Thermo-catalytic bleaching may constitute a risk factor for the development of cervical root resorption.

## References

1. HATTAB FN, QUDEIMAT MA, AL-RIMAWI HS. Dental discoloration: an overview. *J Esthet Dent* 1999;**11**:291–310.
2. MARTIN PD, BARTOLD PM, HEITHERSAY GS. Tooth discoloration by blood: an *in vitro* histochemical study. *Endod Dent Traumatol* 1997;**13**:132–8.
3. ATTIN T, PAQUE F, AJAM F, LENNON M. Review of the current status of tooth whitening with the walking bleach technique. *Int Endod J* 2003;**36**:313–29.
4. KOCKAPAN C, WETZEL WE. SEM study and clinical observations of 'Turner teeth' (in German). *Dtsch Z Mund Kiefer Gesichtschir* 1990;**14**:395–400.
5. WATTS A, ADDY M. Tooth discoloration and staining: a review of the literature. *Brit Dent J* 2001;**190**:309–15.
6. TRUMAN J. Bleaching of non-vital discolored anterior teeth. *Dent Times* 1864;**1**:69–72.
7. HOWELL RA. Bleaching discolored root-filled teeth. *Brit Dent J* 1980;**148**:159–62.
8. SPASSER HF. A simple bleaching technique using sodium perborate. *NY State Dent J* 1961;**27**:332–4.
9. NUTTING EB, POE GS. A new combination for bleaching teeth. *J South Calif Dent Assoc* 1963;**31**:289–91.

10. HAYWOOD VB, HEYMANN HO. Nightguard vital bleaching. *Quintessence Int* 1989;**20**:173–6.

11. HAYWOOD VB. Nightguard vital bleaching, a history and product update. Part I. *Esthet Dent Update* 1991;**2**:63–6.

12. HÄGG G. *General and inorganic chemistry*. Stockholm: Almqvist & Wiksell Förlag AB, 1969.

13. BUDAVARI S, O'NEIL MJ, SMITH A, HECKELMAN PE. *The Merck index. An encyclopedia of chemicals, drugs, and biologicals*. Rahway, NJ: Merck & Co. Inc., 1989.

14. GREGUS Z, KLAASSEN CD. Mechanisms of toxicity. In: Klaassen CD. ed. *Cassarett and Doull's toxicology, the basic science of poisons*. New York: McGraw-Hill, 1995;35–74.

15. COTTON FA, WILKINSON G. Oxygen. In: Cotton FA, Wilkinson G. eds. *Advances in inorganic chemistry. A comprehensive text*. New York: Interscience Publisher, 1972;403–20.

16. SUN G. The role of lasers in cosmetic dentistry. *Dent Clin North Am* 2000;**44**:831–50.

17. MARTIN JH, BISHOP JC, GUENTHENMAN RH, DORMAN HL. Cellular responce of gingiva to prolonged application of dilute hydrogen peroxide. *J Periodontol* 1968;**39**:208–10.

18. WEITZMAN SA, WEITBERG AB, STOSSEL TP, SCHWARTZ J, SHKLAR G. Effects of hydrogen peroxide on oral carcinogenesis in hamsters. *J Periodontol* 1986;**57**:685–8.

19. LEONARD RH, HAYWOOD VB, PHILLIPS C. Risk factors for developing tooth sensitivity and gingival irritation associated with nightguard vital bleaching. *Quintessence Int* 1997;**28**:527–34.

20. TAM L. Clinical trial of three 10% carbamide peroxide bleaching products. *J Can Dent Assoc* 1999;**65**:201–5.

21. CHERRY DV, BOWERS DE, THOMAS L, REDMOND AF. Acute toxicological effects of ingested tooth whiteners in female rats. *J Dent Res* 1993:**72**:1298–303.

22. REDMOND AF, CHERRY DV, BOWERS DE JR. Acute illness and recovery in adult female rats following ingestion of a tooth whitener containing 6% hydrogen peroxide. *Am J Dent* 1997;**10**:268–71.

23. DAHL JE, BECHER R. Acute toxicity of carbamide peroxide and a commercially available tooth bleaching agent in rats. *J Dent Res* 1995;**74**:710–14.

24. ITO R, KAWAMURA H, CHANG HS, TODA S, MATSUURA S, HIDANO T, et al. Safety study on hydrogen peroxide: acute and subacute toxicity. *J Med Soc Toho* 1976;**23**:531–7.

25. WEINER ML, FREEMAN C, TROCHIMOWICZ H, DE GERLACHE J, JACOBI S, MALINVERNO G, et al. 13-week drinking water toxicity study of hydrogen peroxide with 6-week recovery period in catalase-deficient mice. *Food Chem Toxicol* 2000;**38**:607–15.

26. KAWASAKI C, KONDO M, NAGAYAMA T, TAKEUCHI Y, NAGANO H. Effects of hydrogen peroxide on the growth of rats. *J Food Hygienic Soc Jap* 1969;**10**:68–72.

27. KLEIN-SZANTO AJP, SLAGA T. Effects of peroxide on rodent skin: epidermal hyperplasia and tumor promotion. *J Invest Dermatol* 1982;**79**:30–4.

28. SCIENTIFIC COMMITTEE ON COSMETIC PRODUCTS AND NON-FOOD PRODUCTS INTENDED FOR CONSUMERS. Hydrogen peroxide and hydrogen peroxide releasing substances in oral health products. SCCNFP/0058/98. Adopted on 17. February 1999. Summary on http://europa.eu.int/comm/health/ph_risk/committees/sccp/docshtml/sccp_out61_en.htm

29. INTERNATIONAL AGENCY ON RESEARCH ON CANCER. *Monographs on the evaluation of carcinogenic risks to humans. Re-evaluation of some organic chemicals, hydrazine and hydrogen peroxide*. Vol 71. Lyon: 1999.

30. DAHL JE, PALLESEN U. Tooth bleaching – a critical review of the biological aspects. *Crit Rev Oral Biol Med* 2003;**14**:292–304

31. ATTIN T, HANNIG C, WIEGAND A, ATTIN R. Effect of bleaching on restorative materials and restorations – a systematic review. *Dent Mater* 2004;**20**:852–61.

32. DISHMANN MV, COVEY DA, BAUGHAN LW. The effects of peroxide bleaching on composite to enamel bond strength. *Dent Mater* 1994;**9**:33–6.

33. HOMEWOOD C, TYAS M, WOODS M. Bonding to previously bleached teeth. *Austr Orthodont J* 2001;**17**:27–34.

34. TITLEY KC, TORNECK CD, RUSE ND, KRMEC D. Adhesion of a resin composite to bleached and unbleached human enamel. *J Endod* 1993,**19**:112–15.

35. CAVALLI V, REIS AF, GIANNINI M, AMBROSANTA GM. The effect of elapsed time following bleaching on enamel bond strength of resin composite. *Oper Dent* 2001;**26**:597–602.

36. LIM KC. Consideration in intracoronal bleaching. *Aust Dent J* 2004;**30**:69–73.

37. BARATIERI LN, RITTER AV, MONTEIRO S, DE ANDRADA MAC, VIEIRA LCC. Nonvital tooth bleaching: guidelines for the clinician. *Quintessence Int* 1995;**26**:597–608.

38. HOLMSTRUP G, PALM AM, LAMBJERG-HANSEN H. Bleaching of discolored root-filled teeth. *Endod Dent Traumatol* 1988;**4**:197–201.

39. VACHON C, VANEK P, FRIEDMAN S. Internal bleaching with 10% carbamide peroxide in vitro. *Pract Periodontics Aesthet Dent* 1998;**10**:1145–8, 1150, 1152.

40. LIM MY, LUM SOY; POH RSC, LEE GP, LIM KC. An *in vitro* comparison of the bleaching efficacy of 35% carbamide peroxide with established intracoronal bleaching agents. *Int Endod J* 2004;**37**:483–8.

41. LIEBENBERG WH. Intracoronal lightening of discolored pulpless teeth: a modified walking bleach technique. *Quintessence Int* 1997;**28**:771–7.

42. CAUGHMAN WF, FRAZIER KB, HAYWOOD VB. Carbamide peroxide whitening of nonvital single discolored teeth: case reports. *Quintessence Int* 1999;**30**:155–61.

43. FRECCIA WF, PETERS DD, LORTON L, BERNIER WE. An *in vitro* comparison of nonvital bleaching techniques in the discolored tooth. *J Endod* 1982;**8**:70–7.

44. HO S, GOERIG AC. An *in vitro* comparison of different bleaching agents in the discolored tooth. *J Endod* 1989;**15**:106–11.

45. MARTIN PD, HEITHERSAY GS, BRIDGES TE. A quantitative comparison of traditional and non-peroxide bleaching agents. *Endod Dent Traumatol* 1998;**14**:64–7.

46. ROTSTEIN I, ZALKIND M, MOR C, TARABEAH A, FRIEDMAN S. *In vitro* efficacy of sodium perborate preparations used for intracoronal bleaching of discolored non-vital teeth. *Endod Dent Traumatol* 1991;**7**:177–80.

47. ROTSTEIN I, MOR C, FRIEDMANN S. Prognosis of intracoronal bleaching with sodium perborate preparations *in vivo*: 1-year study. *J Endod* 1993;**19**:10–12.

48. ARI H, ÜNGÖR M. *In vitro* comparison of different types of sodium perborate used for intracoronal bleaching of discolored teeth. *Int Endodont J* 2002;**35**:433–6.

49. GLOCKNER K, HULLA H, EBELESEDER K, STÄDTLER PS. Five-year follow-up of internal bleaching. *Braz Dent J* 1999;**10**:105–10.

50. FRIEDMAN S, ROTSTEIN I, LIBFELT H, STABHOLZ A, HELING I. Incidence of external root resorption and esthetic results in 58 bleached pulpless teeth. *Endod Dent Traumatol* 1988;**4**:23–26.

51. BROWN G. Factors influencing successful bleaching of the discolored root-filled tooth. *Oral Surg Oral Med Oral Pathol Oral Radiol Endod* 1965;**20**:238–44.

52. ABOU-RASS M. Long-term prognosis of intentional endodontics and internal bleaching of tetracycline-stained teeth. *Compend Contin Educ Dent* 1998;**19**:1034–44.

53. HEITHERSAY GS. Invasive cervical resorption: An analysis of potential predisposing factors. *Quintessence Int* 1999;**30**:83–95.

54. HEITHERSAY GS, DAHLSTROM SW, MARIN PD. Incidence of invasive cervical resorption in bleached root-filled teeth. *Austr Dent J* 1994;**39**:82–7.

55. ANITUA E, ZABALEGUI B, GIL J, GASCON F. Internal bleaching of severe tetracycline discolorations: Four-year clinical evaluation. *Quintessence Int* 1990;**21**:783–8.

56. MADISON S, WALTON R. Cervical root resorption following bleaching of endodontically treated teeth. *J Endod* 1990;**16**:570–4.

57. ROTSTEIN I, FRIEDMAN S, MOR C, KATZNELSON J, SOMMER M, BAB I. Histological characterization of bleaching-induced external root resorption in dogs. *J Endod* 1991;**17**:436–41.

58. HELLER D, SKRIBER J, LIN LM. Effect of intracoronal bleaching on external root resorption. *J Endod* 1992;**18**:145–8.

59. CVEK M, LINDVALL A-M. External root resorption following bleaching of pulpless teeth with oxygen peroxide. *Endod Dent Traumatol* 1985;**1**:56–60.

60. LADO EA, STANLEY HR, WEISMAN MI. Cervical resorption in bleached teeth. *Oral Surg Oral Med Oral Pathol* 1983;**55**:78–80.

61. ROTSTEIN I. In vitro determination and quantification of 30% hydrogen peroxide penetration through dentin and cementum during bleaching. *Oral Surg Oral Med Oral Pathol* 1991;**72**:602–6.

62. ROTSTEIN I, TOREK Y, LEWINSTEIN I. Effect of bleaching time and temperature on the radicular penetration of hydrogen peroxide. *Endod Dent Traumatol* 1991;**7**:196–8.

63. ROTSTEIN I, TOREK Y, LEWINSTEIN I. Effect of cementum defects on radicular penetration of 30% $H_2O_2$ during intracoronal bleaching. *J Endod* 1991;**17**:230–23.

64. KOULAOUZIDOU E, LAMBRIANIDIS T, BELTES P, LYROUDIA K, PAPADOPOULOS C. Role of cementoenamel junction on the radicular penetration of 30% hydrogen peroxide during intracoronal bleaching *in vitro*. *Endod Dent Traumatol* 1996;**12**:146–50.

65. HELING I, PARSON A, ROTSTEIN I. Effect of bleaching agents on dentin permeability to Streptococcus faecalis. *J Endod* 1995;**21**:540–2.

66. GREVSTAD T. Bleaching of root-filled teeth (in Norwegian). *Nor Tannlægeforen Tid* 1981;**91**:527–31.

67. LEWINSTEIN I, HIRSCHFELD Z, STABHOLZ A, ROTSTEIN I. Effect of hydrogen peroxide and sodium perborate on the microhardness of human enamel and dentin. *J Endod* 1994;**20**:61–3.

68. LAI YL, YANG ML, LEE SY. Microhardness and color changes of human dentin with repeated intracoronal bleaching. *Oper Dent* 2003;**28**:786–92.

69. CHNG HK, PALAMARA JEA, MESSER HH. Effect of hydrogen peroxide and sodium perborate on mechanical properties of human dentin. *J Endod* 2002;**28**:62–7.

70. BARGHI N. Making a clinical decision for vital tooth bleaching: at-home or in-office? *Compend Contin Educ Dent* 1998;**19**:831–8.

71. PAPATHANASIOU A, KASTALI S, PERRY RD, KUGEL G. Clinical evaluation of a 35% hydrogen peroxide in-office whitening system. *Compend Contin Educ Dent* 2002;**23**:335–8, 340, 343–4.

72. LUK K, TAM L, HUBERT M. Effect of light energy on peroxide tooth bleaching. *J Am Dent Assoc* 2004;**135**:194–201.

73. TAVARES M, STULTZ J, NEWMAN M, SMITH V, KENT R, CARPINO E, GOODSON JM. Light augments tooth whitening with peroxide. *J Am Dent Assoc* 2003;**134**:167–75.

# 34

# Economic Aspects of Traumatic Dental Injuries

U. Glendor, L. Andersson & J. O. Andreasen

Traumatic dental injuries (TDI) frequently occur, especially in childhood and adolescence, with consequences for time and cost (1–6). Though increased research during recent decades has enhanced our knowledge of clinical and biological aspects of tooth and bone healing, the knowledge of spent resources in time and costs on dental trauma has been given little attention. Until now only a few population based studies from Scandinavia, including urban and rural populations treated by hospital and public dental health clinics, have addressed this matter (1–4, 7–10). TDI often affects different tissues in a young and growing individual. Thus, long, time-consuming and costly treatments in childhood will often continue into adulthood.

## Costs of traumatic dental injuries

In a prospective and longitudinal study carried out in Sweden, a total cost (including direct and indirect costs) of US$ 3.3–4.4 million was estimated per million individuals per year in the age interval 0–19 years (4). In Denmark, the annual cost of treatment of TDI ranges from US$ 2–5 million per million inhabitants per year irrespective of age (11). Health care service costs and total costs of the emergency visit and for each subsequent visit in Sweden is presented in Table 34.1. The results indicate that the emergency visit is the most expensive visit concerning both health care service cost and total costs. This probably depends on the character of the emergency visit (unplanned) and also the involvement of parents or other companions, compared with subsequent visits.

## Degree of severity

To calculate resources spent on TDI on a population basis, relevant information must be presented in a simple and representative manner. One of the most important pieces of information is the severity of the injury, e.g. whether the injury is *uncomplicated* or *complicated*. An injury should be regarded as complicated when there is an *increased risk of*

*complications* (e.g. pulp necrosis or root resorption) such as when the pulp has been exposed by fracture or the periodontal membrane has been injured by dislocation of the tooth (12–15) (Fig. 34.1). Thus, each traumatic episode should be grouped according to the most severe diagnosis (9, 16–17), for example a tooth with intrusion and crown fracture without pulpal exposure should be grouped as a tooth with intrusion alone (10–11, 18). If there has been more than one traumatic episode, all episodes should be grouped according to the most severe episode (1). The classification into degree of severity (16, 19), and into uncomplicated and complicated traumas (1–4, 6, 10–11, 18, 20) has been used earlier. Studies have shown that a complicated trauma, especially to permanent teeth, is of major significance with respect to time and costs (1–3, 6, 10–11).

Estimated average health care service costs for uncomplicated and complicated traumatized primary and permanent teeth are shown in Table 34.2. The results from Glendor et al. (3) are presented per injured patient during a period of two years in the age interval 0–19 years, while Borum and Andreasen (11) presented their results per injured tooth during a period of 11 years irrespective of age, and Wong and Kolokotsa (6) during a median number of eight visits in the age interval 7–18 years. Despite differences in material and methodology between these three studies, it is clear

Table 34.1 Health care service cost and total costs in US$ in Sweden of the emergency visit and mean cost of subsequent visits of TDI to primary and permanent teeth in the age interval 0–19 years. From GLENDOR et al. (2, 3) 2000, 2001.

| Dentition | Type of costs | Emergency visit ($) | Per subsequent visit ($) |
|---|---|---|---|
| Primary | Health care service cost | 42 | 35 |
| | Total costs[1] | 85 | 75 |
| Permanent | Health care service cost | 81 | 54 |
| | Total costs[1] | 133 | 81 |

[1] Total costs include direct and indirect costs (for definition see How to present costs, p. 865).

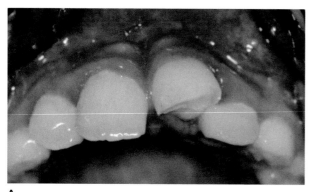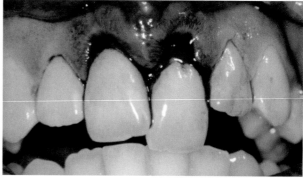

**A**                                              **B**

**Fig. 34.1** Uncomplicated (A) and complicated (B) trauma injuries.

**Table 34.2** Estimated average treatment costs in US$ to uncomplicated and complicated traumatized primary and permanent teeth.

| Authors | Year | Country | | Uncomplicated | | Complicated | |
|---|---|---|---|---|---|---|---|
| | | | | Primary dentition ($) | Permanent dentition ($) | Primary dentition ($) | Permanent dentition ($) |
| Glendor et al. (3) | 2001 | Sweden | | 68 | 200 | 114 | 606 |
| Borum & Andreasen (11) | 2001 | Denmark | 'Standard' estimate[1] | 60 | 110 | 200 | 926 |
| | | | Pessimistic estimate[2] | | 420 | | 1490 |
| Wong & Kolokotsa (6) | 2004 | UK | | Permanent incisor: 858[3] | | | |

[1] Survival of the tooth and pulp, and restoration with composite, [2] Pulp extirpation or endodontic treatment, including fixed restoration or extractions,
[3] £1 = US$ 1.65 (in year 2003).

that complicated traumas to permanent teeth are the most expensive. The average treatment costs in Denmark and Sweden correspond well, taking into account that in the Swedish study more than one tooth could have been injured per patient during a shorter period with an increase of costs, and that in the Danish study there were probably several re-treatments per injured permanent tooth throughout childhood, adolescence and adulthood. In the Danish study this was a 'pessimistic' estimate. Treatment costs also differ according to treatment regimens thus most treatments in Denmark were performed at the hospital trauma center (University Hospital, Copenhagen), in the United Kingdom at a dental hospital, and in Sweden both public dental health clinics and specialist clinics in hospitals were involved.

Borum and Andreasen (11) calculated the final treatment (health care service) costs for traumatized primary and permanent teeth in Denmark (Table 34.3). Treatment costs for TDI to primary and permanent teeth vary between dentitions and type of injuries. The acute trauma treatment (health care service cost) of both primary and permanent teeth correspond well with the results from Sweden (see Table 34.1).

### Sports injuries are expensive

TDI in sports can be very expensive. A conservative estimate of the minimum initial cost per dentist's referral for treatment of a serious dental injury in sport is US$ 1000 (21). Lifetime dental costs of total tooth avulsions have been estimated at US$ 10 000–15 000 per tooth (22). Lang et al. (23)

interviewed members of amateur and semi-professional handball leagues regarding their opinion of life-long subsequent costs for a lost front tooth. The figures varied substantially. On the average, estimates amounted to US$ 10 689 in Germany and US$ 5373 in Switzerland.

### Time and costs

Resources spent on TDI can be presented in time and costs. The difference between time and costs is that time could be regarded as 'universal' for most countries, given the same type of treatment, while costs depend on each country's own market. In some countries treatment costs can be regarded as high, while in others they appear to be moderate. The difference can be due to different welfare systems. Another problem is that it is difficult to present relevant information regarding costs for both patient and society with respect to time. To overcome this, treatment time is more suitable for comparing resources spent both within and between countries. After comparison between countries, time can again be translated to costs for comparison within a country. In Sweden, for example, health care service costs of TDI were found to represent 65% of total costs for the treatment of permanent teeth and 48% for primary teeth respectively, compared to 16% and 11% respectively for treatment time (2, 3). The difference is due to the fact that health care service costs, despite shorter time, are more expensive than companions' costs from loss of production or leisure.

**Table 34.3** Estimated final treatment costs in US$ for traumatized primary and permanent teeth in Denmark treated at a major trauma center. From BORUM & ANDREASEN (11) 2001.

|  | Estimated cost per tooth ($) |
|---|---|
| *Primary dentition* | |
| Acute trauma treatment | 60* |
| Extraction of primary tooth | 35 |
| *Permanent successor* | |
| Composite resin | 50 |
| Crown treatment | 700** |
| Tooth replacement | 2200*** |
| *Permanent dentition* | |
| Acute trauma treatment | 60 |
| Composite resin | 50 |
| Crown or veneer | 700** |
| Endodontics + crown restoration | 1000** |
| Tooth replacement | 2100*** |

\* The estimated yearly cost of running the trauma center divided by the average no. of injured teeth treated per year. \*\* In this amount one composite resin restoration prior to final treatment is included. \*\*\* Average of implant ($2900), conventional bridge ($2400) and resin-bridge ($1000) (Andreasen (62) 1992).

A Canadian study has presented treatment time and cost of permanent incisor replantation during one year (5). Mean treatment time per individual was estimated to be 7.2 hours in the first year and the approximate cost was CAD$ 1465 (1US$ = 1.5CAD$ in year 2000). The mean first year cost of a replantation/extraction case including interim prosthesis was CAD$ 1780. Ninety per cent of patients and 86% of parents reported loss of school and work time. Wong and Kolokotsa (6) have estimated the average cost for treating a patient with a traumatized incisor to be US$ 858, taking into account an average of eight visits (Table 34.2).

When the cost of the parents accompanying the child to receive treatment was considered, this cost increased to US$ 1412.

The differences between costs presented in many studies are due to the difference in local costs and also in population material. Some studies presenting costs for TDI are population based (3, 7–10), while others are hospital based (5–6, 11). The main reason for the high costs in hospital clinics is probably related to the fact that those clinics often receive complicated dental trauma cases on a 24 hour basis, and are also often teaching clinics.

## Resources presented in time

Patients with complicated injuries to the permanent dentition have been shown to stay in treatment over a long time, whereas patients with uncomplicated injuries finish treatment more quickly (2). In Fig. 34.2, total time is stratified according to severity of trauma for patients with TDI to permanent teeth. The proportion of patients remaining in treatment for a two-year period following initial trauma is shown for uncomplicated and complicated trauma.

In Table 34.4 treatment time and number of visits per individual of complicated traumatic injuries to the *primary dentition* is much higher than for uncomplicated trauma. This is because treatment of uncomplicated injuries to primary teeth consists primarily of information and follow-ups, while, beyond information, surgery (extraction), sometimes including sedation and follow-ups, is often the result in complicated injuries. In the *permanent dentition*, treatment time and number of visits increase significantly when

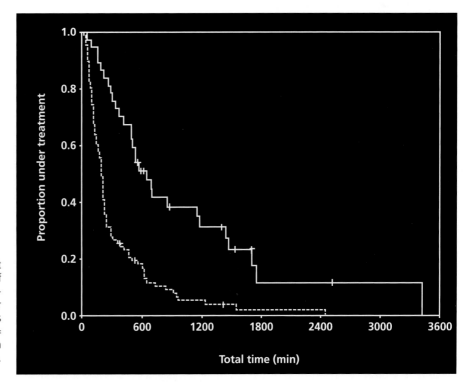

**Fig. 34.2** Total time for permanent teeth, stratified according to severity of trauma. Proportion of patients remaining in treatment for the two-year period following initial trauma is shown for uncomplicated trauma (n = 86) ----, and for complicated trauma (n = 37) —. Censored observations = +. From GLENDOR et al. (2) 2000.

**Table 34.4** The average treatment time in hours and number of visits per individual with uncomplicated (U) and complicated (C) traumatic injuries to primary and permanent teeth in urban (UR) or rural (RU) territories. Treatment is performed by either hospital (HO) and/or public dental health service (PU). Range within parentheses.

| Author | Territory/ Caregiver | Dentition | Age years | Type of injury | Period years | Total treatment time[1] | No. of visits |
|---|---|---|---|---|---|---|---|
| Josefsson & Lilja Karlander (63) 1994 | RU, PU | Permanent | 7–17 | – | 10 | 1.2 (0.1–11.2) | 2.9 (1–9) |
| Solli et al. (9) 1996 | UR, RU, HO, PU | Permanent | 6–18 | – | 1 | 0.9 | 1.9 |
| Glendor et al. (1) 1998 | UR, RU, HO, PU | Primary | 2–6 | U<br>C | 2 | 0.8 (0.3–3.3)<br>1.6 (0.4–4.4) | 2.5 (1–9)<br>4.3 (1–12) |
| | | Permanent | 7–18 | U<br>C | 2 | 3.2 (0.3–11.0)<br>8.5 (1.7–20.5) | 9.2 (1–27)<br>16.4 (1–24) |
| Borssén et al. (10) 2002 | UR, RU, HO, PU | Primary<br>Permanent<br>Permanent | 1–6<br>7–16<br>7–16 | –<br>–<br>C | 15<br>15<br>15 | 0.6 (0.1–4)<br>1.6 (0.3–27.5)<br>8.0* | 2.2 (0–12)<br>4.1 (1–41) |
| Nguyen et al. (5) 2004 | UR, HO | Permanent | 6–18 | C | 1 | – | 9.1 (4–15) |
| Al-Jundi (64) 2004 | UR, HO | Prim & Perm | ? | – | 3 | – | 3–17.2 |
| Wong & Kolokotsa (6) 2004 | UR, HO | Permanent | 7–18 | – | 7 | – | 10.4 (3–27) |

* Children treated by their regular dentist as well as by a specialist had a mean treatment time of 8 h.

the injury is complicated, with a spectrum of various therapies and follow-ups, compared to uncomplicated injuries, where restorations and follow-ups dominate (1). The number of follow-ups in uncomplicated injuries to permanent teeth is probably higher than needed with respect to the low risk of complications. A lower number of follow-ups could be considered when planning treatment (1, 10). Almost 50% of all different treatments for TDI to primary teeth are performed in connection with non-trauma-related dental treatment, but only less than 30% for permanent teeth (1). This reflects the unique character of treatment of traumatic injuries to permanent teeth.

Treatment time in permanent dentition has also been found to increase if the first injury occurred before the age of 11 (10). This conclusion, coupled with the fact that there is an increased risk of sustaining multiple dental injuries to permanent teeth if the first trauma episode occurred before the age of 11 (20), highlights the 'pre-teenage child' at special risk of high costs in the event of a TDI.

## Traumatic dental injuries involve several people

Traumatic dental injuries to children and adolescents generally involve one or more professionals and one or more companions, mostly family members, but also neighbors, teachers or sports leaders (2–3, 5, 24). Only 4 studies to date have analyzed the costs associated with the involvement of people accompanying patients to dental visits, as well as resources spent, e.g. in transportation, lost working or leisure time and actual costs for damaged personal equipment incurred by traumatic dental injuries to primary and permanent teeth (2–3, 5, 6). On average, 1.4 (range 0–3) people except health care professionals were involved with each trauma episode, and in 93% of the cases they were parents (2).

## Dental injuries more expensive than outpatient non-oral injuries

Compared to many other outpatient injuries, TDI seems to be more time consuming and costly. The average number of visits treated on an outpatient basis due to TDI to permanent teeth during one year range from 1.9 to 9.1 visits (1, 5, 9), and exceeds the average number of 1.5 visits due to other accidental bodily injuries also treated on an outpatient basis during one year (25). A comparison of bicycle injuries with oral and non-oral injuries showed that of those with oral injuries, 61% had more than one medical visit, compared to 27% with non-oral injuries (26).

The average cost of treatment of accidental non-oral injuries has been shown to vary between US$ 506 to US$ 1000 in Sweden, the Netherlands and the USA (25, 27, 28). Medical payments per child treated for accidental body injuries in the USA have been estimated to be US$ 800, compared to US$ 506 in a Swedish investigation (25, 27). A study in the Netherlands estimated the total direct medical costs of injury for all ages to be an average of €1000 (1€ ≈ 1US $ in 1997) (28). These 3 studies included inpatient and outpatient care from other non-oral accidental injuries. A comparable figure for outpatient care of accidental injuries for all ages in the Swedish study was US$ 88, which is low compared with the costs of TDI in Tables 34.2 and 34.3. This makes costs of TDI high compared to other bodily injuries, especially for complicated TDI to permanent teeth.

Considering that most studies of costs of TDI have used a relatively short post-trauma period in their reporting methods, and that very few treatments of dental trauma can be regarded as definitive, the costs presented must be regarded as minimum costs. Seen over a lifetime, costs of a dental trauma may rise far over those presented during the last 5–10 years, and in many cases to high levels when including the time spent by the patient and companions in

Table 34.5 Mean values of number of types of treatment per patient in 6–17-year old patients with repeated traumatized permanent teeth related to 2 or 4–7 episodes per patient. Standard deviations in parentheses. From Glendor et al. (20) 2000.

| Pattern of treatment | Mean values of number of types of treatment | |
| --- | --- | --- |
| | 2 episodes | 4–7 episodes |
| Information | 1.1 (0.3) | 2.9 (1.3) |
| Filling therapy | 0.8 (0.6) | 4.0 (5.4) |
| Endodontics | 1.3 (4.1) | – |
| Surgery | 0.3 (1.0) | – |
| Prosthetics | – | – |
| Consultations, etc | 0.4 (0.7) | 1.1 (1.6) |
| Follow-ups | 2.8 (2.1) | 7.9 (5.7) |
| Total | 6.7 (6.1) | 15.9 (10.1) |

travel and treatment. A six-unit fixed bridge in the front, probably replaced several times during a lifetime, may become an extremely costly treatment (29).

## Other factors contributing to increase in cost

Multiple dental trauma episodes (MDTE) (20, 30–38), and repeated TDI to the same teeth (20, 39–40) have been shown to jeopardize the ongoing healing of injuries to pulpal and periodontal tissues (41). Factors such as patient information, filling therapy and follow-ups, especially when the same teeth are traumatized again, contribute to increased cost (20) (Table 34.5).

Poor knowledge of how to manage dental trauma among lay people (32, 42–45), physicians, medical students or physical education teachers (46–47) may also contribute to the high cost of TDI. Other contributing factors may include inadequate emergency care (48–53) and lack of patient satisfaction with the care provided (48, 54), which can result in frequent reconstructions, with extended costs, e.g. of composite fillings (54).

An increase in costs could also be caused by delay in patients seeking treatment (55–56), and for some dental injuries, e.g. avulsion injuries, this could be an economic disaster, as a good prognosis is highly dependent upon prompt emergency treatment (57).

## Economic evaluations

During the past 10 years, no study addressing costs of TDI on a population level could be regarded as a true economic evaluation. The reason for this is that these studies have not considered clinical outcomes. A true economic evaluation can be defined as 'the comparative analysis of alternative courses of action in terms of both their costs and consequences' (58). The studies presented in this chapter could instead be defined as cost-of-illness studies presenting the economic burden of TDI to a defined population. However, the important benefits of these cost-of-illness studies are that they act as points of reference for economic analyses

and provide information for health care policy-makers (59). Cost-of-illness studies should not be confused with other economical studies, such as comparison of different treatments, factors influencing the survival of e.g. resin-retained bridges, cost-effectiveness of dental restorations, cost–benefit of mouthguard protection, and comparison between cost effectiveness of different treatment solutions for anterior tooth loss.

## How to present costs

Assessing costs involves four steps, which are identical in all forms of economic assessment (59). These are:

- Identify the relevant resources used, regardless of whether they can be measured or not.
- Quantify these resources in physical units, such as hospital days, surgical procedures, physician visits, tests.
- Put a value on the different resources used.
- Deal with uncertainty and time (discounting).

Costs can be presented as *direct*, *indirect* and *intangible* costs:

- Direct medical costs (e.g. costs of drugs, analytical procedures required, hospitalization costs, staff time, equipment)
- Direct non-medical costs (e.g. patients' out-of pocket expenses, transportation costs, community support services)
- Indirect costs (e.g. production losses) due to patients or others being off work
- Intangible costs (e.g. pain, suffering) associated with therapy.

Intangible costs are often omitted from many analyses as they are difficult to measure and value. To measure intangible costs, one must assess the use of quality of life instruments, or direct measurements within the framework of willingness to pay assessments.

To be a true economic evaluation, the outcomes should be measured as health improvements, expressed in one or more natural units (health effects), utilities (preference weights), or associated economic benefits (gains or savings).

## Future research

In times of economic constraints, the need for knowledge of health economics is even more important as a basis for judging health gain in curative and preventive care within dental traumatology as well as assessing epidemiological tools for evaluating the consequences of TDI. Among care providers and insurance companies interest has grown in the total costs of traumatic dental injuries.

A wish for the future would be that economic research in dental traumatology could also include prospective economic evaluations concerning both inputs and outcomes of a dental health care program (58, 60–61). During recent years, research in dental traumatology has presented evidence based guidelines on how to manage traumatic dental injuries to both the primary and permanent dentitions. An interesting strategy would be to study those guidelines with respect to how they change time and costs of TDI. Cost–benefit studies, or even better, economic evaluations of emergency services, mouthguards and the like should relate the service to cost to the society.

## Essentials

### Degree of severity

- Uncomplicated
- Complicated

### Sports injuries

### Time and costs

- Time is universal
- Cost is unique

### People involved

- Patient
- Companions

### Dental and non-oral injuries

- Outpatient oral injuries

### Other factors increasing cost

- Multiple dental trauma episodes
- Low level of lay knowledge of TDI
- Inadequate emergency care
- Lack of patient satisfaction

### Economic evaluations

- Cost of illness
- Clinical outcome
- True economic evaluation

### How to present costs

- Direct medical costs
- Direct non-medical costs
- Direct costs
- Indirect costs
- Intangible costs

### Future research

- Prospective economic evaluations
- Inputs
- Outputs
- Evidence based guidelines
- Emergency services
- Mouthguards

## References

1. GLENDOR U, HALLING A, ANDERSSON L, ANDREASEN JO, KLITZ I. Type of treatment and estimation of time spent on dental trauma. A longitudinal and retrospective study. *Swed Dent J* 1998;**22**:47–60.
2. GLENDOR U, HALLING A, BODIN L, ANDERSSON L, NYGREN Å, KARLSSON G, KOUCHEKI B. Direct and indirect time spent on care of dental trauma: a 2-year prospective study of children and adolescents. *Endod Dent Traumatol* 2000;**16**:16–23.
3. GLENDOR U, JONSSON D, HALLING A, LINDQVIST K. Direct and indirect costs of dental trauma in Sweden: a 2-year prospective study of children and adolescents. *Community Dent Oral Epidemiol* 2001;**29**:150–60.
4. GLENDOR U. On dental trauma in children and adolescents. *Swed Dent J Suppl* 2000;**140**:1–52. http://www.ep.liu.se/diss/med/06/24/index.html
5. NGUYEN P-MT, KENNY DJ, BARRET EJ. Socio-economic burden of permanent incisor replantation on children and parents. *Dent Traumatol* 2004;**20**:123–33.
6. WONG FSL, KOLOKOTSA K. The cost of treating children and adolescents with injuries to their permanent incisors at a dental hospital in the United Kingdom. *Dent Traumatol* 2004;**20**:327–33.
7. ANDREASEN JO, ANDREASEN FM. Dental traumatology: quo vadis. *Tandlaegebladet* 1989;**11**:381–4.
8. ANDREASEN JO, ANDREASEN FM. Dental traumatology: Quo vadis? Opening remarks at the Second International Conference of Oral Trauma, Stockholm, Sweden. September 21, 1989. *Endod Dent Traumatol* 1990;**6**:78.
9. SOLLI E, NOSSUM G, MOLVEN O. Ressursbruk ved behandling av tannskader hos norske 6–18 åringer. (In Norwegian) *Nor Tannlaegeforen Tid* 1996;**328**–33.
10. BORSSÉN E, KÄLLESTÅL C, HOLM AK. Treatment time of traumatic dental injuries in a cohort of 16-year-olds in northern Sweden. *Acta Odontol Scand* 2002;**60**:265–70.
11. BORUM MK, ANDREASEN JO. Therapeutic and economic implications of traumatic dental injuries in Denmark: an estimate based on 7549 patients treated at a major trauma centre. *Int J Paediatr Dent* 2001;**11**:249–58.
12. ANDREASEN FM, VESTERGAARD PEDERSEN B. Prognosis of luxated permanent teeth – the development of pulp necrosis. *Endod Dent Traumatol* 1985;**1**:207–20.
13. ANDREASEN FM, YU Z, THOMSEN BL, ANDERSEN PK. The occurrence of pulp canal obliteration after luxation injuries in the permanent dentition. *Endod Dent Traumatol* 1987;**3**:103–15.
14. ANDERSSON L. Dentoalveolar ankylosis and associated root resorption in replanted teeth. Experimental and clinical studies in monkey and man. *Swed Dent J Suppl* 1988;**56**:1–75.
15. FEIGLIN B. Dental pulp response to traumatic injuries – a retrospective analysis with case reports. *Endod Dent Traumatol* 1996;**12**:1–8.
16. JÄRVINEN S. On the causes of traumatic dental injuries with special reference to sports accidents in a sample of Finnish children. A study of a clinical patient material. *Acta Odontol Scand* 1980;**38**:151–4.
17. HOLLAND TJ, O'MULLANE DM, WHELTON HP. Accidental damage to incisors amongst Irish adults. *Endod Dent Traumatol* 1994;**10**:191–4.

18. GLENDOR U, HALLING A, ANDERSSON L, EILERT-PETERSSON E. Incidence of traumatic tooth injuries in children and adolescents in the county of Västmanland, Sweden. *Swed Dent J* 1996;**20**:15–28.

19. ENGELHARDTSEN S, JACOBSEN I, MOLVEN O, MYRHAUG I, NYSETHER S, OKSTAD A, RÖYNESDAL K, STÖEN GKB, STÖRMER K, THORGERSEN A. *Tannskader hos barn og ungdom. En undersökelse i Nord-Tröndelag og Oslo i 1992/93* (in Norwegian) IK-2600. Oslo: Statens Helsetilsyn, 1988.

20. GLENDOR U, KOUCHEKI A, HALLING A. Risk evaluation and type of treatment of multiple dental trauma episodes to permanent teeth. *Endod Dent Traumatol* 2000;**16**:205–10.

21. LABELLA CR, SMITH BW, SIGURDSSON A. Effect of mouthguards on dental injuries and concussions in college basketball. *Med Sci Sports Exerc* 2002;**34**:41–4.

22. NATIONAL YOUTH SPORTS FOUNDATION FOR THE PREVENTION OF ATHLETIC INJURY INC. *Dent Inj Fact Sheet* Needham: Mass, 1992.

23. LANG B, POHL Y, FILIPPI A. Knowledge and prevention of dental trauma in team handball in Switzerland and Germany. *Dent Traumatol* 2002;**18**:329–34.

24. WOOD EB, FREER TJ. A survey of dental and oral trauma in south-east Queensland during 1998. *Aust Dent J* 2002;**47**:142–6.

25. LINDQVIST KS, BRODIN H. One-year economic consequenses of accidents in a Swedish municipality. *Accid Anal Prev* 1996;**28**:209–19.

26. EILERT-PETERSSON E, SCHELP L. An epidemiological study of bicycle-related injuries. *Accid Anal Prev* 1997;**29**:363–72.

27. DANSECO ER, MILLER TR, SPICER RS. Incidence and costs of 1987–1994 childhood injuries: demographic breakdowns. *Pediatrics* 2000;**105**:E27.

28. MULDER S, MEERDING WJ, VAN BEECK EF. Setting priorities in injury prevention: the application of an incidence based cost model. *Inj Prev* 2002;**8**:74–8.

29. COHEN BD, COHEN SC. Realistic monetary evaluation of dental injuries (a current view). *J N J Dent Assoc* 1998;**69**:37, 59.

30. ONETTO JE, FLORES MT, GARBARINO ML. Dental trauma in children and adolescents in Valparaiso, Chile. *Endod Dent Traumatol* 1994;**10**:223–7.

31. KASTE LM, GIFT HC, BHAT M, SWANGO PA. Prevalence of incisor trauma in persons 6 to 50 years of age: United States, 1988–1991. *J Dent Res* 1996;**75**:696–705.

32. HAMILTON FA, HILL FJ, MACKIE IC. Investigation of lay knowledge of the management of avulsed permanent incisors. *Endod Dent Traumatol* 1997;**13**:19–23.

33. BORSSÉN E, HOLM AK. Traumatic dental injuries in a cohort of 16-year-olds in northern Sweden. *Endod Dent Traumatol* 1997;**13**:276–80.

34. CHEN YL, TSAI TP, SEE LC. Survey of incisor trauma in second grade students of Central Taiwan. *Chang Gung Med J* 1999;**22**:212–19.

35. VANDERAS AP, PAPAGIANNOULIS L. Incidence of dentofacial injuries in children: a 2-year longitudinal study. *Endod Dent Traumatol* 1999;**15**:235–8.

36. CUNHA RF, PUGLIESI DMC, VIEIRA AED. Oral trauma in Brazilian patients aged 0–3 years. *Dent Traumatol* 2001;**17**:210–12.

37. ROCHA MJC, CARDOSO M. Traumatized permanent teeth in Brazilian children assisted at the Federal University of Santa Catarina, Brazil. *Dent Traumatol* 2001;**17**:245–9.

38. CARDOSO M, ROCHA MJC. Traumatized primary teeth in children assisted at the Federal University of Santa Catarina, Brazil. *Dent Traumatol* 2002;**18**:129–33.

39. HEDEGÅRD B, STÅLHANE I. A study of traumatized permanent teeth in children aged 7–15 years. Part I. *Swed Dent J* 1973;**66**:431–50.

40. STOCKWELL AJ. Incidence of dental trauma in the Western Australian School Dental Service. *Community Dent Oral Epidemiol* 1988;**16**:294–8.

41. BAKLAND LK, ANDREASEN JO. Examination of the dentally traumatized patient. *J Calif Dent Assoc* 1996;**2**:35–44.

42. OSUJI OO. Traumatised primary teeth in Nigerian children attending University Hospital: the consequences of delays in seeking treatment. *Int Dent J* 1996;**46**:165–70.

43. SAE-LIM V, CHULALUK K, LIM LP. Patient and parental awareness of the importance of immediate management of traumatised teeth. *Endod Dent Traumatol* 1999;**15**:37–41.

44. ADEKOYA-SOFOWORA CA. Traumatized anterior teeth in children: a review of the literature. *Niger J Med* 2001;**10**:151–7.

45. SAE-LIM V, LIM LP. Dental trauma management awareness of Singapore pre-school teachers. *Dent Traumatol* 2001;**2**:71–6.

46. CHAN AWK, WONG TKS, CHEUNG GSP. Lay knowledge of physical education teachers about the emergency management of dental trauma in Hong Kong. *Dent Traumatol* 2001;**17**:77–85.

47. HOLAN G, SHMUELI Y. Knowledge of physicians in hospital emergency rooms in Israel on their role in cases of avulsion of permanent incisors. *Int J Paediatr Dent J* 2003;**13**:13–19.

48. HAMILTON FA, HILL FJ, HOLLOWAY PJ. An investigation of dento-alveolar trauma and its treatment in an adolescent population. Part 1: The prevalence and incidence of injuries and the extent and adequacy of treatment received. *Br Dent J* 1997;**182**:91–5.

49. HAMILTON FA, HILL FJ, HOLLOWAY PJ. An investigation of dento-alveolar trauma and its treatment in an adolescent population. Part 2: Dentists' knowledge of management methods and their perceptions of barriers to providing care. *Br Dent J* 1997;**182**:129–33.

50. KAHABUKA FK, WILLEMSEN W, VAN'T HOF M, NTABAYE MK, BURGERSDIJK R, FRANKENMOLEN F. Initial treatment of traumatic dental injuries by dental practitioners. *Endod Dent Traumatol* 1998;**14**:206–9.

51. KAHABUKA FK, WILLEMSEN W, VAN'T HOF M, NTABAYE MK, PLASSCHAERT A, FRANKENMOLEN F, BURGERSDIJK R. Oro-dental injuries and their management among children and adolescents in Tanzania. *East Afr Med J* 1999;**76**:160–2.

52. MARCENES W, AL BEIRUTI N, TAYFOUR D, ISSA S. Epidemiology of traumatic injuries to the permanent incisors of 9–12-year-old schoolchildren in Damascus, Syria. *Endod Dent Traumatol* 1999;**15**:117–23.

53. MAGUIRE A, MURRAY JJ, AL-MAJED I. A retrospective study of treatment provided in the primary and

secondary care services for children attending a dental hospital following complicated crown fracture in the permanent dentition. *Int J Paediatr Dent* 2000;**10**: 182–90.

54. ROBERTSON A, NOREN JG. Subjective aspects of patients with traumatized teeth. A 15-year follow-up study. *Acta Odontol Scand* 1997;**55**:142–7.

55. OULIS CJ, BERDOUSES ED. Dental injuries of permanent teeth treated in private practice in Athens. *Endod Dent Traumatol* 1996;**12**:60–5.

56. SAROGLU I, SÖNMEZ H. The prevalence of traumatic injuries treated in the pedodontic clinic of Ankara University, Turkey, during 18 months. *Dent Traumatol* 2002;**18**:299–303.

57. ANDREASEN JO, ANDREASEN FM, SKEIE A, HJØRTING-HANSEN E, SCHWARTZ O. Effect of treatment delay upon pulp and periodontal healing of traumatic dental injuries – a review article. *Dent Traumatol* 2002;**18**:116–28.

58. JÖNSSON B. Economic evaluation of health care technologies. A review paper. *Acta Endocrinol* 1993;**128**:50–4.

59. KOBELT G. *Health economics. An introduction to economic evaluation.* London: Office of Health Economics, 1996.

60. DRUMMOND MF, STODDART GL, TORRANCE GW. *Methods for the economic evaluation of health care programmes.* Oxford: Oxford University Press, 1987.

61. EISENBERG JM. Clinical economics: A guide to the economic analysis of clinical practices. *J Am Med Assoc* 1989;**262**:2879–86.

62. ANDREASEN JO. Third International Conference on Dental Trauma. *Endod Dent Traumatol* 1992;**8**:69–70.

63. JOSEFSSON E, LILJA KARLANDER E. Traumatic injuries to permanent teeth among Swedish school children living in a rural area. *Swed Dent J* 1994;**18**:87–94.

64. AL-JUNDI SH. Type of treatment, prognosis, and estimation of time spent to manage dental trauma in late presentation cases at a dental teaching hospital: a longitudinal and retrospective study. *Dent Traumatol* 2004;**20**:1–5.

# 35

# Information to the Public, Patients and Emergency Services on Traumatic Dental Injuries

## M. T. Flores

Traumatic injuries affecting the teeth and surrounding tissues have not been widely recognized as severe lesions which carry with them esthetic problems, economic burden, prolonged periods of treatment and sometimes needing psychological support. Self-image is affected, resulting in low self-esteem and other adverse emotional consequences that go beyond the structural damage to the dentition (see Chapter 6). Moreover, most people fail to grasp the economic impact of such injuries because of their high cost of treatment and rehabilitation (1) (see Chapter 34).

Furthermore, those who have suffered the unfortunate experience of a broken or displaced tooth are not usually well informed on how to prevent or anticipate a traumatic injury.

In most cases, emergency treatment must focus on limiting damage. The urgent need to publicize and promote preventive measures and first aid practices – with the joint objectives of reducing emotional impact, preserving dentition, and reducing short- and long-term costs – cannot be overstated. The rapid advance in knowledge gained through dental research has redirected the professional role toward more preventive and conservative tasks. Hence, the dentist has an ethical duty to provide the community with the necessary information to allow each individual to take responsibility for his or her own dental care by limiting damage and improving outcome through appropriate first aid.

Because so little public health education has addressed issues related to dental trauma, educational campaigns focused on the prevention of life-threatening accidents should also include comprehensive awareness of dental injuries. Campaigns must present their message clearly (2), making the population aware of its role in saving teeth in case of injury. Target groups in this effort would be those exposed to a high risk of accident. Children, adolescents and the adult population should be included in this task (3).

This could be done via picture storybooks (4, 5) (Fig. 35.1), manuals, information included in natural science books, posters, brochures, TV programs, TV and radio talk shows, the local press and multimedia.

Because dental injuries may result from so many varied causes, educational campaigns must encourage appropriate first aid and promotion of mouthguards in contact sports and cycling. Even though the use of mouthguards, helmets and facemasks has been widely recommended, there is still insufficient evidence of their effectiveness in reducing the frequency of sports-related injuries to the head, face and mouth (6) (see Chapter 30). Injury prevention campaigns addressing the need for protective devices in sports and bicycling can increase awareness and use. This can rapidly be achieved through legislation or regulation (7).

The Internet is now the fastest mode of trauma education and prevention. It is a rapid form of dissemination of knowledge and accessible at low cost for many potential users. One of its weaknesses, however, is that the information provided does not always provide scientific references (8). Several organizations provide information related to dental trauma but there is a high variability in the quality of their contents. Thus, it is necessary to identify instruments to be used to rate the quality of such information. From a search of different websites, many organizations follow the avulsed tooth treatment guidelines recommended by the International Association of Dental Traumatology (IADT) (9–12). Many web addresses have a commercial interest and information is provided in a direct and entertaining manner to the general public.

## Developing a public awareness campaign

Many countries have made special efforts to reach the public with educational material in the form of brochures, posters

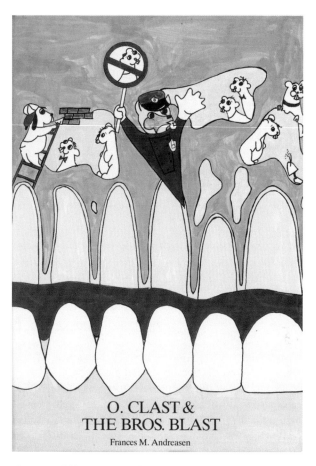

**Fig. 35.1** Children's story book used to inform children what happens after dental trauma.

and informative campaigns (Figs 35.2 and 35.3). Furthermore, the IADT has developed and collected brochures and posters which can be obtained at the website: http://www.iadt-dentaltrauma.org.

The objectives of a dental trauma campaign could be:

- To inform the community about the importance of preventing dental trauma and treating it promptly
- To identify specific methods, appropriate for different age groups, by which dental trauma can be prevented
- To recommend appropriate first aid to be given immediately following dental trauma.

The general public perceives dental trauma as a common accident in children and yet, at the same time, recognizes the lack of knowledge of appropriate first aid in these situations. Because accidents usually occur at weekends, parents are receptive to educational brochures about injuries to the teeth: useful information, such as where to seek treatment and emergency telephone numbers are appreciated. Dentists who are trained in biologically based emergency treatments should be willing to be on call outside usual working hours.

Educational campaigns help the public understand the importance of oral health and recognize the profession's commitment in teaching the community preventive and first aid measures. At the same time, these campaigns help improve the image of the profession, which is still regarded with fear and anxiety by most people.

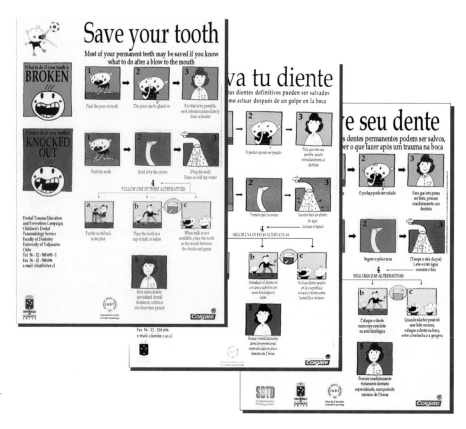

**Fig. 35.2** 'Save your Tooth' poster available in a number of languages.

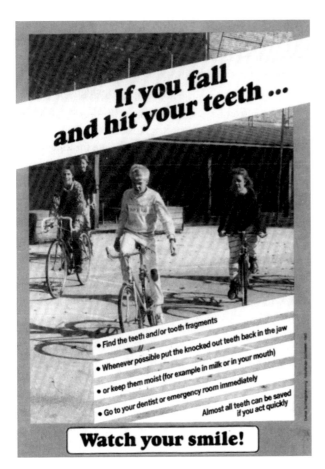

**Fig. 35.3** Poster giving treatment advice after a trauma.

tions can be avoided if people understand that some simple steps may save teeth at the time of an accident.

## For government departments of health and sports organizations

Promote the compulsory use of mouthguards in high-risk contact sports (e.g. ice hockey and rugby). Teach first aid practices at schools, gymnasiums, sport centers, and other organized athletic groups.

## Prevention of sports-related dental trauma

The *International Dental Federation* (FDI) has classified sports in two categories with regard to their risk of causing injury:

- *High-risk sports*: American football, hockey, martial sports, rugby, and skating
- *Medium-risk sports*: basketball.

Several types of mouthguard are available; but the most comfortable and the most protective devices are custom made for each individual.

Dentists must be aware of which mouthguards are available on the market and their manufacturing process. Likewise, he or she must educate the community as to the importance of their use and promote them actively among sport participants of all ages (13–16) (see Chapter 30).

## Recommendations for specific groups

### For government agencies and universities

Keep records of traumatic dental injuries of patients who attended emergency rooms. A complete registration will give important information for promoting preventive measures. Age, cause of injury, place of injury, diagnosis and emergency treatment offered should be registered.

### For insurance companies

Evaluate medical and dental injuries separately and determine treatment costs based on realistic approaches (i.e. worst case scenario in cases with doubtful prognosis). If various treatment approaches are possible, choose the biologically best procedure with minimal intervention (17) (see Chapter 29).

### For the media, government departments of health and education, insurance companies and accident prevention organizations

Educational campaigns must be implemented to increase public awareness of dental trauma. Many serious complica-

## Guidelines to the public: first aid and treatment of trauma to primary teeth

Recommendations to the public when responding to dental trauma in young children include the following measures:

- Dental trauma often includes injuries to the adjacent soft tissue. Therefore, wash the wound with plenty of running water.
- Stop bleeding by compressing the injured area with gauze or cotton for five minutes.
- Seek emergency treatment from a pediatric dentist.

### Guidelines for pediatric dentists responding to emergency injury-related visits include the following regarding primary teeth

- Intrusion and avulsion pose the greatest danger to the development of permanent teeth.
- In cases of intrusion, the direction in which the primary root is displaced must be determined. In most cases, the root is displaced toward the lip, away from the developing permanent incisor. In this situation, the tooth generally re-erupts spontaneously within 2–4 months.

- In cases of avulsion, primary teeth should not be replanted to avoid damage to the developing permanent dentition. It should be verified that the missing tooth has not been swallowed, inhaled or completely intruded.
- Good tooth hygienic control must be maintained during the healing phase. Parents should be instructed in careful brushing and the topical use of chlorhexidine in the affected area.

## Guidelines to the public: first aid and treatment of trauma to permanent teeth

Tooth fractures (broken tooth), luxation (loosened or displaced teeth) and avulsion (complete loss of the tooth) are the most frequent injuries to the permanent teeth. These injuries could have an improved outcome if the public were well informed about appropriate first aid measures.

### Guidelines to the public: first aid following crown fracture

In a crown fracture, the broken piece of tooth may be repositioned using dental adhesives and composite resins. This is a conservative, recommended treatment, especially in adolescents.

- Find the tooth fragment and keep it wet. (Note to the dentist: we know that a tooth fragment is different from an avulsed tooth. But in the heat of the situation, the lay public doesn't. Therefore, as general information, avulsed teeth and tooth fragments should be stored in a physiological medium (e.g. physiological saline, saliva, milk). However, an enamel-dentin tooth fragment need only be kept wet – and for this purpose, tap water will do.)
- Seek dental treatment immediately.

### Guidelines to the public: first aid following tooth avulsion

Often a permanent tooth can be saved through appropriate first aid response and immediate treatment.

- Keep the patient calm.
- Find the tooth and pick it up by the crown.
- If the tooth is dirty, wash it briefly (10 seconds) under cold running water and reposition it.
- If this is not possible, place the tooth in a glass of milk. The tooth can also be transported in the mouth, keeping it between the molars and the inside of the cheek. **Avoid storage in water.**
- Seek emergency dental treatment immediately.

## Information to emergency services

Dental trauma occurs at all hours of the day or night. When it happens – at night or week-ends – and the emergency service staff is contacted, precise questions to the patient or parent can pinpoint the problem and help the clinician decide when a trauma must be treated on an acute basis or when it can be delayed. A poster in the emergency room can serve as a guideline for these queries (28) (see Fig. 35.4).

- Injuries requiring immediate (*acute*) treatment include: extrusive luxation, lateral luxation (intrusion), avulsions of permanent teeth, fractures of the alveolar process, jaw fractures, gingival lesions and penetrating lip lesions.
- Injuries which do not require acute treatment (i.e. can wait until the next day, or *non-acute*) include: complicated and uncomplicated crown fractures, crown-root fractures, lateral luxation and intrusion of primary teeth, concussions and subluxations.

## Information to patients

When the dentist is faced with an emergency, it is of the utmost importance to give emotional support to the patient as well as to the stressed and anxious parents. Simple explanations of diagnosis, purpose of the emergency treatment and prognosis will be reassuring.

- Inform the patient and/or parents about the consequences of the trauma.
- Instruct the patient and/or parents on the importance of good oral hygiene techniques.
- Instruct the patient and/or parents about the importance of follow-up examinations.
- Advise the patient and/or parents about dental insurance coverage and the need to file a claim immediately after injury. Particularly with very young patients (i.e. primary tooth injuries affecting the developing permanent dentition) and adults (i.e. simple luxation injuries), post-traumatic complications may show up years later. Most companies will not cover an injury if the injury is reported when complications later appear.
- Information concerning specific types of injuries can be provided on a pre-printed form.

### Primary tooth injuries

Inform about possible complications so that treatment can be sought:

- Appearance of swelling, fever or an abscess
- Changes of crown color.

In case of intrusion, limit the use of pacifiers and feeding bottles in order to allow spontaneous re-eruption of the intruded tooth (18).

Inform the patient if severe primary tooth injuries might damage the developing permanent successors.

### Tooth fractures

Immediate treatment consisting of reattachment of the tooth fragment will usually be successful; alternatively a bandage of a white tooth filling material will protect the

# DUTY INSTRUCTIONS FOR EMERGENCY SERVICES

## CONDITIONS NOT DEMANDING IMMEDIATE TREATMENT

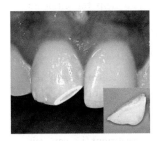

**Crown fracture with exposed dentin** S 02.5*
Exposed yellow dentin is seen. Missing crown fragment should be sought and placed in saline or water until rebonding.

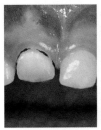

**Lateral luxation and intrusion of primary teeth** S 02.5
The laterally luxated milk tooth is displaced orally (photo to left) The intruded milk tooth is forced up into the jaw (photo to right).

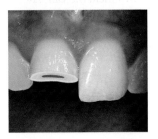

**Crown fracture with exposed pulp** S 02.5
A red and bleeding pulp is seen in the fracture surface.

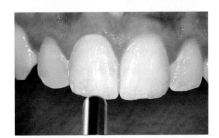

**Concussion** S 03.2
The tooth is tender to percussion, touch and chewing. The tooth is not loose. There is not change in position and the bite is normal.

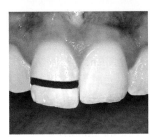

**Crown-root fracture** S 02.5
The fracture extends under the edge of the gingiva. There is usually pain from biting.

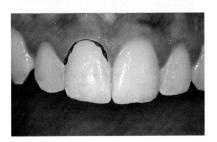

**Subluxation** S 03.2
The tooth is loose. There is sometimes bleeding from the edge of the gingiva. The tooth hasn't been displaced from normal position. The patient can bite normally.

## CONDITIONS DEMANDING IMMEDIATE TREATMENT

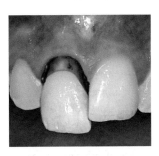

**Extrusion** S 03.2
Note that the tooth is loose and appears longer than adjacent teeth. The patient can't bite together normally.

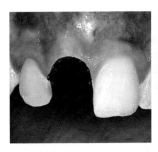

**Avulsion (permanent tooth)** S 03.2
The tooth is replanted after saline rinse, so that the root surface is clean. This should be done immediately and therefore performed by the physician on duty.

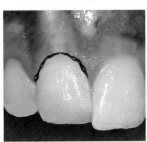

**Lateral luxation** S 03.2
The tooth is angled in relation to adjacent teeth. The patient can't bite together normally.

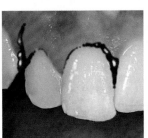

**Fracture of the alveolar process** S 02.4 (left)
Several teeth are displaced and the entire fragment can be moved by palpation.
**Jaw fracture** S 02.4 (right)
The fracture is exposed to the oral cavity and the patient can't bite together normally.

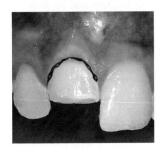

**Intrusion** S 03.2
The tooth appears too short compared to adjacent teeth. The tooth is firm in its new position.

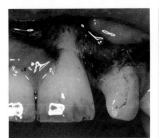
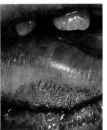

**Gingival lesion** S 01.5 (left)
The gingiva is displaced and root surface and bone are exposed.
**Penetrating lip lesion** S 01.5 (right)
The teeth have been forced through the lip. Corresponding cutaneous and mucosal wounds are seen. The wound often contains tooth fragments.

**Fig. 35.4** Instructions for emergency room personnel used at the Trauma Center, University Hospital Copenhagen, Denmark. * WHO registration code (see Chapter 8, p. 217).

nerve in the tooth. Later, the tooth can be restored with composite resin or porcelain. In cases where the dental nerve is exposed, coverage of the nerve for some time will help the nerve heal and allow later restoration of the tooth crown (20, 21).

## Loosened or displaced permanent teeth

The tooth should be put back in place in the jaw and a splint applied to protect the loosened tooth in the healing period. This splint will be removed after 1–12 weeks, depending on the type of injury (19). Chewing is permitted, but hard foods should be avoided. If the splint becomes loose, it should be re-cemented. During the healing period, when traumatized teeth are splinted, the patient should avoid playing contact sports.

In some cases, loosening of the tooth means that the nerve dies. The dead nerve must be removed and replaced by a root filling. The patient should be reassured that this treatment does not hurt.

### Diet

A soft diet will be prescribed for the first 14 days, to protect the injured teeth. A soft diet means no hard foods, but not necessarily a liquid diet.

### Oral hygiene

Meticulous cleansing of the teeth and gums is necessary to promote healing (18, 23–25). It is necessary to show the patients how to perform a gentle and effective toothbrushing, mainly to reduce the anxiety that this procedure may hurt or endanger healing.

Daily oral hygiene includes the following:

(1) Rinse mouth thoroughly with one tablespoon of chlorhexidine twice a day for one week. For children under 7 years, topical use of chlorhexidine is indicated.
(2) Careful toothbrushing after each meal with a soft toothbrush, working from the gums to the teeth.
(3) After toothbrushing, make sure that splints and teeth are completely clean.
(4) If there are associated lip injuries, recommend lip balm during the healing period to avoid dryness.

### Follow-up examination

Some patients will require the first the day after injury, depending on the severity of injuries. A good recommendation is to see the patient in a week's time, in order to evaluate healing, oral hygiene and control of infection (26).

Radiographs will be taken 3 or 6 weeks and one year after injury to control healing. Radiographs will allow diagnosis of possible late healing complications, such as root canal infection.

### Prognosis of treatment

When treatment has been carried out, the patient and/or parents must receive information about prognosis for the injured teeth (22).

### Injury report

A written report of the accident, including cause, type of injury, treatment and prognosis must be completed for school-related accidents and occupational injuries.

Also, this report will be useful for a court trial when dental injuries are result of violence, assaults or traffic accidents.

## Insurance

Dental needs and dental casualty insurance differ from one country to another. An underlying issue affecting access to care and delivery of services is the cost of care. The dentist should have a general knowledge about dental insurance coverage following accidents. In many countries there are children without effective dental coverage. Thus, they are at greater risk for experiencing complications of untreated traumatic injuries (27).

## Essentials

## Developing public dental trauma awareness

Dental injuries demand long time treatment, high costs and emotional support.

Dentists should agree on a standard first aid message to be delivered to the public.

According to high risks groups, first aid information should be continuously promoted.

### High risks groups and etiology

- Children 18–30 months
- Adolescents
- Young adults

As long as the public is well informed about dental trauma, the prognosis of injuries may be improved, as correct first aid of avulsed teeth and retrieval of tooth fragments may be performed prior to the patient reaching the dental clinic.

## First aid and treatment of trauma to primary teeth

- Wash the wound with plenty of running water. Often, dental traumas include injuries to the adjacent soft tissue.
- Stop bleeding by compressing the injured area with gauze or cotton for five minutes.
- Do not replace a primary tooth that has been knocked out.
- Seek emergency treatment from a pediatric dentist.

## First aid for a crown fracture

- Find the tooth fragment and keep it wet.
- The broken piece of tooth may be repositioned using dental adhesives and composite resins.
- Seek dental treatment immediately.

## First aid for an avulsed tooth

- Find the tooth and pick it up by the crown.
- If the tooth is dirty, wash briefly (10 seconds) under cold running water and reposition immediately.
- If this is not possible, place the tooth in a glass of cold milk. The tooth can also be transported in the mouth, keeping it between the teeth and the inside cheek. **Do NOT store the tooth in water.** This will damage vital cells on the root surface.
- If available, place the tooth in special storage media.
- Seek emergency dental treatment immediately.

## References

1. GLENDOR U, JONSSON D, HALLING A, LINDQVIST K. Direct and indirect costs of dental trauma in Sweden: a 2-year prospective study of children and adolescents. *Community Dent Oral Epidemiol* 2001;**29**:150–60.
2. NATIONAL CANCER INSTITUTE. *Clear and simple: developing effective print materials for low-literate readers.* 2003. Available at: URL: http://cancer.gov/aboutnci/oc/clear-and-simple/allpages.
3. NATIONAL CANCER INSTITUTE. *Theory at a glance: a guide for health promotion practice.* 2003. Available at: URL: http://www.cancer.gov/aboutnci/oc/theory-at-a-glance/allpages.
4. ANDREASEN FM. *O. Clast and Bros. Blast.* Fribourg: Mediglobe SA, 1988.
5. TSUKIBOSHI M. *If you know it, you can save the tooth on trauma.* Tokyo: Quintessence Publishing Co, 1996.
6. Recommendations on selected interventions to prevent dental caries, oral and pharyngeal cancers, and sports-related craniofacial injuries. *Am J Prev Med* 2002;**23**:(1 Suppl):16–20.
7. US DEPARTMENT OF HEALTH AND HUMAN SERVICES. *Oral health in America: A report of the surgeon general.* Chapter 7: Community and other approaches to promote oral health and prevent oral disease. 2000. Available at: URL: http://www.nidcr.nih.gov/sgr/sgrohweb/7.htm.
8. GAGLIARDI A, JADAD AR. Examination of instruments used to rate quality of health information on the internet: chronicle of a voyage with an unclear destination. *Brit Med J* 2002;**324**:569–73.
9. HONG KONG DENTAL ASSOCIATION. *Traumatic injury.* 2003. Available at: URL: http://www.hkda.org/Traumatic.htm.
10. SERVICIO TRAUMATOLOGÍA DENTAL INFANTIL UNIVERSIDAD DE VALPARAÍSO. *Traumatismo Dental Infantil. Información práctica y primeros auxilios.* 2003

Available at: URL: http://www.uv.cl/stdi/pages/folleto/folleto5.htm.
11. AMERICAN ASSOCIATION OF ENDODONTISTS. *Saving a knocked-out tooth.* 2004. Available at: URL: http://www.aae.org/patients/avulsed.htm.
12. AMERICAN DENTAL ASSOCIATION. *Dental emergencies and injuries.* 2005. Available at: URL: http://www.ada.org/public/manage/emergencies.asp#broken.
13. AMERICAN ASSOCIATION OF ORAL AND MAXILLOFACIAL SURGEONS. *Sports safety.* 1999. Available at: URL: http://www.aaoms.org/public/Pamphlets/SportsSafety.pdf.
14. ACADEMY FOR SPORTS DENTISTRY. *Frequently asked questions?* 2004. Available at: URL: http://www.sportsdentistry-asd.org/faqs.asp
15. AMERICAN DENTAL ASSOCIATION. *Mouthguards.* 2005. Available at: URL: http://www.ada.org/public/topics/mouthguards.asp.
16. AMERICAN ACADEMY OF PEDIATRIC DENTISTRY. *Mouth protectors.* 2005. Available at: URL: http://www.aapd.org/publications/brochures/mouthpro.asp.
17. ANDREASEN FM, ANDREASEN JO. Treatment of traumatic dental injuries. Shift in strategy. *Int J Technol Assess Health Care* 1990;**6**:588–602.
18. HOLAN G, RAM D. Sequelae and prognosis of intruded primary incisors: a retrospective study. *Pediatr Dent* 1999 July;**21**:242–7.
19. FLORES MT, ANDREASEN JO, BAKLAND LK, et al. Guidelines for the evaluation and management of traumatic dental injuries. *Dent Traumatol* 2001;**17**:97–102.
20. MJÖR IA. Pulp-dentin biology in restorative dentistry. Part 5: Clinical management and tissue changes associated with wear and trauma. *Quintessence Int* 2001;**32**:771–88.
21. MJÖR IA, FERRARI M. Pulp-dentin biology in restorative dentistry. Part 6: Reactions to restorative materials, tooth-restoration interfaces, and adhesive techniques. *Quintessence Int* 2002;**33**:35–63.
22. ROBERTSON A, NOREN JG. Subjective aspects of patients with traumatized teeth. A 15-year follow-up study. *Acta Odontol Scand* 1997;**55**:142–7.
23. HARDING AM, CAMP JH. Traumatic injuries in the preschool child. *Dent Clin North Am* 1995;**39**:817–35.
24. FLORES MT, ANDREASEN JO, BAKLAND LK, et al. Guidelines for the evaluation and management of traumatic dental injuries. *Dent Traumatol* 2001;**17**:1–4.
25. FLORES MT, ANDREASEN JO, BAKLAND LK, et al. Guidelines for the evaluation and management of traumatic dental injuries. *Dent Traumatol* 2001;**17**:49–52.
26. ANDREASEN JO, JACOBSEN I. Traumatic injuries – follow-up and long term prognosis. In: Koch G, Poulsen S. eds. *Pediatric dentistry. A clinical approach.* Copenhagen: Munksgaard, 2001:381–97.
27. THE NATIONAL INSTITUTE OF DENTAL AND CRANIOFACIAL RESEARCH. *A plan to eliminate craniofacial, oral, and dental health disparities.* 2002. Available at: URL: http://www.nidr.nih.gov/research/healthdisp/hdplan.pdf.
28. ANDREASEN JO, ANDREASEN FM, SKEIE A, HJØRTING-HANSEN E, SCHWARTZ O. Effect of treatment delay upon pulp and periodontal healing of traumatic dental injuries – a review article. *Dent Traumatol* 2002;**18**:116–28.

# Appendix 1

**Emergency record for acute dental trauma**

| | |
|---|---|
| Patient's name<br>Birth date | |

| | |
|---|---|
| Date of examination:<br>Time of examination: | Referred by:<br>Referring diagnosis: |

| | | |
|---|---|---|
| *General medical history*: any serious illness?<br>If *yes*, explain. | yes | no |
| *Any allergy?*<br>If *yes*, explain. | yes | no |
| *Have you been vaccinated against tetanus?*<br>If *yes*, when? | yes | no |

| | | |
|---|---|---|
| *Previous dental injuries*:<br>*If yes,*<br>    When?<br>    Which teeth were injured?<br>    Treatment given and by whom? | yes | no |

| |
|---|
| *Present dental injury:*<br>    Date:                 Time:<br>    Where?<br>    How? |

| | | |
|---|---|---|
| Have you had or have now *headache*? | yes | no |
| Have you had or have now *nausea*? | yes | no |
| Have you had or have now *vomiting*? | yes | no |
| Were you *unconscious* at the time of injury?<br>If *yes*, for how long (minutes)?<br>Can you *remember* what happened before,<br>during or after the accident? | yes<br><br>yes | no<br><br>no |

The emergency record is constructed so that wherever a question is answered by *yes*, more details must be provided. Finally, the last question in the record is whether the examiner has re-read the chart. This is a reminder to check that all relevant points have been registered.

876

**Emergency record for acute dental trauma (*continued*)**

| | |
|---|---|
| Is there pain from *cold air*? <br> If yes, *which teeth*? | yes  no |

| | |
|---|---|
| Is there pain or tenderness from *occlusion*? <br> If yes, *which teeth*? | yes  no |

| | |
|---|---|
| Is there *constant pain*? <br> If yes, *which teeth*? | yes  no |

| | |
|---|---|
| *Treatment elsewhere*? <br> If yes, *what treatment*? | yes  no |

After *avulsion*, the following information is needed:
*Where* were the teeth found (dirt, asphalt, floor, etc.)?
*When* were the teeth found?
Were the teeth *dirty*?
How were the teeth *stored*?
Were the teeth *rinsed* and *with what* prior to replantation?
*When* were the teeth replanted?
Was *tetanus antitoxoid* given?
Were *antibiotics* given?
   *Antibiotic*?
   *Dosage*?

**Objective examination** – Extraoral findings

| | |
|---|---|
| Is the patient's general condition affected? | yes  no |
| If yes, *pulse* <br>     *blood pressure* <br>     *pupillary reflex* <br>     *cerebral condition* | |
| Objective findings beyond the head and neck? | yes  no |
| If yes, *type* and *location* | |
| Objective findings within the head and neck? | yes  no |
| If yes, *type* and *location* | |

**Emergency record for acute dental trauma (*continued*)**

**Objective examination** – Extraoral findings (*continued*)

| | |
|---|---|
| Bleeding from nose, or rhinitis | yes  no |
| Bleeding from external auditory canal | yes  no |
| Double vision or limited eye movement | yes  no |
| Palpable signs of fracture of facial skeleton | yes  no |

If yes, *location of fracture*

---

**Objective examination** – Intraoral findings

| | |
|---|---|
| *Oral mucosa lesions* | yes  no |
| If yes, *type* and *location* | |
| *Gingival lesion* | yes  no |
| If yes, *type* and *location* | |
| *Tooth fracture* | yes  no |
| If yes, *type* and *location* | |
| *Alveolar fracture* | yes  no |
| If yes, *type* and *location* | |

Supplemental information:

---

**General condition of the dentition**

| | | | |
|---|---|---|---|
| Caries | poor | fair | good |
| Periodontal status | poor | fair | good |
| Horizontal occlusal relationship | under bite | over jet | normal |
| Vertical occlusal relationship | deep | open | normal |

---

**Radiographic findings**

Tooth dislocation

Root fracture

Bone fracture

Pulp canal obliteration

Root resorption

**Photographic registration**    yes  no

**Emergency record for acute dental trauma** (*continued*)

**Diagnoses** (check appropriate boxes and designate tooth no. or indicate correct anatomical region)

☐ Infraction

☐ Complicated crown fracture

☐ Uncomplicated crown fracture

☐ Complicated crown-root fracture

☐ Uncomplicated crown-root fracture

☐ Root fracture

☐ Alveolar fracture

☐ Mandibular fracture

☐ Maxillary fracture

☐ Concussion

☐ Subluxation

☐ Extrusion

☐ Lateral luxation

☐ Intrusion

☐ Avulsion

☐ Skin abrasion

☐ Skin laceration

☐ Skin contusion

☐ Mucosal abrasion

☐ Mucosal laceration

☐ Mucosal contusion

☐ Gingival abrasion

☐ Gingival laceration

☐ Gingival contusion

*Supplementary remarks*:

**Treatment plan**

*At time of injury*:
Repositioning (time finished)
Fixation (time finished)
Pulpal therapy (time finished)
Dentinal coverage (time finished)

*Final therapy*:

*Chart re*-read by examining dentist?                                                      yes   no

# Appendix 2

**Clinical examination form for the time of injury and follow-up examinations**

| | | Tooth no. | | | | | | | | |
|---|---|---|---|---|---|---|---|---|---|---|
| **T I M E  O F  I N J U R Y** | Date | | | | | | | | | |
| | Tooth color<br>   normal<br>   yellow<br>   red<br>   gray<br>   crown restoration | | | | | | | | | |
| | Displacement (mm)<br>   intruded<br>   extruded<br>   protruded<br>   retruded | | | | | | | | | |
| | Loosening (0–3) | | | | | | | | | |
| | Tenderness to percussion (+/–) | | | | | | | | | |
| | Pulp test (value) | | | | | | | | | |
| | Ankylosis tone (+/–) | | | | | | | | | |
| | Occlusal contact (+/–) | | | | | | | | | |
| **C O N T R O L** | Fistula (+/–) | | | | | | | | | |
| | Gingivitis (+/–) | | | | | | | | | |
| | Gingival retraction (mm) | | | | | | | | | |
| | Abnormal pocketing (+/–) | | | | | | | | | |

Each column represents an examination of a given tooth. The first column for each tooth gives the values from the time of injury. *Only* the parameters listed in the top half of the form ('Time of injury') are to be recorded at the time of injury. The information from this examination as well as the information collected on the emergency record are used to determine the final diagnoses for the injured teeth. Those parameters *and* the last four (fistula, gingivitis, gingival retraction, abnormal pocketing) are to be registered at all follow-up controls.

# Appendix 3

**Summary of treatment and follow-up procedures and recall schedule following the various trauma types**

| Post-traumatic interval* | Radiographic exposure for various trauma types | | |
| --- | --- | --- | --- |
| | Luxation of 21** | Replantation of 21 | Root fracture of 21 |
| Time of injury | OI 11,21***<br>BI 12,11,21,22 | OI 11,21<br>BI 12,11,21,22 | OI 11,21<br>BI 12,11,21,22 |
| 1 week | | BI 21,22[a,b] | |
| 2–3 weeks | OI 11,21[a,b] | BI 21,22 | OI 11,21 |
| 6–8 weeks | BI 12,11,21,22[a] | BI,12,11,21,22 | BI 12,11,21,22 |
| 3 months | | BI 21,22 | BI 11,21 |
| 6 months | | BI 21,22 | |
| 1 year | BI 12,11,21,22 | BI 12,11,21,22 | BI 12,11,21,22 |
| 2, 3, 4 years | | BI 21,22 | |
| 5, 10, 15 years | BI 12,11,21,22 | BI 12,11,21,22 | BI 12,11,21,22 |

* All examinations include radiographs as well as information from the clinical examination form (see Appendix 2).

** Tooth designation is according to the FDI two-digit system.

*** Regarding radiographic exposure, OI implies 'occlusal identical', or occlusal exposures; BI implies 'bisecting identical'. Both designations imply the use of standardized techniques and filmholder.

[a] Removal of fixation. The following fixation periods are suggested. The reader is referred to the respective chapters for details: Replantation, 1–2 weeks; Extrusion, 2 weeks; Lateral luxation, 4 weeks (depending on radiographic findings); Intrusion, see Chapter 16; Root fracture, 4 weeks.

[b] Begin endodontic therapy: Replantation, after 1 week; Intrusion, after 2–3 weeks.

# Appendix 4

Comparison between cost/effectiveness of different treatment solutions for anterior tooth loss

|  | Orthodontics | Implants | Resin-retained bridges | Conventional bridges | Autotransplants |
|---|---|---|---|---|---|
| Cost | +++ | +++ | + | +++ | + |
| Long-term service | +++ | +++ | + | ++ | +++ |
| Use in growing individuals | +++ | 0 | +++ | 0 | +++ |
| Bone-inducing potential | + | 0 | 0 | 0 | +++ |

Scale used: 0 = not to be used or non-existent; + = minimum (low); ++ = medium (moderate); +++ = maximum (high).

# Index